WITHDRAWN

Infertility

A COMPREHENSIVE TEXT

Machelle M. Seibel, MD
Associate Professor of Obstetrics and Gynecology
Harvard Medical School
Chief, Division of Reproductive Endocrinology and Infertility
Director, In Vitro Fertilization Program
Beth Israel Hospital
Boston, Massachusetts

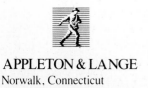

APPLETON & LANGE
Norwalk, Connecticut

0-8385-4024-4

Copyright © 1990 by Appleton & Lange
A Publishing Division of Prentice Hall

90 91 92 93 94 / 10 9 8 7 6 5 4 3 2 1

Prentice Hall International (UK) Limited, *London*
Prentice Hall of Australia Pty. Limited, *Sydney*
Prentice Hall Canada, Inc., *Toronto*
Prentice Hall Hispanoamericana, S.A., *Mexico*
Prentice Hall of India Private Limited, *New Delhi*
Prentice Hall of Japan, Inc., *Tokyo*
Simon & Schuster Asia Pte. Ltd., *Singapore*
Editora Prentice Hall do Brasil Ltda., *Rio de Janeiro*
Prentice Hall, *Englewood Cliffs, New Jersey*

Library of Congress Cataloging-in-Publication Data
Infertility : a comprehensive text / [edited by] Machelle M.
Seibel.
    p. cm.
  ISBN 0-8385-4024-4
  1. Infertility. I. Seibel, Machelle M.
  [DNLM: 1. Infertility. WP 570 I43]
RC889.I556   1989
616.6'92—dc20
DNLM/DLC
for Library of Congress   89-671
                                               CIP

Acquisitions Editor: R. Craig Percy
Production Editor: Christopher J. Bacich
Designer: Steven M. Byrum
Cover Design: Michael J. Kelly

PRINTED IN THE UNITED STATES OF AMERICA

Contributors

Eli Y. Adashi, MD
Professor of Obstetrics and Gynecology
Director, Division of Reproductive Endocrinology
Departments of Obstetrics and Gynecology and
  Physiology
University of Maryland
Baltimore, Maryland

Lori B. Andrews, JD
American Bar Foundation
Chicago, Illinois

D. Randall Armant, PhD
Assistant Professor of Obstetrics and Gynecology
  (Physiology and Biophysics)
Harvard Medical School
Director, In Vitro Fertilization Laboratory
Beth Israel Hospital
Boston, Massachusetts

Joel H. Batzofin, MD
Associate Director, Department of Obstetrics and
  Gynecology
Division of Reproductive Endocrinology and
  Infertility
Cedars-Sinai Medical Center
University of California, Los Angeles School of
  Medicine
Los Angeles, California

Steven R. Bayer, MD
Instructor in Obstetrics and Gynecology
Harvard Medical School
Beth Israel Hospital
Boston, Massachusetts

John D. Biggers, DSc, PhD
Professor of Physiology
Laboratory of Human Reproduction and
  Reproductive Biology
Harvard Medical School
Boston, Massachusetts

Richard E. Blackwell, MD
Associate Professor of Obstetrics and Gynecology
University of Alabama
Birmingham, Alabama

Richard A. Bronson, MD
Division of Human Reproduction
Cornell University Medical College
North Shore University Hospital
Manhasset, New York

William J. Butler, MD
Department of Obstetrics and Gynecology
Albany Medical Center
Albany, New York

R. Jeffrey Chang, MD
Associate Professor of Obstetrics and Gynecology
Division of Reproductive Biology and Medicine
University of California, Davis
Sacramento, California

Augusto P. Chong, MD
Director, Division of Reproductive Endocrinology
  and Infertility
Mt. Sinai Hospital
Hartford, Connecticut

Paul Claman, MD
Assistant Professor, Department of Obstetrics and
  Gynecology
Director, In Vitro Fertilization Program
Ottawa Civic Hospital
Ottawa, Ontario
Canada

John Collins, MD
Professor and Chairman, Department of Obstetrics
  and Gynecology
McMaster University
Hamilton, Ontario
Canada

Jeffrey R. Cragun, MD
Professor of Obstetrics and Gynecology
Division of Reproductive Biology and Medicine
University of California, Davis
Sacramento, California

Carolyn B. Coulam, MD
Center for Reproduction and Transplantation
  Immunology
Methodist Hospital of Indiana
Indianapolis, Indiana

F. Czyglic
Laboratories d'Histologie-Embryologie
CECOS
Centre Hospitalier Kremlin Bicetre
France

Alan H. DeCherney, MD
John Slade Eli Professor of Obstetrics and
  Gynecology
Department of Obstetrics and Gynecology
Yale University School of Medicine
New Haven, Connecticut

Michael P. Diamond, MD
Mellon Fellow in the Reproduction Sciences
Department of Obstetrics and Gynecology
Yale University School of Medicine
New Haven, Connecticut

David Diaz, MD
Instructor in Obstetrics and Gynecology
Fellow, Reproductive Endocrinology
Beth Israel Hospital
Boston, Massachusetts

Alexander M. Dlugi, MD
Assistant Professor of Obstetrics and Gynecology
Harvard Medical School
Assistant Director, In Vitro Fertilization Program
Beth Israel Hospital
Boston, Massachusetts

Alice D. Domar, MD
Section of Behavioral Medicine
New England Deaconess Hospital
Boston, Massachusetts

W. Page Faulk, MD
Center for Reproduction and Transplantation
  Immunology
Methodist Hospital of Indiana
Indianapolis, Indiana

Rene Frydman, MD
Laboratoire d'Histologie-Embryolgie
CECOS
Centre Hospitalier Kremlin Bicetre
France

G. John Garrisi, PhD
Division of Reproductive Endocrinology
Department of Obstetrics and Gynecology
Mt. Sinai Medical Center
New York, New York

Lawrence Grunfeld, MD
Division of Reproductive Endocrinology
Department of Obstetrics and Gynecology
Mt. Sinai Medical Center
New York, New York

David S. Guzick, MD
Associate Professor of Obstetrics and Gynecology
Acting Director, Division of Reproductive
  Endocrinology
Department of Obstetrics and Gynecology
McGee Hospital
Pittsburgh, Pennsylvania

Andrew G. Herzog, MD
Assistant Professor of Neurology
Harvard Medical School
Director, Neuroendocrinology Unit
Department of Neurology
Beth Israel Hospital
Boston, Massachusetts

Robert B. Hunt, MD
Clinical Instructor of Obstetrics and Gynecology
Harvard Medical School
Boston, Massachusetts

Amy S. Jaeger, JD
American Bar Foundation
Chicago, Illinois

Sharon Heim Jette, RN, MS
Infertility and Adoption Counselor
Andover, Massachusetts

Pierre Jouannet, MD
Laboratoire d'Histologie-Embryolgie
CECOS
Centre Hospitalier Kremlin Bicetre
France

Eugene Katz, MD
Assistant Professor of Obstetrics and Gynecology
University of Maryland
Baltimore, Maryland

Neri Laufer, MD
Director, In Vitro Fertilization Program
Department of Obstetrics and Gynecology
Mt. Sinai Medical Center
New York, New York

Gad Lavy, MD
Department of Obstetrics and Gynecology
Yale University School of Medicine
New Haven, Connecticut

Larry I. Lipshultz, MD
Department of Urology
Baylor College of Medicine
Houston, Texas

Randall A. Loy, MD
Department of Obstetrics and Gynecology
Beth Israel Hospital
Boston, Massachusetts

Bruno Lunenfeld, MD
Institute of Endocrinology
Chaim Sheba Medical Center
Bar-Ilan University
Ramat Gan
Israel

Eitan Lunenfeld, MD
Department of Obstetrics and Gynecology
Soroka Medical Center
Beer Sheva
Israel

Colin R. McArdle, MD
Assistant Professor of Radiology
Harvard Medical School
Director, Ultrasound Department
Beth Israel Hospital
Boston, Massachusetts

Paul G. McDonough, MD
Professor of Obstetrics and Gynecology
Acting Director, Human Genetics Institute
Medical College of Georgia
Augusta, Georgia

John A. McIntyre, PhD
Center for Reproduction and Transplantation
  Immunology
Methodist Hospital of Indiana
Indianapolis, Indiana

Clarke F. Millette, PhD
Laboratory of Human Reproduction and
  Reproductive Biology
Harvard Medical School
Boston, Massachusetts

Gilles R.G. Monif, MD
Professor of Obstetrics and Gynecology
Director, Infectious Diseases
Creighton University School of Medicine
Omaha, Nebraska

David Navot, MD
Jones Institute for Reproductive Medicine
Eastern Virginia Medical School
Norfolk, Virginia

Zev Rosenwaks, MD
Director, Jones Institute for Reproductive Medicine
Professor of Obstetrics and Gynecology
Eastern Virginia Medical School
Norfolk, Virginia

Machelle M. Seibel, MD
Associate Professor of Obstetrics and Gynecology
Harvard Medical School
Acting Chief, Division of Reproductive
  Endocrinology and Infertility
Director, In Vitro Fertilization Program
Beth Israel Hospital
Boston, Massachusetts

Sherman J. Silber, MD
Urologist, Reproductive Microsurgeon
St. Louis, Missouri

Patrick J. Taylor, MB
Deputy Director, Bourn Hall Clinic
Cambridge
United Kingdom

Jacques Testart, PhD
Hospital Antoine Beclere
Trivauz, Clamart
France

Judith L. Vaitukaitis, MD
Director, General Clinical Research Centers,
  Program Branch
Division of Research Resources
National Institutes of Health
Bethesda, Maryland

E. Van den Abbeel
Academic Hospital VUB
Brussels, Belgium

A. Van Steirteghem
Academic Hospital VUB
Brussels, Belgium

Anne Colston Wentz, MD
Professor of Obstetrics and Gynecology
Director, Division of Reproductive Endocrinology
Vanderbilt University School of Medicine
Nashville, Tennessee

Robert M.L. Winston, MB, FRCOG
University of London
Hammersmith Hospital
London
United Kingdom

Stephen J. Winters, MD
Associate Professor of Medicine
University of Pittsburgh School of Medicine
Montefiore Hospital
Pittsburgh, Pennsylvania

J.P. Wolf
Laboratoire d'Histologie-Embryologie
CECOS
Centre Hospitalier Kremlin Bicetre
France

Contents

Foreword

The burgeoning field of infertility investigation and treatment tends to be daunting to most physicians, whether generalist or specialist, novice or seasoned, in training or in practice. This is largely the result of the rapid development of basic and applied information being generated from animal, laboratory, and clinical experimental investigations. It is gratifying, therefore, that this authoritative book has been compiled to help bring systematic logic to an important area of clinical gynecology that has too long been cloaked in mystique, dogma, and empiricism. The contributions of leading figures in the discipline are gathered in this collaborative effort to provide, in a single resource, practical material with clinical value supported by objective data elucidating both facts and concepts. The authors were chosen not only for their reputations with regard to their depth of knowledge and special skills, but for their ability to convey their thoughts with directness and clarity.

This book clearly satisfies the unmet need for a textbook that combines and gives approximately equivalent weight to the medical, endocrinologic, pharmacologic, and surgical management of male and female aspects of infertility. It is comprehensive, thorough, and encyclopedic. The material is presented in suitable depth and will prove readily assimilable into clinical practice. The text is intended to be a functional, working book. Because the underlying basis for each recommendation is given, where known, physicians who adopt them will be in an advantageous position to modify their approaches as new information is developed in this rapidly changing field.

Several special attributes about this book deserve to be emphasized. It concentrates on reproductive endocrinology as a tool for assessing and treating infertility, rather than the reverse. It deals extensively with the wide array of reproductive technologies, many already fully accepted and others still being developed and perfected. Equally important, but unfortunately neglected heretofore, it addresses critical issues evolving as a result of infertility and the care of afflicted couples, such as emotional, legal, and ethical associations, consequences, and repercussions. Where appropriate, decision trees have been incorporated and elaborated on to help clarify the stepwise sequences of evaluation and management. The consistently systematic approach is especially worthy of note. I am confident that readers will be duly and amply rewarded.

Emanuel A. Friedman, MD, ScD

Preface

Few areas in medicine have evolved so rapidly or evoked so many emotional, ethical, and legal considerations as infertility and its treatment. Nevertheless, there are few textbooks that provide interested persons a single comprehensive resource. That is the goal of this textbook: to incorporate both the endocrinologic and surgical aspects of male and female infertility into one volume. In contrast to many excellent reproductive endocrinology texts that relegate infertility to a single chapter, my goal was to discuss reproductive endocrinology as a vehicle for understanding and treating infertility.

The major parts begin with a chapter on basic physiology. The subsequent chapters in each part are clinically relevant to infertility. Every ovulation-inducing agent is given an entire chapter, and one whole section is devoted to reproductive technology. Several specific categories of infertility are also discussed in detail, including those relating to immunologic factors, infections, genetics and molecular biology, unexplained infertility, and recurrent pregnancy loss. Chapters are also devoted to neurologic considerations, emotional, legal, and ethical aspects of infertility, adoption, and statistical analysis of infertility data.

I am very proud of and grateful to each of my contributors. Many of their names are synonymous with the topic they wrote about; all were chosen because of their ability to write and convey their knowledge and experience. Each has done a superb job.

Where applicable, many of the authors contributed a decision tree for the beginning of their chapter. In addition to the chapters that I either wrote or coauthored, the decision trees for Chapters 4, 6, 16, 17, 18, 20, 28, 29, 34, 35, and 36 were either written or substantially contributed to by me and may reflect slight variations in approach from those of the authors. This is particularly so in Chapter 28, on operative laparoscopy. Dr. Hunt performs open laparoscopy on all patients. I wrote a second decision tree, therefore, that assumes that closed laparoscopy will be performed. I feel that these decision trees will serve as useful learning tools and teaching devices.

The end result is a current, authoritative, and comprehensive textbook written for the medical student, resident, fellow, or practicing clinician in numerous specialties interested in infertility. It is my express hope that readers will find it a useful and stimulating resource.

Machelle M. Seibel, MD

Acknowledgments

I would like to thank my wife, Dr. Sharon Glazier Seibel, who sacrificed countless hours of evenings and weekends both helping me and allowing me the necessary time to work on this book. Special thanks must be given to Ms. Sarah Jeffries whose exceptional editorial skills contributed so greatly to the uniformity of the chapters. I would also like to acknowledge Ms. Sue Lee of Beth Israel Biomedical Photography Department who drew virtually all of the illustrations with the exception of those in Chapters 7, 12, 17, 21, and 27–31, and who constructed almost every table in all chapters. Ms. Bette McNamee worked tirelessly typing manuscripts and coordinating my efforts with others involved with the text. I would also like to thank Mr. Craig Percy of Appleton & Lange who believed in this project. Special thanks must also be given to my contributing authors who produced outstanding chapters in a timely fashion which allowed the book to be current. Finally, I would like to express a special debt of gratitude to Dr. Alvin LeBlanc, Vice President for Hospital Affairs, of the University of Texas Medical Branch and Dr. John D. Thompson, Past Chairman and Professor of Gynecology and Obstetrics, Emory University, who have guided and directed my professional development throughout my medical career.

Machelle M. Seibel, MD

PART I

Evaluation of Infertility

CHAPTER 1

Workup of the Infertile Couple

Machelle M. Seibel

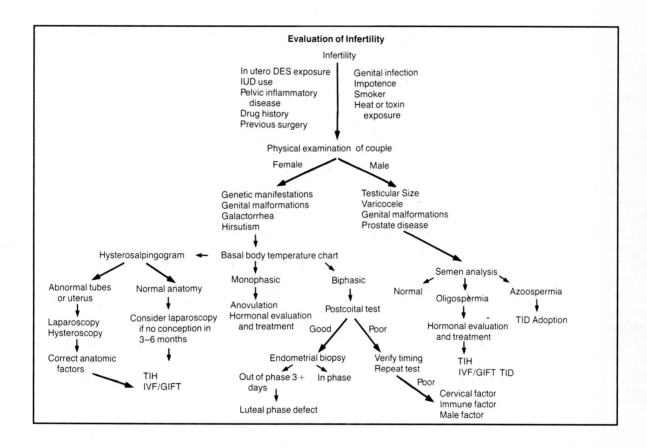

Few areas of medicine have been so exciting since the early 1980s as reproductive biology and its translation into the treatment of infertility. Advances in technology and techniques have become common news items; however, physicians not specifically trained in infertility may be left with the perception that evaluation of the infertile couple requires a subspecialist. This is compounded by the fact that experts disagree as how best to conduct an infertility evaluation. Furthermore, studies often conflict and controls are inconsistently included; however, there is no reason why obstetrician-gynecologists or family practitioners cannot perform the major portion of the workup if

they are conscientious and have a clear understanding of the general principles involved. Almost all of the evaluation can be carried out in an ambulatory setting.

GENERAL PRINCIPLES OF INFERTILITY CARE

Definition

Fertility denotes the ability of a man and woman to reproduce. Conversely, *infertility* denotes lack of fertility, an involuntary reduction in the ability to produce children. Infertility is relative; *sterility* is total inability to reproduce. The definitions of these words are different from those of most other medical conditions because normal fertility requires a variable period of time for pregnancy to occur. Therefore, infertility has an element of time in its definition. Although the actual incidence of infertility can only be estimated, it is believed that of the 28 million couples in the United States of reproductive age in the late 1980s, 3.0 million are conclusively sterile, 2.8 million are subfertile, and 1.2 million required a long wait before conception occurred.[1]

The widely accepted definition proposed by the American Fertility Society states that "a marriage is to be considered barren or infertile when pregnancy has not occurred after a year of coitus without contraception." This definition was based on studies such as those of Tietze, who found that 90% of 1727 couples with planned pregnancies became pregnant in the first year after discontinuing birth control methods.[2] Such a study suggests that a couple not achieving pregnancy after 1 year has a 90% chance of being outside of the norm. An investigation of these individuals would have an excellent chance of uncovering a significant and potentially correctable cause of the infertility.

Conversely, other studies caution physicians against too early an intervention. Pregnancy rates in unselected populations follow a predictable pattern (Fig. 1–1). Half of the nulliparous patients achieve pregnancy within the first 5 months of unprotected intercourse, and half of those remaining nonpregnant at the beginning of each subsequent 5 months will do so.[3] Therefore, if one observes 1,000 unselected nulliparous women, 500 will remain nongravid after 5 months, 250 after 10 months, and 125 after 15 months. Note that women who have already completed one or more pregnancies follow a similar, more rapid predictable pattern.

From these figures it follows that if patients were considered to have an infertility problem after only 5 or even 10 months, a large cure rate could be obtained without any treatment. It is therefore imperative to share this information with couples at their initial interview. It also underscores the need for necessary controls in all treatment of infertility. Finally, it implies that at least 5 months are required for any treatment regimen to be considered as having been given a reasonable trial toward correcting a problem contributing to infertility.

The Couple as a Unit

To evaluate adequately the potential of a couple to achieve pregnancy, the physician must from the very outset view the couple as a unit. Individuals are often neither "fertile" nor "infertile," but for a number of reasons their fertility may be reduced to varying degrees. For instance, a man with a somewhat low fertility potential whose partner is very fertile may never require medical attention. In contrast, that same male, if his partner has a somewhat low fertility potential, may have an infertility problem. Similarly, a woman who has oligoovulation but whose partner is very fertile will not be aware of her condition. Indeed, as a couple these partners are not infertile.

The concept of the couple as a unit may affect patient care in several other ways. First, it establishes the need for evaluating both partners, a practice that is not always carried out in infertility workups. Second, it necessitates that when two physicians are taking care of each partner separately, they must maintain a close liaison in order to evaluate the significance of their findings. This communication is particularly important during therapy so that the relative fertility of the partners will be increased simultaneously, thus enhancing the couple's overall fertility.

Even when the partners are being cared for by separate physicians, they should be interviewed together at the initial visit. The information that is obtained from talking with both of them tells much about their dynamics as a couple. Medical, marital, and sexual histories should be obtained from the couple both together and separately, so that important facts or events that one partner may not wish revealed to the other may be elicited. The physician may also ascertain whether one partner is significantly more motivated or saddened by the infertility, or conversely, whether one is indifferent or resistant to participating in the evaluation. Finally, one can determine the degree of stress the couple is experiencing as a result of infertility. It is imperative to be aware that since fertility may be due to problems relating to one partner, he or she may feel "guilty" or

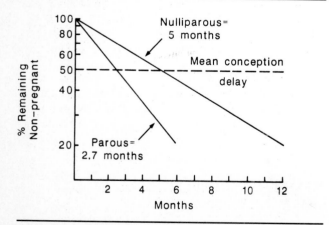

Figure 1–1. Pregnancy rates in unselected populations for nulliparous and parous women. (From Stewart and Glazer.[3] Reproduced with permission.)

at fault. In this fashion, infertility may devastate the person's self-esteem.[4] Working together with the pair as a team can help sustain them through what may be a long battery of inconvenient and painful tests and treatment. Even if they do not conceive, if they work together they will more readily accept that they have tried their utmost, and, in active cooperation with their physician, have been offered the best of medical science and compassionate understanding.

Multiplicity of Factors

Reduced fertility in many cases is brought about by a number of individual factors, each in itself not significant enough to prevent pregnancy, but when added together, sufficient to cause reproductive failure. Therefore, a rational approach has been to put each partner through a basic minimum workup. This generally uncovers the vast majority of the possible contributing factors. In this fashion, simultaneous therapy in both the man and woman may be initiated, thereby reducing the percentage of patients who ultimately require more complicated and extensive testing. Furthermore, testing for and treating one factor at a time while others are being ignored can be avoided.

AN APPROACH TO THE INITIAL INFERTILITY INVESTIGATION

The initial evaluation is often perceived as a stressful experience. Couples may have waited many months for their appointment and have hoped that somehow pregnancy would occur before the visit. The couple should be seen together. It is helpful and saves time to have a questionnaire for them to fill out upon arrival, which includes a menstrual history, documentation of previous pregnancies, birth control history, tests and surgeries previously performed and results, as well as general medical information. The age of the couple, how long they have been married or living together, whether they had previous partners, and how long they have been trying to conceive, should be ascertained. This information helps determine the degree of urgency they are experiencing. It also provides an opportunity to point out the statistical probability that pregnancy may occur without intervention if the infertility has been of relatively short duration. The questionnaire is not intended to replace the history, but merely to serve as a basis for review and further questioning.

Careful questioning concerning ethanol and drug consumption must be obtained because of the frequency with which these substances are abused in our society and the potential deleterious effects they may have on reproduction.[5] A history of abortion, veneral disease, impregnating a previous partner,

and discord between them must always be sought. Frequently, more accurate information will be obtained if these questions are asked separately during the individual examinations. After the answers are obtained, a more directed history should be elicited.

Ovulatory Factors

Ovulatory factors account for approximately 25% of infertility. Ovulation can be affected by a multitude of factors. The three most common ones are (1) excessive weight loss or weight gain, (2) excessive exercise, and (3) extreme emotional stress. Twenty percent above or below ideal body weight may affect ovulation. Furthermore, it must be remembered that obese individuals may in fact be protein deficient and thin individuals may be eating quite well. Therefore a dietary history is essential.

Although an exercise history is easily obtained, factors affecting stress are often not apparent. For example, many individuals hold several jobs to improve their lifestyle. The stress inherent in such a schedule is compounded by the need to leave work frequently for infertility testing. The death of a parent or other loved one might have precipitated the desire to conceive; many couples relocate and have no support base in their new homes. Either of these factors may result in sufficient stress to impair fertility.

Other important information to request of the woman includes age of menarche, menstrual history, and if and when menstrual cyclicity changed. Questioning the patient regarding preference for hot or cold weather, changes in mood and energy, hair loss, and changes in bowel habits may help uncover subtle thyroid disease. She must always be asked directly about excessive hair growth. Hirsute women may spend hours daily removing unwanted hair and thus appear not to have a problem. Acne and oily skin are other clues of androgen excess. Information concerning galactorrhea must be obtained because of its frequent association with ovulatory dysfunction.[6] Several diverse etiologies of infertility such as seizure disorders may also greatly affect ovulatory function.[7]

Peritoneal Factors

Peritoneal factors are uncovered in approximately 25% of infertility evaluations. Pertinent history includes a history of appendicitis, particularly if the appendix ruptured,[8] and abdominal or pelvic surgery. The patient must be asked if she has ever been treated for pelvic inflammatory disease either as an inpatient or outpatient.[9] Unfortunately, as many as 30% of women with pelvic adhesions and who are seropositive for chlamydial infection have a negative history for pelvic inflammatory disease. Previous intrauterine device (IUD) use is also associated with as much as a fourfold increase risk for acquiring pelvic adhesions.[10] Premenstrual spotting, dysmenorrhea, and dyspareunia are all associated with endometriosis.[11]

Cervical Factors

Cervical factors are present in less than 5% of persons with infertility. Because the cervix is a necessary passage for sperm, however, a careful evaluation is important. Factors that reduce either the quantity or quality of cervical mucus may reduce sperm viability and ultimately, fertility. Previous surgery on the cervix—particularly overzealous cryosurgery, cautery, or cone biopsy—may cause cervical stenosis or absent cervical glands with resultant scant mucus. A postpartum dilatation and curettage (D&C) or previous abortion could result in either cervical stenosis or incompetence and habitual abortion. A history of prenatal exposure to diethylstilbestrol must be elicited because of the associated stenosis and other cervical abnormalities.[12]

A chronic vaginal discharge or spotting is suggestive of chronic cervicitis. Infection may destroy cervical glands or contaminate the mucus with leukocytes. Additional information regarding douching and use of vaginal lubricants must be obtained because both are associated with potential spermicidal effects.[13]

Uterine Factors

Uterine factors are revealed in approximately 5% of infertility investigations. They are commonly associated with a history of prenatal diethylstilbestrol exposure,[14] which causes a T-shaped uterus (Fig. 1–2). Other pertinent historical information includes a previous D&C or therapeutic abortion, which could result in intrauterine synechiae (Fig. 1–3). Patients with this problem may complain of reduced quantity of menstrual flow. Spontaneous abortion, particularly if it is recurrent, could signify uterine fibroids (Fig. 1–4) or a congenital abnormality of the uterus (Fig. 1–5). Both uterine fibroids and polyps (Fig. 1–6) are commonly associated with increased menstrual bleeding.

Smoking and Reproduction

Despite the increasing realization of the many potentially harmful effects of smoking, almost one-third of men and women of reproductive age in the United States smoke, and the percentage of adolescents and teenage girls who do so is increasing.[15] Cigarette smoke is known to contain hundreds of toxic substances, including nicotine, carbon monoxide, and the recognized carcinogens and mutagens radioactive polonium, benzo-(α)-pyrine, dimethylbenz-(α)-anthracene, dimethylnitrosamine, naphthalene, and

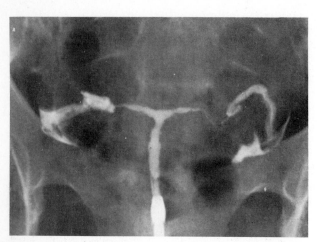

A

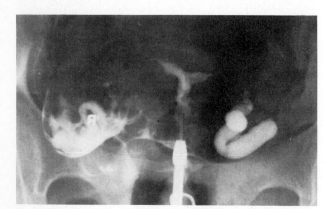

B

Figure 1–2. Hysterosalpingograms of two women (**A** and **B**) prenatally exposed to diethylstilbestrol. Note the characteristic T shape of the uteri. **B**. Patient (**B**) also has a left hydrosalpinx. She delivered a 5-lb, 6-oz daughter at 36 weeks' gestation despite the small uterine size.

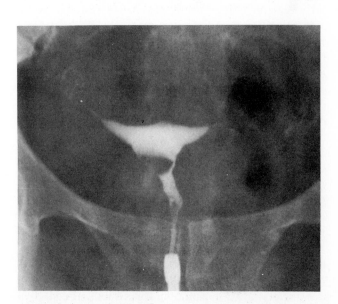

Figure 1–3. Intrauterine synechiae typical of Asherman's syndrome.

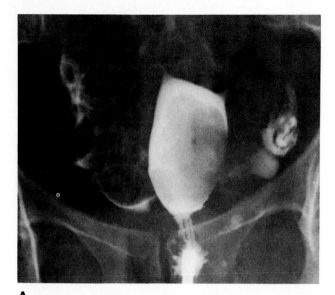

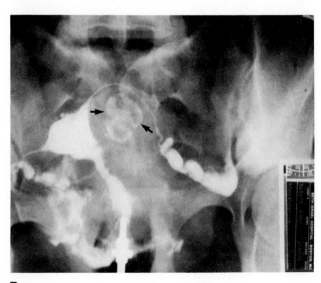

Figure 1–4. A. Uterine cavity markedly distorted by fibroid. **B**. Arrows point to an intraligamentous fibroid, which changes the course of the left fallopian tube and deviates the uterine fundus to the right.

fertility of light smokers (up to 20 cigarettes/day) was 75% that of nonsmokers, and the fertility of heavy smokers (more than 20 cigarettes/day) fell to 57% of that of nonsmokers. Infertility has been reported in up to 46% more smokers than nonsmokers.[21]

Smoking affects reproduction in many and varied ways. Cigarette smoke has been shown to increase uterotubal wave amplitude and tonus, probably secondary to nicotine.[22] This could partially explain the significant increase of ectopic gestation among smokers compared with controls,[23] and the finding that women with both cervical factor and

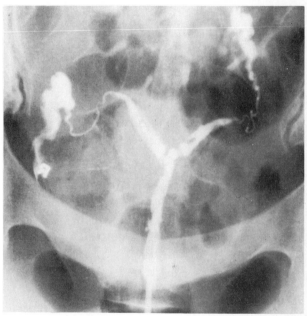

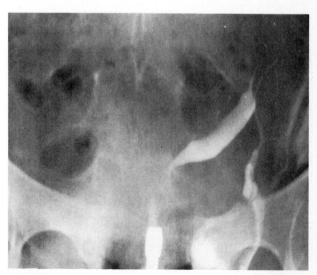

Figure 1–5. Hysterosalpingograms demonstrate (**A**) bicornuate uterus (note Asherman's syndrome) and (**B**) unicornuate uterus.

methylnaphthalene.[16] It has been estimated that an average of 5.5 minutes of life are lost for each cigarette smoked, on the basis of an average reduction in life expectancy for cigarette smokers of 5 to 8 years.[17]

The impact of smoking on reproduction has been less emphasized, but is covered in detail elsewhere.[18] Epidemiologic studies have demonstrated a consistent and highly significant trend of decreased fertility with increasing number of cigarettes per day, especially in women smoking more than 16 cigarettes a day.[19] The trend toward a dose–response effect of heavier smoking on fecundity was observed[20]: the

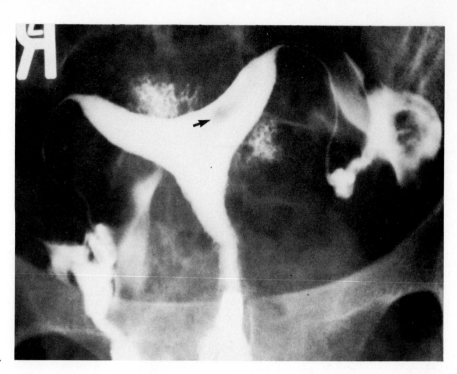

Figure 1–6. Intrauterine polyp.

tubal disease are likely to have been smokers.[24] Nicotine has also been demonstrated to impair decidualization in the pseudopregnant rat,[25] and to cause delays in conceptus cleavage from 2 to 4-cell stage, entry of the conceptus into the uterus, blastocyst formation, shedding of the zona pellucida, and implantation.[26] The effects are probably amplified due to the fact that nicotine is ten times more concentrated in the uterine fluid than it is in plasma.[27]

Smokers have also been shown to have a high frequency of amenorrhea and menstrual abnormalities. The findings appear to be dose related, being most common among persons smoking 20 or more cigarettes a day.[28] These effects may be centrally mediated by nicotine through enhancement of vasopressin, which can diminish levels of luteinizing hormone (LH),[29] or peripherally due to the reduction of aromatase in granulosa cells.[30]

Cigarette smoking may also adversely effect male reproduction. Sperm density is reduced on average 22% among smokers, while sperm motility and morphology are less consistently affected.[18] Cigarette smoke, nicotine, and polycyclic aromatic hydrocarbons are able to produce testicular atrophy, block spermatogenesis, and alter sperm morphologic features in experimental animals.[29] Furthermore, smokers with testicular varicoceles have a frequency of oligospermia ten times greater than that in men who smoked but who did not have testicular varicocele.[31] Therefore, in couples with unexplained infertility, who smoke, or in men whose semen values are marginal, the importance of stopping smoking cannot be overemphasized.

The Influence of Age on Reproduction

Since the 1950s the tendency to delay childbearing until the later reproductive years has increased. Factors such as available contraception, particularly the birth control pill; increasing numbers of working women; changing sexual mores; and the social acceptability of delayed marriage; all contribute to this phenomenon. The end result is that many couples are faced with a relatively shorter period of time in which to conceive.[32] This fact has been enhanced by both lay and medical publications emphasizing significantly reduced fecundity in persons over age 35. One of the earlier of these studies reported that among 2,193 women who were receiving therapeutic insemination with donor sperm (TID) and whose husbands were azoospermic, the probability of success of TID and 12 cycles was 74% for those below age 31, 61% for women age 31 to 35, and 54% for women older than 35.[33] Similar data have been found among patients treated with donor insemination in our institution (Fig. 1–7).[34]

Reduction in fecundity with increasing age is not limited to women. Only one third of males over 40 impregnate their women within 6 months, compared with males under age 25 (Fig. 1–8). This graph does not correct for the age of the woman; therefore it is possible that the reduction in conception is in part due to the compound effect of paternal and maternal age. These data also do not correct for frequency of intercourse. It was argued that fecundity declines linearly from age 20 through age 40 due almost entirely to the progressive decline in the frequency of

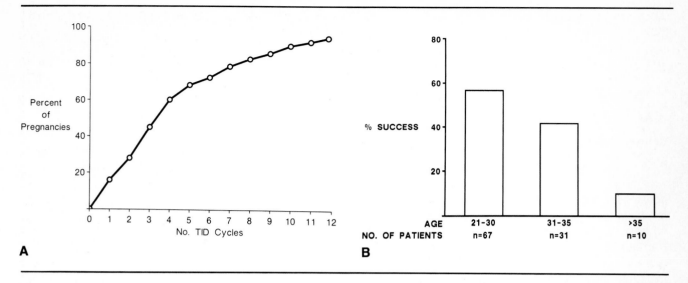

Figure 1–7. Pregnancy rates for patients receiving donor insemination (**A**) regardless of age (from Yeh and Seibel.[34] with permission) and (**B**) according to age (from Seibel, unpublished data)

intercourse.[35] Although frequency of coitus in all probability is not totally accountable for decreased fertility, it is clear that less frequent intercourse substantially reduces the percentage of conceptions within a 6-month interval (Fig. 1–9.)[36] Therefore a sexual history is of particular importance when interviewing infertile couples, particularly among reproductively older patients.

Changes in the endocrinology of reproductively older women also contribute to reduced fertility. When levels of estradiol, progesterone, LH, and follicle-stimulating hormone (FSH) were measured in regularly cycling women aged 40 and 41 years, the hormonal profiles did not differ from those of women aged 18 to 30. Women older than 45 with regular menses did reflect altered endocrine function.[37] Fol-

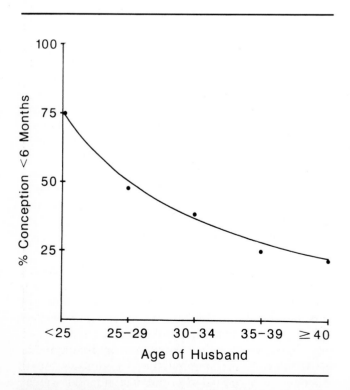

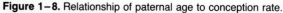

Figure 1–8. Relationship of paternal age to conception rate.

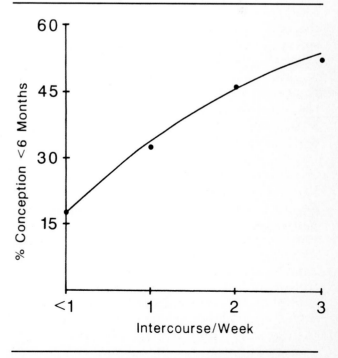

Figure 1–9. Relationship of intercourse frequency to conception rate.

TABLE 1–1. CHANGES IN CYCLE LENGTH WITH INCREASED AGE

Age (yrs)	No. of Patients	Total Cycle Length	Follicular Phase	Luteal Phase
18–30	10	30.0±3.6	16.9±1.8	12.9±1.8
40–45	7	25.4±2.3	10.4±2.9	15.0±0.9
46–56	8	23.2±2.9	8.2±2.8	15.9±1.3

From reference 37. Reproduced with permission.

licular-phase midcycle and luteal phase estradiol levels were lower in the women over 45 years of age, whereas early follicular-phase FSH levels were substantially elevated compared with those of younger women. These data are reflected in the increasingly irregular cycle length with advancing age (Table 1–1)[37] and the resultant reduction in ovulatory frequency. Such changes are due in part to aging of the ovaries and the hypothalamus–pituitary axis, and to altered neurotransmitters.[38–40] That the uterus itself is also affected by advancing age is reflected by the increasing risk of spontaneous abortion (Table 1–2).[41]

The risk of congenital abnormalities among older women is well established (Table 1–3). In addition, the absolute frequency of autosomal dominant disease due to new mutations among offspring of fathers 40 years or older is at least 0.3 to 0.5%.[42] This risk is many times greater than that for children of young fathers, and is similar in magnitude to the risk of Down's syndrome among the offspring of mothers aged 35 to 45. For these reasons, amniocentesis or chorionic villus biopsy must be discussed with respect to a potential pregnancy when either partner is biologically older.

Males also demonstrate endocrinologic and anatomic changes with advancing age. Involution of testicular function, decreased levels of free and total testosterone, decreased sperm production and quality, and maturation arrest of spermatogenesis, have

TABLE 1–2. RISK OF SPONTANEOUS ABORTION WITH INCREASED AGE

Maternal Age (yrs)	Spontaneous Abortion (%)
15–19	9.9
20–24	9.5
25–29	10.0
30–34	11.7
35–39	17.7
40–44	33.8
≥45	53.2

From reference 41. Reproduced with permission.

TABLE 1–3. RISK OF CHROMOSOMAL ABNORMALITY BY MATERNAL AGE

Maternal Age (yrs)	Risk for Down Syndrome	Total Risk for Chromosomal Abnormalities
20	1/1,667	1/526
21	1/1,667	1/526
22	1/1,429	1/500
23	1/1,429	1/500
24	1/1,250	1/476
25	1/1,250	1/476
26	1/1,176	1/476
27	1/1,111	1/455
28	1/1,053	1/435
29	1/1,000	1/417
30	1/952	1/385
31	1/909	1/385
32	1/769	1/322
33	1/602	1/286
34	1/485	1/238
35	1/378	1/192
36	1/289	1/156
37	1/224	1/127
38	1/173	1/102
39	1/136	1/83
40	1/106	1/66
41	1/82	1/53
42	1/63	1/42
43	1/49	1/33
44	1/38	1/26
45	1/30	1/21
46	1/23	1/16
47	1/18	1/13
48	1/14	1/10
49	1/11	1/8

Source: From reference 70. Reproduced with permission.

all been reported.[43–45] These changes underscore the need to view the couple as a unit.

Despite all of these concerns, a report on women over 40 demonstrated that they could expect a good pregnancy outcome.[46] This was particularly true in women whose weight was below 67.5 kg and those who were of low parity. Nevertheless, when either partner is reproductively older, the infertile couple deserves an expedited and complete workup.

Male Factors

A careful history of the male is essential. Prenatal exposure to diethystilbestrol has been associated with anatomic abnormalities such as epididymal cysts, microphallus, and hypertrophy of the prostatic utricle. Reproductive dysfunctions including altered semen analysis are also well documented.[47] A history of childhood diseases or undescended testes is also important. It has been shown that the overall semen quality of men born with either unilateral or bilateral undescended testes is lower than that of normal men regardless of time of orchipexy.[48] Furthermore, in the presence of a unilateral undescended testis, spermatogenesis is impaired in the descended as well as undescended gonad. A history of mumps prepubertally does not appear harmful. After the onset of puberty, however, mumps results in unilateral orchitis in 30% and bilateral orchitis in 10% of affected males.[49] Such men often have markedly atrophic gonads.

A history of surgery on the bladder neck or prostate must be sought, particularly in men with reduced seminal volume and azoospermia or oligospermia. Similarly, a history of testicular cancer must be explored. Return of sperm production after radiation therapy or chemotherapy may require 4 to 5 years, and when it does occur it is generally reduced in quantity.[50] Decreased ejaculate volume may be a clue to diabetes mellitus. If the disease is associated with peripheral neuropathy, a lack of emission or retrograde ejaculation may also occur. Delayed sexual maturation may be a clue to hypogonadotropic hypogonadism (Kallmann's syndrome).

Special care must be taken to inquire about ethanol, smoking, and drug use.[5] Environmental toxins such as pesticides, and occupational exposure to toxins such as agent orange, may reduce semen values. Removal from these toxins often reverses the adverse effects. Medications such as sulfasalazine,[51] cimetidine, and nitrofurantoin may be gonadotoxic. Androgenic steroids are occasionally administered to improve gonadal function, and young athletes more and more commonly are taking anabolic steroids. These substances should be stopped, as they inhibit gonadotropin secretion and interfere with normal spermatogenesis.[48]

Finally, the physician must ask the male if he has difficulty achieving or maintaining an erection or in ejaculating. Problems of this nature are often embarrassing, and may best be asked about separately of both partners.

Physical Examination

After the infertility history is complete, a careful physical examination of both partners is performed. The female's head should be examined for temporal balding, acne, or hirsutism, all of which are signs of androgen excess. Similarly, increased facial hair at the angle of the jaw, chin, or upper lip should be noted. Care is taken to evaluate the size of the thyroid gland. Galactorrhea is evaluated by attempting to express discharge from the nipples.[6] Presternal hair or acne, as well as hair or acne on the back, an increase in suprapubic hair, and a male escutcheon, are additional clues to androgen excess.

The presence of clitoromegaly should be determined. Visualization of the cervix includes inspection of the cervical mucus. Copious amounts suggest either impending ovulation or estrogen excess associated with conditions such as polycystic ovary disease. In the presence of cervical mucus, a postcoital test should be performed if intercourse has

occurred within the last 3 days. Occasionally, abundant sperm will be found in this initial visit, and further testing of the cervix can be eliminated. Attention must be paid to the position of the uterus and whether it is fixed or mobile. The size and mobility of the ovaries should also be determined. A rectovaginal examination must always be done to determine the presence of uterosacral nodularity or tenderness suggestive of endometriosis.[11]

The male's examination includes emphasis on the genitalia. General body habitus and limb length should be noted to evaluate genetic conditions such as Klinefelter's syndrome. Decreased body hair, gynecomastia, and eunuchoid proportions may suggest inadequate virilization. The location of the urethral meatus is determined to ensure proper placement of the ejaculate in the vagina. The scrotal contents are carefully palpated with the patient standing, to determine testicular consistency and testicular size to the nearest millimeter. Alternatively, the volume of the testes can be estimated with an orchidometer. The long measurement should be at least 4 cm and the volume at least 20 mL.[48] A decrease in testicular size is often associated with impaired spermatogenesis. The epididymis is palpated for induration or cystic changes, and the vas deferens palpated for nodularity. The presence of a varicocele, vascular engorgement of the pampiniform plexus, can easily be established by asking the patient to perform a Valsalva's maneuver while standing.

In addition to the obvious physical information obtained, these individual examinations provide the opportunity to obtain brief separate interviews, which are often invaluable in treating and understanding the couple as a unit. On completion of these examinations, the couple is asked to return to the consultation room, where an evaluation plan is described.

BASIC INFERTILITY TESTS

The basic workup as outlined by the American Fertility Society and followed by most specialists consists of history and examination of the female partner with evaluations of insemination (postcoital test), hormonal (endometrial biopsy), and tubal factors (hysterosalpingogram); and history and examination of the male partner, with two semen analyses 4 to 6 weeks apart. Incomplete evaluations, such as only one or two tests, or immediately performing a laparoscopy, often do not explain the cause of infertility. Typically, the basic minimum workup can be completed in 2 to 3 months.

After the tests that are to be performed have been explained to the couple, they are asked to speak with the fertility nurse, who gives the man a semen-collection container with printed instructions, and explains to the woman how to take and record her basal body temperature (BBT). The woman is asked to call the nurse at the start of her next menstrual flow (or on Monday if her period begins on a weekend) and to begin keeping a BBT at that time. She is then given appointments for a hysterosalpingogram and endometrial biopsy. She is asked to bring in a semen sample for her partner during one of these appointments to avoid their both having to miss work. She mails in her temperature chart at the onset of her next menstrual period, and at that time appointments for a postcoital test and another consultation are made. Some physicians prefer to give their patients detailed instructions and have them call to set up their own appointments for these tests. The postcoital test is optimally done in a cycle separate from the endometrial biopsy so as to reduce the chances of the biopsy inadvertently interrupting a pregnancy. A second semen sample is usually brought in on the day of the consultation appointment.

The Cervical Factor

The importance of sperm survival in the cervix after coitus was first described by J. Marian Sims in 1888.[52] His findings were further expanded by Huhner in 1913.[53] Since that time, the Sims-Huhner postcoital test has been widely accepted as an important tool in infertility diagnosis.

Functions of the Cervix. During most of the menstrual cycle, the cervical mucus is thick and tenacious. Under the influence of rising levels of estrogen in the preovulatory period, however, it becomes thin and watery, with the consistency of eggwhite. This midcycle mucus is rich in mucin, glycoproteins, and salts,

and relatively free of endocervical cells. It develops increased elasticity, called spinnbarkeit. The drying of mucus at this time results in the development of aborization, or ferning (Fig. 1–10). In addition, the cervical os and probably the endocervical canal become dilated.

At this stage in the cycle the cervical mucus serves as a passageway for spermatozoa. It also acts both as a filter to remove abnormal sperm and as a reservoir for sperm, which continuously make their way to the distal end of the fallopian tubes during the periovulatory period.[54,55]

Postcoital Test

Timing in the Cycle. Except during the preovulatory period, sperm routinely do not live well in the cervical canal. In the 1 to 2 days before ovulation, however, they have the capacity to live for many hours, if not days, in the cervical mucus. For that reason, in a 28-day cycle, the best time to do the postcoital test is day 12 to day 14, which should correspond with or precede by a day or two the low point in the temperature chart. In women with more irregular cycles, it may be necessary to repeat the test at 2-day intervals. In women with extremely irregular cycles, it may be necessary to prescribe an ovulatory agent such as clomiphene citrate to regulate the cycle in order to prevent the need for repeated office visits.

Timing after Coitus. There is considerable confusion as to when after coitus the postcoital test should be performed. Many authors state that 2 hours after intercourse is the optimum time; however, this recommendation does not take into consideration the function of the cervix as a reservoir. To ensure a high

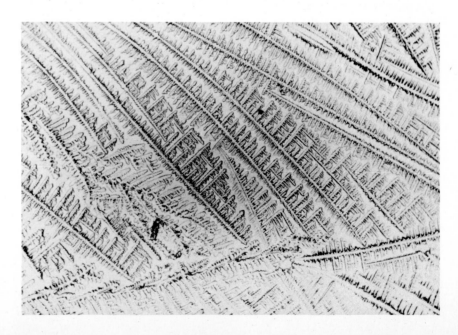

Figure 1–10. Ferning pattern of cervical mucus.

rate of fertilization, active spermatozoa must be, and normally are, available for a 24-hour period.

Therefore, the postcoital test should be performed approximately 12 hours after intercourse. This serves two functions. First, it allows the physician to ascertain whether the sperm are living for an extended period of time after intercourse; this answers the question of whether the cervical mucus functions as an adequate reservoir. Second, it allows the couple to have relations in preparation for the test under relatively natural circumstances and with less time pressure.[56]

Procedure. With the patient in the lithotomy position, a bivalve speculum, lubricated only with warm water, is placed into the vagina. A large dressing forceps and a cotton ball are used to remove vaginal secretions from the exocervix. The closed forceps are then inserted about 1 cm into the cervical canal, opened, rotated 180 degress, closed tightly, and withdrawn. The mucus is placed on a microscope slide.

The amount of mucus is classified as scant, moderate, or profuse. The degree of clarity is noted. The sample is tested for spinnbarkeit by placing a glass coverslip on the mucus, slowly drawing it from the slide, and noting number of centimeters the mucus stretches: 6 to 10 cm suggests impending ovulation. Using the metal dressing forceps instead of the glass coverslip to determine the number of centimeters of spinnbarkeit gives a falsely low reading.

Under the microscope the degree of cellularity is noted, and the number of sperm is evaluated. It is best first to scan the slide under low microscopic power until a representative field has been found. One can then switch to high power and count the number of active, sluggishly motile, and nonmotile sperm per high-power field (hpf). Although one would assume that the more sperm present, the better the chance of pregnancy, this relationship has not been proved. Only two numbers are important in the postcoital test: more than 20 sperm/hpf, which has been positively correlated with pregnancy; and 0, which suggests faulty sperm production in the male, poor coital technique, or antibodies destroying the sperm in situ (Fig. 1–11). Sperm found shaking in place but not moving progressively are also associated with immunologic infertility. After the slide is read, it is dried with an alcohol lamp and evaluated for fern formation. The person performing the postcoital test must recognize the significance of the results to patients, who often feel a poor outcome suggests that they have "failed their love-making test," or that they are "allergic" to each other.

Special Tests. Fractional postcoital tests have been described in which samples are taken at three levels

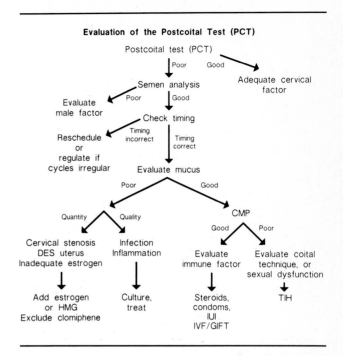

Evaluation of the Postcoital Test (PCT)

Figure 1–11. Decision tree for evaluating a poor postcoital test.

of the endocervical canal by means of a special polyethylene catheter. Although a significant correlation has been noted between sperm count and the number of motile sperm at various levels, no correlation with conception has been found. Other studies have shown that sperm distribution is uniform throughout the cervical canal.[57] Therefore, fractional tests do not appear to be a more reliable method than the Sims-Huhner test.

In vitro sperm-migration tests are recommended when the semen analysis is normal but results of the postcoital test are poor. The physician must first make absolutely certain that the postcoital test was performed at the appropriate time and that the mucus was preovulatory. This is best done by reviewing the temperature chart from the cycle in which the test was performed. Assuming the timing was appropriate, a sperm-penetration test should be performed. The first penetration test was described in 1928 by Kurzrok and Miller.[54] It is performed by placing a small drop of cervical mucus on a slide with a coverslip over it. The corners of the coverslip are supported by small pillars of petrolatum jelly. Semen is applied to the edge of the coverslip and allowed to flow around the cervical mucus. The slide is then placed in a moist chamber at room temperature and read after 3 to 4 hours as follows: degree 0, sperm found only in peripheral parts of the mucus; degree 1, the majority of sperm have invaded the periphery and some are present in the center of the mucus; degree 2, sperm are equally distributed throughout the mucus.

The capillary tube mucus-penetration test described by Kremer is a more widely used in vitro test.[58] Mucus is taken from the cervix as for the postcoital text. It is placed on a microscope slide and, with a flat capillary tube, suctioned with negative pressure by the mouth; the mucus is drawn into the capillary tube, with care taken to ensure that no air bubbles are present. The capillary tube is then placed vertically into a test tube containing 1 mL of the male partner's sperm, and this tube is placed in a rack for 1 hour. At the end of that time, the distance the spermatozoa have traveled is measured (Fig. 1–12). It is important to compare sperm penetration of the patient's mucus to that of donor mucus from another woman. This is made simple by the commercial availability of bovine cervical mucus already drawn in flat capillary tubes. In general, failure to penetrate the mucus implies an immune factor, as does the presence of immotile sperm. Motile sperm seen throughout the 30-mm column of mucus implies normal migration.

Sperm antibody testing should be performed when no sperm or predominately nonmotile sperm are found in the presence of a well-timed postcoital test with abundant cervical mucus. Immune testing is also indicated when results of a mucus-penetration test are poor or sperm are noted to be shaking in place on the postcoital test.

The Tubal Factor

Functions of the Fallopian Tubes. The fallopian tube is not merely a conduit. It is highly sophisticated organ capable of ovum pickup, and involved in sperm transport, fertilization, and ultimately, transport of the zygote into the uterine cavity. The fallopian tube is approximately 9 cm long. Its widest diameter, which is at the fimbriated end, is approximately 2 cm. This narrows to an interstitial diameter of 0.5 mm.

Although it is known that the fallopian tubes play an important role in sperm and ovum develop-

ment, and that cilia and muscular activity are important elements in ovum transport, diagnostic evaluation is limited to determining tubal patency or nonpatency. Two nonsurgical methods are available for this purpose: tubal insufflation with carbon dioxide gas, and hysterosalpingography.

Tubal Insufflation with Carbon Dioxide. Tubal insufflation with carbon dioxide gas was originally described by Rubin in 1920.[59] This test should always be performed in the preovulatory phase so as not to interfere with a newly fertilized ovum. The position of the uterus is ascertained, a tenaculum is placed on the anterior lip of the cervix, and a hollow cannula with an acorn tip is placed into the cervix. An instrument for recording the speed and pressure of flow of the carbon dioxide gas is required. This recording instrument can produce either a permanent record on a graph or temporary marks on a screen to be visualized by the operator. The insufflation is carried out slowly, 25 to 35 mL/minute. The flow is maintained for 1 minute, after which the cannula is removed and reinserted twice more. Subsequently, the patient is asked to sit up. If she feels shoulder pain due to phrenic irritation, the carbon dioxide has passed through the fallopian tubes and into the peritoneal cavity.

Although this test has been performed for over half a century as a screening procedure to rule out complete blockage, it is less widely used now because it gives no information about unilateral or bilateral patency. In addition, comparison of the Rubin's test results with findings of direct visualization of the tubes at laparoscopy has shown that the former are negative when tubes are patent approximately 25% of the time. Nevertheless, it is rare for tubal insufflation to suggest patency when the fallopian tubes are closed, so the procedure can be used as an initial screen in patients with a negative history for tubal disease.

Hysterosalpingography. The hysterosalpingogram (HSG) is an integral part of the infertility evaluation.

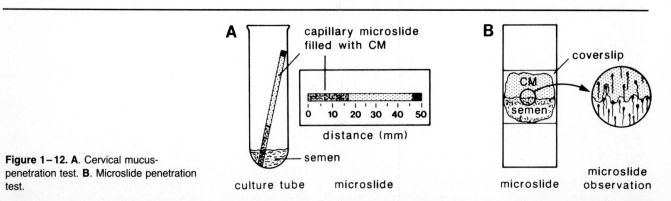

Figure 1–12. **A**. Cervical mucus-penetration test. **B**. Microslide penetration test.

It is performed in the first half of the menstrual cycle after bleeding has stopped and before ovulation. This timing is designed to prevent reflux of endometrial tissue and thus eliminate a potential source of endometriosis. In addition, it precludes the possibility of the test interfering with conception in the uterus or causing an ectopic pregnancy by pushing a conception from the fallopian tube into the peritoneal cavity.

Any history of pelvic inflammatory disease warrants determination of the patient's sedimentation rate. If it is elevated, it is good practice to have the patient take prophylactic antibiotics beginning on the day of the HSG and continuing for 2 or 3 days afterward. In general, tetracycline, 250 mg four times a day for 5 days, is adequate. If tenderness or a pelvic mass is found on pelvic examination prior to the HSG, the procedure should be cancelled.

The procedure is carried out in a radiologic setting, but it is helpful to have a gynecologist perform the instrumentation. First, having her own physician present may decrease the patient's anxiety.

Second, gynecologists are usualy more adept than other physicians at instrumentation of the uterus.

The patient is placed in the dorsal lithotomy position, and a plastic speculum is introduced into the vagina. It is important for the speculum to be plastic; a metal speculum will preclude radiologic visualization of the cervix. Several methods may be used for instrumentation of the uterus, which follows cleansing of the vaginal cavity with an aseptic substance such as benzalkonium chloride (Zephiran) or povidone-iodine (Betadine). A paracervical block placed on the anterior lip of the cervix at the 4 o'clock and 8 o'clock positions is helpful in diminishing discomfort. Prostaglandin inhibitors taken 1 to 2 hours before the procedure have been found effective in reducing discomfort.[60] A Jarco cannula in association with a tenaculum on the anterior lip of the cervix, or special suction devices that grasp the cervix through negative pressure, may be used. A Foley catheter often interferes with visualization of the endometrial cavity and does not allow for adequate traction (Fig. 1–13).

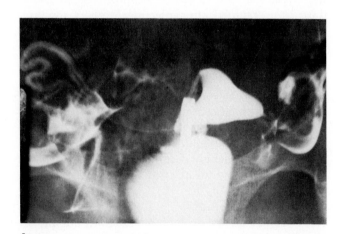

A

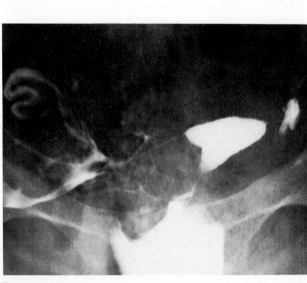

B

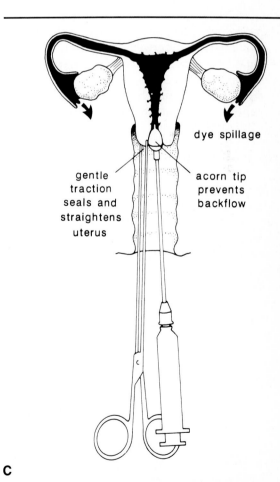

C

Figure 1–13. Retroverted uterus (**A**) before and (**B**) after traction is applied to cervix. **C.** Schematic drawing depicts salient technical points.

Both water-soluble and oil-soluble contrast materials are available, each with its advantages and disadvantages (Tables 1–4 and 1–5).[61] Oil-soluble material is generally associated with a slightly increased risk of granulomatous formations in the peritoneal cavity. It is also poorly absorbed from occluded tubes and thus may remain there until surgery, although the exact significance of this has not been determined. The positive aspect of oil-soluble medium is that it is associated with an increased pregnancy rate. Under no circumstance, however, should the HSG be considered a therapeutic test. It is primarily a diagnostic test that has a slight short-term association with improved outcome.

A more serious concern with oil-soluble medium is embolization, which was reported in 1% of patients in one series.[62] Intravasation produces a spiderweb appearance adjacent to the uterus, with opacified streaks extending toward the pelvic sidewall (Fig. 1–14). The reported frequency of lymphatic or venous intravasation is between 0 and 6%. Factors predisposing to intravasation include excessive pressure during instillation, direct trauma to uterine mucosa, surgically altered cervix or endometrium, and organic or congenital anomalies of the uterine cavity. Should the spiderweb pattern be seen, the HSG should be stopped at once to prevent embolization.

Water-soluble medium has the disadvantage of being slightly more irritating than oil-soluble medium. It is reabsorbed quickly, however, and does not appear to be associated with adhesion formation in the peritoneal cavity.

Regardless of which medium is used, the most important feature is its slow injection. The uterine cavity is a potential space of only 4 or 5 mL. Rapid injection of more than this quantity will only distend the uterus and cause cramping and pain. If pain does occur, temporarily pausing often proves helpful.

Fluoroscopy with an image intensifier is the recommended radiologic equipment. An experienced radiologist using a spot film system can often differentiate between medium in the tubo-ovarian gutter and medium trapped by peritubal adhesions. If

TABLE 1–5. COMPARISON OF WATER SOLUBLE AND OIL SOLUBLE MEDIUM: DIAGONOSING PERITUBAL ADHESIONS

HSG	Laparoscopy	Water-Soluble Medium No.(%)	Oil-Soluble Medium No.(%)	Combined No.(%)
Present	Present	4(9)	8(24)	12(15.5)
Absent	Absent	24(55)	9(27)	33(43)
Absent	Present	14(32)	15(46)	29(37.5)
Present	Absent	2(4)	1(3)	3(4)
Totals		44(100)	33(100)	77(100)

From reference 61. Reproduced with permission.

fluoroscopy is not possible, no more than three or four films should be taken. A preliminary film is obtained before dye is injected. A second film after the injection of 1 mL of medium outlines uterine contour and defines intrauterine pathology such as polyps. Air bubbles are occasionally mistaken for intrauterine polyps or fibroids; they are differentiated by asking the patient to shift positions, which causes the bubbles to rise to a new location (Fig. 1–15). A third film obtained after injecting 5 mL of medium should determine tubal patency.

A final follow-up film should be taken to look for the spread of dye through the peritoneal cavity. If oil-soluble medium is used, a follow-up film is taken 24 hours later; if water-soluble medium is used, it may be performed in 10 to 20 minutes. Accumulation of contrast medium in the pelvis indicates that peritubal adhesions have trapped the medium. This final film is an essential part of the procedure. Failure to obtain it constitutes an inadequate HSG.

The Ovulatory Factor

The presence or absence of ovulation and the quality of corpus luteum function, both important factors in infertility, may be evaluated in three ways: (1) determining basal body temperature, (2) performing endometrial biopsy, and (3) measuring progesterone levels in the blood. These approaches yield only presumptive evidence of ovulation, all dependent on the secretion of progesterone by the corpus luteum. Occasionally, a luteinized unruptured follicle (LUF) secretes progesterone, imitating ovulation.[63]

Basal Body Temperature Chart. The BBT chart, first described in 1904, is the simplest and most inexpensive method of assessing the presence or absence of ovulation. A biphasic chart, characterized by a sustained rise of at least 0.4°F for 12 to 15 days, is typical of ovulation and an adequate luteal phase.

It is generally accepted that ovulation occurs on the day of the lowest temperature and is followed by a sustained rise in temperature. This may actually vary as much as 2 days. Since one cannot predict the

TABLE 1–4. COMPARISON OF WATER SOLUBLE AND OIL SOLUBLE MEDIUM. DIAGNOSING TUBAL PATENCY

HSG	Laparoscopy	Water-Soluble Medium No.(%)	Oil-Soluble Medium No.(%)	Combined No.(%)
Patent	Patent	27(61)	14(42.5)	41(53)
Occlusion	Occlusion	5(11)	11(33.5)	16(21)
Patent	Occlusion	3(7)	1(3)	4(5)
Occlusion	Patent	9(21)	7(21)	16(21)
Totals		44(100)	33(100)	77(100)

From reference 61. Reproduced with permission.

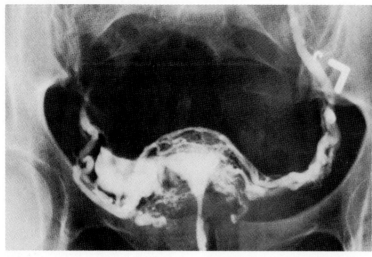

A

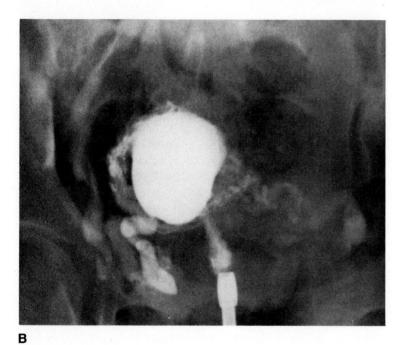

B

Figure 1–14. Spiderweb appearance of intravasation into uterine lymphatics.

day of ovulation, it is poor practice to use the temperature chart to time intercourse. If sperm count and motility as well as cervical mucus are normal, sperm will remain viable in the cervix for at least 48 hours. Thus, for partners who have coitus two or three times a week, there are many times during a year in which sperm will be waiting for the ovum to be released. Furthermore, since the temperature chart may show a number of small dips before the so-called crucial dip, it is not possible to know in advance which dip is the crucial one. Ovulation may occur well before this event, and sometimes there is no dip at all.

For these reasons, emphasis on the temperature chart for coital timing is unwarranted. In fact, when the male partner's semen is of borderline quality,

repeated intercourse based on the temperature chart may actually lead to reduced fertility.

Despite these negative aspects, 3 or 4 months of recording the temperature gives suggestive evidence of ovulation as well as information on the quality of ovulation. Most important, the BBT helps the physician estimate the timing of ovulation for insemination, evaluate the effectiveness of ovulation-inducing compounds, and consider therapy for a luteal phase deficiency. It is of utmost importance for tests to be performed at the appropriate time in the cycle (Fig. 1–16).

The BBT can also be of diagnostic help in luteal phase deficiency. Ovulation occurs in this condition, but due to the reduced function or shortened life of the corpus luteum, the progesterone level is low.

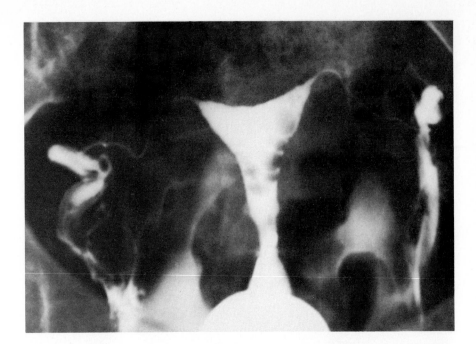

Figure 1–15. Air bubbles give the appearance of intrauterine polyps or fibroids. Note metal speculum, which can obliterate the view of the lower uterine segment.

Deficiency is suggested on the basis of one of three BBT patterns: luteal phase duration of less than 12 days, sluggish rise in luteal phase temperature, and luteal phase temperature of 12 or more days' duration but with a rise of less than 0.4°F. Temperature changes should be confirmed by endometrial biopsy or progesterone assay.

Endometrial Biopsy. Sampling the endometrium to assess progesterone production by the corpus luteum gives indirect evidence of the presence or absence of ovulation. After ovulation, the progesterone secreted by the corpus luteum causes the endometrium to develop progressively and predictably.[64] The first change is subnuclear vacuolization, followed by increasing tortuosity of the glands, edema, and menstruation. So predictable are these changes that the endometrial sample can reveal how many days previously ovulation occurred.

The patient is asked to keep a temperature chart. The day of the endometrial biopsy should be as close to the time of menstruation as possible and may be performed up to 18 hours after the onset of the menstrual flow. Local anesthesia of the cervix and a paracervical block minimize pain.

Before the endometrial biopsy is done, a pelvic examination is performed and the position of the uterus noted. A speculum is then introduced into the vagina and an aseptic solution used to clean the cervix. A Meigs or Novak curette may be used; disposable curettes also are popular. The biopsy curette is passed through the internal os into the fundus. Since most conceptions occur on the posterior wall, the sample should be taken from high on the fundus of the uterus and from the lateral walls to diminish the chance of interrupting a pregnancy (Fig. 1–17).

The results are interpreted in relation to the onset of the menstrual period that follows the test.

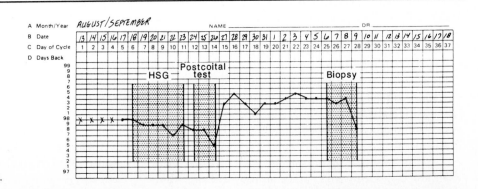

Figure 1–16. Basal body temperature chart demonstrates schedule for testing.

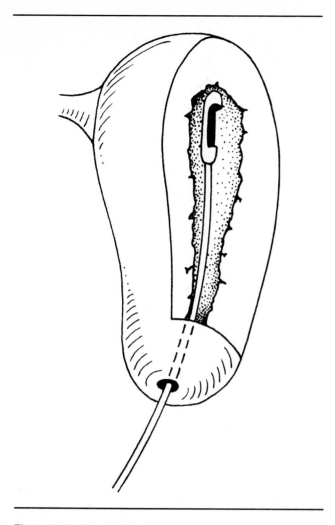

Figure 1–17. Endometrial biopsy.

The first day of menses is considered day 14 of the luteal phase. The endometrial sample is dated as postovulatory or secretory day 1 to 14, according to the number of days that have elapsed since ovulation. The gynecologist then counts backward from day 14 to the day on which the biopsy was performed, and the actual postovulatory day is compared with the apparent postovulatory day determined by the biopsy. No more than a 2-day discrepancy should exist between these numbers. A discrepancy of 3 days or more signifies a luteal phase deficiency. It is prudent to know who is reading the biopsy, as precision and accuracy may vary greatly among individuals.

The advantage of performing the endometrial biopsy after the onset of menstruation is that there is no possibility of interrupting a pregnancy. Furthermore, the os is usually open at this time, making it slightly easier to insert the curette. Should the biopsy be performed in the luteal phase of a cycle in which conception has occurred, a slight chance exists that the pregnancy will be interrupted. Most of these

pregnancies continue without difficulty; however, obtaining a pregnancy test immediately prior to the procedure substantially reduces the risk of pregnancy interruption.

Progesterone Level. A serum progesterone level of 4 ng/mL is evidence that ovulation has occurred.[65] This does not evaluate the quality of the luteal phase. According to some investigators, three samples totaling 15 ng/mL constitute a normal luteal phase; according to others it is a level of greater than 10 ng/mL 1 week after ovulation. Because progesterone levels vary considerably and no sharp demarcation exists between what is normal and what is abnormal on any given day, this assessment is not as useful as endometrial biopsy.

The Male Factor

Semen Analysis. Because the male may be a factor in infertility in as many as one third of all couples, it is imperative that he not be neglected during the workup. If the couple lives near a urologist who is interested in infertility, it is appropriate for the man to be examined by that physician. Usually, however, it is the gynecologist who first examines the woman and thus has the responsibility of ensuring that the male is properly evaluated and treated. A postcoital test alone is not sufficient; it is necessary to do both a history and a physical examination of the male, as well as two semen analyses. One must bear in mind that there is a circannual rhythm in human sperm counts, with a trend toward highest values between February and March and the lowest during September (Fig. 1–18).[66]

The semen should be collected in a small, clean, wide-mouthed, 1 to 2-ounce glass jar. Use of a larger jar often results in the specimen drying along the sides while it is being transported to the office or laboratory. The preferred method of sperm collection is masturbation, but if this is objectionable, coitus withdrawal may be used; a portion of the semen will be lost by this method. Condoms that contain a spermicidal agent should never be used. Latex condoms without spermicidal agents are commercially available.

The male should abstain from sexual relations for approximately 48 hours before collecting the specimen. The specimen should reach the laboratory within 2 to 3 hours; it is not necessary to examine the sperm immediately after collection. During transportation it should be kept as near to room temperature as possible. In cold weather it can be held close to the body. After delivery to the laboratory, the specimen is evaluated for viscosity and volume. Normally, semen is ejaculated as a coagulum, but it liquefies in

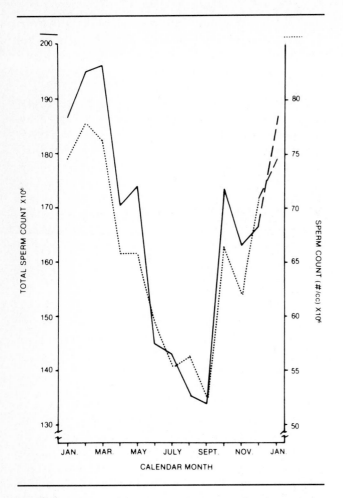

Figure 1–18. Circannual rhythm in human total sperm count and concentration.

5 to 20 minutes, after which it flows easily and freely. Continuation of the viscous state is abnormal and may reduce fertility.

Volume between 2.5 and 8 mL is considered normal. Less than 2.5 mL often results in poor cervical insemination. If the small ejaculatory volume is oligospermic or azoospermic and is alkaline, a postejaculation urine sample should be examined to exclude retrograde ejaculation. This is particularly likely in men with a past history of prostate or bladder surgery. A volume of greater than 8 mL is usually accompanied by diminished sperm density. That finding is an indication for the use of homologous insemination with a split ejaculate.

After thorough mixing, a drop of semen is placed on a microscope slide, and the number of leukocytes and the presence of agglutination are assessed. The percentage of motility is determined by dividing the mean of the number of active forms by the number of inactive forms in four or five hpf. As sperm longevity may be another important factor in conception, a second evaluation of motility should be carried out approximately 5 to 6 hours after ejaculation.

Well-mixed semen is drawn up to the 0.5 mark on a pipette used to count white blood cells. The pipette is then filled with tap water and thoroughly shaken, and the cells are counted in the red blood cell field of a hemocytometer. All the cells lying within 5 blocks of the 16 cells each are counted. The total number of sperm cells counted gives the count in millions per mL. If the count is low, the semen should be brought to the 1.0 mark of the pipette (1:10 dilution) and the number of cells doubled to give the count in millions. This reduces the counting error in cases of severe oligospermia. A chamber has been developed in which direct counting is made from an undiluted sample. Counting the number of sperm heads in 10 squares of the grid immediately provides their concentrations as millions per mL.[67]

Sperm morphology is evaluated as a routine part of the semen analysis.[68] This is done from a sample representing the sperm population as a whole. In general, morphology is normal in at least 40% of sperm. A high percentage of tapering forms has been associated with varicocele. It has been reported that abnormal forms are twice as frequent in nonmotile sperm as they are in motile ones.[69]

Although there is no absolute standard of fertility, certain guidelines for semen analysis have been established. In general, semen is considered fertile if the count is greater than 40 million/mL, the percentage of motility at 6 hours is greater than 50%, and morphology is normal in more than 60%. An infertile specimen is one with a count of less than 20 million, motility at 6 hours of less than 35%, and less than 60% normal forms. Counts and motility percentages between these two levels (20 and 40 million, and 35 and 50%, respectively) constitute a state of relative infertility and deserve to be treated. Obviously, these values are not absolute. Computerized sperm analyzers are available that provide precise quantification of sperm motility, speed, and motion patterns. Although they offer exciting potential for the future, they do not appear to provide more useful data for improving pregnancy outcome than an experienced technician.

FINAL STEPS OF THE BASIC WORKUP

Consultation

After the basic minimum workup is completed, the couple returns to discuss the test results and to determine how best to procede. This consultation is extremely important. The results of all previous tests are reviewed, with verification that they were obtained at the correct time in the cycle. This task is made simpler with the use of a summary sheet. Alternatively, using rubber stamps for each proce-

```
┌─────────────────────────────────────┐
│                 HSG                  │
│  History_____       │
│                                       │
│  Uterus _____       │
│                                       │
│  Tubes  R _____       │
│                                       │
│         L _____       │
│                                       │
│  Dye used _____       │
│                                       │
│  Comments _____       │
└─────────────────────────────────────┘
A
```

```
┌─────────────────────────────────────┐
│  AI _____        │
│  Fresh/frozen                        │
│  Meds _____         │
│                                       │
│  Cycle day_____          │
│                                       │
│  Mucus amt. _____          │
│                                       │
│       F _____ SB _____      │
│                                       │
│  Specimen _____ % Motility     │
└─────────────────────────────────────┘
B
```

```
┌─────────────────────────────────────┐
│          POST COITAL TEST            │
│                                       │
│  Day of cycle_____     │
│                                       │
│  Meds _____        │
│                                       │
│  Hours P.C. _____         │
│                                       │
│  Mucus Amt. _____          │
│                                       │
│  F _____SB _____         │
│                                       │
│  No. Sperm/hpf _____          │
│                                       │
│      %Motile _____          │
└─────────────────────────────────────┘
C
```

```
┌─────────────────────────────────────┐
│           PRENATAL VISIT             │
│                                       │
│  BP _____ WT _____ Urine _____  │
│                                       │
│  LMP_____ EDC_____        │
│                                       │
│  Dates _____ Size _____     │
└─────────────────────────────────────┘
D
```

Figure 1–19. Stamps used for office visits.

dure that highlight the test results of the workup also helps when reviewing the data (Fig. 1–19). Problem areas are explained and discussed, and a treatment plan is outlined.

It is of utmost, importance to establish a timetable for treatment. Because infertility has usually been a problem of long standing, failure to do so often results in couples perceiving that their treatment plan is open ended, which may cause them to feel out of control.

Laparoscopy

With few exceptions, a laparoscopy should be planned only after the basic minimum workup is completed. If there is any suggestion that laparoscopic surgery will be performed, it is advantageous to schedule the procedure for an adequate period of time to perform it completely and meticulously, and to book the appropriate instruments with the operat-

ing room. This also allows the physician the opportunity to discuss operative laparoscopy with the couple ahead of time.

Some physicians prefer to schedule laparoscopy in the follicular phase to avoid either inadvertant rupturing and bleeding of a corpus luteum, or confusing a corpus luteum with an endometrioma. Others prefer performing the procedure in the luteal phase in order to document ovulation. Most prefer to avoid menses if possible to prevent retrograde flux of menstrual endometrium, which may theoretically result in endometriosis.

The patient is placed in the dorsal lithotomy position under general anesthesia. A subumbilical incision is made and a Verres needle inserted to introduce carbon dioxide insufflation. While the abdomen is filling, the bladder is emptied. A tenaculum is applied to the cervix and a Jarco cannula inserted. It saves time to perform this step while the abdomen is filling. After adequate insufflation, the trochar sheath and laparoscope are introduced. If the patient has had a previous midline incision, performing an open laparoscopy under direct vision reduces the potential risk of inadvertent injury to the bowel or other pelvic viscera when inserting the trochar.

A second suprapubic puncture is an essential part of the infertility laparoscopy. Using a blunt probe to sweep away bowel from the cul-de-sac and elevating the ovaries to view their medial aspects preclude overlooking adhesions or endometriosis. The second puncture also allows scissors and other operative instruments to be inserted with ease. To ensure that minimal endometriosis is seen, the laparoscope should be placed close to the peritoneal surface to take advantage of the magnification provided by the instrument.

Prior to completing the laparoscopy, a dilute solution of dye is inserted through the Jarco cannula. Indigo carmine is preferable to methylene blue because it does not stain. Also, confusion can occasionally occur if methylene blue passes through one tube and stains the fimbriae of the other, suggesting patency when in fact the contralateral tube is occluded.

If a D&C is to be performed it should be done after insufflation of dye to prevent retrograde flow of endometrial fragments loosened by the curettage. The uterus should also be sounded to document its depth in case in vitro fertilization requires that measurement for embryo transfer.

After the procedure is completed, the operative note should be dictated immediately and a handwritten note placed in the patient's record in case the operative is lost. Care must be taken to describe in detail the tubal anatomy. If a hydrosalpinx is encountered, the diameter of the ampulla is noted. The lengths of tubal segments are also recorded in cases of tubal resection. Because of the magnification properties of the laparoscope, it is useful to use the graded probe as a ruler to ensure accurate measurements. Patients with endometriosis should be staged according to American Fertility Society classification, thus avoiding rough guesses of amount of disease. The percentage of ovarian surface visible and the mobility of the ovaries are also described. Finally, tubal patency and endometrial depth are documented. These details enhance consultations with colleagues and prevent the need to duplicate the procedure. If a uterine anomaly is suggested by the HSG, a hysteroscopy should be performed as part of the laparoscopy.

SUMMARY

This chapter describes the author's approach to the basic infertility workup. It is designed to determine

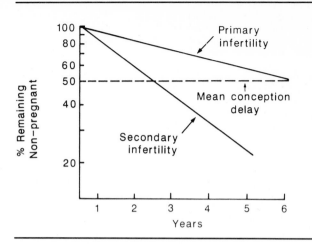

Figure 1–20. Timetable of expected pregnancy for patients with unexplained infertility.

the etiology of infertility and suggest therapy in more than 90% of instances if the physician is conscientious and has a clear understanding of the basic principles involved. If no cause is found, the couple is designated as having unexplained infertility, and a discussion of expectant management versus treatment is in order (Fig. 1–20). Conversely, once a diagnosis is established, a well-planned timetable of treatment is imperative either to help the couple achieve a successful pregnancy in a timely fashion, or help them bring their pursuit of a biologic child to a close or consider adoption. Because of the significance of the outcome to patients receiving infertility care, the importance of the workup cannot be overestimated.

REFERENCES

1. Menning BE: The psychology of infertility, in Aimen J (ed): *Infertility: Diagnosis and Management*. New York, Springer-Verlag, 1984, pp 17–29.
2. Tietze C, Guttmacher AF, Rubin S: Time required for conception in 1727 planned pregnancies. *Fertil Steril* 1:338, 1950.
3. Fundamental considerations, in Keller DW, Strickler RC, Warren JC (eds): *Clinical Infertility*. East Norwalk, CT, Appleton-Century-Crofts, 1984, p 2.
4. Cook EP: Characteristics of the biopsychosocial crisis of infertility. *J Counseling Development* 65:465, 1987.
5. Smith CG, Asch RH: Drug abuse and reproduction. *Fertil Steril* 48:355, 1987.
6. Blackwell RE, Chang RJ: Report of the national symposium on the clinical management of prolactin-related reproductive disorders. *Fertil Steril* 45:607, 1986.
7. Herzog AG, Seibel MM, Schomer D, Vaitukaitis JL, Geschwind N: Reproductive endocrine disorders in men with partial seizures of temporal lobe origin. *Arch Neurol* 43:347, 1986.
8. Mueller BA, Daling JR, Moore DE, et al: Appendectomy and the risk of tubal infertility. *N Engl J Med* 315:1506, 1986.
9. Seibel MM: Infection and infertility, in DeCherney AH (ed): *Reproductive Failure*. New York, Churchill Livingstone, 1986, p 203.
10. Cramer DW, Schiff I, Schoenbaum SC, et al: Tubal infertility and the intrauterine device. *N Engl J Med* 312:941, 1985.
11. Bayer SR, Seibel MM: Endometriosis: clinical symptoms and infertility, in Rolland R, Chadha DR; Willemsen WNP (eds): *Gonadotropin Down-Regulation in Gynecological Practice*. New York, Liss, 1986, p 103.
12. Burke L, Antonioli D, Friedman EA: Evolution of diethylstilbestrol-associated genital tract lesions. *Obstet Gynecol* 57:79, 1981.

13. Goldenberg R, White R: The effects of vaginal lubricants on sperm motility in vitro. *Fertil Steril* 26:872, 1975.

14. Kaufman RH, Adam E, Bender GL, Gerthoffer E: Upper genital tract changes and pregnancy outcomes in offspring exposed in utero to diethylstilbestro. *Am J Obstet Gynecol* 137:299, 1980.

15. U.S. Department of Health and Human Services: The health consequences of smoking: A report of the Surgeon General. Washington DC, U.S. Government Printing Office, 1984.

16. Stedman RL: The chemical composition of tobacco and tobacco smoke. *Chem Rev* 68:153, 1968.

17. Fielding JE: Smoking: health effects and control. *N Engl J Med* 313:491, 1985.

18. Stillman RJ, Rosenberg MJ, Sachs BP: Smoking and reproduction. *Fertil Steril* 46:545, 1986.

19. Howe G, Westhoiff C, Vessey M, Yeates D: Effects of age, cigarette smoking, and other factors on fertility: Findings in a large prospective study. *BR Med J* 290:1697, 1985.

20. Baird DD, Wilcox AJ: Cigarette smoking associated with delayed conception. *JAMA* 253:2979, 1985.

21. Tokutata GM: Smoking in relation to infertility and fetal loss. *Arch Environ Health* 17:353, 1968.

22. Neri A, Marcus SL: Effect of nicotine on the motility of the oviducts in the rhesus monkey: A preliminary report. *J Reprod Fertil* 31:91, 1972.

23. Campbell OM, Gray RH: Smoking and ectopic pregnancy: A multinational case-control study, in Rosenberg MJ (ed): *Smoking and Reproductive Health*. Littleton, MA, PSG, 1986.

24. Phipps WR, Cramer DW, Schiff I, et al: The association between smoking and female infertility as influenced by cause of the infertility. *Fertil Steril* 48:377, 1987.

25. Card JP, Mitchell JA: The effects of nicotine administration on deciduoma induction in the rat. *Biol Reprod* 19:326, 1978.

26. Yoshinaga K, Rice C, Krenn J, Pilot RL: Effects of nicotine on early pregnancy in the rat. *Biol Reprod* 19:326, 1978.

27. McLachlan JA, Dames NM, Sieber SM, Fabro S: Accumulation of nicotine in the uterine fluid of the six-day pregnant rabbit. *Fertil Steril* 27:1204, 1976.

28. Hammond EC: Smoking in relation to physical complaints. *Arch Environ Health* 3:28, 1961.

29. Mattison DR: The effects of smoking on fertility from gametogenesis to implantation. *Environ Res* 28:410, 1982.

30. Barbieri RL, McShane PM, Ryan KJ: Constituents of cigarette smoke inhibit granulosa cell aromatase. *Fertil Steril* 46:232, 1986.

31. Klaiber EL, Broverman DM, Pokoly TB, et al: Interrelationships of cigarette smoking, testicular varicoceles, and seminal fluid indexes. *Fertil Steril* 47:481, 1987.

32. Gindoff PR, Jewelewicz R: Reproductive potential in the older woman. *Fertil Steril* 46:989, 1986.

33. Federation CECOS, Schwartz D, Mayaux MJ: Female fecundity as a function of age: Results of artificial insemination in 2193 nulliparous women with azoospermic husbands. *N Engl J Med* 306:404, 1982.

34. Yeh J, Seibel MM: Artificial insemination with donor sperm: A review of 108 patients. *Obstet Gynecol* 70:313, 1987.

35. James W: The causes of the decline in fecundability with age. *Soc Biol* 26:330, 1979.

36. MacLeod J, Gold RZ: The male factor in fertility and infertility. VI. Semen quality and certain other factors in relation to ease of conception. *Fertil Steril* 4:10, 1953.

37. Sherman B, Korenman S: Hormonal characteristics of the human menstrual cycle throughout reproductive life. *J Clin Invest* 55:699, 1975.

38. Cooper R, McNamara C, Linnoila M: Catecholaminergic-serotonergic balance in the CNS and reproductive cycling in aging rats. *Neurobiol Aging* 7:9, 1986.

39. Sopelak V, Butcher R: Contribution of the ovary versus hypothalamic–pituitary to termination of estrous cycles in aging rats using ovarian transplants. *Biol Reprod* 27:29, 1982.

40. Wise, P: Aging of the female reproductive system. *Rev Biol Res Aging* 1:1945, 1983.

41. Warburton D, Kline J, Stein Z, Strobino B: Cytogenetic abnormalities in spontaneous abortions of recognized conceptions, in Porter IH, Willey A (eds): *Perinatal Genetics: Diagnosis and Treatment.* New York, Academic Press, 1986, p 133.

42. Friedman JM: Genetic disease in the offspring of older fathers. *Obstet Gynecol* 57:745, 1981.

43. Paniagua R, Martin A, Nistal M, Amat P: Testicular involution in elderly men: comparison of histologic quantitative studies with hormone patterms. *Fertil Steril* 47:671, 1987.

44. Warner BA, Dufau ML, Santen RJ: Effects of aging and illness on the pituitary–testicular axis in men: Qualitative as well as quantitative changes in luteinizing hormone. *J Clin Endocrinol Metab* 60:263, 1985.

45. Schwartz D, Mayaux MJ, Spira A, et al: Semen characteristics as a function of age in 833 subfertile men. *Fertil Steril* 39:530, 1983.

46. Spellacy WN, Miller SJ, Winegar A: Pregnancy after 40 years of age. *Obstet Gynecol* 68:452, 1986.

47. Stillman RJ: In utero exposure to diethylstilbestrol: Adverse effects on the reproductive tract and reproductive performance in male and female offspring. *Am J Obstet Gynecol* 142:905, 1982.

48. Lee RL, Lipshultz LI: Evaluation and treatment of male infertility, in Hammond MG, Talbert LM (eds): *Infertility: A Practical Guide for the Physician,* ed 2. Oradell, NJ, Medical Economics Books, 1985, pp 42–63.

49. Werner CA: Mumps orchitis and testicular atrophy. I. Occurrence. *Ann Intern Med* 32:1066, 1950.

50. Damewood MD, Grochow LB: Prospects for fertility after chemotherapy or radiation for neoplastic disease. *Fertil Steril* 45:443, 1986.

51. Cann PA, Holdsworth CD: Reversal of male infertility on changing treatment from sulphasalazine to 5-aminosalicylic acid. *Lancet* 2:1119, 1984.

52. Sims JM: Sterility and value of the microscope in diagnosis and treatment. *Trans Am Gynecol Soc* 13:291, 1888.

53. Huhner M: *Sterility in the Female and its Treatment.* New York, Rebman, 1913.

54. Kurzrok R, Miller E: Biochemical studies of the human and its relation to mucus of the cervix uteri. *Am J Obstet Gynecol* 15:56, 1928.

55. Settlage DSF, Motoshima M, Treadway DR: Sperm transport from the external cervical os to the fallopian tubes in women: A time and quantitation study. *Fertil Steril* 24:655, 1973.

56. Seibel MM, Taymor ML: Emotional aspects of infertility. *Fertil Steril* 37:137, 1982.

57. Drake TS, Tredway DR, Buchanan GC: A reassessment of the fractional post-coital test. *Am J Obstet Gynecol* 133:382, 1979.

58. Kremer J: A simple sperm penetration test. *Int J Fertil* 10:209, 1965.

59. Rubin IC: Nonoperative determination of patency of fallopian tubes in sterility: A preliminary report. *JAMA* 74:1017, 1920.

60. Owens OM, Schiff I, Kaul AF, Cramer DC, Burt RAP: Reduction of pain following hysterosalpingogram by prior analgesic administration. *Fertil Steril* 43:146, 1985.

61. Loy RA, Weinstein FG, Seibel MM, Hysterosalpingography in perspective: The predictive value of oil soluble versus water soluble contrast media. *Fertil Steril* 51:170, 1989.

62. Nunley WC, Bateman BG, Kitchin JD, Pope TL: Intravasation during hysterosalpingography using oil-base contrast medium—A second look. *Obstet Gynecol* 70:309, 1987.

63. Schenken RS, Werlin LB, Williams RF, Prihoda TJ, Hogden GD: Histological and hormonal documentation of the luteinized unruptured follicle syndrome. *Am J Obstet Gynecol* 154:839, 1986.

64. Noyes RW, Hertig AT, Rock J: Dating the endometrial biopsy. *Fertil Steril* 1:3, 1950.

65. Seegar Jones G, Aksel S, Colston Wentz A: Serum progesterone values in the luteal phase defects: Effects of chorionic gonadotropin. *Obstet Gynecol* 44:33, 1974.

66. Tjoa WS, Smolensky MH, Hoi BP, Steinberger E, Smith KD: Circannual rhythm in human sperm count revealed by serially independent sampling. *Fertil Steril* 38:454, 1982.

67. Makler A: The improved 10 µm chamber for rapid sperm count and motility evaluation. *Fertil Steril* 33:337, 1980.

68. Freund M: Standards for rating of human sperm morphology—A cooperative study. *Int J Fertil* 11:97, 1966.

69. Makler A: Distribution of normal and abnormal forms among motile, nonmotile, live and dead spermatozoa. *Int J Fertil* 3:620, 1980.

70. Antenatal diagnosis of genetic disorders. ACOG Technical Bulletin, no 108, Sept 1987.

CHAPTER 2

Emotional Aspects of Infertility

Alice D. Domar, Machelle M. Seibel

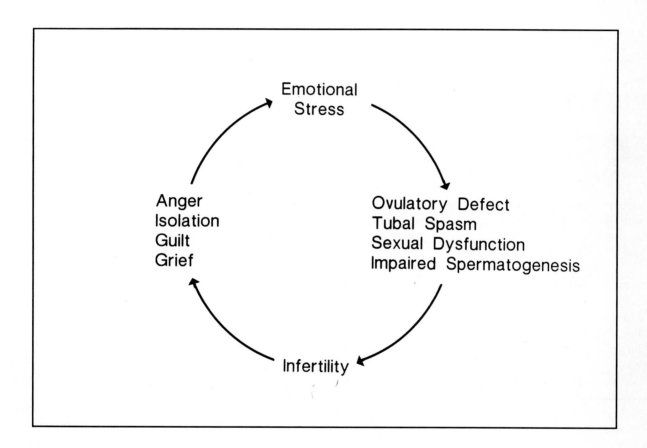

Infertility

The simple union of man and wife
    in love creates a brand new life.
A child to cherish, play with, and be
    their link with immortality.

What bliss and joy they anticipate!
    Unless infertility becomes their fate
and shatters dreams which die within
    as they mourn their child who might have been.
                    M. M. Seibel, 1988

It is estimated that infertility affects 15% of the childbearing age population in the United States, or approximately 10 million couples. Numerous factors, including postponement of childbearing and the rising frequency of venereal disease, use of certain contraceptive methods such as the intrauterine device (IUD), and the number of therapeutic abortions, are contributing to increased numbers of infertile couples.[1-3] Because infertility results in the loss of something that has never been, however, its impact often goes unnoticed by the general population. For these reasons, infertile couples have been termed by some as the most neglected and silent minority in the country.[4]

The study of the emotional aspects of infertility must incorporate three major shifts in emphasis that have occurred during the past 10 years. First, the general concept of psychogenic infertility has been reversed so that, with few exceptions, distress is now seen as the result, not the cause, of infertility. Nevertheless, psychologic, physiologic, and neuroendocrine factors are interactive and interdependent. Second, the evaluation and treatment of infertility have evolved from being viewed exclusively as a woman's problem; physiologic male factors are also being extensively studied. The emotional impact on men is considered as well, but less intensively. Finally, the emphasis on treating infertility as an individual matter has changed to treating the couple as a unit, with both partners viewed as enduring a personal and a family crisis.[5]

Infertility may be experienced as an emotional loss in many ways. For some, it is similar to the amputation of a limb or the diagnosis of a chronic illness. For all, the diagnosis represents being denied the choice of having a biologic child.[6] Although as recently as the late 1960s, 50% of infertility cases were classified as emotionally determined, improved methods in diagnosing defects in reproductive endocrinology and infertility rule out emotional causes in all but 5% of cases.[7,8] Nonetheless, the physical and mental consequences of the infertility workup, subsequent treatment, and lack of success may cause or contribute to a psychologic problem. Thus it is incumbent on physicians who treat infertile couples to be aware of the enormous stresses that infertility places on both partners, and to understand the psychologic interventions that are effective in alleviating some of these stresses.

THE WORKUP

For many couples, infertility has come to be viewed as a physical disease awaiting appropriate medical or surgical therapy.[9] The workup becomes a consuming, long-term preoccupation. It also can be psycho-logically, socially, physically, and financially devastating. The timing of certain tests and sexual relations is so critical that other aspects of living become subordinate.[1] Coitus is no longer an expression of affection or closeness. Instead, couples stop making love and start trying to make babies.[8] This problem has been exacerbated by the widespread use of home ovulation-detection kits. Couples purchase these kits to gain control over their cycles, only to feel required to have intercourse when the indicator dot turns blue. It is not surprising that many express personal distress. In one study of 51 infertile couples, 10% demonstrated some degree of midcycle sexual dysfunction.[10] Contributing factors included the "this-is-the-night" syndrome, the change in the purpose of sexual intercourse, the stress of testing by a third party, and self-doubt of the adequacy of future performance. Some patients cope with their anxiety by avoiding medical assessments, as suggested by repeated cancellations of the postcoital test.

During the initial evaluation, the requisite sexual review may be seen by some patients as embarrassing, intrusive, inappropriate, and demeaning. Questions that focus on sexual habits and patterns may themselves cause sexual dysfunction, thus further contributing to infertility.[9,11] The simplest manner in which psychologic factors can be thought of as causing infertility is through their effect on sexual performance: reduced frequency can contribute to infertility.[12] The pressures of having sex during ovulation may have a significant negative impact on desire; sex for pleasure fades away into a job of procreation.[13]

Treatment for infertility can continue for more than a decade. Many couples marshall all of their strength and stamina in the belief that the condition can be corrected. As long as they are receiving active therapy, they usually put aside crucial decisions about career, life plans, and adoption, and delay confronting childlessness.[2] Despite such outward appearances of stalwart determination, however, living with infertility means working through complex emotional reactions, often with little outside assistance.[11,13]

THE PSYCHOLOGIC IMPACT ON WOMEN

Some women consider the infertility investigation to be the worst experience of their lives. Infertility becomes an all-encompassing focus of their existence, affecting nearly every aspect of their lives. Many feel controlled by the drive to achieve conception and find it hard to concentrate on long-term goals when taking medications, recovering from surgery, dealing with their emotional reactions, and living with the daily hope that it will end soon.[14] Job security and advancement are often affected; women may turn down promotions that require relocating because they are so invested in their physician, and avoid career changes that might interfere with the freedom to continue treatment. Taking time off from work for endless doctor's appointments, blood tests, operations, and other procedures may endanger job security.

In addition to the many practical stresses, a woman's desire to have a child is so powerful that the emotional toll of infertility is enormous. When questioned why they wanted to have a child, the most common answer given by a group of women was, "It is just a feeling." Conception is frequently viewed as the ultimate expression of love between a man and a woman.[15] Furthermore, because of the emphasis society places on parenthood, infertile women feel unfeminine. This is particularly true for those with conditions such as polycystic ovary disease, in which hirsutism and an excess of male hormones add to the problem.

Women may feel guilty for upsetting their partner and disappointing their families. The guilt may focus on sexual behaviors such as early promiscuity, premarital or extramarital sex, past abortion, homosexual experiences, masturbation, prior contraceptive use, or even taking pleasure in sex.[16,17] For some, continued painful or stressful treatments may represent atonement for past behaviors.[17] Anger and sadness are also common emotions. Anger is connected to a sense of unfairness and may be stimulated by seeing pregnant women or babies, resulting in envy or jealousy. Sadness can be pervasive, and is associated with helplessness, lack of control, despair, and grief.[5]

The continued pressures can eliminate self-confidence, a sense of competence, and a sense of control These losses can lead to a decreased feeling of security, compromised health, and interference with close relationships, and destroy hopes and goals for the future.[14]

THE PSYCHOLOGIC IMPACT ON MEN

The major emphasis in the literature on the psychologic impact of infertility has been on women. A review of 121 articles published between 1948 and 1985 revealed that only 18% emphasized the male partner, and these were primarily written since the late 1960s.[18] Prior to 1970, knowledge of male responses to infertility was virtually nonexistent; physiology, not psychology, was emphasized.[19] The main problem in assessing the emotional response to infertility has been men's lack of availability and

willingness to undergo evaluations. Many associate the inability to impregnate a woman with reduced masculinity and virility, and appear threatened when psychologic factors are brought up.[17] One report noted that when a psychiatrist was introduced to investigate psychogenic components of infertility, husbands dropped out of the program rapidly.[20] Many men who willingly submit to semen analysis and elaborate physical examinations consider discussing psychogenic impotence to be humiliating and devasting.

The infertility workup can be extremely stressful to men based on performance appraisal and expectation. The postcoital test seems markedly to increase anxiety. Men are unaccustomed to being told exactly when they have to make love; the knowledge that their performance will be assessed by a third party and given a grade results in many finding it difficult or impossible to perform.[21] Thus sexual dysfunction and impotence can occur as a direct result of the infertility workup.

The popular concept of male responsibilities during the infertility assessment focuses on giving support to the partner. The man is viewed as the stable, calm partner who tries his best to help the woman through painful and stressful treatments. When it is he being treated, however, his responses may be very different. He must cope with his own physical pain, frequent medical appointments, attitudes of others, and his own plus his partner's emotional responses. In addition to shouldering his own complex feelings, he may feel responsible for denying his partner the opportunity to have a child.[14] Therefore, infertile men must deal with many of the same emotions as infertile women.

The desire to have a child may not be less in men than in women, although it may be expressed differently. When questioned why they wanted to have a child, the most frequent response given by infertile men was, "To make life worth living."[15] The fact that most men shun the suggestion of psychologic intervention does not mean that the psychologic impact is any less severe.

THE COUPLE

Although the psychologic burden of infertility may not be experienced equally by both partners, it is certainly experienced together. Most of the literature focuses on the individual rather than on the couple as a unit, despite the fact that psychologic issues are important to both.[5]

Infertile couples face a number of issues that affect their relationship. One of the hardest to deal with is their individual perceptions of infertility. Women are often more emotionally expressive than men. They often cope by talking about their anxiety and depression with their partners who may feel powerless to help. Men may feel a need to contain their emotions, not only to maintain the stoicism expected to them, but out of a sense of responsibility to be the stable one in the relationship. A woman may interpret silence as lack of concern and may escalate her complaints, causing the man to retreat further. This can lead to her feeling abandoned, him feeling overwhelmed, and both feeling resentment. Thus, at a time when the two individuals most need support from each other, they may instead grow apart.[14,17,20]

Guilt and blame may strain the couple's relationship. If an organic factor is identified in one partner, that person may feel guilty at depriving the other of parenthood. Conversely, the unaffected member may feel anger toward the other while at the same time feeling guilty at being impatient with the partners' depression. As the investigation continues, the man may grow to resent the continued scheduling of sexual activity. Tests such as the zona-free hamster egg-penetration test can be particularly significant. He may feel that in addition to being unable to impregnate his partner, he is unable even to impregnate an animal egg. These feelings may lead to his unwillingness either to continue with the investigation or to comply with intercourse at the prescribed time. These stresses often lead to anger, which may account for reports of atypical sexual behavior during the infertility workup.[21]

Most infertile couples experience marked isolation. The social unacceptability of childlessness may result in real or perceived stress from family, friends, acquaintances, and even strangers, which results in reluctance to reveal their infertility. Because others may consider that the couple has experienced no tangible loss and find it difficult to empathize, the couple concludes that no one truly understands. In addition, they may isolate themselves based on a self-protective impulse as outsiders in a fertile world. In a series of interviews with infertile couples, all expressed feelings of abnormality, rejection, abandonment, and being outcast and unlovable.[5,14,22] Finally, they may isolate themselves because social contact is seen as an extra demand. Their time and energy are drained by procedures and physical regimens to such an extent that social interactions are not worth the effort they entail.

THE CRISIS OF INFERTILITY

Although many patients who are treated for infertility do eventually become pregnant, virtually half must come to terms with the fact that they will never be the parents of a biologic child. The subsequent psychologic impact was described as the ''crisis'' of infertility.[4] Patients typically evolve through a series of stages, including surprise, denial, anger, isolation, guilt, grief, and finally resolution. The crisis is biopsychosocial; it affects all areas of life including psychologic, moral, and religious, and may exacerbate existing biologic, emotional, and social problems.[11,23]

One of the most important aspects of the infertility crisis is the sense of losing control. In our society, increasing numbers of individuals rely on birth control until their individual circumstances are optimal for childbearing. Thus, they have a sense of control over their bodies and over procreation. When faced with the loss of the choice of having a baby, the sense of order in their world is disturbed.[13]

Only a few formal investigations have assessed the reaction to infertility. In one study, 48 women were interviewed in an unstructured manner during their infertility treatment.[24] In addition to loss of control, the most common themes among them were ambiguity centering around the reason for the infertility and toward the physician, floundering in the pursuit of life goals, uncertainty about the efficacy and safety of treatment, and suspicion about future fertility. Another theme centered around the need for a time frame for everything, including sexual relations, basal body temperature, and all treatments. The women also acknowledged a sense of otherness, feeling unfairly singled out, left out, and defective, and not being understood by others. Private practice patients reported more distress than clinic patients.

A second study surveyed 500 infertile couples.[4] Most reported sexual dissatisfaction or dysfunction; however, actual sexual dysfunction was not more common than in fertile patients. The female partners felt less need to achieve orgasm; they were more concerned with becoming pregnant than in enhancing pleasure. In a third study, 24 infertile couples were interviewed one month before and two years after reconstructive tubal surgery.[25] over the two-year period, there was a nonsignificant trend for the relationship to deteriorate, as partners' feelings became significantly more negative. Women had significantly more emotional effects than men, but over the 2 years the mens' feelings of grief and depression increased. Women reported avoiding children, while the men reported increasing contact. None of the individuals had been offered professional help prior to the study, while at the end, half of the women reported that they had needed help in solving problems with their partner, sexual relations, crisis reactions, or anxiety.

In one study of 16 couples who had recently been informed of the man's sterility, 63% of the men reported a period of impotence lasting from 1 to 3 months after learning of the diagnosis.[26] Five men suffered from insomnia and depressed mood, and one had exacerbation of peptic ulcer symptoms. Only 3 of the 16 men reported no change in sexual patterns or mood. None of the women reported decreases in sexual desire, although 6 of the 16 felt anger toward their partner. The author recommended that all men diagnosed with azoospermia receive therapy to assure them that impotence is common and typically resolves over the ensuing months.

THE PHYSICIAN'S ROLE

The physician's role in treating infertile couples is extremely complex and challenging. He or she must simultaneously provide state-of-the-art medical and/or surgical management, while never losing sight of the need for empathy and compassionate listening and understanding. By the time a couple first requests an infertility evaluation, the partners are already emotionally charged. The deep desire to have a child makes them dependent on the physician. The resulting relationship may become characterized by a high degree of affection for and confidence in the physician, with willingness to be helped. Alternatively, the physician may become a convenient target for frustration and anger that evolve to overdependence or noncompliance.[11,27]

The physician must be aware of the psychologic and social repercussions of the infertility workup in order to reduce or modify the couple's stress and facilitate adaptation. It is important to consider the additional tensions that are created by tests and treatment.[23,28] For example, the temperature chart may serve as a constant daily reminder of infertility. Not only can it be viewed as a sexual report card, but often results in the couple having sex on schedule, which can lead to decreased sexual desire, impotence, or ejaculatory failure.[9] Therefore, physicians must emphasize that the purpose of the temperature chart is to evaluate the timing of tests, not intercourse. Some experts feel that with the exception of the basic workup or during ovulation induction, it is a mistake to ask patients to take their temperature daily for extended periods of time. With each patient, the medical information versus the stress resulting from a daily reminder of their infertility must be weighed.[29]

There are a number of ways in which the physician can help the couple cope during this time. The first is to treat the infertility as a problem of both partners. This is established by requesting that both attend the initial interview. In addition, the plan of tests and treatments should be developed with the couple as active participants; rationales, explanations goals, and time frames should be shared. To increase their sense of control, the physician should provide

as many treatment choices as possible, encouraging the partners to share responsibility in making decisions.[17]

Starting with the initial interview, the physician should make an effort to provide specific medical information in order to reduce anxiety. Anxious patients cannot hear or understand subsequent information, so this must be a top priority. In relaying such information, however, medical terms should be chosen carefully. Terms such as "hostile mucus," "habitual aborter," "blighted ovum," and "pregnancy wastage" should be avoided since they may be misunderstood, contributing to feelings of inadequacy, guilt, and worthlessness.[16,20]

An open atmosphere must be established for asking questions. For example, many patients may secretly fear that performing sex incorrectly is the cause for their infertility, and the opportunity to discuss these fears must be provided. Such questions allow the physician to recognize feelings of inadequacy, hopelessness, and depression. Some patients may hide their feelings because they are self-conscious, afraid of being criticized or thought of as crazy. The physician must be alert for changes in personality, alterations in appetite or sleep patterns, loss of friends, sexual difficulties, excessive crying, or serious employment problems.[14] Optimistic assessments should not be substituted for direct confrontations of such emotional difficulties.

Although not all patients need psychiatric help, the physician must provide emotional support and education, and offer adequate time for ventilation. If a psychiatric referral is indicated, it should be made carefully so as not to give the patient the impression that she or he is crazy, or worse, is being abandoned.[4,30,31]

THE EFFECT OF EMOTIONS ON FERTILITY

Psychoneuroendocrinology of Infertility

In the past, indirect evidence associated infertility with secretion of biogenic amines and hypothalamic gonadotropin-releasing hormone (GnRH). Medications that interfered with catecholamine synthesis, metabolism, reuptake, or receptor binding were noted to disturb gonadotropin release and subsequently result in anovulation. Common examples include reserpine, a catechol-depleting antihypertensive medication; d-methyl-p-tyrosine, an antihypertensive medication that inhibits tyrosine hydroxylase and depletes dopamine and norepinephrine; and phenothiazine, a dopamine receptor blocker that frequently causes amenorrhea or chronic anovulation.

Norepinephrine has been measured in human plasma during the periovulatory period and its level been found to rise sharply either immediately proceeding or simultaneously with the luteinizing hormone (LH) surge.[32] In rats, the depletion of norepinephrine during diestrus prevents the growth of ovarian follicles and the release of LH expected during proestrus and estrus.[33]

Large accumulations of catecholamines in the mammalian brain have been localized in the median eminence with cell bodies arising outside the basal hypothalamus. In the rhesus monkey this part of the brain has been shown to be the necessary nucleus in the pulsatile gonadotropin center[34] and the predominant location of GnRH. Neurons carrying catecholamines are distinct from those carrying GnRH. Using ovariectomized monkeys, adrenergic-blocking agents immediately inhibited the pulsatile pattern of gonadotropin release.[35] Both norepinephrine and epinephrine are present in axons and nerve terminals in the arcuate nucleus, preoptic area, and other regions of the hypothalamus. The arcuate-median eminence regions of the hypothalamus also contain the highest concentration of β-endorphins (endogenous opioids) in the human brain. Furthermore, estradiol and dihydrotestosterone are concentrated in the nuclei of catecholaminergic neurons in the medial basal hypothalamus, and the target neurons of those two steroids are surrounded by catecholaminergic terminals.[36] Other workers localized axo-axonic interaction between dopamine and GnRH nerve terminals in the rat median eminence. This information is supported by the finding of a transient depression in circulatory LH after the administration of L-dopa, a precursor of dopamine. In addition, opiate receptors exist on dopamine neurons, and the naloxone-induced release of LH is abolished by dopamine.[37]

The mammalian pineal gland is innervated by the superior cervical ganglia. Activation of this network by the sympathetic nervous system may excite the pineal to secrete melatonin, which inhibits LH and stimulates prolactin. The mode and site of action of melatonin are still incompletely understood, but most studies suggest that melatonin suppresses pituitary function either by suppressing the pituitary response to GnRH[38] or by inhibiting the frequency and amplitude of GnRH pulses.[39] We showed that the preovulatory LH surge occurs when serum melatonin levels are rapidly falling, suggesting that the early-morning onset of the LH surge may be related to the concurrent decline in melatonin secretion, as is the case in lower animals.[40] Serotonin, from which melatonin arises, also stimulates prolactin in laboratory rodents.[41] Serotonin may counteract the actions of the catecholamines by inhibiting GnRH. It has also been shown to stimulate prolactin in humans. Melatonin in human beings has been shown to have

highest levels 12 days before ovulation and lowest levels at the time of ovulation.[42] Furthermore, norepinephrine has been shown to stimulate the pineal gland of some animals to secrete melatonin. In one report, ovulation was induced in a group of formerly anovulatory women after procaine blockade of their superior cervical ganglia.[43] Therefore strong evidence exists that gonadotropin secretion is intimately associated with biogenic amines.

Depression has also been found to be related to disorders of turnover or metabolism of central biogenic amines.[44] Others[45] postulated that an alteration of central catecholamine function may be causative in the development of acyclicity in patients with stress-induced, hypothalamic, chronic anovulation. Normogonadotropic patients with amenorrhea and discernible psychologic disturbances were evaluated. Basal pituitary and ovarian hormone levels and the diurnal rhythm of cortisol, were within normal limits. The pituitary–ovarian system was fully operational in those patients. They responded normally to GnRH and spontaneous reversal of amenorrhea occurred after appropriate counseling. Subsequent studies showed that impairment of GnRH secretion is the likely underlying cause, since in general, the frequency and amplitude of LH pulses are diminished.[46]

There is also evidence for increased dopaminergic and opioid activity in patients with hypothalamic hypogonadotropic amenorrhea.[47] The study was based on the knowledge that opioid substances inhibit LH and augment prolactin secretion by the hypothalamic–pituitary system, and that naloxone, an opioid receptor antagonist, could competitively inhibit these effects. These data tied in nicely with previous reports showing that endogenous opioids increase pituitary prolactin levels through their interaction with opiate receptors located on dopamine nerve terminals in the median eminence. A significant elevation of circulating LH levels occurred in response to both a dopamine receptor antagonist (metoclopramide) and an opiate receptor antagonist (naloxone). These findings suggest that LH inhibition was due to increased hypothalamic opiate or dopamine activity. Since these patients responded normally to exogenous GnRH, it is reasonable to assume that this effect was mediated through an increased inhibitory effect of endogenous opiates on GnRH rather than on the pituitary directly.

Several other studies similarly showed strong indirect evidence that psychologic trauma can lead to alterations in central catecholamines and endorphins, resulting in anovulation. Endorphins have also been shown to decrease appetite. Thus, it may be that they are responsible for the low basal gonadotropin levels in persons with anorexia nervosa. Neuropharmacologic data suggest that excess dopamine and possibly norepinephrine are responsible for the clinical aspects of anorexia nervosa[48]: (1) dopamine induces anorexia and weight loss; (2) amphetamine, a drug that increases brain catecholamines by inhibiting the reuptake of dopamine and epinephrine and affecting their release, leads to anorexia and weight loss in habitual users; (3) apomorphine, a dopamine agonist, produces similar effects; (4) apomorphine and amphetamine both cause hypothermia; and (5) central catecholamine changes may be the cause of amenorrhea.

Hormonal studies provide a different theoretical role as to how emotional factors affect infertility. Stress has been shown to stimulate the adrenal cortex to produce hirsutism and acne in certain women.[49] In addition, whereas exercise induces a response of the sympathetic nervous system, psychologic stress has been shown to induce primarily an adrenal response.[50] Some authors suggested that the most important neuroendocrine response to stress is that of the adrenocorticotropic hormone (ACTH)–adrenal axis with the subsequent release of glucocorticoids and catecholamines.[51] In addition to releasing ACTH, corticotropin-releasing factor (CRF), together with vasopressin and oxytocin, modulates mood, behavior, and learning. It stimulates central noradrenergic activity, which in turn activates peripheral norepinephrine release and adrenomedulary secretion of epinephrine.[45] When CRF reaches the portal circulation it stimulates the anterior pituitary to release ACTH and β-endorphin. The resulting release of cortisol can affect metabolism, the immune system, and mood. Corticotropin-releasing factor also affects reproductive functions. Castrated rats exposed to noxious stimulation demonstrated both an inhibited pulsatile pattern of LH release and markedly lower plasma concentrations. The central administration of a CRF antagonist reversed the inhibitory action of stress. Neither peripheral nor intraventricular injection of an inactive CRF analog was effective.[52] The CRF that is secreted by the brain during stress also inhibits GnRH secretion into the hypophyseal portal circulation.[52] It has been shown that a high proportion of patients with hypothalamic chronic anovulation had psychosexual problems and socioenvironmental trauma occurring either before or around the time of puberty.[45] It is therefore possible that chronic and recurrent tension, or even the normal stress of adolescence, might affect adrenal steroidogenesis. The resultant excess androgens could upset the balance of LH and follicle-stimulating hormone secretion, resulting in chronic anovulation and polycystic ovaries.

Another aspect of stress and amenorrhea can be found in the relationship between stress and hyperprolactinemia. Follicular prolactin concentrations of greater than 25 ng/mL were shown to suppress the normal follicular steroidogenic response to gonadotropins.[53] Women with hypothalamic amenorrhea may have increased dopaminergic levels. Patients with hyperprolactinemic amenorrhea are also believed to have increased dopamine activity. In addition, increased prolactin levels have been shown to suppress gonadotropins. This could certainly provide an additional mechanism whereby stress could inhibit ovulation and ultimately lead to amenorrhea. Further evidence of the role of prolactin is gained by the fact that hyperprolactinemic, amenorrheic women treated with bromocriptine, a dopamine receptor agonist, resume normal gonadal function as long as prolactin levels are reduced. This finding adds support to the concept that prolactin inhibits gonadotropin release, and that dopamine plays an important role in the hypothalamic–pituitary control of ovulation.

Autonomic Control of the Reproductive Tract

The rich autonomic innervation of the pelvic viscera helps explain mechanisms through which emotional stress might theoretically affect ovulation, uterotubal function, or pregnancy maintenance (Fig. 2–1).[54] Sympathetic centers in the lower thoracic segments (T-10 to T-11) supply the ovary and part of the oviduct, and the remainder of the oviduct, the uterus, and the vagina are supplied by T-12 to L-2. The human cervix is innervated from three plexuses of the pelvic autonomic nervous system, the superior, middle, and inferior hypogastric. Norepinephrine is the major sympathetic neurotransmitter, although dopamine, epinephrine, acetylcholine, and prostaglandins are also involved. Two types of receptors, α and β, exist for the catecholamines. Alpha-receptors are most responsive to epinephrine and are usually excitatory, causing uterine contractions. Conversely, β-receptors are inhibitory and usually relax the uterus. It is by this mechanism that β-mimetic drugs such as ritodrine and terbutaline suppress uterine contractility in premature labor. The parasympathetic fibers arise from S-2 to S-4. The major neurotransmitter is acetylcholine. The ovary itself contains a few nerve bundles and small nonmyelinated adrenergic fibers in the parenchyma. These nerves transmit impulses to vascular smooth muscles within the ovary and could influence the hemodynamic state of blood vessels around the follicle. In this fashion, the relative amount of hormones reaching the follicle could be affected and thus alter ovulation. In addition, distributed throughout the stroma are adrenergic and cholinergic fibers that terminate in neuromuscular connections in the theca interna. Stress-related circumstances could modulate steroid production directly in this fashion.

Other fibers are also located around follicles in all stages of growth, particularly graafian follicles, which

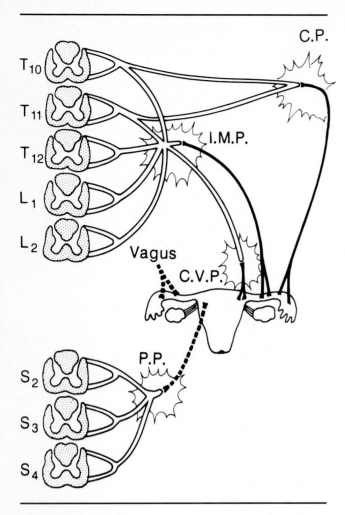

Figure 2–1. Autonomic control of the female reproductive tract. Preganglionic fibers are shown in white, sympathetic postganglionics in solid black, and parasympathetic postganglionics in broken lines. CP = coeliac plexus; IMP = inferior mesenteric plexus; CVP = cervico-vaginal plexus; PP = pelvic plexus (parasympathetic). (From reference 54. Reproduced with permission.)

contain smooth muscle cells in the theca interna.[55] This allows the follicles to display spontaneous motor activity both in vivo and in vitro. Contractions are mediated both by α-adrenergic receptors and by muscarinic cholinergic receptors. Relaxation is mediated by β-receptors.[56] The nerve supply does not cross the basement membrane of the follicles. Hence, the proximity of adrenergic and cholinergic nerve fibers with smooth muscle fibers located throughout the stroma and theca interior resembles a neuromuscular system.[57] This anatomic relationship controlled by normal stimuli might be responsible for ovulation. Both norepinephrine and acetylcholine have induced contractions in follicular walls and increased intrafollicular pressure; dibenzylene, and α-adrenergic blocker, has been shown to inhibit ovulation in rabbits. Despite the interesting conjecture, sufficient evidence to the contrary has also been reported to cast doubt on ovarian contractility as the sole mechanism of ovulation.[58] One might theorize, however, that excessive catecholamines resulting from stress might in some way affect ovulation.

Stress-related catecholamine excess might also affect oviductal activity.[59] In the human, the ampulloisthmic junction and the uterotubal junction are richly endowed with adrenergic nervous innervation. Both α and β-receptors have been found in the circular muscle of the isthmus and ampulloisthmic junction. In the rabbit, excitatory, α-receptors that are stimulated by norepinephrine have been identified in both circular and longitudinal muscles. Inhibitory β-receptors are located in the circular muscle, whereas longitudinal muscle possesses inhibitory β-receptors.

Steroids have been shown to influence receptor properties. Estrogen enhances and progesterone reduces the activity of excitatory receptors in the rabbit oviduct, and the inhibitory action of β-receptors is stronger in the luteal phase. During the luteal phase in humans, norepinephrine similarly causes inhibitory responses in the oviduct. This change in sensitivity of α-adrenergic receptors has led some workers to speculate that high levels of midcycle estrogen result in the isthmus functioning as a sphincter at that time. As progesterone rises over the next few days, β-adrenergic receptors are stimulated and the isthmic sphincter relaxes. This mechanism may be very important in ovum transport.[58] Further evidence supporting the isthmus as a factor in egg transport comes from recordings of pressure differences on either side of the ampulloisthmic junction. These differences are understandable, since the isthmus is richly innervated, in contrast to the sparse innervation of the ampulla. In addition, the isthmus is more sensitive than the ampulla to norepinephrine. Due to the rich innervation of the uterus, the tubes, and the ovaries by the autonomic nervous system, stress-related excess catecholamine secretion has a sound neurologic basis by which it could affect ovulation, ovum transport, and implantation.

These comments are not intended to be all-inclusive, but only to provide an overview of the enormous interplay between the psychologic and the physiologic.

It has been known since ancient times that a relationship exists between the menstrual cycle and the psyche. The study of the emotional aspects of infertility is rapidly moving from considerations of psychologic presets, psychic trauma, and developmental influences to investigating the production, reception, and effects of transmitter amines in brain centers associated with emotions and reproduction. The best-known brain transmitters are dopamine and norepinephrine, which are catecholamines, serotonin, and indolamine. The most notable direct effects of emotional stress on infertility involve these biogenic amines.

Other Psychogenic Factors

Psychogenic infertility has been documented also in males. Decreased libido and impotence are obvious sequelae of psychologic problems. Evidence also shows that stress may result in retrograde and sham ejaculation due to malfunctions in the sympathetic nervous system. Possible explanations include closure of the posterior sphincter of the urethra during orgasm, abnormal response to sympathetic stimuli in seminal vesicles and the ampulary part of the vasa deferentia, and a spastic permanent contraction of the ejaculatory duct. There is also evidence that psychologic stress can lead to abnormal spermatogenesis through aberrant regulation of the hypothalamic–hypophysial axis.[60]

Despite the solid biochemical evidence on the effects of stress on the reproductive system, the question remains of underlying psychopathology as the root of infertility. Experts in analytic psychology propose that an unconscious psychologic defense mechanism defends the ego against the physiologic process of motherhood, which is basically feared. The majority of the reports in the literature do not support a psychopathologic basis for infertility, however. A review of 235 papers written between 1935 and 1963 revealed no conclusive evidence that specific psychologic factors alter fertility.[61] Other work continues to support this hypothesis.[62] All of these studies and theories fail to take into account the stress that infertility itself places on the couple. It is quite possible that infertility results in emotional problems, instead of the opposite.

Conception After Adoption

It is commonly assumed, especially among laypeople, that infertile couples frequently conceive after adoption. This concept was studied by several authors, with conflicting results. One author reported that in couples in whom organic factors were adequately treated and in whom continuing emotional tensions were present, adoption facilitated conception.[63] He reported evidence that adoption relieves emotional stress and thus results in conception. In contrast, several other groups refuted these claims. A study of 100 adopting couples determined that adoption was responsible for conception among only 4%.[64]

In many studies the diagnosis of definite infertility was not adequately controlled. Of 388 couples who adopted, less than 3% of subsequent pregnancies could be attributed to adoption.[65] A comparison of 249 adoptive infertile parents and 113 nonadoptive infertile couples revealed no evidence that adoption increased the tendency to conceive.[66] Thus the statistical evidence documents that adoption itself does not appear to increase the chances of conception beyond that expected over time. Alternatively, those pregnancies that did occur could possibly be explained by

a reduction in stress altering the neuroendocrinologic characteristics of the couple.[5]

PSYCHOLOGIC TREATMENT OF THE INFERTILE COUPLE

It is probably true that all individuals experiencing the stress of infertility could benefit from some form of counseling. There are three times when such intervention is particularly beneficial: (1) concurrently with starting an infertility workup, (2) when a psychiatric indication is present, and (3) at the termination of unsuccessful treatment.

Unfortunately, few clinics and private practitioners routinely require contact with a counselor prior to or concurrent with the commencement of an infertility workup. At the minimum, however, the impact of the diagnostic and therapeutic procedures should be addressed. An initial interview with a mental health professional should focus on identifying and explaining possible sources of anxiety, preparing the couple for future tests and treatments, and exploring sexual and marital problems, concerns, and unrealistic beliefs. Ideally, the couple should be seen both together and individually, preferably with a counselor of the same sex.[5] It must be remembered, however, that despite the degree of emotional stress experienced by couples at the initial visit, they are usually quite resistant to therapy at this point because of their optimism that at long last their problem will soon be solved.

Many patients become overwhelmed by the anxiety and stress that accompany infertility therapy. This is particularly true if treatment has been prolonged. At this point, therapy can help the couple to increase the feeling of control over their lives and to lessen the impact of the medical and surgical interventions.

A psychiatric referral must be made when patients express inability to cope with their emotions, or if they display depressive or suicidal symptoms, exacerbated alcohol or drug use, signs of unresolved grief, or sexual disorders. It is critical to explain to patients that a referral to a mental health professional does not mean the termination of medical care; the reasons for referral should be clarified.[13] Patients are often resistant, however, because of the additional appointments for which they must miss work, the added costs, or the added perceived loss of control over their minds as well as their bodies.

The termination of unsuccessful treatment represents a crisis for most couples and is an appropriate time for short-term counseling. This is a critical period in which self-image, sexuality, and life plans must be reassessed. Patients must close an important chapter in their lives. Those who are told that they cannot bear children may require help mourning that loss. The most effective therapy is an educating process to modify the emotional conflicts. Couples should be assisted in recognizing that just because they are infertile does not imply that they are defective as human beings. They require help to maintain feelings of self-worth, self-esteem, and equanimity. Again, most couples resist therapy based on the feeling that they can "handle it themselves." The more likely reason, however, is the desire of one or both partners not to give up, because the reality is too painful to accept.

Most patients who receive a mental health referral either do not follow through to obtain services, or delay calling the therapist for months or even years. In one study of 212 infertile couples who had been offered counseling services, only 62 attended any sessions.[67] At the end of the therapy, all 62 couples received a questionnaire concerning the frequency of psychologic symptoms and the response to counseling. The 50% who responded reported that counseling enhanced the quality of life; the women were more overtly affected than the men, but both benefited. Long-term counseling appeared to be more beneficial than short-term. Unfortunately, since only half of the couples responded, the results could represent self-selection of patients; however, as those who did respond reported therapy to be beneficial, at least half, if not more, of the couples who accepted counseling benefited.

In a small study of 10 infertile couples referred for instruction in transcendental meditation, only 2 completed the course and both reported decreased anxiety levels.[68] This study is primarily important in demonstrating that even nonconventional forms of therapy may prove beneficial for these highly stressed couples. It is also important to note that only 2 of the 10 couples actually followed through with the suggested intervention.

Group therapy is very valuable with infertile patients because so many of them report that they feel alone in the world. Groups demonstrate that they are not alone and that they can share thoughts, problems, experiences, and concerns with others in similar circumstances. In addition, participants can give support, which is often beneficial and rewarding. Group therapy can lead to improved communication with physicians as patients become aware of specific needs and learn to ventilate their frustrations at medical interventions. It is also cost-effective, and good results can be obtained without expensive, intensive psychotherapy.[69]

In one report, a group of 5 infertile women met with a registered nurse.[70] All women reported initial dissatisfaction with medical treatment and took their anxiety out on their husbands. At the outset of group therapy the overwhelming impressions were a great amount of pressure and marked sense of personal failure. At the end of the group work, all patients reported that the main value was a release of pressure and frustration, plus deeper insight into their own situation, and a general increased sense of well-being and security. Three years later two of the patients had a live birth, one had a miscarriage, one refused to have tubal reconstructive surgery, and one was lost to follow-up.

In another group for infertile patients the emphasis was on attempting to internalize the patients' locus of control.[31] The participants shared feelings, did role-playing, explored free associations, used sentence completions, and searched for alternative patterns of behavior. In addition, they had discussions of societal pressure, blame and guilt, fears of medical testing and treatment, anger, feelings of family incompletion, sexual dysfunction, and alternatives to biologic parenting. These sessions led to tremendous decreases reported in fear, anxiety, isolation, and depression, as well as resolving feelings of blame and guilt.

Another study of infertile couples required both partners to complete a battery of psychologic tests prior to starting a six-session group counseling program.[71] The discussions covered denial, guilt, anger, depression, and self-concept in large and small groups, and included role-playing. The women experienced significant decreases in grief, depression, and anger, and increases in self-concept. Similar benefits are often informally reported by patients simultaneously going through ovulation induction or in-vitro fertilization, as a result of meeting daily in the ultrasound or phlebotomy waiting areas.

In general, there is a lack of systematic appraisal of the impact of psychotherapy on infertile patients. Most of the literature is based on clinical assertions rather than precise evaluations of the problems experienced by couples or the methods employed to resolve them. It is clear that infertility is stressful, and emotional support is beneficial, but patients are resistant to receiving psychologic care.

IDIOPATHIC INFERTILITY

In the 1960s it was estimated that 30% of all infertile patients suffered from idiopathic infertility. By the 1980s that number had been reduced to 5% or less. As biomedical knowledge increases, it is possible that anatomic, neuroendocrinologic, or pathophysiologic causes may eventually be found to explain all infertility. Since evidence increasingly supports a biochemical connection between stress and the neuroendocrine system, a psychosomatic mechanism may operate in mediating some cases of infertility. Thus, when dealing with two apparently healthy but infertile partners, there are two possible explanations: the sophistication of modern testing is inadequate and undiagnosed organic abnormalities exist; or, alternatively but not exclusively, psychologic factors are operating. There may be a feedback loop mechanism to incorporate both hypotheses; delayed conception for an unknown reason leads to anxiety, leading to physiologic changes that delay conception even more. Thus stress can be both cause and effect of infertility (see flow diagram at the beginning of this chapter).

A woman is assumed to be psychogenically infertile if all known organic reasons have been excluded. In a study that compared 22 couples with unexplained infertility with 10 fertile control couples, the former had higher mean anxiety scores for all emotional factors.[72] In another study 19 women with unexplained infertility were compared with 19 fertile women. No significant differences were noted on assessment of traditional sex roles. The infertile patients had significantly more guilt than the control patients, but there were no other significant differences on attitudes toward sexuality. As previously stated, it is not known which comes first in these patients. It would seem logical that unexplained infertility could cause anxiety and guilt about the inability to become pregnant, rather than the psychologic factors causing the infertility. A review of the claims that psychologic factors cause nonorganic female infertility concluded that the available data do not support the hypothesis.[73]

Despite the lack of evidence supporting the impact of psychologic factors on idiopathic infertility, numerous studies have documented increased conception rates after various psychologic interventions. One group followed 16 patients with unexplained infertility and depressive illness for 3 years.[74] The length of infertility ranged from 2 to 11 years. Seven patients had depressive symptoms of long duration and 9 reported such symptoms only after becoming aware of their infertility. Nine patients consented to undergo psychiatric treatment. Of the 5 with long-standing depression who underwent therapy, 3 became pregnant. None of the other patients became pregnant over the next 3 years. In another study women who had unexplained infertility for a minimum of 3 years met in group sessions for 4 to 6 weeks.[69] Discussions included marriage, sex, infertility tests, husbands, childlessness, and clarification of medical questions. In addition to marked improvement in psychologic variables, attitudes toward medical treatment, and sexual functioning, 21% became pregnant within the first 3 months and a total of 26.5% had become pregnant by the end of 6 months. In a second group therapy study, 5 patients with unexplained infertility participated in a discussion group.[70] They acknowledged guilt, inadequacy, and problems with the marital relationship. All expressed

benefits from the group sessions and felt they had achieved deeper insight into their own situation. Three of the 5 patients became pregnant, with 2 of these pregnancies resulting in live births.

A two-part study further documented the effects of stress in infertility.[75] Initially, 42 women with unexplained infertility completed a psychologic battery prior to intensive medical treatment. During follow-up, 12 became pregnant. All 12 showed significant decreases in measured anxiety prior to pregnancy. Thus, anxiety seemed to predict pregnancy. It was not anxiety as a general trait, however, but as it related to infertility. In the second part of the study, 14 of the women who had not become pregnant were randomly assigned to a behavioral treatment group or to a waiting list control group. The 16 weekly behavioral sessions included relaxation training, cognitive restructuring, modeling of positive self-verbalizations, stress-inoculation training, anxiety management training, and self-instructional management. Patients were asked to do progressive relaxation daily. Of the 7 women receiving behavioral treatment, 4 became pregnant within 3 months. None of the 7 control patients became pregnant. The author concluded that situational anxiety may be an important antecedent variable contributing to unexplained infertility. In addition, it is apparent that behavioral therapy may be highly effective.

Thus, although few data document that psychologic factors cause idiopathic infertility, four studies that examined the effects of psychologic interventions revealed subsequent pregnancy rates ranging from 26.5 to 60%. In the majority of these studies, the patients had long-standing histories of documented unexplained infertility. Three of the four interventions involved group treatment. It appears that group therapy provides effective management for patients suffering from unexplained infertility; not only does it apparently provide major psychologic benefits, it may serve to increase the chance of conception.

IVF:
A PSYCHOLOGIC CHALLENGE

In-vitro fertilization (IVF) has received a great deal of publicity since the birth of the first "test-tube" baby in 1978. More than 3,000 babies have been born through IVF, and at least 100 centers are using the procedure in the United States.[76] This technique condenses substantial stress into a short period of time.[77] One of the main reasons is that it often represents the last hope of ever achieving pregnancy. This "last-chance" concept not only leads to increased emotional pressure, it contributes to unrealistic expectations for success.[3,78] Almost every couple entering an IVF program hopes to be the exception to the fact that the odds are very much against them.

Many fears and anxieties are associated with participating in an IVF program, such as the time spent waiting to begin, the expense that is often not covered by insurance, and the possibility of failure at each stage of the cycle, including ovulation induction, oocyte retrieval, fertilization and cleavage, and embryo transfer. Many patients find the most anxious time to be between embryo transfer and pregnancy confirmation. This can be due to a perceived lack of support from the IVF team, since there is no daily contact as during the first half of the cycle, and the unrelenting fear that the transferred embryo(s) will be lost. Furthermore, patients also realize that the outcome beyond this point is not only out of their control, but out of the control of their physician as well.

In addition, the emphasis is often on technology, while the human aspects are frequently ignored. The IVF team may unintentionally focus on monitoring the physiologic aspects of the cycle, leaving patients caught between trying to understand the significance of daily hormone levels and ultrasound examinations, and simultaneously experiencing the tremendous emotional turmoil caused by the process. Failures during the cycle may be interpreted differently by the couple. For example, failure to ovulate or to produce sufficient sperm may result in self-blame, which can be devastating when superimposed on the emotional, physical, and financial expense of the process.[79]

Psychologic interventions for patients undergoing IVF should be at two levels: (1) psychosocial assessment prior to entering the program and (2) counseling and support during and after each cycle. The initial psychologic evaluation should address ambivalence, anxiety, and unrealistic expectations, and assess abilities to tolerate stress and the potential for disappointment.[78] During this initial session, enough time is needed to establish a relationship, provide information, and set appropriate goals.[77] Counseling should be continued throughout each cycle to aid patients in dealing with the emotional roller coaster that accompanies IVF.

When counseling is offered on a voluntary basis, few patients choose to participate. Thus, contact with a mental health professional is mandatory at many IVF centers.[77] One reason that this support is needed is that many couples become so distressed during the process that they drop out of the program, often at great personal and financial cost.[78] In a survey of women who had dropped out of an IVF program, the most cited reason was cost, followed by anxiety and depression.[80] It appears obvious that patients need advice on how to deal with the stress prior to or simultaneously with being admitted to the program.

Since there has been no thorough investigation of the psychologic characteristics and perceived needs of couples entering IVF programs, it is difficult to plan adequate support systems. In one study of 200 couples entering an IVF program, 49% of the women considered being infertile as the most upsetting experience of their lives.[81] Because group therapy has achieved such high levels of success with infertile patients in general, it may serve as a beneficial form of treatment with those undergoing IVF. Not only would group therapy help foster a sense of camaraderie to reduce the sense of isolation that many patients report, especially during the second half of the cycle, but it would serve as a forum to discuss feelings of fear, stress, anxiety, and hope.[82]

Acknowledgments. The authors thank Dr. Herbert Benson for his support, and Catherine Imbasciati and Mary Boyne for their help with the manuscript preparation. Supported in part by grant HL-07374 from the National Heart, Lung, and Blood Institute, National Institutes of Health, Washington, DC.

REFERENCES

1. Mazor M: Barren couples. *Psychol Today* May, 1979.
2. McGuire L: Psychologic management of infertile women. *Postgrad Med* 57(6):173, 1975.
3. Stewart S, Glazer G. Expectations and coping of women undergoing in vitro fertilization. *Matern Child Nurs J* 15(2):103, 1986.
4. Menning B: The emotional needs of infertile couples. *Fertil Steril* 34(4):313, 1980.
5. Seibel MM, Taymor ML: Emotional aspects of infertility. *Fertil Steril* 37(2):137, 1982.
6. Williams L, Power P: The emotional impact of infertility in single women: Some implications for counseling. *JAMA* 32(9):327, 1977.
7. Moghissi K, Wallach E: Unexplained infertility. *Fertil Steril* 39(1):5, 1983.
8. Mozley P: Psychophysiologic infertility: An overview. *Clin Obstet Gynecol* 19(2):407, 1976.
9. Keye W: Psychosexual responses to infertility. *Clin Obstet Gynecol* 27(3):760, 1984.
10. Drake T, Grunert G: A cyclic pattern of sexual dysfunction in the infertility investigation. *Fertil Steril* 32(5):542, 1979.
11. Cook E: Characteristics of the biopsychosocial crisis of infertility. *J Counseling Dev* 65:465, 1987.
12. Berger D: The role of the psychiatrist in a reproductive biology clinic. *Fertil Steril* 28(2)141, 1977.
13. Honea-Fleming P: Psychosocial components on obstetric/gynecologic conditions with a special consideration of infertility. *Ala J Med Sci* 23(1):27, 1986.
14. Mahlstedt P: The psychological component of infertility. *Fertil Steril* 43(3):335, 1985.
15. Lalos A, Jacobsson L, Lalos O, von Schoultz B: The wish to have a child: A pilot study of infertile couples. *Acta Psychiatr Scand* 72:476, 1985.
16. Clapp D: Emotional responses to infertility: Nursing interventions. *JOGN Nurs* Nov/Dec:32S, 1985.
17. Spencer L: Male infertility: Psychological correlates. *Postgrad Med* 81(2):223, 1987.
18. Bents H: Psychology of male infertility—A literature survey. *Int J Androl* 8(4):325, 1985.
19. Pantesco V: Nonorganic infertility: Some research and treatment problems. *Psychol Rep* 58:731, 1986.
20. Farrer-Meschan R: Importance of marriage counseling to infertility investigation. *Obstet Gynecol* 38(2):316, 1971.
21. Walker H: Psychiatric aspects of infertility. *Urol Clin North Am* 5(3):481, 1978.
22. Daniels K, Gunby J, Legge M, Williams T, Wynn-Williams D: Issues and problems for the infertile couple. *NZ Med J* 97:185, 1984.

23. Taymor M, Bresnick E: Emotional stress and infertility. *Infertility* 2(1a):39, 1979.
24. Sandelowski M, Pollock C: Women's experiences of infertility. *Image* 18(4):140, 1986.
25. Lalos A, Lalos O, Jacobsson L, von Schoultz B: The psychosocial impact of infertility two years after completed surgical treatment. *Acta Obstet Gynecol Scand* 64(7):599, 1985.
26. Berger D: Impotence following the discovery of azoospermia. *Fertil Steril* 34(2):154, 1980.
27. Frick-Bruder C, Braendle W, Bettendorf G: Doctor–patient relationship during treatment of infertility, in Insler V, Bettendorf G (eds): *Advances in Diagnosis and Treatment of Infertility.* Amsterdam, Elsevier North-Holland, 1981.
28. Hertz D: Infertility and the physician–patient relationship: a biopsychosocial challenge. *Gen Hosp Psychiatry* 4(2):95, 1982.
29. Fisher I: Psychogenic aspects of sterility. *Fertil Steril* 4(6):466, 1953.
30. Dorfman W: Psychosomatics, psychopharmacology, psychotherapy, and sterility. *J Reprod Med* 3(4):39, 1969.
31. Rosenfeld D, Mitchell E: Treating the emotional aspects of infertility: Counselling services in an infertility clinic. *Am J Obstet Gynecol* 135(2):177, 1979.
32. Rosner J, Nagle C, deLaborde N, et al: Plasma levels of norepinephrine (NE) during the periovulatory period and after LH-RH stimulation in women. *Am J Obstet Gynecol* 124:567, 1976.
33. Terabawa E, Bridson W, Davenport J, Coy R: Role of brain monamines in release of gonadotropin before proestrus in the cyclic rat. *Neuroendocrinology* 18:345, 1975.
34. Belchetz P, Plant T, Nakai Y, Keogh E, Knobil E: Hypophyseal responsiveness to continuous and intermittent delivery of hypothalamic gonadotropin-releasing hormone. *Science* 202:631, 1978.
35. Bhattacharya A, Dierschke O, Yamaji T, Knobil E: The pharmalogic blockade of the circhoral mode of LH secretion on the ovariectomized rhesus monkey. *Endocrinology* 90:778, 1972.
36. Heritage A, Stumpf W, Sar M, Grant L: Brainstem catecholamine neurons are target sites for sex steroid hormones. *Science* 207:1377, 1980.
37. Yen S: Neuroendocrine control of hypophyseal function, in Yen S, Jaffe R (eds): *Endocrinology,* ed 2. Philadelphia, Saunders, 1986.
38. Martin J, Sattler C: Selectivity of melatonin pituitary inhibition for luteinizing-hormone releasing hormone. *Neuroendocrinology* 34:112, 1982.
39. Bittman E, Kaynard A, Olster D, et al: Pineal melatonin mediates photoperiodic control of pulsatile luteinizing hormone secretion in the ewe. *Neuroendocrinology* 40:409, 1985.
40. Brzezinski A, Lynch H, Wurtman R, Seibel M: Possible contribution of melatonin to the timing of the luteinizing hormone surge. *N Engl J Med* 316:1550, 1987.
41. Lu K, Meites J: Effects of serotonin precursors and melatonin on serum prolactin release in rate. *Endocrinology* 93:152, 1973.
42. Webley G, Leidenberger F: The circadian pattern of melatonin and its positive relationship with progesterone in women. *J Clin Endocrinol Metab* 63:323, 1986.
43. Novak E, Woodruff J: *Gynecologic and Obstetric Pathology with Clinical and Endocrine Relations.* Philadelphia, Saunders, 1974.
44. Schildkrant J: Biogenic amines and affective disorders. *Annu Rev Med* 25:333, 1974.
45. Yen S: Chronic anovulation due to CNS–hypothalamic pituitary dysfunction, in Yen S, Jaffe R (eds): *Reproductive Endocrinology,* ed. 2. Philadelphia, Saunders, 1986.
46. Crowley W, Felicori M, Spratt D, Santoro N: The physiology of gonadotropin-releasing hormone (GnRH) secretion in men and women. *Recent Prog Horm Res* 41:473, 1985.
47. Quigley M, Sheehan, K, Casper R, Yen S: Evidence for increased dopaminergic and opioid activity in patients with hypothalamic hypogonadotropic amenorrhea. *J Clin Endocrinol Metab* 50:949, 1980.
48. Barry V, Klawans H: On the role of dopamine in the pathophysiology of anorexia nervosa. *J Neural Transm* 38:107, 1976.
49. Karahasanglu A, Barglow P, Growe G: Psychological aspects of infertility. *J Reprod Med* 9:241, 1972.
50. Dimsdale J, Moss J: Plasma catecholamines in stress and exercise. *JAMA* 243:340, 1980.
51. Axelrod J, Reisine T: Stress hormones: Their interactions and regulation. *Science* 224:452, 1984.
52. Rivier C, Rivier J, Vale W: Stress-induced inhibition of reproductive function: Role of endogeneous corticotropin-releasing factor. *Science* 231:607, 1986.
53. McNatty K, Sawers R, McNeilly A: A possible role for prolactin control of steroid secretion by the human graafian follicle. *Nature* 250:653, 1974.
54. Pauerstein CJ: Anatomy, in Powerstein CJ: *The Fallopian Tube: A Reapraisal.* Philadelphia, Lea & Febiger, 1974.
55. Amsterdam A, Lindner H, Groschel-Stewart U: Localization of actin and myosin in the rat oocyte and follicle wall by immunofluorescence. *Anat Rec* 187:311, 1977.
56. Yoshimura Y, Wallach E: Studies on the mechanism(s) of mammalian ovulation. *Fertil Steril* 47:22, 1987.
57. Edward R: The adult ovary, in Edwards R (ed): *Conception in the Human Female.* London, Academic Press, 1980.
58. Espey L: Ovarian contractility and its relationship to ovulation: A review. *Biol Reprod* 19:540, 1978.
59. Edwards R: The female reproductive tract, in Edwards R (ed): *Conception in the Human Female.* London, Academic Press, 1980.
60. Walker H: Sexual problems and infertility. *Psychosom Med* 19(8):477, 1978.
61. Noyes R, Chapnick E: Literature on psychology and infertility: A critical analysis. *Fertil Steril* 15(5):543, 1964.
62. Brand H: Psychological stress and infertility. II. Psychometric test data. *Br J Med Psychol* 55(4):385, 1982.
63. Sandler B: Conception after adoption: A comparison of conception rates. *Fertil Steril* 16(3):313, 1965.
64. Tyler E, Bonapart J, Grant J: Occurrence of pregnancy following adoption. *Fertil Steril* 11(6):581, 1960.
65. Aronson H, Glienke C: A study of the incidence of pregnancy following adoption. *Fertil Steril* 14(5):547, 1963.
66. Rock J, Tietze C, McLaughlin H: Effect of adoption on infertility. *Fertil Steril* 16(3):305, 1965.
67. Bresnick E, Taymor ML: The role of counseling in infertility. *Fertil Steril* 32(2):154, 1979.
68. Harrison R, O'Moore A, Mosurski K, O'Moore R, Cranny A: Intermittent hyperprolactinemia and the unexplained infertile couple. A placebo-controlled study of combined clomiphene citrate, bromocriptine therapy. *Infertility* 9:1, 1986.
69. Arbanel A, Bach G: Group psychotherapy for the infertile couple. *Int J Infertil* 4(2):151, 1959.
70. Wilchins S, Park R: Use of group "rap sessions" in the adjunctive treatment of five infertile females. *J Med Soc NJ* 1(12):951, 1974.
71. Lukse M: The effect of group counseling on the frequency of grief reported by infertile couples. *JOGN Nurs* Nov/Dec:67S, 1985.
72. Harrison R, O'Moore A, O'Moore R, McSweeney J: Stress profiles in normal infertile couples: Pharmacological and psychological approaches to therapy, in Insler V, Bettendorf G (eds): *Advances in Diagnosis and Treatment of Infertility.* Amsterdam, Elsevier North-Holland, 1981.
73. Denber H: Psychiatric aspects of infertility. *J Reprod Med* 20(1):23, 1978.
74. Ellenberg J, Koren Z: Infertility and depression. *Int J Infertil* 27(4):219, 1982.
75. Rodriguez B, Bermudez L, Ponce de Leon E, Castro L: The relationship between infertility and anxiety: Some preliminary findings. Presented at the second world congress of behavior therapy, Washington, Dec, 8–11, 1983.
76. Seibel MM: A new era in reproductive technology: In vitro fertilization, gamete intrafallopian transfer, and donated gametes and embryos. *N Engl J Med* 318:828, 1988.
77. Seibel MM, Levin S: A new era in reproductive technologies: The emotional stages of in vitro fertilization. *JIVF/ET* 4(3):135, 1987.
78. Greenfeld, D, Haseltine F: Candidate selection and psychosocial considerations of in-vitro fertilization procedures. *Clin Obstet Gynecol* 29(1):119, 1986.
79. Dennerstein L, Morse C: Psychological issues in IVF. *Clin Obstet Gynecol* 12(4):835, 1985.
80. Mao K, Wood C: Barriers to treatment of infertility by in-vitro fertilization and embryo transfer. *Med J Aust* 140(9):532, 1984.
81. Freeman E, Boxer, A, Rickels K, Tureck R, Mastroianni L: Psychological evaluation and support in a program of in vitro fertilization and embryo transfer. *Fertil Steril* 43(1):48, 1985.
82. Shrednick A: Emotional support programs for the vitro fertilization. *Fertil Steril* 49(5):704, 1983.

PART II

Endocrinology of Female Infertility

CHAPTER 3

Oocyte Maturation and Follicle Development

Machelle M. Seibel

Ovarian Physiology

Oocyte Maturation
Follicle Development
    The Effect of LH on Theca Cells
    The Effect of FSH on Granulosa Cells
Follicular Microenvironment
    Inhibin
    Follicle-Regulatory Protein
    Prostaglandins
    Melatonin
    Steroids, Gonadotropins, and Prolactin

OOCYTE MATURATION

Oocyte maturation is a process that begins early in fetal life and is not completed until fertilization occurs in the adult female, often more than two decades later. The main purpose of this process is to provide the means by which a diploid germ cell (2n), which has four times the necessary chromatin (4c), can exchange genetic material and ultimately result in a genetically distinct gamete that is haploid (1n) and contains only the necessary amount of chromatin (1c).

Three weeks after conception, the primordial germ cells can be identified in the epithelium of the yolk sac near the developing allantois.[1] These germ cells progress by ameboid action through the tissues of the yolk sac and the gut to the region of the developing kidneys (mesonephros), and finally into the adjacent genital ridge, which will ultimately become the gonad.[2] Beginning at about 5 weeks' gestation, some of the primordial cells begin replication by mitosis and are called oogonia. Each of these oogonia is diploid (2n) and contains 46 chromosomes. By 5 to 6 months this process will result in 6 to 7 million oogonia (Fig. 3–1). During mitosis, two daughter cells genetically identical to the parent cell are produced. The oogonia undergoing mitosis pass through the four stages of cell life: G 1 (the stage in which a cell carries out its primary function), S (synthesis of DNA), G 2 (chromosome replication), and M (mitosis, including prophase, metaphase, anaphase, and telophase). As a result of DNA synthesis and chromosome replication, each oogonium still has 46 chromosomes, but has produced twice the amount of chromatin or DNA in anticipation of dividing into two genetically identical daughter cells during mitosis. Beginning at 11 to 12 weeks, however, some of the oogonia with twice the amount

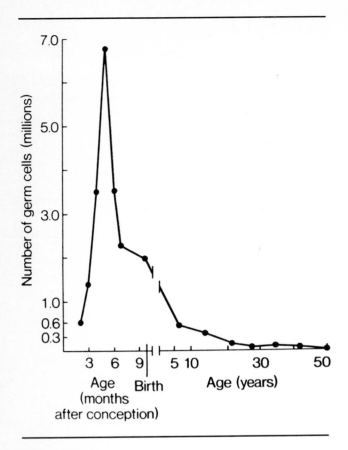

Figure 3–1. Number of germ cells at various ages after conception. (From Baker and Wai Sum.[4] Reproduced with permission.)

of chromatin stop entering mitosis and instead enter prophase of the first meiotic division.[3] These oogonia are now called primary oocytes, and progress through the stages of meiotic prophase (Fig. 3–2).

Meiosis is a form of cell division that occurs only in gametes. During the leptotene stage of meiotic prophase, the 46 chromosomes containing twice the needed DNA are decondensed and appear as 46 single, slender threads. During the next stage, zygotene, the homologous chromosomes align parallel to each other in synapses forming 23 bivalent pairs. Each of the pairs has twice the needed DNA. Therefore, each bivalent represent two times (2n) the haploid number of chromosomes and four times (4c) the needed amount of chromatin or DNA. At this point each chromosome splits longitudinally except at points of junction, called centromeres. The four chromatids are now called tetrads. It is during the ensuing pachytene stage that the chromatids break and recombine, resulting in the exchange of genetic material. In the next stage of prophase, diplotene, the pairs of chromatids demonstrate mutual repulsion from each other except at the chaismata, where "crossing over" has occurred.

Due to atresia, the nearly 7 million germ cells present at midterm have declined to about 2 million.[4] This phase is in general completed by or shortly after birth. At this point, most of the oocytes have entered the first of two resting phases called the dictyate or dictyotene stage. This stage is exceedingly long and lasts from the time of birth until after puberty, when ovulation occurs. Although apparently inert, oocytes in the dictyate stage do grow and do show evidence of protein synthesis. Chromosomes decondense, forming lateral projections that resemble lamp brushes and that primarily produce DNA-dependent RNA polymerase. During this period the oocyte also secretes three different sulfated glycoproteins that are laid down to produce the zona pellucida.[5] The ZP-3 protein is a species-specific receptor for sperm binding.

It is during the process of ovulation that resumption of meiosis occurs[6] (Fig. 3–3). At the onset of the luteinizing hormone (LH) surge the egg is still a primary oocyte; RNA synthesis ceases. The chromosomes become short and thick. This is called the germinal vesicle, or diakinesis, stage of meiosis, and the first meiotic prophase becomes complete. The nuclear membrane breaks down and the tetrads align themselves on the equator of the metaphase I plate. Tetrads rotate 90 degrees and pull apart. One of the chromosomes still containing twice the necessary chromatin pinches off in a small blob of cytoplasm called the polar body. The polar body is located in the perivitelline space and contains one chromosome (1n) and a double amount of chromatin (2c). The oocyte is also now haploid (1n) but contains twice the necessary chromatin (2c). This stage is called metaphase II and the egg is called a secondary oocyte. This is the stage at the time of ovulation[7] (Fig. 3–4).

Metaphase II is the second resting phase of meiosis. The oocyte will remain in this stage unless fertilization occurs. Should fertilization occur, the remaining chromosome containing twice the chromatin (2c) splits longitudinally, and half the chromatin pinches off to the second polar body. The oocyte is now haploid and contains the proper amount of chromatin (1n, 1c), Therefore, the process of meiosis, which begins in the early fetus, becomes complete only in the adult when fertilization occurs.

FOLLICLE DEVELOPMENT

During fetal life the follicle also develops. At approximately 8 weeks some of the primary oocytes become surrounded by a single layer of spindle-shaped cells derived from mesonephric tissue that migrates to the genital ridge,[2] and are the precursors of granulosa and theca cells. These cells develop cytoplasmic processes that project to the plasma membrane of the

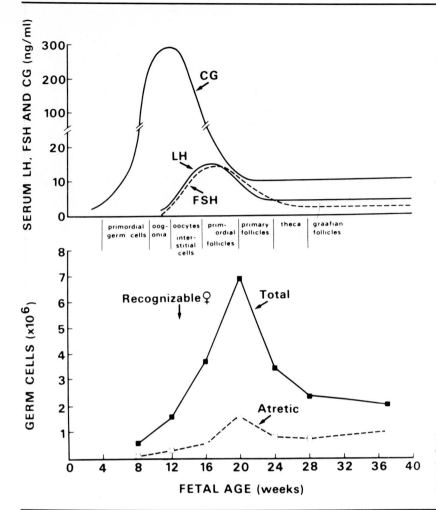

Figure 3–2. Oocyte and follicle maturation and gonadotropin levels at various fetal ages. Gonadotropin values approximate the menopausal range at approximately 16 weeks. From Winter et al.[81] Reproduced with permission.

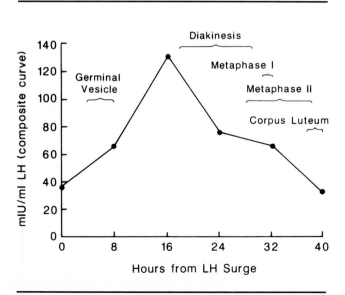

Figure 3–3. Oocyte maturation at various time intervals after the LH surge. From Seibel et al.[7] Reproduced with permission.

oocyte. The oocyte and adjacent granulosa cells become surrounded by a basal lamina, which separates this complex, now called a primordial follicle, from the stroma (Fig. 3–5). During the fifth to sixth gestational month some of the spindle-shaped granulosa cells become cuboidal and begin to divide. This unit is called a primary follicle and it is the first evidence of recruitment.[8] During this transition the oocyte and surrounding granulosa cells become electrically and metabolically coupled by the development between them of small gap junctions, which increase in number during this developmental stage and remain throughout the remainder of folliculogenesis.[9,10] In this fashion the oocyte and its surrounding environment are capable of communicating. Granulosa cell proliferation results in numerous layers of granulosa cells that contribute greatly to increasing follicle diameter. Although up to four layers of granulosa cell proliferation are believed to be independent of gonadotropin control, and may be due to ovarian paracrine mechanisms, gonadotropins

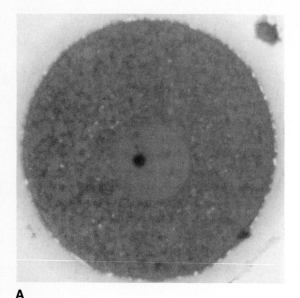

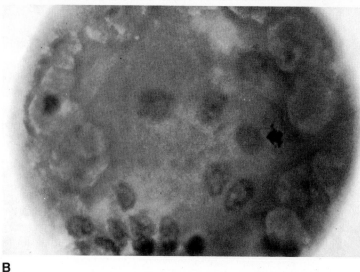

B

A

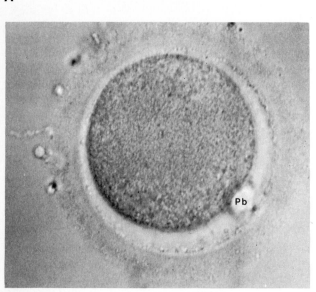

Pb

C

Figure 3–4. Various stages of oocyte maturation. **A.** Germinal vesicle stage oocyte. Note the intact and well-defined nuclear membrane. **B.** A metaphase I oocyte with arrow pointing to chromatin plate. Notice absence of nuclear membrane and absence of a polar body. **C.** A metaphase II oocyte with a polar body (Pb) present in the periviteline space.

are definitely necessary to go beyond this point.[11] The oocyte and its early surrounding layers of granulosa cells is called a secondary follicle. The cytoplasmic process from the granulosa cells traverses the zona pellucida and maintains intimate association with the plasma membrane of the oocyte. At about 7 months' gestation some of the primary follicles form an antrum and thus become known as tertiary, or graafian, follicles. The oocyte is located eccentrically within the antrum surrounded by two to three layers of granulosa cells called the cumulus oophorus. Those cells comprising the cumulus that are contiguous with the wall of the follicle are known as the membranum granulosum. At the time of ovulation, cleavage occurs between the cumulus and the membranum granulosum, and the oocyte and its cumulus are extruded.

The Effect of FSH on Granulosa Cells

During the process of folliculogenesis, the granulosa, theca, and oocyte must acquire the structural and functional properties necessary to accomplish their specialized tasks.[12] The first significant step in granulosa cell autodifferentiation is their transformation from squamous to cuboidal in shape. During this transition specific follicle-stimulating hormone (FSH) receptors appear. The absolute number of receptors per granulosa cell does not increase beyond this early stage of follicle growth. It is only through mitosis and the incremental increase in the number of granulosa cells that the number of FSH receptors is increased. With advancement of follicular development to late secondary and early tertiary stages, receptors for estradiol, progesterone, testosterone, and glucocorti-

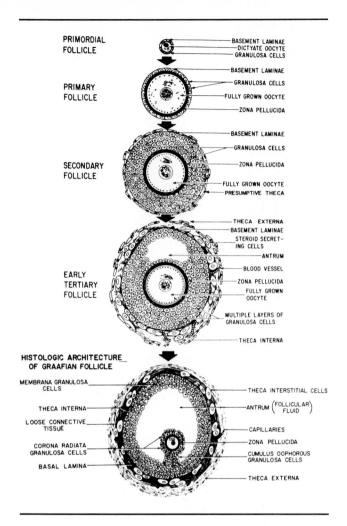

PRIMORDIAL FOLLICLE — BASEMENT LAMINAE / DICTYATE OOCYTE / GRANULOSA CELLS

PRIMARY FOLLICLE — BASEMENT LAMINAE / GRANULOSA CELLS / FULLY GROWN OOCYTE / ZONA PELLUCIDA

SECONDARY FOLLICLE — BASEMENT LAMINAE / GRANULOSA CELLS / ZONA PELLUCIDA / FULLY GROWN OOCYTE / PRESUMPTIVE THECA

EARLY TERTIARY FOLLICLE — THECA EXTERNA / BASEMENT LAMINA / STEROID SECRETING CELLS / ANTRUM / BLOOD VESSEL / ZONA PELLUCIDA / FULLY GROWN OOCYTE / MULTIPLE LAYERS OF GRANULOSA CELLS / THECA INTERNA

HISTOLOGIC ARCHITECTURE OF GRAAFIAN FOLLICLE

MEMBRANA GRANULOSA CELLS / THECA INTERNA / LOOSE CONNECTIVE TISSUE / CORONA RADIATA GRANULOSA CELLS / BASAL LAMINA — THECA INTERSTITIAL CELLS / ANTRUM (FOLLICULAR FLUID) / CAPILLARIES / ZONA PELLUCIDA / CUMULUS OOPHOROUS GRANULOSA CELLS / THECA EXTERNA

Figure 3–5. Architecture and classification of ovarian follicles during folliculogenesis. From Erickson.[9] Reproduced with permission.

coids appear.[9] From this point onward, however, further development requires FSH. The hormone crosses the basal lamina, binds to granulosa cell membrane FSH receptors, and activates adenylate cyclase, which results in synthesis of the intracellular second messenger cyclic adenosine 3', 5'-monophosphate (cAMP).[13] The cAMP binds to a regulatory protein subunit of protein kinase, resulting in the phosphorylation of regulatory proteins. Estrogen amplifies FSH action by enhancing FSH-stimulated cAMP and cAMP-dependent protein kinase formation. In this fashion granulosa cells are capable of a maximal response to a minimal concentration of follicular fluid FSH. Furthermore, FSH is only detectable in follicular fluid when the estrogen:androgen ratio is above 1. In contrast, when FSH is not detected, androgen levels predominate.[14] Follicle-stimulating hormone stimulates mitosis, which increases the number of granulosa cells. Estradiol has the ability to increase the number of its own receptors and therefore exerts a direct mitogenic effect on

granulosa cells that is independent on FSH. By acting synergistically with FSH to stimulate granulosa cell proliferation, FSH together with estradiol promotes an increase in the number of FSH receptors. Epidermal growth factor and fibroblast growth factors have also been found to have potent mitogenic capabilities on human granulosa cells.[15] Insulin and insulinlike growth factor I receptors have also been identified on human granulosa cells.[16,17] Their physiologic role is the subject of further investigation.

In a time and dose-dependent manner, FSH is also responsible for the induction of aromatase enzyme and LH receptors.[18] Aromatase acts to convert androgens to estrogens. Receptors for LH are present only in the dominant follicle and are essential for the follicle to respond to the LH surge and release the oocyte. The presence of LH receptors on granulosa cells is also responsible for progesterone production.[19,20] Normally, LH is not found in follicular fluid until onset of the surge. Low levels of LH receptors and aromatase appear about day 7 of the follicular phase when estradiol levels are beginning to rise. Under the influence of FSH, LH receptors reach a maximum about day 12, which is coincidental with the preovulatory peak of estradiol. Therefore, estradiol appears to act synergistically initially with FSH to promote FSH receptors and later to enhance the ability of FSH to increase and maintain LH receptors. In the absence of estrogen synthesis by the ovary, follicle maturation will arrest at the stage of a small graafian follicle no greater than 2.2 mm in diameter.[21]

The importance of FSH in folliculogenesis is best summarized by the statement that once a granulosa cell has received FSH stimulation, it must continue to be stimulated by FSH or all FSH and LH receptors and aromatase enzyme will be lost and the granulosa cell will die.[22] Selection of the dominant follicle results in part due to this fact. The preovulatory estradiol rise results in a negative feedback effect on pituitary FSH secretion.[23] The preovulatory follicle maintains normal development because its microcirculation is twice as abundant as that of other antral follicles, and because it has a greater number of granulosa cells, and therefore greater aromatizing capacity and more FSH receptors. The remainder of the cohort of developing follicles succumb to the reduced FSH levels and undergo atresia. Modulation of FSH on granulosa cells can also occur through the inhibitory effects of prolactin,[24] glucocorticoids,[25] progesterone, and growth factors, or by the stimulatory effects of estrogen,[26] insulin, and platelet-derived growth factors on aromatase and LH receptor formation.[27] Therefore FSH, the principal hormone of folliculogenesis, may be affected positively or negatively by a vast number of hormonal variations. Follicular physiology is further complicated by the finding that only the membrana granulosa cells appear capable of developing aromatase and LH and prolactin receptors in response to FSH.[27] This finding in combination with the realization that FSH increases intragranulosa cell communication by increasing both the number and size of gap junctions between granulosa cells further develops the concept of the granulosa cells and their surrounded oocyte as a complex system of intracellular communication dominantly influenced by FSH.

The Effect of LH on Theca Cells

By the time follicular development progresses to the secondary follicle stage, two important morphologic events have occurred. The first is the migration of mesenchymal cells to the basement lamina where they align in a radial fashion around the entire follicle. These cells will ultimately become the theca interna and externa. The second morphologic event is the development of an independent blood supply, which is responsible for bringing the necessary hormonal stimulation for follicular growth and development.[9] The theca interna contains theca interstitial cells on all tertiary and graafian follicles. These cells develop specific receptors for LH but not for FSH, and also the enzyme complex 3β-hydroxy-steroid dehydrogenase Δ4-5 isomerase. In response to LH, these theca interstitial cells transform from elongated mesenchymal cells into large epithelial-like cells capable of androgen production, predominantly androstenedione.[18] This is accomplished immediately by LH stimulating cAMP and the second messenger system.[8] Long-term androstenedione biosynthesis requires gene transcription that codes for cholesterol side chain cleavage, the 3β-hydroxy-steroid dehydrogenase, the 17α-hydroxylase, and the 17,20-ylase enzymes.[9]

Androstenedione is the principal precursor of follicle estradiol production and therefore highly significant to follicular outcome. Excessive androgen levels overwhelm the limited capacity of aromatization and induce atresia of the oocyte. Furthermore, granulosa cells derived from human preantral follicles placed in vitro into an androgen-rich environment favor the conversion of androstenedione into more potent androgens instead of estrogens.[28] This process appears to be due to the presence of the enzyme 5α-reductase and the resultant formation of the nonaromatizable androgens dihydrotestosterone and androstenedione. With follicular maturation, granulosa cells from preovulatory follicles are quite capable of aromatizing androgens into estrogens, which diffuse into the follicular fluid.[29] Low levels of androgens appear further to enhance aromatase activity, which can be blocked by preventing nuclear translocation of the androgen-receptor complex.[18] Although the theca is capable of estrogen formation

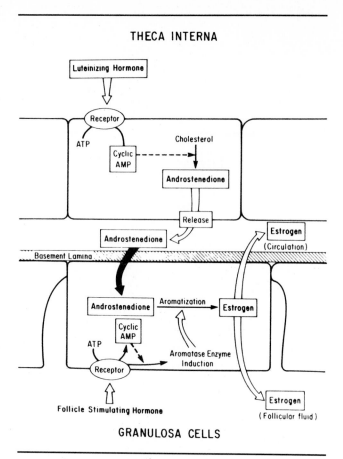

Figure 3–6. Diagram of two-cell–two-gonadotropin concept of follicle estrogen production. (From Erickson.[9] Reproduced with permission.)

from androgen precursors, combining theca and granulosa cells potentiates estrogen production in vitro.[30] This is the basis of the two-cell theory (Fig. 3–6). Theca interstitial cells, like granulosa cells, are modulated by other hormones. Prostaglandins, lipoproteins, insulin, and catecholamines amplify estradiol. Prolactin growth factors, and gonadotropin-releasing hormone (GnRH), inhibit the effects of LH[9] (Fig. 3–7).

FOLLICULAR MICROENVIRONMENT

There has been continued interest in the ovarian follicular microenvironment for nearly 50 years; however, great strides have taken place only in the 1980s. What has evolved is an appreciation that follicular fluid contains in addition to steroids and pituitary hormones, enzymes, plasma proteins, placental proteins, glycosaminoglycans, and nonsteroidal ovarian factors. The concentration of some of those substances changes with follicular growth and oocyte maturation. Although the presence of many of the

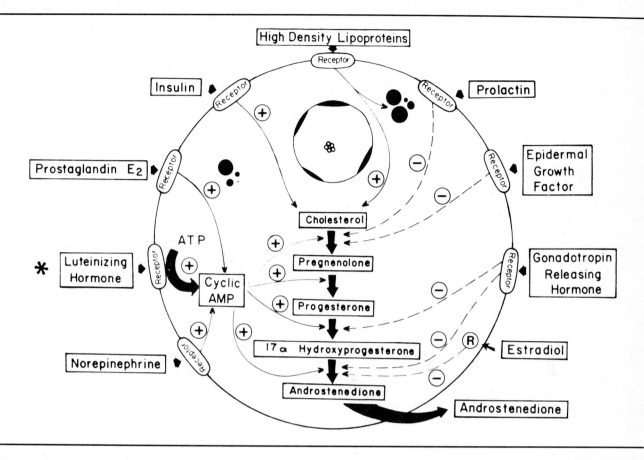

Figure 3–7. Diagram shows current concepts of hormonal control of ovarian interstitial cell steroidogenic activity. (From Erickson.[9] Reproduced with permission.)

substances is newly recognized and their precise role has not yet been explicitly determined, a brief summary of some of the salient nonsteroidal substances other than pituitary hormones found in follicular fluid is of interest.

Inhibin

Inhibin is a gonadal protein that specifically inhibits the secretion of pituitary FSH. Two forms, A and B, have been purified from porcine follicular fluid and characterized as heterodimers with a molecular weight of 32,000. Each inhibin is comprised of an identical β-subunit of MW 18,000 and a distinct but related β-subunit of 13,800 linked by interchain disulfide bonds. In the male, the Sertoli cells of the testis secrete inhibin. Granulosa cells, the ovarian counterpart of the Sertoli cells, but not theca cells, are also capable of producing inhibin.[31–33] The inhibin activity in follicular phase follicular fluid is greater than that in fluid sampled during the luteal phase,[34] and ovulation induction with human menopausal gonadotropins in women with normal cycles increases this activity fourfold.[35] It has also been shown that progesterone inhibits and androgens stimulate granulosa cell inhibin secretion.[32,35] This latter fact may explain the finding of higher inhibin levels in

follicular fluid obtained from patients with polycystic ovary disease than from healthy women.[36]

An FSH-releasing substance has been identified in porcine follicular fluid.[37,38] It is heterodimeric protein composed of the two β-subunits of inhibins A and B linked by interchain disulfide bonds. It has been suggested that this substance be called activin.[37] It is not GnRH. Unlike GnRH, activin has no effect on LH. While GnRH acts immediately to stimulate gonadotropin release, activin requires 4 hours to stimulate FSH release and 24 hours for maximum effect. Activin acts independently of the GnRH receptor and increases stored as well as released FSH.[38] The intriguing notion set forth by these findings is the possibility that a complex regulatory system may exist in which the association of different subunits can give rise to dimers with opposite biologic effects. Conversely, abnormal concentrations or proportions of either inhibin or activin could contribute to the pathophysiology of certain hormonal conditions.

Follicle-Regulatory Protein

In 1983 follicle-regulatory protein was identified and found to be secreted from human[39] and porcine granulosa cells.[40] It does not inhibit FSH secretion by pituitary cells in vitro,[41] and is therefore different from inhibin. Follicle-regulatory protein has been shown to inhibit aromatase activity in porcine granulosa cells from medium but not large-sized follicles, and therefore may play a role in follicular fluid androgen levels and ultimately in atresia. Testosterone appears to sensitize granulosa cells to the action of follicle-regulatory protein on steroid secretion, an effect that can be overcome by FSH.[42] This apparently occurs because follicle-regulatory protein inhibits FSH induction of adenylate cyclase.[43] Therefore, it may play an important role as a paracrine regulatory substance involved in folliculogenesis.

Prostaglandins

An important role for prostaglandins (PG) in preovulatory follicles has been suggested. Much of the information is based on animal studies, which reported increasing levels of PGE_2 and $PGF_{2\alpha}$ just before ovulation in vivo and in vitro studies when preovulatory follicles were incubated with LH. Human follicular tissue has been shown to synthesize $PGF_{2\alpha}$ in vitro under the influence of either naturally secreted or endogenous gonadotropins.[44] We found that follicular fluid levels of $PGF_{2\alpha}$ increase in a time-related sequence from the onset of the LH surge[45] (Fig. 3–8). This association implies that LH may play an important role in follicular prostaglandin accumulation either directly or indirectly by some mediator such as cAMP.[44]

Prostaglandins are also thought to have a potentially significant role in cumulus expansion and oocyte maturation. Prostaglandin E_2 has been shown to stimulate cumulus expansion in vitro in the mouse. Using indomethacin to block ovulation in the rabbit

ovary perfused in vitro, oocytes continue to mature but display increased degeneration at the metaphase II stage.[46] This degeneration could be prevented by supplemental $PGF_{2\alpha}$. In the mouse, indomethacin was also effective in preventing germinal vesicle breakdown and oocyte maturation, events that could be prevented by the administration of prostaglandin. Increasing levels of $PGF_{2\alpha}$ 30 or more hours after the onset of the LH surge and associated with advancing stages of oocyte maturation supports the notion that prostaglandins play a role in ovulation, oocyte maturation, and/or the maintenance of healthy oocytes.

Melatonin

Melatonin, the major hormone of the pineal gland, has been shown to influence reproductive function in many mammalian species.[47] Administration of melatonin to female rats diminished ovarian weight, blocked ovulation, and suppressed the vaginal estrus cycle. During periods of prolonged darkness, which results in prolonged melatonin synthesis, gonadal function is suppressed in several mammalian species.[47] Subsequently, melatonin was reported to be involved in such human reproductive processes as puberty[48] and the menstrual cycle.[49,50]

It has generally been thought that melatonin exerted its antigonadotropic effect predominantly at the level of the brain and pituitary.[51] However, exogenous melatonin has been found to be concentrated in the ovaries of both rats and cats, and specific melatonin receptors have been reported in ovarian tissue obtained from the hamster, rat, and human.[52] Furthermore, melatonin added in vitro has been reported to manifest direct effects on ovarian steroidogenesis.[53,54]

These studies led to the investigation and discovery of melatonin in human preovulatory follicular fluid.[55] The mean follicular fluid concentration was 36.5 ±4.8 pg/mL, which was substantially higher than that concurrently found in serum (10 ±1.4 pg/mL) (Fig. 3–9). To date it is unknown whether this melatonin is sequestered or produced in the follicle, although sequestration appears more likely. The physiologic significance of melatonin to follicular maturation may be quite extensive. Certainly the hormone's central effects, such as suppressing pituitary responsiveness to GnRH[51] and inhibiting of pulsatile hypothalamic GnRH secretion,[56] are best recognized. Melatonin is concentrated in the ovary, however. It causes a dose related stimulation of progesterone synthesis by human corpus luteum[53] and granulosa cells[57] in vitro, and increases the ovarian incorporation of (I-^{14}C) acetate into androstenedione. A positive correlation between melatonin and progesterone levels has also been suggested due to apparently higher luteal phase levels of melatonin. Other investigators[54] reported that hu-

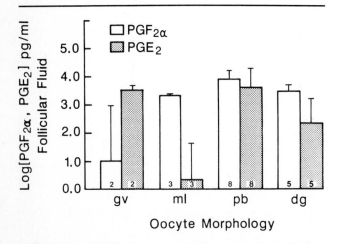

Figure 3–8. Prostaglandin $F_{2\alpha}$ and E_2 levels at various stages of oocyte maturation. Gv = germinal vesicle; ml = metaphase I; pb = polar body or metaphase II; dg = degenerating oocytes. (From Seibel et al.[45] Reproduced with permission.)

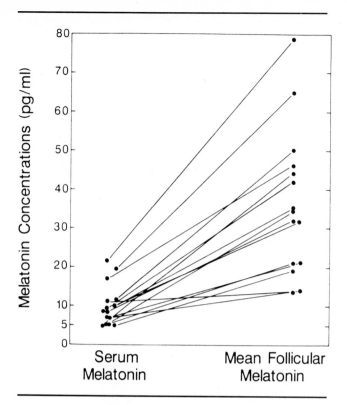

Figure 3–9. Melatonin concentrations obtained from serum and preovulatory follicles measured at the time of oocyte retrieval. (From Brzezinski et al.[55] Reproduced with permission.)

man chorionic gonadotropin (HCG) stimulation of rabbit ovarian follicles was blocked by melatonin, and that rat testicular androgen synthesis was inhibited when melatonin was added to the culture medium.[54] Future investigations will be required to establish the extent of involvement of melatonin on follicular development and oocyte maturation.

Steroids, Gonadotropins, and Prolactin

Early reports describing human antral fluid steroid concentrations used follicular fluid either aspirated at laparotomy or obtained from follicles dissected from ovaries or ovarian fragments excised at various stages of the menstrual cycle.[58–62] The course of the midcycle LH surge was not considered, and in only one of these studies[61] were steroid levels in antral fluid correlated with the degree of follicular normality and atresia. Several investigators measured human follicular fluid (ff) hormone levels immediately prior to ovulation in an attempt to correlate these values with the fertilizability of oocytes obtained.[63–67] All of these studies obtained oocytes and follicular fluid approximately 35 to 37 hours after the injection of human HCG, when ovulation was anticipated to be near. The pattern of ff hormone secretion at various times after triggering ovulation was not considered. We

recently compiled data from follicular fluid aspirated during laparoscopy in unstimulated cycles at various times after the onset of an endogenous LH surge when HCG was not administered.[68] Steroid levels in antral fluids were correlated with the stage of maturation of the oocyte obtained.

Follicular fluid E_2 concentrations demonstrate an increase from 911 ±469 ng/mL to 1,896 ±677 ng/mL as the oocyte resumes meiosis and proceeds from germinal vesicle (gv) to mI (Fig. 3–10). This is followed by a relative decline to 1,100 ±427 ng/mL as mII is achieved. These levels compare favorably to those reported by McNatty and associates[61] for healthy preovulatory follicles defined as containing more than 50% of their complement of granulosa cells, as well as to those obtained in the preovulatory phase of the natural menstrual cycle.[58] They are higher than those reported in ff obtained from follicles stimulated by human menopausal gonadotropins (HMG).[69] The overall rise in E_2 levels with oocyte maturation is in contrast to the data reported by Bomsel-Helmreich and associates,[62] who noted a 30% drop in ff E_2 levels from the time intervals between the E_2 and LH peaks (9.0 ±4.2 pmol/μL) to that between the LH peak and ovulation (3.0 ±1.8 pmol/μL). Those authors, however, did not report the stage of oocyte maturation. Furthermore, the exact time of follicle aspiration in relation to the onset of the LH surge was not defined. Although our results demonstrate an initial rise in ff E_2 levels, a 42% ($p > 0.05$) fall in E_2 levels is seen as the oocyte matures from mI to mII. Thus it is possible that Bomsel-Helmreich and associates[62] retrieved ff from follicles whose oocytes were already beyond the mI stage. The decline in E_2 concentrations may reflect a

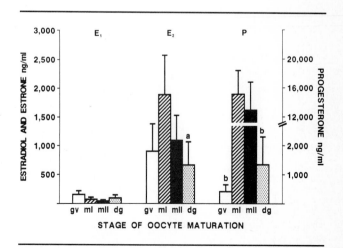

Figure 3–10. Follicle fluid levels of E_1, E_2, and P at various stages of oocyte maturation in unstimulated cycles. (From Seibel et al.[68] Reproduced with permission.)

shift in steroidogenesis as the follicle begins the process of luteinization. A decline in aromatase activity with progressive follicular maturity has been reported.[70] The (E_2) was significantly ($p < 0.05$) lower in fluids containing degenerating (dg) oocytes. This is consistent with the results of studies describing the hormonal microenvironment of atretic follicles.[61,62] Follicular fluid E_1 concentrations did not differ among the different stages of oocyte maturation and were markedly lower than the (E_2), a finding that was reported previously.[58]

Follicular fluid progesterone (P) concentration increases from 431 ±219 ng/mL in the gv stage to 15,340 ±3,220 ng/mL in mII. These levels are much higher than those reported for ff (P) in the follicular phase[58,61,71] and are consistent with the findings in unstimulated cycles of both animals and humans, in whom a shift in preovulatory follicular steroidogenesis from androgen and estrogen biosynthesis to progesterone occurs.[72–74] The (P) is significantly ($p < 0.0001$) higher in ff associated with mI and mII oocytes as compared to gv and dg oocytes, and compares favorably to the increase in ff (P) after the LH peak as previously reported.[62] This may reflect a time-dependent potentiation of progesterone biosynthesis as oocyte maturation occurs.

In this regard, it is interesting to note that the ff LH is also significantly higher in mI (87 ±32 mIU) and mII (129 ±26 mIU) as compared to gv (823 ±9 mIU) ($p < 0.05$) and dg (26 ±3 mIU) ($p < 0.01$) oocyte-associated follicles (Fig. 3–11). It has been proposed that LH inhibits 17,20 desmolase and aromatase activity, thus promoting progesterone synthesis. Although (E_2) in our study was higher in mI and mII than in gv, it should be realized that ff measurements

reflect the cumulative results of steroidogenesis and may not accurately reflect the acute synthetic processes under way in the granulosa luteal cells.[75,76] Thus, the high (E_2) may represent the results of previous steroidogenic activity while the increased (P) may represent the response to the acquisition of new LH receptors or an enhanced responsiveness to LH per se. Alternatively, the increased (P) with time after the LH surge may be due to the relocation of the subcellular organelles involved in low-density lipoprotein metabolism and steroidogenesis, resulting in a more efficient post-receptor processing of the lipoprotein.[77]

Of further interest is the finding of significantly higher ($p < 0.001$) prolactin levels in ff of mI (15 ±3 ng/mL) and mII (21 ±3 ng/mL) follicles as compared to gv (11 ±3 ng/mL) and dg (26 ±3) follicles. These values are comparable to those previously reported in preovulatory follicles of unstimulated cycles,[78] but markedly lower than those found in HMG-stimulated cycles.[79] It has been suggested that prolactin induces LH receptors and modulates steroidogenesis by increasing pregnenolone biosynthesis and increasing the activity of 3 β-01-hydroxysteroid dehydrogenase.[80] Furthermore, low levels of prolactin have been demonstrated to enhance progesterone biosynthesis in in-vitro granulosa cell culture systems.[78] Thus, the higher prolactin and LH levels in mI and mII follicles may together promote the increased progesterone biosynthesis reflected in the higher progesterone levels in the fluid of these more mature follicles.

Concomitant with the higher (P) and (E_2) in mI and mII ff, the $P:E_2$ ratio is also significantly ($p < 0.05$) higher in the ff of these follicles than in those associated with gv or dg oocytes (Fig. 3–12). The ff $P:E_2$ ratio is the steroid value that correlates best with morphologic maturity and, in the case of in-vitro fertilization cycles, subsequent fertilizability.[66]

Follicular fluid androstenedione and testosterone concentrations are both significantly greatest in follicles containing dg oocytes (Fig. 3–13). This finding is in agreement with previously reported data.[61,62,66,71] The androgen levels in the ff of the healthy follicles are comparable to those reported by Lobo,[66] Brailly,[71] and their associates, but are much lower than those reported by McNatty and associates,[61] who may have obtained ff from follicles at an earlier stage of maturation. The (T) is significantly ($p < 0.05$) higher in gv ff as compared to mII. Similarly, there is a trend toward a decrease in (A) as oocyte maturation progresses from gv (244 ±163 ng/mL) to mII (31 ±10 ng/mL). The significance of these findings is unclear. Both androgens may serve as precursors of follicular estrogen. Thus, one might expect an increased level of E_2 in these follicles, as previous investigators have demonstrated the retention of aromatase activity in

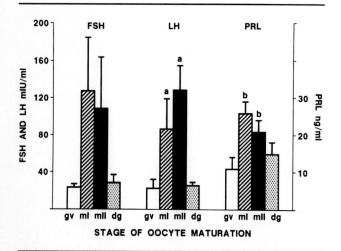

Figure 3–11. Follicle fluid levels of LH, FSH, and prolactin at various stages of oocyte maturation in unstimulated cycles. (From Seibel et al.[68] Reproduced with permission.)

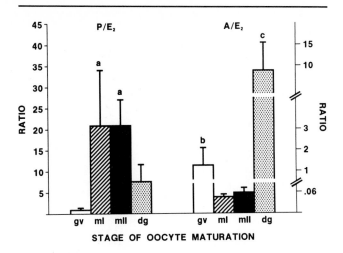

Figure 3–12. Follicle fluid $P:E_2$ and $A:E_2$ ratios at various stages of oocyte maturation in unstimulated cycles. (From Seibel et al.[68] Reproduced with permission.)

granulosa luteal cells as much as 36 hours after the injection of an ovulatory dose of HCG.[76] Nevertheless, the (E_2) is lower in gv ff as compared to the later stages of maturation.

The $A:E_2$ is highest in the ff of follicles containing dg oocytes (see Fig. 3–12). In addition, the ratio in gv follicular fluid is significantly ($p < 0.05$) higher compared to that of mI ff. Again, the explanation for this finding is unclear. While a high $A:E_2$ ratio is certainly an indication of follicular atresia,[61,62,66] it may also reflect the relative immaturity of an otherwise healthy preovulatory follicle.

In summary, these data define the changing preovulatory follicular fluid hormonal microenviron-

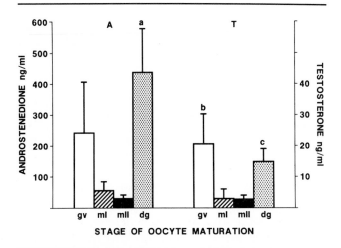

Figure 3–13. Follicle fluid A and T levels at various stages of oocyte maturation in unstimulated cycles. (From Seibel et al.[68] Reproduced with permission.)

ment in the natural cycle. Maturational development of the oocyte at various time intervals after the onset of the LH surge in the unstimulated menstrual cycle was used as a marker. These values from the natural cycle provide a valuable reference point for comparison with ff obtained from stimulated cycles intended for IVF.

REFERENCES

1. Eddy EM, Clark JM, Gong D, Fenderson BA: Review article: Origin and migration of primordial germ cells in mammals. *Gamete Res* 4:333, 1981.
2. Zamboni L, Bezard J, Mauleon P: The role of the mesonephros in the development of the sheep fetal ovary. *Ann Biol Anim Biochem Biophys* 19:1153, 1979.
3. Gondos B, Westergaard L, Byskov AG: Initiation of oogenesis in the human fetal ovary: Ultrastructural and squash preparation study. *Am J Obstet Gynecol* 155:189, 1986.
4. Baker TG, Wai Sum O: Development of the ovary and oogenesis. *Clin Obstet Gynecol* 3:3, 1976.
5. Bleil JD, Wassarman PM: Synthesis of zona pellucida proteins by denuded and follicle-enclosed mouse oocytes during culture in vitro. *Proc Natl Acad Sci USA* 77:1029, 1980.
6. Seibel MM: Timing of ovulation, in Studd JWW (ed): *Progress in Obstetrics and Gynaecology.* London, Churchill Livingstone, 1987, vol 6.
7. Seibel MM, Smith D, Levesque L, Borten M, Taymor ML: The temporal relationship between the luteinizing hormone surge and human oocyte maturation. *Am J Obstet Gynecol* 142:568, 1982.
8. Hodgen GD: The dominant ovarian follicle. *Fertil Steril* 38:281, 1982.
9. Erickson GF: An analysis of follicle development and ovum maturation. *Semin Reprod Endocrinol* 4:233, 1986.
10. Burghardt RC, Matheson RL: Gap junction amplification in rat ovarian granulosa cells. I. A direct response to FSH. *Dev Biol* 94:206, 1982.
11. Wolff-Exalta AE: Influence of gonadotropins on early follicle cell development and early oocyte growth in the immature rat. *J Reprod Fertil* 66:537, 1982.
12. Hsueh AJW, Adashi EY, Jones PBC, Welsh TH: Hormonal regulation of the differentiation of cultured ovarian granulosa cells. *Endocr Rev* 5:76, 1948.
13. Richards JS, Sengal N, Tash JS: Changes in content and cAMP-dependent phosphorylation of specific proteins in granulosa cells of preantral and preovulatory ovarian follicles and in corpora lutea. *J Biol Chem* 258:5227, 1983.
14. McNatty KP, Smith DM, Makris A, Osathanondh R, Ryan KJ: The microenvironment of the human antral follicle: interrelationships among the steroid levels in antral fluid, the population of granulosa cells, and the status of the oocyte in vivo and in vitro. *J Clin Endocrinol Metab* 49:851, 1979.
15. Hammond JM, English HF: Regulation of deoxyribonucleic acid synthesis in cultured porcine granulosa cells by growth factors and hormones. *Endocrinology* 120:1039, 1987.
16. Poretsky L, Grigorescu F, Seibel M, Moses A, Flier JS: Distribution and characterization of insulin and insulin-like growth factor I receptors in normal human ovary. *J Clin Endocrinol Metab* 61:728, 1985.
17. Gates GS, Bayer S, Seibel M, et al: Characterization of insulin-like growth factor binding to human granulosa cells obtained during in vitro fertilization. *J Recept Res*, 7:885, 1987.
18. Erickson GF, Magoffin DA, Dyer CA, Hofeditz C: The ovarian androgen-producing cells: A review of structure/function relationships. *Endocr Rev* 6:371, 1985.
19. Yamoto M, Nalcano R, Iwasaki M, Ikoma H, Furukawa K: Luteinizing hormone receptors in human ovarian follicles and corpora lutea during the menstrual cycle. *Obstet Gynecol* 68:200, 1986.
20. Hill GA, Herbert CM, Wentz AC, Osteen KG: Use of individual human follicles to compare oocyte in vitro fertilization to granulosa cell in vitro luteinization. *Fertil Steril* 48:258, 1987.
21. Araki S, Chikazawa K, Sekiguchi I, et al: Arrest of follicular development in a patient with 17α-hydroxylase deficiency: Folliculogenesis in association with a lack of estrogen synthesis in the ovary. *Fertil Steril* 47:169, 1987.
22. Uilenbroek JTH, Woutersen PJA, Van der Shoot P: Atresia of preovulatory follicles: gonadotropin binding and steroidogenic activity. *Biol Reprod* 23:219, 1980.

23. Zeleznik AJ: Premature elevation of systemic estradiol reduces serum levels of follicle-stimulating hormone and lengthens the follicular phase of the menstrual cycle in rhesus monkeys. *Endocrinology* 109:352, 1981.

24. Dorrington J, Gore-Langton RE: Prolactin inhibits estrogen synthesis in the ovary. *Nature* 290:600, 1981.

25. Schoonmaker JN, Erickson GF: Glucocorticoid modulation of follicle-stimulating hormone-medited granulosa cell differentiation. *Endocrinology* 113:1356, 1983.

26. Adashi EY, Hsueh AJW: Estrogens augment the stimulation of ovarian aromatase activity by follicle-stimulating hormone in cultured rat granulosa cells. *J Biol Chem* 257:6077, 1982.

27. Oxberry BA, Greenwald GS: An autoradiographic study of the binding of ^{125}I-labeled FSH, hCG and prolactin to the hamster ovary throughout the estrous cycle. *Biol Reprod* 27:505, 1982.

28. Hillier SG, VanDen Boogaard AMJ, Reichert LE, Van Hall EV: Intraovarian sex steroid hormone interactions and the regulation of follicular maturation: aromatization of androgens by human granulosa cells in vitro. *J Clin Endocrinol Metab* 50:640, 1980.

29. Hillier SG, DeZwart FA: Evidence that granulosa cell aromatase induction/activation by follicle stimulating hormone is an androgen receptor-regulated process in vitro. *Endocrinology* 109:1303, 1981.

30. McNatty KP, Makris A, DeGrazia C, Osathanondh R, Ryan KJ: Steroidogenesis by recombind follicular cells from the human ovary in vitro. *J Clin Endocrinol Metab* 51:1286, 1980.

31. Findlay J: The nature of inhibin and its use in the regulation of fertility and diagnosis of infertility. *Fertil Steril* 46:770, 1986.

32. Channing CP, Anderson LD, Hoover DJ, et al: The role of nonsteroidal regulators in the control of oocyte and follicular maturation. *Recent Prog Horm Res* 38:331, 1982.

33. Franchimont P: Inhibin: from concept to reality. *Vitam Horm* 37:243, 1979.

34. Chappel SC, Holt JA, Spies HG: Inhibin: Differences in bioactivity within human follicular fluid in the follicular and luteal stages of the menstrual cycle. *Proc Soc Exp Biol Med* 163:310, 1980.

35. Marrs RP, Lobo JD, Campeau JD, et al: Correlation of human follicular fluid inhibin activity with spontaneous and induced follicle maturation. *J Clin Endocrinol Metab* 58:704, 1984.

36. Tonabe K, Gagliano P, Channing CP, et al: Levels of inhibin-F activity and steroids from human follicular fluid from normal women and from women with polycystic ovary disease. *J Clin Endocrinol Metab* 57:24, 1983.

37. Ling N, Shao-Yao Y, Veno N, et al: Pituitary FSH is released by a heterodimer of the β subunits from the two forms of inhibin. *Nature* 321:779, 1986.

38. Vale W, Rivier J, Vaughan J, et al: Purification and characterization of an FSH-releasing protein from porcine ovarian follicular fluid. *Nature* 321:776, 1986.

39. DiZerega GS, Marrs RR, Roche PC, Campeau JD, Kling OR: Identification of proteins in pooled human follicular fluid which suppresses follicular response to gonadotropins. *J Clin Endocrinol Metab* 56:35, 1983.

40. Kling OR, Roche PC, Campeau JD, et al: Identification of a porcine follicular fluid fraction which suppresses follicular response to gonadotropins. *Biol Reprod* 30:564, 1984.

41. DiZerega GS, Campeau JD, Vjita EL, Marrs RP, Lobo RA: Correlation of inhibin and follicle regulatory protein activities with follicular fluid steroid levels in anovulatory patients. *Fertil Steril* 41:849, 1984.

42. Ono T, Campeau JD, Holmberg EA, et al: Biochemical and physiological characterization of follicle regulatory protein: A paracrine regulator of folliculogenesis. *Am J Obstet Gynecol* 154:709, 1986.

43. Vjita EL, Campeau JD, diZerega GS: Inhibition of FSH augmented adenylate cyclase activity in porcine granulosa cells by ovarian protein. *Mol Cell Endocrinol*, in press.

44. Plunkett ER, Moon YS, Zemecnik J, Armstrong DT: Preliminary evidence of role for prostaglandin F in human follicular function. *Am J Obstet Gynecol* 123:391, 1975.

45. Seibel MM, Swartz SL, Smith DM, Levesque L, Taymor ML: In vivo prostaglandin concentrations in human preovulatory follicles. *Fertil Steril* 42:482, 1984.

46. Yoshimura Y, Wallach EE: Studies of the mechanism(s) of mammalian ovulation. *Fertil Steril* 47:22, 1987.

47. Brzezinski A, Wurtman RJ: The pineal gland: Its possible roles in human reproduction. *Obstet Gynecol Surv* 43:197, 1988.

48. Waldhuser F, Weissenbacher G, Zeitlhuber U, Waaldhuser M, Wurtman RJ: Fall in nocturnal serum melatonin levels during prepuberty and pubescence. *Lancet* 1:362, 1984.

49. Brzezinski A, Lynch HJ, Wurtman RJ, Seibel MM: Possible contribution of melatonin to the timing of the luteinizing hormone surge. *N Engl J Med* 316:1550, 1987.

50. Webley GE, Leindenberger F: The circadian pattern of melatonin and its positive relationship with progesterone in women. *J Clin Endocrinol Metab* 63:323, 1986.

51. Martin JE, Sattler C: Selectivity of melatonin pituitary inhibition for luteinizing hormone-releasing hormone. *Neuroendocrinology* 34:112, 1982.

52. Cohen M, Roselle D, Chabner B: Evidence for a cytoplasmic melatonin receptor. *Nature* 274:894, 1978.

53. Macphee AA, Cole FE, Rice BF: The effect of melatonin on steroidogenesis by the human ovary in vitro. *J Clin Endocrinol Metab* 40:688, 1974.

54. Younglai EV: In vitro effects of melatonin on hCG stimulation of steroid accumulation by rabbit ovarian follicles. *J Steroid Biochem* 10:714, 1979.

55. Brzezinski A, Seibel MM, Lynch HF, Deng M-H, Wurtman RJ: Melatonin in human preovulatory follicular fluid. *J Clin Endocrinol Metab* 64:865, 1987.

56. Bittman EL, Kaynard AH, Olster DH, et al: Pineal melatonin mediates photoperiod control of pulsatile luteinizing hormone secretion in the ewe. *Neuroendocrinology* 40:409, 1985.

57. Webley GE, Luck MR: Melatonin directly stimulates the secretion of progesterone by human granulosa cells. *Acta Endocrinol* (Copenh) (Suppl) 108:91, 1985.

58. Sanyal MK, Berger MJ, Thompson IE, Taymor ML, Horne HW: Development of graafian follicles in adult human ovary. I. Correlation of estrogen and progesterone concentrations in antral fluid with growth of follicles. *J Clin Endocrinol* 38:828, 1977.

59. Fowler RE, Chan STH, Edwards RG, Walters DE, Steptoe PC: Steroidogenesis in human follicles approaching ovulation as judged from assays of follicular fluid. *J Endocrinol* 72:259, 1977.

60. McNatty KP, Baird DT: Relationship between follicle-stimulating hormone, androstenedione and estradiol in human follicular fluid. *J Endocrinol* 76:527, 1978.

61. McNatty KP, Smith DM, Makris A, Osathanondh R, Ryan K: The microenvironment of the human antral follicle: Interrelationships among the steroid levels in antral fluid, the population of granulosa cells, and the status of the oocyte in vivo and in vitro. *J Clin Endocrinol Metab* 49:851, 1979.

62. Bomsel-Helmreich O, Gougeon A, Thibault A, et al: Healthy and atretic human follicles in the preovulatory phase: differences in evolution of follicular morphology and steroid content of follicular fluid. *J Clin Endocrinol Metab* 48:686, 1979.

63. Wramsby H, Kullander S, Liedholm P, Sundstrom P, Thorell J: The success rate of in vitro fertilization of human oocytes in relation to the concentration of different hormones in follicular fluid and peripheral plasma. *Fertil Steril* 36:448, 1981.

64. Carson RS, Trounson AO, Findlay JK: Successful fertilization of human oocytes in vitro: Concentration of estradiol-17β, progesterone and androstenedione in the antral fluid of donor follicles. *J Clin Endocrinol Metab* 55:798, 1982.

65. Fishel SB, Edwards RG, Walters DE: Follicular steroids as a prognosticator of successful fertilization of human oocytes in vitro. *J Endocrinol* 99:335, 1983.

66. Lobo RA, diZerega GS, Marrs RP: Follicular fluid steroid levels in dysmature and mature follicles from spontaneous and hyperstimulated cycles in normal and anovulatory women. *J Clin Endocrinol Metab* 60:81, 1985.

67. Uehara S, Naganuma T, Tsuiki A, et al: Relationship between follicular fluid steroid concentrations and in vitro fertilization. *Obstet Gynecol* 66:19, 1985.

68. Seibel MM, Smith DM, Dlugi AM, Levesque L: Periovulatory follicular fluid hormone levels in unstimulated human cycles. *J Clin Endocrinol Metab* In press.

69. Boteros-Ruiz W, Laufer N, DeCherney AH, et al: The relationship between follicular fluid steroid concentrations and successful fertilization of oocytes in vitro. *Fertil Steril* 41:820, 1984.

70. Polan ML, Laufer N, Ohkawa R, et al: The association between granulosa cell aromatase activity and oocyte-cumulus-corona complex maturity from individual human follicles. *J Clin Endocrinol Metab* 59:170, 1984.

71. Brailly S, Gougeon A, Milgrom E, Bomsel-Helmreich O, Papiernik E: Androgens and progestins in the human ovarian follicle: Differences in the evolution of preovulatory, healthy non-ovulatory, and atretic follicles. *J Clin Endocrinol Metab* 53:128, 1981.

72. Moor RM: The ovarian follicle of the sheep: Inhibition of oestrogen secretion by LH. *J Endocrinol* 61:455, 1974.

73. Leung PCK, Armstron DT: Interactions of steroid and gonadotropins in the control of steroidogenesis in the ovarian follicle. *Annu Rev Physiol* 42:71, 1980.

74. Hillier SG, Reichert LE Jr, Van Hall EV: Control of pre-ovulatory follicular estrogen biosynthesis in the human ovary. *J Clin Endocrinol Metab* 52:847, 1981.

75. Bjersing L, Cortenseu H: Biosynthesis of steroids by granulosa cells of the porcine ovary in vitro. *J Reprod Fertil* 14:101, 1967.

76. Dlugi AM, Laufer N, Polan ML, et al: 17 β-estradiol and progesterone production by human granulosa-luteal cells isolated from human menopausal gonadotropin-stimulated cycles for in vitro fertilization. *J Clin Endocrinol Metab* 59:986, 1984.

77. Golos TG, Soto EA, Tureck RW, Strauss JF III: Human chorionic gonadotropin and 8-Bromo-adenosine 3',5'-monophosphate stimulate (I^{125}) low-density lipoprotein uptake and metabolism by luteinized human granulosa cells in culture. *J Clin Endocrinol Metab* 61:633, 1985.

78. McNatty KP, Sawers RS, McNeilly AS: A possible role for prolactin in control of steroid secretion by the human graafian follicle. *Nature* 250:653, 1974.

79. Laufer N, Botero-Ruiz W, DeCherney AH, et al: Gonadotropin and prolactin levels in follicular fluid of human ova successfully fertilized in vitro. *J Clin Endocrinol Metab* 58:430, 1984.

80. Hsueh AJW, Adashi EY, Jones PBC, Welsh TH: Hormonal regulation of the differentiation of cultured ovarian granulosa cells. *Endocr Rev* 5:76, 1984.

81. Winter JSD, Faiman C, Reyes FI: The gonadotropins of the fetus and neonate: Their ontogeny, function and regulation, in Flamigni C, Givens JR (eds): *The Gonadotropins: Basic Science and Clinical Aspects in Females.* New York, Academic Press, p 160, 1982.

CHAPTER 4

Anovulation and Amenorrhea

Judith L. Vaitukaitis

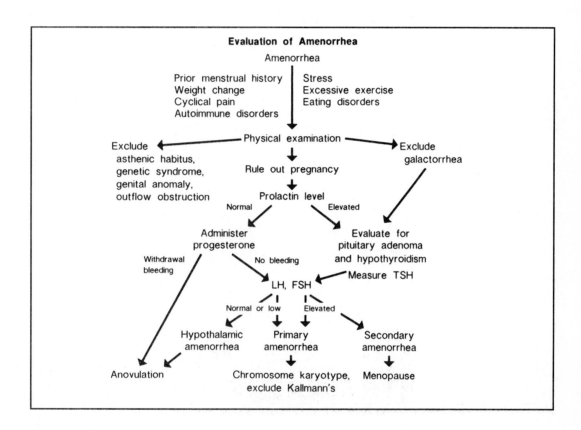

Evaluation of Amenorrhea

The normal menstrual cycle reflects carefully regulated interactions among the hypothalamus, pituitary, and ovaries. Modulators of gonadotropin secretion include sex steroids, secreted by the ovaries, and gonadotropin-releasing hormone (GnRH), a decapeptide synthesized and secreted by hypothalamic peptidergic neurons. In addition, a host of other peptide and biogenic amines modulate GnRH neuron function.[1-3] Nutrition, stress, physical activity, abnormalities of the central nervous system, and systemic illness may adversely affect gonadotropin secretion through poorly defined mechanisms, and induce menstrual dysfunction ranging from an irregular menstrual pattern to anovulation to amenorrhea.[4-7]

FETAL OVARIAN DEVELOPMENT

Early in fetal life, germ cells migrate to the primitive ovary and proliferate so that by the tenth week of fetal life the ovary contains 5 to 7 million oogonia. To protect oogonia from accelerated degeneration and

This chapter was written by Dr. Vaitukaitis in her private capacity. Official support or endorsement by the Division of Research Resources is not intended, nor should it be inferred.

atresia, a layer of progranulosa cells must surround the oocyte, forming a primordial follicle. With stimulation by follicle-stimulating hormone (FSH), the layer of flattened granulosa cells becomes cuboidal and forms a structure known as a primary follicle. Once follicles are formed, they undergo atresia even with the protective layer of granulosa cells. At birth only 1 to 2 million follicles persist. Atresia continues, so that by the expected time of onset of spontaneous menses, only 300,000 to 400,000 follicles remain. When no gonadotropin-responsive follicles remain in the ovaries, primary gonadal failure results and usually signals menopause.[8,9]

In the Western world, spontaneous menopause occurs in the early to middle 50s. Women who develop primary ovarian failure prior to age 40 have premature menopause.[10,11]

ONSET OF HYPOTHALAMIC–PITUITARY–OVARIAN FEEDBACK

Coincident with the formation of primordial follicles by the 20th week of gestation, fetal pituitary gonadotropin synthesis is evident and fetal FSH blood levels approach castrate levels. With differentiation of primordial follicles to those with several layers of granulosa cells, fetal circulating FSH concentrations decline, signaling the onset of negative feedback between the hypothalamic–pituitary axis and the ovaries.[12] Gonadotropin synthesis and secretion decrease thereafter, but ovarian follicles continue to undergo growth and atresia. Fetal ovarian follicular growth is dependent on fetal gonadotropin stimulation, since ovaries of the anencephalic fetus contain only primordial and primary follicles, reflecting abnormal hypothalamic–pituitary function in the anencephalic.[13]

Cells of ovarian follicles synthesize a host of peptides, which some investigators suggest may modulate pituitary gonadotropin secretion. More than likely, they modulate ovarian function locally through a paracrine mechanism. Those peptides include inhibin, epidermal growth factor, and GnRH-like peptide.[14–16]

NEONATAL AND PREPUBERTAL GIRL

At birth only 1 to 2 million ovarian follicles remain. For the first 1 to 2 years after birth, girls have slightly elevated levels of circulating gonadotropin and sex steroids.[17] The physiologic mechanism responsible for the increased hypothalamic–pituitary–ovarian activity is unknown. After that first year or two,

circulating gonadotropin levels remain tonically low until the onset of puberty.

PUBERTY

In the United States and other Western countries, menarche, or the onset of the first menses, occurs at a mean age of 13.5 years, with 95% confidence limits of 11 to 16 years. If menarche occurs prior to age 10, an abnormality exists and the patient has precocious puberty. If the onset of menses is delayed beyond the 16th year, the girl has a form of primary amenorrhea. Menarche is one pubertal milestone. Puberty reflects a closely orchestrated series of dynamic physiologic events integrated among the hypothalamic–pituitary axis and higher central nervous system sites. Puberty occurs over 3 to 5 years. The first sign is usually breast budding, normally observed at a mean age of 11 years. Approximately 6 months after breast budding, pubic hair develops. For approximately 20% of normal girls, pubic growth is the first sign of puberty. Table 4–1 summarizes the stages of puberty in girls, with the expected mean age and age range for onset. Whenever a young patient is amenorrheic, the clinician should document Tanner staging[18] of breast and pubic hair development, especially if she is a teenager. A disparity in Tanner staging by more than one stage for breast and pubic hair development may be a clinical clue to an underlying development defect of the internal genitalia or, alternatively, a sign of abnormal sex steroid synthesis or action.

With the onset of normal puberty, daytime or nighttime sleep-induced secretion of both FSH and luteinizing hormone (LH) is observed.[19,20] The frequency of LH secretory pulses ranges between 75 and 100 minutes, similar to that for the REM–NREM sleep cycle[19] (Fig. 4–1). The increased gonadotropin levels are the result of increased amplitude and frequency of gonadotropin secretory pulses. The anatomic site of the "neuronal switch" that mediates gonadotropin pulsatile secretion with sleep during

TABLE 4–1. STAGING OF PUBERTAL EVENTS IN GIRLS

Event	Mean Age (yrs)	Range
Breast budding	11.2	9–13.5
Pubic and axillary hair growth	11.7	9–14.5
Menarche	13.5	11–16
Adult-pattern pubic hair	14.4	
Adult breast development	15.3	

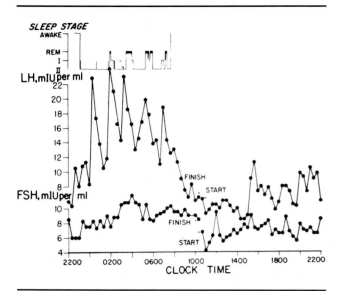

Figure 4–1. Plasma LH and FSH levels sampled during nocturnal sleep and after awakening. Sleep-associated increased gonadotropin secretion is apparent. Sleep stage is indicated at the top of the figure. Note the linking with REM–NREM sleep stage. (From Boyar et al.[20] Reproduced by permission of the *New England Journal of Medicine.*)

puberty is unknown. With completion of puberty sleep-induced release of gonadotropin subsides. That pattern may return with selected pathophysiologic states, for example, anorexia nervosa. Circulating levels of gonadotropin undergo significant changes in peripheral blood levels over short segments of time. That pattern reflects pulsatile gonadotropin secretion and has been called *circhoral* secretion, reflecting the approximately hourly pulses of gonadotropin released into the peripheral circulation. Probably GnRH undergoes pulsatile variation in portal blood, based on studies in nonhuman primates.[21]

MENSTRUAL CYCLE

The normal menstrual cycle is divided into two parts, the follicular and luteal phases. By convention, the follicular phase begins with the first day of menses and extends to the midcycle or preovulatory surge of LH. Blood LH levels progressively increase during the follicular phase and culminate in a preovulatory surge that divides the menstrual cycle into the follicular and luteal phases. In contrast, circulating FSH levels increase during the first half of the follicular phase, but decrease in the second half. In most normal women there is a concordant preovulatory or midcycle surge of both LH and FSH. Ovulation occurs approximately 36 to 38 hours after onset of the midcycle LH surge. Based on studies in nonhuman primates, the follicle, destined to become

the dominant or graafian follicle, is selected and becomes the primary source of circulating estradiol during the second half of the follicular phase.[22] The rising estradiol blood levels exert a negative feedback effect on pituitary FSH synthesis and secretion, resulting in decreased FSH levels during the second half of the follicular phase. Moreover, the increased estradiol levels observed during the second half of the follicular phased exert a positive feedback effect on gonadotropin secretion and contribute to the midcycle surge of gonadotropin. Other hypothalamic modulators undoubtedly contribute to the preovulatory surge but the sites of their effects are unknown.

At the time of ovulation, the ovum and its surrounding cells are extruded from the graafian follicle. The remainder of the follicle is subsequently transformed into a corpus luteum, predominantly an organ responsive to LH and human chorionic gonadotropin (hCG). The corpus luteum secretes progesterone, estradiol, and 17-hydroxyprogesterone. As a result of increased secretion of estradiol and progesterone during the luteal phase, circulating levels of both LH and FSH decrease. The luteal phase encompasses that part of the menstrual cycle from the LH preovulatory surge up to the first day of menses. Figure 4–2 characterizes changes in circulating gonadotropin and sex steroid levels during the normal menstrual cycle.[23]

The pulse frequency and amplitude of both immunoreactive and bioactive LH vary during the normal menstrual cycle.[2,24,25] In the follicular phase, pulse frequency varies between 60 and 90 minutes; LH pulse amplitude and frequency increase progressively. Pulse frequency decreases during the luteal phase and ranges from 100 minutes in the early phase to 250 to 300 minutes in the late phase. In general, as pulse frequency decreases, LH pulse amplitude increases. Pulsatile release of both immunoreactive and bioactive LH is similar throughout the menstrual cycle.[24] Both bioactive and immunoreactive LH are secreted in discrete pulsations, but significant discordance exists between bioactive and immunoreactive pulses. Those relationships are summarized in Figure 4–3.

With the development of the corpus luteum and its concomitant secretion of progesterone, a thermogenic shift in basal body temperature results. Progesterone produces that effect by interacting with a hypothalamic thermoregulatory site. The luteal phase generally lasts between 11 and 15 days, with most women having a luteal phase of 13 to 14 days.[11] It is the luteal phase that is the most constant part of the normal menstrual cycle. In contrast, the follicular phase is more variable. With prolonged intermenstrual intervals, the follicular phase is markedly lengthened. Circulating levels of progesterone usually exceed 10 ng/mL 5 to 8 days after the midcycle

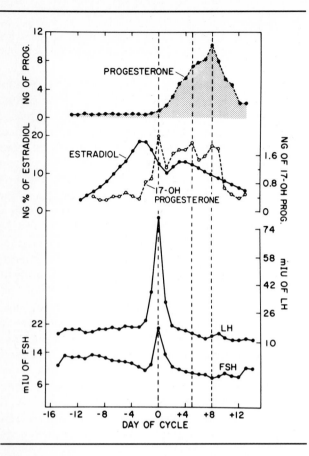

Figure 4–2. Gonadotropin and sex steroid levels during a presumptively ovulatory menstrual cycle. Levels are synchronized about the LH midcycle or preovulatory surge and designated day 0 of the cycle. (From Vaitukaitis & Ross.[23] Reproduced with permission.)

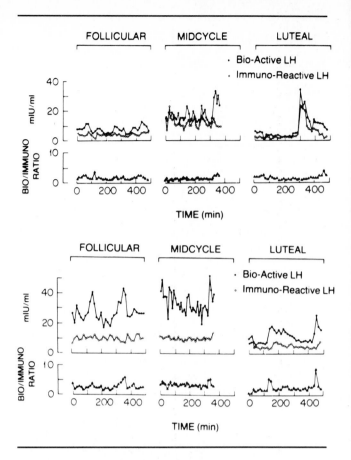

Figure 4–3. Immunoreactive and bioactive LH in samples of two different women sampled during the follicular, midcycle, and luteal phases. Note the lack of synchronization of activities for many of the LH pulses. (From Veldhuis.[24] Reproduced with permission.)

surge of LH. During the reproductive years, the median intermenstrual interval is approximately 28 days.[11]

The extremes of the reproductive life cycle are accompanied by a higher frequency of anovulatory or inadequately ovulatory cycles. Moreover, the intermenstrual intervals during these extremes vary widely. Postmenarcheal adolescents manifest considerable variability in LH secretory profiles, which contributes to the higher frequency of anovulatory menstrual cycles in this age group.[2,26] Healthy adult women exhibit nocturnal slowing of LH secretory pulses during the follicular phase[2,27] (Fig. 4–4). As women approach their late 20s and early 30s, the intermenstrual interval decreases by a few days.

During the several years prior to permanent cessation of spontaneous menses, there is a disproportionate increase in circulating FSH levels and lower circulating estradiol concentrations during the menstrual cycle compared with earlier reproductive years.[28] Investigators have attributed the increased FSH levels to decreased ovarian inhibin secretion[28]; however, no evidence exists for a direct effect of

inhibin on pituitary FSH secretion in a physiologic state. The waning years of the reproductive life span have been referred to as perimenopause, but that is a misnomer since it alludes to premenopausal changes. Menopause is characterized by high circulating LH and FSH levels, reflecting primary gonadal failure. A few follicles may be present in the postmenopausal ovary but they are apparently not gonadotropin responsive.

PATHOPHYSIOLOGY OF THE MENSTRUAL CYCLE

Amenorrhea

The word amenorrhea simply connotes the absence of menses and does not indicate the anatomic site of a possible abnormality. Classification of amenorrhea as primary and secondary may be misleading, since the same abnormalities may induce either the primary or secondary condition. That classification, however, is helpful since patients with primary amenorrhea have a 35 to 40% probability of having

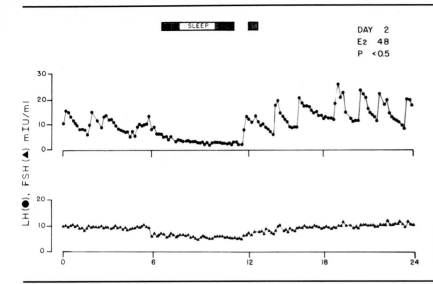

Figure 4–4. Immunoreactive LH levels of a young woman sampled over 24 hours. (From Crowley et al.[2] Reproduced with permission.)

either primary ovarian failure or a developmental defect of the fallopian tubes, uterus, or vagina. Primary amenorrhea is characterized by the failure of onset of spontaneous menses by age 16 years.

Secondary amenorrhea is characterized by the cessation of spontaneous menses for at least 4 consecutive months. The most common cause is pregnancy. Whether a patient has primary or secondary amenorrhea, one can localize the site of abnormality by measuring circulating levels of estradiol and gonadotropin. Measuring FSH alone suffices and is cost-effective. Hypothalamic–pituitary abnormalities are characterized by tonically low gonadotropin and estradiol levels, comparable to or lower than those of the normal early follicular phase. Primary gonadal dysfunction is characterized by high gonadotropin levels and low estradiol levels. Whenever a woman is amenorrheic, pregnancy should be excluded by measuring hCG in a specific hCG β-subunit assay. As with any other medical disorder, a careful history and physical examination are important in the differential diagnosis of menstrual dysfunction, as the condition is an early warning for systemic illness.[4] Table 4–2 presents the definitions of amenorrhea as well as the biochemical differences between central and peripheral causes of menstrual dysfunction.

Primary Amenorrhea. The most common cause of primary amenorrhea is gonadal dysgenesis, usually due to a genetic defect. Patients with classic Turner's syndrome have a 45,XO karyotype. Genetic mosaicism is common among patients with Turner's syndrome; several different karyotypes may be encountered and may include 45,XO, 46,XX, and ringed X chromosomes. Phenotypically, patients demonstrate linear growth abnormalities resulting in short stature, cardiovascular abnormalities including coarctation of the aorta, developmental abnormalities of the genitourinary tract, high arched palate, increased freckling, and a shield chest. Of interest, individuals with Turner's syndrome are endowed with a normal cohort of primordial follicles in utero.[29,30] Those follicles undergo atresia at an accelerated rate, however, so that by the time of menarche, none persist.[30] Consequently, the patients have primary amenorrhea. If the rate of atresia is slower in some affected individuals, young girls with Turner's syndrome may have secondary amenorrhea together with other classic somatic abnormalities. In fact, some women with Turner's syndrome have conceived and delivered normal term babies.[29]

The second most common cause of primary amenorrhea is a defect of müllerian duct differentiation, resulting in aberrant development of the fallopian tubes, uterus, or vagina. Ovarian function remains intact. Consequently, young women with this abnormality have normal secondary sex characteristics, reflecting normal ovarian function, but have primary amenorrhea because of the absence or incomplete development of the uterus vagina, or both.

TABLE 4–2. TYPES OF AMENORRHEA

Type	Description
Primary	No spontaneous menses by age 16 yrs
Secondary	Cessation of spontaneous menses for ≥4mo
Central	Low basal gonadotropin levels, low blood estradiol concentrations (<50 pg/ml)
Peripheral	High basal gonadotropin levels, low estradiol levels (<25 pg/ml)

Graded developmental abnormalities may be observed. Some affected girls may have abdominal pain monthly, but no external gential bleeding because the menstruum cannot be sloughed due to a lack of a vagina or functional connection between the uterus and the vagina. On physical examination, enlarged fallopian tubes (filled with sloughed blood) and an enlarged uterus filled with blood may be found. Other young women may have fully developed secondary sex characteristics and primary amenorrhea because of an imperforate hymen.

Intense exercise begun several years before the expected age of menarche may result in delayed puberty and primary amenorrhea. Swimmers and runners who begin training prior to the expected onset of menarche have an increased risk of having amenorrhea or irregular menses.[31] The effect of training on menses is discussed in more detail later. In general, menarche may be delayed 0.4 years for each year of intense premenarcheal training.[32] A variety of other acquired congenital abnormalities of the hypothalamic–pituitary axis may result in primary amenorrhea, including defects in hypothalamic synthesis of GnRH, together with developmental abnormalities of the olfactory nerve, craniofacial abnormalities that may result in a cleft palate or harelip, and developmental abnormalities of the genitourinary tract. Affected women have the syndrome as olfactogenital dysplasia, the female counterpart of Kallmann's syndrome in males.

Secondary Amenorrhea. Pregnancy must be excluded by either physical examination, or by measuring urinary or blood hCG levels by specific assay prior to subjecting the patient to further testing. Secondary amenorrhea results from primary gonadal dysfunction as well as from abnormalities of the hypothalamic–pituitary axis. Hypothalamic amenorrhea is a diagnosis of exclusion and simply reflects a functional defect of the hypothalamic–pituitary axis. It is characterized by absent cyclic gonadotropic secretion and levels of circulating estradiol that are comparable to or lower than those encountered in the early follicular phase of a normal menstrual cycle. Patients with secondary amenorrhea have a high frequency of prolactin secretory abnormalities. Prolactin levels should be determined in blood samples obtained in a truly basal, nonstressed state. When elevated, the patient should be evaluated for a pituitary adenoma. Hypothyroidism should also be excluded by obtaining a blood sample for thyroid-stimulating hormone (TSH), since with extreme hypothyroidism both serum TSH and prolactin are increased. In the presence of normal prolactin levels, elevated nocturnal plasma melatonin levels have been reported in women with secondary hypothalamic amenorrhea, suggesting that the hormone may

be involved in the neuroendocrine pathology underlying this disorder (Fig. 4–5).[33] A precise mechanism has not been elucidated.

Among young women in the United States, the most common contributors to hypothalamic amenorrhea are rapid weight loss with or without excessive physical conditioning. Athletes who begin training after menarche may have a 50% frequency of irregular menses, including amenorrhea.[34] It should be remembered, however, that those who develop amenorrhea with exercise may have an underlying organic defect. The intensity and duration of physical exercise, independent of body weight, may directly influence the occurrence of amenorrhea. Of interest, amenorrheic athletes may resume menstrual function during states of inactivity, despite little change in weight.[35] Well-designed studies found a higher frequency of anovulatory cycles than previously suspected among women undergoing supervised, graded-intensity training.[36]

Some women undergo voluntary weight loss too rapidly and develop amenorrhea. Those with anorexia nervosa may experience rapid, marked weight loss to levels 50% of their ideal body weight. They may have bradycardia, constipation, lanugo-like hair growth on the trunk and legs, leukopenia, and hypothalamic abnormalities that result in altered thermoregulation and partial diabetes insipidus. The partial diabetes insipidus, the thermoregulatory alterations, and amenorrhea are hypothalamic abnormalities reversible with weight gain. Restoration toward normal or normalization of hypothalamic function usually occurs after a variable length of time after restoring weight to the "ideal" range.

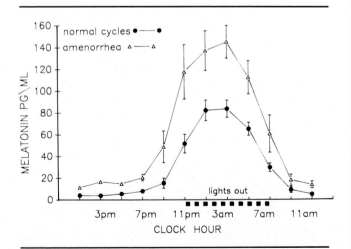

Figure 4–5. Mean (±SE) plasma melatonin levels in 14 healthy women (mean of all 3 study days) and 7 women with hypothalamic amenorrhea. To convert pg/mL melatonin to pmol/L, multiply by 4.31. (From Brzezinski et al.[33] Reproduced with permission.)

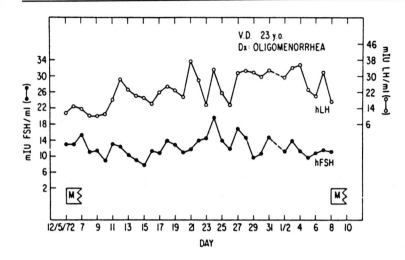

Figure 4–6. The LH and FSH levels of a woman with a prolonged intermenstrual interval. M = menses.

Some women with amenorrhea may require endocrinologic intervention with clomiphene citrate to restore cyclic menses. Others may require more heroic therapeutic measures with exogenous GnRH or exogenous gonadotropin stimulation to induce ovulation if they wish to conceive.

Autoimmune disorders may induce transient or permanent ovarian dysfunction; women may have

TABLE 4–3. CAUSES OF MENSTRUAL DYSFUNCTION

Disorder	Comment	Hormone Levels
Hypothalamic amenorrhea	Diagnosis of exclusion. Functional defect of gonadotropin secretion induced by rapid weight loss or gain, systemic illness, intense exercise, stress. May be preceded by luteal phase insufficiency and anovulation.	Gonadotropin tonically low; estradiol low.
Pregnancy	Most common cause of secondary amenorrhea. Patient may be asymptomatic early in gestation.	Specific HCG (β-subunit) assay positive; FSH low or undetectable; LH high because of cross-reactivity with HCG antiserum.
Turner's syndrome	Most commonly causes short stature and primary amenorrhea; may result in secondary amenorrhea. May have congenital developmental anomalies of the genitourinary tract, cardiovascular system, skeletal system. May be 46, XX/45, XO, ringed X chromosome, or some other genetic variant.	Gonadotropin high and estradiol low, signaling primary gonadal failure.
Polycystic ovary	Most common endocrinologic cause of infertility. May cause regular or irregular menstrual pattern including amenorrhea. Signs of androgen excess.	Gonadotropin may be low or LH may be inappropriately high and FSH tonically low. Androgen may be normal or increased.
Drug/irradiation	Opiates suppress gonadotropin secretion and may be associated with amenorrhea or irregular menses. Chemotherapeutic agents may induce transient or permanent gonadal failure. Ethanol induces both primary gonadal and hypothalamic defects. Irradiation may destroy ovarian follicles and induce amenorrhea.	Gonadotropin and estradiol low with amenorrhea. Chemotherapeutic agents associated with high gonadotropin and low estradiol. Alcohol may suppress gonadotropin secretion. Irradiation associated with high gonadotropin and low estradiol transiently or permanently.
Congenital abnormalities of vagina, uterus, or fallopian tubes	Secondary sex characteristics normal but women have primary amenorrhea. May have pelvic mass. Normal secondary sex characteristics.	Normal gonadotropin and sex steroid for menstrual cycle.
Premature menopause	Cessation of menses permanently before age 40 May be induced chemically or through an autoimmune mechanism. No genetic abnormality in most. May be familial disorder.	Gonadotropin high, estradiol low.

(Continued)

TABLE 4-3. (CONTINUED)

Pituitary tumor	May cause regular or irregular menses, or amenorrhea. If tumor large, may have signs of suprasellar extension (e.g., visual field abnormalities, diabetes insipidus) May have signs of hormonal secretion by tumor (e.g., Cushing's, acromegaly).	Gonadotropin usually tonically low, comparable to early follicular phase levels; estradiol low. Prolactin increased in most.
Hypothalamic tumor or cyst	Irregular or absent menses. Young girls may have precocious puberty or delayed menarche or arrested pubertal development.	Gonadotropin and estradiol low.
Infiltrative disorders of pituitary stalk or hypothalamus (tuberculosis, sarcoidosis, histiocytosis X)	Irregular or absent menses. Signs and symptoms of underlying disorder.	Gonadotropin and estradiol low.

either primary or secondary amenorrhea.[37] The latter is more common. Autoimmune pluriglandular endocrine gland failure may be a familial disorder.[38] Convincing evidence now exists for autoimmune-induced ovarian failure. Perifollicular lymphocytic infiltrates, circulating antibody to components of the ovarian follicle, and the presence of other autoimmune disorders in the same patient constitute that evidence. Patients may have discernable circulating antibody to several endocrine glands—thyroid, adrenal, pancreatic, and ovarian tissues—in addition to antibodies to other tissues, such as the acetylcholine receptor in patients with myasthenia gravis.[37-39] Other associated immunologic disorders include systemic lupus erythematosus, rheumatoid arthritis, and Sjögren's syndrome.

In the early stages of ovarian autoimmune involvement, follicles undergo accelerated atresia, probably as a result of ovarian cytotoxic antibodies. Since affected ovaries may have lymphocytic infiltrates, clinicians have treated some patients with glucocorticoids, but with little therapeutic benefit. Affected women have elevated levels of circulating gonadotropin and low levels of estradiol, consistent with primary gonadal failure. Some of those individuals resume spontaneous menses with normalization of circulating gonadotropin levels, however. Other women have been treated with oral contraceptive formulations that contain both estrogen and progestins; some have conceived.[40] Similarly, women undergoing systemic chemotherapy for an underlying malignancy develop secondary amenorrhea with elevated gonadotropin and low estradiol levels, consistent with primary gonadal failure. After a variable time, sometimes years, they may resume spontaneous cyclic menses and even conceive. Longitudinal studies suggest that women who undergo chemotherapy during their younger reproductive years may experience menopause at a younger age. A wide array of environmental agents may induce transient or permanent primary ovarian failure[41]

Anovulation

The word *anovulation* is confusing. In everyday parlance, it is used interchangeably with ovulation of an immature egg from an incompletely developed graafian follicle. Technically, anovulation occurs only when no graafian follicle develops. Inadequate gonadotropin stimulation or a defect of steroidogenesis that precludes the synthesis of sex steroids may induce abnormal development of the graafian follicle. If a follicle is underdeveloped, the corpus luteum derived from that structure will also be abnormal and secrete lower than normal levels of progesterone. Sufficient levels of progesterone may be secreted, and that amount of progesterone may induce a significant increase in basal body temperature. In general, many of the acquired causes of amenorrhea are also associated with anovulation. In fact, anovulatory menstrual cycles with or without an irregular menstrual interval may precede the onset of amenorrhea. Women with well-documented irregular intermenstrual intervals may have both ovulatory and anovulatory cycles. The frequency of anovulation is greater among those with intermenstrual intervals of 35 to 40 days than among women with a history of "regular" monthly intermenstrual intervals.

Figure 4-6 depicts circulating gonadotropin levels in a woman with anovulation and an irregular menstrual interval. It is obvious that the gonadotropin pattern is markedly different from that of a normally cycling woman.

Table 4-3 provides a summary of the more common causes of menstrual dysfunction and their clinical features.

REFERENCES

1. Vaitukaitis JL: Neuroendocrine control of gonadotropin secretion in women, in Taymor MD, Nelson JH Jr (eds): *Progress in Gynecology*. New York, Grune & Stratton, 1983, pp 3–19.
2. Crowley WF Jr, Filicori M, Spratt DI, Santoro NF: The physiology of gonadotropin-releasing hormone (GnRH) secretion in men and women. *Recent Prog Horm Res* 41:473, 1985.
3. Lachelin GCL, Yen SSC: Hypothalamic chronic anovulation. *Am J Obstet Gynecol* 130:825, 1978.
4. Morley JE, Melmed S: Gonadal dysfunction in systemic disorders. *Metabolism* 28:1051, 1979.
5. Herzog AG, Seibel MM, Schomer DL, Vaitukaitis JL, Geschwind N: Reproductive endocrine disorders in women with partial seizures of temporal lobe origin. *Arch Neurol* 43:341, 1986.
6. Henley K, Vaitukaitis JL: Exercise-induced menstrual dysfunction. *Annu Rev Med* 39:443, 1988.
7. Warren MP, Vande Wiele RL: Clinical and metabolic features of anorexia nervosa. *Am J. Obstet Gynecol* 117:435, 1973.
8. Baker TG: A quantitative and cytological study of germ cells in human ovaries. *Proc R Soc Lond* 158:417, 1963.
9. Peters H: The human ovary in childhood and early maturity. *Gynecol Reprod Biol* 9:137, 1979.
10. MacMahon B, Worcester J: *Age at Menopause: United States 1900–1962*. Washington, DC, U.S. Government Printing Office, 1966.
11. Treloar AE, Boynton RE, Behn BG: Variation of the human menstrual cycle through reproductive life. *Int J Fertil* 12:77, 1967.
12. Kaplan SL, Grumbach MM, Aubert ML: The ontogenesis of pituitary hormones and hypothalamic factors in the human fetus: Maturation of central nervous system regulation of anterior pituitary function. *Recent Prog Horm Res* 32:161, 1976.
13. Baker TG, Scrimgeour JB: Development of the gonad in normal and anencephalic human fetuses. *J Reprod Fertil* 60:193, 1980.
14. Li CH, Ramasharma K, Yamashiro D, Chung D: Gonadotropin-releasing peptide from human follicular fluid: Isolation, characterization, and chemical synthesis. *Proc Nat Acad Sci USA* 84:959, 1987.
15. Khan-Dawood FS: Human corpus luteum: Immunocytochemical localization of epidermal growth factor. *Fertil Steril* 47:916, 1987.
16. Demoulin A, Guichard A, Mignot TM, et al: Inhibin concentration in the culture media of human oocyte-cumulus-corona cell complexes is not related to subsequent embryo cleavage. *Fertil Steril* 46:1150, 1986.
17. Swerdloff RS: Physiological control of puberty. *Med Clin North Am* 62:351, 1978.
18. Marshall WA, Tanner JM: Variations in patterns of pubertal changes in girls. *Arch Dis Child* 44:291, 1969.
19. Boyar R, Finkelstein J, Roffwarg H, et al: Synchronization of augmented luteinizing hormone secretion with sleep during puberty. *N Engl J Med* 287:582, 1972.
20. Boyar RM, Finkelstein JW, David R, et al: Twenty-four-hour patterns of plasma luteinizing hormone and follicle-stimulating hormone in sexual precocity. *N Engl J Med* 289:282, 1973.
21. Carmel PW, Araki S, Ferin M: Pituitary stalk portal blood collection in rhesus monkeys: Evidence for pulsatile release of gonadotropin-releasing hormone (GnRH). *Endocrinology* 99:243, 1976.
22. Goodman AL, Hodgen GD: The ovarian triad of the primate menstrual cycle. *Recent Prog Horm Res* 39:1, 1983.
23. Vaitukaitis JL, Ross GT: Clinical studies of gonadotropin in the female. *Pharmacol Ther* 1:317, 1976.
24. Veldhuis JD, Beitins I, Johnson ML, Serabian MA, Dufau M: Biologically active luteinizing hormone is secreted in episodic pulsations that vary in relation to stage of the menstrual cycle. *J Clin Endocrinol Metab* 58:1050, 1984.
25. Santen RJ, Bardin CW: Episodic luteinizing hormone secretion in man. *J Clin Invest* 52:2617, 1973.
26. Apter D, Raisanen I, Ylosalo P, Vihko R: Follicular growth in relation to serum hormonal patterns in adolescent compared with adult menstrual cycles. *Fertil Steril* 47:82, 1987.
27. Soules MR, Steiner RA, Cohen NL, Bremner WJ, Clifton DK: Nocturnal slowing of pulsatile luteinizing hormone secretion in women during the follicular phase of the menstrual cycle. *J Clin Endocrinol Metab* 61:43, 1985.
28. Sherman BN, West JH, Korenman SG: The menopausal transition of LH, FSH, estradiol and progesterone concentrations during menstrual cycles of older women. *J Clin Endocrinol Metab* 42:629, 1976.
29. Nielsen J, Sillesen I, Hansen KB: Fertility in women with Turner's syndrome: A case report and review of the literature. *Br J Obstet Gynaecol* 86:833, 1979.
30. Singh RP, Carr DH: The anatomy and history of XO human embryos and fetuses. *Anat Rec* 155:369, 1966.
31. Warren MP: The effect of exercise on pubertal progression and reproductive function in girls. *J Clin Endocrinol Metab* 51:1150, 1980.
32. Frisch RE, Gotz-Welbergen AV, McArthur JW, et al: *JAMA* 246:1559, 1981.
33. Brzezinski A, Lynch HJ, Seibel MM, et al: The Circadian rhythm of plasma melatonin during the normal menstrual cycle and in amenorrheic women. *J Clin Endocrinol Metab* 66:891, 1988.
34. Cumming DC, Rebar RW: Exercise and reproductive function in women. *Am J Indust Med* 4:113, 1983.
35. Abraham SF, Beaumont PJV, Fraser IJ, Llewellyn-Jones D: Body weight, exercise and menstrual status among ballet dancers in training. *Br J Obstet Gynaecol* 89:507, 1982.
36. Bullen BA, Skrinar GS, Beitins IZ, et al: Induction of menstrual disorders by strenuous exercise in untrained women. *N Engl J Med* 312:1349, 1985.
37. Coulam CB: The prevalence of autoimmune disorders among patients with primary ovarian failure. *Am J Reprod Immunol* 4:63, 1983.
38. Alper MA, Garner PR, Seibel MM: Premature ovarian failure: Current concept. *J Reprod Med* 31, 699, 1986.
39. Coulam CB, Kempers RD, Randall RV: Premature ovarian failure: Evidence for the autoimmune mechanism. *Fertil Steril* 36:238, 1981.
40. Shangold MM, Turksoy RN, Bashford RA, Hammond CB: Pregnancy following the "insensitive ovary syndrome." *Fertil Steril* 28: 1179, 1977.
41. Verp MS: Environmental causes of ovarian failure. *Semin Reprod Endocrinol* 1:101, 1983.

CHAPTER 5

Polycystic Ovary Disease

Machelle M. Seibel

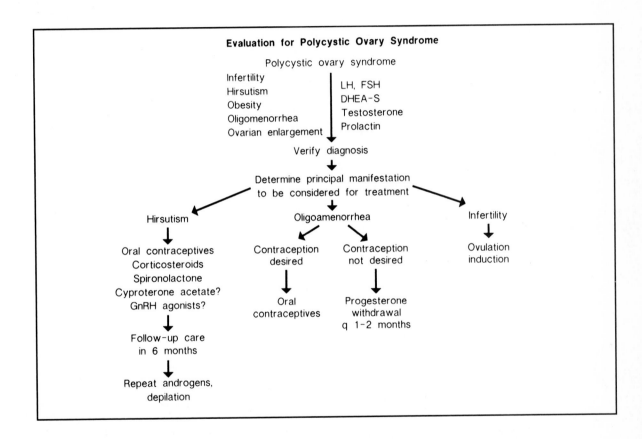

Polycystic ovary syndrome (PCO) has been a subject of interest and investigation for over 50 years. Because it is not a discrete disease, however, but rather a spectrum of symptomatology, pathology, and laboratory findings, a complete description of its etiology and pathogenesis has not been elucidated. What has evolved is the concept of PCO as a self-perpetuating cycle in which the hypothalamus, pituitary, ovaries, and adrenals all contribute to an endocrine imbalance that is usually associated with oligoovulation, hirsutism, and infertility.*

HYPOTHALAMIC–PITUITARY RELATIONSHIP

The characteristically elevated levels of luteinizing hormone (LH) in association with normal to low normal levels of follicle-stimulating hormone (FSH) and chronic anovulation initially led many investigators to suspect that the primary disturbance in PCO was in the hypothalamic regulation of gonadotropins.[1] This was later found not to be an inherent defect, but rather a functional de-

---

*This concept has been extensively reviewed by Loy and Seibel. See reference 184.

rangement.[2] Frequent blood sampling for LH and FSH revealed exaggerated pulsatile levels of LH associated with low or low normal FSH, which did not display a discernible pulsatile pattern. This pattern could not be due to a defect of the negative feedback effect of estrogen, because estradiol-17β (E_2) infusion resulted in reduced levels of LH but not of FSH. The positive feedback effect of estrogen also appeared intact, as clomiphene citrate elicited an LH rise similar to that in healthy controls.[1] What did appear to be the reason for the exaggerated pulsatile pattern of LH release with resultant elevated LH levels was a heightened pituitary responsiveness to gonadotropin-releasing hormone (GnRH).[3] Studies in women with PCO reveal that mean LH pulse frequencies are indistinguishable from those of healthy controls. The mean LH pulse amplitude in patients with PCO (12.2 ±2.7 mIU/mL) is higher ($p <$ 0.05) than that in healthy women in either the early (6.2 ±0.8 mIU/mL) or midfollicular (6.4 ±0.6 mIU/

mL) phase[4] (Fig. 5–1). This difference in amplitude may be due to a relative increase of bioactive LH over immunoreactive LH in those with PCO.[5]

This does not, however, explain the disparity between the high LH levels and the low or low normal FSH levels. Several theories have been suggested, including a preferential inhibitory effect of estrogen on FSH, a relative insensitivity of FSH to GnRH,[3] and elevated circulating levels of inhibin.[6] Adaptation of work in the rhesus monkey has provided another explanation.[7]

Radio frequency destruction of the arcuate nucleus in these animals resulted in a precipitous drop in gonadotropins owing to elimination of endogenous secretion of GnRH. Subsequently, GnRH was administered intravenously in a series of experiments in which both its frequency and amplitude were varied. Once the appropriate frequency and amplitude were established to duplicate the normal conditions, administering GnRH continuously reduced both LH and FSH levels (Fig. 5–2). Increasing the amplitude of GnRH while maintaining a constant pulse frequency resulted in a reduction of the peripheral levels of FSH with little effect on LH levels (Fig. 5–3), and a gonadotropin ratio similar to the one that exists in PCO. Widening the pulse interval while maintaining the same GnRH dosage reduced LH levels. Similar studies have been conducted in humans (Fig. 5–4).[8]

Additional support is found in a study demonstrating higher peripheral levels of immunoreactive GnRH pulses in patients with PCO than in healthy controls.[9] Abnormalities in the diurnal variation of

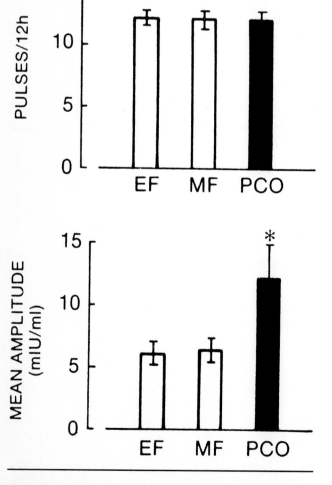

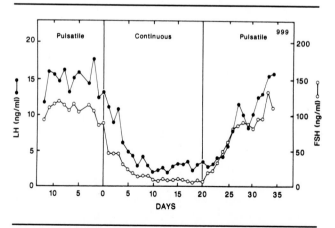

Figure 5–2. Inhibition of gonadotropin secretion in a rhesus monkey with a hypothalamic lesion when an intermittent gonadotropin-releasing hormone (GnRH) replacement regimen (lμg/min for 6 minutes every hour) was replaced by a continuous infusion of GnRH beginning on day 0. This inhibition was gradually reversed when the pulsatile mode of GnRH was reinstituted on day 20. (From Knobil et al.[7] Reproduced with permission.)

Figure 5–1. Comparison of LH pulse frequency and amplitude demonstrates increased LH pulse amplitude among patients with PCO. (From Kazer et al.[4] Reproduced with permission.)

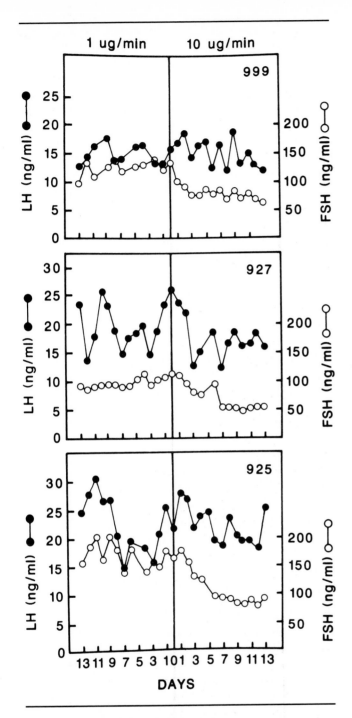

Figure 5–3. Suppression of plasma follicle-stimulating hormone (FSH) levels by increasing the amplitude of GnRH from 1μg/min to 10μg/min for 6 minutes every hour. Plasma luteinizing hormone (LH) levels remained essentially unchanged. (From Knobil.[7] Reproduced with permission.)

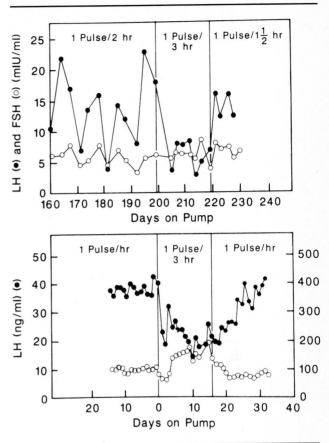

Figure 5–4. Disparate responses to pulsatile GnRH are created by widening the pulse interval. The upper panel represents data from a woman with Kallmann's syndrome. The lower panel is taken from the work of Knobil[8] performed in the rhesus monkey. (From Seibel et al.[8] Reproduced with permission.)

the frequency and amplitude of GnRH secretion. For this reason, hormones that affect GnRH secretion must also be considered in the pathophysiology or pathogenesis of PCO.

Endogenous Opioids in PCO

Endogenous opioids may affect hypothalamic GnRH. Inferences of brain opioid activity in PCO have been made on the basis of LH measurements in response to infusions of the opioid antagonist naloxone. Levels of LH in patients with PCO failed to respond to naloxone infusions.[12] Similar studies performed in women with PCO and healthy controls in midfollicular phase, in whom estradiol levels were similar, demonstrated no difference in central opioid tone between the two groups.[13] Pretreatment with dopamine infusion can abolish the naloxone-induced LH release in men and healthy women,[14,15] but subjects with PCO pretreated with L-dopa/cabidopa, which crosses the blood–brain barrier, respond to naloxone with an increase in LH, while controls do not.[16] In addition, β-endorphin does not suppress

LH secretion have also been reported in PCO (Fig. 5–5).[10] The normal pubertal diurnal pattern of LH secretion was reversed in four of five postmenarcheal teenagers with classic PCO. Since diurnal rhythmicity is believed to be under hypothalamic control,[11] the inappropriate gonadotropin secretion so commonly associated with PCO appears due to disturbances of

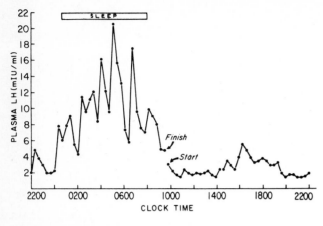

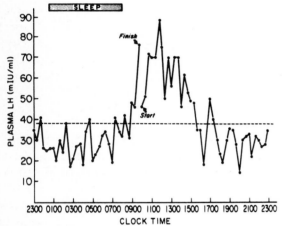

Figure 5–5. Frequent blood samples for LH demonstrate an abnormal circadian rhythm among pubertal girls with PCO. (From Zumoff et al.[10] Reproduced with permission.)

the elevated LH levels in PCO,[12] although it is effective in inhibiting LH release in healthy males and females.[17] It has been demonstrated that β-endorphins decrease hypothalamic and increased striatal dopamine turnover.[17,18] Enkephalin also has been shown to block dopamine-induced GnRH release from the rat mediobasal hypothalamus.[19] These findings suggest either an interaction among dopamine, opioid peptides, and GnRH secretion,[14,15] or a functional dissociation of opioid neuronal activity in PCO.

Peripheral levels of β-endorphin have also been found to be significantly high in patients with PCO (Fig. 5–6).[20] Furthermore, patients who weighed more demonstrated even higher levels. Other investigators found a naloxone-induced LH release only in oligomenorrheic women with PCO who were overweight, but not in those who were of normal weight, or in hypogonadotropic women, with the exception of those with prolactin-secreting adenomas.[21] Both β-endorphin and adrenocorticotropic hormone (ACTH) are derived from the same precursor, proopiomelanocortin (POMC), and it is known

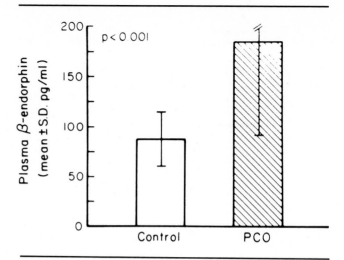

Figure 5–6. Peripheral values of β-endorphins in healthy women and those with PCO. (From Aleem et al.[20] Reproduced with permission.)

that β- endorphin is increased in conditions with increased ACTH production (Fig. 5–7).[22] However, ACTH levels and cortisol production are normal in PCO.[23] It is known that stress increases peripheral β-endorphin levels,[24] and that patients with PCO have a significantly higher level of psychologic stress than ovulatory controls.[25]

In addition, a β-endorphinlike peptide has been identified in the same islet cell clusters that produce insulin.[26,27] This pancreatic opioid is two to four times more potent than β-endorphin and 50 times more potent than morphine. Its effects are reversed by naloxone. This substance may account for some of the peripherally elevated opioids demonstrated in PCO. Animal studies have demonstrated both increased pituitary content and circulating levels of β-endorphin in genetically obese mice.[28] Naloxone inhibits overeating in these mice and suggests that β-endorphin may have a role in the genesis of obesity. These studies may help explain the association of β-endorphins, hyperinsulinemia, and obesity associated with PCO, and may ultimately prove the disease to be a metabolic disorder.

Neurologic Considerations

Neurologic factors may also modulate GnRH and contribute to the pathophysiology of PCO. In particular, patients with temporal lobe epilepsy (TLE) have a high prevalence of reproductive dysfunction.[29,30] One study of 50 women with TLE reported a 20% occurrence of PCO, which is much higher than that in the general population.[30] The relationship between TLE and PCO is based on anatomic factors. Seizures of temporal lobe origin generally involve limbic portions of the lobe. The amygdala is an anatomically distinct portion of the limbic structures, and has

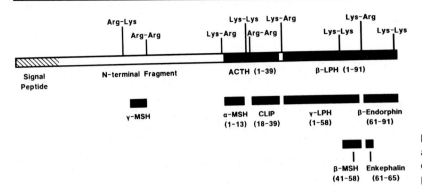

Signal Peptide

N-terminal Fragment

ACTH (1–39)

β-LPH (1–91)

γ-MSH

α-MSH (1–13) CLIP (18–39)   γ-LPH (1–58)   β-Endorphin (61–91)

β-MSH (41–58)   Enkephalin (61–65)

Figure 5–7. Schematic drawing of proopiomelanocortin. Both β-endorphin and ACTH as well as other hormones are derived from this common precursor. (Modified from Kreiger & Martin.[33])

extensive, direct, anatomic connections with the ventromedial and preoptic hypothalamic nuclei, which are involved in regulating and secreting GnRH.[31] Bilateral amygdalectomy in the adult female monkey induces amenorrhea and hypogonadal vaginal changes.[32] Furthermore, previous studies described satiety centers for food intake in the ventromedial nucleus.[33] This interrelationship could contribute to the obesity associated with PCO. In addition, β-endorphins levels, which are known to be elevated in PCO, have been shown to induce epileptiform activity in the limbic cortex when administered into cerebrospinal fluid of rats.[34] This activity is induced by doses that are devoid of analgesic activity, and the epileptiform activity is not associated with discernible effects on behavior. Stimulation of the amygdala has been shown capable of inducing elevations of pituitary and serum LH levels.[35]

As is discussed below, elevated prolactin levels are also associated with PCO. Altered concentrations of dopamine and homovanillic acid have been documented in the brains of animals with kindled amygdaloid seizures[36] and in the spinal fluid of patients with TLE.[37] For these reasons, epileptic discharges in medical temporal limbic structures may modulate hypothalamic dopamine as well as GnRH, and contribute, in some patients, to the pathophysiology of PCO.[38]

Prolactin and PCO

Other factors that affect GnRH secretion must also be considered in the pathogenesis of PCO; in this context, the association with galactorrhea and hyperprolactinemia has been of particular interest.[39] Sommers and Wadman[40] studied pituitary glands from unselected autopsies of 7 to 16 women with bilateral polycystic ovaries and found all 7 to have unusual numbers of normally granulated basophils collected into hyperplastic nodules. Other reports associated patients with PCO who were also found to have hyperprolactinemia and pituitary tumors.[41,42] The authors concluded that in some cases an association

may exist between PCO and prolactin-producing adenomas.[41] Falaschi and associates[39] felt that the hyperprolactinemia and enhanced prolactin released in PCO were due to estrogen and the dopaminergic system. They postulated that the peripheral conversion of androgens to estrogens in PCO sensitized the lactotrope cells whether or not hyperprolactinemia was present. In support of this theory, their patients with PCO who had normal or elevated prolactin levels exhibited exaggerated responses to thyroid-releasing hormone (TRH). Similar observations were made during the use of the dopamine receptor antagonist metoclopramide, whether or not basal prolactin levels were elevated.[43] Such studies imply a central defect or deficiency in the inhibitory influence of hypothalamic dopamine.

Whether this defect or deficiency of hypothalamic dopamine is primary or secondary is not known; however, it may be responsible for the exaggerated pulsatile amplitude of GnRH activity in PCO. Administration of dopamine results in a prompt and sustained decline in circulating LH levels in many of these patients (Fig. 5–8).[44,45] The role of estrogen is once again implied, as the dopamine-induced reduction in LH was similar in patients with PCO and in healthy controls during the LH surge, both conditions with high endogenous estrogens.

Animal models have provided evidence that elevated estrogen levels modulate dopamine neurons by enhancing LH inhibition by dopamine. Cyclic changes in dopamine turnover occur during the estrous cycle,[46] and labeled E_2 has been localized inside dopamine nerve terminals.[47] Furthermore, significant data suggest that the tuberoinfundibular dopaminergic system inhibits the neuronal activity of GnRH in the lateral palisade zone of the median eminence by a mechanism that is distinct from prolactin regulation.[48]

These series of studies suggest a mechanism whereby deficient hypothalamic dopamine could modulate LH secretion through its effect on GnRH, resulting in higher amplitudes of LH secretion. At the

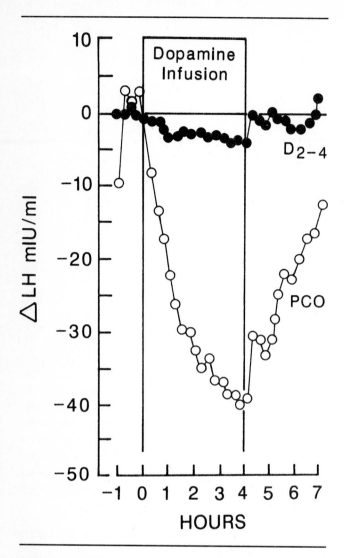

Figure 5–8. Mean net (Δ) decrement in serum LH levels before, during, and after dopamine (DA) infusion (4 μg/kg/min) for 4 hours in 8 patients with PCO (opened circles) and 6 healthy women studied between days 2 and 4 of the menstrual cycle (closed circles). (From Quigley et al.[44] Reproduced with permission.)

same time, a basis for the relationship between hyperprolactinemia and PCO is provided. Additional evidence is drawn from a study demonstrating a synchrony between endogenous pulses of LH and prolactin.[49] Furthermore, the administration of bromocriptine, a dopamine agonist, decreased both prolactin and the integrated LH secretion of patients with PCO.[50] Replacement of the deficient dopamine or its agonist theoretically would provide a physiologic basis for correction of the biochemical imbalance so typical of PCO.

OVARIAN CONTRIBUTIONS TO PCO

By its very name, PCO incriminates the ovaries in its pathophysiology. Bilaterally enlarged ovaries with

multiple 2 to 6-mm follicles lying beneath a smooth, glistening capsule are typical (Figs. 5–9 and 5–10). These follicles are generally in various stages of growth and atresia, with hyperplastic theca interna. This increased rate of atresia, coupled with high levels of intrafollicular androstenedione (A) and low E_2, led investigators to suspect an inherent defect in steroidogenesis within the polycystic ovary as the explanation for the inappropriate hormone levels.[51] Granulosa cells cultured from normal 8 to 15-mm follicles were compared with those cultured from 4 to 6-mm follicles originating from both normal and polycystic ovaries (Fig. 5–11). Granulosa cells from the 8 to 15-mm follicles displayed a dose-related increase in estrogen production when incubated with the aromatase substrate A. Since the follicles in PCO usually range from 2 to 6 mm, they probably did not possess aromatase. However, this does not appear due to an inherent defect in the granulosa cells from 4 to 6-mm polycystic ovarian follicles. The addition of FSH to their culture media that also contained A resulted in a 24-fold increase in estrogen production even in the PCO follicles (Fig. 5–12). Addition of LH had little or no effect. These findings demonstrated that the granulosa cells of polycystic ovaries are inherently capable of responding to FSH with the production of aromatase. Apparently, in PCO local concentrations of FSH are deficient, and the follicles never grow to a size sufficient to develop aromatase.

Inhibin, a hormone with FSH-suppressing activity, has been demonstrated in human follicular fluid, particularly in patients with PCO.[6] The accumulation of follicles not undergoing maturation can result in increased quantities of inhibin and additional sup-

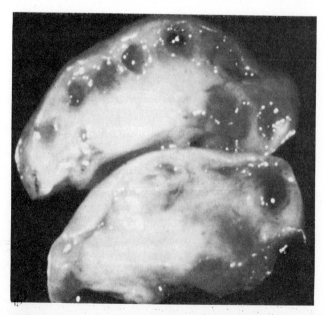

Figure 5–9. Gross pathology specimen typical of polycystic ovary disease. Numerous 2 to 6-mm subcapsular cysts are demonstrated.

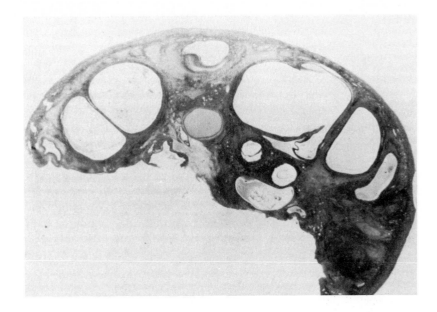

Figure 5–10. Microscopic section of ovary from a patient with PCO.

pression of FSH secretion. It would therefore seem reasonable that long-term administration of FSH to patients with PCO would result in a physiologic reduction in the increased local levels of androgens and in decreased follicular atresia.

The Role of Insulin

An association between insulin resistance and PCO is now well established.[52] In fact, several clinical conditions associating insulin resistance and ovarian hyperandrogenism currently exist. These include (1) type A insulin resistance due to either an inherited deficiency of insulin receptors or to postbinding abnormalities in the insulin action, abnormalities such as tyrosine–kinase activity of the insulin recep-

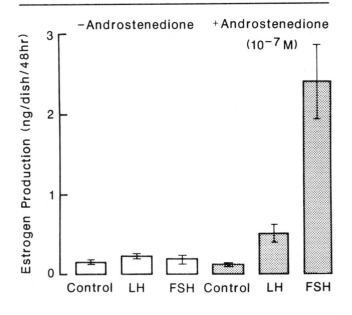

Figure 5–11. Effect of gonadotropins on estrogen production by cultured PCO granulosa cells isolated from 4 to 6-mm follicles of a patient with classic Stein-Leventhal syndrome. The addition of FSH plus the androgen precursor androstenedione resulted in significant estrogen production. Similar results were achieved when granulosa cells from a 6-mm follicle from a control patient at the midluteal phase of the cycle were cultured in the same way. (From Erickson et al.[51] Reproduced with permission.)

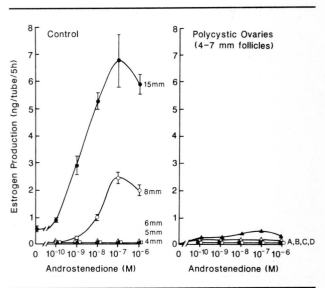

Figure 5–12. Relationship between aromatase substrate and estrogen production in granulosa cells from normal (control) follicles of various sizes and PCO follicles. Neither granulosa cells from small control follicles nor small PCO follicles appear to have acquired aromatase, whereas larger control follicles have acquired the aromatase enzyme. (From Erickson et al.[51] Reproduced with permission.)

tor β-subunit; (2) type B insulin resistance due to insulin receptor autoantibodies[53–55]; (3) lipoatrophic diabetes[56]; and (4) PCO. Patients who are type A insulin resistant are typically thin and develop PCO or hyperthecosis during their teenage years, whereas those who are type B insulin resistant are usually older and have evidence of autoimmune disease.[57]

Despite the well-established association between hyperinsulinemic insulin-resistant states and ovarian hyperandrogenism, different views of the possible cause and effect have been expressed. Because the great majority of women who have PCO are obese, their insulin resistance has been presumed on the basis of obesity; however, they have higher basal insulin levels than weight-matched controls.[58] In addition, insulin levels are elevated in patients with PCO who are not obese and who do not have evidence of acanthosis nigricans.[59,60]

Hyperinsulinemia has also been associated with hyperandrogenism,[61] but this does not establish cause and effect. In humans, there is no direct evidence implicating androgens in insulin resistance. Synthetic androgens have been reported to cause hyperinsulinemia, but this was coincident with weight gain in each case.[62] In addition, the administration of an oral contraceptive containing both estrogen and progesterone to a patient with PCO caused remission of insulin resistance.[63] Furthermore, nonobese, insulin-resistant patients treated with a GnRH agonist to suppress ovarian androgen secretion demonstrated no change in insulin resistance, suggesting that such resistance in PCO is unrelated to ovarian hyperandrogenism.[64]

Conversely, another study implicated hyperinsulinemia as playing a potential pathogenic role in the hyperandrogenemia of PCO.[65] Insulin was infused into nonobese and obese females, and females with insulin resistance, hirsutism, and acanthosis nigricans. Significant augmentation of androstenedione concentrations occurred in all three groups. Insulin infusion does not appear to augment testosterone or dehydroepiandrosterone sulfate (DHEAS) production.[65,66] These clinical findings are compatible with in vitro studies demonstrating that insulin both potentiates the androgenic activity of porcine theca cells, particularly androstenedione,[67] and is synergistic with LH.[68] The clinical findings, however, are in conflict with in vitro studies showing insulin capable of stimulating the accumulation of androstenedione, testosterone, progesterone, and estradiol in theca cell incubations, and of androstenedione, testosterone, and dihydrotestosterone in stroma cell incubations.[69] Furthermore, insulin stimulates steroidogenesis in porcine and bovine granulosa cells,[70] and has also been found to be one of the most potent factors studied for promoting granulosa cell proliferation in tissue culture.[71]

The probable mechanism by which this occurs has now been clarified. Specific insulin-binding sites have been identified in polycystic ovary tissue that was largely stroma.[72] These initial studies were extended to normal ovarian tissue in which insulin receptors were identified in stroma, theca, and granulosa cells.[73,74] Insulin in high concentrations also interacts with receptors.[75] Insulin and IGF1 are structurally similar. Positions 1 to 29 of the IF1 molecules are homologous to the insulin β chain; positions 42 to 62 are homologous to the α chain. The three-dimensional structures of the two peptides are virtually identical.[62] The receptors of insulin and IGF1 are also similar structurally. Receptors for IGF1 have been identified in both ovarian stroma and purified human granulosa cells.[73,76] Because ovarian stroma is capable of producing a wide variety of steroids, these facts become important. It also helps to explain the insulin resistance among patients with PCO. While Scatchard analysis has revealed these patients to possess similar receptor numbers, ID_{50} values demonstrate their decreased receptor affinity.[60] Whether or not hyperandrogenism in fact alters insulin receptor affinity has not been fully determined.

Insulin also appears to be important in oocyte maturation.[77] Animal studies have shown that insulin stimulates pig oocyte maturation beyond metaphase I,[78] and facilitates germinal vesicle breakdown in *Rana pipiens*.[79] It also stimulates porcine granulosa cell formation of LH/human chorionic gonadotropin (HCG) receptors, and granulosa cell luteinization[80] and steroid secretion.[70,71]

In humans, insulin further augments FSH-induced aromatase activity by granulosa cells.[81] It has also been identified in follicular fluid of some but not all patients.[82] Whether it is secreted or sequestered has not been determined. Insulin was found to correlate with follicular fluid progesterone levels but not with estradiol and androstenedione.[82]

Although not yet completely defined, the role of insulin in PCO may be substantial. In addition to its direct action on ovarian tissue, it may stimulate gonadotropin secretion at a pituitary or hypothalamic level. Adashi and associates showed that GnRH stimulation of LH from rat pituitary cells is enhanced by insulin at physiologic concentrations.[83] Furthermore, circulating insulin has been shown capable of entering the hypothalamus and binding to specific receptors localized to the arcuate nucleus and median eminence.[84,85] In female rats with streptozotocin-induced diabetes, the median eminence content of GnRH was low and plasma LH response to GnRH was inadequate.[86] The arcuate nucleus and the median eminence contained numerous degenerate axons, and LH gonadotroph cells were altered. The authors hypothesized that the abnormalities were caused by insulin deficiency. It is therefore possible that the insulin resistance associated with PCO leads to increased peripheral insulin levels, resulting in enhanced release of LH, and both directly and indirectly augments ovarian androgen production.[87,88] Since elevated levels of both androgens and LH are associated with follicular atresia, the negative effects of excessive insulin might outweigh the beneficial effects of insulin at more physiologic levels.

In addition, follicular fluid insulin and progesterone levels are correlated.[82] Because insulin enhances pituitary–hypothalamic LH secretion[83,84] and LH induces a switch in theca cell function from an androgen to a progesterone-secreting tissue,[89] another component of hyperinsulinemia and PCO may be a dramatic decrease in the available androgen for aromatization, resulting in reduced follicular estrogen and ultimately, follicular atresia. Furthermore, progesterone itself has also been shown to have an inhibitory effect on oocyte maturation.[90] There is little doubt that insulin plays an important role in the pathophysiology of PCO. The precise cause and effect are under intensive investigation.

ADRENAL CONTRIBUTION TO PCO

The adrenal glands are thought to play a significant role in the pathogenesis of PCO. The extent of the contribution is still unknown, since both the ovaries and the adrenals have in common the synthesis of androgens and their precursors. Approximately 60% of peripheral androstenedione is of adrenal origin, while only 40% is derived from the ovaries.

The adult adrenal gland is composed of a centrally located medulla surrounded by an external cortex.[91] The medulla responds to sympathetic stimulation by secreting epinephrine and norepinephrine. The adrenal cortex makes up 90% of the gland and consists of three zones: (1) the zona glomerulosa, which produces mineralocorticoids such as aldosterone; (2) the zona fasciculata, which produces glucocoricoids such as cortisol; and (3) the innermost zona reticularis, which secretes sex steroids such as androstenedione and testosterone.

The adrenal cortex produces all steroid hormones from cholesterol. The majority of the cholesterol is obtained from plasma, although some may be formed in the adrenals de novo from acetate.[92] The first step in steroid metabolism is the side chain cleavage from cholesterol yielding pregnenolone (Fig. 5–13). This step is under the direct control of ACTH in the fasciculata and reticularis cells, and is the rate-limiting step for cortisol biosynthesis.[91] A relative deficiency of cortisol production due to congen-

ital enzyme deficiency will lead to increased ACTH release. Depending on the severity of the enzyme deficiency, serum cortisol may or may not be normalized by the increased ACTH. Depending on the location of the enzyme block, precursor hormones may be elevated, which leads to hirsutism, acne, oligoamenorrhea, infertility, and the appearance of PCO. These defects are discussed in great detail elsewhere.[91,92]

A hypothalamic–pituitary–adrenal negative feedback axis exists that is similar to the hypothalamic–pituitary–ovarian axis. Hypothalamic corticotropin-releasing factor (CRF), a 41-aminoacid peptide, is secreted into the hypophyseal portal system. Adrenocorticotropin (ACTH), together with β-lipotropin (βLPH) and β-endorphin are derived from a precursor molecule proopiomelanocortin (POMC) within the corticotroph of the anteromedial region of the anterior pituitary gland[93] (see Fig. 5–7). Corticotropin-releasing factor is capable of releasing both ACTH and β-endorphins from the pituitary,[94] as well as inhibiting GnRH secretion into the hypophyseal portal circulation.[95] All of these peptide hormones have a short half-life of less than 10 minutes and follow a circadian periodicity.

Chang and associates[96] measured endogenous ACTH levels in healthy women and in women with PCO. The levels were not significantly different in these groups, although women with PCO demonstrated higher levels of LH, DHEAS, DHEA, testosterone, and androstenedione. The DHEAS:ACTH ratio was similar in both groups. This study indicates that pituitary ACTH secretion is normal in PCO, but that adrenal androgen excess might arise from either altered adrenal responsiveness to ACTH, owing to a functional or relative enzyme deficiency, or from abnormal stimulation by factor(s) other than ACTH. This latter concept is strengthened by a report demonstrating reduced levels of DHEAS but not ACTH and cortisol levels in postmenopausal women and in other low-estrogen states.[97]

In this context, another hormone that may prove to be significant in the adrenal contribution to PCO is prolactin.[98] Levels of DHEAS but not testosterone and androstenedione are significantly higher in hyperprolactinemic women than in controls. This selective increase in adrenal Δ^5 androgens appears to be due a direct effect of prolactin on the adrenal cortex in the presence of ACTH.[99] Since hyperprolactinemia is associated with elevated DHEAS levels, and whereas a reduction in serum prolactin levels is followed by a reduction in DHEAS, a possible modulating role of prolactin on DHEAS is suggested. Elevated prolactin levels have been associated with PCO,[100] as have elevated levels of DHEAS. In addition, PCO has been experimentally induced in rats by the administration of DHEA.[101] It is therefore possible that the associa-

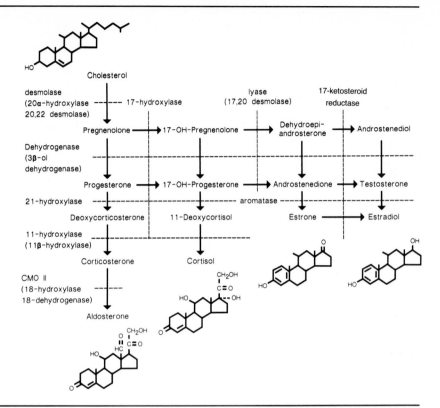

Figure 5–13. Biochemical pathway of steroid metabolism.

tion between increased prolactin levels or from increased prolactin reserve[39,43] and increased DHEAS is important in the pathophysiology of PCO.

In this regard, patients with TLE must again be mentioned. Prolactin elevation consistently follows temporal lobe seizures but does not occur after seizures that do not involve those areas.[102] Furthermore, electrical stimulation of the human amygdala, but not sham stimulation, significantly increases serum prolactin.[103] Levels of DHEAS are often measured as part of a battery of endocrine tests diagnosing PCO, since that is the most abundant steroid in the circulation and arises primarily from the adrenal cortex.[104] Since PCO appears to be overrepresented among women with TLE,[31,38] there is a reasonable chance that DHEAS levels may be inadvertently measured in patients receiving antiseizure medications. We have demonstrated that antiseizure medication falsely lowers serum DHEAS levels among treated patients with TLE (Fig. 5–14).[105] For this reason, a careful medication history must be obtained before establishing that these levels are in fact within the normal range.

PERIPHERAL EXTRAGLANDULAR CONTRIBUTIONS TO PCO

The realization that circulating levels of estrogens do not originate exclusively from glandular secretion has added much to our understanding of the pathogenesis of PCO.[106] Androgen precursors are metabolized to estrogen peripherally in extraglandular tissues. In conditions such as PCO in which increased androgen precursors are available, extrahepatic aromatization in the skin, brain, and adipose tissue may be substantial.

Several studies have sought to expand our knowledge of the role of extraglandular aromatization. Forney and co-workers[107] found that estrone was the sole estrogenic product identified in incubations in which androstenedione was used as a substrate, whereas estradiol-17β was the exclusive estrogen when using testosterone. The same group subsequently reported that only 14% of the aromatase activity of the adipose tissue resided in the adipocyte; the remaining 86% was found to reside in the stromal and vascular fraction of the culture.[108] This information is of particular interest in PCO, especially when coupled with the fact that the fractional conversion of plasma androstenedione to estrone in obese subjects is not decreased after weight loss (PCO is associated with, although not exclusively limited to, obese patients). It may be on this basis that women who are not presently obese may still develop or manifest PCO.

Another extraglandular mechanism may also be operational in PCO.[109] Patients were found to have normal levels of total E_2 but increased levels of unbound E_2 compared with controls. This results in part from lowered sex hormone-binding globulin-binding capacity (SHBG-BC).[110] Elevated unbound E_2

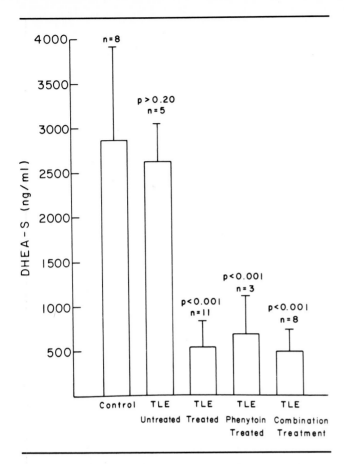

Figure 5–14. Serum levels of DHEAS in healthy controls and in women with TLE. Note the significant reduction in DHEAS levels among treated patients. (From Levesque et al.[105] Reproduced with permission.)

induction. Because it is easily administered and relatively safe, it is particularly popular among physicians treating the ovulatory dysfunction associated with PCO. Clomiphene citrate is an orally active, nonsteroidal, weak estrogen that is distantly related to diethylstilbestrol. Its mechanism of action involves competitive inhibition with the estrogen receptor in both the hypothalamus and anterior pituitary gland. As a result of the negative feedback, GnRH is functionally reduced, resulting in the secretion of gonadotropins by the anterior pituitary. As a result, follicular development ensues; serum estradiol levels increase, resulting in a positive feedback on the hypothalamus and pituitary; and an endogenous LH surge follows. Ovulation can be anticipated in approximately 85% of cycles, only half of which will result in pregnancy.[113–115] Patients who demonstrate withdrawal bleeding after progestin therapy (medroxyprogesterone acetate 10 mg/day for 5 days) are most likely to respond to the medication. It is imperative to obtain a negative pregnancy test before administering either clomiphene citrate or progestins. Clomiphene citrate is available in 50-mg tablets. Typically, patients are initiated at dosages of 50 mg daily for days 5 to 9 of a spontaneous or induced menstrual cycle. There is nothing magical about beginning the medication on day 5, however, and in fact the medication may be initiated on any day from 3 through 7. Because patients with PCO typically demonstrate an increased sensitivity to clomiphene, the lowest dosage should be used initially, and even dosages of 25 mg daily for 5 days may

correlated with high LH:FSH ratios in women with PCO.[109] One explanation of these findings might be that elevated unbound estradiol levels act at the hypothalamic–pituitary level to increase the LH responsiveness to GnRH. An alternative, or additional, explanation might be that the elevated unbound estradiol reduces hypothalamic dopamine, as has been shown in experimental animals.[111] Furthermore, administration of estrone benzoate to subjects with PCO was shown to reduce FSH levels without altering LH release.[112] Under these sets of conditions, one can visualize the last segment of a self-perpetuating vicious cycle culminating in inappropriate gonadotropin secretion and PCO (Fig. 5–15).

TREATMENT OF POLYCYSTIC OVARY DISEASE

Ovulation Induction

Clomiphene Citrate. Clomiphene citrate is one of the most common medications used for ovulation

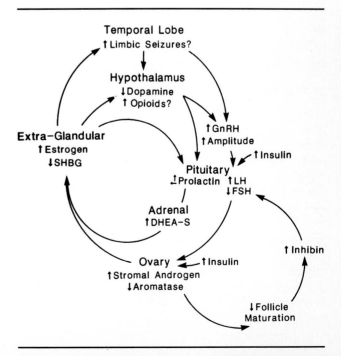

Figure 5–15. Proposed mechanism for the pathogenesis of PCO.

successfully induce ovulation. Nevertheless, dosages as high as 250 mg daily are occasionally required. The medication should be increased in 50-mg increments only if ovulation fails to occur. Once an ovulatory dosage has been established, there is no benefit from increasing the dosage further. An LH surge usually occurs 7 to 10 days after the last clomiphene tablet.[116] In my experience, the majority of both the singleton conceptions and the multiple births occur at the lowest dosage of the medication.

A frequently observed finding in patients with PCO who receive clomiphene citrate therapy is a relatively high frequency of luteal phase inadequacy defined as a luteal phase length of 12 days or less[117] This may in part explain the discrepancy between the high ovulation rate and the lower conception rates observed with clomiphene usage.[113,114] Furthermore, the associated luteal phase inadequacy may account for the elevated spontaneous abortion rate.[118] Because most of the conceptions using clomiphene citrate occur within six ovulatory cycles,[119] failure to conceive in this period of time demands more intensive evaluation to exclude other correctable infertility factors.[115]

Patients who fail to ovulate on clomiphene citrate alone may benefit from the addition of HCG. An intramuscular injection of 5,000 to 10,000 IU of HCG is administered when the lead follicle is 18 to 20 mm in diameter. This regimen has been reported to decrease the rate of spontaneous abortion and increase the rates of both ovulation and pregnancy.[118,120,121] It is important to realize that HCG administered at inappropriate times in the periovulatory period may result in down-regulation of the LH receptors and premature luteinization. Therefore, HCG should not be used without the benefit of ultrasound monitoring of follicular diameter. Otherwise, one can anticipate no advantage over the use of clomiphene citrate alone.

Clomiphene citrate has also been used in combination with either dexamethasone, 0.25 to 0.5 mg daily,[112] or prednisone, 5 to 10 mg daily at bedtime, in an attempt to blunt the nocturnal ACTH peak. This form of treatment works best in individuals who have an elevated level of DHEAS.[122,123]

Glucocorticoids. Glucocorticoids are one of the oldest medications used to induce ovulation. Early reports using cortisol in ovulatory dysfunction were published in the early 1950s. As mentioned earlier, prednisone and dexamethasone are the two most common corticosteroids in clinical use for PCO. Although the primary site of action of glucocorticoids is the adrenal gland, some ovarian suppression of androgen production occurs as well.[124–126]

Testosterone, which is primarily an ovarian androgen, has been associated with prolongation of the follicular phase and a decrease in luteal phase length.[127] Both dexamethasone and prednisone are capable of lowering free testosterone in the early follicular phase. This may explain the mechanism by which follicular maturation and increased luteal phase length occurs.[128–131] In my opinion, if ovulation does not result within 2 months of commencing therapy, this form of treatment should be discontinued as more successful alternative therapies are now available. Because of the nocturnal rise in ACTH, corticosteroids exert a greater effect if administered at bedtime. Dexamethasone dosages exceeding 0.5 mg daily increase the risk of creating cushingoid side affects.[132] Patients should also be advised that aseptic necrosis of the femoral head is a rare side effect that is not dose related. Patients diagnosed with adult-onset congenital adrenal hyperplasia and who demonstrate clinical findings typical of PCO are particularly suited to corticosteroid therapy.

Human Menopausal Gonadotropins. Human menopausal gonadotropin (HMG) is a liophilized preparation containing equal units of LH and FSH that is extracted from the urine of postmenopausal women. Each ampule contains either 75 or 150 IU of both gonadotropins. Patients should not receive HMG unless clomiphene citrate fails to result in ovulation. Many physicians will not administer HMG unless clomiphene dosages of 250 mg daily for 5 days fail to result in ovulation. It is my preference to suggest HMG when patients fail to respond to 150 mg daily of clomiphene citrate. As with clomiphene citrate, patients with PCO are frequently sensitive to HMG and care must be taken to avoid developing ovarian hyperstimulation syndrome with this medication. Patients who are observed to have numerous small follicles at the onset of HMG treatment are at particular risk for ovarian hyperstimulation. The dosage should be initiated at one ampule daily.

Ovulation rates have been reported between 76 and 95% and pregnancy rates of 28% can be anticipated.[133–136] Approximately two thirds of patients who fail to ovulate with clomiphene citrate respond to HMG. Approximately one third of patients with PCO treated with HMG develop a multiple pregnancy. The spontaneous abortion rates with this medication is slightly under 25%.

Patients with PCO treated with HMG are particularly challenging to monitor. Daily serum estradiol levels and pelvic ultrasounds at regular intervals are mandatory. Estradiol levels typically rise exponentially in a matter of 1 to 2 days, and in contrast to patients with hypothalamic amenorrhea, patients with PCO may ovulate spontaneously with an endogenous LH surge even if HCG is withheld. It is my practice to withhold HCG when estradiol levels exceed 1,800 pg/mL or more than three preovulatory follicles of 15 mm in diameter or greater are detected. Although multiple follicles do not ensure multiple births, patients with PCO are at particularly high risk.[137]

Purified FSH. The availability of purified FSH has been an exciting addition to the treatment of PCO. Laboratory basis for the use of this medication stems from in-vitro studies of granulosa cells obtained from patients.[51] These granulosa cells have been shown to be capable of converting androgen precursors to estrogens, clearly demonstrating that their basic cellular components are intact. If the proper hormonal environment is made available, granulosa cells from patients with PCO can respond normally. The clinical interest in purified FSH stems from the fact that while HMG may be successful for ovulation induction in patients with PCO, there is often an increased frequency of ovarian hyperstimulation and multiple gestations.[134]

Several earlier reports in the literature indicated limited success using pure FSH to induce ovulation. The first report described one patient with PCO successfully stimulated with pure FSH prior to the use of HCG.[138] The FSH preparation that was used in fact contained substantial and varied amounts of FSH and was administered in relatively high dosages. Subsequently, a more purified preparation of FSH was used, resulting in fewer side effects and fewer multiple births than HMG.[139,140] That study also administered FSH in relatively high doses for a short duration of time in conjunction with HCG.

During the last decade, substantial refinements have occurred in the administration of FSH to patients with PCO. Pituitary (National Pituitary Agency, Baltimore, MD) FSH was administered for a long duration in a low dosage of 40 to 80 IU/day, without HCG. The goal was to correct endogenously the biochemical imbalance in PCO. Ovulation occurred in four of six cycles and pregnancy followed in three. Levels of LH dropped immediately prior to ovulation and coincidental with a rise in E_2. This was subsequently followed by an endogenous LH surge (Fig. 5–16).[141] Only a single dominant follicle 15 mm or greater was noted in all cycles in which ultrasound was used.[142] This study provided clinical evidence that the self-perpetuating state of biochemical imbalance so characteristic of PCO could be interrupted in a physiologic way. No patient experienced evidence of ovarian hyperstimulation, and only a single dominant follicle developed in each patient despite the presence of several smaller follicles.

A subsequent study used a urinary preparation of FSH (Urofollitropin, Serono Laboratories, Randolph, MA).[143] Ten patients were studied for a total of 11 cycles. Five of these 11 cycles were ovulatory. Among these patients, a single preovulatory follicle

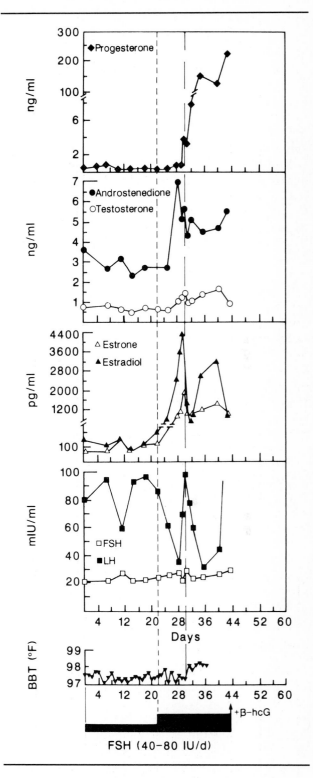

Figure 5–16. Pattern of hormonal response observed in a patient with PCO treated with long-term, low-dose pituitary FSH. (From Kamrava et al.[141] Reproduced with permission.)

developed in 4 cases, and 2 preovulatory follicles were noted in 1 cycle. In 3 cycles we noted that despite a preovulatory rise in E_2 and the development of preovulatory follicles, the preovulatory LH surge was blunted and no luteal phase rise in progesterone levels was noted. Similar findings have also been reported in the intact rhesus monkey treated with preparations of urinary FSH.[144]

The combined information from these early studies suggests that both pituitary and urinary FSH may be used in low dosages for long duration to correct the biochemical imbalance and induce ovulation in PCO. However, the finding of a blunted LH surge in some patients receiving urinary FSH suggested that HCG might be necessary to stimulate ovulation consistently in these patients. For this reason, we have incorporated an ovulatory dosage of HCG to ensure a more consistent ovulatory frequency.[145]

Urinary FSH became commercially available in November 1986 (Metrodin, Serono Laboratories, Randolph, MA). It is derived from HMG by extracting LH using immunochromatography. Each ampule of Metrodin contains 75 IU of FSH and less than 1 IU of LH activity. We have obtained optimum results by initiating treatment on cycle days 4 to 6 (Fig. 5–17). An initial dosage of 1 ampule (75 IU) intramuscularly is administered daily for 6 days. A pelvic ultrasound is then performed and serum estradiol level measured. If the follicular diameter is 10 mm or smaller, or serum estradiol levels are 200 pg/mL or below, the dosage of FSH should be increased by 1 ampule daily

for 3 additional days. Otherwise the same dosage is maintained for an additional 3 days and the ultrasound and estradiol level repeated. If the largest follicle is smaller than 13 mm or serum estradiol levels are below 300 pg/mL at that time, the dosage should be increased to 3 ampules daily for 3 days. Three ampules of FSH are then continued daily until 1 or 2 follicles reach a diameter of 17 mm or larger. If at least 1 follicle is larger than 15 mm and less than 17 mm and the E_2 level is above 1200 pg/mL, additional FSH can be withheld and HCG 5,000 to 10,000 IU can be administered 24 hours later. Ideally, HCG should be administered when the lead follicle exceeds 17 mm and E_2 levels are between 400 and 1,800 pg/mL. It should be withheld for one day if more than 3 follicles 17 mm or greater are noted or if estradiol levels exceed 1,800 pg/mL. Should this protocol not result in preovulatory follicle development, the initial dosage of FSH should be increased to 2 ampules daily for 6 days and the same outline followed. Similarly, if a poor response is observed with this dosage, the initial treatment cycle should begin with 3 ampules daily. We have found it unnecessary to administer more than 3 ampules daily or to extend treatment beyond 3 weeks. In my opinion, patients who fail to ovulate within these guidelines typically will not respond to FSH.

Dopamine Agonists. Because PCO has been associated with both hyperprolactinemia[146] and an increased sensitivity to dopamine,[44] dopamine or its agonists have been considered a logical approach to interrupting its self-perpetuating cycle (Table 5–1). Results using these agents have not been consistent. Part of this has to do with the patient selection in the various studies. Dopamine infused into male and female volunteers reduced both LH and prolactin levels.[147] Administering L-dopa in the early follicular phase also resulted in a reduction in LH levels.[148] However, neither of these studies took into account the potential modulating role of the E_2 levels. When dopamine was given on cycle day 14, the inhibitory

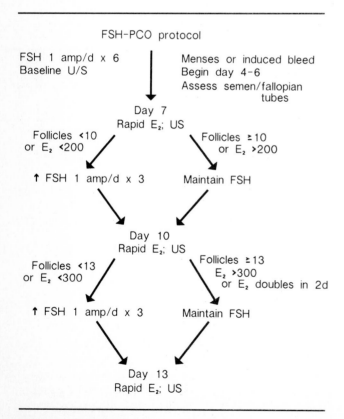

Figure 5–17. Proposed protocol for ovulation induction with FSH for patients with PCO.

TABLE 5–1. RESPONSE OF LH TO DOPAMINE AGONISTS

Reference	Agent	Finding
147	DA	↓ LH in normal females and males
148	L–dopa	↓ LH in normal females
	BCT	↓ LH in hyperprolactinemic females
149	DA	↓ LH in normal females (day 14 > days 2–12)
44	DA	↓ LH in PCO > in normal females
160	BCT	↓ LH rise in postcastration females
156	BCT	↓ LH in PCO ovulators
		↑ LH in PCO anovulators
159	BCT	↓ LH in PCO after 3 months
158	BCT	↓ LH response to GnRH in PCO
161	BCT	↓ LH/FSH in hyperprolactinemic PCO

DA = dopamine; BCT = bromocriptine

effect on LH and prolactin was substantially increased.[149] Since dopamine has no direct effect on pituitary LH release in vitro,[150] it is possible that it exerts its action at least in part essentially through its effect on LH pulsation.

An example of the effect of bromocriptine (Parlodel, Sandoz Pharmaceutical, East Hanover, NJ) on LH pulsation in a patient with PCO in the early follicular phase is shown in Figure 5–18. Whether this is due to a central defect or deficiency in dopamine, or whether it reflects indirect modulation of LH by its effects on GnRH, demands further delineation.

As a result of these studies, several authors attempted to determine the effect of bromocriptine on ovulation induction in healthy prolactinemic patients with amenorrhea. Several studies achieved ovulation in 50 to 60% of patients,[151–153] but subsequent ones obtained comparable results using placebo.[154,155] All of these reports used patients with either hypothalamic amenorrhea or amenorrhea occurring after the cessation of oral contraceptives. In a study performed in our institution, healthy normoprolactinemic patients with PCO who had failed to conceive with clomiphene citrate were administered low-dose bromocriptine.[156] Seven patients were treated for a total of 9 cycles. Ovulation occurred in 4 cycles, and 2 of these patients conceived. No ovulation occurred in 5 cycles.

Among ovulatory cycles, prolactin levels declined, but not to undetectable levels. There was also a periovulatory drop in DHEAS. Levels of LH either dropped immediately or rose modestly and then dropped to below baseline after ovulation. Among anovulatory cycles, prolactin fell to undetectable levels and DHEAS was unaffected, while LH rose to more than twice baseline and remained elevated throughout the treatment cycle. In both ovulatory and anovulatory cycles, FSH levels remained low. Although no specific biochemical response to bromocriptine could be demonstrated to explain its precise mechanism of action of in PCO, consistent and disparate gonadotropin alterations were described between ovulatory and anovulatory women. These variable effects probably reflect the diverse etiologic components in the pathophysiology of PCO or inappropriate dosages of the agent. The latter explanation is less likely, since variable responses to bromocriptine in hyperprolactinemic women have been reported with comparable serum levels of the drug.[157] Administering bromocriptine to patients with PCO resulted in a significant fall in the serum LH response to GnRH.[158] Similarly, long-term administration has been shown capable of reducing serum LH levels in PCO,[159] and of reducing the postcastration LH rise in menopausal women.[160] A subsequent controlled clinical trial administered bromocriptine to normoprolactinemic and hyperprolactinemic patients with PCO.[161] Both groups experienced a significant drop in prolactin, LH:FSH ratio, testosterone, and estrone, and a significant increase in estradiol after treatment. These results further suggest that dopamine deficiency contributes to the pathophysiology of PCO.

Although bromocriptine would appear to be an ideal medication to treat PCO, its variable effect on ovulation does not currently make it a first-line choice in the treatment of normoprolactinemic women with PCO. Further delineation of which patients will respond may increase its usefulness.

GnRH and Analog. Because of the difficulty in achieving ovulation for all patients with PCO, pulsatile GnRH has been used as an alternative treatment.[162–166] It was hoped that the mechanical infusion of exogenous GnRH might override the abnormal endogenous release of that hormone released from a dysfunctional hypothalamic–pituitary system. At the present time, experience using pulsa-

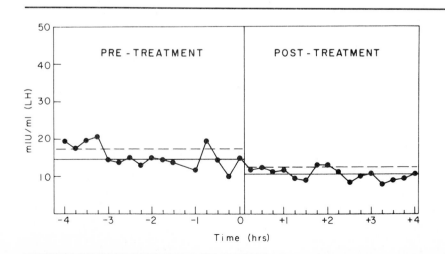

Figure 5–18. Follicular phase LH levels at 15-minute intervals from a patient with PCO before and after administration of 2.5 mg of bromocriptine. Altered levels may reflect a central defect or deficiency of dopamine, or indirect modulation of LH through dopaminergic affects on GnRH. (From Seibel.[2] Reproduced with permission.)

tile GnRH for PCO is still relatively limited. The two main areas of controversy surround the optimum dosage and the most efficacious route of administration (subcutaneous versus intravenous).

In my experience, the subcutaneous route of administration is much less effective in patients with PCO than it is in patients with hypothalamic amenorrhea. We have achieved ovulation in over 93% of patients with hypothalamic amenorrhea.[167] In contrast, among patients with PCO we have only achieved ovulation in 20% of cycles. Furthermore, ovarian hyperstimulation is occasionally encountered with this treatment.[165] Other investigators treating PCO with subcutaneous pulsatile GnRH have achieved similarly disappointing results.[168–170]

Pulsatile GnRH administered intravenously to patients with PCO has yielded somewhat better results. Ovulatory rates appear to be improved; however, pregnancy rates are nonetheless inconsistent.[171] Therefore, the data do not support pulsatile GnRH as being superior to either HMG or FSH in inducing ovulation in these patients. Should pulsatile GnRH be employed, I would clearly recommend using the intravenous route. Effective pulse dosages of 5 to 40 μg intravenously at 60, 90, or 120-minute intervals have all been used successfully. Treatment should be initiated with a dosage of 5 μg at 90-minute intervals for 1 week. If the response is poor, the dosage can be increased in 5-μg units. After ovulation, pulsatile GnRH may be discontinued and HCG, 1,500 to 2,500 IU, administered intramuscularly every 3 days to ensure luteal phase adequacy.[172] It must be remembered that the intravenous catheter does carry with it potential hazards of thrombophlebitis[173] and sepsis.[168] Nevertheless, it has been my practice to allow the catheter to remain in place for up to 1 week unless redness or tenderness occurs. It is highly unusual to encounter serious side effects if the patient is carefully informed. Finally, it must also be remembered that multiple pregnancies and hyperstimulation may both occur after GnRH treatment.[173] For this reason, it is wise to assume that careful monitoring is necessary, particularly among patients with PCO.

Long-acting, highly potent GnRH agonists (GnRHa) have been used in women with PCO. The down-regulation of the pituitary gland of these agonists results in a "medical oophorectomy" and arrested follicular development. Therefore, the several follicles typically present in various stages of atresia and development should be prevented from being stimulated by an ovulation-inducing agent. The desired goal is a reduction in ovarian hyperstimulation and multiple births. Endocrinologically, circulating levels of ovarian androgens, estrogens, and progestins are reduced to levels comparable to those in oophorectomized patients acting as controls. In contrast to the ovarian steroid suppression, the adrenal hormones DHEA and DHEAS are unaffected by GnRHa administration. This is true even with longer-term (6 months) administration.[174]

Based on these antigonadotropic effects, several investigators have pretreated patients with GnRHa prior to ovulation induction. The hope has been that by suppressing the pituitary gland, these women could be converted to hypothalamic amenorrhea and be expected to accomplish a safer and more efficient response to ovulation induction. In one study of 6 patients with PCO, D-Ser (TBU)^6-DES-GLY-NH2^{10} GnRH ethylamide (Buserelin, Hoechst, Holland, NY) was administered intranasally at a dosage of 1,000 μg daily.[175,176] Luteal phase insufficiency was noted in 2 of 4 patients treated. Similar ovulation-induction protocols have been employed by others.[177] Eight clomiphene-resistant patients with PCO were treated with D-TRP^6-GnRH analog, 100 μg subcutaneously daily, to produce suppression of pituitary gonadotropins. Once this was accomplished HMG was simultaneously administered with the GnRHa.[178] Despite a 94% ovulation rate among 33 cycles, several follicles developed in each cycle. Furthermore, luteal phase insufficiency occurred in 3 of the 31 ovulatory cycles. A total of 5 pregnancies occurred, resulting in a pregnancy rate of 17.8% per normal ovulatory cycle.

Our experience using GnRHa for down-regulation of PCO has been similar. To reduce ovarian steroid production to undetectable levels, 30 to 90 days of ovarian suppression may be required. When either HMG or FSH is then simultaneously continued with the GnRHa to achieve follicle development, hyperstimulation occurs with an alarming frequency of 75%.[178,179] Furthermore, what is of most concern is the fact that even severe hyperstimulation can occur when ovulation is triggered with HCG at estradiol levels that would be considered safe in other circumstances.[179] For these reasons, it must be appreciated that these protocols are still experimental and potentially dangerous, and the ovulation induction in patients with PCO remains a difficult challenge for the clinician.

Wedge Resection

Because of the difficulty in achieving ovulation in all patients with PCO, ovarian wedge resection remains a seldom-used but still necessary treatment. Wedge resection results in regular cycles in 6 to 95% of women (mean 80%), and pregnancy rates from 13 to 89% (mean 63%).[180] A subsequent survey revealed a 75% resumption of regular menstrual cycles postoperatively, with a corrected live birth rate of 56%.[181] Four types of wedge resection operations were included in this survey: laparoscopic wedge resection, culdoscopic cortico-wedge with follicular puncture, classic wedge resection, and hialar resection with minimal stromal excision. The classic was the least successful.

After wedge resection, testosterone and androstenedione levels decrease significantly. The reduction in testosterone is sustained, whereas androstenedione levels rise to prepoperative levels within 1 month.[182] Although the mechanism of resumed postoperative ovulation is unknown, it is presumed that the local ovarian blood flow after surgery results in increased gonadotropin delivery to the follicles, and that the local androgen levels that have an inhibitory effect on follicular maturation are reduced.[178] It is also theoretically possible that the wedge excision reduces local levels of inhibin, which allows for a postoperative increase in FSH secretion.

One of the concerns surrounding ovarian wedge resection is the potential for postoperative peritubal adhesions. This may account in part for the disparity between postoperative ovulation rates and pregnancy rates. In a report of 173 patients who had previously undergone wedge resection and who were currently undergoing a laparoscopy or laparotomy for infertility, 59 (34%) of 173 were found to have adhesions.[183] Studies such as this suggest that if conception does not occur in the first postoperative year, it is not likely to occur at all. It is hoped that the risk of peritubal and periovarian adhesions will decline as the use of microsurgical techniques increases.[184] Despite the fact that wedge resection continues to be performed to achieve ovulation in patients with PCO, it must be recognized as a final mode of therapy due to its potentially serious risks.

Electrocautery

In an effort to reduce the surgical risk of wedge resection, a less extensive surgical procedure was described to cauterize the ovary laparoscopically.[185] The ovary was grasped with forceps and electrocautery scissors were used to create 8 to 10 cautery points of 3 to 4 mm diameter in each ovary. The cautery was continued until both the capsule and the cortex of the ovary were penetrated.

The initial report of 35 patients with PCO resulted in a 92% ovulation rate within 3 months of surgery and an overall pregnancy rate of 69%.[185] The endocrine response after electrocautery of the ovary and after wedge resection are similar.[186] Within 1 month of surgery, 72% of 58 women with PCO achieved ovulation. Immediately after cautery, serum LH and FSH levels increased significantly and subsequently declined gradually to below pretreatment levels. Testosterone, dihydrotestosterone, and androstenedione also decreased, while E_2 levels increased significantly and progesterone levels remained unchanged. A smaller subsequent series confirmed these findings.[187] Over the next few years laser vaporization will probably replace electrocautery as the laparoscopic method of wedge resection.

CONCLUSIONS

Polycystic ovary disease is a self-perpetuating spectrum of clinical and biochemical entities. Despite our many advances in unraveling this disease, the factors that initiate this sequence of events is at present unknown. As our understanding of the pathogenesis of PCO continues to grow, more physiologic methods of interrupting this self-perpetuating cycle should be discovered, providing safer and more effective forms of treatment.

REFERENCES

1. Rebar R, Judd HL, Yen SSC, et al: Characterization of the inappropriate gonadotropin secretion in polycystic ovary syndrome. J Clin Invest 57:1320, 1976.
2. Seibel MM: Toward understanding the pathophysiology and treatment of polycystic ovary disease. Semin Reprod Endocrinol 2:297, 1984.
3. Patton WC, Berger MJ, Thompson IE, et al: Pituitary gonadotropin responses to synthetic luteinizing hormone-releasing hormone in patients with typical and atypical polycystic ovary disease. Am J Obstet Gynecol 121:282, 1975.
4. Kazer RR, Kessel B, Yen SSC: Circulating luteinizing hormone pulse frequency in women with polycystic ovary syndrome. J Clin Endocrinol Metab 65:233, 1987.
5. Lobo RA, Kletzky OA, Campeau JD, diZerega GS: Elevated bioactive luteinizing hormone in women with polycystic ovary syndrome. Fertil Steril 39:674, 1983.
6. Tanabe K, Gagliano P, Channing CP, et al: Levels of inhibin-F activity and steroids from human follicular fluid from normal women and women with polycystic ovary disease. J Clin Endocrinol Metab 57:24, 1983.
7. Knobil E: The neuroendocrine control of the menstrual cycle. Recent Prog Horm Res 36:53, 1980.
8. Seibel MM, Claman P, Oskowitz SP, et al: Events surrounding the initiation of puberty with long-term subcutaneous pulsatile gonadotropin-releasing hormone in a female patient with Kallmann's syndrome. J Clin Endocrinol Metab 61:575, 1985.
9. Ravnikar VA, Elkind-Hirsch K, Schiff I, Tulchinsky D, Ryan KJ: Peripheral immunoreactive LH-RH concentrations in polycystic ovary disease. Presented at the meeting of the Society for Gynecologic Investigation, Washington, DC, March 17–20, 1983.
10. Zumoff B, Freeman R, Coupey S, et al: A chronobiologic abnormality in luteinizing hormone secretion in teenage girls with polycystic ovary syndrome. N Engl J Med 309:1206, 1983.
11. Brzezinski A, Lynch HJ, Wurtman RJ, Seibel MM: Possible contribution of melatonin to the timing of the luteinizing hormone surge. N Engl J Med 316:1550, 1987.
12. Cummings DC, Reid RL, Quigley ME, et al: Evidence for decreased endogenous dopamine and opioid inhibitory influences on LH secretion in polycystic ovary syndrome. Clin Endocrinol 20:643, 1984.
13. Barnes RB, Lobo RA: Central opioid activity in polycystic ovary syndrome (PCO) with and without dopaminergic modulation. J Clin Endocrinol Metab 61:779, 1985.
14. Elitala G, Devilla L, Musso NR: On the role of dopamine receptors in the naloxone-induced hormonal changes in man. J Clin Endocrinol Metab 56:118, 1983.
15. Ropert JD, Quigley ME, Yen SSC: The dopaminergic inhibition of LH secretion during the menstrual cycle. Life Sci 34:2067, 1984.
16. Barnes RB, Lobo RA: Endogenous opioids in polycystic ovary syndrome. Semin Reprod Endocrinol 5:185, 1987.
17. Reid RL, Hoff JD, Yen SSC, et al: Effects of exogenous β-endorphin on pituitary hormone secretion and its disappearance rate in normal human subjects. J Clin Endocrinol Metab 52:1179, 1981.
18. Van Loon GR: Brain opioid peptide regulation of autonomic function, in Givens J (ed): The Hypothalamus. Chicago, Year Book, 1984, p. 39.
19. Rotsztejn WH, Drouva SV, Pattou E, Kordon C: Met-enkephalin inhibits dopamine-induced LH-RH release from mediobasal hypothalamus of male rats. Nature 274:281, 1978.
20. Aleem FA, McIntosh T: Elevated plasma levels of β-endorphin in a group of women with polycystic ovary disease. Fertil Steril 42:686, 1984.

21. Petraglia F, D'Ambrogio G, Comitini G, et al: Impairment of opioid control of luteinizing hormone secretion in menstrual disorders. *Fertil Steril* 43:534, 1985.

22. Hollt V, Muller OA, Fahbush R: β-Endorphin in human plasma: Basal and pathologically elevated levels. *Life Sci* 25:37, 1979.

23. Chang RJ, Mandel FP, Wolfsen AR, et al: Circulating levels of plasma adrenocorticotropin in polycystic ovary disease. *J Clin Endocrinol Metab* 54:1265, 1982.

24. Colt SWD, Wardlaw SL, Franz AG: The effect of running on plasma β-endorphin. *Life Sci* 28:1637, 1981.

25. Lobo RA, Granger LR, Paul WL, et al: Psychological stress and increases in urinary norepinephrine metabolites, platelet serotonin, and adrenal androgens in women with polycystic ovary syndrome. *Am J Obstet Gynecol* 145:496, 1983.

26. Kimball CD: Do opioid peptides mediate appetites and love bonds? *Am J Obstet Gynecol* 156:1463, 1987.

27. Houck JC, Kimball CD: Pancreatic beta-endorphin-like polypeptide. *Pharmacology* 23:1423, 1981.

28. Margules DL, Moisset B, Lewis MJ, Shibrija H, Pert CB: β-Endorphin in association with overeating in genetically induced mice (ob/ob) and rats (l lla). *Science* 202:988, 1978.

29. Herzog AG, Seibel MM, Schomer DL, Vaitukaitis JL, Geschwind N: Reproductive endocrine disorders in men with partial seizures of temporal lobe origin. *Arch Neurol* 43:341, 1986.

30. Herzog AG, Seibel MM, Schomer DL, Vaitukaitis JL, Geschwind N: Reproductive endocrine disorders in women with partial seizures of temporal lobe origin. *Arch Neurol* 43:347, 1986.

31. Renaud LP: Influence of amygdala stimulation on the activity of identified tuberoinfundibular neurones in the rat hypothalamus. *J Physiol* 260:237, 1976.

32. Erickson LB, Wada JA: Effects of lesions in the temporal lobe and rhinencephalon on reproductive function in adult female rhesus monkeys. *Fertil Steril* 21:434, 1970.

33. Kreiger DT, Martin JB: Brain peptides. *N Engl J Med* 304:876, 1981.

34. Henriksen SJ, Bloom FE, McLoy F, Ling N, Guillemin R: β-Endorphin induces nonconvulsive limibic seizures. *Proc Natl Acad Sci USA* 75:5221, 1978.

35. Zolovnik AJ: Effects of lesions and electrical stimulation of the amygdala on hypothalamic–hypophyseal regulation, in Eleftheriou (ed): *The Neurobiology of the Amygdala*. New York, Plenum, 1972, pp 745–762.

36. Sato M, Nakashima T: Kindling: Secondary epileptogenesis, sleep and cathecholamines. *Cam J Neurol Sci* 2:349, 1975.

37. Papeschi R, Molina-Negro P, Sourkes TL, et al: The concentration of homovanillic and 5-hydroxyindoleacetic acid in ventricular and lumbar CSF. *Neurology* 22:1151, 1972.

38. Herzog A, Seibel MM, Schomer D, Vaitukaitis JL, Geschwind N: Temporal lobe epilepsy: An extrahypothalamic pathogenesis for polycystic ovary syndrome? *Neurology* 34:1389, 1984.

39. Falaschi P, Del Pozo E, Rocco A, et al: Prolactin release in polycystic ovary. *Obstet Gynecol* 55:579, 1980.

40. Sommers SC, Wadman PJ: Pathogenesis of polycystic ovaries. *Am J Obstet Gynecol* 72:160, 1956.

41. Futterweit W, Krieger DT: Pituitary tumors associated with hyperprolactinemia and polycystic ovary disease. *Fertil Steril* 31:608, 1979.

42. Futterweit W: Pituitary tumors and polycystic ovarian disease. *Obstet Gynecol* 62:74s, 1983.

43. Alger M, Vasquez-Matute L, Mason M, et al: Polycystic ovarian disease associated with hyperprolactinemia and defective metoclopramide response. *Fertil Steril* 34:70, 1980.

44. Quigley ME, Rakoff JS, Yen SSC: Increased luteinizing sensitivity to dopamine inhibition in polycystic ovary syndrome. *J Clin Endocrinol Metab* 52:231, 1981.

45. Barnes RB, Mileikowsky GN, Cha KY, et al: Effects of dopamine and metoclopramide in polycystic ovary syndrome (PCO) *J Clin Endocrinol Metab* 63:506, 1986.

46. Lofstrom A: Catecholamine turnover alterations in discrete areas of the median eminence of the 4 and 5 day cycling rat. *Brain Res* 120:113, 1977.

47. Grant LD, Stumpf WE: Localization of 3H estradiol and catecholamines in identical neurons in the hypothalamus. *J Histochem Cytochem* 21:404, 1973.

48. McNeill TH, Sladek JR Jr: Fluorescence immunocytochemistry: simultaneous localization of catecholamines and gonadotropin-releasing hormone. *Science* 200:72, 1978.

49. Cetel NS, Yen SSC: Concomitant pulsatile release of prolactin and luteinizing hormone in hypogonadal women. *J Clin Endocrinol Metab* 56:1313, 1983.

50. Falaschi P, Rocco A, Del Pozo E: Inhibitory effect of bromocriptine treatment of luteinizing hormone secretion in polycystic ovary syndrome. *J Clin Endocrinol Metab* 62:348, 1986.

51. Erickson GF, Hsueh AJW, Quigley ME, Regar RW, Yen SSC: Functional studies of aromatase activity in human granulosa cells from normal and polycystic ovaries. *J Clin Endocrinol Metab* 49:514, 1979.

52. Poretsky L, Kalin MF: The gonadotropic function of insulin. *Endocr Rev* 8:132, 1987.

53. Kahn CR, Flier JS, Bar RS, et al: The syndromes of insulin resistance and acanthosis nigricans. Insulin-receptor disorders in man. *N Engl J Med* 294:739, 1976.

54. Flier JS, Kahn CR, Jarrett DB, Roth J: Characterization of antibodies to the insulin receptor. A cause of insulin-resistant diabetes in man. *J Clin Invest* 58:1442, 1976.

55. Flier JS, Kahn R, Roth J: Receptors, antireceptor antibodies and mechanisms of insulin resistance. *N Engl J Med* 300:413, 1979.

56. Taylor SI: Receptor defects in patients with extreme insulin resistance. *Diabetes/Metab Rev* 1:171, 1985.

57. Givens JR, Kurtz BR: Understanding the polycystic ovary syndrome, in Rolland R, Chada DR, Willemsen WNP (eds): *Gonadotropin Down-Regulation in Gynecologic Practice*. New York, Liss, 1986, pp 355–376.

58. Stuart CA, Peters EJ, Prince MJ, et al: Insulin resistance with acanthosis nigricans: The role of obesity and androgen excess. *Metabolism* 35:197, 1986.

59. Chang RJ, Nakamura RM, Judd HL, Kaplan SA: Insulin resistance with acanthosis nigricans: The role of obesity and androgen excess. *Metabolism* 35:197, 1987.

60. Jialal I, Naiker P, Reddi K, Moodley J, Joubert SM: Evidence for insulin resistance in nonobese patients with polycystic ovarian disease. *J Clin Endocrinol Metab* 64:1066, 1987.

61. Burghen GA, Givens JR, Kitabchi AE: Correlation of hyperandrogenism with hyperinsulinism in polycystic ovarian disease. *J Clin Endocrinol Metab* 50:113, 1980.

62. Barbieri RL, Ryan KJ: Hyperandrogenism, insulin resistance, and acanthosis nigricans syndrome: A common endocrinopathy with distinct pathophysiologic features. *Am J Obstet Gynecol* 147:90, 1983.

63. Cole C, Kitabachi AE: Remission of insulin resistance with Orthonovum in a patient with polycystic ovarian disease and acanthosis nigricans (abstr). *Clin Res* 26:412A, 1978.

64. Geffner ME, Kaplan SA, Bersch N, et al: Persistence of insulin resistance in polycystic ovarian disease after inhibition of ovarian steroid secretion. *Fertil Steril* 45:327, 1986.

65. Stuart CA, Prince MJ, Meyer WJ: Hyperinsulinemia and hyperandrogenemia: In vivo androgen response to insulin infusion. *Obstet Gynecol* 69:921, 1987.

66. Nestter JE, Clove JN, Strauss JF, Blackard WG: The effects of hyperinsulinemia on serum testosterone, progesterone, dehydroepiandrosterone sulfate and cortisol levels in normal women and in a woman with hyperandrogenism, insulin resistance, and acanthosis nigricans. *J Clin Endocrinol Metab* 64:180, 1987.

67. Barbieri RL, Makris A, Ryan KJ: Effects of insulin on steroidogenesis in cultured porcine ovarian theca. *Fertil Steril* 40:237, 1983.

68. Barbieri RL, Makris A, Randall RW, et al: Insulin stimulates androgen accumulation in incubations of ovarian stroma obtained from women with hyperandrogenism. *J Clin Endocrinol Metab* 62:904, 1986.

69. Barbieri RL, Makris A, Ryan KJ: Insulin stimulates androgen accumulation in incubations of human ovarian stroma and theca. *Obstet Gynecol* 64:735, 1984.

70. Veldhuis JD, Kolp LA, Toaff ME, Strauss JF, Demers LM: Mechanisms subserving the trophic actions of insulin on ovarian cells. In vitro studies using swine granulosa cells. *J Clin Invest* 72:1046, 1983.

71. Savion N, Lui GM, Laherty R, et al: Factors controlling proliferation and progesterone production by bovine granulosa cells in serum-free medium. *Endocrinology* 109:409, 1981.

72. Poretsky L, Smith D, Seibel M, et al: Specific insulin-binding sites in human ovary. *J Clin Endocrinol Metab* 59:809, 1984.

73. Poretsky L, Grigorescu F, Seibel M, Moses AC, Flier JS: Distribution and characterization of insulin and insulin-like growth factor I receptors in normal human ovary. *J Clin Endocrinol Metab* 61:728, 1985.

74. Jarrett JC, Ballijo G, Tsibris JCM, Spellacy WN: Insulin binding to human ovaries. *J Clin Endocrinol Metab* 60:460, 1985.

75. Zapf J, Schmid CH, Froesch ER: Biological and immunological properties of insulin-like growth factors (IGF) I and II. *Clin Endocrinol Metab*

13:3, 1984.

76. Gates GS, Bayer S, Seibel MM, et al: Characterization of insulin-like growth factor binding to human granulosa cells obtained during in vitro fertilization. *J Recept Res* 7:885, 1987.

77. Pellicer A, Diamond MP, DeCherney AH, Naftolin F: Intraovarian markers of follicular and oocyte maturation. *J IVF/ET* 4:209, 1987.

78. Tsafiri A, Channing CP: Influence of follicular maturation and culture conditons on the meiosis of pig oocytes in vitro. *J Reprod Fertil* 43:149, 1975.

79. Lessman CA, Schuetz AW: Role of follicle wall in meiosis reinitiation induced by insulin in *Rana pipiens* oocytes. *Am J Physiol* 241:E51, 1981.

80. May JV, Schomberg DW: Granulosa cell differentiation in vitro: Effect of insulin on growth and functional integrity. *Biol Reprod* 35:421, 1981.

81. Garzo G, Dorrington JH: Aromatase activity in human granulosa cells during follicular development and the modulation by follicle-stimulating homone and insulin. *Am J Obstet Gynecol* 148:657, 1984.

82. Diamond MP, Webster BW, Carr RK, Wentz AC, Osteen KG: Human follicular fluid insulin concentrations. *J Clin Endocrinol Metab* 61:990, 1985.

83. Adashi EY, Hsueh AJW, Yen SSC: Insulin enhancement of luteinizing hormone and follicle-stimulating hormone release by cultured pituitary cells. *Endocrinology* 108:1441, 1981.

84. Van Houten M, Posner BI, Kopriwa BW, et al: Insulin enhancement of luteinizing hormone and follicle-stimulating hormone release by cultured pituitary cells. *Endrocrinology* 108:1441, 1981.

85. Van Houten M. Posner BI, Kopriwa BM, et al: Insulin binding sites localized to nerve terminals in rat median eminence and arcuate nucleus. *Science* 207:1081, 1980.

86. Bestetti G, Locatelli V, Tirone F, Rossi GL, Muller EE: One month of streptozotocin-diabetes induces different neuroendocrine and morphological alterations in the hypothalamus–pituitary axis of male and female rats. *Endocrinology* 117:208, 1985.

87. Scarmuzzi RJ, Davidson WG, Van Hook PFA: Increasing ovulation rate in sheep by active immunization against an ovarian steroid androstenedione. *Nature* 269:817, 1979.

88. Terranova PF, Greenwald GS: Increased ovulation rate in the cycling guinea pig after a single injection of an antiserum to LH. *J Reprod Fertil* 61:37, 1981.

89. Terranova PF: Steroidogenesis in experimentally induced atretic follicles in the hamster: A shift from estradiol to progesterone synthesis. *Endocrinology* 108:1885, 1981.

90. Downs SM, Eppig JJ: Cyclic adenosine monophosphate and ovarian follicular fluid act synergistically to inhibit mouse oocyte maturation. *Endocrinology* 114:418, 1984.

91. Brodie BL, Wentz AC: Late-onset congenital adrenal hyperplasia: a gynecologist's perspective. *Fertil Steril* 48:175, 1987.

92. White PC, New MI, Dupont B: Congenital adrenal hyperplasia. *N Engl J Med* 316:1519, 1987.

93. Krieger DT: Pathophysiology of Cushing's disease. *Endocr Rev* 4:22, 1983.

94. Bruhn TD, Sutton RE, Rivier CL, Vale W: Corticotropin-releasing factor regulates proopiomelanocortin messenger ribonucleic acid levels in vivo. *Neuroendocrinology.* 39:170, 1984.

95. Rivier C, Rivier J, Vale W: Stress-induced inhibition of reproductive functions: Role of endogenous corticotropin-releasing factor. *Science* 231:607, 1986.

96. Chang RJ, Mandel FP, Wolfson AR, et al: Circulating levels of ACTH in polycystic ovary disease. *J Clin Endocrinol Metab* 54:1265, 1982.

97. Cumming DC, Rebar RW, Hopper BR, Yen SSC: Evidence of an influence of the ovary on circulating dehydroepiandrosterone sulfate levels. *J Clin Endocrinol Metab* 54:1069, 1982.

98. Lobo RA, Kletzky OA, Kaptein EM, Goebelsman U: Prolactin modulation of dehydroepiandrosterone sulfate secretion. *Am J Obstet Gynecol* 138:632, 1980.

99. Higuchi K, Niwata H, Maki T, et al: Prolactin has a direct effect on adrenal androgen secretion. *J Clin Endocrinol Metab* 59:714, 1984.

100. Falaschi P, Fragese G, Rocco A, et al: Polycystic ovary syndrome and hyperprolactinemia. *J Steroid Biochem* 8:13, 1977.

101. Knudsen JF, Costoff A, Mahesh VB: Dehydroepiandrosterone- induced polycystic ovaries and acyclicity in the rat. *Fertil Steril* 26:807, 1975.

102. Sperling MR, Pritchard PB, Engel J Jr, Daniel C, Sagel J: Prolactin in partial epilepsy: An indicator of limbic seizures. *Ann Neurol* 20:716, 1986.

103. Parra A, Velasco M, Cervantes C, et al: Plasma prolactin increase following electric stimulation of the amygdala in humans. *Neuroendo-*

crinology 31:60, 1980.

104. Vande Wiele RL, MacDonald PC, Gurpide E, Lieberman S: Studies on the secretion and interconversion of the androgens. *Recent Prog Horm Res* 19:275, 1963.

105. Levesque LA, Herzog AG, Seibel MM: The effect of phenytoin and carbamazepine on serum dehydroepiandrosterone sulfate in men and women who have partial seizures with temporal lobe involvement. *J Clin Endocrinol Metab* 63:243, 1986.

106. Siiteri PK, MacDonald PC: Role of extraglandular estrogen in human endocrinology, in Greep RO, Astwood EB (eds): *Handbook of Physiology.* Washington, DC: American Physiology Society, 1973, vol 2, pp 615–629.

107. Forney JP, Milewich L, Chen GT, et al: Aromatization of androstenedione to estrone by human adipose tissue in vitro: Correlation with adipose tissue mass, age, and endometrial neoplasia. *J Clin Endocrinol Metab* 53:192, 1981.

108. Ackerman GE, Smith ME, Mendelson CR, et al: Aromatization of androstenedione by human adipose tissue stromal cells in monolayer culture. *J Clin Endocrinol Metab* 53:412, 1981.

109. Lobo RA, Granger L, Goebelsmann U, Mishell DR: Elevations in unbound serum estradiol as a possible mechanism for inappropriate gonadotropin secretion in women with PCO. *J Clin Endocrinol Metab* 52:156, 1981.

110. Anderson DC: Sex-hormone binding globulin. *Clin Endocrinol* 104:419, 1979.

111. Cramer DM, Parker CR, Porter JC: Estrogen inhibition of dopamine release into hypophyseal portal blood. *Endocrinology* 104:419, 1979.

112. Chang RJ, Mandel FP, Lu JKH, Judd HL: Enhanced disparity of gonadotropin secretion in women with polycystic ovarian disease. *J Clin Endocrinol Metab* 54:490, 1982.

113. Raj SG, Thompson IE, Berger MJ, Taymor ML: Clinical aspects of the polycystic ovary syndrome. *Obstet Gynecol* 49:552, 1977.

114. Gorlitsky GA, Kase NG, Speroff L: Ovulation and pregnancy rates with clomiphene citrate. *Obstet Gynecol* 51:265, 1978.

115. Gysler M, March CM, Mishell DR Jr, Baily EF: A decade's experience with an individualized clomiphene treatment regimen including its effect on the postcoital test. *Fertil Steril* 37:161, 1982.

116. Wu CH: Plasma hormones in clomiphene citrate therapy. *Obstet Gynecol* 49:443, 1977.

117. Yen SSC, Vela P, Ryan KJ: Effect of clomiphene citrate in polycystic ovarian syndrome: Relationship between serum gonadotropin and corpus luteum function. *J Clin Endocrinol Metab* 31:7, 1970.

118. Garcia JE, Jones GS, Wentz AC: The use of clomiphene citrate. *Fertil Steril* 28:707, 1977.

119. MacGregor AH, Johnson JE, Bunde CA: Further clinical experience with clomiphene citrate. *Fertil Steril* 19:616, 1968.

120. Poliak A, Smith JJ, Romney SL: Clinical evaluation of clomiphene, clomiphene and human chorionic gonadotropin, and estrogens in anovulatory cycles. *Fertil Steril* 24:921, 1973.

121. Talbert LM: Clomiphene citrate induction of ovulation. *Fertil Steril* 39:742, 1983.

122. Lobo RA, Paul W, March CM, Granger L, Kletzky OA: Clomiphene and dexamethasone in women unresponsive to clomiphene alone. *Obstet Gynecol* 60:497, 1982.

123. Daly DC, Walters CA, Soto-Albors CE, Tohan N, Riddick DH: A randomized study of dexamethasone in ovulation induction with clomiphene citrate. *Fertil Steril* 41:844, 1984.

124. Kirschner MA, Jacobs JB: Combined ovarian and adrenal vein catheterization to determine site(s) of androgen overproduction in hirsute women. *J Clin Endocrinol Metab* 33:199, 1977.

125. Maroulis GB: Evaluation of hirsutism and hyperandrogenemia. *Fertil Steril* 36:273, 1981.

126. Rittmaster R, Loriaux DL, Cutler GB Jr: Sensitivity of cortisol and adrenal androgens to dexamethasone suppression in hirsute women. *J Clin Endocrinol Metab* 61:462, 1985.

127. Smith KD, Rodriguez-Rigau LJ, Tcholakian PK, Steinberger E: The relation between plasma testosterone levels and the lengths and phases of the menstrual cycle. *Fertil Steril* 32:402, 1979.

128. Bardin CW, Hembree WD, Lipsett MB: Suppression of testosterone and androstenedione production rates with dexamethasone in women with idiopathic hirsutism and polycystic ovaries. *J Clin Endocrinol Metab* 28:1300, 1968.

129. Horton R, Niesler J: Plasma androgens in patients with polycystic ovary syndrome. *J Clin Endocrinol Metab* 28:479, 1968.

130. Moroulis GB: Polycystic ovarian disease and dexamethasone. *Semin*

Reprod Endocrinol 2:263, 1984.

131. Rodriguez-Rigau LJ, Smith KD, Tcholakian PK, Steinberger E: Effect of prednisone on plasma testosterone levels and on duration of phases of the menstrual cycle in hyperandrogenic women. *Fertil Steril* 32:408, 1979.

132. Boyers SP, Buster JE, Marshall JR: Hypothalamic–pituitary–adrenocortical function during long-term low-dose dexamethasone therapy in hyperandrogenized women. *Am J Obstet Gynecol* 142:330, 1982.

133. Wang CF, Gemzell C: The use of human gonadotropins for the induction of ovulation in women with polycystic ovarian disease. *Fertil Steril* 33:479, 1980.

134. Gindoff PR, Jewelewicz R: Polycystic ovarian disease. *Obstet Gynecol Clin North Am* 14:931, 1987.

135. Schwartz M, Jewelewicz R: The use of gonadotropins for induction of ovulation. *Fertil Steril* 35:3, 1981.

136. Franks S, Adams J, Mason H, Polson D: Ovulatory disorders in women with polycystic ovary syndrome. *Clin Obstet Gynecol* 12:605, 1985.

137. Seibel MM, McArdle C, Thompson IE, Berger MJ, Taymor ML: The role of ultrasound in ovulation induction: a critical appraisal. *Fertil Steril* 36:573, 1981.

138. Gemzell C: Induction of ovulation with human gonadotropins. *Recent Prog Horm Res* 21:179, 1965.

139. Raj SG, Berger MJ, Grimes EM, Taymor ML: The use of gonadotropins for the induction of ovulation in women with polycystic ovarian disease. *Fertil Steril* 28:1280, 1977.

140. Schoemaker J, Wentz AC, Jones GS, Dubin NH, Sapp KC: Stimulation of follicular growth with "pure" FSH in patients with anovulation and elevated LH levels. *Obstet Gynecol* 51:270, 1978.

141. Kamrava M, Seibel MM, Berger MJ, Thompson IE, Taymor ML: Reversal of persistent anovulation in polycystic ovarian disease by administration of chronic low-dose follicle-stimulating hormone. *Fertil Steril* 37:520, 1982.

142. Seibel MM, Kamrava MM, McArdle C, Taymor ML: Treatment of polycystic ovary disease with chronic low-dose follicle-stimulating hormone: biochemical changes and ultrasound correlation. *Int J Fertil* 29:39, 1984.

143. Seibel MM, McArdle C, Smith D, Taymor ML: Ovulation induction in polycystic ovary syndrome with urinary follicle-stimulating hormone or human menopausal gonadotropin. *Fertil Steril* 43:703, 1985.

144. Schenken RS, Hodgen GD: Follicle-stimulating hormone blocks estrogen-positive feedback during the early follicular phase in monkeys. *Fertil Steril* 45:556, 1986.

145. Claman P, Seibel MM, McArdle C, Berger MJ, Taymor ML: Comparison of intermediate-dose purified urinary follicle-stimulating hormone with and without HCG for ovulation induction in polycystic ovarian syndrome. *Fertil Steril* 46:518, 1986.

146. Falaschi P, Del Pozo E, Rocco A, et al: Prolactin release in polycystic ovary. *Obstet Gynecol* 55:579, 1980.

147. LeBlanc H, Lachelin GCL, Abu-Fadil S, Yen SSC: Effects of dopamine infusion on pituitary hormone secretions in humans. *J Clin Endocrinol Metab* 43:668, 1976.

148. Lachelin GCL, LeBlanc H, Yen SSC: The inhibitory effects of dopamine agonists on LH release in women. *J Clin Endocrinol Metab* 44:728, 1977.

149. Judd SJ, Rakoff JS, Yen SSC: Inhibition of gonadotropin and prolactin release by dopamine: Effect of endogenous estradiol levels. *J Clin Endocrinol Metab* 47:494, 1978.

150. Yen SSC: Neuroendocrine regulation of gonadotropin and prolactin secretion in women: Disorders in reproduction, in Vaitukaitis JL (ed): *Clinical Reproductive Neuroendocrinology*. New York, Elsevier, 1982, p 140.

151. Seppala M, Hirvonen E, Ranta T: Bromocriptine treatment of secondary amenorrhea. *Lancet* 1:1154, 1976.

152. Tolis G, Naftolin F: Induction of menstruation with bromocriptine in patients with euprolactinemic amenorrhea. *Am J Obstet Gynecol* 126:426, 1976.

153. Van der Steeg HJ, Coelingh Bennink HJTR: Bromocriptine for induction of ovulation in normoprolactinemic post-pill ovulation. *Lancet* 1:502, 1977.

154. Crosignani PG, Reschini E, Lombroso GC, et al: Comparison of placebo and bromocriptine in the treatment of patients with normoprolactinemic amenorrhea. *Br J Obstet Gynaecol* 85:773, 1978.

155. Coelingh Bennink HJT, Van der Steeg HJ: Failure of bromocriptine to restore the menstrual cycle in normoprolactinemic post-pill amenorrhea. *Fertil Steril* 39:238, 1983.

156. Seibel MM, Oskowitz S, Kamrava M, Taymor ML: Bromocriptine response in normoprolactinemic patients with polycystic ovary disease: A preliminary report. *Obstet Gynecol* 64:213, 1984.

157. Thorner MO, Schran HF, Evans WS, Rogol AD, MacLeod RM: A broad spectrum of prolactin suppression by bromocriptine in hyperprolactinemic women: A study of serum prolactin and bromocriptine levels after acute and chronic administration of bromocriptine. *J Clin Endocrinol Metab* 50:1026, 1980.

158. Buvat J, Buvat-Herbant M, Marcolin G, et al: A double-blind controlled study of the hormonal and clinical effects of bromocriptine in the polycystic ovary syndrome. *J Clin Endocrinol Metab* 66:119, 1986.

159. Spruce BA, Kendall-Taylor P, Dunlop W, et al: The effect of bromocriptine in the polycystic ovary syndrome. *Clin Endocrinol (Oxf)* 20:643, 1984.

160. Melis GB, Paoletti AM, Mais V, et al: Inhibitory affect of the dopamine agonist bromocriptine on the postcastration gonadotropin rise in women. *J Clin Endocrinol Metab* 53,530, 1981.

161. Tabbakh GHE, Loutfi IA, Azab I, et al: Bromocriptine in polycystic ovarian disease: A controlled clinical trial. *Obstet Gynecol* 71:301, 1988.

162. Burger CW, Korsen TJM, Hompes PGA, et al: Ovulation induction with pulsatile luteinizing releasing hormone in women with clomiphene citrate-resistant polcystic ovary-like disease: Clinical results. *Fertil Steril* 46:1045, 1986.

163. Coelingh Bemink HJT, Weber HW, Alsbach HPJ, Thijssen JHH: Induction of ovulation by pulsatile intravenous administration of GnRH in polycystic ovarian disease. *Fertil Steril* 41:34S, 1984.

164. Molloy BG, Hancock KW, Glass MR: Ovulation induction in clomiphene non-responsive patients: the place of pulsatile gonadotropin-releasing hormone in clinical practice. *Fertil Steril* 43:26, 1985.

165. Saffan D, Seibel, MM: Ovulation induction with subcutaneous pulsatile gonadotropin-releasing hormone in various ovulatory disorders. *Fertil Steril* 45:475, 1986.

166. Ory SJ, London SN, Tyrey L, Hammond CB: Ovulation induction with pulsatile gonadotropin-releasing hormone administration in patients with polycystic ovarian syndrome. *Fertil Steril* 43:20, 1985.

167. Seibel MM, Kamrava M, McArdle C, Taymor ML: Ovulation induction and conception using subcutaneous pulsatile luteinizing hormone-releasing hormone. *Obstet Gynecol* 161:292, 1983.

168. Tucker M, Adams J, Mason WP, Jacobs HS: Infertility megaloblastic and polycystic ovaries: Differential response to LH-RH therapy. *Ups J Med Sci* 89:43, 1984.

169. Loucopoulos A, Ferin M, Vande Wiele RL, et al: Pulsatile administration of gonadotropin-releasing hormone for ovulation. *Am J Obstet Gynecol* 148:895, 1984.

170. Hurwitz A, Rosenn B, Palti Z, et al: The hormonal response of patients with polycystic ovarian disease to subcutaneous low-frequency pulsatile administration of luteinizing hormone-releasing hormone. *Fertil Steril* 46:378, 1986.

171. Jansen RPS, Handelsman DJ, Boylan LM, et al: Pulsatile intravenous gonadotropin-releasing hormone for ovulation-induction in infertile women. II. Analysis of follicular and luteal responses. *Fertil Steril* 48:39, 1987.

172. Weinstein FG, Seibel MM, Taymor ML: Ovulation induction with subcutaneous pulsatile gonadotropin-releasing hormone: The role of supplemental human chorionic gonadotropin in the luteal phase. *Fertil Steril* 41:546, 1984.

173. Berg D, Mickan H, Mickael S, et al: Ovulation and pregnancy after pulsatile administration of gonadotropin-releasing hormone. *Arch Gynecol* 233:205, 1983.

174. Steingold K, DeZiegler D, Cedars M, et al: Clinical and hormonal effects of chronic gonadotropin-releasing hormone agonist treatment in polycystic ovarian disease. *J Clin Endocrinol Metab* 65:773, 1987.

175. Armitage M, Wilkin T, Dewbury K: Successful treatment of infertility due to polycystic ovary disease using a combination of luteinizing hormone releasing hormone agonist and low-dosage menotrophin. *Br Med J* 29:96, 1987.

176. Hompes PGA, Van Weissenbruch MM, Burger CW, et al: The additional use of Buserelin in hMG-hCG ovulation induction in PCO: A double-blind controlled study, in Rolland R, Chadha DR, Willemsen WNP (eds): *Gonadotropin Down-Regulation in Gynecological Practice*. New York, Liss, 1986, p 391.

177. Fleming R, Haxton MJ, Hamilton MPR, et al: Successful treatment of infertile women with oligomenorrhea using a combination of an LH-RH agonist and exogenous gonadotropins. *Br J Obstet Gynaecol* 92:369, 1985.

178. Charbonnel B, Krempf M, Blanchard P, Dano P, Delage C: Induction of ovulation in polycystic ovary syndrome with a combination of a luteinizing hormone-releasing hormone analog and exogenous gonadotropins. *Fertil Steril* 47:920, 1987.

179. Bayer S, Claman P, Garner P, Seibel M: Hyperstimulation complicating ovulation induction in polycystic ovary patients pretreated with a GnRH agonist. Presented at the 44th annual meeting of the American Fertility Society, Atlanta, 6–10, 1988.

180. Goldzieher JW, Axelrod LR: Clinical and biochemical features of polycystic ovarian disease. *Fertil Steril* 14:631, 1963.

181. Cohen MB: Surgical management of infertility in the polycystic ovary syndrome, in Givens J (ed): *The Infertile Female.* Chicago, Year Book, 1979, p 273.

182. Judd HL, Rigg LA, Anderson DC, Yen SSC: The effects of ovarian wedge resection on circulating gonadotropin and ovarian steroid levels in patients with polycystic ovary syndrome. *J Clin Endocrinol Metab* 43:347, 1976.

183. Buttram VC Jr, Vaquero C: Post-ovarian wedge resection adhesive disease. *Fertil Steril* 26:874, 1975.

184. Loy RA, Seibel MM: Evaluation and treatment of polycystic ovary syndrome, in Mahajan DK (ed): *Endocrinology and Metabolism Clinics of North America.* Philadelphia, Saunders, 1988.

185. Gjonnaess H: Polycystic ovarian syndrome treated by ovarian electrocautery through the laparoscope. *Fertil Steril* 41:20, 1984.

186. Aakvaag A: Hormonal response to electrocautery of the ovary in patients with polycystic ovarian disease. *Br J Obstet Gynaecol* 92:1258, 1985.

187. Greenblatt E, Casper RF: Endocrine changes after laparoscopic ovarian cautery in polycystic ovarian syndrome. *Am J Obstet Gynecol* 156:279, 1987.

CHAPTER 6

Luteal Phase Inadequacy

Anne Colston Wentz

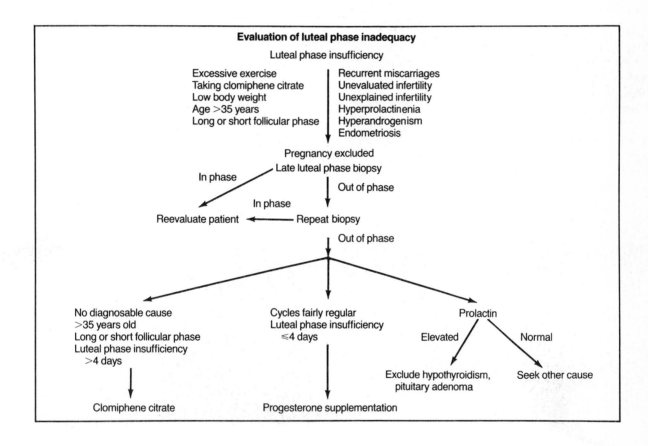

Luteal phase inadequacy (LPI) does exist. The problem for the clinician is to determine its importance as a cause of either infertility or recurrent miscarriage, and its impact on the evaluation of infertility. Defects in corpus luteum function can be responsible for inappropriate hormonal output and an abnormal pattern of endometrial development as ascertained from evaluation of biopsy material. Over the years, we have identified clinical situations in which LPI can be demonstrated, and have illustrated how to make the diagnosis.[1-14] An early article[4] pointed out three groups of patients—recurrent aborters, clomiphene-

treated patients, and women over age 35 years—who were at risk for LPI; at present, 11 clinical conditions can be identified.

Making the diagnosis does not speak to the impact of LPI, however. A few studies have evaluated its prevalence and some have found it high, but the condition has never been shown to be the *cause* of infertility in a great percentage of patients. If it is diagnosed, however, and is not the reason for the infertility, other and more important causes may be overlooked. The criteria for making the diagnosis may be misinterpreted, and the role of LPI in infertility overemphasized. To avoid these problems, we adhere to a consistent approach to diagnosis, maintaining that criteria should be defined and upheld, and that the rules of diagnosis should be stringent.

Over the past 6 years in my clinical practice I have taken approximately 1,000 endometrial biopsies from patients with infertility, of which about 160 have been diagnosed to be 2 or more days out of phase. Approximately 80% of these, or 128 (12.8%) of my patient population, have had consistent LPI; these results are taken from women who were primarily referred, often *because* of their luteal inadequacy. During this time, with a consistent approach to diagnosis and treatment, it has not been possible to demonstrate that these patients have benefited, from the standpoint of pregnancy initiation and outcome. In women with recurrent abortion, however, treatment of LPI does result in a significantly increased rate of live births. Therefore, my experience suggests that LPI, although present in the population, may not be a significant factor causing infertility.

Perhaps, if strict criteria are used to identify the condition, and collaborative studies are instituted, it may be possible to demonstrate that LPI is associated with infertility, and that its diagnosis and treatment are important in the care of these patients. At this writing, such assurance is not available.

PATHOPHYSIOLOGY OF LUTEAL INADEQUACY

Abnormalities of corpus luteum function, either in absolute hormone output or in the ratio of steroid hormone levels, may be reflected by abnormalities of endometrial development; conversely, local endometrial or uterine pathology may prevent the endometrium from responding normally to adequate hormone production. Both situations result in failure of the endometrium to mature and develop normally, which could prevent the initiation or maintenance of pregnancy. Maturation is not simply morphologic but rather biochemical and physiologic development of the capacity to synthesize proteins, among other functions. It has been illustrated how decidual prolactin production can be a marker of endometrial response.[15,16] Similarly, a serum protein, progestogen-associated endometrial protein has been used to indicate normal progesterone output during the luteal phase.[17] A normal histologic response of the endometrium appears to reflect, in a qualitative manner, the stimulation from normal steroid hormone output and ratio. This use of the endometrium as a bioassay of luteal function is a clinical tool that has shown, first, that measurement of hormonal output cannot conveniently be used to make the diagnosis; and second, that luteal inadequacy should

be defined in terms of endometrial inadequacy, since an endometrial defect can exist in the presence of normal hormone output. These concepts were initially described in 1949, in a discussion of endometrial inadequacy with or without the presence of an abnormal progesterone output.[18]

DETERMINANTS OF NORMAL OVULATORY FUNCTION

The ovarian cycle begins with the rise of follicle-stimulating hormone (FSH) intercycle initiating the process of folliculogenesis, continues with the generation of the luteinizing hormone (LH) surge that induces ovulation, and culminates in the function of the corpus luteum, at the demise of which another follicular stimulation begins. The concept that follicular development predetermines the adequacy of corpus luteum function was initially described by Ross[19] and McNatty[20]; these earlier works should be read and appreciated, not only for their concepts, most of which remain true today, but also for their detail of basic morphologic and physiologic mechanisms.

The factor that results in early maturational growth of the primordial follicles is unknown. The process is known to be gonadotropin independent, but it is not clear whether the initiating signal is stimulatory or inhibitory. An adequate increase in FSH prior to menstruation seems to stimulate growth from the secondary follicle stage on, and an estrogenic milieu is needed to stimulate granulosa cell proliferation and the appearance of FSH receptors on these cells. Induction of aromatase enzyme activity, synthesis of LH receptors on granulosa cells, formation of the antrum, and stimulation of the production of certain constituents of the follicular fluid, are primary functions of FSH working at the ovarian level. Sufficient estradiol synthesis prepares target tissues in other parts of the body, induces local intraovarian mechanisms, and stimulates the LH surge. An adequate LH surge results in ovulation; luteinization of granulosa cells, which is reflected by progesterone output by the corpus luteum; and reinitiation of the first meiotic division, allowing the oocyte to continue to mature. The final determinant of adequate luteal activity is the continued pulsatile stimulation of granulosa cells by LH, resulting in progesterone synthesis.

Interference with these and other processes clearly can occur, suggesting many mechanisms for the development of LPI. The follicle must contain sufficient numbers of granulosa cells with a capacity to produce sufficient progesterone during the luteal phase. In the final analysis, both granulosa and theca cells must be responsive to LH. Cell physiology, including enzyme and receptor systems and hormone production, must be functional for normal corpus luteum function to occur.

CELLS OF THE CORPUS LUTEUM

Two types of progesterone-secreting cells—small and large—have been demonstrated in the cow[21] and sheep.[22] They are derivatives of theca and granulosa cells. In the sheep, the small luteal cells are five times more numerous than the large cells. The LH receptors are primarily found on the small cells, which respond to LH stimulation by releasing progesterone. The large cells have few LH receptors, do not respond to either LH or cyclic adenosine monophosphate,[23] and are responsible for baseline progesterone production. When there is no LH stimulation, there is no significant difference between the total amount of progesterone production by the two cell types; however, with LH stimulation, the small luteal cells produce substantially more progesterone and are the main source of luteal progesterone. Receptors for prostaglandin E_2 and $PGF_{2\alpha}$ are found only on large cells, and $PGF_{2\alpha}$ has an inhibitory effect on progesterone output.[24]

As the corpus luteum develops,[25] the small cells differentiate into large cells, with the result that the majority of luteal cells are of thecal origin and respond to LH stimulation. If pregnancy occurs, the granulosa-derived luteal cells disappear entirely while the theca-derived cells persist. It is suggested that LH-stimulated progesterone production by small cells is dependent on the presence of large cells.[26] In addition, the large cells may have other functions, including production of oxytocin, the physiologic significance of which is not known,[27] and perhaps inhibin.

The cells of the human corpus luteum cannot be separated as easily as those in the ovine and bovine corpora lutea.[28] Nevertheless, if an analogous developmental pattern occurs in the human corpus luteum, the inability of the early corpus luteum to respond to human chorionic gonadotropin (HCG), as in the Wilks test,[29] could be explained by the few LH receptors on the large granulosa cells, and the few theca-derived cells present in the developing corpus luteum. As the number of small luteal cells increases, however, the response to LH stimulation increases markedly, resulting in the large, pulsatile progesterone output typical of the luteal phase. By perhaps 10 to 12 days into the luteal phase, $PGF_{2\alpha}$-induced luteolysis may affect the large cell; as the small cell differentiates into a large cell, it may require a continued pulsatile stimulation to maintain steroidogenesis. Without pregnancy, a continued response is impossible and luteal demise results. To date, the human corpus luteum has not been shown

to be composed of the two cell types; however, the analogy may be appropriate and help our understanding of normal corpus luteum function.

DETERMINANTS OF ABNORMAL OVULATORY FUNCTION

Deficient progesterone output might be caused by a defect in any of the factors responsible for normal, ovulatory, menstrual function. As we previously summarized,[5,6] an inadequate increase of intercycle FSH could result in inadequate proliferation of granulosa cells, insufficient numbers of both FSH and LH receptor sites on granulosa cells, and insufficient induction of the aromatase enzyme necessary for estradiol synthesis. Less-than-optimal LH stimulation of theca cells could result in decreased androstenedione secretion, with less substrate for aromatization. An inadequate LH surge could inhibit ovulation or cause suboptimal luteinization of granulosa cells, decreasing their progesterone output. Any interruption of pulsatile LH stimulation could also induce inadequate progesterone output. The corpus luteum appears to have a built-in mechanism responsible for its longevity,[30,31] but inhibitory factors that could decrease its output of progesterone or estradiol might exert their influence prematurely, resulting in a defective corpus luteum response. Thus, inadequate FSH output or granulosa cell response, a poor quantitative LH surge, and suboptimal LH stimulation during the luteal phase, could all result in inadequate formation or function of the corpus luteum.

From a teleologic standpoint, normal corpus luteum function is essential to fertility; however, this particular point has been difficult to establish clinically in an infertile population. Diagnosis and treatment of luteal phase inadequacy did not improve pregnancy rates or outcome in one infertile population, although patients with recurrent abortion were benefited.[32] Another group did not separate patients on the basis of pregnancy rate and recurrent abortion, although their overall population was benefited by treatment.[33] Compelling evidence permitting the conclusion that identifying and treating luteal phase (endometrial) inadequacy improves either the rate of initiation of pregnancy or its maintenance in an infertile population is still lacking.

CLINICAL CONSIDERATIONS

Inadequate Luteal Phase

For clinical purposes, our definition of luteal phase inadequacy is based solely on endometrial dating. Ideally, cycle length and ovulatory pattern should be normal. Abnormalities such as significant oligoovulation should be dealt with before luteal phase adequacy is assessed. One group proposed that the diagnosis of LPI be made only if endometrial development lags 2 days behind the date expected according to ovulation and the onset of menses; at least two biopsies should confirm these findings, and for proper histologic evaluation, the endometrium should be taken from high in the fundus because the response of the lower uterine segment to progesterone is not typical.[34] These researchers confirmed a predictable endometrial response to steroid hormone stimulation. We have consistently used these definitions in our studies of LPI. Some other centers define LPI as a discrepancy of 3 or more days.

Short Luteal Phase

The short luteal phase was originally described as being 8 days or less from the LH peak to onset of flow in otherwise healthy women.[35] Individuals with short luteal phase may have deficient luteal secretion of both estradiol and progesterone associated with defective follicular maturation or a defect in FSH output.[36] Progesterone secretion[37] and the endometrial response may be totally normal, however, so the difference between inadequate and short luteal phase must be emphasized. A biopsy is taken during a short luteal phase with the expectation that the endometrial pattern will be normal and not need treatment.

The short luteal phase is not usually associated with either infertility or miscarriage,[38] and does not occur more frequently in women with unexplained infertility. Attempts are frequently made to "improve" the cycle; progesterone therapy is usually effective in lengthening the luteal phase, but benefit is difficult to prove.

Aluteal Cycle

The aluteal cycle is a clinical syndrome characterized by regular menses, no history of menorrhagia, and occasional pregnancy with abortion. Aluteal cycles might ordinarily be diagnosed as anovulatory, but in fact are ovulatory and represent the most severe form of luteal phase defect.[39,40] A monophasic basal body temperature chart is usually observed in women with 25 to 35-day cycles, and a secretory endometrial pattern is documented within 2 or 3 days of the occurrence of bleeding. Probably the aluteal cycle represents an intermediate stage between the classic anovulatory pattern and LPI.

Occult Miscarriage (Now Called "Chemical Pregnancy")

The development of highly sensitive assays for measuring HCG has led to the identification of subclinical spontaneous abortion or occult pregnancy; early but failed implantation is not infrequently observed among patients undergoing at-

tempts at in-vitro fertilization (IVF), and the term *chemical pregnancy* has come into clinical usage. Most infertile women do not have blood for sensitive pregnancy tests drawn before the missed menses, but the concept is essentially the same: pregnancy in terms of fertilization and cleavage may occur, implantation begins with HCG production, but the implantation process fails. Menses may be slightly heavier or "different." Without a sensitive pregnancy test, the history is that of irregularly ovulatory cycles with variable bleeding patterns.

"Infertile" patients may conceive and miscarry so early that both the pregnancy and the miscarriage are unrecognized, suggesting that the true incidence of spontaneous abortions may be somewhat higher than the 15 to 20% reported. These women have abnormally low serum HCG concentrations for the estimated length of gestation, reflecting defective trophoblastic function. Progesterone levels have not been reported in these patients.

A higher frequency of occult miscarriage in clomiphene-treated patients might be anticipated. Based on biopsy criteria a 49% prevalence of luteal phase inadequacy was reported,[41] indicating an abnormal endometrial implantation site; however, occult miscarriage has not been identified as more frequent in clomiphene-treated patients, although overall pregnancy failure may increase.

To summarize, there are various forms of LPI, not all of which are associated with infertility or miscarriage, and not all of which are pathologic.

CLINICAL FEATURES

Normal Progesterone Levels

In some clinical conditions "normal" luteal estradiol and progesterone levels are documented and still the endometrial pattern is abnormal. Inadequate vascularization of the developing endometrium or local abnormalities preventing a normal response are among the usual explanations. Examples in which LPI would be diagnosed by endometrial biopsy in the presence of normal progesterone output are septate uterus; local endometrial abnormalities, including polyps, endometritis, and Asherman's syndrome; submucous myomata; first cycle after stopping danazol or oral contraceptives; and progesterone receptor defect. The mechanisms involved in these conditions are discussed elsewhere in considerable detail.[42]

The clinical relevance of a submucous myoma or a septate uterus should be obvious, and emphasizes the necessity of performing a hysterogram with any patient diagnosed by endometrial biopsy to have an out-of-phase endometrial pattern. The diagnosis of endometritis or polyps is easily made by histologic evaluation; alternatively, polyps may be diagnosed by hysterogram, and treated by hysteroscopy or curettage. The history should identify patients who have just discontinued the use of danazol or oral contraceptives who might be expected to have a poorly stimulated endometrial pattern; this finding has led to the recommendation that such patients complete a cycle or two using barrier contraception before attempting pregnancy.

A "dysharmonic luteal phase" has been described in which delayed endometrial maturation is found in conjunction with normal progesterone levels, perhaps due to a delay in the postovulatory rise of progesterone, or a defect in the endometrial progesterone receptor.[43] Of interest, endometrial asynchrony was not incompatible with normal nidation and gestation; 6 cases of successful pregnancy were followed among patients with a dysharmonic luteal phase.

Endometrial inadequacy can be found in the presence of normal progesterone levels. This makes a strong point in favor of using endometrial biopsy, and not hormonal measurements, to diagnose luteal inadequacy: without the biopsy, other significant findings—for example, endometritis—would likely be missed.

Progesterone Inadequacy

Clinicians dealing with a large infertile population have come to recognize that luteal phase endometrial inadequacy can be identified more readily in certain groups of patients, including (1) those with recurrent miscarriage; (2) those who have been treated with clomiphene citrate and other agents to induce ovulation; (3) women with hyperprolactinemia; (4) patients at the extremes of reproductive life (postmenarcheal and perimenopausal); (5) women who undertake long-term, stressful exercise programs; (6) those of low body weight; (7) patients whose infertility is unexplained; (8) those with a long follicular phase; (9) patients with hyperandrogenism of adrenal etiology; (10) women undergoing follicular aspiration (in IVF– gamete–intrafallopian transfer, or GIFT, cycles); and (11) patients with endometriosis, although this last is controversial. Each of these groups will now be discussed.

Recurrent Miscarriage. The frequency of LPI diagnosed by endometrial criteria was 4% in fertile and 12.9% in infertile women, and 28.3% in women with recurrent miscarriage.[32] This last figure compares favorably with 23[44] and 35%[45] reported by two other groups, although less than 67% noted by others.[46] Recurrent abortion is the only condition in which statistical significance could be attached to the diagnosis and treatment of LPI in terms of benefit to the patient.

Treatment with Clomiphene Citrate and Other Ovulation-Induction Agents. Biopsy-proved LPI has been described repeatedly in patients undergoing ovulation stimulation with clomiphene citrate.[41,47] When administered to normally ovulating women, clomiphene induces increased estrogen output and abnormal endometrial biopsy patterns.[47] In anovulatory women, there is no guarantee that the FSH increase induced by clomiphene will result in normal folliculogenesis and corpus luteum function. Luteal phase estradiol levels in clomiphene-treated patients are higher than in nontreated women[48]; such an abnormal estradiol:progesterone ratio could be expected to result in a deranged endometrial pattern.

The endometrial pattern and the frequency of LPI after ovulation induced by clomiphene citrate has been well described, but little information exists about the endometrium when ovulation is induced using other modalities. A short interval from HCG administration to menstruation was noted in gonadotropin-treated patients, but preovulatory estradiol levels did not correlate with the short luteal phase, and neither luteal hormone levels nor endometrial bioposies were taken.[49] Earlier, investigators concluded that endometrial biopsy in gonadotropin-treated cycles led to increased frequency of early abortion[50]; therefore the procedure has not been used to evaluate luteal function in these cycles. Nevertheless, some information suggests that ovarian hyperstimulation with human menopausal gonadotropin (HMG) and human chorionic gonadotropin (HCG) may result in pituitary dysfunction, hyperprolactinemia, and LPI. Elevated prolactin, estradiol, testosterone, and sex hormone-binding globulin levels, and lowered FSH levels, were documented; and pituitary hormone output in response to metoclopramide, thyroid-releasing hormone (TRH), and gonadotropin-releasing hormone (GnRH), were abnormal compared to natural cycles.[51] When normally ovulating women superovulated in response to several different stimulation protocols,[52] including pulsatile pure FSH administered by pump,[53] lower midluteal serum progesterone values and shorter luteal phase correlated with preovulatory estradiol levels; the higher the endogenous estradiol, the shorter the luteal phase.

Hyperprolactinemia. The increased dopamine output in response to hyperprolactinemia can suppress gonadotropin output and alter folliculogenesis by a central mechanism. Prolactin itself has effects on the granulosa cell; it is controversial whether these effects are stimulatory or inhibitory in vivo, but both changes can be observed with varying conditions in vitro.[54,55] Ovulatory patients with hyperprolactinemia may have an increased frequency of deranged endometrial pattern on biopsy; conversely, an out-of-phase biopsy reading dictates the need to document the serum prolactin level.

Primary hypothyroidism is associated with hyperprolactinemia due to prolactin stimulation by the increased TRH. Therefore, in patients who are documented to have LPI by endometrial biopsy, measuring serum prolactin level is always recommended. If elevated, serum TSH should be evaluated.

Extremes of Reproductive Life. Postmenarchal oligomenorrhea is common during the development of normal corpus luteum function. The transition from prepubertal anovulation to normal function includes a period during which progesterone output decreases shortly after menarche and the luteal phase is of short duration.[56] Luteal phase inadequacy, although demonstrable, is ordinarily clinically irrelevant and short lived.

Clinical observation suggests that patients between the ages of approximately 35 and 40 years have a short luteal phase, cycles typically 25 to 26 days in duration, and an increased frequency of LPI. After age 40 years, cycle length is again normal, although in later years a shortened follicular phase may result in a shortened overall cycle.[57]

LPI in Exercising Women. Joggers, runners, marathon runners, ballet dancers, gymnasts, and other individuals who regularly undertake stressful exercise are likely to have LPI if their cycles continue.[58,59] Ordinarily, this is clinically irrelevant, but infertile women who exercise should be considered at risk for the condition.

Low Body Weight. Some women with low body weight who do not exercise regularly may have LPI. This is simply a phase between regular ovulatory menstruation and anovulation, as shown by longitudinal measurements. The only study to approach this question found unexplained infertility in low-weight women.[60]

Unexplained Infertility. Before endometrial biopsy became relatively accepted for diagnosis, several investigators measured serial plasma steroid and gonadotropin levels in ovulatory but infertile women,[61,62] and found subtle abnormalities including decreased progesterone output and abnormal progesterone:estradiol ratios during the luteal phase. The duration of progesterone secretion and the maximum progesterone concentration during the luteal phase were shown to be significantly less in patients with unexplained infertility.[63] The authors were not convinced that the defect was repetitive or responsible for infertility. Subtle abnormalities of follicular development and hormonal profile in women with unexplained infertility were indeed

noted to be repetitive,[64] in contrast to findings by others.[65]

This debate over LPI in unexplained infertility is irrelevant in our view, as all patients undergo endometrial biopsy in the routine infertility evaluation, and no woman's fertility would be diagnosed as unexplained unless she had had a normal inphase biopsy.

Long Follicular Phase. Assuming that a long follicular phase implies some abnormality of folliculogenesis, the question is whether it is associated with abnormalities of luteal function, and if so, when to institute therapy and of what type. Luteal adequacy was documented when follicular phase length, as measured from the first day of menstruation to and including the day of the LH surge, was greater than 16 days, with ovulation intervals of 34 to 40 days.[65,66] No difference was noted in the fertility potential in patients with long cycles,[66] and no abnormality was found in hormone levels measured.[67] When follicular phase duration exceeded 20 days, however, endometrial luteal phase deficiency was 39.4%.[68] In 10 of 13 patients, progesterone levels were totally normal, suggesting that cycles with delayed ovulation have a high frequency of endometrial inadequacy, and that the endometrium is a better indicator of endometrial adequacy than plasma progesterone levels.

Hyperandrogenism of Adrenal Etiology. In hyperandrogenic patients, an inverse ratio was noted between the length of follicular and luteal phases, and the fertility potential appeared to be less in those with a long follicular phase.[69] Previously, the length of the follicular phase was positively associated with hyperandrogenism, and suppression of the condition returned follicular length to normal.[70] Thus the possibility exists that a long follicular phase in association with hyperandrogenism is associated with decreased fertility.

Follicular Aspiration in IVF and GIFT Cycles. A short luteal phase has been noted in cycles of deliberate hyperstimulation, as in IVF and GIFT. Aspiration of the oocyte induces a significant disruption of the integrity of the follicle, with removal of granulosa cells and follicular fluid. Whether LPI in terms of decreased progesterone output is caused by this traumatic occurrence has been investigated with conflicting and controversial results.[71-73] Most agree that progesterone levels are decreased immediately after aspiration and during the luteal phase, and most agree that HCG stimulation increases progesterone output during the luteal phase. No difference in pregnancy rates has been documented with or without intramuscular progesterone administration.[74] Most IVF and GIFT programs, however, support the luteal phase with progesterone administration. Interesting therefore is a publication by authors who sampled the endometrium at the time of embryo transfer and found that the pattern was unpredictable, even showing proliferative endometrium in some biopsies.[75] The finding of a secretory endometrium was most likely to be associated with pregnancy. This traumatic procedure did not exclude viable pregnancy.

Late luteal phase endometrial biopsies, timed to be 9 to 11 days after laparoscopy or 11 to 12 days after HCG administration, were performed in 25 nontransferred patients, and only 6 had in-phase endometrial biopsy patterns.[76] Nineteen (76%) had luteal phase defects ranging from 3 to 7 days, most with immature endometria, while in only 1 was the phase advanced. In this study, women who had significantly higher mean estradiol levels on the day of HCG or LH surge had a total luteal phase that was significantly longer and were more likely to have endometrial biopsies that were in phase. Four of 6 patients with estradiol levels greater than 1,000 pg/mL had in-phase endometrial biopsies, while only 4 (26%) of 15 with out-of-phase biopsies had an estradiol level greater than 1,000 pg/mL on the day of HCG or LH. Therefore the earlier suggestion that elevated estradiol in the preovulatory part of the cycle predisposes to a shorter luteal phase was not confirmed. These results suggest that progesterone support to the endometrium in the luteal phase is necessary in the majority of patients undergoing hyperstimulation for IVF regardless of circulating hormonal levels.

Endometriosis. Pregnanediol output was shown to be lowest early in the luteal phase in patients ultimately diagnosed to have endometriosis, although the decrease was not maintained for the total duration of the luteal phase.[77] Serum progesterone levels were not lower, so the authors postulated that progesterone metabolism was altered.[78] Peripheral vein and ovarian vein progesterone levels were elevated in the follicular phase of the next cycle, suggesting that failure of adequate luteolysis and ovulatory asynchrony were involved in the infertility of mild endometriosis.[79] When endometrial biopsy results were correlated with the diagnosis of mild to severe endometriosis, a higher frequency of abnormal endometrial patterns was not demonstrated.[8,80,81]

FREQUENCY OF LPI

The frequency of LPI depends entirely upon the clinical population sampled, the criteria used for diagnosis, and the rigidity of one's definition. Luteal phase inadequacy was identified in only 3.5% of 550 private patients with primary infertility when the diagnosis was based on the results of two biopsies.[82] When 1,174 endometrial biopsies obtained from 1,084 patients from two institutions were evaluated, 10.9 and 9.6%, respectively, were out of phase.[83] One of the rare studies with a control group[32] found biopsy-proved luteal inadequacy in 1 (4%) of 25 fertile women and in 46 (12.9%) of 355 infertile women (not a significant difference), suggesting that luteal inadequacy may *not* be an important cause of infertility.

Referral bias makes our own frequency figures invalid, and the literature cannot be reviewed adequately to give a true prevalence of repetitive endometrial inadequacy. Although a "best guess" suggests that it may exist as a repetitive entity in about 10% of infertile women, there are reports of 45[84] and 43%.[85] A plea is made for consistency of diagnostic criteria.

DIAGNOSIS OF LPI

Whether the diagnosis of LPI should be sought at all is a major decision to be made by the clinician, since the condition may be completely irrelevant with respect to human infertility. Perhaps only patients at risk for the condition should be screened, although proper diagnosis and appropriate treatment have not altered pregnancy rates in patients with infertility. On the other hand, for women with recurrent miscarriage, diagnosis and treatment of LPI significantly benefit the ultimate pregnancy outcome; clearly, those with two or more early miscarriages should be screened and the diagnosis either made or ruled out.

Diagnostic Approaches

Numerous approaches to diagnosis of LPI have been attempted. Several methods or combinations have been used, but when a particular one is recommended, its efficacy is rarely compared to that of other modalities. Those frequently described include (1) plasma progesterone and estradiol measurements, (2) salivary sex steroid measurements, (3) urinary pregnanediol and total estrogen output, (4) endometrial biopsy, (5) measurement of endometrial estrogen and progesterone receptors, (6) measurement of estradiol dehydrogenase and other enzyme activities, (7) endometrial prolactin and other protein production, (8) basal body temperature chart, (9) pulsatile LH output, and (10) measurement of endometrial thickness by ultrasonography. Discussion of each of these in terms of diagnostic efficacy and clinical utility is beyond the scope of this chapter. Most clinicians use what is readily available, primarily progesterone measurements and endometrial biopsy.

Measurement of Serum Progesterone

Measurement of serum progesterone levels during the luteal phase cannot be used to diagnose LPI because of the pulsatile nature of LH and progesterone output at that time. Although serial progesterone measurements in patients known to have LPI are low,[2] measuring several levels is neither logical nor clinically convenient. Urinary pregnanediol output, collected serially, is shown to be decreased in some patients, but few laboratories are equipped to do this assay, and few patients are likely to cooperate. Salivary progesterone measured daily can be used to diagnose luteal inadequacy, but is inconvenient and requires a special laboratory effort.

Measuring three progesterone levels at 2 to 3-day intervals was suggested as giving convincing evidence of luteal phase inadequacy.[86] Patients with LPI established by endometrial biopsy criteria may not necessarily be identified by the pooling of these three blood levels, however.[2]

Combining a midluteal phase progesterone level with endometrial biopsy evidence has been used, with some indication that the two measurements together may aid in diagnosis.[87,88] Since our patients are rarely seen in the midluteal phase, we have not used this approach, and have no evidence that an additional office visit would substantially change our findings.

Endometrial Biopsy

Dating of the endometrial biopsy has been both recommended[7,9,12,89–92] and condemned as irrelevant[93,94] in the diagnosis of LPI. The concept of dating the endometrium from the *next*, not the *last*, menstrual period was proposed.[34] Seventy-eight percent of secretory phase biopsy specimens were correctly dated, allowing one day of error in interpretation, when histologic assessment was related to basal body temperature. Subsequently, in 1,007 secretory phase biopsies,[95] the results correlated with basal body temperature and the date of subsequent menses within 1 day in 60% and within 2 days in 80%. These figures suggest that perhaps 20% of endometrial biopsies are out of phase on initial determination. In one study,[94] 19% of biopsies were out of phase, with no other values measured to establish luteal phase normalcy. Using progesterone levels for diagnosis failed to detect up to 21.5% of abnormal patterns.[96] This finding has been confirmed.[97] In a referral population, 19% of LPI was diagnosed on the basis of two out-of-phase biopsies.[7]

Thus, although endometrial dating alone is used with confidence by a majority of investigators, its adequacy in diagnosing LPI has been questioned. Most important, several authors[32,93] found no difference in the cumulative pregnancy rate of all infertile patients whether or not endometrial inadequacy was

diagnosed. Only one group[33] established by life table analysis a difference between pregnancy rates in individuals diagnosed to have LPI who responded to treatment, and those who did not respond to progesterone administration. Evidence that diagnosis and treatment are beneficial is convincing in patients who experience recurrent abortion.[12,32,44]

Timing and Technique of Biopsy. Much of the problem with diagnosis appears to revolve around the timing and technique of taking the endometrial biopsy. This is a quite reproducible diagnostic method, and although not quantitative, does indicate the pattern of hormone influence on the endometrial implantation site. The procedure should be performed premenstrually, preferably in relation to temperature elevation, and ideally on the 27th day of a 28-day cycle (or 1 to 2 days before expected menses). The patient is examined to determine uterine position; the uterus may be sounded, but this is not essential if a prior examination for uterine position has been performed. The Novak curette or other instrument is introduced into the endocervical canal, pushed to the fundus, and then turned such that either the anterior or posterior wall may be biopsied. The tissue is taken by a firm and rapid scraping of the curette down the wall of the uterus. It is blown out onto a paper towel (not a gauze square, as it sticks) and examined. It should measure at least 2 cm in length and be cylindric. The tissue must be fixed immediately, as autolysis can occur rapidly.

The biopsy is evaluated by the criteria of Noyes and associates[34] and its histologic dating is recorded. The results cannot be interpreted in relation to the patient's cycle until the date of her next menstrual period is known, which is arbitrarily called day 28. Because a biopsy taken 2 days before the onset of the next period should appear similar in all women, the time of the next period is then the reference date, and the patient is instructed to report the first day of her next menstrual period so that the biopsy can be interpreted. Since day 28 has been assigned as the day of menstruation, a biopsy obtained 2 days before the menses should have the appearance of secretory day 26 endometrium.

Histologic dating is simple if the biopsy is taken within 2 to 3 days of the next menstrual period. At ideal day 23, periarteriolar cuffing is seen, which at day 24 extends out from the vessels. At ideal day 25, the pseudodecidual pattern is first seen under the surface epithelium or capsule, and develops over the next several days until it encompasses the whole subcapsular area. Glands may be hypersecretory or lined with flattened epithelium. The sweeping decidual pattern is qualitative evidence of adequate progesterone stimulation.

To make the diagnosis of LPI, the biopsy date

must be out of phase by 2 days or more from the expected date as judged from the next menstrual period; for example, secretory day 23 or 24 on ideal day 26. Thus, the dating of the endometrium depends on the onset of the next menstrual period, and the diagnosis and dating are both unrelated to the onset of the previous menstrual period and, for all practical purposes, the time of ovulation, which may be difficult to judge.

TREATMENT OF LPI

Treatment of LPI can be either by stimulating hormone output or by substituting for the deficiency. The first translates to an attempt to improve folliculogenesis, realizing that corpus luteum function is predetermined by follicular events. The second is to change the abnormal pattern of endometrial development by supplementation with progesterone.

If the etiology of LPI can be identified, this should be treated first, followed by documentation that the treatment corrected the defect. For example, if hyperprolactinemia due to hypothyroidism if found, treatment of the hypothyroidism should result in a return to normal prolactin levels and resumption of normal ovulatory in-phase cycles. If a long follicular phase is associated with deranged follicular development and subsequent luteal inadequacy, follicular stimulation might be improved by therapy with clomiphene citrate, and the resultant increased FSH should result in normalization of LPI.

There should be no paradox in the observation that clomiphene citrate can both improve and induce LPI. When the agent is given to induce ovulation in oligoovulatory or anovulatory patients, the subsequent hormonal output may not be entirely normal, and in fact is reflected by a high frequency of LPI. This induced endometrial abnormality can be treated by increasing the dosage of clomiphene, which may increase FSH stimulation, enhance folliculogenesis, and normalize the hormonal output. This approach may result in diminishing returns, however, as too high a dosage of clomiphene may have significant antiestrogenic effects[98] and fail to correct, or even worsen, the LPI.

In patients with hyperprolactinemia-induced ovulatory dysfunction, bromocriptine is the treatment of choice. Patients with a significantly deformed endometrial cavity, with submucous myomata, or with exposure to diethylstilbestrol who may have an abnormal endometrial pattern because of the anatomic defect, may be helped by a surgical approach. Polyps, endometritis, Asherman's syndrome, and perhaps an infectious process such as *Mycoplasma* or *Ureaplasma* infection should all be treated by the appropriate modality, as there is no reason to expect

that the endometrial derangement will be improved by progesterone supplementation.

We have tended to use progesterone supplementation as the treatment of choice in carefully selected patients, that is, those who have no clearly diagnosable cause of LPI. Additional criteria for progesterone supplementation are (1) age below 35 years, (2) normal follicular phase length, (3) normoprolactinemia, and (4) a normal hysterogram. Progesterone supplementation administered to such patients usually results in correction of the endometrial inadequacy, ordinarily at a dosage of 25 mg twice daily. For patients who do not fulfill the strict criteria, clomiphene citrate or some other approach to correcting the cause of LPI is appropriate.

Progesterone Supplementation

Plasma progesterone levels obtained after vaginal, rectal, or intramuscular administration are comparable to those seen during the normal luteal phase.[99] Synthetic progestins have been used in the treatment of LPI, but in the United States they are not cleared for use in pregnancy. Therefore dehydrogesterone (Duphaston), which has been evaluated thoroughly,[100-102] and other preparations containing synthetic progestins do not offer a therapeutic alternative.

For successful therapy of a luteal phase defect, an accurate basal temperature recording is needed to determine proper timing of the onset of supplementation. If progesterone is begun too early, it may block ovulation, and the elevated oral temperature it maintains may be misinterpreted as an early pregnancy. Successful therapy must be begun in the cycle in which ovulation is related to the pregnancy, because normal endometrial development is required to allow normal implantation and maintenance of an early pregnancy. Especially in patients with recurrent miscarriage, therapy begun after missed menses is inadequate and does not reliably prevent implantation failure.

Progesterone Suppositories. Substitution therapy using progesterone vaginal suppositories is our primary approach because of its simplicity, lack of complications, and good results. The patient should begin substitution after at least 3 days of temperature rise (for most patients) above 97.8°F. Therapy should be continued until menses, and ordinarily menstruation is not delayed. An occasional patient will have a persistently elevated temperature in the follicular part of her cycle, which does not drop to low levels until shortly before ovulation; therefore it is then only after basal temperature has risen.

Correction of the defect must be documented by endometrial biopsy in the first treatment cycle. At least 13% of patients will have a persistent defect despite treatment.[12] If the defect persists, a higher progesterone dose or an alternative treatment approach may be required.

Oral Progesterone. The use of an oral progesterone preparation has been investigated over the years as to its efficacy in the treatment of various gynecologic disorders. Several formulations of micronized progesterone are absorbed rapidly, but also are metabolized so rapidly that frequent dosing appears to be necessary. Most studies[103-105] have investigated oral progesterone absorption and metabolism in postmenopausal women. Progesterone in a dosage of 100 to 200 mg orally every 8 to 12 hours can result in an increase in circulating progesterone, but a comparative study during the follicular phase in ovulatory women showed that absorption was better in rectal than in sublingual, oral, and vaginal routes of administration.[106] Response is extremely varied, which might be expected to be reflected at the endometrial level. The bioeffects of oral or sublingual progesterone administration at the level of the endometrium must be studied carefully before this formulation can be recommended to replace suppositories for the therapy of LPI.

Pure FSH

In 1976 Wilks and co-workers[107] concluded that inappropriate FSH:LH ratios during the follicular phase of the menstrual cycle could result in impaired corpus luteum function. Pure FSH might therefore be useful in the treatment of LPI by correcting the problem at its etiology or source. An FSH-rich gonadotropin preparation (3:1 FSH:LH) was used to reverse the negative effects of porcine follicular fluid, which contains inhibin, on folliculogenesis in the monkey.[108] Later, 15 women were treated with pure FSH for 45 cycles, which resulted in improved endometrial biopsy pattern in 20 of 38 cycles.[109]

Although this application of FSH may be effective, it appears to be an arduous and expensive approach to treating an entity that may be clinically irrelevant.

LPI AND PREGNANCY

There is no disagreement that progesterone is needed during the luteal phase to induce a secretory endometrial change and to maintain early pregnancy. It was shown that luteectomy performed 19 days after missed menses resulted uniformly in abortion, which could be entirely prevented by progesterone supplementation alone (estrogen supplementation did not work, and estrogen was not necessary as progesterone alone would maintain the pregnancy).[110]

From a theoretical standpoint, if the endo-metrium is normal in pattern, implantation can occur, and corpus luteum function should be stimulated by increasing HCG. Progesterone supplementation might then be discontinued at the time of a positive pregnancy test. Generally, however, patients who have the diagnosis of LPI and who have been treated with progesterone supplementation are unwilling to discontinue the supplementation until fetal heart activity is seen on ultrasound.

The debate continues as to the effects of sex hormones in early pregnancy. At present, the Food and Drug Administration has not cleared progesterone as supplementation during the luteal phase and in pregnancy. A review of the Johns Hopkins experience revealed no undue frequency of congenital anomalies, and the establishment of a progesterone registry was recommended.[111] As progesterone is likely to be administered as a luteal supplement in all patients undergoing IVF and GIFT attempts, this appears even more important. Several other studies have subsequently confirmed these findings,[112-115] and the debate from an epidemiologic standpoint continues.[116-121]

Progesterone is a potent antiandrogen that could induce an antiandrogenic effect on the male genitourinary tract, resulting in developmental errors such as hypospadias. It was observed that maternal progestin therapy could be a cause of hypospadias.[122] Progesterone itself was not on the list of agents associated with hypospadias, although hydroxyprogesterone caproate and medroxyprogesterone acetate both were. Others[123] were unable to verify these data; in a sample of 3,602 male newborns, of whom 33 were found to have hypospadias, only 8 had been exposed to progestins, which was not a significant proportion. The circulating progesterone levels achieved by supplementation using progesterone suppositories 25 mg twice daily are significantly less than are achieved later in pregnancy from placental output alone. Clearly, the possibility of inducing hypospadias with levels of progesterone as administered is small.

CONCLUSION

The clinical relevance of LPI remains, at best, controversial. Although it can be diagnosed, whether it needs to be diagnosed is another question. Only consistency in diagnosis and treatment will permit these questions and doubts to be resolved.

REFERENCES

1. Jones GS, Wentz AC: The structure and function of the corpus luteum. *Clin Obstet Gynaecol* 3:43, 1976.
2. Jones GS, Aksel S, Wentz AC: Serum progesterone values in the luteal phase defects. Effect of chorionic gonadotropin. *Obstet Gynecol* 44:26, 1974.

3. Wentz AC: Treatment of luteal phase defects. *J Reprod Med* 18:159, 1977.

4. Wentz AC: Physiologic and clinical considerations in luteal phase defects. *Clin Obstet Gynecol* 22:169, 1979.

5. Wentz AC: Pathophysiology of luteal phase inadequacy, in Tozzini R, Reeves G, Pineda RI (eds): *Endocrine Physiopathology of the Ovary*. Amsterdam, Elsevier Biomedical, 1980.

6. Wentz AC: Progesterone therapy of the inadequate luteal phase, in Givens JR (ed): *Clinical Use of Sex Steroids*. Chicago, Year Book, 1980.

7. Wentz AC: Endometrial biopsy in the evaluation of infertility. *Fertil Steril* 33:121, 1980.

8. Wentz AC: Premenstrual spotting: Its association with endometriosis but not luteal phase inadequacy. *Fertil Steril* 33:605, 1980.

9. Wentz AC: Diagnosing luteal phase inadequacy. *Fertil Steril* 37:334, 1982.

10. Wentz AC: Progesterone therapy of the inadequate luteal phase. *Curr Probl Obstet Gynecol* 6:1, 1982.

11. Wentz AC, Martens P, Wilroy RS Jr: Luteal phase inadequacy and a chromosomal anomaly in recurrent abortion. *Fertil Steril* 41:142, 1984.

12. Wentz AC, Herbert CH, Maxson WS, Garner CH: Outcome of progesterone treatment of luteal phase inadequacy. *Fertil Steril* 41:856, 1984.

13. Wentz AC, Herbert CM, Maxson WS, Hill GA, Pittaway DE: Cycle of conception endometrial biopsy. *Fertil Steril* 46:196, 1986.

14. Wentz AC: Luteal phase inadequacy, in Behrman SJ, Kistner RW (eds): *Progress in Infertility*. Boston, Little, Brown, 1987.

15. Daly DC, Maslar IA, Rosenberg SM, Tohan N, Riddick DH: Prolactin production by luteal phase defect endometrium. *Am J Obstet Gynecol* 140:587, 1981.

16. Ying YK, Walters CA, Kuslis S, et al: Prolactin production by explants of normal, luteal phase defective, and corrected luteal phase defective late secretory endometrium. *Am J Obstet Gynecol* 151:801, 1985.

17. Joshi SG, Rao R, Henriques EE, Raikar RS, Gordon M: Luteal phase concentrations of progestagen-associated endometrial protein (PEP) in the serum of cycling women with adequate or inadequate endometrium. *J Clin Endocrinol Metab* 63:1247, 1986.

18. Jones GES: Some newer aspects of the management of infertility. *JAMA* 141:1123, 1949.

19. Ross GT: Preovulatory determinants of human corpus luteum function. *Eur J Obstet Gynecol Reprod Biol* 6:147, 1976.

20. McNatty KP: Follicular determinants of corpus luteum function in the human ovary, in Channing CP, Marsh JM, Sadler WA (eds): *Ovarian Follicular and Corpus Luteum Function*. New York, Plenum, 1979.

21. Koos RD, Hansel W: The large and small cells of the bovine corpus luteum: Ultrastructural and functional differences, in Schwartz NB (ed): *Dynamics of Ovarian Function*. New York, Raven, 1981.

22. Fitz TA, Mayan MH, Sawyer HR, Niswender GD: Characterization of two steroidogenic cells types in the ovine corpus luteum. *Biol Reprod* 27:703, 1982.

23. Hoyer PB, Fitz TA, Niswender GD: Hormone-independent activation of adenylate cyclase in large steroidogenic ovine luteal cells does not result in increased progesterone secretion. *Endocrinology* 114:604, 1984.

24. Fitz TA, Mock EJ, Mayan MH, Niswender GD: Interactions of prostaglandins with subpopulations of ovine luteal cells. II. Inhibitory effects of PGE_{2a} and protection by PGE_2. *Prostaglandins* 28:127, 1984.

25. Alila HW, Hansel W: Origin of different cell types in the bovine corpus luteum as characterized by specific monoclonal antibodies. *Biol Reprod* 31:1015, 1984.

26. Rodgers RJ, O'Shea JD, Findlay JK: Do small and large luteal cells of the sheep interact in the production of progesterone? *J Reprod Fertil* 75:85, 1985.

27. Rodgers RJ, O'Shea JD, Findlay JK, Flint APF, Sheldrick EL: Large luteal cells the source of luteal oxytocin in the sheep. *Endocrinology* 113:2302, 1983.

28. Mori T, Nihnobu K, Takeuchi S, Onho Y, Tojo S: Interrelation between luteal cell types in steroidogenesis in vitro of human corpus luteum. *J Steroid Biochem* 19:811, 1983.

29. Wilks JW, Noble AS: Steroidogenic responsiveness of the monkey corpus luteum to exogenous chorionic gonadotropin. *Endocrinology* 113:1256, 1983.

30. Hutchison JS, Zeleznik AJ: The corpus luteum of the primate menstrual cycle is capable of recovering from a transient withdrawal of pituitary gonadotropin support. *Endocrinology* 1117:1043, 1985.

31. Hutchison JS, Kubik CJ, Nelson PB, Zeleznik AJ: Estrogen induces premature luteal regression in rhesus monkeys during spontaneous menstrual cycles, but not in cycles driven by exogenous gonadotropin-releasing hormone. *Endocrinology* 121:466, 1987.

32. Balasch J, Creus M, Marquez M, Burzaco I, Vanrell JA: The significance of luteal phase deficiency on fertility: a diagnostic and therapeutic approach. *Hum Reprod* 1:145, 1986.

33. Daly DC, Walters CA, Soto-Albors CE, Riddick DH: Endometrial biopsy during treatment of luteal phase defects is predictive of therapeutic outcome. *Fertil Steril* 40:305, 1983.

34. Noyes RW, Hertig AT, Rock J: Dating the endometrial biopsy. *Fertil Steril* 1:3, 1950.

35. Strott CA, Cargille CM, Ross GT, Lipsett MB: The short luteal phase. *J Clin Endocrinol* 30:246, 1970.

36. Sherman BM, Korenman SG: Measurement of plasma LH, FSH, estradiol and progesterone in disorders of the human menstrual cycle: the short luteal phase. *J Clin Endocrinol Metab* 38:89, 1974.

37. Smith SK, Lenton EA, Cooke ID: Plasma gonadotropin and ovarian steroid concentrations in women with menstrual cycles with short luteal phase. *J Reprod Fertil* 75:363, 1985.

38. Smith SK, Lenton EA, Landgren BM, Cooke ID: The short luteal phase and infertility. *Br J Obstet Gynaecol* 91:1120, 1984.

39. Moraes-Ruehsen MD, Jones GS, Burnett LS: The aluteal cycle. *Am J Obstet Gynecol* 103:1059, 1969.

40. Aksel S, Wiebe RH, Tyson JE, Jones GS: Hormonal findings associated with aluteal cycles. *Obstet Gynecol* 48:598, 1976.

41. Garcia J, Jones GS, Wentz AC: The use of clomiphene citrate. *Fertil Steril* 28:707, 1977.

42. Wentz AC: Luteal phase inadequacy, in Behrman SJ, Kistner RW (eds): *Progress in Infertility*. Boston, Little, Brown, 1987.

43. Zorn JR, Cedard L, Nessman C, Savale M: Delayed endometrial maturation in women with normal progesterone levels. *Gynecol Obstet Invest* 17:157, 1984.

44. Tho PT, Byrd JR, McDonough PG: Etiologies and subsequent reproductive performance of 100 couples with recurrent abortion. *Fertil Steril* 32:389, 1979.

45. Jones GES, Delfs E: Endocrine patterns in term pregnancies following abortion. *JAMA* 146:1212, 1951.

46. Grant A, McBride WG, Moyes JM: Luteal phase defects in abortion. *Int J Fertil* 4:323, 1959.

47. Cook CL, Schroeder JA, Yussman MA, Sanfilippo JS: Induction of luteal phase defect with clomiphene citrate. *Am J Obstet Gynecol* 149:613, 1984.

48. Taubert HD, Dericks-Tan JSE: High doses of estrogens do not interfere with the ovulation-inducing effect of clomiphene citrate. *Fertil Steril* 27:375, 1976.

49. Olson JL, Rebar RW, Schreiber JR, Vaitukaitis JL: Shortened luteal phase after ovulation induction with human menopausal gonadotropin and human chorionic gonadotropin. *Fertil Steril* 39:284, 1983.

50. Jacobson A, Marshall JR: Detrimental effect of endometrial biopsies on pregnancy rate following human menopausal gonadotropin/human chorionic gonadotropin-induced ovulation. *Fertil Steril* 33:602, 1980.

51. Martikainen H, Ronnberg L, Ruokonen A, Kauppila A: Anterior pituitary dysfunction during the luteal phase following ovarian hyperstimulation. *Fertil Steril* 47:446, 1987.

52. Messinis JE, Templeton A, Baird DT: Luteal phase after ovarian hyperstimulation. *Br J Obstet Gynaecol* 94:345, 1987.

53. Messinis IE, Templeton AA: Disparate effects of endogenous and exogenous oestradiol on luteal phase function in women. *J Reprod Fertil* 79:549, 1987.

54. Hunter MG: Prolactin stimulates steroidogenesis by human luteal tissue in vitro. *J Endocrinol* 103:107, 1984.

55. Lee MS, Ben-Rafael Z, Meloni F, Mastroianni L Jr, Flickinger GL: Effects of prolactin on steroidogenesis by human luteinized granulosa cells. *Fertil Steril* 56:32, 1986.

56. Apter D, Raisanen I, Ylostoalo P, Vihko R: Follicular growth in relation to serum hormonal patterns in adolescent compared with adult menstrual cycles. *Fertil Steril* 47:82, 1987.

57. Sherman BM, West JH, Korenman SG: The menopausal transition: analysis of LH, FSH, estradiol, and progesterone concentrations during menstrual cycles of older women. *J Clin Endocrinol Metab* 42:629, 1976.

58. Loucks AB, Horvath SM: Athletic amenorrhea: A review. *Med Sci Sports Exerc* 17:56, 1985.

59. Ellison PT, Lager C: Moderate recreational running is associated with lowered salivary progesterone profiles in women. *Am J Obstet Gynecol* 154:1000, 1986.

60. Bates GW, Bates SR, Whitworth NS: Reproductive failure in women who practice weight control. *Fertil Steril* 37:373, 1982.

61. Cooke ID, Lenton EA, Adams M, et al: Some clinical aspects of pituitary–ovarian relationships in women with ovulatory infertility. *J Reprod Fertil* 51:203, 1977.

62. Lenton EA, Adams M, Cooke ID: Plasma steroid and gonadotropin profiles in ovulatory but infertile women. *Clin Endocrinol* 8:241, 1978.

63. Driessen F, Kremer J, Alsbach GPJ, deKroon RA: Serum progesterone and oestradiol concentrations in women with unexplained infertility. *Br J Obstet Gynaecol* 87:619, 1980.

64. Lewinthal D, Furman A, Glankstein J, et al: Subtle abnormalities in follicular development and hormonal profile in women with unexplained infertility. *Fertil Steril* 46:833, 1986.

65. Polan ML, Totora M, Caldwell BV, et al: Abnormal ovarian cycles as diagnosed by ultrasound and serum estradiol levels. *Fertil Steril* 37:342, 1982.

66. Broom TJ, Matthews CD, Cooke ID, et al: Endocrine profiles and infertility status of human menstrual cycles of varying follicular phase length. *Fertil Steril* 36:194, 1981.

67. Aksel S: Hormonal characteristics of long cycles in fertile women. *Fertil Steril* 36:521, 1981.

68. Balasch J, Creus M, Vanrell JA: Luteal function after delayed ovulation. *Fertil Steril* 45:342, 1986.

69. Rodriguez-Rigau LJ, Shenoi PN, Smith KD, Steinberger E: The relationship between the lengths of the follicular and luteal phases of the menstrual cycle and the fertility potential of the female. *Fertil Steril* 39:856, 1983.

70. Rodriguez-Rigau LJ, Smith KD, Tcholakian RK, Steinberger E: Effect of prednisone on plasma testosterone levels and on duration of phases of the menstrual cycle in hyperandrogenic women. *Fertil Steril* 32:408, 1979.

71. Vargyas J, Kletzky O, Marrs RP: The effect of laparoscopic follicular aspiration on ovarian steroidogenesis during the early preimplantation period. *Fertil Steril* 45:221, 1986.

72. Taylor PJ, Trounson A, Besanko M, Burger HG, Stockdale J: Plasma progesterone and prolactin changes in superovulated women before, during, and immediately after laparoscopy for in vitro fertilization and their relation to pregnancy. *Fertil Steril* 45:680, 1986.

73. Huang KE, Muechler EK, Schwarz KR, Goggin M, Graham MC: Serum progesterone levels in women treated with human menopausal gonadotropin and human chorionic gonadotropin for in vitro fertilization. *Fertil Steril* 46:903, 1986.

74. Leeton J, Trounson A, Jessup D: Support of the luteal phase in in vitro fertilization programs: results of a controlled trial with intramuscular proluton. *J IVF/ET* 2:166, 1985.

75. Abate V, DeCorato R, Cali A, Stinchi A: Endometrial biopsy at the time of embryo transfer: Correlation of histological diagnosis with therapy and pregnancy rate. *J IVF/ET* 4:173, 1987.

76. Graf MJ: Histologic evaluation of the luteal phase in women following follicle aspiration for oocyte retrieval. *Fertil Steril* 49:616, 1987.

77. Cheesman KL, Ben-Nun I, Chatterton RT Jr, Cohen MR: Relationship of luteinizing hormone, pregnanediol-3-glucuronide, and estriol-16-glucuronide in urine of infertile women with endometriosis. *Fertil Steril* 38:542, 1982.

78. Cheesman KL, Cheesman SD, Chatterton RT Jr, Cohen MR: Alterations in progesterone metabolism and luteal function in infertile women with endometriosis. *Fertil Steril* 40:590, 1983.

79. Ayers JWT, Birenbaum DL, Menon RKJ: Luteal phase dysfunction in endometriosis: Elevated progesterone levels in peripheral and ovarian veins during the follicular phase. *Fertil Steril* 47:925, 1987.

80. Pittaway DE, Maxson WS, Daniell J, Herbert C, Wentz AC: Luteal phase defects in infertility patients with endometriosis. *Fertil Steril* 39:712, 1983.

81. Balasch J, Vanrell JA: Mild endometriosis and luteal function. *Int J Fertil* 30:4, 1985.

82. Jones GS, Pourmand K: An evaluation of etiologic factors and therapy in 555 private patients with primary infertility. *Fertil Steril* 13:398, 1962.

83. Wild RA, Sanfilippo JS, Toledo AA: Endometrial biopsy in the infertility investigation. The experience at two institutions. *J Reprod Med* 31:954, 1986.

84. Huang KE: The primary treatment of luteal phase inadequacy: progesterone versus clomiphene citrate. *Am J Obstet Gynecol* 155:824, 1986.

85. Cumming DC, Honore LH, Scott JZ, Williams KP: The late luteal phase in infertile women: Comparison of simultaneous endometrial biopsy and progesterone levels. *Fertil Steril* 43:715, 1985.

86. Abraham GE, Maroulis GB, Marshall JR: Evaluation of ovulation and corpus luteum function using measurements of plasma progesterone. *Obstet Gynecol* 44:522, 1974.

87. Cook CL, Rao CV, Yussman MA: Plasma gonadotropin and sex steroid hormone levels during early, midfollicular, and midluteal phases of women with luteal phase defects. *Fertil Steril* 40:45, 1983.

88. Shangold M, Berkeley A, Gray J: Both midluteal serum progesterone levels and late luteal endometrial histology should be assessed in all infertile women. *Fertil Steril* 40:627, 1983.

89. Soules MR, Wiebe RH, Aksel S, Hammond CB: The diagnosis and therapy of luteal phase deficiency. *Fertil Steril* 28:1033, 1977.

90. Rosenfeld DL, Chudow S, Bronson RA: Diagnosis of luteal phase inadequacy. *Obstet Gynecol* 56:193, 1980.

91. Balasch J, Vanrell JA, Creus M, Marquez M, Gonzalez-Merlo J: The endometrial biopsy for diagnosis of luteal phase deficiency. *Fertil Steril* 44:699, 1985.

92. Annos T, Thompson I, Taymor ML: Luteal phase deficiency and infertility: Difficulties encountered in diagnosis and treatment. *Obstet Gynecol* 55:705, 1980.

93. Driessen F, Holwerda PJ, Putte SCJ, Kremer J: The significance of dating an endometrial biopsy for the prognosis of the infertile couple. *Int J Fertil* 25:112, 1980.

94. Johannisson E, Parker RA, Landgren BM, Diczfalusy E: Morphometric analysis of the human endometrium in relation to peripheral hormone levels. *Fertil Steril* 38:564, 1982.

95. Noyes R, Haman JO: Accuracy of endometrial dating: Correlation of endometrial dating with basal body temperature and menses. *Fertil Steril* 4:504, 1953.

96. Balasch J, Vanrell JA, Marzuez M, Rivera F, Gonzalez-Merlo J: Luteal phase in infertility: Problems of evaluation. *Int J Fertil* 27:60, 1982.

97. Rosenfeld DL, Garcia CR: A comparison of endometrial histology with simultaneous plasma progesterone determinations in infertile women. *Fertil Steril* 27:1256, 1976.

98. Maxson WS, Pittaway DE, Herbert CM, Garner CH, Wentz AC: Antiestrogenic effect of clomiphene citrate: Correlation with serum estradiol concentrations. *Fertil Steril* 42:356, 1984.

99. Nillius VJ, Johansson EDB: Plasma levels of progesterone. *Am J Obstet Gynecol* 110:470, 1971.

100. Balasch J, Vanrell JA, Rivera F, Gonzalez-Merlo J: The effect of postovulatory administration of dehydrogesterone on plasma progesterone levels. *Fertil Steril* 34:21, 1980.

101. Balasch J, Vanrell JA, Marquez M, Burzaco I, Gonzalez-Merlo J: Dehydrogesterone versus vaginal progesterone in the treatment of the endometrial luteal phase deficiency. *Fertil Steril* 37:751, 1982.

102. Balasch J, Vanrell JA, Marquez M, Gonzalez-Merlo J: Dehydrogesterone treatment of endometrial luteal phase deficiency after ovulation induced by clomiphene citrate and human chorionic gonadotropin. *Fertil Steril* 40:469, 1983.

103. Whitehead MI, Townsend PT, Gill DK, Collins WP, Campbell S: Absorption and metabolism of oral progesterone. *Br Med J* 280:825, 1980.

104. Maxson WS, Hargrove JT: Bioavailability of oral micronized progesterone. *Fertil Steril* 44:622, 1985.

105. Padwick ML, Endacott J, Matson C, Whitehead ML: Absorption and metabolism of oral progesterone when administered twice daily. *Fertil Steril* 46:402, 1986.

106. Chakmakjian ZH, Zachariah NY: Bioavailability of progesterone with different modes of administration. *J Reprod Med* 32:443, 1987.

107. Wilks JW, Hodgen GD, Ross GT: Luteal phase defects in the rhesus monkey: The significance of serum FSH:LH ratios. *J Clin Endocrinol Metab* 43:1261, 1976.

108. DiZerega GS, Hodgen GD: Follicular phase treatment of luteal phase dysfunction. *Fertil Steril* 35:428, 1981.

109. Huang KE, Muechler EK, Bonfiglio TA: Follicular phase treatment of luteal phase defect with follicle-stimulating hormone in infertile women. *Obstet Gynecol* 64:32, 1984.

110. Csapo AI, Pulkkinen M: Indispensability of the human corpus luteum in the maintenance of early pregnancy luteectomy evidence. *Obstet Gynecol Surv* 22:69, 1978.

111. Rock JA, Wentz AC, Cole KA, et al: Fetal malformations following progesterone therapy during pregnancy: A preliminary report. *Fertil Steril* 44:17, 1985.

112. Resseguie LJ, Hick JF, Bruen JA, et al: Congenital malformations among offspring exposed in utero to progestins, Olmsted County, MN, 1936–1974. *Fertil Steril* 43:514, 1985.

113. Katz Z, Lancet M, Skornik J, et al: Teratogenicity of progestogens given during the first trimester of pregnancy. *Obstet Gynecol* 65:775, 1985.

114. Check JH, Rankin A, Teichman M: The risk of fetal anomalies as a result of progesterone therapy during pregnancy. *Fertil Steril* 45:575, 1986.

115. Wiseman RA, Dodds-Smith IC: Cardiovascular birth defects and antenatal exposure to female sex hormones: A reevaluation of some base data. *Teratology* 30:359, 1984.

116. Oakley GP: Comment: Teratogenicity of progestational agents. *Teratology* 29:131, 1984.

117. Nora JJ, Nora AH: Teratogenicity of progestational agents: Comments on Dr. Ferencz's paper. *Teratology* 29:133, 1984.

118. Ferencz C: Teratogenicity of progestational agents: Response to the Drs. Nora. *Teratology* 29:135, 1984.

119. Wilson PD: Sample size and power in case-control studies: Response to the Drs. Nora. *Teratology* 29:137, 1984.

120. Nora JJ: Teratogenicity of progestational agents: Comments on Dr. Schardein's paper. *Teratology* 29:139, 1984.

121. Schardein JL: Teratogenicity of progestational agents: Response to Dr. Nora. *Teratology* 29:145, 1984.

122. Aarskog D: Maternal progestins as a possible cause of hypospadias. *N Engl J Med* 300:75, 1979.

123. Mau G: Progestins during pregnancy and hypospadias. *Teratology* 24:285, 1981.

CHAPTER 7

Prolactin Disorders in Infertility

Richard E. Blackwell, R. Jeffrey Chang, and Jeffrey R. Cragun

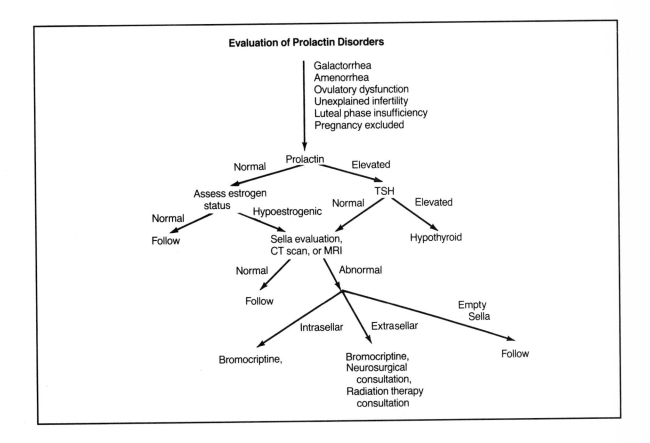

The association of hyperprolactinemia and suboptimal reproductive function has long been recognized in both animals and humans. In the earliest accounts it was noted that lactating mammals failed to conceive as long as intermittent suckling persisted. In 1855, several women with puerperal atrophy of the uterus, amenorrhea, and persistent lactation were reported in the literature. This condition was redescribed in 1882 and bears the name Chiari-Frommel syndrome. In 1953 a second syndrome was described by Argonz and del Castillo, which was characterized by estrogen insufficiency, galactorrhea, and decreased urinary estrogen levels. One year later Albright and Forbes reported the clinical association of galactorrhea, amenorrhea, and low urinary follicle-stimulating hormone levels as a syndrome that bears their names. Although the measurement of human prolactin could not be accomplished until 1972, we now know that these disruptions in reproduction function can occur in association with abnormal release of this hormone.

PHYSIOLOGY OF PROLACTIN SECRETION

Hypothalamic–Pituitary Axis

Historically, prolactin was considered to be unique compared to other anterior pituitary hormones in that its release was governed primarily by an inhibitory influence from the hypothalamus. This concept arose from studies that demonstrated persistent prolactin secretion when the pituitary gland was transplanted in vivo to a site removed from the base of the brain or maintained in organ culture.[1] It has been thought that a single prolactin-inhibitory factor served as the sole regulator of prolactin secretion. Despite many attempts, however, no such factor has been isolated from the hypothalamus.

Instead, prolactin seems to be regulated by a host of chemical signals, both inhibitory and stimulatory, that interact at all levels of the hypothalamic–pituitary axis. The principal inhibitory agent appears to be dopamine. This neurotransmitter inhibits prolactin secretion promptly in vitro and in vivo.[2,3] In vivo studies in the rat demonstrated that dopamine produced in the median eminence and secreted into the hypothalamic portal vessels accounts for most of the inhibition. These conclusions were reached after dopamine was measured in hypophyseal portal blood. Subsequently, those concentrations were simulated by infusing similar levels of dopamine into animals that had been pretreated with an inhibitor of dopamine synthesis, α-methylparatyrasine. Seventy percent of prolactin secretion could be blocked in animals with such pretreatment; the remaining 30% appeared to rise from the neurophypophyseal lobe. Such studies were confirmed in monkeys but not in humans.[4]

Further evidence for dopamine as a principal regulator of prolactin secretion stems from suckling experiments in monkeys and rats. A brief decrease in exogenous dopamine infusion in primates leads to a large increase in prolactin secretion. In the rat, a similar small decrease in hypothalamic dopamine secretion can be observed during simulated suckling[5,6]; however, this results in a limited increase of prolactin. Whether or not the transient decline of dopamine is sufficient to account for the suckling-induced prolactin rise is unclear.

At a cellular level, dopamine appears to act on lactotropes by way of both cyclic adenosine 3′,5′-monophosphate (cAMP) and calcium-dependent mechanisms. High-affinity dopamine receptors have been demonstrated on lactotrope membranes, and after establishment of the dopamine receptor complex, the inhibition of adenyl cyclase is thought to occur.[7] Such inhibition brings about a reduction in cAMP production in calcium-dependent prolactin release. Furthermore, it has been demonstrated that dopamine inhibits prolactin synthesis at transcription, and this effect is amplified by cAMP.

A second agent that may play a role in inhibiting prolactin secretion is gamma-aminobutyric acid (GABA). It has been shown that GABA is secreted into the portal blood, and receptors for GABA have been located on pituitary lactotropes.[8] The inhibitory effect of dopamine is far greater than that of GABA, and it has been suggested that these two agents serve different inhibitory functions within the lactotrope. For example, dopamine induces the storage of newly synthesized prolactin, which may be rapidly released after the withdrawal of dopamine. Such a response is not seen with GABA.

Although the major control of prolactin secretion appears to be one of inhibition, several factors can bring about the short-term release of this hormone. These include thyrotropin-releasing hormone (TRH),[9] vasoactive intestinal polypeptide (VIP),[10] and angiotensin II (Ang II).[11] TRH has been shown to stimulate both synthesis and release of prolactin in in-vitro and in-vivo systems. As a potent stimulator of prolactin release in primates, TRH also provokes a concomitant release of thyroid-stimulating hormone (TSH), and the circulating levels of both T3 and T4 modify the response. Despite this apparent obligatory interaction, prolactin secretion may occur independent of that of TSH. For example, the short-term release of prolactin after suckling is not accompanied by an increase in TSH secretion.[12] Therefore, while under certain clinical circumstances TRH might function as a prolactin-releasing factor, it has a relatively minor role in the normal physiologic control of prolactin.

Vasoactive intestinal polypeptide, purified from porcine duodenum, is a 28-amino-acid polypeptide present throughout the nervous system. This hormone has been measured in hypothalamic portal blood samples and its release appears to be prostaglandin mediated.[13] Studies have demonstrated that VIP may be produced by the pituitary gland. Although a precise role has not been defined, it has been proposed that VIP may serve as an intrahypophyseal regulator of prolactin secretion.

Angiotensin II has also been shown to stimulate prolactin release both in vivo and in vitro. That Ang II receptors are found on lactotropes implies a direct action.[14] Ang II is an octapeptide that has been identified throughout the brain; its injection brings about a rapid release of prolactin that is, in fact, of far greater magnitude than that produced by TRH. This response has been blocked by the Ang II antagonist saralasin.

Several other transmitters appear to be involved in the control of prolactin secretion. Administration of serotonin precursors caused a significant increase in prolactin level, while the administration of cyproheptadine, a serotonin antagonist, blocked the pro-lactin-releasing effect of these precursors.[15] It has been proposed that endogenous opioids modify prolactin secretion by inhibiting dopamine turnover and release. Histamine, a hypothalamic neurotransmitter, has been shown to stimulate prolactin release by binding H_1 receptors, and to inhibit prolactin release through H_2 receptor interaction. Both neurotensin, a tridecapeptide, and substance P, a unidecapeptide, demonstrated a stimulatory effect on prolactin secretion.[16] The precise role of these neuropeptides in controlling prolactin secretion is unclear at the present time.

Autoregulation and Paracrine Control of Prolactin Secretion

Although the principal regulatory pathway appears to emanate from the median eminence to the pituitary, either humorally or by neurotransmission, several intricate mechanisms seem to augment the control of prolactin secretion. First, retrograde flow has been demonstrated in the hypothalamic portal system, which supports the concept that prolactin regulates its own secretion by a short feedback loop.[17] For instance, in rats it was shown that intraventricular injection of prolactin results in an increase of dopamine turnover in the median eminence. A similar high rate of turnover was demonstrated both during lactation and pregnancy, and may be decreased by hypophysectomy or treatment with bromocriptine. These data may account for the observation that autographs of prolactin-secreting tumors have been associated with reduced pituitary prolactin content. Second, intrahypophyseal mechanisms appear to be involved in the self-regulation of prolactin secretion. It was demonstrated that VIP can be synthesized from radiolabeled amino acid added to pituitary cell cultures, and subsequently it stimulates prolactin release.[18] When antibodies to VIP were introduced into these cultures, prolactin secretion was inhibited. These findings are consistent with clinical studies that show that administration of VIP antagonists inhibited release of prolactin. Thus VIP may function as an autocrine regulator of prolactin synthesis and release.

Several reports have appeared suggesting that gonadotropes may exert a regulatory influence on the secretion of prolactin from lactotropes in vivo and in vitro. Synthetic gonadotropin-releasing hormone (GnRH) was shown to release prolactin in vitro using rat superfusion and human pituitary monolayer culture systems.[19] Incubation of GnRH with lactotropes separated from large gonadotropes failed to increase prolactin secretion, whereas coaggregation of these two cell types restored the stimulatory effect of GnRH on prolactin. In human pituitary monolayer cell culture systems, coincubation of a potent GnRH antagonist with native GnRH inhibited the release of prolactin, whereas coincubation of this antagonist with synthetic GnRH failed to alter the release of the hormone.[20] In another study, incubating a luteinizing hormone (LH) with fetal rat lactotropes stimulated differentiation of these cell types.[21] Incubation of β-LH or follicle-stimulating hormone (FSH) with human pituitary cells in vitro failed to stimulate prolactin secretion consistently; however, coincubation of antisera to β-LH and FSH inhibited the GnRH-mediated release of prolactin.[22] Gonadotropin-releasing hormone-associated peptide (GAP), a peptide component of the precursor to GnRH, was reported to inhibit prolactin secretion in the rodent model.[23] These observations have not been confirmed.

Prolactin and Ovarian Function

It has been speculated that the menstrual dysfunction in patients with hyperprolactinemia may be secondary to a direct effect on the ovary in addition to or instead of central inhibition. Possible mechanisms include atresia of the developing dominant follicle, inhibition or interruption of ovulation and normal corpus luteum development, and premature destruction of the corpus luteum. Such speculation is supported by the finding that in the rat fetus, ovarian interstitial cells contain a single class of specific high-affinity prolactin receptors.[24] In this system prolactin acts as a potent inhibitor of LH median androgen synthesis. Since most androgen substrate is derived from theca cells, a decrease in its production secondary to hyperprolactinemia could reduce estrogen synthesis. In addition, high-affinity prolactin receptors have been demonstrated on the surface membranes of granulosa cells.[25] These receptors have been located near the basal lamina and it is these same cells that contain aromatase enzyme. Follicle-stimulating hormone induces aromatase enzyme activity in vitro, and this effect is completely blocked by coincubation of granulosa cells with high levels (100 ng/mL) of prolactin. In-vivo prolactin blocks aromatase activity in rat preovulatory follicles. These observations support the contention that prolactin disrupts both the synthesis of androgen precursors and the induction of aromatase enzyme, which results in both decreased estrogen synthesis and reduced induction of FSH receptors. In the rat, the oocyte seems to have intracellular prolactin activities.[26] Both prolactin and its receptor are concentrated heavily in the cytoplasm. Whether these findings have a bearing on folliculogenesis and health of the oocyte is unknown.

Although prolactin may alter ovarian function in the rat, similar evidence in humans is less clear. First, it has been demonstrated that prolactin is present in the microenvironment of follicles in vitro.[27] In the early follicular phase of the cycle a fourfold to sixfold increase of prolactin is found in the fluid of developing follicles compared to concentrations in the blood. Most follicles with high concentrations of prolactin were noted to have low concentrations of estradiol. Second, in patients with hyperprolactinemia exceeding 100 ng/mL, 100% of follicles in the ovaries were atretic.[28] Third, high levels of prolactin block both basal and human chorionic gonadotropin (HCG)-stimulated estradiol synthesis in human follicles perfused in vitro. These observations imply that, in humans, prolactin in excessive amounts may disrupt normal follicular development. Whether this process leads to interruption of ovulation has not been specifically defined.

The role of prolactin in corpus luteum function appears to be even less clear, with most evidence coming from the rat. Prolactin both stimulates and inhibits corpus luteum function. On the positive side, it is involved in the induction of LH receptors to stimulate progesterone synthesis.[29] Apparently, this action of prolactin is necessary for the completion of luteinization. In-vitro experiments in humans, however, have shown that very high levels of prolactin have an inhibitory effect on both progesterone and estradiol synthesis.[30] Therefore it is evident that hyperprolactinemia may produce an alteration in normal reproductive physiologic function that would result in infertility.

Prolactin and Testicle Function

Prolactin has been shown to affect the male hypothalamic–pituitary–gonadal axis. Classic studies demonstrated that crude prolactin extracts decreased testicle size in the adult pidgeon.[31] In fact, prolactin has been shown to affect almost every aspect of male reproduction, including gonad function, sexual behavior, seminal plasma, accessory reproductive glands, and the central nervous system. In some species it is essential in maintaining fertility. Its effect on the central axis has been manifested by impairment of LH release such that the frequency of pulsation is increased and the amplitude is altered. It has been speculated that prolactin alters the presence of basal and GnRH-induced pituitary GnRH receptors.[32] It has also been demonstrated that administration of pulsatile GnRH to hypogonadal men with prolactinomas restores LH pulsatility and testosterone concentrations.[33]

Although hyperprolactinemia may have a central effect on male reproductive function, prolactin receptors (as in the ovary) have been demonstrated in testicular homogenates.[34] Prolactin receptors were found on rat Leydig cells, although they have not been documented in human testes. They appear to have high affinity and low capacity as in other tissues, and are subject to both up and down-

regulation by prolactin. Luteinizing hormone also has been shown to regulate testicular prolactin receptors, as injection of ovine LH caused a rise of receptor content in rat testes.[35]

Luteinizing hormone-stimulated steroidogenesis also may be inhibited by chronic hyperprolactinemia, which leads to a decrease in testosterone production in adult animals and humans.[36] It was proposed that the ability to enhance steroidogenesis is explained by prolactin-induced up-regulation of LH receptors in animal models,[37] however, the mechanism by which prolactin inhibits LH-stimulated steroidogenesis is less clear. It appears that in the absence of LH, prolactin has no effect on basal testosterone production. Even with LH, the effect on testosterone production is variable and dose dependent. Similarly, no change in numbers of LH receptors has been demonstrated, suggesting that the inhibitory effect may be at the post-LH-receptor-binding site. For instance, in the rat, pituitary graft-induced hyperprolactinemia stimulated α-reductase activity but decreased 17-hydroxylase activity.[38] In addition, 5α-reductase activity is reported to be inhibited by sulpiride-induced hyperprolactinemia in humans. Prolactin also has been shown to increase 3β-hydroxysteroid dehydrogenase in the mouse and accumulation of esterified cholesterol in Leydig cells.

As with the Leydig cells, prolactin seems to have an effect on the tubular compartment of the testes.[39] Superphysiologic concentrations are associated with numerous defects in spermatogenesis in human and animal models.[40] These include seminiferous epithelial disorganization, germ cell exfoliation, increased tubule wall thickness, and abnormal lipid content of Leydig cells. Testicular biopsy confirms the presence of tubule wall thickness and Sertoli cell disorganization in humans. It should be noted that no prolactin receptors have been identified in the testes outside the interstitial compartment.

It seems clear that, as in the female, prolactin has a major impact on male reproduction. Hyperprolactinemia affects prolactin receptors and testicular enzyme activity as well as spermatogenesis. These interactions with the gonads, in addition to the central effects discussed previously, lead to a clear understanding of the importance of prolactin in reproductive dysfunction.

THE ROLE OF HYPERPROLACTINEMIA IN INFERTILITY

The clinical spectrum of prolactin-related infertility includes galactorrhea, amenorrhea, oligomenorrhea, luteal insufficiency, and possibly, subtle follicular dysfunction, all of which occur as a result of hyperprolactinemia.[41] These features are commonly encountered in women with primary disorders of prolactin metabolism, namely, prolactin-secreting pituitary tumors, or prolactinomas.[42] Idiopathic or functional hyperprolactinemia and the empty sella syndrome are also included in this group.

Another form of prolactin-related infertility that might classify as a primary disorder is intermittent or transient hyperprolactinemia. This is an extremely subtle phenomenon and its precise impact on fertility remains to be elucidated.

Secondary disorders of prolactin-related infertility are those in which the mechanism of infertility is associated with, but not necessarily dependent on, hyperprolactinemia. Examples include polycystic ovary syndrome and primary hypothyroidism.[43] In general, these clinical entities represent the major disorders of prolactin metabolism, and as such should be considered in the diagnosis and management of hyperprolactinemic infertility.

Prolactinomas and Infertility

Infertility in patients with a prolactinoma generally has been a consequence of hyperprolactinemia rather than of tumor size, with the exception of massive lesions. As stated previously, persistent hyperprolactinemia may act at the level of the gonad or the hypothalamic–pituitary axis to cause infertility. Since hyperprolactinemic infertility generally causes amenorrhea, disruption of pituitary gonadotropin secretion is not necessarily unexpected. In addition to loss of the midcycle gonadotropin surge, attenuation of episodic secretion has been documented. These alterations occurred despite, in some instances, the lack of change in basal LH and FSH concentrations.

Anovulation is likely related to decreased GnRH secretion, as implied by reduced pulsatile gonadotropin release. Conceptually, the presence of a prolactin-secreting neoplasm results in an increase of hypothalamic dopamine by a short loop feedback mechanism. Increased dopamine inhibits the release of GnRH, which in turn is responsible for decreased gonadotropin secretion and anovulation. This concept is supported by the restoration of ovulation after resolution of hyperprolactinemia by surgical extirpation or administration of bromocriptine.

As is the case with microadenomas, anovulation in patients with macroadenomas commonly results from hyperprolactinemia.[44] On occasion, an extensive lesion occupies or extends beyond the sellar space and destroys the entire pituitary gland, including gonadotropes. Eradication of such a tumor or resolution of hyperprolactinemia will not restore ovulation; instead, treatment with human menopausal gonadotropin is necessary.

Increased prolactin secretion in the absence of a demonstrable pituitary neoplasm is functional or idiopathic. In most cases, serum prolactin levels are minimally or moderately elevated and do not exceed 200 ng/mL. If the patient is amenorrheic, the mechanism of anovulatory infertility is similar to that in women with microprolactinomas. In some instances, however, patients are oligomenorrheic or have regular menstrual cycles. It has been suggested that in these cases infertility may result from an adverse effect of prolactin on follicle development, or disruption of corpus luteum function leading to a luteal phase defect. In humans, little clinical evidence supports a direct action of prolactin on the follicle. On the other hand, abnormal corpus luteum development may be a direct consequence of prolactin effect or an indirect result of inadequate follicular maturation. A lack of corpus luteum support is reflected by diminished progesterone production and incomplete endometrial development in the luteal phase. This alteration may preclude implantation or lead to increased pregnancy wastage and habitual abortion. Clinically, a luteal phase defect secondary to hyperprolactinemia is corrected by treatment with bromocriptine.[45]

The empty sella syndrome may be viewed as either primary or secondary disorder of prolactin metabolism.[46] Not infrequently, this condition is associated with a pituitary tumor. In theory, the lesion has previously expanded the sella turcica, and in doing so, has widened the aperture in the sellar diaphragm through which passes the infundibulum. As a result, herniation of the arachnoid membrane into the sellar cavity occurs, and the pituitary is displaced to the side. Radiologic evaluation reveals a clear area in the expanded sella, which represents the arachnoid membrane filled with cerebrospinal fluid. The prolactinoma, which may be difficult to detect radiologically due to compression effect, continues to release excess prolactin, and anovulation persists. In rare situations the defect of the sellar diaphragm is congenital, and hyperprolactinemia does not result from a pituitary neoplasm. Instead, the fluid-filled hernia sac impinges on the infundibulum to interrupt the inhibitory control of prolactin, which leads to increased prolactin secretion. If the expansion of the hernia is substantial, compression of the optic chiasm may occur, with compromise of visual fields.

The concept of intermittent hyperprolactinemia emerged from several studies in which bromocriptine was used to treat unexplained infertility. Although initial impressions suggested that bromocriptine was beneficial in the management of these patients, studies to support this contention were lacking. For example, evaluation of follicular-phase prolactin levels in 40 ovulatory infertile and 25 fertile women failed to demonstrate a significant difference.[47] Subsequently, two double-blind studies yielded the same results.[48,49] In addition, in one of the studies, more pregnancies occurred during the 12-month follow-up period than during treatment cycles with bromocriptine.

In what was perhaps the first study suggesting that intermittent hyperprolactinemia might be associated with infertility, 94% of the patient population had transient preovulatory hyperprolactinemia.[50] This elevation coincided with the estrogen peak and lasted from 1 to 3 days. Forty percent of patients receiving bromocriptine conceived within 3 months after initiating therapy, compared to 1% prior to treatment. The relevance of such episodic hyperprolactinemia has to be questioned, since administration of a dopamine antagonist, metoclopramide, for 6 days during the preovulatory period had no apparent detrimental effect on ovulation.[51] If hyperprolactinemia was induced in the early follicular phase, however, ovulation was disrupted in 60% of women. Others have noted that patients with sulpiride-induced hyperprolactinemia exhibited smaller follicles, with lower estradiol concentrations and higher testosterone levels than euprolactinemic controls with similar-size follicles.

Transient hyperprolactinemia is often associated with ovulation induction and in-vitro fertilization (IVF) stimulation protocols.[52] It occurs with the use of clomiphene, human menopausal gonadotropin (HMG), or a mixture of the two agents. In IVF programs, preanesthetic serum prolactin levels are correlated to follicular fluid prolactin levels and are inversely related to pregnancy rate. Since the percentage of oocytes fertilized is not correlated to preanesthetic prolactin values, however, any change in pregnancy rate does not appear to be due to disordered fertilization. In the monkey, treatment with HMG increases luteal phase prolactin levels. The administration of bromocriptine-suppressed prolactin levels but did not change the length of the menstrual cycle or luteal phase in these animals. Luteal phase progesterone and estrogen levels are also increased in such therapy.[53]

Despite the seeming lack of correlation of intermittent hyperprolactinemia with the response to treatment and pregnancy, three subsets of patients might benefit from bromocriptine therapy. First, a variety of heterogeneous forms of prolactin have been described that are present in both healthy and hyperprolactinemic patients.[54] An iso-B-prolactin was described in patients with unexplained infertility; suppression of iso-B-prolactin with bromocriptine resulted in pregnancy in a significant number of these women.[55] Second, in a subpopulation of women with high psychologic stress scores associated with intermittent elevations of prolactin, autogenic training lowered psychologic stress markers.[56] Combined bromocriptine and clomiphene therapy was reported

to produce significantly higher pregnancy rates than placebo. Third, women with galactorrhea and euprolactinemia as measured by conventional radioimmunoassay were treated with bromocriptine.[57] This resulted in a significant increase in pregnancies compared to clomiphene and vitamin B_6 administered to matched controls. Therefore subgroups of patients with various forms of hyperprolactinemia might benefit from bromocriptine therapy. As a rule, however, it appears clear that the empiric use of bromocriptine in infertile patients is *unwarranted*.

Secondary disorders of prolactin metabolism associated with infertility include polycystic ovary syndrome (PCO) and primary hypothyroidism. Serum prolactin levels are reported to be elevated in about 30% of patients with PCO.[58] In addition, in the absence of overt hyperprolactinemia, prolactin concentrations are increased within the normal range compared to weight-matched ovulatory women.[59] The same study also showed that the prolactin response to TRH stimulation in women with PCO was significantly greater than that of healthy controls. The increased production of prolactin has been logically attributed to the hyperestrogenism associated with this syndrome and possibly a deficiency of hypothalamic dopamine; however, confirmatory evidence for these mechanisms is lacking.

First, long-term suppression of estrogen secretion in patients with PCO treated with a GnRH agonist for 6 months failed to reduce circulating prolactin levels (R.J. Chang, unpublished data). Second, several attempts to document a hypothalamic dopamine deficiency all have provided inconclusive results. That hyperprolactinemia is primarily responsible for anovulation in PCO seems unlikely. Rather, available evidence suggests that prolactin has a possible contributory role, and anovulation is a result of a more central disturbance.

An effect of prolactin on adrenal androgen production was suggested in this syndrome by the dehydroepiandosterone sulfate (DHEAS) response to bromocriptine or dopamine administration.[60] Treatment with bromocriptine decreased prolactin levels and reduced DHEAS concomitantly. In addition, it was demonstrated that the rate of prolactin production falls and metabolic clearance rate increases during treatment.[61] It has not been established whether these results are due to changes in prolactin or to a direct effect of bromocriptine on steroidogenesis. Treatment of PCO with bromocriptine has yielded variable results with respect to ovulation and pregnancy.[62] While this therapy generally reduces prolactin and DHEAS levels, gonadotropin levels and menstrual status are unaltered in all but a small subset of patients.[63]

Normal thyroid function has long been thought

necessary to maintain synchronous menstrual cycles; however, the precise mechanism of this relationship has not been determined. In thyroid disease, alteration of menstrual cyclicity and disruption of reproductive function have been attributed to abnormal peripheral steroid metabolism.[64] In primary hypothyroidism, irregular vaginal bleeding may occur in part as a result of hyperprolactinemia. In this disorder, elevated TSH levels presumably are stimulated by increased TRH, which could account for increased prolactin secretion. Moreover, studies in animals and humans indicate that the prolactin response to TRH is greater than that of TSH, its accepted target hormone. Unfortunately, the clinical findings in untreated primary hypothyroidism have not consistently supported this concept. In one study, patients with untreated disease had an exaggerated prolactin response to TRH stimulation that reverted to normal after appropriate thyroid replacement.[65] On the other hand, in a study of 49 patients, 30% demonstrated some degree of hyperprolactinemia, whereas only 1 patient had galactorrhea.[66] In another study, patients with untreated disease had an exaggerated prolactin response to TRH stimulation, which reverted to normal after appropriate thyroid replacement.

These observations suggest that in primary hypothyroidism, an increase of prolactin production may not necessarily be associated with an increase in circulating levels. The rates of menstrual irregularity and infertility have not been assessed in this condition. Conversely, in infertile couples with menstrual irregularity, the rate of thyroid dysfunction has not been established. Because routine thyroid evaluation in these patients seldom reveals thyroid disease, the prevalence generally has been thought to be low. Thus, despite extensive evidence that thyroid diseases, in particular primary hypothyroidism, can influence prolactin release, the clinical significance of these findings remains in question.

DIAGNOSIS OF HYPERPROLACTINEMIA

The patient with menstrual irregularity or galactorrhea must undergo a serum prolactin determination (see flow diagram). If the level is elevated, it should be measured a second time because of the known erratic pattern of secretion. It should be recalled that prolactin is a dynamic hormone that is influenced by a variety of physiologic stimuli such as stress, exercise, food intake, and sleep.[67] Therefore care must be taken to avoid these confounding features in choosing an optimal time of sampling. For example, blood should be obtained either in the morning after an overnight fast and well removed from awakening, or

just before lunch provided there has not been a midmorning snack. In the patient with hyperprolactinemia, T4 and TSH levels should be measured to rule out the presence of compensated hypothyroidism. In these patients thyroxin levels are often normal while TSH is markedly elevated.[68]

The patient with an abnormal basal body temperature chart, several low midluteal serum progesterone levels, consistent out-of-phase endometrial biopsies, or poor folliculogenesis patterns as measured by sonography, should be investigated for hyperprolactinemia. It has been claimed that up to 20% of patients with such findings have elevated prolactin levels, although the condition was found in 15 of 130 infertile patients with regular menstrual cycles and no galactorrhea.[69] In the same study, luteal phase levels of progesterone and estrogen were similar in both hyperprolactinemic and euprolactinemic patients. In fact, significantly higher instances of inadequate luteal phase histology were noted in euprolactinemic than in hyperprolactinemic women. It was concluded that the role of elevated serum prolactin in patients with apparent luteal phase defects was minimal.

The patient with hyperprolactinemia documented on several occasions should undergo radiographic evaluation,[70] but at what point this should be instituted is controversial. Some reproductive endocrinologists recommend computerized tomographic (CT) scans or magnetic resonance imaging (MRI) when any elevation is found, while others choose to proceed depending on a specific maximal concentration such as 50 or 100 ng/mL. Almost without exception, once a prolactin level of 100 ng/mL has been determined on several occasions, advanced radiographic surveillance is recommended (Fig. 7–1). Patients with serum prolactin levels greater than 50 ng/mL have a 20% frequency of harboring a prolactinoma; those with 100 ng/mL value are at a 50% risk; and levels greater than 100 ng/mL are almost diagnostic for the presence of at least a microadenoma.[71] If a prolactinoma is detected, visual field examinations by Goldman-bowl perimetry might be undertaken if the lesion is 10 mm or greater (Fig. 7–2). There is little indication for visual field surveillance, since most subtle defects (superior bitemporal hemianopsia) are not detected until the prolactinoma extends out of the sella and compresses the optic chiasm.

The choice of radiologic procedure has evolved with time. Cone down view of the sella was once used to detect lesions 10 mm or larger. This gave way to linear and hypocycloidal tomography, which have been all but abandoned due to the fact that they are best used to detect erosion of bone. Unfortunately, the normal sella shows great variation, making the

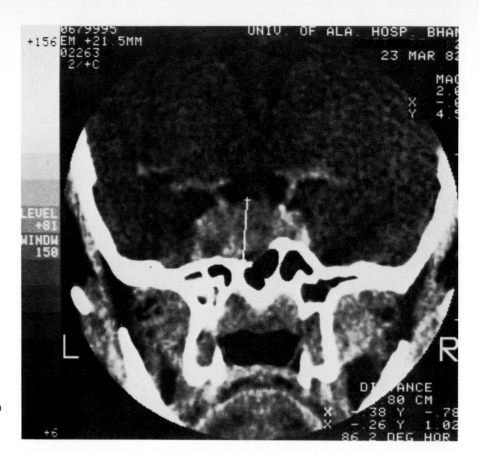

Figure 7–1. CT scan of a patient with an initial prolactin level of 566 ng/mL. Note extrasellar extension.

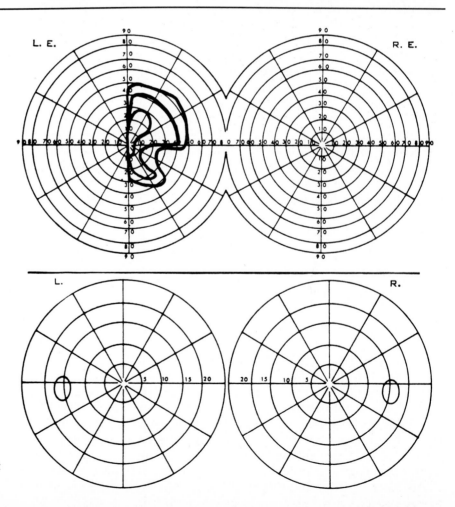

Figure 7–2. Visual field defect in a patient with a macroadenoma.

rate of false positive and false negative results for adenoma detection high. Computerized tomographic scans with metrisemide enhancement can be used to detect lesions as small as 2 mm, and currently are the most common radiologic technique. Magnetic reso-

nance imaging appears to be superior to all previous forms of pituitary surveillance (Figs. 7–3 and 7–4). The images generated by these machines in the hands of a skilled technician and experienced radiologist are vastly superior to CT scans. Moreover, the

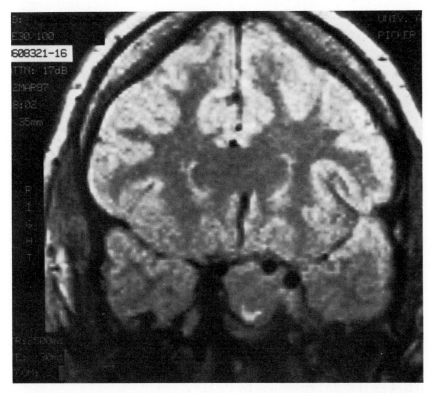

A

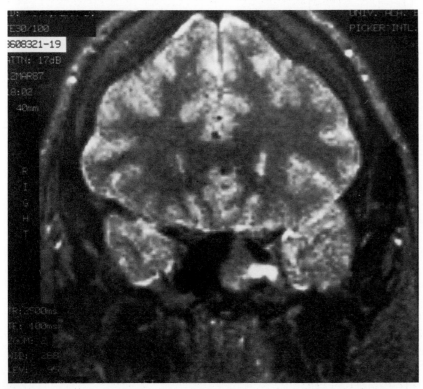

B

Figure 7–3. A. MRI scan of a macroadenoma (35 mm). **B.** MRI scan of the same patient. Note that the lesion (40 mm) involves the carotid artery.

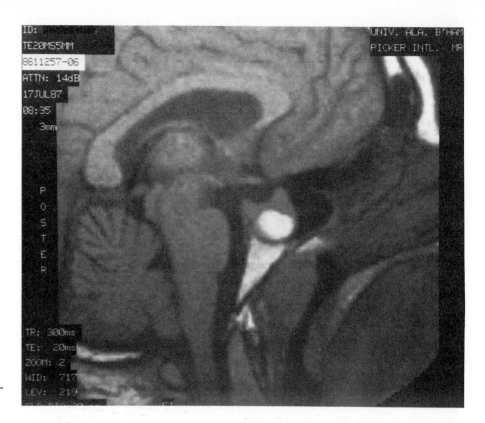

Figure 7–4. MRI scan shows cystic degeneration of a macroadenoma.

patient is not exposed to irradiation. Although slower to perform and more expensive than CT scans, MRI continues to evolve as the state-of-the-art technique for the radiologic evaluation of the pituitary in the infertile patient with hyperprolactinemia.

TREATMENT OF HYPERPROLACTINEMIC INFERTILITY

Historically, radiation therapy and surgery were used exclusively to treat patients with prolactinomas. In the absence of a pituitary lesion, infertile women with hyperprolactinemic anovulation of a functional nature were subjected to ovulation induction with either clomiphene citrate or HMG. Patients with microprolactinomas were treated by selective extirpation during transsphenoidal surgery. Consideration of radiation therapy was limited by the potential risk of hypopituitarism and damage to surrounding structures.

The response to surgery was generally marked by resumption of ovulatory menses in greater than 70% of cases and a corresponding increase in the frequency of pregnancy. Intraoperative complications were minimal since the tumors were small, and mortality was rare. Initial follow-up studies appeared to justify surgical management of microadenomas. Extended long-term follow-up has revealed a sub-

stantial recurrence of hyperprolactinemia, however, and, even more disturbing, reappearance of the tumor.[72] Nevertheless, operative intervention remains one treatment choice.

The development of synthetic dopamine agonists and bromocriptine has been of clear benefit in the treatment of infertility in these patients. Bromocriptine provides at least equivalent clinical responses with respect to ovulation and pregnancy compared to those achieved by surgical therapy.[73] In addition, the medication has proved to be well tolerated, with minimal side effects. With the success of dopamine agonist therapy, there seems to be little indication for the surgical resection of small pituitary tumors in these patients.

The treatment of the macroadenoma is more complicated and may involve surgery, irradiation, use of a dopamine agonist, or a combination. Unfortunately, the failure rate after transsphenoidal resection of these lesions has been reported as high as 70%. This lack of success is related to tumor size, as a direct correlation exists between surgical failure and increased size of the lesion.[74] Similarly, patients with prolactin levels greater than 200 ng/mL have a poorer outcome than those with lower levels.[75] It is understandable that surgical resection of a macroadenoma is associated with increased morbidity and mortality compared to operative removal of a microadenoma. Radiation therapy delivered by either linear cobalt mode or BRAGG peak proton beam has been used as

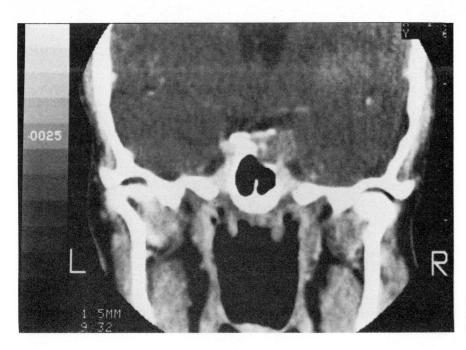

Figure 7–5. CT scan demonstrates expansion of a macroadenoma during pregnancy in an untreated patient.

a primary method of treating macroprolactinomas. Most commonly it is employed in patients who have undergone surgery and exhibit evidence of persistent disease. Proton beam therapy has posed the risk of panhypopituitarism, and the necessity of hormone replacement such as thyroid, cortisone, sex steroids, and vasopressin must be considered. Dopamine agonists, although not uniformly successful in suppressing prolactinoma growth, have substantial effects on the vast majority of large lesions.[76] In 50 to 75% of cases, significant reduction in tumor size has been demonstrated, and in 25 to 30% the neoplasm resolves totally. Adjunctive use of a dopamine agonist as preoperative treatment has been suggested, although clinical benefit has not been evident in all instances.

A consideration of pregnancy should be made in all patients with prolactinomas should therapy result in the return of prolactin levels to normal and resumption of regular ovulatory menses. In the case of a microadenoma, very few complications have been reported as a result of tumor expansion during pregnancy.[77,78] Furthermore, at least three major studies examined the development of children exposed in utero to bromocriptine and determined that no abnormalities have arisen as a result of drug administration.[79] There is no contraindication to breast-feeding in the postpartum woman with a microadenoma.

In patients with macroadenomas there is more concern relative to the side effects of tumor growth (Fig. 7–5). If left untreated, approximately 30% of patients have required medical, surgical, or radiation therapy during pregnancy.[80] This is opposed to patients with microadenoma, of whom less than 1%

require any therapy during gestation. As mentioned earlier, lactotrope hypertrophy and hyperplasia occur normally in pregnancy as a result of increased estrogen secretion. In most women the increased pituitary size is rarely symptomatic. Preexisting macroadenomas have been known to expand rapidly during pregnancy, however, causing major vision disturbances and headache. It has been suggested that if necessary, bromocriptine therapy be continued throughout or instituted during pregnancy if clinically indicated. The ability to breast-feed postpartum is contingent on the continued need for bromocriptine therapy.

Precise assessment of tumor size in pregnancy is difficult, as methods of evaluation are limited and indirect. For instance, serum prolactin levels in an individual rise in a progressive but erratic fashion throughout pregnancy, reaching a peak between 200 and 500 ng/mL, and it is generally accepted that these levels do not provide useful information in pregnancy. Visual field examination with Goldman-bowl perimetry has been the most sensitive and noninvasive management technique. Performing CT scans during pregnancy is to be discouraged, and the utility of MRI, with its possible effects of magnetism on the fetus, is as yet unclear. Therefore, the physician is usually faced with making the clinical decision based on limited data.

SUMMARY AND CONCLUSION

Hyperprolactinemia is clearly associated with infertility in both men and women. It may affect numerous tissue sites (brain, pituitary, ovaries, testes) and alter their physiologic roles in reproduction. As a result, increased prolactin production is associated with a number of pathologies, including polycystic ovary syndrome and thyroid and pituitary disease. The etiology of hyperprolactinemia must be determined and suppression of one condition carefully confirmed so as to facilitate appropriate management and eliminate empiric use of bromocriptine, particularly in infertile patients.

Medical therapy is preferred for both males and females with hyperprolactinemic infertility, regardless of whether or not a pituitary tumor is present. Reestablishment of normal ovulation predisposes to conception, and during pregnancy, therapy may be discontinued in all patients except those with macroprolactinomas. These individuals may require therapy throughout pregnancy.

Evidence indicates no deleterious effects of bromocriptine on mother or fetus. Although bromocriptine is the mainstay of the medical therapy for the patient with hyperprolactinemia, a new generation of drugs, both ergoline and nonergoline dopamine agonists, are in the final phases of development. These agents offer once-a-day therapy, have few side effects, and should expand our therapeutic alternatives.

Acknowledgment. The authors are grateful to Elizabeth Perry for her excellent secretarial assistance in the preparation of this manuscript.

REFERENCES

1. Blackwell RE, Guillemin R: Hypothalamic control of adenohypophyseal secretions. *Annu Rev Physiol* 35:357, 1973.
2. MacLeod RM: Influence of norepinephrine and catecholamine-depleting agents on the synthesis and release of prolactin and growth hormone. *Endocrinology* 85:916, 1969.
3. Leblanc H, Lachelin G, Abu-Fadil S, Yen SSC: Effects of dopamine infusion on pituitary hormone secretion in humans. *J Clin Endocrinol Metab* 43:669, 1976.
4. Gibbs OM, Neill JD: Dopamine levels in hypophyseal stalk blood in the rat are sufficient to inhibit prolactin secretion in vitro. *Endocrinology* 102:1895, 1978.
5. Plotsky PM, deGreef WF, Neill JD: In situ voltametric microelectrodes: Application to the measurement as median eminence catecholamine release during simulated suckling. *Brain Res* 250(2):251, 1982.
6. Plotsky PM, Neill JD: Interactions of dopamine and thyrotropin-releasing hormone in the regulation of prolactin release in lactating rats. *Endocrinology* 111:168, 1982.
7. Schettini G, Cronin MJ, MacLeod RM: Adenosine 3′,5′-monophosphate (cAMP) and calcium–calmodulin interrelation in the control of prolactin secretion: Evidence for dopamine inhibition of cAMP accumulation and prolactin release after calcium mobilization. *Endocrinology* 112:1801, 1983.
8. Grossman A, Delitala G, Yeo T, Besser GM: GABA and muscimol inhibit the release of prolactin from dispersed rat anterior pituitary cells. *Neuroendocrinology* 32:145,1981.
9. Vale W, Blackwell RE, Grant G, Guillemin R: TRF and thyroid hormones on prolactin secretion by rat pituitary cells in vitro. *Endocrinology* 93:26, 1973.
10. Matsushita N, Kato Y, Shimatsu A, et al: Effects of VIP, TRH, GABA and dopamine on prolactin release from superfused rat anterior pituitary cells. *Life Sci* 32:1263, 1983.
11. Dufy-Barbe L, Rodriguez F, Arsaut J, Verrier D, Vincent JD: Angiotensin II stimulates prolactin release in the rhesus monkey. *Neuroendocrinology* 35:242, 1982.
12. Gerhengorn MC: Thyrotropin-releasing hormone: A review of the mechanisms of acute stimulation of pituitary hormone release. *Mol Cell Biochem* 45:163, 1982.
13. Shimatsu A, Kao Y, Matsushita N, et al: Effect of prostaglandin E on vasoactive intestinal polypeptide release from the hypothalamus and on prolactin secretion from the pituitary in rats. *Endocrinology* 113:2059, 1983.
14. Aguilera G, Hyde CL, Catt KJ: Angiotensin II receptors and prolactin release in pituitary lactotrophs. *Endocrinology* 111:1045, 1987.
15. Clemens JA, Roush ME, Fuller RW: Evidence that serotonin neurons stimulate secretion of prolactin-releasing factor. *Life Sci* 22:2209, 1978.
16. Knigge U, Dejgaard A, Wollesen F, Thuesen B, Christiansen PM: Histamine regulation of prolactin secretion through H_1-H_2-receptors. *J Clin Endocrinol Metab* 55:118, 1982.
17. Bergland R, Page R: Can the pituitary secrete directly to the brain? (Affirmative anatomical evidence.) *Endocrinology* 102:1325, 1978.
18. Hagen TC, Arnaout MA, Scherzer WJ, Martinson DR, Garthwaite TL: Antisera to vasoactive intestinal polypeptide inhibit basal prolactin release from disbursed anterior pituitary cells. *Neuroendocrinology* 43(6):641, 1986.
19. Denef C, Andries M: Evidence for panacine interaction between gonadotrophs and lactotrophs in pituitary cell aggregates. *Endocrinology* 112:813, 1983.
20. Blackwell RE, Rodgers-Neame NT, Bradley EL, Asch RH: Regulation of human prolactin secretion in gonadotropin releasing hormone in vitro. *Fertil Steril* 46:26, 1986.
21. Begeot M, Hemming FJ, DuBois PM: Induction of pituitary lactotrope difference by luteinizing hormone alpha subunit. *Science* 226:566, 1984.
22. Blackwell RE, Garrison PN: Inhibition of prolactin secretion by antiserum to the α- and β-subunits of gonadotropin. *Am J Obstet Gynecol* 156:863, 1987.
23. Nikolics K, Mason AJ, Szonyl E, Ramachandran JR, Seeburg PH: A prolactin-inhibiting factor within the precursor for human gonadotropin-releasing hormone. *Nature* 316(6028):511, 1985.
24. Magoffin DA, Erickson GF: Prolactin inhibition of LH stimulated androgen synthesis in ovarian interstitial cells cultured in defined medium: Mechanism of action. *Endocrinology* 111:2001, 1982.
25. Ben-David M, Schenker JG: Human ovarian receptors to human prolactin: Implications in infertility. *Fertil Steril* 38:182, 1982.
26. Dunaif AE, Zimmerman EA, Friesen HG, Frantz AG: Intracellular localization of prolactin receptor and prolactin in the rat ovary by immunocytobiochemistry. *Endocrinology* 110:1465, 1982.
27. McNatty KP, Sawers RS, McNeilly AS: A possible role for prolactin in control of steroid secretion by the human graafian follicle. *Nature* 250:653, 1974.
28. McNatty KP: Relationship between plasma prolactin and the endocrine microenvironment of the developing human antral follicle. *Fertil Steril* 32:433, 1979.
29. Wang C, Hsueh AJW, Erickson GF: Prolactin inhibition of estrogen production by cultured rat granulosa cells. *Mol Cell Endocrinol* 20:136, 1980.
30. Tan GJS, Biggs JSG: Effects of prolactin on steroid production by human luteal cells in vitro. *J Endocrinol* 96:499, 1983.
31. Bates RW, Riddle O, Lahr EL: The mechanism of the antigonadal action of prolactin in adult pigeons. *Am J Physiol* 119:610, 1937.
32. Marchetti B, Labrie F: Prolactin inhibits pituitary luteinizing hormone (LH)-releasing hormone receptors in the rat. *Endocrinology* 111:1209, 1982.
33. Bouchard P, Lagoguey M, Barilly S, Schaison G: Gonadotropin-releasing hormone pulsatile administration restores luteinizing hormone pulsatility and normal testosterone levels in males with hyperprolactinemia. *J Clin Endocrinol Metab* 60:258, 1985.
34. Posner BI, Kelly PA, Shiu RPC, Friesen HG: Studies of insulin, growth hormone and prolactin binding tissue distribution, species variation and characterization. *Endocrinology* 95:521, 1974.
35. Kelly PA, Seguin C, Cusan L, Labrie F: Stimulatory effect of luteinizing hormone and human chorionic gonadotropin on testicular prolactin receptor levels. *Biol Reprod* 23:924, 1980.
36. Murray FT, Cameron DF, Ketchum C: Return of gonadal function in man with prolactin-secreting pituitary tumors. *J Clin Endocrinol Metab* 59:79, 1984.
37. Bohnet HG, Friesen HG: Effect of prolactin and GH on prolactin and LH receptors in dwarf mouse. *J Endocrinol Fertil* 48:307, 1976.

38. Ngareda T, Takeyama M, Ueda T, et al: Hyperprolactinemia enhances LH-L stimulated 4-ene-5 alpha-reductase activity but inhibits LH-induced 17-hydroxylase activity in testes of hypophysectomized immature rats. *J Steril Biochem* 24:1199, 1985.

39. Bartke A, Lloyd CW: Influence of PRL and pituitary isografts on spermatogenesis in dwarf mice and hypophysectomized rats. *J Endocrinol* 46:321, 1982.

40. Katovich MJ, Cameron DF, Murray FT, Gunsalus GL: Alterations of testicular function induced by hyperprolactinemia in the rat. *J Androl* 6:179, 1985.

41. Blackwell RE: Diagnosis and treatment of hyperprolactinemic syndromes. *Fertil Steril* 43:5, 1985.

42. Keye WR, Chang RJ, Wilson CB, Jaffe RB: Prolactin-secreting pituitary adenomas. III. Frequency and diagnosis of amenorrhea-galactorrhea. *JAMA* 244:1329, 1980.

43. Blackwell RE, Chang RJ: Report of the national symposium on the clinical management of prolactin-related reproductive disorders. *Fertil Steril* 45:607, 1986.

44. Pepperell RJ: Prolactin and reproduction. *Fertil Steril* 35:267, 1981.

45. Daly DC, Walters CA, Soto-Albors CE, Riddick DH: Endometrial biopsy during treatment of luteal phase defects is predictive of therapeutic outcome. *Fertil Steril* 40:305, 1983.

46. Hsu TH, Shapiro JR, Tyson JE, Leddy AL, Paz-Guevera AT: Hyperprolactinemia associated with empty sella syndrome. *JAMA* 235:2002, 1976.

47. Lenton EA, Sobowale OS, Cooke ID: Prolactin concentrations in ovulatory but infertile women: Treatment with bromocriptine. *Br Med J* 2: 1179, 1977.

48. Wright CS, Steele SJ, Jacobs HS: Value of bromocriptine in unexplained primary infertility: A double-blind controlled trial. *Br Med J* 1:2037, 1979.

49. McBain JC, Pepperell RJ: Use of bromocriptine in unexplained infertility. *Clin Reprod Fertil* 1:145, 1982.

50. Ben-David H, Schenker JG: Transient hyperprolactinemia: A correctable cause of idiopathic female infertility. *J Clin Endocrinol Metab* 57:442, 1983.

51. Ylikorkala O, Kauppila A: The effects on the ovulatory cycle of metoclopramide-induced increased prolactin levels during follicular development. *Fertil Steril* 35:588, 1981.

52. Tang LC, Ho PC: Transient hyperprolactinemia in human menopausal gonadotropin induction of ovulation. *Int J Fertil* 29:236, 1984.

53. Collins RL, Williams RF, Hodgen GD: Human menopausal gonadotropin-human chorionic gonadotropin-induced ovarian hyperstimulation with transient hyperprolactinemia: Steroidogenesis enhanced during bromocriptine therapy in monkeys. *J Clin Endocrinol Metab* 59:727, 1984.

54. Suh HK, Frantz AG: Size heterogeneity of human prolactin in plasma and pituitary extract. *J Clin Endocrinol Metab* 39:928, 1974.

55. Ben-David M, Chrambach A: A method for isolation by gel electrofocusing of isohormones B and C of human prolactin from amniotic fluid. *J Endocrinol* 84:125, 1980.

56. Harrison FR, O'Moore A, Mosurski K, O'Moore R, Cranny A: Intermittent hyperprolactinemia and the unexplained infertile couple: A placebo-controlled study of combined clomiphene citrate, bromocriptine therapy. *Infertility* 9:1, 1986.

57. DeVane G, Guzick D: Bromocriptine therapy in normoprolactinemic women with unexplained infertility and galactorrhea. *Fertil Steril* 46:1026, 1986.

58. Corenblum B, Taylor PJ: The hyperprolactinemic polycystic ovary syndrome may not be a distinct entity. *Fertil Steril* 38:549, 1982.

59. Shoupe D, Lobo RA: Prolactin response after gonadotropin releasing hormone in the polycystic ovary syndrome. *Fertil Steril* 43:549, 1985.

60. Steingold KA, Lobo RA, Judd HL, Lu JKH, Chang RJ: The effect of bromocriptine on gonadotropin secretion in polycystic ovarian disease. *J Clin Endocrinol Metab* 62:1048, 1986.

61. Schiebinger RJ, Chrousos GP, Cutler GB, Loriaux DL: The effect of serum prolactin on plasma adrenal androgens and the production and metabolic clearance rate of dehydroepiandrosterone sulfate in normal and hyperprolactinemic subjects. *J Clin Endocrinol Metab* 62:202, 1986.

62. Suginami H, Hamada K, Yano K, Kuroda G, Matsuura S: Ovulation induction with bromocriptine in normoprolactinemic anovulatory women. *J Clin Endocrinol Metab* 62:899, 1986.

63. Seibel MM, Oskowitz S, Kamarara M, Taymor ML: Preliminary observations on the response of low-dose bromocriptine in normoprolactinemic patients with polycystic ovary disease. *Obstet Gynecol* 64:213, 1984.

64. Gordon GG, Southren AL, Tochimoto S, Rand JJ, Olivo J: Effect of hyperthyroidism and hypothyroidism on the metabolism of testosterone and androstenedione in man. *J Clin Endocrinol* 29:164, 1969.

65. Snyder PJ, Jacobs LS, Utiger RD, Daughaday WH: Thyroid hormone inhibition of the prolactin response to thyrotropin-releasing hormone. *J Clin Invest* 52:2324, 1973.

66. Honbo KS, Van Herle AJ, Kellett KA. Serum prolactin levels in untreated primary hypothyroidism. *Am J Med* 65:782, 1978.

67. Dollar J, Blackwell R: Diagnosis and management of prolactinomas. *Cancer Metastasis Rev* 5:125, 1986.

68. Yamamoto K, Saito K, Takai T, Naito M, Yoshida N: Visual field defects and pituitary enlargement in primary hypothyroidism. *J Clin Endocrinol Metab* 67:283, 1983.

69. Vanrell JA, Balasch J: Prolactin in the evaluation of luteal phase in infertility. *Fertil Steril* 39:30, 1983.

70. Chang RJ, Keye WR, Monroe SE, Jaffe RB: Prolactin-secreting pituitary adenomas in women. IV. Pituitary function in amenorrhea associated with normal or abnormal serum prolactin and sellar polytomography. *J Clin Endocrinol Metab* 51:830, 1980.

71. Blackwell RE, Boots LR, Goldenberg RL, Younger JB: Assessment of pituitary function in patients with serum prolactin levels greater than 100 ng/ml. *Fertil Steril* 32:177, 1979.

72. Serri O, Rasio E, Beauregard H, Hardy J, Somme M: Recurrence of hyperprolactinemia after selective transsphenoidal adenomectomy in women with prolactinoma. *N Engl J Med* 309:280, 1983.

73. Molitch ME, Elton RL, Blackwell RE, et al: Bromocriptine as primary therapy for prolactin-secreting macroadenomas: Results of a prospective multicenter study. *J Clin Endocrinol Metab* 60:698, 1985.

74. Domingue JN, Richmond IL, Wilson CB: Results of surgery in 114 patients with prolactin-secreting pituitary adenomas. *Am J Obstet Gynecol* 137:102, 1980.

75. Faria MA, Tindall GT: Transsphenoidal microsurgery for prolactin-secreting pituitary adenomas: Results in 100 women with the amenorrhea–galactorrhea syndrome. *J Neurosurg* 56:38, 1982.

76. Blackwell RE, Bradley EL, Kline LB, et al: Comparison of dopamine agonists in the treatment of hyperprolactinemic syndrome: A multicenter study. *Fertil Steril* 39:744, 1983.

77. Corenblum B: Successful outcome of ergocryptine-induced pregnancies in twenty-one women with prolactin-secreting pituitary adenomas. *Fertil Steril* 32:183, 1979.

78. Divers WA, Yen SSC: Prolactin-producing microadenomas in pregnancy. *Obstet Gynecol* 61:425, 1978.

79. Turkalj I, Braun P, Krupp P: Surveillance of bromocriptine in pregnancy. *JAMA* 247:1589, 1982.

80. Magyar DM, Marshall JR: Pituitary tumors and pregnancy. *Am J Obstet Gynecol* 132:739, 1978.

PART III

Endometriosis

CHAPTER 8

Endometriosis: Pathophysiology and Treatment

Steven R. Bayer, Machelle M. Seibel

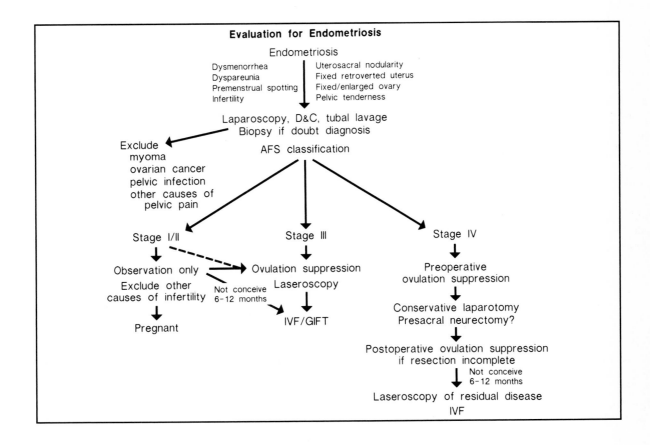

Endometriosis is one of the most prevalent diseases encountered in gynecology. Although it was previously thought to be confined to Caucasian women of older reproductive age, it is now recognized that women of all ages and races are potentially at risk for this disease. Its symptoms are vast and varied, but infertility and dysmenorrhea are by far the most common. Endometriosis can be diagnosed easily by laparoscopy, but its pathogenesis and pathophysiology are poorly understood, and the treatment in many instances is controversial.

PATHOPHYSIOLOGY OF INFERTILITY DUE TO ENDOMETRIOSIS

The pathophysiology of the infertility associated with endometriosis is complex. Endometriosis is associated with several alterations of reproductive physiology that can potentially prevent conception. These include (1) mechanical factors, (2) a toxic peritoneal environment, (3) immunologic abnormalities, and (4) endocrinologic alterations.

Mechanical Factors

In advanced stages, endometriosis can result in the formation of endometriomas and pelvic adhesions that distort normal pelvic anatomy. Peritubal and periovarian adhesions can alter crucial tubo-ovarian relationships that are necessary for ovum pickup. Although distal tubal obstruction rarely occurs, proximal tubal obstruction has been associated with endometriosis. A previous study confirmed that 14% of patients undergoing tubal-cornual anastomosis for proximal tubal obstruction had histologic confirmation of endometriosis in resected tubal segments.[1] This finding was then tested clinically. Several studies reported that some patients with proximal tubal obstruction (with or without pelvic endometriosis) showed resolution of the obstruction after medical treatment with danazol.[2,3] Subsequent pregnancy rates after medical treatment have not been established, however. Nevertheless, it does appear that endometriosis can be the cause of cornual obstruction even when the disease is not present in the pelvis. For this reason, conservative medical management of cornual obstruction may prove efficacious and obviate the need for more aggressive surgical treatment.

Endometriosis commonly involves the ovary. Small endometriotic implants on the surface are of questionable detriment. If the endometriosis has invaded the substance of the ovary, however, an endometrioma can develop and destroy normal tissue. Furthermore, these endometriomas may cause ovarian dysfunction, which can interfere with follicular development and subsequent ovulation. The ovary many times becomes fixed to the pelvic sidewalls which interferes with the normal ovum pickup mechanism.

It is apparent that extensive disease is likely to result in the creation of a mechanical barrier to conception; however, the etiology of the infertility associated with mild or minimal endometriosis is less clear. This has forced investigators to focus their research on more subtle abnormalities associated with endometriosis that may play a role in the overall process.

Peritoneal Fluid Environment

The ovaries and fallopian tubes are bathed in peritoneal fluid. The volume of the fluid varies during the menstrual cycle and reaches a peak of 20 mL at the time of ovulation.[4] In patients with endometriosis the volume is reported to be increased, and it has been suggested that this may be a prognostic indicator for eventual pregnancy. In a previous report, patients with endometriosis with less than 14 cc of peritoneal fluid had a higher pregnancy rate than those with larger volumes.[5]

Not only is endometriosis associated with an increased volume of peritoneal fluid, evidence also suggests that the fluid environment may be embryotoxic. This toxicity can be extrapolated from well-designed animal studies. In one study, peritoneal fluid obtained from rabbits with surgically induced endometriosis was injected into the peritoneal cavity of normal rabbits 1 day prior to insemination.[6] This resulted in significant reduction in the number of normal fetuses. In another study, hamster oviducts were placed in tissue culture with peritoneal fluid from patients with endometriosis and were found to have decreased ability to pick up mouse oocytes compared to controls.[7] These studies strongly suggest that the peritoneal fluid associated with endometriosis is toxic and may potentially interfere with many aspects of the reproductive process. There is evidence that peritoneal prostaglandins and macrophages contribute in part to the toxicity of the peritoneal fluid environment associated with endometriosis.

Prostaglandins. Prostaglandins are potent modulators of a wide variety of physiologic actions. These molecules have a short half-life and generally exert their biologic action near their site of production. Thromboxane B and 6-keto-PGF (stable breakdown products of thromboxane A and prostacyclin) have been noted to be present in high concentrations in peritoneal fluid of patients with endometriosis.[8] Furthermore, these levels have been shown to be proportional to the severity of the disease.[9] The source of these prostaglandins remains unknown; however, macrophages,[10] peritoneal epithelium,[11] and endometriotic tissue[12] have the potential to produce them.

Elevated levels of peritoneal prostaglandins may adversely affect fertility in a number of ways. Prostaglandins have been shown to alter the state of smooth muscle contractility. In-vitro studies demonstrated that prostacyclin relaxes the smooth muscle of the fallopian tube.[13] Conversely, thromboxane A has been shown to induce smooth muscle contraction.[14] Thus the elevated levels of peritoneal prostaglandins associated with endometriosis could potentially alter the normal state of tubal musculature and interfere with ovum pickup, or tubal transport of the ovum or fertilized embryo. In addition, prostaglandins play important roles in ovulation and luteal regression.[15] Theoretically, elevated peritoneal prostaglandin levels could interfere with these ovarian processes as well.

Macrophages. Peritoneal fluid contains 0.5 to 2.0 million leukocytes/mL, of which 85% are macrophages.[16] Macrophages are attracted to sites of inflammation and participate in cell-mediated immunity. Increased concentrations of macrophages are found in the peritoneal fluid of women with endometriosis. An increased number of peritoneal macrophages also was reported in infertile women with unexplained infertility.[17] It is possible that patients with unexplained infertility have microscopic implants of endometriosis not grossly seen. Alternatively, they may be a subset of patients destined to acquire endometriosis.

In addition, the concentration of peritoneal macrophages seems to be influenced by tubal patency. Peritoneal fluid from women with tubal occlusion contains fewer macrophages than that from controls with patent fallopian tubes.[18] This suggests that peritoneal macrophages may originate either in the fallopian tube or the endometrium. Not only are these macrophages associated with endometriosis increased in quantity, they appear to be qualitatively different. They have increased ability to survive in vitro[19] and are better able to phagocytize sperm (Fig. 8–1).[20] These altered peritoneal macrophages may not be the result of endometriosis, but could play a role in its pathogenesis.

Macrophages in patients with endometriosis are capable of producing increased levels of fibrinectin.[21] Since the number of endometrial cells in peritoneal fluid of women with and without endometriosis is the same,[22] increased fibrinectin levels may explain the mechanism by which endometrial cells implant on peritoneal surfaces.

The prostaglandins and macrophages present in the peritoneal fluid of patients with endometriosis may create a hostile peritoneal environment capable of interfering with tubal, ovarian, or gamete function. It is difficult to determine whether this altered environment is the result or the cause of endometri-

osis. Further research should help to clarify these uncertainties.

Immunologic Aspects

Preventing infection and disease requires a competent immune system capable of identifying and destroying foreign antigens. Implantation of the embryo and successful pregnancy, however, are dependent on the immune system's restraint in rejecting the conceptus, which actually represents an allograft. Therefore, the uterine cavity offers a unique immunologic milieu that is necessary for the establishment of pregnancy.

Immunoglobulins have been identified in endometrial tissue. Their quantity varies throughout the menstrual cycle, reaching a peak during the secretory phase.[23] Levels of endometrial IgG, IgM, and IgA in patients with endometriosis and in healthy controls do not differ.[24] The concentration of immunoglobulins in patients with endometriosis, however, are negatively correlated with the severity of disease. Complement was identified in endometrial samples taken from patients with endometriosis; however, it was not identified in samples from controls.[25] These findings were not confirmed by other investigators.[24]

Evidence is increasing that endometriosis may be an autoimmune disease. In one report, all patients with endometriosis studied had antibodies directed against endometrial tissue.[26] These findings were extended by immunoelectrophoresis, which identified a line of precipitate at the interface between endometrial homogenates and serum from patients with endometriosis.[27] This finding was not confirmed

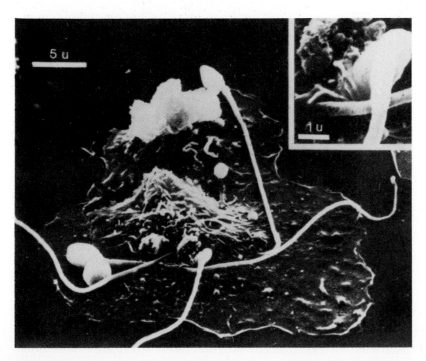

Figure 8–1. Scanning electron micrograph of a human peritoneal macrophage phagocytizing sperm. (From Muscato et al.[20] Reproduced with permission.)

in healthy controls. These results suggest that patients with endometriosis may have autoantibodies directed against normal endometrial tissue.

Additional evidence that endometriosis may represent an autoimmune disease was substantiated by a study of 59 patients[28] of whom 29% had positive antinuclear antibody (ANA) titers, 46% were positive for lupus anticoagulant, and almost 50% demonstrated IgM and IgG autoantibodies. Furthermore, patients with endometriosis are at increased risk for systemic lupus erythematosus.[29]

If indeed autoimmunity is associated with endometriosis, theoretically, antibodies directed against endometrial tissue may create an unfavorable uterine environment that interferes with implantation. It is difficult to determine whether an immunologic derangement precedes or follows the development of the disease.

Endocrinologic Alterations

Successful ovulation, fertilization, and implantation are dependent on intricate endocrinologic interactions in the hypothalamic–pituitary–ovarian axis. Several studies suggested that endometriosis may be associated with endocrinologic alterations that could interfere with conception. Abnormal secretion of prolactin and gonadotropins has been associated with this disease.

Prolactin Secretion. Prolactin is necessary for normal corpus luteal function; however, hyperprolactinemia may interefere with the physiology of the menstrual cycle at any level of the hypothalamic–pituitary–ovarian axis. Abnormal prolactin secretion has been associated with endometriosis.[30] This clinical finding was extended in an investigation of women with and without endometriosis.[31] Although baseline levels were essentially the same in both groups, their rise was significantly greater after stimulation with thyroid-releasing hormone (TRH) among the patients with endometriosis (Fig. 8–2). These finding suggest that prolactin secretion may be altered in patients with endometriosis.

Gonadotropin Secretion. One of the most intriguing areas of endometriosis research is that of altered gonadotropin secretion. Daily levels of urinary luteinizing hormone (LH), estriol-16-glucuronide, and pregnanediol-3-glucuronide were measured in groups of infertile women with and without endometriosis.[32] A single urinary LH peak was noted in the group without endometriosis; however, 26 of 29 patients with endometriosis had two urinary LH peaks that were from 2 to 3 days apart. In addition, separation of LH peaks was greater in those with more severe disease. Pregnanediol-3-glucuronide levels did not rise until after the second LH peak.

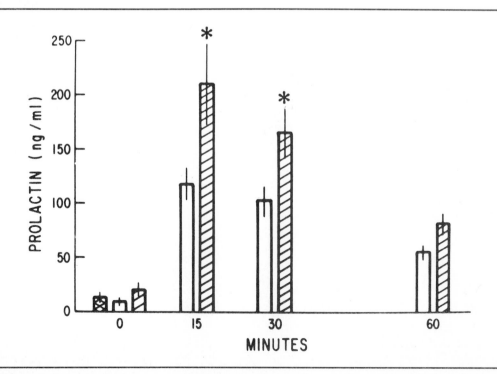

Figure 8–2. Baseline prolactin concentrations (time 0) and the prolactin response to TRH in women without endometriosis (clear bar, n = 10) and in patients with endometriosis (crossed bar, n = 14). (From Muse et al.[31] Reproduced with permission.)

We attempted to repeat this work measuring LH in serum samples from patients with endometriosis.[33] The LH surge was investigated in 20 women with and 39 women without the disease. Blood samples from all patients were obtained at 3 to 4-hour intervals at the time of the suspected LH surge. No differences were observed between patients with and without endometriosis in the frequency of several LH peaks or mean LH values. Additional studies determined that the onset of the surge tended to occur in the early morning hours in patients with endometriosis. In the group without endometriosis, however, the onset of the surge tended to be more heterogeneous (Fig. 8–3). These studies suggest that endometriosis may be associated with a central defect that causes abnormal release of gonadotropins.

Several clinical correlates give additional validity to the endocrinopathy associated with endometriosis, including the luteinized unruptured follicle syndrome, luteal phase inadequacy, and spontaneous abortion.

Luteinized Unruptured Follicle Syndrome. The widespread use of ultrasound to monitor follicle growth for ovulation induction has resulted in the realization of a new etiology for infertility—the luteinized unruptured follicle syndrome (LUF). This condition is defined as lack of physical expulsion of the ovum from the follicle at the time of presumed ovulation despite other indirect signs of ovulation, including a biphasic basal body temperature chart, the development of secretory endometrium, and elevated luteal phase serum progesterone levels. The diagnosis of LUF is substantiated by (1) absence of ovulatory stigmata noted at laparoscopy during the luteal phase, (2) periovulatory ultrasound examinations that fail to demonstrate follicle collapse, or (3) absence of elevated estradiol and progsterone levels in the peritoneal fluid during the luteal phase. Although the criteria appear straightforward, controversy surrounds the diagnosis.

Studies have shown that at laparoscopy, ovulatory stigmata are identified in only 53 to 94% of healthy, fertile patients.[34–36] In addition, elevated levels of peritoneal fluid estradiol and progesterone in patients with ovulatory stigmata have not been consistently reported.[34] Nevertheless, an apparent increased frequency of LUF is reported in association with endometriosis. Evidence of ovulation was found in 94% of control women undergoing laparoscopy, but only in 21% of patients with endometriosis.[37] The prevalence of LUF appears higher among those with more severe stages of endometriosis; however, one cannot exclude the possibility that the fixation of the adnexa that occurs with advanced disease precludes adequate visualization of ovulatory stigmata.

Others suggest that LUF may be a cause rather than the result of endometriosis. Retrograde menstruation is thought by most to be a prerequisite to the development of endometriosis, although it is known to be a common occurrence in most women.[38] Furthermore, it was observed that comparable numbers of viable endometrial cells are present in the peritoneal fluid of infertile women with and without endometriosis.[22] The progesterone in the peritoneal fluid may suppress ectopic implantation of endometrial tissue. Additional studies are necessary to establish the prevalence and significance of LUF and endometriosis.

Luteal Phase Inadequacy. As with LUF, the association of luteal phase inadequacy with endometriosis is far from conclusive. In a study comparing women with endometriosis with healthy controls,[39] no differences were found in cycle length, luteal phase length, and luteal phase serum progesterone levels. However, 4 (18%) of 22 women in the control group and 24 (67%) of 36 in the endometriosis group had endometrial biopsies that were out of phase. Furthermore, luteal phase secretion of pregnanediol-3-glucuronide, the major urinary metabolite of progesterone, was delayed in those with endometriosis. In another study, patients with endometriosis had shorter luteal lengths and had no increase in serum progesterone

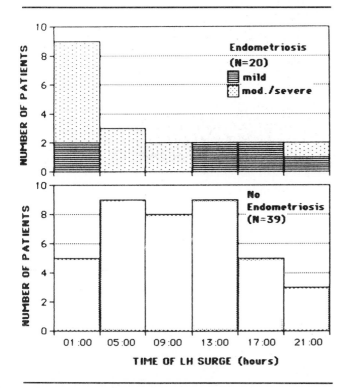

Figure 8–3. Timing of the LH surge onset in a group of patients with endometriosis (*n* = 20) and a control group (*n* = 39). (From Alper and Seibel.[33] Reproduced with permission.)

level the day after the LH peak.[37] In contrast, other investigators were unable to find a correlation between endometriosis and luteal phase deficiency.[40]

Spontaneous Abortion. Spontaneous abortion among the healthy population is a common occurrence, with its frequency estimated at 15 to 20%. Rates in patients with endometriosis have been reported to be higher than in the healthy population, ranging from 10 to 51%.[41-44]

The association of endometriosis and spontaneous abortion has been strengthened by studies demonstrating decreased rates of the latter after treatment for the former. However, a major criticism of these studies has been the lack of a control group for comparison. On 139 infertile patients who had a combined spontaneous abortion rate of 63.1%, 95 underwent conservative surgical treatment for endometriosis and 44 opted for expectant management.[45] None (0%) of the 32 pregnancies in the treated group and 6 (18.7%) of 32 pregnancies in the control group resulted in abortion. The rate of spontaneous abortion was reduced after treatment, and a statistically significant reduction was noted in the untreated group.

DIAGNOSIS

Endometriosis is suspected in any patient who has dysmenorrhea, dyspareunia, premenstrual spotting, or infertility. Findings on pelvic examination such as uterosacral nodularity, bilaterally enlarged adnexae, or a fixed, retroverted uterus, raise the suspicion of this disease. The diagnosis can be made with certainty only by visual or histologic confirmation at the time of laparoscopy or laparotomy. When performing a diagnostic laparoscopy it is important to carry out meticulous inspection of both the anterior and posterior cul-de-sacs, as well as the pelvic sidewalls. Special care also must be taken to elevate both ovaries (Fig. 8–4). If the ovaries cannot be mobilized, endometriosis should be strongly suspected.

Endometriotic implants look like irregularly shaped powder burns and appear black or tobacco-stained. Although pigmented endometriosis is by far the most common type, a nonpigmented variety has also been described. Histologic evidence of endometriosis was found in white, fleshy-appearing, and red, flamelike peritoneal lesions.[46] It was also evident in periovarian adhesions when there was no other visual evidence of pelvic inflammatory disease or pelvic endometriosis.[46] These abnormal variations may often be overlooked at the time of routine laparoscopy. If the diagnosis of endometriosis is in doubt, it is prudent to biopsy any suspicious lesions for histologic examination.

Once the diagnosis is made, the extent of disease should be assessed. When dictating operative notes or reports it is important to avoid the use of imprecise terms. The revised American Fertility Society classification of endometriosis[47] is the accepted staging reference (Fig. 8–5). It is based on scoring the extent of disease and the degree of pelvic adhesions. The summation of the scores allows endometriosis to be classified into one of four stages—minimal, mild, moderate, and severe. Although the classification system allows physicians to describe the severity of a patient's disease in a standard fashion, it also provides clinical investigators with a standard by which to compare success rates after various treatment modalities. Staging forms can be obtained from the American Fertility Society, 2131 Magnolia Avenue, Suite 201, Birmingham, AL 35256.

Although direct visualization has remained the hallmark for diagnosing endometriosis, a noninvasive screening test would be most helpful to aid clinicians in identifying patients who are at risk for this disease. One such method uses CA-125, which is a membrane antigen of epithelial origin that can be measured in the serum. Levels of CA-125 are elevated in women with epithelial ovarian cancer as well as neoplasms of other pelvic organs. Mild elevations have been reported in women with endometriosis.[48,49] Levels have been shown to be increased in proportion to the severity of endometriosis, but they may be normal in women with less severe disease. Although the ultimate value of CA-125 as a screening test for endometriosis is yet to be determined, future studies may demonstrate its utility as a marker for assessing response to treatment.

TREATMENT

As many uncertainties surround the pathophysiology of the infertility associated with endometriosis, it is difficult to prescribe a specific or ideal form of treatment. The past and present goal of treatment has been to eradicate all active disease in hope of providing symptomatic improvement as well as enhancing fertility. This can be accomplished through either medical or surgical modalities.

The primary indications for medical management include (1) the desire to defer pregnancy, (2) recurrent endometriosis after conservative surgery, (3) preoperative therapy for extensive disease or cornual obstruction, and (4) failed observation for minimal endometriosis. Progestational treatment, including gestrinone, medroxyprogesterone acetate, and continuous administration of oral contraceptives, has been used widely in the past. Although these agents have received widespread use, they have largely been superceded by danazol. Gonadotropin-

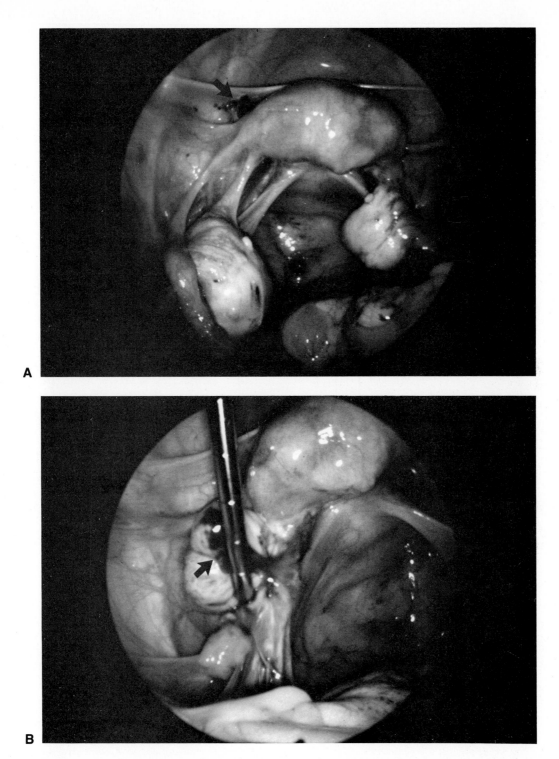

Figure 8–4. Laparoscopic view of the pelvis shows endometriosis on anterior bladder flap and in cul-de-sac. Endometriosis beneath the left ovary cannot be seen with the single puncture **(A)** but is easily seen with the use of a probe through a second puncture **(B)**.

releasing hormone agonists (GnRHa) have become available for clinical study and appear to yield promising results.

Danazol

Danazol was first introduced in 1971.[50] Its use has been widespread not only for the dysmenorrhea and infertility associated with endometriosis, but for the treatment of diseases more obscure to the gynecologist, such as angioneurotic edema,[51] idiopathic thrombocytopenic purpura,[52] and fibrocystic breast disease.[53] Although danazol has been available for clinical use for some time, it is only since the early 1980s that it has been more fully appreciated.

THE AMERICAN FERTILITY SOCIETY
REVISED CLASSIFICATION OF ENDOMETRIOSIS

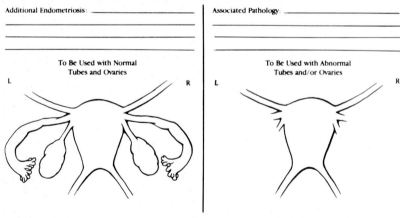

Patient's Name _____ Date_____

Stage I   (Minimal) · 1-5
Stage II (Mild)   · 6-15   Laparoscopy_____ Laparotomy_____ Photography_____
Stage III (Moderate) · 16-40   Recommended Treatment_____
Stage IV (Severe)   · >40
Total_____   Prognosis_____

PERITONEUM	**ENDOMETRIOSIS**		<1cm	1-3cm	>3cm
		Superficial	1	2	4
		Deep	2	4	6
OVARY	R	Superficial	1	2	4
		Deep	4	16	20
	L	Superficial	1	2	4
		Deep	4	16	20

	POSTERIOR CULDESAC OBLITERATION	Partial	Complete
		4	40

	ADHESIONS		<1/3 Enclosure	1/3-2/3 Enclosure	>2/3 Enclosure
OVARY	R	Filmy	1	2	4
		Dense	4	8	16
	L	Filmy	1	2	4
		Dense	4	8	16
TUBE	R	Filmy	1	2	4
		Dense	4*	8*	16
	L	Filmy	1	2	4
		Dense	4*	8*	16

*If the fimbriated end of the fallopian tube is completely enclosed, change the point assignment to 16.

Additional Endometriosis: _____   Associated Pathology: _____
_____   _____
_____   _____

| To Be Used with Normal | To Be Used with Abnormal |
| Tubes and Ovaries | Tubes and/or Ovaries |

Figure 8–5. Revised AFS classification of endometriosis.

For additional supply write to: The American Fertility Society, 2131 Magnolia Avenue, Suite 201, Birmingham, Alabama 35256

Pharmacology. Danazol is an isoxazole derivative of the synthetic steroid 17-α-ethinyl testosterone (Fig. 8–6). It is well absorbed by the gastrointestinal tract and is rapidly metabolized by the liver. Over 60 metabolites have been identified by thin-layer chromatography.[54] The pharmacokinetics of danazol follow an open, one-compartment body model. After an oral dose of 400 mg, serum drug levels peak 2 hours later and are undetectable 8 hours after administration. Doubling the dose has been shown to increase the serum concentration by only 35 to 40%.[55] The serum half-life is 4.5 hours, and this emphasizes that the agent should be administered every 6 to 8 hours to obtain maximum serum concentrations.

Mechanisms of Action. Endometriosis is dependent on ovarian hormones for its sustenance. Danazol creates a hypoestrogenic, hypoprogestational state called a pseudomenopause that theoretically results in atrophy of endometriosis. The agent induces this altered hormonal state by numerous actions.

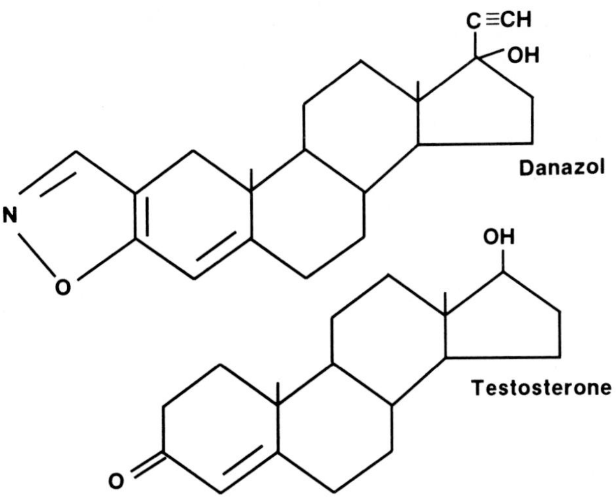

Figure 8–6. Structural formulas of danazol and testosterone.

Antigonadotropic Effect. Based on early animal studies, danazol was initially thought to exert its action solely as an antigonadotropin. This assumption was based on experiments demonstrating that danazol prevented the compensatory gonadal hypertrophy in hemicastrated rats.[56,57] However, this effect could be overridden by the administration of gonadotropins. A major criticism of these early reports was that gonadotropins were not measured, and thus a direct effect of danazol on the gonads could not be excluded. In follow-up studies the agent was shown to reduce gonadotropin levels in castrated animals.[58] This is not a distinct feature of danazol, however, as estradiol, testosterone, and dihydrotestosterone have also been shown to reduce these levels in similar fashion.[58]

Subsequent studies were carried out in humans, with comparable results. Danazol reduced follicle-stimulating hormone (FSH) and LH levels in postmenopausal women.[59,60] Premenopausal women showed no change in basal levels of gonadotropins, but rather a diminution of the midcycle FSH and LH surge.[61,62] Thus danazol does not induce a hypogonadotropic state in premenopausal females, but prevents the preovulatory gonadotropin surge of FSH and LH.

Steroid Receptors. Danazol interferes with hormone action by binding to steroid receptors. After it binds to the androgen receptors, the substrate-receptor complex is translocated into the nucleus and induces synthesis of androgen-specific messenger RNA.[63] Although binding to progesterone receptors has been demonstrated, the complex is translocated poorly

into the nucleus and is unable to initiate protein synthesis.[64] Finally, danazol does not bind to estrogen receptors.[65]

Sex-Hormone-Binding Globulin. Approximately half of serum estradiol and testosterone are bound to sex-hormone-binding globulin (SHBG), which is a carrier protein produced by the liver. The remaining estradiol and testosterone are almost entirely bound to albumin, with only a small percentage circulating in the unbound or free state. Only these unbound fractions are able to exert a physiologic effect at the cellular level. Danazol displaces testosterone and estradiol from SHBG, as well as progesterone and cortisol from corticosteroid-binding globulin.[66] This increases the free fraction of these hormones, thereby increasing their metabolic clearance rates.[67] Even though the circulating fractions of both free testosterone and estradiol are increased, it is the hyperandrogenic state that is most notable. Danazol compounds this state by reducing the synthesis of SHBG, which further increases the free testosterone level.

Direct Gonadal Effect. Evidence suggests that danazol may have a direct effect on the ovaries. In-vitro experiments demonstrated that danazol inhibits several enzymes of the steroid pathways, including 20-22-desmolase, 3-β-hydroxysteroid dehydrogenase, 17-β-hydroxysteroid dehydrogenase, 17-α-hydroxylase, 17-20-lysase, and 11-hydroxylase.[68] It inhibits these enzymes by direct competition with the steroid substrates. Danazol has no effect on aromatase.

Studies demonstrated that danazol may also have an effect on the adrenal glands. Inhibition of 11-hydroxylase and 21-hydroxylase[69] enzymes was confirmed in human adrenal tissue. This suggests that danazol interferes with corticosteroid synthesis; however, patients taking the agent have been shown to have normal serum cortisol levels and in addition, demonstrate a normal response to the metyrapone test.[70]

The direct effect of danazol on the ovary was documented in vivo.[71] When administered to primates in the luteal phase, it both decreased progesterone production and shortened the luteal phase.

Side Effects. The hyperandrogenic state that complicates danazol treatment results in many common undesirable side effects, including weight gain, acne, hirsutism, and decreased breast size. Deepening of the voice is less common but more serious. A study documented the persistence of the decreased fundamental frequency of the voice in a patient 12 months after completion of therapy, suggesting that this side effect may be irreversible.[72] Other commonly reported side effects, including muscle cramps, hot flushes, mood changes, and occasional diaphoresis, are the result of hypoestrogenism. Despite the high frequency of these symptoms, over 90% of patients continue treatment.

The majority of patients, although not all, who receive high doses of danazol become amenorrheic. When dosages less than 400 mg/day are prescribed, however, cyclic menstrual bleeding can occur. In rare instances, pregnancy has occurred during danazol treatment. The agent readily crosses the placental barrier, and a case of female pseudohermaphroditism complicating therapy was reported.[73] Therefore, patients should be advised to use barrier methods of contraception while taking the drug. This is particularly true during the first few months of therapy and when lower dosages are prescribed.

Perhaps the most potentially serious side effect of danazol therapy is the metabolic derangement of the blood lipoprotein system. There is a marked decrease in high-density lipoprotein (HDL) cholesterol, although levels of total plasma, low-density lipoprotein (LDL), and very LDL (VLDL) cholesterols are unchanged during treatment.[74,75] Fortunately, all effects on the lipoprotein system are reversed within 3 to 5 months after discontinuation of therapy. Nevertheless, concern is increasing over the role of blood lipids in the pathogenesis of atherosclerosis. Both LDL and VLDL cholesterols seem to promote the process, while HDL cholesterol offers protection. Because the HDL cholesterol level is decreased during danazol administration, there is a theoretical increase in the risk of atherosclerosis and subsequent heart disease. The risk may be minimal when therapy is for only 6 months. Prolonged use of the drug for extended periods of time is undesirable.

Alteration in thyroid function may also occur during danazol administration.[76] Typically, T_4 is depressed while T_3 RU is elevated. The TSH and free thyroxine index are normal, confirming a euthyroid state. The alteration of the measured thyroid hormones may be explained by the hyperandrogen state, which decreases the hepatic synthesis of thyroid-binding globulin. In addition, danazol induces mild elevation of liver enzymes, including creative phosphokinase, LDH, and serum transaminases (SGOT and SGPT).[77]

Therapeutic Effects. Reported pregnancy rates after danazol treatment range from 28 to 72%.[78-84] It is difficult to make a conclusion regarding the agent's effectiveness because most earlier studies made no distinction regarding the severity of the disease. In addition, many of these studies used varying doses of medication as well as variable lengths of follow-up.

In more advanced disease in which ovarian endometriomas are commonly encountered, danazol has little or no effect when the endometrioma exceeds 1 cm in diameter.[85] This is not unlike chemotherapy for malignancy, in that tumor masses require debulking prior to successful medical management. In addition, more severe stages of endometriosis may be associated with dense adhesions that do not respond to medical treatment. Thus, in extensive disease, surgical treatment is preferable, such as lysing adhesions and resecting ovarian endometriomas, in hope of restoring normal pelvic anatomic relationships. Nevertheless, danazol may have a role as an adjunctive therapy either preoperatively or postoperatively.

Minimal and mild endometriosis associated with infertility present a clinical dilemma. In these cases, the pelvic anatomy is preserved and there is no mechanical barrier to conception. One major criticism of most investigations studying the effectiveness of danazol treatment, particularly for minimal endometriosis, has been the lack of a control population to be used for comparison. The assumption has been that infertile patients with even small amounts of endometriosis require treatment; however, this is not true. In one report, the investigators found that 11 (64.7%) of 17 patients with minimal endometriosis became pregnant over a 2-year period without treatment.[86] Another investigation prospectively followed 31 couples with minimal endometriosis who received no treatment.[87] Nineteen couples (61.3%) achieved pregnancy within 18 months. These studies suggest that patients with minimal disease may be subfertile, but not necessarily infertile (Table 8–1).

We reported the first prospective, randomized study on the effectiveness of danazol treatment for minimal endometriosis.[88] Patients were randomized to receive either 6 months of danazol or no treatment at all. Observation for pregnancy started immediately after laparoscopy in the untreated group and after completion of danazol in the treated group. In that preliminary report, 6 (30%) of the 20 danazol-treated and 14 (50%) of 28 untreated patients conceived after 6 months' observation, thus questioning the efficacy of danazol treatment for minimal endometriosis. This study was subsequently expanded to include additional patients and to extend the observation period from 6 to 12 months. Using life table analysis, the cumulative pregnancy rate at the end of the 12 months was 37.2% in the danazol-treated group and 57.4% in the untreated group (NS;$p > 0.10$).[89] The lower pregnancy rate in the treated group suggests a possible detrimental effect of danazol and categorically demonstrates that the agent is not beneficial for minimal disease (Fig. 8–7). Medical treatment is expensive, is associated with side effects, and, most important, postpones opportunity for conception. Our results conclusively show that medical treatment with danazol does not enhance fertility in patients with minimal endometriosis over doing nothing at all, and suggests that a period of observation is warranted before that agent is instituted.

TABLE 8–1. PREGNANCY RATES OF PATIENTS WITH MINIMAL ENDOMETRIOSIS AFTER DANAZOL TREATMENT OR NO TREATMENT

Reference	N	Treated Group Number of Pregnancies (%)		N	Untreated Group Number of Pregnancies (%)		Follow-up (months)
82	44	23	(53)	—	—	—	37
84	10	3	(30)	—	—	—	12
79	22	11	(50)	—	—	—	18
116	10	4	(40)	—	—	—	1–10
85	111	52	(47)	—	—	—	6
117	10	4*	(40)	—	—	—	16–34
89	37	13	(35)	36	17	47	12
111	52	18	(35)	56	21	38	30
118	59	29	(49)	10	3	30	—
119	14	6	(42)	17	9	52	—
87	—	—	—	31	19	61	18
86	—	—	—	17	11	65	24
Cumulative	369	163	44	167	80	48	

*Two pregnancies were ectopic.

Dosage. Danazol is available in 200-mg tablets. The standard dosage is 800 mg every day given in two divided doses for 6 to 9 months. As previously stated, a 6-hour interval would theoretically be optimum. At an average cost of $2 per tablet, a 6-month course may cost in excess of $1,400.00. To help minimize the side effects, which are dose related, and to reduce the cost, some have suggested that lower dosages may be effective in the treatment of endometriosis. Results of a randomized, double-blind study using 100, 200, 400, or 600 mg daily revealed that even patients with severe endometriosis had symptomatic improvement with lower dosages.[84] In those treated with lower dosages, however, an increased frequency of persistent disease was noted at the time of repeat laparoscopy. Although lower dosages may be adequate in the treatment of minimal disease, increased amounts appear to be necessary for the treatment of moderate or severe endometriosis.

The presence of amenorrhea has been used as an indication of adequate treatment but does not ensure resolution of the disease. One group treated patients with mild, moderate, and severe endometriosis with danazol.[90] Those with moderate disease who showed complete resolution at the time of repeat laparoscopy had an average serum estradiol level below 40 pg/mL with danazol, and those with severe endometriosis who demonstrated complete resolution had an average level of below 20 pg/mL. Patients with amenorrhea had an average serum estradiol of only 57 pg/mL. These investigators also found that the decrease in serum estradiol was inversely correlated with the patient's weight and the frequency of danazol administration. In women who received 400 mg every 12 hours, the average level was 61 pg/mL, while in those who received 200 mg every 6 hours, it was 37 pg/mL. These authors concluded that measuring serum estradiol levels may be helpful in guiding medical treatment. They suggested that the initial dosage of danazol should be 200 mg every 8 hours; in the presence of extensive disease or a patient weighing over 150 pounds, it should be 200 mg every 6 hours.

Recurrence Rates. Danazol arrests but does not cure endometriosis. Once the medication has been stopped, the disease may return and cause recurrence of symptoms. Recurrence rates after danazol range from 33 to 39%.[78–80,83] One study of 100 patients who completed a 6-month course of danazol

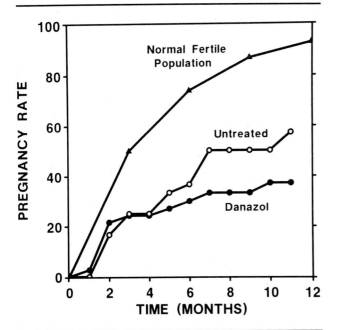

Figure 8–7. Pregnancy rates in danazol-treated and untreated patients with minimal endometriosis. (From Bayer et al.[89] Reproduced with permission.)

cited a recurrence rate of 15% in the first year and an additional 5% for each year thereafter.[89] Most recurrences are manifest between 6 and 12 months after treatment is terminated.

GnRH Analog

Over the past several years GnRH analogs have become available for clinical investigation. These agents induce a hypogonadotropic, hypoestrogenic state called medical castration that may be efficacious in the treatment of a number of gynecologic conditions, including precocious puberty, uterine fibroids, premenstrual syndrome, dysfunctional uterine bleeding, and endometriosis.

The classic work of Knobil[91] confirmed that the secretion of pituitary gonadotropins is dependent on the pulsatile release of GnRH by the hypothalamus. Conversely, GnRH administered in a continuous fashion down-regulates pituitary GnRH receptors and results in a reversible hypogonadotropic state. These low levels of gonadotropins are unable to sustain ovarian steroidogenesis, which may be especially efficacious in the treatment of endometriosis. Obviously, continuous infusion of GnRH is impractical. This obstacle has been overcome with the synthesis of long-acting GnRH analogs.

Pharmacology. Native GnRH is a decapeptide that was structurally characterized in 1971. Its half-life is between 2 and 8 minutes.[92–94] The hormone is rapidly metabolized by endopeptidases that cleave the peptide between glycine[6] and leucine,[7] and at position 9.[95,96] D-amino acid substitutions of native GnRH at position 6 and ethylamide replacement of the C-terminal amino acid of GnRH results in the creation of superagonists. These are more resistant to endopeptidase degradation, thereby increasing their patency. Increased activity of the GnRHa also results from the increased binding of the analog to the GnRH receptor.

The GnRHa are rapidly degraded after oral ingestion; therefore they must be administered by injection or by intranasal inhalation. Subcutaneous injections must be administered on a daily basis to obtain the hypogonadotropic state. A depo form of GnRHa is available that can be given on a monthly basis. Administration of the aerosol form by intranasal inhalation improves patient compliance. Three daily inhalations are typically necessary to achieve therapeutic serum concentrations. Numerous agonists have been synthesized, but two of the most widely evaluated are buserelin (D-Ser-(Bu t)^6-LHRH (1-9) nonapeptide ethylamide) and leuprolide (D-Leu^6-Pro^9-NEt LHRH) (Table 8–2).

The pharmacology of the GnRHa has been reviewed extensively.[97] Serum concentrations of buserelin remain elevated for 6 hours after a 1000-μg

TABLE 8–2. CHEMICAL STRUCTURES OF GONADOTROPIN-RELEASING HORMONE AND FIVE GONADOTROPIN-RELEASING HORMONE AGONISTS

Name	Structure									
	1	2	3	4	5	6	7	8	9	10
GnRH	ProGlu	His	Trp	Ser	Tyr	Gly	Leu	Arg	Pro	Gly-NH₂
Leuprolide						D-Leu			Pro-NEt	
Buserelin					D-Ser(tBu)				Pro-NEt	
Nafarelin						D-Nal				
Zoladex					D-Ser(tBu)					Aza-Gly
Lutrelin						D-Trp	Me-Leu		Pro-NEt	

subcutaneous injection, and its half-life is 78 to 86 minutes.[98] Urinary secretion of buserelin after subcutaneous injection is 10 times greater than after an equal dose taken by intranasal spray. This finding confirms the relatively limited absorption of the analog by way of the intranasal route. A therapeutic level of the agent can be achieved more rapidly if several subcutaneous injections precede the initiation of intranasal administration.

Actions. The initial response to the administration of a GnRHa is accentuation of gonadotropin release. Several weeks of treatment are required before down-regulation of the GnRH receptors occurs, resulting in a reduction of gonadotropin secretion by the pituitary. The drop in serum FSH levels is more precipitous than the decrease in serum LH levels, which may not decrease below baseline levels (Fig. 8–8). The ratio of bioactive to immunoreactive LH decreases with the duration of GnRHa administration. The increased levels of measured immunoreactive LH

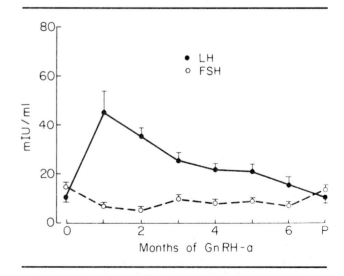

Figure 8–8. Levels of LH and FSH before, during, and after 6 months of GnRHa therapy. (From Steingold et al.[100] Reproduced with permission.)

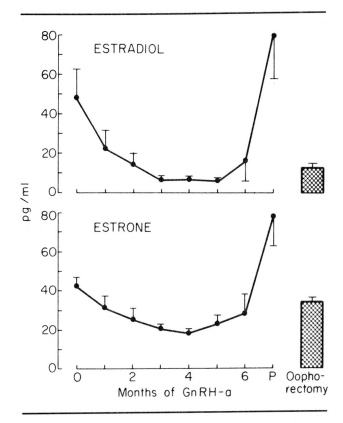

Figure 8–9. Mean ± SE levels of estradiol and estrone before, during, and after 6 months of GnRH therapy, compared with concentrations in 10 oophorectomized women. (From Steingold et al.[100] Reproduced with permission.)

represent the increased production of the LH α-subunit, whereas the production of the LH β-subunit remains unchanged during therapy.[99]

The resolution of endometriosis after medical treatment is correlated with the degree of hypoestrogenism that is attained.[100] The analogs are very effective in reducing serum estrogen levels (Fig. 8–9). Fourteen women were treated with a GnRHa 9 (Imbzl[10]-D-His[6], Pro[9]-NEt)-GnRH, 100 μg a day subcutaneously. The average baseline estradiol level was 49 pg/mL, which decreased to 22, 15, and 7 pg/mL at 1, 2, and 3 months, respectively, after beginning therapy.[100] Although administration of GnRHa decreases estrogen levels, the rapidity with which the hypoestrogenic state is attained depends on the stage of the menstrual cycle when the analog is begun. Lower levels of estradiol are achieved more rapidly if it is begun in the late luteal phase than in the follicular phase.[101]

The pituitary is the major site of action of GnRHa; however, evidence suggests that GnRHa may also have an affect at the level of the ovaries. In the rat model, GnRH has an initial stimulatory effect on steroid biosynthesis; however, sustained stimulation results in an inhibitory affect on steroid production.[102] Receptors for GnRH have been con-

firmed in the human corpus luteum.[103,104] In-vitro studies with human granulosa cells demonstrated that GnRH decreases progesterone production.[105,106] Therefore the hypoestrogenic, hypoprogestational state that occurs after GnRHa therapy might result from the combined down-regulation of GnRH receptors in the ovaries as well as the pituitary.

Side Effects. The predominant side effects of GnRHa result from hypoestrogenism. As compared to danazol, most if not all patients complain of hot flashes 1 month after beginning treatment. Other commonly reported side effects include vaginal dryness, decreased libido, breast tenderness, and depression. Also, in contrast to danazol, the blood lipoprotein system appears to be unaltered during therapy (Fig. 8–10).[107] Calcium excretion during analog treatment increases to a rate similar to that in postmenopausal women.[100] The significance of this finding over a 6 to 9-month course of treatment remains to be determined.

Therapeutic Effects. Preliminary studies confirm that most patients experience improvement in the painful symptomatology associated with endometriosis after starting GnRHa treatment. Investigators treated patients with a 7 to 8-month course of buserelin, 400 μg three times a day by intranasal spray, preceded by 200 μg daily administered subcutaneously for 5 days.[108] Seven of 8 patients had no pelvic tenderness on pelvic examination after completion of treatment. In another study, 14 women who completed a 6-month course of a GnRH analog had a significant reduction in the endometriosis pain score.[100] Resolution of painful symptoms does not guarantee resolution of the disease, however. In the latter study,[100] despite 78% reduction of visible endometriosis after GnRHa treatment, 10 of 14 patients still had visible endometriosis at the time of follow-up laparoscopy.

More reports are forthcoming and will help to further establish the efficacy of GnRHa therapy in the treatment of the painful symptomatology of endometriosis. Despite promising preliminary results, insufficient data are available to determine absolutely the effectiveness of GnRHa for the treatment of the associated infertility. Pregnancy rates comparable to those achieved with danazol appear likely.

The GnRHa seem to offer many advantages over danazol, which has been the mainstay of medical treatment of endometriosis. Resolution of the disease is dependent on the degree of hypoestrogenism, and GnRHa accomplish this to a greater extent than danazol. Although hot flashes and vaginal dryness are common side effects of both agents, GnRHa therapy is not complicated by the androgenic side effects that are common with danazol. As mentioned

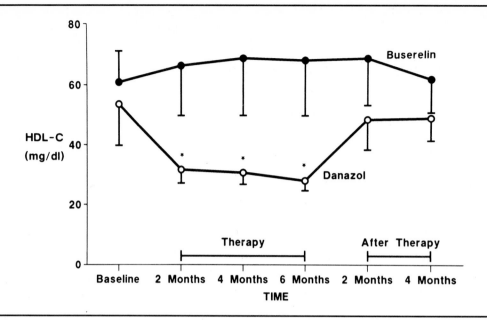

Figure 8–10. The mean plasma HDL levels are shown in a group of patients with endometriosis who were treated with buserelin or danazol. (From Dlugi et al.[107] Reproduced with permission.)

above, GnRHa do not alter the blood lipoprotein system. The analogs are still considered investigational drugs; however, once approved they will most likely become the preferred medical therapy for endometriosis.

Surgery

The mainstay of treatment has traditionally been surgical. In the past, cold knife excision and cauterization were used to resect and destroy endometriotic implants. Laser vaporization of the lesions has emerged as an effective treatment. Theoretically, the laser may be especially useful since it reduces injury to the normal surrounding peritoneum. Regardless of the modality, the goals of surgical therapy are to eradicate all active disease and to lyse adhesions in hope of restoring normal pelvic anatomy. Indications for surgical treatment include (1) ovarian enlargement, (2) pain unresponsive to medical treatment, (3) desire for pregnancy in a biologically older woman to avoid prolonged medical management, and (4) infertility due to distortion of tubo-ovarian pickup or significant adhesive disease. Even if the surgeon is able to resect all visible disease, however, the patient cannot be considered cured. Biopsies of adjacent, uninvolved peritoneal surfaces from patients with endometriosis revealed 26% frequency of microscopic disease (Fig. 8–11).[109] This suggests that surgical eradication of all visible disease is not curative, but cytoreductive at best.

Pregnancy rates after surgical treatment of mild, moderate, and severe disease were reported to be 66,

53, and 42%, respectively.[110] These results are encouraging; however, the lack of control groups for comparison prevent conclusions from being made. This is particularly true in less advanced stages of disease. Pregnancy rates after conservative surgery in patients with endometriosis were compared with those in well-matched controls.[111] Surgical therapy did not improve the rates in women with mild and moderate disease; the only group to benefit from surgery were those with severe endometriosis. These conclusions were substantiated in a study that reported comparable pregnancy rates in women with mild endometriosis who either received no treatment or underwent surgical therapy.[112] These controlled studies suggest that surgery may improve pregnancy rates only in patients with extensive disease.

Nevertheless, many times surgery is performed not only to enhance fertility, but also to correct incapacitating dysmenorrhea or pelvic pain. In such instances, in addition to ablation of endometriosis, a presacral neurectomy (if laparotomy is performed) or transection of the uterosacral ligaments (if laser laparoscopy is performed) may be indicated.

The laser has increased enthusiasm for a surgical approach to the treatment of endometriosis. Laser vaporization of the disease and lysis of adhesions can many times be accomplished through the laparoscope, making this form of treatment especially attractive. Once again, controlled studies are necessary to demonstrate its effectiveness. It must be emphasized also that the results of the most skilled laser-laparoscopists cannot necessarily be reproduced by individuals with less experience and skills.

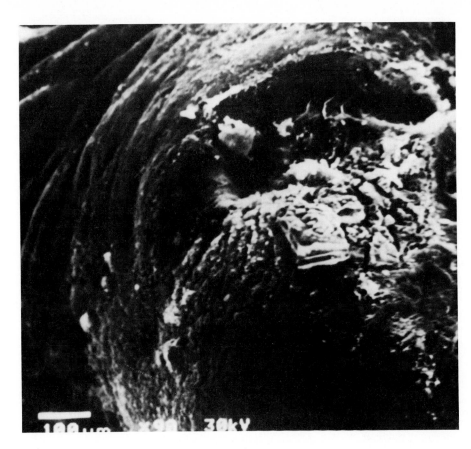

Figure 8–11. Scanning electronmicrograph of uninvolved peritoneal surfaces from a patient with endometriosis. This low-power view (magnification 90×) reveals an endometriotic gland orifice with normal mesothelium surrounding it. (From Murphy et al.[109] Reproduced with permission.)

In-Vitro Fertilization

In-vitro fertilization (IVF) is an option available to infertile patients with endometriosis who fail to conceive after either medical or surgical treatment. Theoretical benefits of IVF include the ability both to bypass potential infertility etiologies such as faulty ovulation, and the removal of both the ovum and sperm from a potentially toxic peritoneal environment. Studies reported decreased fertilization rates of oocytes obtained from women with endometriosis.[113] However, a subsequent report failed to confirm these findings.[114]

In another investigation,[115] three groups of patients with endometriosis undergoing IVF were studied: (1) those with a history of endometriosis but no active disease at the time of oocyte retrieval, (2) women with active mild and moderate endometriosis, and (3) patients with active severe endometriosis at the time of oocyte retrieval. The highest pregnancy rate was noted in those with mild to moderate endometriosis (60%) compared to the group with inactive disease (33%). The lowest pregnancy rate occurred in patients with active severe disease (6%). The difference could be explained in part by the smaller number of oocytes obtained from women with severe endometriosis, which was thought to be due to technical problems at the time of retrieval. This study suggests that IVF is much more successful in patients with lesser degrees of endometriosis. Whether women with severe disease may benefit from surgical or medical treatment immediately prior to IVF is implied but not known.

CONCLUSION

It is hoped that with further research we will acquire a beter understanding of the pathophysiology of the infertility associated with endometriosis. Until this is accomplished, treatment will remain imprecise and we can only attempt to eradicate active disease through medical or surgical modalities. Well-designed, randomized, controlled investigations should allow us to determine which forms of treatments are truly efficacious.

REFERENCES

1. Haney AF, Fortier KJ: Observations on the pathophysiology of uterine–tubal junction obstruction. *Fertil Steril* 37:293, 1982.
2. Ayers JWT: Hormonal therapy for tubal occlusion: danazol and tubal endometriosis. *Fertil Steril* 38:748, 1982.
3. Claman P, Taymor ML, Berger MJ, Seibel MM: Danazol therapy for proximal obstruction of the oviduct. *J Reprod Med* 31:687, 1986.
4. Maathuis JB, Van Look PFA, Michie EA: Changes in volume, total protein and ovarian steroid concentrations of peritoneal fluid throughout the human menstrual cycle. *J Endocrinol* 76:123, 1978.
5. Syrop CH, Halme JH: A comparison of peritoneal fluid parameters of

infertile patients and the subsequent occurrence of pregnancy. *Fertil Steril* 46:631, 1986.

6. Hahn DW, Carraher RP, Foldesy RG, McGuire JL: Experimental evidence for failure to implant as a mechanism of infertility associated with endometriosis. *Am J Obstet Gynecol* 155:1109, 1986.

7. Suginami H, Yano K, Watanabe K, Matsuura S: A factor inhibiting ovum capture by the oviductal fimbriae present in endometriosis peritoneal fluid. *Fertil Steril* 46:1140, 1986.

8. Drake TS, O'Brien WF, Ranwell PW, Metz SA: Peritoneal fluid thromboxane B and 6-keto-prostaglandin F in endometriosis. *Am J Obstet Gynecol* 140:401, 1981.

9. Ylikorkala O, Koskimies A, Laatkainen T, et al: Peritoneal fluid prostaglandins in endometriosis, tubal disorders and unexplained infertility. *Obstet Gynecol* 140:401, 1981.

10. Sun F, Chapman J, McQuire J: Metabolism of prostaglandin endoperoxide in animal tissues. *Prostaglandins* 14:1055, 1977.

11. Jerman AG, Claeys M, Moncada S, Vane JR: Biosynthesis of PGE and 12-Hete by pericardium, pleura, peritoneum and aorta of the rabbit. *Prostaglandins* 18:439, 1979.

12. Moon YS, Leung PCS, Ho Yuen B, Gomel V: Prostaglandin F in human endometriotic tissue. *Am J Obstet Gynecol* 141:344, 1981.

13. Omini C, Pasargiklian R, Folco GC, Fano M, Berti F: Pharmacological activity of PGI and its metabolite 6-oxo-PGF on human uterus and fallopian tubes. *Prostaglandins* 15:1045, 1978.

14. Svensson J, Strandberg K, Tuvemo J, et al: Thromboxane A_2: effects on airway and vascular smooth muscle. *Prostaglandins* 14:425, 1977.

15. Seibel MM, Swartz SL, Smith D, Levesque L, Taymor ML: In vivo prostaglandin concentrations in human preovulatory follicles. *Fertil Steril* 4:452, 1984.

16. VanFurth R, Raeburn JA, Vanawet TL: Characteristics of human mononuclear phagocytes. *Blood* 54:485, 1979.

17. Olive DL, Weinberg JB, Haney AF: Peritoneal macrophages and infertility: The association between cell number and pelvic pathology. *Fertil Steril* 44:772, 1985.

18. Halme J, Becher S, Wing R: Accentuated cyclic activation of peritoneal macrophages in patients with endometriosis. *Obstet Gynecol* 148:85, 1984.

19. Syrop CH, Halme J: Peritoneal fluid environment and infertility. *Fertil Steril* 48:1, 1987.

20. Muscato JJ, Haney AF, Weinberg JB: Sperm phagocytosis by human peritoneal macrophage: Possible cause of infertility in endometriosis. *Am J Obstet Gynecol* 144:503, 1982.

21. Kauma S, Clark M, White C. Halme J: Fibronectin production by human peritoneal macrophages in patients with endometriosis. Presented at the 43rd annual meeting of the American Fertility Society, Reno, Sept 28–30, 1987.

22. Koninckx RP, Ide P, Vandenbrouke W, Bosens IA: New aspects of the pathophysiology of endometriosis and infertility. *J Reprod Med* 24:257, 1980.

23. Tourville DR, Ogra SS, Lippes J, Tomasi TB: The human female reproductive tract: Immunological localization of IgA, IgG, IgM, secretory "piece," and lactoferrin. *Am J Obstet Gynecol* 108:1102, 1970.

24. Bartosik D, Viscarello RR, Damjanov T: Endometriosis as an autoimmune disease. *Fertil Steril* 41:215, 1984.

25. Weed JC, Arquembourg PC: Endometriosis: Can it produce an autoimmune response resulting in infertility? *Clin Obstet Gynecol* 23:85, 1980.

26. Mathur S, Peress MR, Williamson HO, et al: Autoimmunity to endometrium and ovary in endometriosis. *Clin Exp Immunol* 50:259, 1982.

27. Badawy SZA, Cuenca V, Stitzel A, Jacobs RDB, Tomar RH: Autoimmune phenomenon in infertile patients with endometriosis. *Obstet Gynecol* 63:271, 1984.

28. Gleicher N, El-Roeiy A, Confino E, Friberg J: Is endometriosis an autoimmune disease? *Obstet Gynecol* 70:115,1987.

29. Grimes DA, Lebolt SC, Grimes KR, et al: Systemic lupus erythematosus and reproductive function: Case control study. *Am J Obstet Gynecol* 153:179, 1985.

30. Hirschowitz JS, Soler NG, Wortsman J: The galactorrhea-endometriosis syndrome. *Lancet* 1:896, 1978.

31. Muse K, Wilson EA, Jawad MJ: Prolactin hyperstimulation in response to thyrotropin-releasing hormone in patients with endometriosis. *Fertil Steril* 38:419, 1982.

32. Cheesman KL, Ben-Nun I, Chatterton RT, Cohen MF: Relationship of luteinizing hormone, pregnanediol-3-glucuronide, and estriol-16-glucuronide in urine of infertile women with endometriosis. *Fertil Steril* 38:542, 1982.

33. Alper M, Seibel MM: Aberrant surge of luteinizing hormone in women with endometriosis. Presented at 33rd meeting of the Society for Gynecologic Investigation, Toronto, March 19–22, 1986.

34. Dhont M, Serreyn R, Duvivier P, et al: Ovulation stigma and concentration of progesterone and estrogen in peritoneal fluid: relation with fertility and endometriosis. *Fertil Steril* 41:872, 1984.

35. Vanrell JA, Balosch J, Fuster JS, Fuster R: Ovulation stigmata in fertile women. *Fertil Steril* 37:712, 1982.

36. Donnez J, Thomas K: Incidence of LUF syndrome in fertile women and in women with endometriosis. *Eur J Obstet Gynaecol Reprod Biol* 14:187, 1982.

37. Brosens IA, Koninckx PR, Corveleyn PA: A study of plasma progesterone, oestradiol, prolactin and LH levels and the luteal phase appearance of the ovaries in patients with endometriosis and infertility. *Br J Obstet Gynaecol* 85:246, 1978.

38. Halme J, Hammond MG, Hulka JF, Raj SG, Talbert LM: Retrograde menstruation in healthy women and in patients with endometriosis. *Obstet Gynecol* 64:151, 1984.

39. Chessman KL, Cheesman SD, Chatterton RT, Cohen MR: Alterations in progesterone metabolism and luteal function in infertile women with endometriosis. *Fertil Steril* 40:590, 1983.

40. Rosenfeld DL, Chudow S, Bronson RA: Diagnosis of luteal phase inadequacy. *Obstet Gynecol* 56:193, 1980.

41. Naples JD, Batt RE, Sadigh H: Spontaneous abortion rates in patients with endometriosis. *Obstet Gynecol* 57:509, 1981.

42. Rock JA, Guzick DS, Sengos C, et al: The conservative surgical treatment of endometriosis: Evaluation of pregnancy success with respect to the extent of disease as categorized using contemporary classification systems. *Fertil Steril* 35:131, 1981.

43. Wheeler JM, Johnston BM, Malinak LR: The relationship of endometriosis and spontaneous abortion. *Fertil Steril* 39:656, 1983.

44. Groll M: Endometriosis and spontaneous abortion. *Fertil Steril* 41:993, 1984.

45. Metzger DA, Olive DL, Stohs GF, Franklin RR: Association of endometriosis and spontaneous abortion: Effect of control group selection. *Fertil Steril* 45:18, 1986.

46. Jansen RPS, Russel P: Non-pigmented endometriosis: clinical, laparoscopic, and pathologic definition. *Am J Obstet Gynecol* 155:1154, 1986.

47. Buttram VC: Evolution of the revised American Fertility Society classification of endometriosis. *Fertil Steril* 43:347, 1985.

48. Barbieri RL, Niloff JM, Bast RC, et al: Elevated serum concentrations of CA-125 in patients with advanced endometriosis. *Fertil Steril* 45:630, 1986.

49. Pittaway DE, Fayez JA: The use of CA-125 in the diagnosis and management of endometriosis. *Fertil Steril* 46:790, 1986.

50. Greenblatt RB, Dmowski WP, Mahesh VB, et al: Clinical studies with an antigonadotropin danazol. *Fertil Steril* 22:102, 1971.

51. Hosea SW, Santaella ML, Brown EJ, et al: Long-term therapy of hereditary antioedema with danazol. *Ann Intern Med* 93:809, 1980.

52. Ahn YS, Harrington WJ, Simon SR, et al: Danazol for the treatment of idiopathic thrombocytopenic purpura. *N Engl J Med* 308:1396, 1983.

53. Asch RH, Greenblatt RB: The use of an impeded androgen—danazol—in the management of benign breast disorders. *Am J Obstet Gynecol* 127:130, 1977.

54. Davison C, Banks W, Fritz A: The absorption, distribution, and metabolic rate of danazol in rats, monkeys, and human volunteers. *Arch Int Pharmacodyn Ther* 221:294, 1976.

55. Potts GO, Schane HP, Edelson J: Pharmacology and pharmokinetics of danazol. *Drugs* 19:321, 1980.

56. Dmowski WP, Scholer HFL, Mahesh VD, Greenblatt RB: Danazol—Synthetic steroid derivative with interesting physiologic properties. *Fertil Steril* 22:9, 1971.

57. Potts GO, Beyler AL, Schane HP: Pituitary gonadotropin inhibitory activity of danazol. *Fertil Steril* 25:367, 1974.

58. Dmowski WP: Biological properties of a new steroid compound (danazol) with alleged antigonadotropic function. PhD dissertation, Medical College of Georgia, 1971.

59. Fanchimont P, Cramilion C: The effect of danazol on anteriorpituitary function. *Fertil Steril* 28:814, 1977.

60. Fraser IS, Thorburn GD: Effects of danazol on pituitary gonadotropins in post-menopausal women. *Aust NZ J Obstet Gynaecol* 18:247, 1978.

61. Floyd WS: Danazol: Endocrine and endometrial effects. *Int J Fertil* 25:75, 1980.

62. Goebel R, Rjosk HK: Laboratory and clinical studies with the new antigonadotropin, danazol. *Acta Endocrinol* 85:134, 1977.

63. Chamness GC, Asch RH, Pauerstein CJ: Danazol binding and translocation of steroid receptors. *Am J Obstet Gynecol* 136:426, 1980.

64. Tamaya T, Furuta N, Motoyama T, et al: Mechanisms of antiprogestational action of synthetic steroids. *Acta Endocrinol* 88:190, 1978.

65. Wood GP, Wu CH, Flichinger GL, et al: Hormonal changes associated with danazol therapy. *Obstet Gynecol* 54:302, 1975.

66. McGinley R, Casey JH: Analysis of progesterone in unextracted serum: A method using danazol—A blocker of steroid binding to proteins. *Steroids* 33:127, 1979.

67. Schwarz S, Tappeiner G, Hintner H: Hormone-binding globulin levels in patients with hereditary angio-oedema during treatment with danazol. *Clin Endocrinol* 14:563, 1981.

68. Barbieri RL, Canich JA, Makris A, et al: Danazol inhibits steroidogenesis. *Fertil Steril* 28:809, 1977.

69. Barbieri RL, Osathanondh R, Canick JA, et al: Danazol inhibits human adrenal 21- and 11-beta-hydroxylation. *Steroids* 35:251, 1980.

70. Wentz AC, Jones GS, Andrews MC, et al: Adrenal function during chronic danazol administration. *Fertil Steril* 26:1113, 1975.

71. Asch RH, Fernandez ED, Siler-Khodr TM, et al: Mechanism of induction of luteal phase defects by danazol. *Am J Obstet Gynecol* 136:932, 1980.

72. Mercaitis PA, Peaper RE, Schwartz PA: Effect of danazol on vocal pitch: A case study. *Obstet Gynecol* 65:131, 1985.

73. Shaw RW: Female pseudohermaphroditism associated with danazol exposure in utero. Case report. *Br J Obstet Gynaecol* 91:386, 1984.

74. Luciano AA, Hauser KS, Chapler FK, et al: Effects of danazol on plasma lipid and lipoprotein levels in healthy women and in women with endometriosis. *Am J Obstet Gynecol* 145:422, 1983.

75. Allen JK, Fraser IS: Cholesterol, high-density lipoprotein and danazol. *J Clin Endocrinol Metab* 53:149, 1981.

76. Graham RL, Gambrell RD: Changes in thyroid function tests during danazol therapy. *Obstet Gynecol* 55:395, 1980.

77. Holt JP, Keller D: Danazol treatment increases serum enzymes. *Fertil Steril* 41:70, 1984.

78. Puleo JG, Hammond CB: Conservative treatment of endometriosis: Analysis of 100 cases with a 4-year follow-up *Fertil Steril* 40:164, 1983.

79. Barbieri RL, Evans S, Kistner RW: Danazol in the treatment of endometriosis: analysis of 100 cases with a 4-year follow-up. *Fertil Steril* 37:737, 1982.

80. Biberoglu KO, Behrman SJ: Dosage aspects of danazol therapy in endometriosis: Short-term and long-term effectiveness. *Am J Obstet Gynecol* 139:645, 1981.

81. Greenblatt RB, Tzingournis V: Danazol treatment of endometriosis: long-term follow-up *Fertil Steril* 32:518, 1979.

82. Dmowski WP, Cohen MR: Antigonadotropin (danazol) in the treatment of endometriosis: Evaluation of post-treatment fertility and three-year follow-up data. *Am J Obstet Gynecol* 130:41, 1978.

83. Dmowski WP, Kaperanakis E, Scommegna A: Variable effects of danazol on endometriosis at 4 low-dose levels. *Obstet Gynecol* 59:408, 1982.

84. Moore EE, Harger JH, Rock JA, et al: Management of pelvic endometriosis with low-dose danazol. *Fertil Steril* 36:15, 1981.

85. Buttram VC, Reiter RC, Ward S: Treatment of endometriosis with danazol: Report of a 6-year prospective study. *Fertil Steril* 43:353, 1985.

86. Garcia CR, David SS: Pelvic endometriosis: Infertility and pelvic pain. *Am J Obstet Gynecol* 129:740, 1977.

87. Portuondo JA, Echanojauregui AD, Herran C, Alijarte I: Early conception in patients with untreated mild endometriosis. *Fertil Steril* 39:22, 1983.

88. Seibel MM, Berger MJ, Weinstein FG, Taymor ML: The Effectiveness of danazol on subsequent fertility in minimal endometriosis. *Fertil Steril* 38:534, 1982.

89. Bayer SR, Seibel MM, Saffan DS, et al: The efficacy of danazol treatment for minimal endometriosis in an infertile population: A prospective randomized study. *J Reprod Med* 33:179, 1988.

90. Dickey RP, Taylor SN, Curole DN: Serum estradiol and danazol. I. Endometriosis response, side effects, administration interval, concurrent spironolactone and dexamethasone. *Fertil Steril* 42:709, 1984.

91. Knobil E: The neuroendocrine control of the menstrual cycle. *Recent Prog Horm Res* 36:53, 1980.

92. Pimstone B, Epstein S, Hamilton SM, LeRoith D, Henricks S: Metabolic clearance and plasma half-disappearance time of exogenous gonadotropin releasing hormone in normal subjects and in patients with liver disease and chronic renal failure. *J Clin Endocrinol Metab* 44:356, 1977.

93. Arimura A, Kastin AJ, Gonzales-Barcena D, et al: Disappearance of LH-releasing hormone in man as determined by radioimmunoassay. *Clin Endocrinol* (Oxf) 3:421, 1974.

94. Miyachi Y, Mecklenburg RS, Hansen JW, Lipsett MB: Metabolism of ^{125}I-luteinizing hormone-releasing hormone. *J Clin Endocrinol Metab* 37:63, 1973.

95. Wilk S, Banuck M, Orlowski M, Marks N: Degradation of luteinizing hormone-releasing hormone (LH-RH) by brain propyl endopeptidase with release of des-glycinamide LH-RH and glycinamide. *Neurosci Lett* 14:275, 1979.

96. Hazum E, Fridkin M, Baram T, Kock Y: Degradation of gonadotropin-releasing hormone by anterior pituitary enzymes. *FEBS Lett* 127273, 1981.

97. Corbin A: From contraception to cancer: A review of the therapeutic applications of LHRH analogues as anti-tumor agents. *Yale J Biol Med* 55:27, 1982.

98. Sandow J, Jerabek-Sandow G, Krauss B, Schmidt-Gollwitzer M: Pharacokinetics and metabolism of LHRH agonists, clinical aspects, in Labrie F, Belanger A, Dupont A (eds): *LHRH and Its Analogs*. Amsterdam, Elsevier 1983, p 123.

99. Meldrum DR, Tsao Z, Monroe SE, et al: Stimulation of LH fragments with reduced bioactivity following GnRH agonist administration in women. *J Clin Endocrinol Metab* 58:755, 1984.

100. Steingold KA, Cedars M, Lu JKH, et al: Treatment of endometriosis with a long-acting gonadotropin-releasing hormone agonist. *Obstet Gynecol* 69:403, 1987.

101. Lemay A, Maheux R, Jean C, Faure N: Efficacy of different modalities of LHRH agonist (buserelin) administration of the inhibition of the pituitary–ovarian axis for the treatment of endometriosis, in Rolland R, Chadha DR, Willemsen HNP (eds): *Progress in Clinical and Biological Research*. New York, Liss, 1986, vol 225, p 157.

102. Fraser HM, Sharpe RM, Popkin RM: Direct stimulatory actions of LHRH on the ovary and testis, in Vickery BH, Nestor JJ, Hafez ESE (eds): *LHRH and Its Analogs—A New Class of Contraceptive and Therapeutic Agents*. Lancaster, MTP Press, 1984, pp 181–195.

103. Bramley TA, Menzies GS: Subcellular fractionation of the human corpus luteum: Distribution of GnRH agonist binding sites. *Mol Cell Endocrinol* 45:27, 1986.

104. Popkin R, Bramley TA, Currie A, et al: Specific binding of luteinizing hormone-releasing hormone to human luteal tissue. *Biochem Biophys Res Commun* 14:750, 1983.

105. Tureck RW, Mastroianni L, Biasco L, Strauss JF: Inhibition of human granulosa cell progesterone secretion by a gonadotropin-releasing hormone agonist. *J Clin Endocrinol Metab* 54:1078, 1982.

106. Aten RF, Williams T, Behrman HR, Wolin DL: Ovarian gonadotropin-releasing hormone-like proteins: Demonstration and characterization. *Endocrinology* 118:961, 1986.

107. Dlugi AM, Rufo S, D'Amico JF, Seibel MM: A comparison of buserelin versus danazol on plasma lipids. *Fertil Steril* 49:913, 1988.

108. Lemay A, Maheux R, Faure N, Jean C, Fazekas ATA: Reversible hypogonadism induced by a luteinizing hormone-releasing hormone (LH-RH) agonist (buserelin) as a new therapeutic approach for endometriosis. *Fertil Steril* 41:863, 1984.

109. Murphy AA, Green R, De LaCruz I, Rock JA: Unsuspected endometriosis documented by scanning electron microscopy in visually normal peritoneum. *Fertil Steril* 46:522, 1986.

110. Buttram VC: Conservative surgery for endometriosis in the infertile female: A study of 206 patients with the implications for both medical and surgical therapy. *Fertil Steril* 31:117, 1979.

111. Hull ME, Moghissi KS, Maguar DF, Hayes MF: Comparison of different treatment modalities of endometriosis in infertile women. *Fertil Steril* 47:40, 1987.

112. Schenken RS, Malinak LR: Conservative surgery versus expectant management for the infertile patient with mild endometriosis. *Fertil Steril* 37:183, 1982.

113. Wardle PG, Mitchell JD, McLaughlin EA, et al: Endometriosis an ovulatory disorder: Reduced fertilization in vitro compared with tubal and unexplained infertility. *Lancet* 2: 236, 1985.

114. Matson PL, Yovich JL: The treatment of infertility associated with endometriosis by in-vitro fertilization. *Fertil Steril* 46:432, 1986.

115. Chilik CF, Acosta AA, Garcia JE, et al: The role of in vitro fertilization in infertile patients with endometriosis. *Fertil Steril* 44:56, 1985.

116. Puleo JG, Hammond CB: Conservative treatment of endometriosis externa: The effects of danazol therapy. *Fertil Steril* 40:164, 1983.

117. Audebert AJM, Larrne-Charlus S, Emperaire JC: Endometriosis and infertility: A review of sixty-two patients treated with danazol. *Postgrad Med* 30:857, 1985.
118. Starks GC, Grimes EM: Clinical significance of local pelvic endometri-osis. *J Reprod Med* 30:481, 1985.
119. Kable WT III, Yussman MA: Fertility after conservative treatment of endometriosis. *J Reprod Med* 30:857, 1985.

PART IV

Male Infertility

CHAPTER 9

Reproductive Physiology of the Male

Clarke F. Millette

Reproductive Physiology of the Male

Pituitary–Testicular Axis of Spermatogenic Regulation
  Structure and Function of Leydig Cells
  Androgen Biosynthesis
  Testosterone Transport and Metabolism
  Pituitary–Leydig Cell Axis: Hormonal Control
Pituitary–Seminiferous Tubule Axis
  Sertoli Cells and FSH
  Inhibin
  Paracrine Regulation of Spermatogenesis
Histology of Spermatogenesis
  Spermatocytogenesis
  Meiosis
  Spermiogenesis
Sperm Maturation in the Epididymis
Sperm Capacitation and Acrosome Reaction
Normal Semen Analysis

To assess infertility in the human male, it is important to appreciate the normal physiology and structural organization of the male reproductive tract. This chapter highlights those areas deemed particularly relevant to clinical manifestations of male infertility. Large areas of interest are ignored or underemphasized because of space limitations. For example, the male accessory organs including the seminal vesicles and prostate are not discussed, and the processes of epididymal sperm maturation and capacitation are touched on only briefly.

PITUITARY–TESTICULAR AXIS OF SPERMATOGENIC REGULATION

The mammalian testis has a dual role. As an exocrine organ it produces gametes; as an endocrine organ it synthesizes and secretes steroid hormones. These two functions are divided anatomically with the interstitial Leydig cells necessary for the synthesis of androgens and the seminiferous tubules containing the various cells involved in spermatogenesis. The anterior pituitary plays an important regulatory role, interacting with both Leydig cells and the seminiferous tubules. Two major gonadotropins secreted by the pituitary act as the key modulators of testicular physiology. Luteinizing hormone (LH) is primarily involved in the pituitary–Leydig cell axis, while follicle-stimulating hormone (FSH) is responsible for interactions with the Sertoli cells of the seminiferous epithelium. These two hormonal axes are considered in sequence here, but it should be remembered that they exist in very close coordination with one another. Moreover, many aspects of the hormonal control of male reproduction, particularly in the human, remain unclear.

Structure and Function of Leydig Cells

The known constituents of the pituitary-Leydig cell axis are the Leydig cells themselves, the hormones gonadotropin-releasing hormone (GnRH), LH, and testosterone, and the blood plasma. Additional elements, including testosterone-binding proteins and blood estrogens, are also important.

Leydig cells are located in the interstitial, connective tissue regions between the seminiferous tubules. They were first described in man by von Kolliker[1] and in other species by Leydig[2]. Very early, they were suspected as the primary source of male sex hormone.[3] Now known to be the most important testicular source of steroid hormones formed de novo from cholesterol, Leydig cells exhibit an ultrastructural morphology consistent with this role.[4] They have large amounts of smooth endoplasmic reticulum, numerous mitochondria that contain tubular cristae, a large Golgi complex, and many lipid droplets. Human Leydig cells also contain specialized crystals in their cytoplasm. Called Reinke crystals, their function has not yet been determined.

Leydig cells are situated in close proximity to blood capillaries of the testicular interstitial stroma. In humans, clusters are scattered randomly in the interstitial space. Since this space contains abundant connective tissue and fluid, the Leydig cells are not always immediately adjacent to a blood vessel. Other species, such as the rodents, have sparse interstitial space, with Leydig cells clustered directly around the capillaries and with prominent lymphatic sinusoids. Finally, in yet other animals, such as the boar and some marsupials, Leydig cells fill almost the entire interstitial regions, leaving little room for the obvious connective tissue noted in humans.[5,6]

Human Leydig cells differentiate and first secrete androgens during the seventh week of fetal development, coincident with the onset of other androgen-dependent differentiations in the male. After birth, the cells appear to regress. This suggests that their initial appearance is stimulated by human chorionic gonadotropin (HGC), a possibility supported by the fact that infants born without pituitary glands still develop functional Leydig cells. The final differentiation of Leydig cells does not occur until puberty, as the levels of plasma-borne gonadotropins increase.

Without active Leydig cells, androgen-dependent differentiation does not occur. Some rats deficient in Leydig cell function have small testes that remain abdominal and show no androgen-dependent development of internal or external genitalia.[7] Such animals are phenotypic females, are classified as pseudohermaphrodites, and have elevated plasma levels of LH and FSH with very low levels of testosterone. The Leydig cells present do not respond to LH or HCG, and it is thought that they lack specific plasma membrane LH receptors. A similar condition has been described in humans,[8] again indicating the importance of an active Leydig cell population in the testis.

The major response by Leydig cells to LH is the production and secretion of testosterone. Testosterone biosynthesis in the cells results from the binding of Lh to specific cell surface receptors. This binding initiates adenylate cyclase catalysis of intracellular cyclic adenosine 3′, 5′-monophosphate (cAMP) synthesis in a process involving three distinct plasma membrane elements: (1) the receptor, which contains the specific LH recognition site; (2) the catalytic unit of adenyl cyclase, which converts adenosine 5′-triphosphate (ATP) to cAMP and pyrophosphate; and (3) the guanyl nucleotide regulatory subunit, which binds guanosine 5′-triphosphate (GTP) and couples the hormone receptor to the adenyl cyclase.[9] Inside the Leydig cell, cAMP releases the regulatory subunit of a protein kinase, which, in turn, activates the kinase catalytic subunit. The kinase catalytic subunit facilitates conversion of cholesterol to pregnenolone. Although total intracellular cAMP rises after LH binding, maximal testosterone synthesis is achieved with less than a 10% cAMP increase. In contrast, a direct correlation exists between steroid biosynthesis and occupancy by cAMP of the regulatory protein kinase subunits.[10]

Regulation of the plasma membrane LH receptors occurs after binding of exogenous LH. Leydig cells stimulated by LH exhibit a desensitivity that is caused by the down-regulation, or loss in numbers, of surface Lh receptors. The loss of sensitivity is proportional to the loss of receptors.[11,12] Leydig cells therefore contain substantial reserve numbers of LH receptors, far above those required for maximum stimulation of testosterone secretion. In the rat, for example, hormone binding increases until an extracellular concentration of 200 ng/mL is attained, even though steroid synthesis is maximized at hormone levels of only 0.5 ng/mL.[13] As a result of the excess number of LH receptors, complete responsiveness of the adenyl cyclase system can recover faster than the number of membrane receptors after LH-induced down-regulation. In addition, testosterone synthesis remains depressed after Leydig cells have regained their increased cAMP response to LH.[14] These findings are consistent with studies demonstrating that patients with highly elevated levels of HCG have decreased testosterone secretion,[15] since HCG can bind to the membrane receptors targeted for LH.

Other factors also result in the down-regulation of Leydig cell LH receptors. Large amounts of exogenous GnRH and analog cause lowered receptor numbers.[16] Also, GnRH decreases the numbers of receptors for FSH and prolactin.[17] Finally, since hypophysectomized animals show many of these same responses,[18] GnRH and analogous hormones may have a direct regulatory function in the testis in addition to their primary role in events mediated by LH.

Androgen Biosynthesis

Most potent androgens are steroids, and it is evident that testosterone is the major androgen synthesized in the testis for secretion into plasma. Although small amounts of other strong androgenic steroids such as dihydrotestosterone are also secreted, these substances do not constitute a significant proportion of total blood androgens in the male. Plasma testosterone levels in males approximate 700 ng/dL, while only 45 ng/dL of dihydrotestosterone is detected. Total androgen levels synthesized are 7,000 ng/day testosterone and 300 ng/day dihydrotestosterone. In the female, however, dihydrotestosterone is a relatively important circulating hormone; circulating levels are approximately 20 ng/dL, compared to only about 45 ng/dL testosterone.

Androstenedione is also secreted by Leydig cells. When secreted, its only known function is to serve as a precursor in plasma for estrogens, although in Leydig cells it is a precursor to testosterone. Still other testosterone anabolites such as 17-hydroxy-progesterone and progesterone are secreted, but have no known physiologic roles.

About 95% of the blood testosterone in males derives from the Leydig cells of the testis.[19] The major pathways for its synthesis are shown in Figure 9–1.[19] Leydig cells synthesize cholesterol either from acetate or from cholesterol formed elsewhere and transported to the testis by the blood. Low-density lipoprotein cholesterol may be used by Leydig cells. The relative proportion of testosterone formed from acetate or cholesterol varies among species, but in any case the acetate is first converted to cholesterol, probably as indicated in Figure 9–2. Acetyl coenzyme A (CoA) molecules combine and combine again with acetyl CoA to yield mevalonic acid. Mevalonic acid is then converted and condensed, with accompanying elongation of the carbon chain until squalene is formed. Squalene, containing 30 carbons, is folded

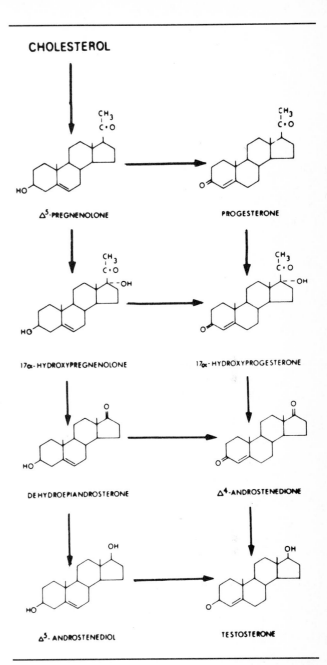

Figure 9–1. The various metabolic pathways from pregnenolone to testosterone, with the right-hand side illustrating the Δ4 pathway and the left-hand side showing the Δ5 pathway. The conversions from left to right columns use an isomerase and 3β-hydroxysteroid dehydrogenase. Vertically, each pair of conversions involves the same enzyme; 17-α-hydroxylase, 17-20 lyase, and 17β- hydroxysteroid dehydrogenase, respectively.

and closed to yield lanosterol, which is converted to cholesterol.

The androgenic testicular steroids do not contain a long side chain attached to the 17-carbon atom, as does cholesterol (Fig. 9–3). A key early step in the conversion of cholesterol to testosterone is, therefore, cleavage of this side chain to form Δ5-pregnenolone. This reaction requires NADPH and occurs in the mitochondria of the Leydig cell. The Δ5-pregneno-

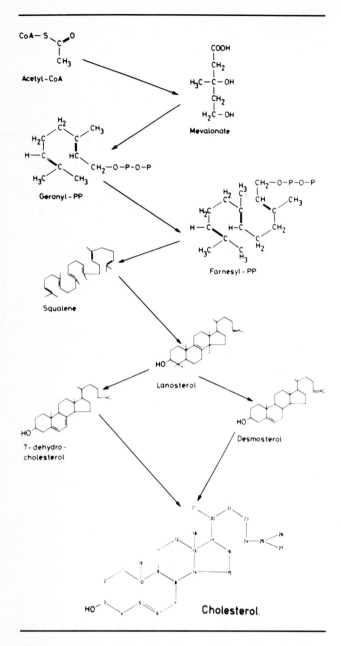

Figure 9–2. A simplified view of the metabolic pathways leading from acetyl CoA to cholesterol.

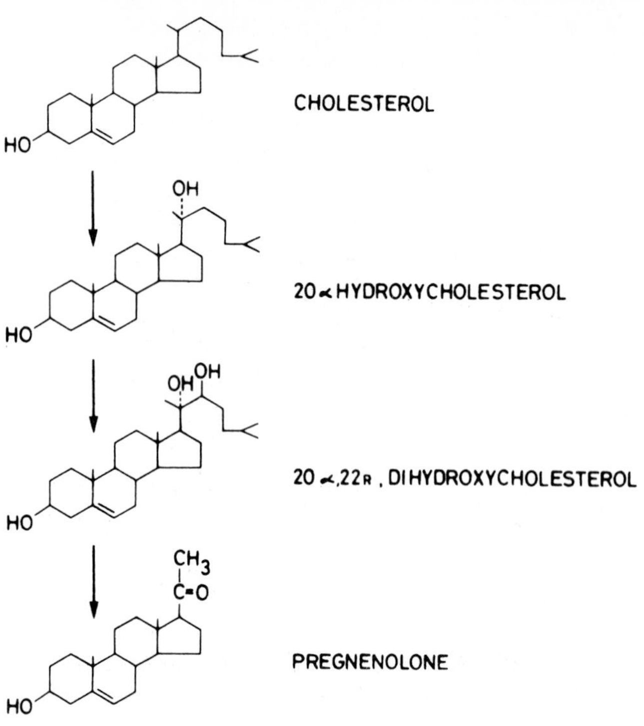

CHOLESTEROL

20 α HYDROXYCHOLESTEROL

20 α,22R , DIHYDROXYCHOLESTEROL

PREGNENOLONE

Figure 9–3. The probable pathway for the formation of pregnenolone from cholesterol. Luteinizing hormone stimulation of Leydig cells exerts a major influence here.

9–1). It is likely that important species-specific differences exist in the relative effectiveness of these alternative pathways. The Δ4 pathway, for example, seems most important in the rat, while in the human the Δ5-pathway predominates.[20]

Although LH regulates a key step in testosterone biosynthesis, and its levels are known to oscillate with a frequency of 2 to 4 every 6 hours, there is little reliable evidence for a corresponding pulsatile secretion of testosterone by Leydig cells. Some data exist describing a daily, that is, circadian, cycle of testosterone secretion with maximum levels at awakening, but the amplitude of the change during each day is small, about 10 to 25%.[21]

Testosterone Transport and Metabolism

Blood transport of testosterone is not a simple process. Due to its highly hydrophobic structure, the steroid is predominantly insoluble in aqueous solutions. Its transport is therefore accomplished by binding to specific plasma proteins. In males, one of the most important of these transport proteins is testosterone-estradiol-binding globulin (TeBG). This protein is a different polypeptide than cortisol-binding globulin, which transports cortisol, corticosterone, and progesterone. It has been isolated in an

lone is an important precursor to all subsequent reactions in the pathway. During the side chain cleavage pathway, successive oxidations of cholesterol to 20α-hydroxycholesterol take place before a second hydroxl group is added to yield 20α-, 20R-dihydrocholesterol. The side chain is finally split off between atoms 20 and 22 by the enzyme C20-C22 lyase to form pregnenolone. It is during these steps of the testosterone biosynthetic pathway that LH, by way of cAMP and the catalytic subunit of protein kinase, modulates testicular androgen levels.

From pregnenolone there are several pathways by which testosterone may be synthesized (see Fig.

active form from blood plasma.[22] It has a molecular weight of 94,000 and contains 30% carbohydrate by weight. It has two subunits, but only one testosterone-binding site per mole.[23] Under hormonal influence, TeBG levels fluctuate significantly. Estrogens increase circulating TeBG concentrations by as much as tenfold, while testosterone causes twofold decreases in TeBG levels. In humans, TeBG is responsible for the binding and transport of about 30% of the total plasma testosterone; only approximately 3% is free, with the remainder being bound to serum albumin and other blood polypeptides. It is probable that testosterone bound to TeBG is inactive, since metabolism of the steroid by target tissues is usually required for physiologic responses. Moreover, the rate of testosterone metabolism measured in humans is directly proportional to the total of free testosterone plus albumin-bound hormone.[24] Not all mammals exhibit TeBG, suggesting that this transport protein may not play an obligatory role in testosterone function.

Metabolism of testosterone accompanies its irreversible removal from the circulation. This removal may be accomplished by steroid entry into a cell, followed by metabolic alteration to another steroid form. The metabolite may be less active and destined for excretion. Alternatively, the metabolized steroid may be more active and may exert a stimulatory influence on the metabolizing cell or a distant target tissue. In the brain, the mammary glands, and elsewhere, testosterone is aromatized to yield estradiol, a strong estrogen. In addition to providing high local estrogen concentrations, this metabolic response results in an important contribution to levels of circulating estrogens in males. Amplification of testosterone activity occurs by way of the enzyme 5α-reductase, which alters testosterone to form dihydrotestosterone (DHT). Dihydrotestosterone is produced in the male reproductive tract and is involved in the modulation of extensive absorptive and secretory activities by the epididymis. In skin and perhaps the epididymis as well, DHT stimulates cell division. Nonandrogenic derivatives of testosterone, including 5α-dihydrotestosterone and etiocholanolone are also produced in humans. They are important in stimulating erythrocyte production in bone marrow.[25] Testosterone in the liver may be metabolized to inactive steroid sulfates and glucuronides for excretion.[26] Approximately 60% of plasma testosterone is cleared by the liver in a single pass. This value is less than that of other steroids, perhaps as the result of testosterone binding to TeBG.

Pituitary–Leydig Cell Axis: Hormonal Control

Blood LH levels are the primary regulator of the rate of testosterone synthesis and the secretion of this androgen into the blood. Increased LH levels cause hypertrophy of Leydig cells and accompanying increased testosterone secretion. Decreased LH levels are determined by the secretory activity of the anterior pituitary. Pituitary secretion of LH is directly responsive to plasma testosterone levels, with a reduction in testosterone inducing increased LH secretion. Maintained high testosterone levels decrease LH secretion by the pituitary (negative feedback). Since LH secretion is under the control of GnRH, the testis, pituitary, and hypothalamus form a functional unit involved with the regulation of spermatogenesis. This axis maintains relatively constant levels of plasma testosterone, except for the slight diurnal variation mentioned previously.

Estrogenic metabolites of testosterone, such as estradiol produced by the brain, also affect LH secretion, but they do so in a manner deferent from that of testosterone. Sudden infusion of estradiol reduces mean LH concentration by lowering the amplitude of each individual LH secretory event. This is accomplished by inhibiting the sensitivity of the anterior hypophysis to GnRH. In contrast, infusion of testosterone reduces the mean LH levels in blood by reducing the frequency of LH secretory events. This effect is not related to any alteration in pituitary responsiveness to GnRH, and suggests that a primary mode of testosterone-mediated inhibition occurs by way of the hypothalamus.

A positive feedback mechanism involved in the hormonal control of the pituitary-Leydig cell axis has also been demonstrated in the male as a response to extended estrogen exposure. In the female, positive feedback is obvious and results in the midcycle LH surge, but in the male this action of estrogen is difficult to establish. Experimental studies have shown that only about one half of men treated with estrogen exhibit positive feedback, and even in these individuals the maximum LH levels achieved after the initial fall rarely exceed pretreatment baseline concentrations. Patients having elevated gonadotropin levels, such as men with either Klinefelter's or the Sertoli-cell-only syndrome, do demonstrate a strong positive feedback response, even in the presence of normal testosterone concentrations. Similarly, positive feedback on LH, caused by estradiol, can be demonstrated in male monkeys after orchiectomy and estrogen exposure.

PITUITARY–SEMINIFEROUS TUBULE AXIS

The important known constituents of the pituitary–seminiferous tubule axis are the Sertoli cells of the seminiferous epithelium, and the hormones FSH and inhibin. In addition, other hormones, such as Sertoli-cell-specific growth factor and opioid peptides, may play regulatory roles.

Sertoli Cells and FSH

The interaction of FSH and Sertoli cells is clearly the most important element regulating the pituitary–seminiferous tubule axis. Like LH, FSH is released from the anterior pituitary in response to GnRH. However, GnRH is only about 20% as active in the release of FSH compared to release of LH, and the details of the FSH secretory response to GnRH are not yet well identified. The existence of a separate FSH-releasing factor has been hypothesized, but it has not been positively identified and isolated in humans.

Both FSH and LH are required for human spermatogenesis, with the effects of LH believed to be directed solely by Leydig cell secretion of testosterone. Surface receptors for LH have not been detected on Sertoli cells or on differentiating male germ cells. In the adult, spermatogenesis may be maintained with testosterone alone, as demonstrated in hypophysectomized animals. In immature animals, or in animals that have undergone hypophysectomy without testosterone replacement therapy, however, both testosterone (or LH) and FSH are needed to initiate spermatogenesis.[27] The testicular alterations that must occur to effect this change in hormonal regulation have not been identified.

Plasma membrane receptors specific for FSH have been described on Sertoli cells.[28–31] These receptors are of high affinity and low capacity, with dissociation constants at or near the physiologic FSH concentration. Sertoli cells respond rapidly to FSH, concomitant with the intracellular stimulation of adenyl cyclase and before other cellular events such as the secretion of specific polypeptides. Receptors for FSH have been studied in enriched preparations of Sertoli cell membranes.[32–35] As a result of FSH binding, Sertoli cell adenylate cyclase is activated,[36] cyclic nucleotide phosphodiesterase is inhibited,[37] and intracellular levels of cAMP increase. Increased cAMP levels have been quantified in immature,[38] hypophysectomized,[39] cryptorchid,[38] and X-irradiated animals,[37,40] and in isolated, cultured Sertoli cells.[36,41] As elsewhere, including the interaction of Lh and Leydig cells, in Sertoli cells cAMP binds to the regulatory subunit of protein kinase, thereby releasing the kinase catalytic subunit. This kinase subunit then phosphorylates a number of proteins, many uncharacterized biochemically, which in turn stimulate increased synthesis of RNA, and the production and secretion of specific proteins.[42] A protein kinase inhibitor (PKI) has been purified from the rat testis,[43] and using immunocytochemistry, shown to be a Sertoli-cell-specific marker enzyme[44,45] The PKI is cAMP dependent and is also synthesized in direct response to FSH binding. Neither testosterone nor LH affects intracellular levels of Sertoli cell PKI[46] Details of the protein kinase–PKI interrelationship in Sertoli cells have not been established.

In Sertoli cells the responses to FSH stimulation are both morphologic and biochemical. All FSH effects seem to be mediated by intracellular increases in cAMP and, presumably, subsequent protein phosphorylation events. Ultrastructural alterations occur after treatment of Sertoli cells with antisera to either LH or FSH.[47,48] Anti-FSH exposure decreases total Sertoli cell volume and increases dilation of the smooth endoplasmic reticulum. In contrast to Sertoli cell morphology after anti-LH exposure, anti-FSH does not result in major changes in the shape of the Sertoli cell nucleus, the total number of mitochondria, the number of lipid inclusions, or the extent of nuclear heterochromatization.

Biochemical responses of Sertoli cells to FSH are manifest and are most probably directly responsible for mediating and coordinating spermatogenesis. It is now well known that androgen-binding protein (ABP) is produced and secreted by Sertoli cells in response to FSH. A secretory protein,[49] ABP is transported through the efferent ductules of the testis to the epididymis. Numerous studies have established that ABP is produced only by Sertoli cells in intact seminiferous tubules and in culture.[50–54] Rat ABP has a molecular weight of 105,000, calculated from its amino acid composition,[55] which agrees with determinations of Mr 94,000 made from sedimentation analysis.[56] Rat ABP in sodium dodecylsulfate (SDS) has two subunits of 47,000 and 41,000 Mr, respectively. The physiologic function of ABP is not clearly understood. In the rat, a species that does not have TeBG, it is thought that the ABP secreted vectorially to the lumen of the epididymis may help to maintain relatively high local concentrations of DHT, important for the synthesis and secretion of epididymal proteins during sperm maturation. In other species, such as the human or rabbit where TeBG does exist, ABP has a slightly smaller molecular weight, and its secretion by Sertoli cells and transport to the epididymis have not been as well delineated.[57] Human ABP and TeBG are definitely different polypeptides, however, as determined using a variety of biochemical assays. So far, human ABP has only been detected in testicular extracts. On the other hand, TeBG has been isolated from serum using affinity chromatographic procedures using concanavalin A.[58–61]

Gamma-glutamyl transpeptidase is another Sertoli cell marker enzyme stimulated by FSH. This protein is a membrane-bound enzyme and is well distributed in many tissues in many mammalian species, including humans.[62] It transfers the gamma-glutamyl group of glutathione and similar com-

Reproductive Physiology of the Male

pounds to amino acid and peptide cofactors. The enzyme is thought to affect the translocation of amino acids across the plasma membrane. Although most experimental data regarding FSH-Sertoli interactions have been obtained of necessity using rodent tissues, a few investigators have demonstrated that human Sertoli cells cultured in vitro contain a gamma-glutamyl transpeptidase, which shows a twofold increase after administration of exogenous FSH.[53,63] Luteinizing hormone and testosterone do not cause similar stimulatory increases and they do not act synergistically with FSH. Other constituents must be operant in this system, however, since the FSH effect on human Sertoli cells was noted only with serum in the in-vitro culture medium. It is also of interest that the human appears to differ here from species such as the rat. Although rat Sertoli cells do contain gamma-glutamyl transpeptidase, in this species the enzyme is not affected by FSH.[54,64] In the rat, the testicular form of the enzyme also seems to be associated exclusively with the Sertoli cell.[54]

Synthesis and secretion of the iron-transporting polypeptide transferrin is also responsive to FSH. Sertoli cells contain two forms of transferrin, one apparently identical to transferrin present in serum and another unique to the Sertoli cell itself. It is now thought, based on both biochemical and morphologic analysis, that Sertoli cells take up iron by way of serum transferrin, dissociate the mineral, and then rebind iron to the testicular transferrin.[65,66] The Sertoli-cell-specific transferrin-iron complex is then secreted vectorially into the adluminal compartment of the testis for probable delivery to the developing spermatogenic cells.[66,67] Although the existence of an FSH-dependent testicular form of transferrin and its vectorial secretory pathway have been deciphered, the exact role of iron metabolism in the testis is still largely unappreciated.

Present data do not allow a well-grounded understanding of the exact roles of FSH and cAMP-dependent Sertoli cell secretory proteins in maintaining and regulating spermatogenesis in human males. The issue is complicated by the fact the Sertoli cell response to FSH is not limited to the new or increased biosynthesis of specific polypeptides. Sertoli cells also respond, for example, by the increased production of intracellular lactate.[68] Differentiating germ cells in the rat and mouse are highly dependent on exogenous lactate and pyruvate for maximum synthesis of both amino acids and proteins.[69-71] Using in vitro cultures of isolated male germ cells, it was demonstrated in the rat that lactate and other low-molecular-weight substances secreted by Sertoli cells are used by pachytene spermatocytes and round spermatids.[72] This form of germ cell–Sertoli cell cooperation therefore provides an additional mechanism by which FSH can exert modulating effects on spermatogenesis.

Similar effects could be operating in the human. Isolated populations of human pachytene primary spermatocytes seem to require exogenous pyruvate for maximal protein synthesis.[73]

The physiology of the Sertoli cell and its relationship to modulating hormones produced by the anterior pituitary is obviously complex. The present state of information may be summarized as follows:

1. Follicle-stimulating hormone binds to specific Sertoli cell plasma membrane receptors and alters adenyl cyclase activity.
2. Intracellular cAMP levels increase due to FSH binding. It should be noted, however, that cAMP levels are also controlled by cAMP phosphodiesterases, which in turn are affected by calcium-dependent calmodulin and other agents.
3. Increased cAMP levels act to stimulate a cAMP-dependent protein kinase, which phosphorylates a variety of Sertoli cell proteins. This step is regulated by the cytoplasmic PKI.
4. Resultant cellular events stimulated by phosphorylation include the synthesis and secretion of numerous Sertoli cell proteins and low-molecular-weight compounds, as well as increased fluid secretion by Sertoli cells. Many of the polypeptides and other substances are believed to act locally to supply differentiating germ cells in the adluminal epithelial compartment with required nutrients and activating agents.
5. Once initiated, most of the FSH-induced events can be maintained by testosterone alone.
6. The role of germ cells is not yet evident, but they can produce cAMP and they possess a germ-cell-unique adenyl cyclase. Data showing that germ cells can alter Sertoli secretory activity have been reported.
7. Paracrine interactions among Sertoli cells, Leydig cells, and germ cells are increasingly attracting the attention of investigators. Examples of such interactions are the secretion of lactate/pyruvate by Sertoli cells for delivery to germinal cells and the possible local role of luteinizing-hormone-releasing hormone (LHRH) in coordinating spermatogenesis.
8. Finally, Sertoli cells also synthesize inhibin, which acts to feed back negatively on the secretion of FSH by the pituitary (Fig. 9–4).

Inhibin

As early as 1932 it was suggested that a water-soluble compound produced in the testis acted to regulate gonadotrophin secretion.[75] This consideration was based on the fact that castrated rats show atrophy of the secondary sex organs and increased gonadotropin concentrations. Administration of fat-soluble testis extracts or testosterone did not reverse the pitu-

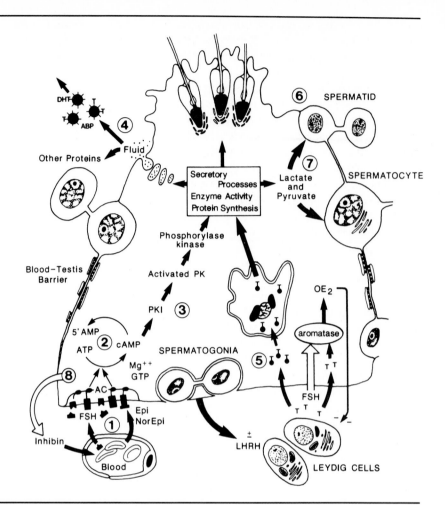

Figure 9–4. A diagram illustrates the physiologic and structural interrelationships of Sertoli cells and germ cells in the mammalian seminiferous tubule. (Modified from Hansson.[74])

itary hyperplasia, although secondary sex organs recovered. Aqueous testis extracts, however, were effective in lowering gonadotropin concentrations, and the factor believed responsible was named inhibin. Evidence for inhibin in humans first became apparent by about 1950 when workers reported increases in urinary gonadotropins in men with absent or damaged seminiferous epithelium due to the Sertoli-cell-only syndrome, irradiation exposure, and idiopathic oligospermia.[76,77]

Positive identification of inhibin was delayed for many years by inability to purify this compound and by the possibility that low, contaminating amounts of hormones such as testosterone were present but unrecognized. A large variety of indirect evidence, however, continually suggested the existence of inhibin. Such data included rises in FSH secretion accompanying damage to the testis induced by irradiation,[78] heat,[79] busulfan and other alkylating compounds,[80] cryptorchidism,[81] and ligation of the efferent ducts leading from the organ.[82] As a result of these and similar studies, intensive attempts to isolate and characterize inhibin were initiated, greatly facilitated by the increasing availability of radioimmu-

noassays for most relevant substances. Most workers attempted to isolate inhibin from porcine follicular fluid, but some reported the apparent purification of the hormone from different male fluids and tissues.[83–90]

Positive isolation and characterization of inhibin were not demonstrated until it was purified from porcine follicular fluid using high-performance liquid chromatography and gel filtration. The protein has a molecular weight of 32,000 and consists of two polypeptide chains, Mr 14,000 and 18,000, which may be separated after reduction. Using an in vitro pituitary cell culture assay, it was shown to have an EC50 of about 0.3 ng/mL (10 pM).[91] In addition, antibodies were raised against the purified molecule and were demonstrated to neutralize inhibin activity in vitro. Continuing these studies, the same workers isolated cDNA clones for inhibin.[92] Oligonucleotide probes synthesized from the determined amino acid sequence of purified inhibin were used to probe a cDNA library from porcine ovary. The DNA clones encoding the 18,000 Mr moiety, the A chain, of inhibin were obtained and applied to isolate similar cDNA probes from a human placental cDNA library.

Based on DNA sequence analysis, the A chain of inhibin is first synthesized as a large precursor and has apparent carbohydrate binding sites. Human inhibin A chain precursor is highly homologous to that of the pig and is also predicted to be glycosylated.[92]

Several antibodies have been prepared recognizing different portions of the A chain of porcine follicular inhibin. Using some of these antibodies, one group reported that inhibin production by cultured rat Sertoli cells is hormonally regulated.[93] Follicular-stimulating hormone, but not HCG or prolactin, causes a dose-dependent increase in both the intracellular and secretory forms of inhibin. Agents known to increase intracellular cAMP levels augment this response, but the addition of DHT or estradiol to the Sertoli cell cultures has no effect. The inhibin secreted by Sertoli cells has been bioassayed and demonstrated to have a molecular weight of approximately 32,000, as expected from previous data.[94-97]

It is therefore firmly established that inhibin is produced by Sertoli cells of the seminiferous epithelium, and that these cells are its only apparent testicular source. The role of inhibin is to feed back negatively on the anterior pituitary in order to maintain functional levels of FSH secretion. Many details of the intricate and intertwined feedback mechanisms governing FSH and LH secretion are reviewed elsewhere.[98-100]

Paracrine Regulation of Spermatogenesis

Both the pituitary–Leydig cell axis and the pituitary–Sertoli cell axis operate over long distances using soluble hormones. Increasing attention, however, is being given to the possibility that paracrine relationships, short-distance hormonal interactions between different testicular cell populations, may also be important in local modulations of spermatogenesis. For example, the relative hypertrophy of Leydig cells was reported to coincide with their individual position relative to particular stages of differentiated germ cells in the seminiferous epithelium of the rat.[101] This morphologic observation may be interpreted to mean that germ cells at specific developmental times, the Sertoli cells that alter morphologically and biochemically in concert with the germ cells, or both, produce diffusable factors that act directly upon the neighboring interstitial cells. Similarly, it was shown that when peritubular myoid cells are co-cultured with Sertoli cells, the myoid cells secrete a protein factor called PMod-S, which acts to stimulate the synthesis of ABP and transferrin by Sertoli cells.[102] The paracrine nature of this activity is indicated by the term PMod-S (peritubular modification of Sertoli cells). Other co-culture studies using germ cells, Sertoli

cells, and Leydig cells have indicated that Sertoli cells can somehow increase the number of HCG receptors on Leydig cells with a corresponding increase in steroidogenic activity.[103] Furthermore, Leydig cells are reported to cause an increase in FSH responsiveness by Sertoli cells.[103] Presumably such effects are the result of secretory cell products, although these have not been described.

Extensive data have been obtained implicating GnRH, or a close analog of this compound, in the paracrine regulation of spermatogenesis.[104-109] Although mostly indirect and not universally accepted, this evidence supports the concept that GnRH secreted locally in the rat testis can alter the permeability of testicular capillaries and the interstitial fluid concentration of testosterone. The testicular source of the GnRH-like hormone has not yet been identified, but could be the Sertoli cell.

Other hormones, or possible paracrine factors, have also been identified. Sertoli cells, for example, produce a specific growth factor whose target tissue remains to be defined, but that could act to coordinate the early mitotic proliferation of spermatogonia in the testis.[110] A number of opioid peptides have been detected in mammalian testis, including β-endorphin.[111-113] Proopiomelanocortin (POMC) mRNA gene transcripts have been detected in the mouse testis and been found to exhibit developmental stage specificity. The POMC messages are found primarily in Leydig cells, with some in situ hybridization also noted in spermatogonia and spermatocytes.[114] The appearance of mRNAs for POMC in the testis seems to be controlled by local interactions between Leydig cells and germ cells as determined by northern blot analysis of mouse strains deficient in spermatogenic cells at different stages of development.[115] Prodynorphin gene mRNAs[116] and those for proenkephalin[117,118] have also been detected. In all instances, the mRNAs are detected only in Leydig cells and/or restricted classes of differentiating germ cells. The physiologic roles of these different opioid peptides in testicular function have not yet been determined, nor is it yet clear that all of the detected mRNA species are actually translated in vivo. These data do, however, support the concept that paracrine interactions among Leydig cells, Sertoli cells, and germinal cells are much more important in the regulation of mammalian spermatogenesis than is recognized.

HISTOLOGY OF SPERMATOGENESIS

Spermatogenesis is the process of sperm differentiation in the testis, beginning with the mitotic proliferation of spermatogonia (*spermatocytogenesis*), proceeding through the development of spermatocytes (*meiosis*), and culminating in the morphologic alteration of a haploid round spermatid into the highly elongated, polarized sperm cell (*spermiogenesis*). This complex cellular transformation occurs in the seminiferous epithelium of the testis. The testicular epithelium is composed of two cell populations, the germ cells at various stages of differentiation, and the somatic, supporting Sertoli cells. Space does not permit a discussion of Sertoli cell morphology and physiology, but these cells are extremely complex and undergo dramatic changes in overall shape during the varying stages of the spermatogenic cycle. Human Sertoli cells are described elsewhere.[119-122]

The Sertoli cells are relatively static in their intratubular position. Germ cells, on the other hand, translocate adluminally in the epithelium as they differentiate. Overall, spermatogenesis is very tightly regulated by a variety of hormonal influences, but it is also evident that cell–cell interactions within the epithelium itself are important in coordinating sperm differentiation. Most morphologic and biochemical experimentation on mammalian spermatogenesis has used tissue from laboratory animals, but detailed morphologic descriptions of human spermatogenesis are available.[123] Reviews of spermatogenesis in mammals[124,125] and particularly in humans[126] may be found elsewhere.

Spermatocytogenesis

Primordial germ cells in man are first detected by the end of the third week of gestation.[127,128] These cells are seen near the yolk sac, from where they migrate by ameboid locomotion to the gonadal ridge. After intensive proliferation, two populations of the primitive germ cells, now termed gonocytes, are seen in humans. Until the sixth week of gestation gonocytes have a round nucleus and a prominent nucleolus. These cells also have sparse mitochondria, with tubular cristae and cytoplasm containing numerous microfilaments. Similar cells are seen throughout gestation. In contrast, a second class of gonocytes containing extensive cytoplasmic glycogen deposits and many mitochondria disappears by the tenth week of gestation.[129,130]

During the third month of development fetal spermatogonia are seen in humans.[131] The origin of these cells and their relation to gonocytes are not clear. Although in other species many early gonocytes fail to mature,[125,132,133] little is understood in detail for humans. Investigators have described the proliferation of surviving gonocytic cells[134] and two populations of germ cells in infantile human testis.[135] Quantitative data were reported on the survival and differentiation of human spermatogonia,[136] but further studies are needed in this area.

Gonocytes differentiate into spermatogonia by mitotic division. Spermatogonia continue to undergo rounds of mitosis and form the permanent, renewing stem population needed to ensure continuous sperm production during an individual's reproductive lifetime. Morphologic studies of human spermatogonia have been reported.[137-141] Three or four different types can be identified based on morphologic differences in the staining of their cytoplasm, the extent of nuclear heterochromatization, and the cellular position with respect to the basement membrane of the seminiferous tubule. The various spermatogonial populations have been called types Ap, Ad, B, and AL, with the last discussed only by Rowley and associates.[138]

Two spermatogonial forms have been described in biopsies of boys aged 3½ months to 13 years.[142,143] Type Ap (type A pale) cells seem most frequent during these ages, with type Ad (type A dark) also present. Fetal-type spermatogonia were detected up to age 4 years. Gonocytes had apparently disappeared by this age, having differentiated into type Ap spermatogonia. Type A spermatogonia eventually differentiate into type B, which are characterized by pale cytoplasm, spheric nucleus, and clumped, peripheral heterochromatin. In addition, human type B cells may contain a crystal of Lubarsch, a cytoplasmic inclusion constituted of packed, parallel, dense filaments and interspersed granules of unknown origin and function.[144] The complete details of the kinetics of spermatogonial proliferation and renewal in animals and humans are not understood. Discussions of this complex problem are available.[145-148]

Meiosis

Type B spermatogonia complete a final mitotic division and differentiate into primary spermatocytes, thereby initiating meiosis. Meiosis involves two successive nuclear divisions with only one accompanying chromosomal division in order to achieve haploidy. The first meiotic prophase is long, enabling the processes of chromosomal condensation, pairing, exchange, and separation.

Preleptotene spermatocytes result from the mitotic division of type B spermatogonia. They are characterized by nuclei smaller than those in the type B cells. These cells are located at the periphery of the seminiferous tubule, often still in contact with the basement membrane. Preleptotene cells duplicate their DNA and start to translocate adluminally, away from the tubule periphery. The spermatocytes then enter the leptotene stage of meiosis, in which the chromosomes are seen as thin filaments. Leptonema is followed by the zygotene stage, during which synapsis of paired genetic material occurs. The synaptonemal complex is first evident at this stage.[125,149-151] Chromosomal thickening, pairing, and exchange continue during the next stage, that of pachytene spermatocytes. Extensive cell growth occurs during the long pachytene stage, both as detected from cell size measurements and from biochemical analysis of isolated germ cells in rodents[152-154] and humans.[73,155,156] After pachynema is complete, the spermatocytes enter the diplotene stage, at which time the paired chromosomes begin to separate and chiasmata (chromosomal bridges) may be seen. Finally, during diakinesis the chromosomes of each bivalent pair continue to separate as the chiasmata move from the centromeres to the chromosomal telomeres. This completes the first meiotic prophase. Description of spermatocyte morphology in humans is published elsewhere.[157]

After diakinesis, the nuclear envelope disintegrates, facilitating alignment of bivalents at the metaphase plate in metaphase I. Anaphase I and telophase I are completed quickly, with daughter chromatids moving to opposite poles of the new cells, called secondary spermatocytes. Each secondary spermatocyte contains a haploid number of chromosomes. Secondary spermatocytes are short-lived cells, much smaller than the earlier primary spermatocytes. They are also characterized by spheric nuclei with pale, granular chromatin. No DNA synthesis occurs prior to the second meiotic reduction division. Meiotic interphase II is short, and cells pass rapidly through metaphase II, anaphase II, and telophase II. Completion of these events yields young spermatids, destined to undergo substantial morphologic and biochemical transformations as they develop into testicular spermatozoa.

Spermiogenesis

Spermiogenesis is the process by which a round spermatid transforms morphologically and biochemically into the elongated testicular spermatozoon. This alteration is accomplished without concomitant cell division, but involves a host of biochemical changes. Numerous investigators have examined the ultrastructure of spermatozoa in mammals, including humans. Several significant reports with emphasis on the human have appeared.[158-167] Differentiating spermatids in humans also have been described in detail.[123,167-170]

The entire process of spermiogenesis is subdivided into four well-described phases: Golgi, cap, acrosome, and maturation. These distinctions are based on the light and electron microscopic morphology of developing spermatids. During the Golgi phase, the new spermatids exhibit an extensive Golgi apparatus in the cytoplasm. The nucleus is spheric, with chromatin condensation not yet initiated. Mitochondria and other normally occurring cytoplasmic organelles are obvious. Soon, proacrosomic granules appear in close juxtaposition to the Golgi apparatus. Containing a variety of lytic enzymes, the acrosomal granules fuse, forming a single, large, cytoplasmic compartment called the acrosomic vesicle. This vesicle contains a dense granule surrounded by diffusely staining material as determined with the electron microscope. The vesicle and granule continue to enlarge, with the intracellular position of this structure determining the anterior pole of the differentiating sperm.

Also during the Golgi phase, mitochondria leave the perinuclear region and assume positions immediately subjacent to the plasma membrane. The plasma membrane itself seems thickened when examined at the ultrastructural level. Paired centrioles migrate to the nuclear pole opposite that occupied by the acrosomic vesicle and start flagellar elongation.

The cap phase involves continued development of the acrosome, which attaches to the anterior pole of the spermatid nucleus and flattens in close association with the nuclear membrane. Eventually, the acrosomic vesicle covers fully one third to one half of the anterior nuclear surface. This is the so-called acrosomal cap.

During the acrosomal phase of spermatid differentiation the cell nucleus first begins to elongate and condense. The anterior-posterior axis of the cell is well defined, and the cytoplasm is displaced adluminally with respect to the long axis of the entire seminiferous tubule. The anterior nucleus with its associated acrosomal cap becomes closely associated with the overlying plasma membrane as the spermatid nucleus continues elongating. Chromatin condensation also continues until most of the genetic material is involved, with only occasional remaining vacuoles. These vacuoles often are more pronounced in humans than in other species. The Golgi apparatus detaches from the developing acrosome and new cytoplasmic organelles appear. The manchette, for example, is composed of microtubules that are aligned parallel to one another and surround the posterior half of the elongating nucleus. Long postulated to be important in shaping the sperm head, a precise role of the manchette is still unknown. At the site of flagellar attachment to the posterior nucleus, or implantation fossa, organellar structures differentiate to form the eventual sperm neck. From this region, thick, outer, dense fibers develop in concert with the lengthening flagellum. These fibers are characteristic of mammalian spermatozoa. They surround the central microtubular pairs that make up the flagellar axoneme itself. In turn, the flagellar fibrous sheath also develops during the cap phase. The fibrous sheath is a ribbed structure interposed between the outer dense fibers and plasma membrane.

Finally, the maturation phase of this complex transformation process features the removal and phagocytosis of most residual spermatid cytoplasm by the neighboring Sertoli cells. Morphologic details of this process have been described, but most of the important biochemical events occurring throughout spermiogenesis have not been determined. Bellvé[125] summarized much of our current understanding of those biochemical changes that have been examined. Figure 9–5 illustrates the important morphologic steps of human spermiogenesis.[167]

The result of spermiogenesis is the morphologically mature spermatozoon. In humans this cell is about 60 μm long and is subdivided structurally into a head and a tail. The head consists of the nucleus with its associated acrosome and is 4.5 μm long, 3.0 μm wide, and about 1 μm deep. Human sperm heads have a flattened, oval shape, contrasted to many experimental species. Joining the head and tail, the sperm neck region contains a pair of centrioles and nine segmented columns forming the beginnings of the flagellar outer dense fibers. The sperm neck region leads directly to the middle piece of the sperm tail. The middle piece, 5 to 7 μm long, consists of the flagellar axoneme and outer dense fibers, surrounded by a spiral sheath of sperm mitochondria. Posterior to the middle piece, the principal piece constitutes the predominant portion of the sperm tail. It is approximately 45 μm long and contains the central axoneme, the outer dense fibers, and the fibrous sheath in concentric arrangement. The fibrous sheath terminates just before the end of the tail, where the outer dense fibers have also disappeared. This most posterior area, the end piece of the sperm tail, is only about 5 μm in length. The entire spermatozoon is covered by a continuous plasma membrane known to be highly polarized in its polypeptide and lipid composition.[171–173]

Organization of the Seminiferous Epithelium. Germ cells in the testis are not placed at random. Instead, they exist as cohorts of cells at exactly the same stage of differentiation. Cell cohorts are first formed during the earliest steps of spermatogonial proliferation when cytokinesis between daughter cells is incomplete, leaving extensive intercellular bridges connecting cells.[174] Incomplete cytokinesis persists throughout all of the mitotic and meiotic cell divisions of male germ cells, yielding cell cohorts numbered in the thousands by the time of sperm release into the lumen of the seminiferous tubule.

Furthermore, germ cells in the mammalian testis are organized into precise cellular associations, wherein certain cohorts of cells early in development are always found with particular cohorts of cells at defined stages of later differentiation. A diagram illustrating the six recognized cell associations in humans is shown in Figure 9–6.[175] In most species each successive association, formed of cohorts slightly later in differentiation than those preceding it, is also organized spatially so that a linear wave of spermatogenesis is formed along the tubule. That is, each defined stage of spermatogenesis occupies a given length of tubule in its full circumference, and successive stages occupy successive portions along the longitudinal axis of the tube.

Such is not true in the human, however. Cell associations in the human testis occupy only a small portion of the epithelium, both in terms of length and circumference. The different stages are placed as patches or plaques, with each individual grouping not extending around the entire circumference of the tubule. As a result, the human testis does not exhibit a morphologic wave of spermatogenesis. It should be noted, however, that differentiating germ cells in humans progress in an orderly fashion through the same cycle of stages as in other species.

Duration of Spermatogenesis. Spermatogenesis in humans takes 74 ±4 days as determined by autoradiographic protocols.[176,177] Each stage of male germ cell differentiation has a characteristic length. For example, it requires 16 days for a human preleptotene spermatocyte to complete all six stages of the seminiferous cycle and to reappear as a pachytene spermatocyte in the same cell association.[177] This is apparently the longest cycle duration known in

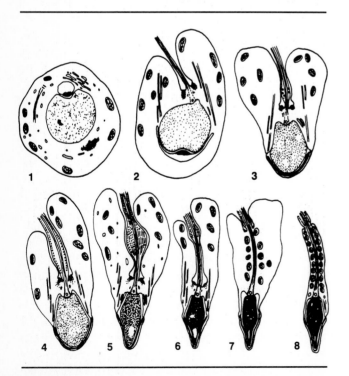

Figure 9–5. The different stages of spermiogenesis in humans. (Modified from Holstein.[168])

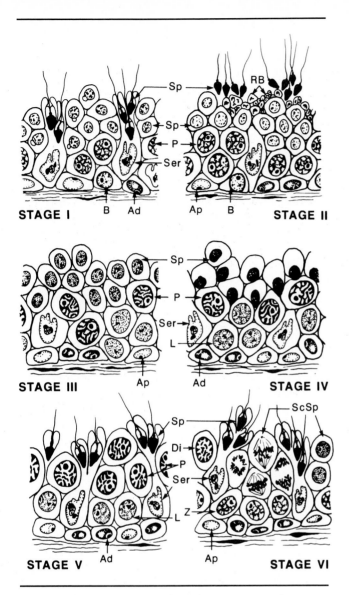

STAGE I   B   Ad   Ap   B   **STAGE II**

STAGE III   Ap   Ad   **STAGE IV**

STAGE V   Ad   Ap   **STAGE VI**

Figure 9–6. The six stages of the spermatogenic cycle in humans. Ser = Sertoli cell nuclei; Ap and Ad = pale and dark type A spermatogonia; B = type B spermatogonia; L,Z,P, Di = leptotene, zygotene, pachytene, and diplotene primary spermatocytes; ScSp = secondary spermatocytes; SP = spermatids at different stages of differentiation; RB = residual bodies. (Modified from Clermont.[175])

mammals.[126] These data, then, show that the entire process of human spermatogenesis takes about 4 to 6 complete cycles (see Fig. 9–6). It requires about 74 days for only the testicular maturation of sperm. This period does not include the added time necessary for sperm maturation in and transport through the epididymis. Epididymal transport time in humans varies, but has usually been estimated at between 20 and 30 days. Therefore, it requires approximately 80 to 100 days for an individual type Ap spermatogonium to mature into an ejaculated spermatozoon capable of fertilization.

SPERM MATURATION IN THE EPIDIDYMIS

Spermatogenesis itself is not sufficient to produce male gametes capable of successful fertilization. After detachment from the seminiferous epithelium, spermatozoa enter the rete testis and pass through the efferent ductules en route to the epididymis. In the epididymis, they undergo an extensive series of biochemical changes that includes alterations of both cell surface and intracellular macromolecules. Interaction with the epididymal epithelium is significant, with it well-established that the epididymal cells both absorb fluid from the epididymal lumen and secrete specific compounds for direct use by spermatozoa. Many of the physiologic responses of the epididymal epithelium are under hormonal control, with DHT coupled to ABP presumed to represent two of the important regulatory elements.

One of the first documented reports of sperm maturation in the epididymis was in the guinea pig.[178] Similar studies followed for many mammalian species, but these events were not reported for humans until the early 1980s.[179,180] Reviews on epididymal sperm maturation may be found elsewhere.[125,181–183]

During epididymal transit, spermatozoa undergo changes in their morphologic structure, composition of their surface membrane, and capacity for active motility. Morphologic alterations occur with varying severity, depending on the species. Usually, the major changes include acrosomal modifications, and the posterior movement and loss of the cytoplasmic droplet, a remaining bit of residual cytoplasm not apparently required for fertilization. Acrosomal changes have been described,[184–186] but few studies have been directly relevant to humans. The physiologic significance, if any, of those morphologic differences between testicular and epididymal sperm are still obscure.

Biochemical differences arising due to epididymal transit, on the other hand, are well-documented and many clearly related directly to sperm activity. Changes include increases in the disulfide linkages and in resistance to sonication detected in sperm constituents of the nucleus, outer dense fibers, fibrous sheath, and mitochondrial membranes.[187–189] Other studies described differences in the lipoprotein composition of bovine spermatozoa taken from different portions of the epididymal tube.[190,191] Subsequently, it has become clear that extensive modifications of sperm lipid composition, including plasma membrane lipids, accompany sperm epididymal transit.[192–196] Some of these lipid differences, including changes in cholesterol and phosphoinositide composition, may result in increased ability of sperm membranes to fuse successfully with plasma membranes of the egg. Morphologic experiments using molecular probes such as filipin, which localize membrane lipid domains, have also been applied to mammalian spermatozoa,[197-199] with notable changes evident in epididymal sperm. Finally, biophysical studies using fluorescence photobleaching also suggest significant modifications of sperm plasma membrane fluidity accompanying sperm maturation.[200,201]

Epididymal sperm in transit also exhibit extensive changes in the polarized distribution of plasma membrane proteins,[172] in the uptake of epididymally secreted polypeptides,[202-204] and in the acquisition of motility.[181,205-207] Although few of these investigations have used human tissue, it is generally accepted that epididymal sperm maturation is an absolute requirement for activation of spermatozoa.

SPERM CAPACITATION AND ACROSOME REACTION

Epididymal spermatozoa must be capacitated in order to fertilize. Normally, sperm are capacitated as they reside in the female reproductive tract. The exact physiologic and biochemical mechanisms constituting capacitation are not well-defined for the human, but the process in mammals has been reviewed by many workers.[208-212] Accordingly, details are not presented here. Depending on the particular species, both the timing and the biochemical events occurring during capacitation vary greatly. Human spermatozoa have been successfully capacitated in a defined tissue culture medium.[210,213] Moreover, with the relatively recent clinical importance of human in vitro fertilization, more investigators are beginning to conduct experimental trials directed at increasing the fertilizing activity of human semen samples.[214,215]

On contact with the ovum and its protective vestments, mammalian spermatozoa undergo the acrosome reaction during which the acrosome vesiculates, yielding hybrid membrane vesicles composed of acrosomal and plasma membrane constituents. The process is exocytic and results in exposure of the egg to the lytic enzymes of the acrosome. These enzymes include hyaluronidase, proteinases, glycosidases, and lipases. Acrosomal hydrolyases are both soluble and attached to the inner acrosomal membrane; in their case they are accessible to the egg and egg vestments after acrosomal vesiculation. The membrane fusion event has an absolute requirement for extracellular calcium and involves a calcium-dependent phospholipase. Guanine nucleotide-binding agents and cyclic nucleotide metabolism are also involved. Increased intercellular pH during the acrosome reaction results from the action of an ATP-dependent proton pump, influx of sodium and calcium, and efflux of hydrogen ions.[216-219] Only sperm that have completed the acrosome reaction can penetrate the zona pellucida surrounding the mature oocyte, but it remains controversial whether the acrosome reaction is needed for passage of sperm through the cumulus oophorus. The role of the acrosome reaction in mammalian fertilization is discussed elsewhere.[220] More research on the precise timing and role of the acrosome reaction in humans is required before detailed hypotheses concerning possible dysfunctions resulting in clinical infertility can be proposed and tested.

NORMAL SEMEN ANALYSIS

Several conditions may result in male infertility. Semen variables that must be considered include abnormal sperm count, sperm motility, fluid volume, fluid viscosity, and the presence of cells other than spermatozoa. Furthermore, one must consider the possible contribution of variocoele, stress, infection, and other similar factors. Both azoospermia and oligozoospermia may be established due to genetic disorders, endocrinopathies, and other disruptions of either spermatogenesis itself or the ductal system of the male reproductive tract. Subnormal sperm motility may be the result of immunologic causes, infection, morphologic defects in spermatozoa, or poor liquefaction of semen. Additional factors are also relevant and discussed elsewhere in this volume.

Extensive variations in normal semen values will be encountered both among individuals and among individual samples taken from particular patients. Therefore it is necessary to perform several semen studies before a definitive diagnosis is stated. At least 2 days of abstinence should be required before collection of sperm by masturbation. More extended periods of time are not necessary. Sperm should be gathered in a clean glass receptacle and brought to the laboratory within 60 to 120 minutes. Samples should not be exposed to temperature extremes. The time of sperm collection, period of abstinence, and any spillage should be noted carefully. To allow for liquefaction, semen should not be examined for at least 30 minutes. Examination after liquefaction should include generally viscosity, color, volume, pH, and the presence of any persistent gel material. An aliquot of the raw semen is then examined under light microscopy (total magnification $\times$ 400 to 600) and assayed for sperm number, agglutination or aggregation, particulate debris, and round cells. The semen must be well mixed, usually with a vortex mixer, prior to microscopic analysis. Samples need not be stained, but with unstained preparations a phase contrast microscope is preferable because of the low inherent contrast of biologic specimens.

Sperm number or concentration should first be estimated in order to determine a proper dilution for final quantification. Using an × 40 objective, the mean number of spermatozoa in several fields is counted. This number multiplied by 10 million provides a rough approximation of the final count. Definitive sperm concentrations may be performed using a hemocytometer, a Makler counter, or one of several computerized electronic instruments. Low sperm counts should be determined with the hemocytometer or Makler counter, as should single samples from which immediate data are required. Samples are diluted as needed in bicarbonate-buffered formalin with gentian violet stain (may be omitted if using phase contrast microscopy), thoroughly mixed, and examined using normal hemocytometer protocols. Only spermatozoa that are seemingly mature and that have attached tails are counted. Using two different dilutions of the same sample, values should not exceed 10% at the low sperm density or 20% at densities greater than 60 million/mL. The concentration is given as the number of sperm per milliliter of semen, while the count describes the total number of sperm in the ejaculate. Sperm concentrations from 20 to 250 million/mL are generally considered normal, but there are many instances of fertile men having values well below this range. The total number of sperm per ejaculate varies as well, but values of 20 to about 80 million are usually considered to be below normal. Azoospermia means complete absence of spermatozoa in the ejaculate.

Sperm motility is also usually assessed microscopically. A single drop (2 to 3 mm diameter) is placed on a slide and covered with an 18 mm² coverslip. The sample must be examined immediately to prevent drying artifacts, and the time and temperature conditions used for these analyses should be standardized. Motility is quantified by observing both motile and immotile cells in at least 10 different, randomly chosen fields. A minimum of 100 sperm per field should be counted, and the percentage of motile sperm calculated from the mean value for all fields assayed and adjusted to the nearest 5%. Forward sperm progression is graded subjectively as follows: "none" indicates absence of forward progression (given a value of 0); "poor" indicates weak forward progression by the majority of sperm (1); "good" indicates moderate progression (2); and "excellent" indicates very active forward movement by most sperm (3). Normal semen samples have 60% or more motile sperm, with most showing good to excellent progression up to 3 hours after ejaculation. Abnormal progression patterns, such as circling movements, should be noted. Samples with less than 40% motility or impaired forward progression should be reassayed using both fresh samples and samples taken after prolonged abstinence from either intercourse or masturbation.

Increasing use is being made of computerized methods to analyze sperm motility. Sophisticated programs allow detailed determinations of the percentage of motile sperm, their average speed, frequency distributions of velocities, and finely graded quantifiable values for forward progression, including figures describing linearity of movement and lateral sperm head displacement from the forward progression track. These procedures have a distinct advantage in that they are free from subjective judgments that could vary from sample to sample or from day to day. It is not yet clear, however, exactly which of the computerized values are most relevant as predictive factors, or what the normal ranges for these values may be. As a result, it remains difficult to recommend complete reliance on these machines, without careful internal standardization of computerized software packages with the ongoing manual methods in individual laboratories. Currently, the relatively high cost of these automated methods is also prohibitive in some instances. It seems clear, however, that these procedures will soon be developed to the point at which they will be the preferred analytic method because of their speed and reproducibility.

Morphologic assessment of spermatozoa and contaminating cells in the ejaculate is also an important test of semen normalcy. A freshly smeared slide of the semen sample is fixed and stained using a variety of protocols. Staining methods used may include fast green, Wright's stain, Giemsa stain, and eosin Y-nigrosin. Other methods are also used, and in some instances may be preferable in order not to confuse true leukocyte contamination from immature spermatogenic cells. The total number and percentage of leukocytes or other round cells in the ejaculate may be easily calculated from the stained slides and

TABLE 9–1. SHAPES AND FREQUENCIES OF SPERM HEADS IN NORMAL HUMAN EJACULATES

Morphology	Mean	Frequency Low	Frequency High	Standard Deviation
Normal	80.5	48.0	98.0	9.7
Large oval head	0.3	0.0	5.2	0.6
Small oval head	1.4	0.0	13.5	1.8
Tapering head	0.4	0.0	6.2	0.9
Pyriform head	2.0	0.0	21.8	2.8
Duplicate head	1.5	0.0	8.3	1.5
Amorphous head	6.5	0.0	24.9	4.0
Tail defect	5.2	0.0	37.4	4.7
Cytoplasmic droplet	2.2	0.0	14.5	2.1

From Schulze.[121] Reproduced with permission.

the hemocytometer counts. Morphology is assayed by examination of at least 100 sperm having tails. Particular attention should be paid to the general shape of the sperm head; the various shapes and their frequencies in normal human ejaculates are given in Table 9–1.[221]

REFERENCES

1. Von Kolliker R: *Beiträge zur Kenntnis der Geschlectsverhältnisse und der Samenflüssigkeit wirbelloser Tiere.* Berlin, 1841
2. Leydig F: Zur Anatomie der männlichen Geschlechtsorgane und Analdrüsen der Säugetiere. *Z Wiss Zool* 2:1, 1850.
3. Bouin P, Ancel P: Recherches sur les cellules interstitielles du testicule des mammiferes. *Arch Zool Exp Gen* 1:437, 1903.
4. Christensen AK: Leydig cells, in Hamilton DW, Greep RD (eds): *Handbook of Physiology. V. Male Reproductive System.* Washington, DC: American Physiological Society, 1975, pp 57–94.
5. Fawcett DW, Neaves WB, Flores MN: Comparative observations on intertubular lymphatics and the organization of the interstitial tissue of the mammalian testis. *Biol Reprod* 9:500, 1973.
6. Setchell BP: Reproduction in male marsupials, in Gilmore DP, Stonehouse B (eds): *Marsupials.* London, Macmillan, 1977, pp 411–457.
7. Bardin CW, Bullock LP, Sherins RJ, Mowszowicz I, Blackburn WR: Androgen metabolism and mechanism of action in male pseudohermaphroditism: A study of testicular feminization. *Recent Prog Horm Res* 29:65, 1973.
8. Berthezene F, Forest MJ, Grimaud JA, Claustrat B, Mornex R: Leydig cell agenesis. *N Engl J Med* 295:969, 1976.
9. Abramowitz J, Iyengar R, Birnbaumer L: Guanyl nucleotide regulation of hormonally responsive adenyl cyclases. *Mol Cell Endocrinol* 16:129, 1979.
10. Catt KJ, Dufau ML: Gonadotrophin receptors and regulation of interstitial cell function in the testis. *Recent Horm Act* 3:291, 1978.
11. Saez JM, Haour F, Cathiard AM: Early hCG-induced desensitization in Leydig cells. *Biochem Biophys Res Commun* 81:552, 1978.
12. Haour F, Sanchez P, Cathiard AM, Saez JM: Gonadotropin receptor regulation in hypophysectomized rat Leydig cells. *Biochim Biophys Res Commun* 81:547, 1978.
13. Catt KJ, Tsuruhara T, Mendelson C, Ketelegers J-M, Dufau, ML: Gonadotropin binding and activation of the interstitial cells of the testis. *Curr Top Molec Endocrinol* 1:1, 1974.
14. Dufau ML, Catt KJ: Gonadotropin receptors and regulation of steroidogenesis in the testis and ovary. *Vitam Horm* 36:461, 1978.
15. Kirschner MA, Widner JA, Ross GT: Leydig cell function in men with gonadotropin-producing testicular tumors. *J Clin Endocrinol Metab* 30:504, 1970.
16. Labrie F, Auclair C, Cusan L, Kelly PA, Pelletier G, Ferland L: Inhibitory effect of LHRH and its agonists on testicular gonadotropin receptors and spermatogenesis in the rat. *Int J Androl (Suppl)* 2:303, 1978.
17. Catt KJ, Baukal AJ, Davies TF, Dufau ML: Luteinizing hormone-releasing hormone-induced regulation of gonadotropin and prolactin receptors in the rat testis. *Endocrinology* 104:17, 1979.
18. Hsueh AJW, Erickson GF: Extrapituitary inhibition of testicular function by luteinising hormone releasing hormone. *Nature* 281:66, 1979.
19. Lipsett MB, Wilson H, Kirschner MA, et al: Studies on Leydig cell physiology and pathology: Secretion and metabolism of testosterone. *Recent Prog Horm Res* 22:245, 1966.
20. Yanahara T, Troen P: Studies of the human testis. I. Biosynthetic pathways for androgen formation in human testicular tissue in vitro. *J Clin Endocrinol Metab* 34:783, 1972.
21. Yen, SSC, Jaffe RB: *Reproductive Endocrinology* Philadelphia, W. B. Saunders, 1986, p. 183.
22. Rosner W, Smith RN: Isolation and characterization of the testosterone-estradiol-binding globulin from human plasma; Use of a novel affinity column. *Biochemistry* 14:4813, 1975.
23. Musto NA, Larrea F, Cheng S-L, et al: Extracellular androgen binding proteins: Species comparison and structure-function relationships. *Ann NY Acad Sci* 383:342, 1982.
24. Vermeulen A, Verdonck L, Van der Straeten M, Orie N: Capacity of the testosterone-binding globulin in human plasma and influence of specific binding of testosterone on its metabolic clearance rates. *J Clin Endocrinol Metab* 29:1470, 1969.
25. Bardin CW, Catterall JR: Testosterone: A major determinant of extragenital sexual dimorphism. *Science* 211:1285, 1981.
26. Baird DT, Horton R, Longcope C, Tait JF: Steroid dynamics under steady state conditions. *Recent Prog Horm Res* 25:611, 1969.
27. Steinberger E: Hormonal control of mammalian spermatogenesis. *Physiol Rev* 51:1, 1971.
28. Means AR, Vaitukaitus J: Peptide hormone ''receptors'': Specific binding of 3H-FSH to testis. *Endocrinology* 90:39, 1972.
29. Bhalla VK, Reichert LE Jr.: Properties of follicle-stimulating-hormone receptor in cell membranes of bovine testis. *J Biol Chem* 249:43, 1974.
30. Desjardins C, Zeleznik AJ, Midgely AR, Reichert LE Jr.: In vitro binding and autoradiographic localization of human chorionic gonadotropin and follicle stimulating hormone in rat testis during development. In Dufau ML and Means AR (eds): *Hormone Binding and Target Cell Activation in Testis.* New York, Plenum, 1974, pp. 221–236.
31. Rabin D: Binding of human FSH and its subunits to rat testis. In Dufau ML and Means AR (eds): *Hormone Binding and Target Cell Activation in Testis.* New York, Plenum, 1974, pp. 193–200.
32. Cheng K-W: Properties of follicle-stimulating-hormone receptor in cell membranes of bovine testis. *Biochem J* 149:123, 1975.
33. Abou-Issa H, Reichert LE Jr.: Solubilization and some characteristics of the follitropin receptor from calf testis. *J Biol Chem* 252:4166, 1977.
34. Orth J, Christensen AK: Localization of 125I-labeled FSH in testes of hypophysectomized rats by autoradiography at the light and electron microscope levels. *Endocrinology* 101:262, 1977.
35. Tindall DJ, Rowley DR, Murthy L, Lipshultz LI, Chang CH: Structure and biochemistry of the Sertoli cell. *Int Rev Cytol* 94:127, 1985.
36. Van Sickle M, Oberwetter JM, Birnbaumer L, Means AR: Developmental changes in the hormonal regulation of rat testis Sertoli cell adenylyl cyclase. *Endocrinology* 109:1270, 1981.
37. Fakunding JL, Tindall DJ, Dedman JR, Mena CR, Means AR: Biochemical actions of follicle-stimulating hormone in the Sertoli cell of the rat testis. *Endocrinology* 98:392, 1976.
38. Dorrington JH, Fritz IB: Effects of gonadotropins on cyclic AMP production by isolated seminiferous tubule and interstitial cell preparations. *Endocrinology* 94:395, 1974.
39. Keuhl FA, Patanelli DJ, Tarnoff J, Humes JL: Testicular adenyl cyclase: Stimulation by the pituitary gonadotropins. *Biol Reprod* 2:154, 1970.
40. Means AR, Huckins C: In Dufau ML and Means AR (eds): Coupled events in the early biochemical; actions of FSH on the Sertoli cells of the testis. *Hormone Binding and Target Cell Activation in Testis,* New York, Plenum, 1974, pp. 145–166.
41. Heindel JJ, Rothenberg R, Robison GA, Steinberger A: LH and FSH stimulation of cyclic AMP in specific cell types isolated from the testis. *J Cyclic Nucleotide Res* 1:69, 1975.
42. Means AR, Tindall DJ: FSH-induction of androgen binding protein in testes of Sertoli cell-only rats, in French FS, Ritzen EM, Nayfeh SN, (eds): *Hormonal Regulation of Spermatogenesis.* New York, Plenum, 1975, pp. 383–398.
43. Beale EG, Dedman JR, Means AR: Isolation and characterization of a protein from rat testis which inhibits cyclic AMP-dependent protein kinase and phosphodiesterase. *J Biol Chem* 252:6322, 1977.
44. Tash JS, Welsh MJ, Means AR: Protein inhibitor of cAMP-dependent protein kinase: production and characterization of antibodies and intracellular localization. *Cell* 21:57, 1980.
45. Tash JS, Welsh MJ, Means AR: Regulation of protein kinase inhibitor by follicle-stimulating hormone in Sertoli cells in vitro. *Endocrinology* 108:427, 1981.
46. Tash JS, Dedman JR, Means AR: Protein kinase inhibitor in Sertoli cell-enriched rat testis. *J Biol Chem* 254:1241, 1979.
47. Dym M, Madhwa Raj HG: Response of adult rat Sertoli cells and Leydig cells to depletion of luteinizing hormone and testosterone. *Biol Reprod* 17:676, 1977.
48. Chemes HE, Dym M, Madhwa Raj HG: Hormonal regulation of Sertoli cell differentiation. *Biol Reprod* 21:251, 1979.
49. French FS, Ritzen EM: A high-affinity androgen binding protein (ABP) in rat testis: Evidence for secretion into efferent duct fluid and absorption by epididymis. *Endocrinology* 95:88, 1973.
50. Steinberger A, Heindel JJ, Lindsey JN, et al: Isolation and culture of FSH response Sertoli cells. *Endocrinol Res Commun* 2:261, 1975.
51. Fritz IB, Rommerts FG, Louis BG, Dorrington JH: Regulation of FSH and dibutyryl cyclic AMP of the formation of androgen-binding protein in Sertoli cell-enriched cultures. *J Reprod Fertil* 46:17, 1976.

REPRODUCTIVE PHYSIOLOGY OF THE MALE 145

52. Welsh MJ, Van Sickle M, Means AR: Possible involvement of cyclic AMP, calcium, and cytoskeleton in control of protein secretion by Sertoli cells, in Steinberger A, Steinberger E (eds): *Testicular Development, Structure, and Function*. New York, Raven, 1980, pp 89–98.

53. Tindall DJ, Rowley DR, Lipshultz LI: Sertoli cell structure and function in vivo and in vitro, in Lipshultz LI, Howards SS (eds): *Infertility in the Male*. New York, Churchill Livingstone, 1983, pp 71–98.

54. Tindall DJ, Rowley DR, Murthy L, Lipshultz LI, Chang CH: Structure and Biochemistry of the Sertoli cell. *Int Rev Cytol* 94:127, 1985.

55. Tindall DJ, Means AR: Properties and hormonal regulation of androgen binding proteins, in Thomas JA, Singhal RL (eds): *Advances in Sex Hormone Research*. Baltimore, Urban & Schwarzenberg, 1980, vol 4, p 295.

56. Hansson V, Djoseland O: Preliminary characterization of the 5-alpha-dihydrotestosterone binding protein in the epididymal cytosol fraction. In vivo studies. *Acta Endocrinol* 71:614, 1972.

57. Mather JP, Gunsalus GL, Musto NA, et al: The hormonal and cellular control of Sertoli cell secretion. *Steroid Biochem* 19:41, 1983.

58. Hsu A-F, Troen P: An androgen-binding protein in the testicular cytosol of human testis. Comparison with human plasma testosterone-estrogen binding globulin. *J Clin Invest* 61:1611, 1978.

59. Lee JA, Yoshida K-J, Hosaka M, et al: Studies of the human testis. XV. Androgen-binding protein and function of Leydig cells and tubules in aged men with prostatic carcinoma. *J Clin Endocrinol Metab* 50:1105, 1980.

60. Gulizia S, Sanborn BM, D'Agata R, Steinberger E: Androgen-binding species in human testes, in D'Agata R, Lipsett MB, Polosa P, van der Molen HJ (eds): *Recent Advances in Male Reproduction: Molecular Basis and Clinical Implications*. New York, Raven, 1983, pp 47–52.

61. Musto N, Gunsalus G, Cheng CY, et al: Identification of androgen-binding proteins and their localization in the testes and male reproductive tract, in D'Agata R, Lipsett MB, Polosa P, van der Molen HJ (eds): *Recent Advances in Male Reproduction: Molecular Basis and Clinical Implications*. New York, Raven, 1983, pp 37–45.

62. Sikka SC, Kalra VK: Gamma-glutamyl transpeptidase-mediated transport of amino acid in lecithin vesicles. *J Biol Chem* 255:4399, 1980.

63. Lipshultz LI, Murthy L, Tindall DJ: Characterization of human Sertoli cells in vitro. *J Clin Endocrinol Metab* 55:228, 1982.

64. Tindall DJ, Rowley DR, Lipshultz LI: Sertoli cell structure and function in vivo and in vitro, in Lipshultz LI, Howards SS (eds): *Infertility in the Male*. New York, Churchill Livingstone, 1983, pp 71–98.

65. Skinner MK, Griswold MD: Sertoli cells synthesize and secrete transferrin-like protein. *J Biol Chem* 255:9523, 1980.

66. Skinner MK, Cosand WL, Griswold MD: Purification and characterization of testicular transferrin secreted by rat Sertoli cells. *Biochem J* 218:313, 1984.

67. Hadley MA, Byers SW, Suarez-Guian CA, Kleinman HK, Dym M: Extracellular matrix regulates Sertoli cell differentiation, testicular cord formation, and germ cell development in vitro. *J Cell Biol* 101:1511, 1985.

68. Jutte NHPM, Jansen R, Grootegoed JA, Rommerts FFG, van der Molen HJ: FSH stimulation of the production of pyruvate and lactate by rat Sertoli cells may be involved in hormonal regulation of spermatogenesis. *J Reprod Fertil* 68:219, 1983.

69. Nakamura M, Hino A, Yasumasu I, Kato J: Stimulation of protein synthesis in round spermatids from rat testis by lactate. *J Biochem Tokyo* 89:1309, 1981.

70. Mita M, Hall PF: Metabolism of round spermatids from rats: Lactate as the preferred substrate. *Biol Reprod* 26:445, 1982.

71. Jutte NHPM, Jansen R, Grootegoed JA, et al: Regulation of survival of rat pachytene spermatocytes by lactate supply from Sertoli cells. *J Reprod Fertil* 65:431, 1982.

72. Grootegoed JA, Oonk RB, Jansen R, van der Molen HJ: Spermatogenic cells utilize metabolic intermediates from Sertoli cells, in Rolland R (ed): *Gamete Quality and Fertility Regulation*. London, Elsevier, 1985, pp 225–237.

73. Nakamura M, Ishida K, Waku M, Okinaga S, Arai K: Stimulation of protein synthesis in pachytene primary spermatocytes from the human testis by pyruvate. *Andrologia* 17:561, 1985.

74. Hansson V: Recent Advances in Male Reproduction: Motecular Basis and Clinical Implications. New York, Raven, 1983.

75. McCullagh DR: Dual endocrine activity of testis. *Science* 76:19, 1932.

76. Del Castillo EB, Trabucco A, de la Balze FA: Syndrome produced by absence of the germinal epithelium without impairment of the Sertoli or Leydig cells. *J Clin Endocrinol* 7:493, 1947.

77. McCullagh EP, Schaffenberg CA: Role of the seminiferous tubules in the production of hormones. *Ann NY Acad Sci* 55:674, 1952.

78. Bain J, Keene J: Further evidence for inhibin: Changes in serum luteinizing hormone and follicle-stimulating hormone levels after X-irradiation of rat testes. *J Endocrinol* 66:279, 1975.

79. Setchell BP, Davies RV, Main SJ: Inhibin, in Johnson AD, Gomes YYR (eds): *The Testis*. New York, Academic press, 1977, vol 4, pp 189–238.

80. Gomes WR, Hall RW, Jain SK, Boots DR: Serum gonadotropin and testosterone levels during loss and recovery of spermatogenesis in rats. *Endocrinology* 93:800, 1973.

81. Swerdloff RS, Walsh PC, Jacobs HS, Odell WD: Serum LH and FSH during sexual maturation in the male rat: Effect of castration and cryptorchidism. *Endocrinology* 88:120, 1971.

82. Setchell BP, Main SJ, Davies RV: The effect of ligation of the efferent ducts of the testis on serum gonadotropins and testosterone. *J Endocrinol* 72:13P, 1977.

83. Lugaro G, Casellato MM, Mazzola G, Fachini G, Carrea G: Evidence for the existence in spermatozoa of a factor inhibiting the follicular-stimulating hormone-releasing hormone synthesis. *Neuroendocrinology* 15:62, 1974.

84. Setchell BP, Jacks F: Inhibin-like activity in rete testis fluid. *J Endocrinol* 62:675, 1974.

85. Franchimont P, Chari S, Hagelstein MT, Duraiswami S: Existence of a follicle-stimulating hormone inhibiting factor, "inhibin," in bull seminal plasma. *Nature* 257:402, 1975.

86. Nandini SG, Lipner H, Moudgal NR: A model system for studying inhibin. *Endocrinology* 98:1460, 1976.

87. Steinberger A, Steinberger E: Secretion of an FSH-inhibiting factor by cultured Sertoli cells. *Endocrinology* 99:918, 1976.

88. Scott RS, Burger HG, Quigg H: A simple and rapid in vitro bioassay for inhibin. *Endocrinology* 107:1536, 1980.

89. Setchell BP, Sirinathsinghji DJ: Antigonadotrophic activity in rete testis fluid, a possible "inhibin." *J Endocrinol* 53:10, 1972.

90. Au CL, Robertson DM, DeKretser DM: In vitro bioassay of inhibin in testes of normal and cryptorchid rats. *Endocrinology* 112:239, 1983.

91. Rivier J, Spiess J, McClintock R, Vaughan J, Vale W: Purification and partial characterization of inhibin from porcine follicular fluid. *Biochem Biophys Res Commun* 13:120, 1985.

92. Mayo KE, Cerelli GM, Spiess J, et al: Inhibin A-subunit cDNAs from porcine ovary and human placenta. *Proc Natl Acad Sci USA* 83:6849, 1986.

93. Bicsak TA, Vale W, Vaughan J, et al: Hormonal regulation of inhibin production by cultured Sertoli cells. *Mol Cell Endocrinol* 49:211, 1987.

94. Le Gac F, DeKretser DM: Inhibin production by Sertoli cell cultures. *Mol Cell Endocrinol* 28:487, 1982.

95. Verhoeven G, Franchimont P: Regulation of inhibin secretion by Sertoli cell-enriched cultures. *Acta Endocrinol* 102:136, 1983.

96. Rich KA, DeKretser DM: Spermatogenesis and the Sertoli cell. *Monogr Endocrinol* 25:84, 1983.

97. Ultree-van Gessel AM, Leemborg FG, deJong FH, van der Molen HJ: In vitro secretion of inhibin-like activity by Sertoli cells from normal and prenatally irradiated immature rats. *J Endocrinol* 109:411, 1986.

98. Franchimont P: Regulation of gonadal androgen secretion. *Horm Res* 18:7, 1983.

99. Steinberger A, Dighe RR, Diaz J: Testicular peptides and their endocrine and paracrine functions. *Arch Bio Med Exp* 17:267, 1984.

100. Rivier C, Rivier J, Vale W: Inhibin-mediated feedback control of follicle-stimulating hormone secretion in the female rat. *Science* 234:205, 1986.

101. Bergh A: Paracrine regulation of Leydig cells by the seminiferous tubules. *Int J Androl* 6:57, 1983.

102. Skinner MK, Fritz IB: Testicular peritubular cells secrete a protein under androgen control that modulates Sertoli cell functions. *Proc Natl Acad Sci USA* 82:114, 1985.

103. Saez JM, Tabone E, Perrard-Sapori MH, Rivarola MA: Paracrine role of Sertoli cells. *Med Biol* 63:225, 1986.

104. Sharpe RM, Fraser HM: HCG stimulation of testicular LHRH-like activity. *Nature* 287:642, 1980.

105. Sharpe RM, Fraser HM, Cooper I, Rommerts FFG: Sertoli–Leydig cell communication via an LHRH-like factor. *Nature* 290:785, 1981.

106. Sharpe RM, Fraser HM, Cooper I, Rommerts FFG: The secretion, measurement, and function of a testicular LHRH-like factor. *Ann NY Acad Sci* 383:272, 1982.

107. Sharpe RM: Intratesticular factors controlling testicular function. *Biol Reprod* 30:29, 1984.

108. Kerr JB, Sharpe RM: Effects and interactions of LH and LHRH agonist on testicular morphology and function in hypophysectomized rats. *J Reprod Fertil* 76:175, 1986.

109. Sharpe RM, Cooper I: Comparison of the effects on purified Leydig cells of four hormones (oxytocin, vasopressin, opiates and LHRH) with suggested paracrine roles in the testis. *J Endocrinol* 113:89, 1987.

110. Feig LA, Bellvé AR, Horbach Erickson N, Klagsbrun M: Sertoli cells contain a mitogenic polypeptide. *Proc Natl Acad Sci USA* 77:4774, 1980.

111. Shu-Dong T, Phillips DM, Halmi N, Krieger D, Bardin CW: Beta-Endorphin is present in the male reproductive tract of five species. *Biol Reprod* 27:755, 1982.

112. Margioris AN, Liotta AS, Vaudry H, Bardin CW, Krieger DT: Characterization of immunoreactive proopiomelanocortin-related peptides in rat testes. *Endocrinology* 113:663, 1983.

113. Gerendai I, Shaha C, Thau R, Bardin CW: Do testicular opiates regulate Leydig cell function? *Endocrinology* 115:1645, 1984.

114. Gizang-Ginsberg E, Wolgemuth DJ: Localization of mRNAs in mouse testes by in situ hybridization: Distribution of alpha-tubulin and developmental stage specificity of pro-opiomelanocortin transcripts. *Dev Biol* 111:293, 1985.

115. Gizang-Ginsberg E, Wolgemuth DJ: Expression of the pro-opiomelanocortin gene is developmentally regulated and affected by germ cells in the male mouse reproductive system. *Proc Natl Acad Sci USA* 84:1600, 1987.

116. Douglass J, Cox B, Quinn B, Civelli O, Herbert E: Expression of the prodynorphin gene in male and female reproductive tissues. *Endocrinology* 120:707, 1987.

117. Kilpatrick DL, Howells RD, Noe M, Bailey CL, Udenfriend S: Expression of preproenkephalin-like mRNA and its peptide products in mammalian testis and ovary. *Proc Natl Acad Sci USA* 82:7467, 1985.

118. Kilpatrick DL, Millette CF: Expression of proenkephalin messenger RNA by mouse spermatogenic cells. *Proc Natl Acad Sci USA* 83:5015, 1986.

119. Bawa SR: Fine structure of the Sertoli cell of the human testis. *J Ultrastruct Res* 9:459, 1963.

120. Nagano T: Some observations on the fine structure of the Sertoli cells in the human testis. *Z Zellforsch* 73:89, 1966.

121. Schulze C: On the morphology of the human Sertoli cell. *Cell Tissue Res* 153:339, 1974.

122. Schulze C, Holstein AF, Schirren C, Korner F: On the morphology of the human Sertoli cells under normal conditions and in patients with impaired fertility. *Andrologia* 8:167, 1976.

123. Holstein AF, Roosen-Runge EC: *Atlas of Human Spermatogenesis*. Berlin, Groose Verlag, 1981.

124. Ewig LL, Davis JC, Zirkin BR: Regulation of testicular function: a spatial and temporal view. *Int Rev Physiol* 22:41, 1980.

125. Bellvé AR: The molecular biology of mammalian spermatogenesis, in Finn CA (ed): *Oxford Reviews of Reproductive Biology*. Oxford, Clarendon Press, 1979, vol I, pp 159–261.

126. Bustos-Obregon E, Courot M, Flechon JE, Hochereau-De-Reviers MT. Holstein AF: Morphological appraisal of gametogenesis: spermatogenic process in mammals with particular reference to man. *Andrologia* 7:141, 1975.

127. Witschi E: Migration of the germ cells of human embryos from the yolk sac to the primitive gonadal folds. *Carnegie Institute Publication* no 575. Washington, DC, Carnegie Institute, 32:67, 1948.

128. Wagenen G. van, Simpson ME: *Embryology of the Ovary and Testis, Homo sapiens and Macaca mulatta.* New Haven, Yale University Press, 1965.

129. Wartenberg H, Holstein AF, Vossmeyer J: Zur Cytologie der pranatalen Gonaden-entwicklung beim Menschen. II. Elektronenmikroskopische Untersuchungen über die Cytogenese von Gonocyten und fetalen Spermatogonien im Hoden. *Z Anat Entwickl* 134:165, 1971.

130. Wartenberg H: Spermatogenese-oogenese: Ein cyto-morphologischer Vergleich. *Verh Anat Ges* 68:63, 1974.

131. Gondos b, Hobel CJ: Ultrastructure of germ cell development in the human fetal testis. *Z Zellforsch Mikrosk Anat* 119:1, 1971.

132. Allen E: Studies on degenerating sex cells in immature mammals. I. An analysis of degeneration in primordial germ cells in male albino rats aged 1–9 days. *J Morphol* 85:405, 1949.

133. Roosen-Rung EC, Leik J: Gonocyte degeneration in the postnatal rat. *Am J Anat* 122:275, 1968.

134. Mancini RI, Narbaitz R, Lavieri JC: Origin and development of the germinative epithelium and Sertoli cells in the human testis: Cytological, cytochemical and quantitative study. *Anat Rec* 136:477, 1960.

135. Vilar O: Histology of the human testis from neonatal period to adolescence, in Rosenberg E, Paulsen CA (eds): *The Human Testis*. New York, Plenum, 1970, pp 95–111.

136. Roosen-Runge EC, Barlow FD: Quantitative studies on human spermatogenesis. I. Spermatogonia. *Am J Anat* 93:143, 1953.

137. Clermont Y: Spermatogenesis in man. A study of the spermatogonial population. *Fertil Steril* 17:705, 1966.

138. Rowley MJ, Berlin JD, Heller CG: The ultrastructure of four types of human spermatogonia. *Z Zellforsch Mikrosk Anat* 112:139, 1971.

139. Fukuda T, Hedinger C: Ultrastructure of developing germ cells in the fetal human testis. *Cell Tissue Res* 161:55, 1975.

140. Wartenberg H: Comparative cytomorphic aspects of the male germ cells, especially of "gonia." *Andrologia* 8:117, 1976.

141. Schulze C: Morphological characteristics of the spermatogonial stem cells in man. *Cell Tissue Res* 198:191, 1979.

142. Seguchi H, Hadziselimovic F: Ultramikroskopische untersuchungen am tubulus seminiferus bei kindern von der geburt bis zur pubertat. I. Spermatogonieentwicklung. *Verh Anat Ges* 68:133, 1974.

143. Hadziselimovic F: Elektronenmikrooskopishce untersuchunen uber die entwicklung des tubulus seminiferus unmittlebar nach der geburt bis zum vollendeten ersten jahr. *Acta Anat* 95:287, 1976.

144. Nagano T: The crystalloid of Lubarsch in the human spermatogonium. *Z Zellforsch* 97:491, 1969.

145. Clermont Y: Kinetics of spermatogenesis in mammals: Seminiferous epithelial cycle and spermatogonial renewal. *Physiol Rev* 52:198, 1972.

146. Huckins C, Oakberg EF: Morphological and quantitative analysis of spermatogonia in mouse testes using whole mounted seminiferous. II. The irradiated testis. *Anat Rec* 192:529, 1978.

147. Bartmanska J, Clermont Y: Renewal of type A spermatogonia in adult rats. *Cell Tissue Kinet* 16:135, 1983.

148. deRooij DG, Lok D, Weenk D: Feedback regulation of the proliferation of the undifferentiated spermatogonia in the Chinese hamster by differentiating spermatogonia. *Cell Tissue Kinet* 18:71, 1985.

149. Moses MJ: Synaptinemal complex. *Annu Rev Genet* 2:363, 1968.

150. Moses MJ, Counce SJ, Paulson DF: Synaptonemal complex complement of man in spreads of spermatocytes, with details of the sex chromosome pair. *Science* 187:363, 1975.

151. Von Wettstein D: The synaptonemal complex and four-strand crossing-over. *Proc Natl Acad Sci USA* 68:851, 1971.

152. Romrell LJ, Bellvé AR, Fawcett DW: Separation of mouse spermatogenic cells by sedimentation velocity. A morphological characterization. *Dev Biol* 49:119, 1976.

153. Bellvé AR, Millette CF, Bhatnagar YM, O'Brien DA: Dissociation of the mouse testis and characterization of isolated spermatogenic cells. *J Histochem Cytochem* 25:480, 1977.

154. Bellvé AR, Cavicchia JC, Millette CF, et al: Spermatogenic cells of the prepubertal mouse. Isolation and morphological characterization. *J Cell Biol* 74:68, 1977.

155. Shepard RW, Millette CF, DeWolf WC: Enrichment of primary pachytene spermatocytes from the human testis. *Gamete Res* 4:487, 1981.

156. Narayan P, Scott BK, Millette CF, DeWolf WC: Human Spermatogenic cell marker proteins detected by two-dimensional electrophoresis. *Gamete Res* 7:227, 1983.

157. Vilar O: Spermatogenesis, in Hafez E, Evans R (eds): *Human Reproduction. Conception and Contraception*. New York, Harper & Row, 1973, pp 12–37.

158. Fawcett DW, Burgos MH: Observations on the cytomorphosis of the germinal and interstitial cells of the human testis. *Ciba Found Colloq Aging* 2:86, 1956.

159. Anberg A: The ultrastructure of the human spermatozoon. *Acta Obstet Gynecol Scand* 36 (suppl 2) 4, 1957.

160. Fawcett DW: The structure of the mammalian spermatozoon. *Int Rev Cytol* 7:195, 1958.

161. Fawcett DW: A comparative view of sperm ultrastructure. *Biol Reprod* 2:90, 1970.

162. DeKretser DM: Ultrastructural features of human spermiogenesis. *Z. Zellforsch* 98:477, 1969.

163. Pedersen H: Ultrastructure of the ejaculated human sperm. *Z Zellsforsch* 94:542, 1969.

164. Burgos MH, Vitale-Calpe R, Aoki A: Fine structure of the testis and its functional significance, in Johnson AD, Gomes Wr, Vandemark NL (eds): *The Testis.* New York, Academic Press, 1970, pp 551–649.

165. Vilar O, Paulsen CA, Moore DJ: Electron microscopy of the human seminiferous tubule. *Adv Exp Med Biol* 10:63, 1970.

166. Pedersen H: The human spermatozoon. *Dan Med Bull* 21 (suppl 1), 3, 1974.
167. Holstein AF: Morphologische Studien an abnormen Spermatiden und Spermatzoen des Menschen. *Virchows Arch [A]* 367:93, 1975.
168. Holstein AF: Ultrastructural observations on the differentiation of spermatids in man. *Andrologia* 8:157, 1976.
169. Holstein AF, Schafer E: A further type of transient cytoplasmic organelle in human spermatids. *Cell Tissue Res* 192:359, 1978.
170. Holstein AF, Eckmann C: Multinucleated spermatocytes and spermatids in human seminiferous tubules. *Andrologia* 18:5, 1986.
171. Millette CF: Distribution and mobility of lectin binding sites on mammalian spermatozoa, in Johnson MHS, Edidin M (eds): *Immunobiology of Gametes.* Cambridge, Cambridge University Press, 1976, pp 51–71.
172. Koehler JK: The mammalian sperm surface: Studies with specific labeling techniques. *Int Rev Cytol* 54:73, 1978.
173. Myles DG, Primakoff P: Localized surface antigens of guinea pig sperm migrate to new regions prior to fertilization. *J Cell Biol* 99:1634, 1984.
174. Dym M, Fawcett DW: Further observations on the numbers of spermatogonia, spermatocytes, and spermatids connected by intracellular bridges in the mammalian testis. *Biol Reprod* 4:195, 1971.
175. Clermont Y: The cycle of the seminiferous epithelium in man. *Am J Anat* 112:35, 1963.
176. Heller CG, Clermont Y: Spermatogenesis in man: An estimate of its duration. *Science* 140:184, 1963.
177. Heller CG, Clermont Y: Kinetics of the germinal epithelium in man. *Recent Prog Horm Res* 20:545, 1964.
178. Young WC: A study of the function of the epididymis. III. Functional changes undergone by the spermatozoa during their passage through the epididymis and vas deferens in the guinea pig. *J Exp Biol* 8:151, 1931.
179. Hinrichsen MJ, Blaquier JA: Evidence suggesting the existence of sperm maturation in the human epididymis. *J Reprod Fertil* 60:291, 1980.
180. Hinrichsen MJ, Blaquier JA: Proceso de maduracion de los espermatozoides, in Otamendi B (ed): *Esterilidad masculina.* Buenos Aires, Lopez Libreros Editores, 1980, pp 31–34.
181. Hamilton DW: The epididymis, in Greep RD, Koblinsky MA (eds): *Frontiers in Reproduction and Fertility Control.* Cambridge, MIT Press, 1977, pp 411–426.
182. Bellvé AR, O'Brien DA: The mammalian spermatozoon: structure and temporal assembly, in Hartmann JF (ed): *Mechanism and Control of Animal Fertilization.* New York, Academic Press, 1983, pp 56–137.
183. Hinrichsen-Kohane AC, Hinrichsen MJ, Schill W-B: Molecular events leading to fertilization—A review. *Andrologia* 16:321, 1984.
184. Fawcett DW, Hollenberg RD: Changes in the acrosomes of guinea pig spermatozoa during passage through the epididymis. *Z Zellforsch Mikrosk Anat* 60:276, 1963.
185. Fawcett DW, Phillips DM: Observations on the release of spermatozoa and on changes in the head during passage through the epididymis. *J Reprod Fertil* 6:405, 1969.
186. Hoffer AP, Shalev M, Frisch DH: Ultrastructure and maturational changes in spermatozoa in the epididymis of the pigtailed monkey, *Macaca nemestrina. J. Androl* 3:140, 1981.
187. Henle W, Henle G, Chambers LA: Studies on the antigenic structure of some mammalian spermatozoa. *J Exp Med* 68:335, 1938.
188. Calvin HI, Bedford JM: Formation of disulphide bonds in the nucleus and accessory structures of mammalian spermatozoa during maturation in the epididymis. *J Reprod Fertil* 13:65, 1971.
189. Bedford JM, Calvin HI: Changes in -S-S-linked structures in the sperm tail during epididymal maturation, with comparative observations in sub-mammalian species. *J Exp Zool* 187:181, 1974.
190. Lavon U, Volcani R, Davon D: The lipid content of bovine spermatozoa during maturation and aging. *J Reprod Fertil* 23:215, 1970.
191. Lavon U, Volcani R, Davon D: The proteins of bovine spermatozoa from the caput and cauda epididymis. *J Reprod Fertil* 24:219, 1971.
192. Evans RW, Setchell BP: Lipid changes in boar spermatozoa during epididymal maturation with some observations on the flow and composition of boar rete testis fluid. *J Reprod Fertil* 57:189, 1979.
193. Parks JE, Hammerstedt RH: Developmental changes occurring in the lipids of ram epididymal spermatozoa plasma membrane. *Biol Reprod* 32:653, 1985.
194. Nikolopoulou M, Soucek DA, Vary JC: Changes in the lipid content of boar sperm plasma membranes during epididmal maturation. *Biochim Biophys Acta* 815:486, 1985.
195. Holt WV, North RD: Determination of lipid composition and thermal phase transition temperature in an enriched plasma membrane fraction from ram spermatozoa. *J Reprod Fertil* 73:285, 1985.
196. Touchstone JC, Alvarez JG, Levin SS, Storey BT: Evidence for diplasmalogen as the major component of rabbit sperm phosphatidylethanolamine. *Lipids* 20:869, 1985.
197. Bearer EL, Friend DS: Anionic lipid domains: Correlation with functional topography in a mammalian cell membrane. *Proc Natl Acad Sci USA* 77:6601, 1980.
198. Bearer EL, Friend DS: Modifications of anionic-lipid domains preceding membrane fusion in guinea pig sperm. *J Cell Biol* 92:604, 1982.
199. Toshimori K, Higashi R, Oura C: Distribution of intramembranous particles and filipin–sterol complexes in mouse sperm membranes: Polyene antibiotic filipin treatment. *Am J Anat* 174:455, 1985.
200. Wolf DE, Voglmayr JD: Diffusion and regionalization in membranes of maturing ram spermatozoa. *J Cell Biol* 98:1678, 1984.
201. Wolf DE, Scott BK, Millette CF: The development of regionalized lipid diffusibility in the germ cell plasma membrane during spermatogenesis in the mouse. *J Cell Biol* 103:1745, 1986.
202. Acott TS, Hoskins DD: Bovine sperm forward motility protein: Binding to epididymal spermatozoa. *Biol Reprod* 24:234, 1981.
203. Klinefelter GR, Hamilton DW: Synthesis and secretion of proteins by perifused caput epididymal tubules, and association of secreted proteins with spermatozoa. *Biol Reprod* 33:1017, 1985.
204. Hamilton DW, Wenstrom JC, Baker JB: Membrane glycoproteins from spermatozoa: Partial characterization of an integral Mr ~ 24,000 molecule from rat spermatozoa that is glycosylated during epididymal maturation. *Biol Reprod* 34:925, 1986.
205. Hoskins DD, Brandt H, Acott TS: Initiation of sperm motility in the mammalian epididymis. *Fed Proc* 37:2534, 1978.
206. Jones R: Comparative biochemistry of mammalian epididymal plasma. *Comp Biochem Physiol B* 61B:365, 1978.
207. Hinrichsen MJ, Blaquier JA: Acquisition of fertilizing capacity of spermatozoa in the human epididymis, in Hafez RSE, Semmk (eds): *Instrumental Insemination.* New York, Elsevier- North Holland, 1982, pp 63–65.
208. Austin CR: Membrane fusion events in fertilization. *J Reprod Fertil* 44:155, 1975.
209. Meizel S: The mammalian sperm acrosome reaction: A biochemical approach, in Johnson MH (ed): *Development in Mammals.* Amsterdam, Elsevier, 1978, vol 3, pp 1–62.
210. Yanagimachi R: Mechanisms of fertilization in mammals, in Mastroianni L, Biggers JD (eds): *Fertilization and Embryonic Development in Vitro.* New York, Plenum, 1981, pp 81–182.
211. Clegg ED: Mechanism of mammalian sperm capacitation, in Hartmann JF (ed): *Mechanism and Control of Animal Fertilization.* New York, Academic Press, 1983, pp 178–212.
212. Langlais J, Roberts KD: A molecular membrane model of sperm capacitation and the acrosome reaction of mammalian spermatozoa. *Gamete Res* 12:183, 1985.
213. Perreault S, Rogers J: Capacitation pattern of human spermatozoa. *Fertil Steril* 38:258, 1982.
214. Barros C, Vigil P, Herrera E, et al: In vitro interaction between human spermatozoa and human cervical mucus. *Micros Electron Y Biol Cell* 7:13, 1983.
215. Berger T, Marrs RP, Moyer DL: Comparison of techniques for selection of motile spermatozoa. *Fertil Steril* 43:268, 1985.
216. Shapiro BM, Shackman RW, Gabel CA: Molecular approaches to the study of fertilization. *Annu Rev Biochem* 50:815, 1981.
217. Trimmer JS, Vacquier VD: Activation of sea urchin gametes. *Annu Rev Cell Biol* 2:1, 1986.
218. Kopf GS, Woolkalis MJ, Gerton GL: Evidence for a guanine nucleotide-binding regulatory protein in invertebrate and mammalian sperm: Identification by islet-activating protein-catalyzed ADP-ribosylation and immunochemical methods. *J Biol Chem* 261:7327, 1986.
219. Endo Y, Lee MA, Kopf GS: Evidence for the role of a guanine nucleotide-binding regulatory protein in the zonna pellucida-induced mouse sperm acrosome reaction. *Dev Biol* 119:210, 1987.
220. Wassarman PM: Early events in mammalian fertilization. *Annu Rev Cell Biol* 3:109, 1987.
221. Belsey MA, Eliasson R, Gallegos AJ, et al. *Laboratory Manual for the Examination of Human Semen and Semen–Cervical Mucus Interaction.* Singapore, Press Concern, 1980, pp 3–42.

CHAPTER 10

The Relationship of Abnormal Semen Values to Pregnancy Outcome

Sherman J. Silber

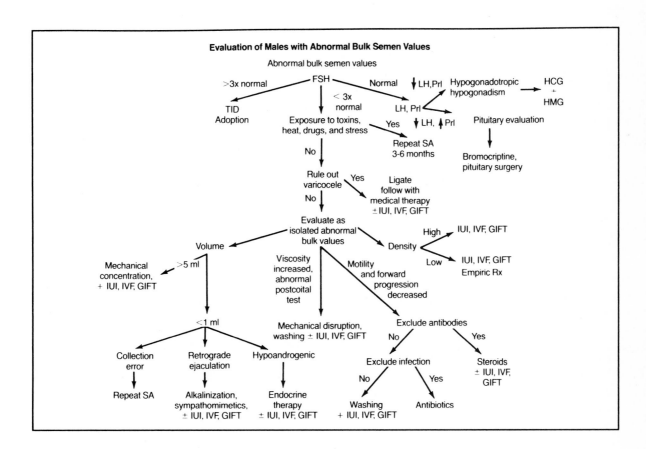

Evaluation of Males with Abnormal Bulk Semen Values

SEMEN ANALYSIS

The time-honored method of evaluating male infertility has been the semen analysis (sperm count). It has been assumed that if a man's sperm count is below a certain arbitrary minimum, he is infertile, and the couple's failure to achieve pregnancy is caused by his infertility. As recently as the early 1970s it was thought that a sperm count of under 40

million/cc meant that men were infertile, and urologists gave these couples a dire prognosis for pregnancy. If pregnancy did occur, it was ascribed to whatever useless treatment was being administered to the "infertile" husband. Since the early 1980s the sperm count thought to indicate infertility has been reduced to 20 million/cc. One group, however, reported pregnancy from a man who had only 50,000 sperm/cc. The man, the mother, and the baby were

149

all carefully blood typed and tissue typed, and it was determined to be 99.99% sure that the husband was genetically the father.[1]

Pregnancies have been reported with the great excitement in couples with very low sperm counts after in vitro fertilization (IVF). Fertilization rates in most IVF centers are clearly poorer in couples with oligospermia, yet in better centers, good rates have been reported even in these couples. The confusion is not helped by the frustrating discrepancy between the results of hamster egg penetration tests and fertilization of the woman's egg by IVF.

LITERATURE REVIEW

Studies Indicating that Low Sperm Counts Indicate Male Factor Infertility

The original correlation of sperm count to fertility was made in a study of 1,000 "fertile" and 1,000 "infertile" men (Table 10–1).[2] The results clearly indicated that among a fertile population, sperm counts in the vast majority are above 40 million/cc, and in only 17% are under that number. Only 5% of fertile men had counts below 20 million/cc. This distribution would make us conclude that a normal count is certainly above 40 million, and, in fact, this has been the assumption over many decades. In the control group of "infertile" men, however, the frequency distribution, although different, was not tremendously different, except for counts below 20 million sperm/cc. Sixteen percent of these so-called infertile men had sperm counts less than 20 million, compared with 5% of "fertile" men whose counts were in that range. It was therefore concluded that any count under 20 million definitely indicated male infertility. We now recognize that such a conclusion based on that population sampling may have been tenuous indeed.

Another group did sperm counts on 1,300 fertile men, but had no infertile controls.[3] They found remarkably similar percentages, with only 7% of fertile men having sperm counts under 20 million/cc, compared with 59% with counts over 60 million. In

TABLE 10–2 FREQUENCY DISTRIBUTION OF QUALITY OF SPERM MOTILITY IN 1300 FERTILE MEN

Motility (grade)	Fertile Men (%)
1	3
2	14
3	58
4	25

Men in the last two grades combined make up 83% of the sample.
From Steinberger and Rodriguez-Rigau.[8]

addition, in 83% of fertile men sperm motility was grades 3 and 4; but what has perhaps not been emphasized enough is that 17% had very poor sperm motility—grades 1 and 2. Similarly, 86% of fertile men had over 40% motile sperm, but in a full 14% the percentage was less than 40%, and in 4% of perfectly fertile men motility was less than 20% (Tables 10–2 through 10–4). Neither of these studies addressed the issue of whether low sperm counts, like high sperm counts, just occurred at one end or the other of the bell-shaped population curve and perhaps might have had nothing to do with the man's fertility—that is, the chance of the woman becoming pregnant.

A study in France reported on sperm counts in almost 3,000 infertile men with a control group of only 190 fertile men.[4] The frequency distribution of counts in both groups was remarkably similar to that of MacLeod and Gold.[2] In almost 70% of fertile men the counts were above 60 million/cc, and in only 6.9% were they below 20 million. Yet in 28% of the "infertile" group the count was below 20 million. Thus once again the inference was that sperm counts of above 40 million/cc indicate a much greater likelihood of fertility.

Studies Indicating that Low Sperm Counts May Be Compatible with Fertility

In 1974 workers reported on 386 fertile men, of whom 20% had sperm counts of below 20 million/cc, and only 28% had counts of above 60 million.[5] These data suggested that low sperm counts are quite compatible

TABLE 10–1. FREQUENCY DISTRIBUTION OF SPERM COUNTS IN 100 FERTILE AND 1000 INFERTILE MEN

Sperm Count (million/cc)	Fertile Men (%)	Infertile Men (%)
<20	5	16
20–39	12	13
40–59	12	11
≥60	71	60

From MacLeod and Gold.[2]

TABLE 10–3. FREQUENCY DISTRIBUTION OF SPERM COUNT IN 1300 FERTILE MEN

Sperm Count (million/cc)	Fertile Men (%)
<20	7
20–39	16
40–59	18
≥60	59

From Rehan et al.[3]

TABLE 10–4. FREQUENCY DISTRIBUTION OF SPERM MOTILITY IN 1300 FERTILE MEN

Motile Sperm (%)	Fertile Men (%)
<20	4
20–39	10
40–59	31
60–79	34
80–100	21

Men with > 40% motile sperm make up 86% of the sample.
From Rehan et al.[3]

TABLE 10–5. MEAN NUMBER OF CYCLES TO CONCEPTION AS RELATED TO SPERM MOTILITY

Motile Count (million/cc)	Number of Cycles to Conception (mean)
<5	11.0
5–20	9.4
20–60	8.0
>60	6.0

From Smith et al.[7]

with fertility, and that indeed a count below 20 or 40 million does not indicate a male factor problem. Another group studied literally thousands of fertile men who requested vasectomy.[6] They noted similar findings: In 23% of fertile men sperm counts were below 20 million/cc, and in only 40% were they above 60 million. Among infertile couples, with no prejudicial preconception as to whether infertility was a male or a female problem, 42% (twice as many) of the men had counts below 20 and 29% below 10 million. Careful inspection of all the data suggests that there is no difference in the chances of a couple being fertile or not at any sperm count above 10 million/cc. It is only when the count goes below that that the risk of infertility would be significantly greater.

These investigators did conclude from their data that sperm count was nonessential in determining male infertility as long as it was over 10 million.[7] Rather, what they did show was the direct relationship of the numerical sperm count to the chances of the couple becoming pregnant (Table 10–5).

Sperm motility correlated both with the chance of pregnancy and with the number of cycles required for the wife to conceive.[8] When the motile sperm count was less than 5 million, a mean of 11 months was required to achieve pregnancy, whereas when the motile count was over 60 million, a mean of only 6 months was required. Nonetheless, the facts that a lower motile sperm count is associated with a longer mean time until pregnancy occurs, that 11% of men who have had all the children they want (and are requiring a vasectomy) have sperm counts under 10 million, and that a man with only 50,000 sperm/cc appears able to impregnate his partner, should cause us to qualify telling a couple that the male is responsible for their infertility.

Further evidence along this line is provided by treatment of large numbers of men with hypogonadotropic hypopituitarism. These azoospermic eunuchoid men require replacement therapy with follicle-stimulating hormone and luteinizing hormone (human menopausal and human chorionic gonadotropins) to induce puberty and stimulate the testes to make androgens and sperm. Despite adequate gona-

dotropin replacement, sperm counts rarely increased above 2 to 5 million/cc. Nevertheless, virtually all of these men (20 of 22) impregnated their wives although their sperm counts appeared extremely dismal.[9]

A review of sperm count and motility indexes in men after vasovasostomy (vasectomy reversal) comparing those who did and did not impregnate their wives (S.J. Silber and co-workers, unpublished observations, 1987) (Table 10–6), revealed the distribution of sperm count, percentage motility, and total motile sperm count per ejaculate to be quite similar to those in previous reports.[6]

Eleven percent of my patients who impregnated their wives after vasovasostomy had total motile sperm counts per ejaculate (not total sperm/cc) of less than 10 million. Sixty-four percent had over 40 million sperm/cc. The differences between this group and the men who remained infertile after vasovasostomy are insignificant, except for those with sperm counts below 10 million ejaculate; that is, 11% successful versus 23% unsuccessful. Most of these 23% actually had fewer than 3 million motile sperm per ejaculate. Thus, sperm count seems to make a difference, but the effect is primarily at the lowest end of the scale. Even then it may not be the only factor, because fully 11% of quite fertile men also fall into this very low category.

TABLE 10–6. FREQUENCY DISTRIBUTION OF MOTILE SPERM AFTER VASOVASOSTOMY IN MEN WHO DID AND DID NOT IMPREGNATE THEIR WIVES

Total Motile Sperm Count/Ejaculate (millions)	Total No.(%) of Patients	No.(%) Pregnant	No.(%) Not Pregnant
1–10	32(12)	25(11)	7(23)
10–20	31(12)	27(12)	4(13)
20–40	32(12)	30(13)	2(7)
40–80	79(31)	68(30)	11(37)
>80	84(33)	78(34)	6(20)
Totals	258	228	30

From S. J. Silber et al, unpublished data, 1987

RELATIONSHIP OF SPERM COUNT TO PREGNANCY RATE

The motile sperm count in infertile couples was compared to the ultimate pregnancy rate over many years of follow-up (assuming the women were treated) (Table 10–7).[7] When the number of motile sperm was below 10 million/cc, approximately 30% of the couples conceived. When the count was greater than 100 million 70% conceived. In general, the higher the motile sperm count the greater the potential for conception. This study assumed that the woman was always treated if contributing infertility factors were found in her. While typically nothing can be done to improve a low sperm count, treatment of the female is often successful, and the better the sperm count, the more likely it is that treatment will succeed. Although the numbers are different, these data are in basic agreement with previous work.[4]

A similar relationship was noted among 1,327 oligospermic men who had a long history of infertility that was assumed, rightly or wrongly, to be simply due to male factors, and whose wives were on a long waiting list to receive therapeutic insemination by donor (TID) (Table 10–8). The data were compiled at a time when there were only a few good TID programs in Europe, which created waiting lists of many years before treatment could be initiated. These pregnancy rates refer to women who conceived either before their names came up on the list (which was several years), or after they had already given up on the idea. Even when the sperm count was below 1 million and as low as 100,000/cc, with no treatment of either partner the pregnancy rate approached 4% in 5 years and 9% in 12 years.

With increasing levels still within the oligospermic range, the pregnancy rate increased, so that when the sperm count was between 15 and 20 million, with no treatment whatsoever, almost 70% of couples eventually conceived in 5 years. These data suggest that with adequate time, even exceedingly low sperm counts are associated with pregnancy and

TABLE 10–8. CORRELATION BETWEEN OLIGOSPERMIA AND PREGNANCY

Motile Sperm Count (millions/cc)	Pregnancy Rate (%) 5 years	12 Years
0.1–1	3.9	8.7
1–5	11.9	26.6
5–10	22.1	34.3
10–15	45.0	58.5
15–20	68.6	82.0

From Schoysman and Gerris.[10]

fertility, and that higher counts within the oligospermic range seem to be associated with higher pregnancy rates.

A discrepancy exists between these two studies with respect to impregnation and motile sperm counts. In general, rates reported by one group were much lower over a longer period of time[10] than those disclosed by the other.[7] It is likely that this discrepancy stems from the fact that all along, female factors may have contributed to the infertility, and treatment of these factors was being delayed until such time as the couples could come to the front of the donor insemination list. Thus, these are rather unique data that could not be duplicated in most other retrospective studies.

Four groups from Australia tabulated their data on infertile couples and oligospermia in a graph that demonstrates the same points (Fig. 10–1).[11-14] In their infertility clinic, in which the women were treated no matter how poor the men's semen, pregnancy rates were compared for couples in which the men had a sperm count (per cc) of less than 5 million, 5 to 20 million, greater than 20 million with less than 50% motile, and greater than 20 million with more than 60% motile. These four groups were then compared to the TID group (presumably highest-quality semen) and the normal pregnancy rate table from Vessey's study.[14] Normal was assumed to be the spontaneous pregnancy rate reported in the early 1950s by MacLeod and Gold.[2]

Again, quite remarkably with fewer than 5 million sperm/cc (this does not mean 5 million motile sperm/cc, but a total of 5 million regardless of motility), the pregnancy rate at 2 years was almost 30% and at 3 years was over 30%. When the sperm count was between 5 and 20 million/cc, the pregnancy rate at 2 years was approximately 43%, and at 3 years was 50%. When the sperm count was over 20 million although less than 60% motile, pregnancy rate at 2 years was very similar to when the count was between 5 and 20 million and a little bit higher than that at 3 years. When the sperm count was essentially normal, that is, over 20 million/cc with greater than

TABLE 10–7. CORRELATION BETWEEN SPERM COUNT AND PREGNANCY IN INFERTILE COUPLES

Motile Sperm Count (million/cc)	Pregnancy Rate (%)
<5.1	33.3
5.1–10.0	27.8
10.1–20.0	52.9
20.1–40.0	57.1
40.1–60.0	60.0
60.1–100.0	62.5
>100	70.0

From Smith et al.[7]

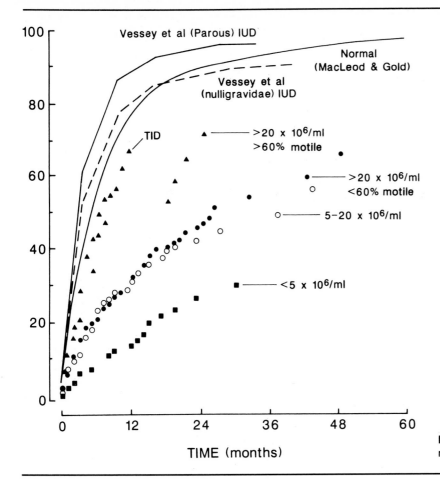

Figure 10–1. Cumulative and life table pregnancy rates. (From Baker and Burger.[11])

60% motility, the pregnancy rate at 2 years was about 72%. When any of these pregnancy rates is compared with that of TID or to a normal curve, it is clear that in an infertile couple no matter how high the sperm count, the pregnancy rate in a life table analysis is somewhat lower than normal.

It would be easy to speculate from such data that the sperm count is relatively constant in oligospermic males and resistant to improvement. Therefore the major variable in the couple's chance for pregnancy probably revolves around the woman. Women appear capable of conceiving with extremely low sperm counts, but the higher the motile sperm count, the greater the chances.

PREGNANCY RATES WITH DONOR INSEMINATION IN WIVES OF OLIGOSPERMIC OR AZOOSPERMIC MEN

In 1982 a group from France published a remarkable observation from their donor insemination program.[15] They classified women undergoing TID as to whether their husbands were azoospermic or oligospermic. The pregnancy rate per cycle in women whose husbands were azoospermic was 11.6%, while that in women whose husbands were oligospermic was only 4.9%. Overall, 61% of women whose husbands were azoospermic conceived after donor insemination as opposed to only 29% of those whose husbands were oligospermic.

A reasonable speculation for this unexpected finding was that the oligospermic men might have impregnated their partners with their small number of sperm if the women themselves did not also have decreased fertility. The wives of azoospermic husbands were less likely to have decreased fertility and more likely to fit into a normal population. Their failure to achieve pregnancy appears more likely to have been due strictly to the complete absence of sperm in the men's ejaculate. Because many oligospermic men are able to impregnate, it is clear that the most fertile partners of relatively infertile men would have become pregnant anyway and never would have undergone TID.

These results provide indirect evidence that a low sperm count is no barrier to pregnancy in very fertile women, and that infertility is commonly caused not simply by male factor alone, but by a combination of male and female factors. Thus, a low sperm count alone is less likely to prevent conception than is widely believed.

Another investigator found that when the husband's sperm count was less than 2 million/cc the life table pregnancy rate after TID was almost 100%.[16] When the sperm count was between 2 and 9 million/cc the rate was only 73%, and when the count, although still in the oligospermia range, was greater than 10 million the rate was only 62%. In 1982 Schoysman from Belgium in reviewing these data was quoted as saying, "A group of couples in whom the male with a low semen output did cause a pregnancy before referral escapes us altogether. Thus it is very well possible that the fertility rate in that group of oligospermic men has a very different distribution . . . the subfertile female reveals the subfertile male."

RELATIONSHIP BETWEEN SPERM COUNT AND FEMALE SUBFERTILITY

In our data of a large number of infertile couples (all of whom were seen only as couples no matter what the prior presumption of which partner was infertile) demonstrated an inverse relationship between sperm count and degree of fertility of the woman.[17] We eliminated women with greater than minimal endometriosis lesions or with pelvic inflammatory disease, and divided the remaining patients as having "good" or "poor" ovulation. Poor ovulation was defined as no ovulation, delayed ovulation, or short luteal phase. When the sperm count was less than 5 million/cc, 33% of the women had poor ovulation and 67% had good ovulation. When the sperm count was between 5 and 20 million/cc (higher, but still in an oligospermic range), the figures were 78% and 22%, respectively. The lower the sperm count in an infertile couple, the less is the chance that the woman will be subfertile. The greater the sperm count, even though it is still within an oligospermic range, the greater the chance that the woman will be subfertile. Again our data indicate that a low sperm count will impregnate a fertile woman, but the higher the sperm count the easier it is for a woman with good ovulation to become pregnant.

A similar relationship was detected in a comparison of pregnancy rates TID using fresh versus frozen semen.[8,18] Women who were receiving TID were divided into two groups: those with normal ovulation requiring no treatment, and those with poor ovulation requiring treatment. Differentiation based on insemination with fresh sperm and frozen sperm was thought to be an excellent model for differences in semen quality. Using fresh semen, the mean time to conception for women who had normal ovulation was only 2.8 cycles, while in those who had poor ovulation requiring treatment it was 6.6 cycles. Clearly, despite the use of fresh semen, poor ovulators required longer to become pregnant than normal ovulators. On the other hand, normal ovulators who were inseminated with frozen semen had a mean time to conception of 5.5 cycles. Thus, despite normal ovulation, the use of frozen semen almost halved the conception rate per cycle. The remarkable finding is that frozen semen in poor ovulators yielded a mean time to conception of 22 months.

Therefore in this model, a moderate male factor alone, and poor ovulation had a measurable, but not clinically significant, effect. In the presence of a combination of male and female factors, the pregnancy rate per cycle was almost one tenth of that when there was normal ovulation and no male factor. This lends credence to the theory that neither a low sperm count in itself nor female subfertility in itself prevents conception, but a combination of the two does.

Data are available from studies in in vitro fertilization (IVF) and gamete intrafallopian transfer (GIFT) that back up the clinical point of view presented here.

In cases of congenital absence of the vas we have aspirated sperm from the epididymis, fertilized the wife's eggs in vitro, and placed the resultant embryos into the fallopian tubes (zygote intrafallopian tube transfer, or ZIFT).[19] Resultant pregnancies lead us to conclude that sperm with reduced motility (so long as there is linear forward progression, however slow) can fertilize the egg if other obstacles are eliminated.

Other investigators carefully evaluated the semen of a large number of couples who did and did not become pregnant with GIFT.[20] They found very poor correlation of pregnancy rate and standard semen variables such as count, velocity, and motility. What was very predictive was the linearity of sperm movement. This means one may be able simply to look at the sperm under the microscope and, regardless of standard values, determine whether pregnancy is likely. If any sperm have linear forward progression, fertilization may be achievable.

A similar finding was reported by a group who very carefully examined morphology of the sperm in husbands of patients undergoing IVF.[21] Any sperm with the slightest defect, such as neck droplets, bent necks, abnormal heads, and the like, were considered of abnormal morphology. It was remarkable that, as long as more than 4% of sperm had absolutely normal morphology, fertilization in vitro was achieved. Once again it is suggested that examining the husband's sperm can provide an excellent view of the likelihood of fertilization, and it requires only small numbers of "fertile" sperm to do so.

Work using GIFT in couples in whom a male factor contributes to infertility supports the concept that even with reduced semen values (including a poor hamster test), improved treatment of the woman can yield normal pregnancy rates (J. Kerin and R. Marrs, personal communication, October 1987). With previous series both of these workers had noted lower pregnancy rates in such couples. With a more recent GIFT cycle, however, they used lupro-lide (TAP Pharmaceuticals, Chicago), a gonadotro-pin-releasing hormone agonist, as part of the stimulation protocol to ensure a synchronized, mature development of follicles. With that improved stimulation regimen, they achieved a 34% pregnancy rate.

Thus the most recent IVF and GIFT data support the concept presented here that even very low sperm counts do not preclude pregnancy, and treatment of the woman can result in pregnancy even when treatment of the man has been ineffective.

REFERENCES

1. Sokol, RZ, Sparkes R: Demonstrated paternity in spite of oligospermia. *Fertil Steril* 47:356, 1987.
2. MacLeod J, Gold RZ: The male factor in fertility and infertility. II. Sperm counts in 1000 men of known fertility and in 1000 cases of infertile marriage. *J Urol* 66:436, 1951.
3. Rehan N, Sobrero AJ, Fertig JW: The semen of fertile men: Statistical analysis of 1300 men. *Fertil Steril* 26:492, 1975.
4. David G, Jonannet P, Boyce AM, Spira A, Schwartz D: Sperm counts in fertile and infertile men. *Fertil Steril* 31:453, 1979.
5. Nelson CMK, Bunge RG: Semen analysis: Evidence for changing parameters of male infertility potential. *Fertil Steril* 25:503, 1974.
6. Zukerman Z, Rodriguez-Rigau LJ, Smith K, Steinberger E: Frequency distribution of sperm counts in fertile and infertile males. *Fertil Steril* 28:1310, 1977.
7. Smith KD, Rodriguez-Rigau LJ, Steinberger E: Relation between indices of semen analysis and pregnancy rate in infertile couples. *Fertil Steril* 28:1314, 1977.
8. Steinberger E, Rodriguez-Rigau LJ: The infertile couple. *J Androl* 4:111, 1983.
9. Sherins R: State-of-the-art lecture. Presented at the meeting of the American Fertility Society, Toronto, Ontario, Canada, 1986.
10. Schoysman R, Gerris J: Fertility potential of sperm with regard to the duration of infertility—The time factor. Presented at the international andrology symposium, Pisa, Italy, 1982.
11. Baker HWG, Burger HG: Male infertility in reproductive medicine, in Steinberger E, Frajese G, Steinberger A (eds): New York, Raven, 1986, pp 187–197.
12. Kovacs AT, Lecton JF, Matthews CD, et al: The outcome of artificial donor insemination compared to the husband's fertility status. *Clin Reprod Fertil* 1:295, 1982.
13. Vessey M, Doll R, Peto R, Johnson B, Wiggins P: A long-term follow-up study of women using different methods of contraception: An interim report. *J Biosoc Sci* 8:373, 1976.
14. MacLeod J, Gold RZ: The male factor in fertility and infertility. VI. Semen quality and other factors in relation to ease of conception. *Fertil Steril* 4:10, 1953.
15. Emperaire JC, Gauzere-Sonmireu E, Andefert AJ: Female fertility and donor insemination. *Fertil Steril* 37:90, 1982.
16. Kremer J: Factors influencing the occurrence of pregnancy following donor insemination. Presented at the 10th world congress on fertility and sterility, Madrid, Spain, July 5–11, 1980.
17. Silber S: Simultaneous treatment of the wife in infertile couples with oligospermia. *Fertil Steril* 4:505, 1983.
18. Smith KD, Rodriguez-Rigau LJ, Steinberger E: The influence of ovulatory dysfunction and timing of insemination on the success of artificial insemination donor (AID) with fresh or cryopreserved semen. *Fertil Steril* 36:496.
19. Silber S, Ord T, Borrero C, Balmaceda J, Asch R: New treatment for infertility due to congenital absence of vas deferens. *Lancet* 2:850, 1987.
20. Rodriguez LJ, Smith K, Steinberger E, Grunert G: Relationship of semen parameters to pregnancy with GIFT. Presented at the meeting of the American Society of Andrologists, Denver, March 1987.
21. Rosenwaks Z: State-of-the-art lecture. Presented at the meeting of the American Fertility Society, Reno, 1987.

CHAPTER 11

Evaluation and Medical Management of Male Infertility

Stephen J. Winters

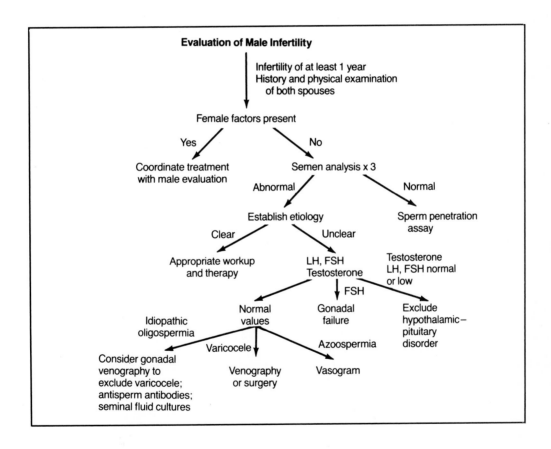

Male factors are estimated to contribute to infertility in 25 to 50% of infertile couples.[1] Therefore a screening evaluation for the male should ideally be performed early in the infertility work-up. For practical purposes, this can be limited to a medical history, physical examination, and direct sperm count. This information, together with results of a similar noninvasive evaluation of the female partner, can be used to direct further efforts at diagnosis and therapy. It is useful for the andrologist as well as the gynecologist to interview both partners. This guarantees a free exchange of information, with the acquisition of important clinical details and identification of possible psychologic and sexual strains between the couple.

The majority of infertile men have oligospermia (reduced sperm output), asthenospermia (poor sperm motility), and/or teratospermia (sperm with abnormal morphology) of unknown etiology. Presumably, spermatogenesis is quantitatively as well as qualitatively abnormal. The men are generally in good health and have a paucity of physical findings. Until the cause(s) of infertility is known, any classification is incomplete. Nevertheless, based on current information, a practical approach must be developed, which entails awareness of the disorders associated with hypospermatogenesis and an honest assessment of the available treatment options.

TESTICULAR DYSFUNCTION

Abnormalities of testicular function can affect the two compartments of the testis, leading to both impaired production of testosterone by the Leydig cells, resulting in under-androgenization, and hypospermatogenesis, with infertility. Studies indicate an extensive paracrine communication among the testicular cell types[2]; however, the complex process of spermatogenesis is more sensitive to disruption than is testosterone biosynthesis. Therefore infertility with apparently normal androgenization often occurs. Testicular dysfunction may result from disorders that primarily affect the testis or from a disturbance of the hypothalamus–pituitary axis, leading to altered gonadotropin stimulation of the testis.

Primary Testicular Failure
Disorders that primarily affect the testis generally result in elevated circulating levels of luteinizing hormone (LH) and follicle-stimulating hormone (FSH). They can be conveniently classified as congenital or acquired (Table 11–1).

Congenital Disorders.   Klinefelter's syndrome and its sex chromosomal variants affect 0.21% of male adults.[3] In one series this diagnosis was made in 4% of infertile men and 11% of azoospermic men. It is characterized clinically by small testes, gynecomastia,

TABLE 11–1. DISORDERS THAT PRODUCE PRIMARY TESTICULAR FAILURE

Congenital	Acquired
Klinefelter's syndrome (47,XXY and variants)	Orchitis (mumps, pyogenic, traumatic)
Cryptorchidism	Malignancy (germ cell, leukemia, lymphoma)
Congenital anorchia (vanishing testis syndrome)	Torsion
	Varicocele
Noonan's syndrome	Spinal cord injury
Myotonic muscular dystrophy	Systemic illness (liver disease, renal failure)
Sickle cell disease	Drugs
	X-irradiation
	Aging

incomplete androgenization, and infertility. The typical histologic changes in the testis are seminiferous tubule hyalinization and an apparent increase in the density of Leydig cells. A buccal smear can be used to identify Barr bodies, and a peripheral blood karyotype is 47,XXY. A subgroup of 10% of these patients have 46,XY/47,XXY mosaicism and generally have less severe physical abnormalities. A testis biopsy is not needed for diagnosis.

Various autosomal abnormalities, including translocations, inversions, and extra marker chromosomes, occur with increased frequency among infertile men. Only about 1 to 2% have identifiable autosomal abnormalities, however.[4] DNA hybridization methods represent a promising new approach to identifying the genes on the Y chromosome responsible for organization of the testis and spermatogenesis, as well as abnormal sequences on the X chromosome or autosomes that may be present among infertile men.[5] Testicular dysfunction is present in men with the congenital disorders myotonic muscular dystrophy and sickle cell disease.

Cryptorchidism was found in 6.4% of men attending a large infertility clinic. Patients with sex chromosome abnormalities or hypogonadotropic hypogonadism may also have cryptorchidism. In most cases, however, there is no clear explanation of why the testes fail to descend into the scrotum. A high rate of infertility is noted in men wth unilateral as well as bilateral cryptorchidism.[6] Spermatogenesis is impaired in the scrotal and in the cryptorchid gonads. Retractile testis may also be a cause of male infertility.[7] In this condition, the testis may be scrotal but is easily withdrawn to an inguinal location. Surgical treatment of cryptorchidism has been recommended for boys 1 to 2 years of age; however, the role of early surgery in preserving fertility remains to be clarified.

Acquired Disorders.   Testicular trauma and inflammation are recognized causes of hypogonadism. Thirty percent of adult men who develop mumps have clinical orchitis; in two thirds of these it is unilateral. Before age 10 years, however, mumps is rarely accompanied by orchitis. The extent of subsequent adult testicular dysfunction may vary from azoospermia and marked androgen deficiency to no fertility disturbance.

Testicular torsion is an acute twisting of the testis occluding its blood supply, which, if untreated, results in testicular atrophy. In some patients, subsequent sperm counts are abnormal, suggesting an underlying testicular disorder or damage to both testes.

Epididymitis and epididymo-orchitis may result from sexually transmitted disease and ascending spread of urethritis. *Neisseria gonorrhoeae* and *Chlamy-*

dia trachomatis are the commonly associated organisms. These men experience rapid onset of pain and swelling of the epididymis. The results of testicular biopsies performed in one study revealed that spermatogenesis was impaired in 20 of 28 patients.[8] Nevertheless, a history of acute epididymo-orchitis is rare among infertile men, and the role of infection in idiopathic human male infertility is uncertain.

Hypogonadotropic Hypogonadism

Testicular dysfunction in men with hypogonadotropic hypogonadism results from inadequate gonadotropin stimulation of the testis (Table 11–2). Both primary pathology within the pituitary gland and a disturbance in secretion of gonadotropin-releasing hormone (GnRH) by the hypothalamus can result in gonadotropin deficiency. These men usually seek medical attention for androgen deficiency and, less commonly, for infertility. Serum levels of testosterone are reduced, and LH levels are in the low normal range with disturbed pulsatile LH release.

Idiopathic Hypogonadotropic Hypogonadism.
Idiopathic hypogonadotropic hypogonadism generally is identified when teenagers fail to enter puberty.[9] They are phenotypic males, because maternal human chorionic gonadotropin (HCG) stimulated the fetal testis to produce testosterone, resulting in masculinization of the genitalia. They produce little or no GnRH, however; therefore pulsatile LH secretion does not occur as teenagers, and prepubertal testicular function persists. Approximately 50% of these individuals have midline defects, including anosmia, which results from hypoplasia of the rhinencephalon.[10] A family history is also positive for similarly affected individuals in nearly 50% of cases, with most kindreds indicating an autosomal dominant mode of inheritance with incomplete penetrance.

Occasionally, men are detected later in life with congenital eunuchoidism and some degree of testicular enlargement. Their circulating testosterone levels that are intermediate between those of prepubertal boys and normal adults. Some of these men have been shown to have fewer than normal spontaneous LH secretory pulses, or pulses of reduced amplitude.[11] This variant, which has been called the fertile eunuch syndrome, may occur with increased frequency among certain ethnic groups.[12] Hypogonadotropic hypogonadism also may occur together with other deficiencies of hypothalamic-releasing factor 5, especially growth-hormone-deficient dwarfism, and is designated idiopathic hypopituitarism.

Acquired Hypogonadotropic Hypogonadism.
Any mass lesion that damages the hypothalamus–pituitary can interfere with the secretion of both gonadotropins and other trophic hormones. These tumors may be functional, as in acromegaly, or nonfunctional, as in craniopharyngioma. Men with sellar and parasellar tumors often have headaches and vision disturbances. Trauma and infiltrative disease of the hypothalamus–pituitary axis may result in acquired gonadotropin deficiency.

Gonadotropin secretion can also be altered by the effects of other hormones. Men with prolactin-producing tumors may experience delayed puberty, poor androgenization, impotence, and infertility. In addition to a mass effect of the prolactinoma on the surrounding normal pituitary, hyperprolactinemia is associated with disturbance of pulsatile LH (and presumably GnRH) secretion, which can be reversed by bromocriptine treatment.[13] Gonadotropin deficiency in men with Cushing's syndrome probably results from cortisol hypersecretion, since reduction in cortisol levels by either bilateral andrenalectomy[14] or treatment with a glucocorticoid antagonist returns testosterone levels to normal. Men with poorly treated congenital adrenal hyperplasia may also have disturbed gonadotropin secretion resulting in infertility, although the pathophysiology remains unclear.[15] No evidence for attenuated 21-hydroxylase deficiency was found among 50 men with unexplained infertility.[16]

Androgen Resistance Syndromes

Complete androgen insensitivity (testicular feminization) is an X-linked disorder in which genotypic males with testes have a female phenotype.[17] This form of male pseudo-hermaphroditism is due to absent or defective androgen receptors. A more limited form of androgen resistance, wth clinical features of variable ambiguity of the external genitalia and impaired peripheral androgenization, has been called incomplete androgen insensitivity. Subsequently, some infertile men with normal external genitalia and normal secondary sex characteristics have been found to have reduced androgen receptor

TABLE 11–2. DISORDERS THAT PRODUCE HYPOGONADOTROPIC HYPOGONADISM

Congenital	Acquired
Isolated hypogonadotropic hypogonadism	Pituitary adenomas
Kallmann's syndrome	Nonfunctional "chromophobe" adenomas
Prader–Willi syndrome	Prolactinomas
Fertile eunuch syndrome	Cushing's syndrome
	Acromegaly
Idiopathic hypopituitarism	Hypothalamic tumors and cysts
Partial	Others
Complete	Head trauma, meningitis, cerebritis, sarcoidosis, acute illness, histiocytosis, hemochromatosis, vasculitis, X-irradiation, anorexia nervosa, autoimmune hypophysitis

binding to skin fibroblasts. Androgen resistance at the level of the hypothalamus–pituitary axis is suggested in certain of these men by the finding of an elevated rate of testosterone production and increased levels of circulating LH. It has been suggested that the product of serum testosterone multiplied by LH be used to identify such patients; however, misleading conclusions may result from this approach. More convincing is the finding of an increased free or non-sex-hormone-binding globulin testosterone level. The prevalence of androgen insensitivity among infertile men has been calculated to range from rare to 19%.[18] Because the methods used for these analyses are complicated, further studies are needed.

Systemic Illnesses Associated with Gonadal Dysfunction

Testicular function is frequently abnormal in men with acute and chronic systemic illnesses.[31] The associated effects of weight loss, malnutrition, and stress no doubt contribute to this abnormality; however, specific endocrine syndromes have been associated with certain systemic disorders.

Gonadal dysfunction is common in men with chronic renal failure. Reduction in libido, impotence, reduced body mass, and impaired androgenization all contribute to the poor quality of life for these patients. Testosterone levels are often low, and LH and FSH levels are either normal or elevated.[19] Pulsatile secretion of LH is markedly attenuated in uremic men, perhaps because of delayed metabolic clearance. Prolactin levels may increase. Semen typically are of poor quality even during dialysis, but improve after successful kidney transplantation.

The reproductive disturbances that occur in women who are anorexic and those who participate in stressful physical conditioning programs such as long-distance running are widely recognized. These changes may be due to loss of body weight or body fat. Men also develop hypogonadotropic hypogonadism in response to the profound weight loss that characterizes anorexia nervosa. Serum testosterone levels declined during fasting[20] and intense exercise in healthy men,[21] although random levels were normal in two studies of male marathon runners.[22,23] In one study,[23] LH pulse frequency and amplitude were less in runners than in healthy nonrunners; however, mean LH levels were normal. In the absence of changes in mean LH or testosterone levels, the significance of these alterations in LH pulsatile secretion are as yet undefined. Serum testosterone levels were also less in college wrestlers during their competitive season than during the off season, at which time their mean weight had increased by 3.5 kg.[24] The results of routine semen analyses performed in 20 self-selected distance runners were normal in 18.[25] Thus, although gonadal hormones are influenced by weight loss and endurance training in men, no evidence exists that currently popular physical fitness programs impair male fertility.

In contrast, hypogonadism is often suspected on clinical grounds in obese men. Serum testosterone levels are subnormal in massively obese men and return toward normal with weight loss.[26] The low total level is best explained by a reduction in serum sex-hormone-binding globulin (SHBG) levels and may not be clinically significant, because most obese men are not hypogonadal. Serum estrone levels are often high due to the aromatization of androgens by fat tissue. Testis size is normal, and the results of one study indicate that sperm density and motility are normal in otherwise healthy obese men.

Thyrotoxicosis may result in gynecomastia and reduced libido and potency.[27] Testosterone levels in hyperthyroid men are often increased due to increased SHBG levels. Serum estradiol levels may rise due to enhanced peripheral conversion of androgenic precursors. There are occasional reports of low sperm counts that improve with antithyroid therapy. Testicular disturbances may also occur in hypothyroid men[28]; however, unsuspected hypothyroidism is rare among healthy infertile men.

Aging is associated with a gradual decline in sexual performance and endocrine testicular dysfunction.[29] The age at which these changes occur is variable; however, serum testosterone levels fall and the total number of Leydig cells in the testes is reduced with aging.[30] Mean testosterone levels in men in the sixth to seventh decade are generally in the low normal range; very low levels suggest additional medical problems. Although one study found that healthy grandfathers had normal sperm production, most studies conclude that seminiferous tubule function declines with age. Levels of FSH and LH may be high normal or slightly increased. The inverse relationship between age and fertility is also influenced by the female partner's age. Low testosterone levels are also found in men after general surgery, and in acutely ill patients such as those with burns, respiratory failure, and head trauma.

Drugs and Toxins that Affect Testicular Function

Several prescription drugs can directly inhibit testicular function or indirectly interfere with gonadotropin secretion, resulting in androgen deficiency, spermatogenic arrest, or both. Drugs may interfere with erection and ejaculation, or impede androgen action at target tissues, affecting libido and producing gynecomastia as well as impotence (Table 11–3).

Prescribed Drugs. Exposure in utero to diethylstilbestrol (DES) has been associated with the presence of epididymal cysts and functional sperm

TABLE 11-3. DRUGS AND TOXINS THAT ALTER REPRODUCTIVE FUNCTION

Exposure	Agent
In utero	Diethylstilbestrol, antiandrogens
Occupational	Carbon disulfide, dibromochlorpropane, lead, estrogens, chlordectone
Prescription drugs	Chemotherapeutic agents, sulfasalazine, androgens
Drugs that alter male sexual function	Testosterone biosynthesis inhibitors (spironolactone, ketoconazole, cyproterone acetate)
	Androgen antagonists (spironolactone, cyproterone acetate, flutamide, cimetidine)
	Inhibitors of erectile function and ejaculation (antihypertensives—methyldopa, reserpine, beta blockers, clonidine; neuroleptics—phenothiazines, butyrophenones, lithium; tricyclic antidepressants; monoamine oxidase inhibitors; anticholinergics)
Recreational	Ethanol, marijuana, opiates, tobacco

abnormalities.[37] Chemotherapeutic agents, particularly the alkalating agents mustargen, cyclophosphamide, and chlorambucil, can damage the testes.[38] Although the mechanism for this damage is not known, FSH levels generally rise, and germinal aplasia is frequently found at biopsy. Dosage and duration of chemotherapy determine the severity of the injury and potential for recovery in these men. Radiation therapy can also affect spermatogenesis. Most boys with acute lymphoblastic leukemia who receive testicular irradiation have permanently low serum testosterone levels.[39] Sulfasalazine, a conjugate of 5-aminosalicylic acid, used in the treatment of ulcerative colitis, has been associated with a reduction in sperm motility and sperm density, which may be reversed upon discontinuation of treatment.[40]

Other medications also result in reproductive disturbances. Spironolactone[41] and ketoconazole[42] impair testosterone biosynthesis. Spironolactone[41] and cimetidine[43] bind to androgen receptors and can impede androgen action. Each of these drugs may produce gynecomastia; however, no consistent convincing detrimental effects on spermatogenesis have been demonstrated. The C-17α-alkyltestosterone derivatives used by athletes as anabolic agents produce profound hypospermatogenesis, which appears to be reversible after discontinuation of steroid treatment.[44] Finally, many drugs, including antihypertensives, antidepressants, and sedatives, can produce impotence based on their mode of action.

Recreational Substances. Substance abuse is another form of drug use that is of increasing importance in our society. Chronic alcoholism is usually associated with infertility, impotence, and signs of reduced androgenization. Changes in the testis, the hypothalamic–pituitary axis, serum sex-hormone-binding globulin, and adrenal steroids all contribute to this complex endocrinopathy, which results from both cirrhosis and the toxic effects of alcohol on the hypothalamic–pituitary–gonadal unit.[32] Serum FSH and LH levels are often increased, but may remain normal. Reductions in testis size, seminal volume, and sperm density, motility, and morphology have also been reported among alcohol abusers.[33] These values may improve after use of alcohol is discontinued.[34,35] Although ethanol administration reduces testosterone production in healthy men,[36] the role of moderate alcohol consumption in male infertility is unknown. Chronic alcohol abuse is toxic to the testis and suppresses gonadotropin secretion. Concomitant liver disease leads to changes in androgen metabolism. Infertility is common among these men. Opiate abuse, is associated with the production of an abnormal ejaculate.[45] By inhibiting gonadotropin secretion, opiate drugs also reduce serum testosterone levels.[46] The observation that opiate antagonists increase LH secretion suggests a physiologic role for endogenous opiates in the regulation of gonadotropin secretion in men.[47] Malnutrition and associated acute and chronic illness may contribute to the effects of both habitual ethanol and opiate abuse.

Another commonly abused substance, marijuana, interferes with gonadotropin secretion in experimental animals and directly inhibits testosterone biosynthesis. Maternal cannabinoid exposure may influence testicular function in offspring.[48] Furthermore, marijuana may directly impair sperm motility. Because of obvious limitations, controlled studies are not possible in humans, and the data available are insufficient to permit any meaningful conclusions. Cigarette smoking has also been associated with a reduction in sperm output and an increase in serum estradiol levels.[49]

Occupational Agents. Considerable efforts have been exerted to identify the role of environmental and occupational toxins in human male infertility.[50] Carbon disulfide, a solvent used in the manufacture of rayon, produces neurotoxicity and has been associated with testicular damage. Dibromochloropropane added to soil to kill nematodes is mutagenic and is cytotoxic to the testes. Its sale and distribution were banned in the United States in 1979. Central nervous system, hepatic, and testicular toxicities were found in a group of workers exposed to the chlorinated hydrocarbon chlordectone (kepone). There is also a clear relationship between reproductive dysfunction in both men and women and toxic lead exposure. Individuals at risk include smelters, painters, battery workers, and those exposed to lead-containing fuels. The role of heat in the workplace as well as the reproductive risks to anesthesiologists remain unclear. Many other agents have been proposed as damaging to the testes; however, results are inconclusive.

OTHER DISORDERS

Genital Tract Obstruction

Obstructive azoospermia has been reported in 3 to 13% of infertile men.[51] This diagnosis should be suspected in the azoospermic man with normal-sized testes and a normal serum FSH level. These clinical findings are not specific, however, because some men with azoospermia due to seminiferous tubule dysfunction have normal serum FSH levels. Testicular biopsy is indicated, and if spermatogenesis is normal, reconstructive surgery may be successful.

The absence of palpable vas deferens on physical examination suggests congenital absence of the vas. Obstructive azoospermia occurs in patients with cystic fibrosis and disorders of mucociliary transport, producing bronchitis and bronchiectasis (Young's syndrome),[52] gonococcal and nongonococcal epididymitis, tuberculosis, surgical trauma, and various tropical diseases.

Immotile Sperm

The syndrome of immotile cilia is associated with a defect in the axoneme of the cilia in the respiratory tract and sperm tail. Affected men produce sperm that are immotile yet normal in density and morphology. They are uniformly sterile. Additional clinical findings include situs inversus, chronic sinusitis, and brochiectasis (Kartagener's syndrome).[53]

Coital Disorders

Retrograde ejaculation and ejaculatory failure are common among men with diabetes mellitus.[54] Neurologic, vascular, and psychophysiologic factors are all believed to contribute to this dysfunction. Endocrine testicular function is normal in most but not all men with diabetes, however.[55]

Men with spinal cord injuries are generally infertile. Ejaculatory failure, genital duct obstruction, and seminiferous tubule dysfunction are all common among these men.[56] Drugs such as narcotics, sedatives, psychotropics, and antiadrenergics may produce anejaculation.

Ejaculatory impotence and associated infertility may also be psychophysiologic, and be treatable by sexual therapy.[57] Although a small semen volume is consistent with androgen deficiency, it may be idiopathic, or could reflect incomplete collection of the ejaculate.

Male Infertility of Uncertain Etiology

Unfortunately, no specific diagnosis can be made in most otherwise healthy men with oligospermia or asthenospermia. If testis biopsies are performed, results are generally abnormal and reveal hypospermatogenesis of variable severity, indicating that the testis is damaged. The genetic or biochemical defects in these men remain unknown. Because of this lack of awareness of the pathophysiology of most cases of male infertility, many additional explanations have been proposed. The following selected disorders remain controversial causes of infertility in the male.

Varicocele. The veins of the scrotal pampiniform plexus are dilated in 20 to 39% of infertile men. Although it is generally believed that sperm production and quality are abnormal in infertile men with varicocele,[58] some reports question the relationship between varicocele and infertility.[59]

Varicocele is believed to result from incompetence of the valves of the gonadal veins, and the predilection for it to occur clinically on the left side has been explained by the asymmetry in renal–gonadal venous anatomy. Results of gonadal venography, however, indicate that right and bilateral varicoceles also occur. In certain cases, the varicocele is not palpable (subclinical), adding one more element of complexity. Varicocele may be identified in asymptomatic adolescents[60] as well as infertile adults. Its natural history is presently unknown, and careful study will produce important insight into this disorder.

Genitourinary Infection. Infection has been proposed to cause male infertility because it is reasonable that inflammation of the genital ducts might alter seminal plasma and render sperm abnormal. Accordingly, antibiotics have been used to treat oligospermia, asthenospermia, elevated semen pH, and poor semen liquefaction. Many contradictory results can be found in the literature; however, most of these studies are difficult to interpret because they used no placebo control group, they were not prospective or randomized, duration of therapy was short, and eradication of infection was uncertain.

Particular interest has surrounded the possible role of infections with *T-strain mycoplasma (Ureaplasma urealyticum).*[61] This organism is frequently present in male and female genital tracts, and treatment of both partners with doxycycline may improve sperm quality and fertility.[62] Results of semen analysis are often unaffected by the presence of *U. urealyticum,* however.[63]

Antisperm Antibodies. Many studies have sought to determine whether antibodies in male serum or semen directed against sperm antigens play a role in male infertility; results have been conflicting. Newer methods of detecting these antibodies, such as immunobead binding and the use of radiolabeled antiglobulins, may be more specific and may allow for more direct identification of immunoglobulins on the sperm surface than do sperm-immobilization or agglutination assays.[64] For example, in the partners of vasectomized men with high levels of sperm-immobilizing antibodies after vasovasostomy, the pregnancy rate was as high as 25%, compared to 56% in men with low antibody titers.[65] In one study using the immunobead-binding assay, antibodies to sperm were found in 24% of infertile men, compared to 7% of fertile men.[64]

Immune infertility may also be more complicated than an all-or-none phenomenon, because relationships have been found between the percentage of sperm binding to antibody, as well as the extent of antibody binding per sperm, and cervical mucus penetration. Furthermore, certain antibodies could produce detrimental effects, and others may not impede fertility. Although the cause of putative immune infertility is presently unknown, infection and inflammation of the testes and epididymis have been proposed to render sperm antigens immunogenic. These antibodies, however, could represent an epiphenomenon, a consequence of sperm abnormality, and not directly relate to the observed male infertility. In this regard, studies of the prevalence of sperm antibodies in men with other identifiable causes for infertility will be of interest.

Antibodies presumably enter semen from blood plasma in the secretions of the seminal vesicles and prostate. These antibodies would not be expected to enter the seminiferous tubules due to the presence of the blood–testis barrier. Therefore the seminiferous tubules might be expected to be normal histologically in men with infertility due to antibodies in seminal plasma. Data to confirm this contention are not currently available.

Thermal Effects on the Testes. The temperature within the scrotum is normally 2 to 3 degrees lower than ambient body temperature. It is generally believed that this lower temperature is necessary for normal testicular function, and experiments in which the testes of experimental animals are heated support this hypothesis. A higher than normal scrotal temperature has been offered as the explanation for the infertility in men with cryptorchidism and varicocele.[66] The possibility that scrotal "hyperthermia" might contribute to idiopathic male infertility has also been considered.[67] The available data are preliminary, and the role of jockey shorts, athletic supporters, hot baths, and saunas in male infertility remains unclear. The temporary decrease in sperm output that follows a significant febrile medical illness is probably due to impaired gonadotropin secretion.

Endocrine Dysfunction. Studies in women indicate that a disturbance in pulsatile gonadotropin secretion may cause hypothalamic amenorrhea. Similarly, an alteration in gonadotropin secretion could produce male infertility. Although a positive correlation between serum LH and testosterone levels had been reported in mildly hypospermatogenic men with normal serum FSH levels,[68] no data confirm this hypothesis. A slight decrease in LH pulse frequency has been reported in a subgroup of men with variable sperm counts and elevated serum FSH levels.[69] However, the cause-and-effect relationships are uncertain.

Rarely, infertile men have normal virilization, normal LH and testosterone levels, and undetectable serum FSH levels.[70] Because serum FSH levels may at times be undetectable in healthy men, the diagnosis of isolated FSH deficiency is difficult. Serum FSH levels measured with an in-vitro bioassay were found to be less elevated than were immunoreactive FSH levels in oligospermic and azoospermic men.[71] These results suggest that in infertile men with increased serum FSH levels, the FSH produced is biochemically modified, altering its bioactivity.

CLINICAL APPROACH TO THE INFERTILE MALE

As in many areas of medicine, a chronologic approach to the medical history is particularly attractive. Maternal illness and drug use (such as DES) have been associated with infertility in offspring. The presence at birth of ambiguous genitalia, microphallus, cryptorchidism, or inguinal hernia is suggestive of congenital hypogonadism. Most chronic illnesses in childhood result in delayed growth and impaired sexual development. Precocious puberty may indicate congenital adrenal hyperplasia, whereas delayed puberty and incomplete pubertal development may result from either primary testicular failure or gonadotropin deficiency.

Hypogonadal adult men may complain of a decrease in libido, impotence, gynecomastia, or symptoms of a sellar or parasellar mass such as headache and vision disturbance. Men with varicocele may complain of scrotal aching. Orchitis, testicular torsion, and epididymitis are characterized by a sudden onset of pain and swelling of the scrotal contents. An occupational and recreational history is important, because environmental toxins such as chlorinated hydrocarbons used as pesticides and lead have been implicated in some cases of male infertility. Medications such as azulfidine and cancer chemotherapeutics adversely affect germ cell development. Alcohol and street drugs may also impair gonad function in adult men. A coital history should identify the timing and technique of intercourse. In evaluating the man with a borderline ejaculate, it is important to determine whether he has children from a previous relationship.

A complete physical examination should be performed. Many systemic illnesses, such as kidney disease, gastrointestinal disorders, and so on, are associated with testicular dysfunction. Exact measurement of the length and width of the testis is important and easily accomplished. Most of the mass of the testis is seminiferous tubules. The testis can also be compared in volume with a series of precalibrated ovoids. Normal median testis length approximates 5.0 cm, which is equivalent to 25 mL in volume. Although testes that measure 4 cm may be normal, the testes of many men with hypospermatogenesis are longer than or equal to 4 cm.

A varicocele may be visible or palpable when the patient assumes the upright posture. It will increase during a Valsalva's maneuver, and will disappear when the patient is recumbent. A reduction in the size of the left testis is common in men with varicocele. Gynecomastia is a frequent finding among men with severe testicular dysfunction.

Laboratory Evaluation

Semen Analysis. Despite its limitations, the direct sperm count is a simple, inexpensive screening test with which to begin the laboratory evaluation for infertility. Three ejaculates should be obtained to provide a representative sample.

If the medical history, physical examination, and semen analyses are normal, attention should be redirected to the female partner before continuing the evaluation of the male (see flow diagram). In certain couples with unexplained infertility, however, the results of a direct semen analysis may be normal and a disorder of sperm function may still be present. Conversely, the direct sperm count may incorrectly identify certain men wth borderline sperm output or motility as abnormal. Newer functional sperm assays, such as the zona-free hamster-egg-penetration assay, may be better indicators of male infertility, and are useful adjunctive tests when neither male nor female factors are identified initially.

Testosterone. The serum or plasma testosterone level should be measured if hypogonadism is suspected clinically or hypospermatogenesis is found. Commercial kits for the direct assay of testosterone in unextracted serum using ^{125}I-labeled testosterone are relatively simple to use, precise, and accurate. Testosterone is present in serum largely bound to SHBG, a high-affinity protein produced by the liver, and albumin. Changes in circulating SHBG concentrations may influence the measured total testosterone concentration. This is particularly common in obese men with low SHBG levels, who are often believed to be hypogonadal. Measurement of non-SHBG or free testosterone can be used to clarify this finding.

Gonadotropins. The pituitary gonadotropins LH and FSH are the major regulators of testicular function. Elevated levels of either or both suggest primary testicular failure. Levels of LH rise when testosterone production falls due to a decline in negative feedback.[72] They are rarely increased in men without a concomitant increase in FSH levels. High FSH levels indicate seminiferous tubule dysfunction, and probably result from a deficiency in the secretion of inhibin as well as sex steroids. High FSH but normal LH levels are often found among infertile men and suggest that the function of Leydig cells is relatively preserved compared to that of seminiferous tubules.[73] Both LH and FSH levels are often normal in infertile men, however, even in those with severe oligospermia.

Both LH and FSH may also be undetectable in normal male serum. Therefore the diagnosis of gonadotropin deficiency cannot be based on the measurement of gonadotropin levels alone. The finding of a low testosterone level together with low or even normal LH and FSH concentrations is suggestive of a disturbance in gonadotropin secretion. A disturbance in pulsatile gonadotropin secretion may be present even when random LH levels are well within the range of normal. Because the proposed clinical approach is to identify recognizable causes of male infertility that are either treatable or untreatable, the suggestion by some that little is gained from measuring gonadotropin levels in infertile men seems counterproductive.

Prolactin. Measurement of prolactin in serum is of great importance in evaluating men with impotence, impaired libido, low semen volume, or a suspected pituitary tumor. In those with prolactinomas, circulating testosterone levels are usually low but may be normal. Prolactin levels may be elevated slightly in men with testicular failure,[74] but they are rarely increased among otherwise healthy men with oligospermia. Both the stress of venipuncture and chest wall stimulation may increase serum levels. Prolactin deficiency is rare, and is without known clinical sequelae.

Estrogens. Estradiol and estrone levels in the sera of healthy men are typically low, and commercial assays frequently overestimate the concentration of estrogens in male serum. Gonadal and adrenal tumors may secrete estradiol and estrone, respectively. Such patients generally have gynecomastia, decreased libido, and low circulating testosterone levels.[75] Circulating estrone levels are often elevated in men with cirrhosis and in those who are obese. The increased secretion of androstanedione by the adrenals during stress, and the presence of aromatase in fat tissue, may contribute to these findings. Estradiol levels are often increased in men with HCG-producing tumors. Measurement of estrogens is not worthwhile in infertile men who have no signs of feminization or normal testosterone levels.

Functional Tests

Response to HCG. Stimulating of testosterone secretion by administering HCG is a useful test of Leydig cell function in prepubertal boys who secrete little or no endogenous gonadotropin. Adult men with Leydig cell failure have elevated basal LH levels. Administration of HCG to them predictably increases circulating testosterone levels less than in healthy men. Because of preexposure of Leydig cells to less than normal LH stimulation, however, short-term administration of HCG also produces an attenuated increase in serum testosterone levels in gonadotropin-deficient men. In these men, the finding that basal LH levels fail to rise with low serum testosterone levels indicates that gonadotropin secretion is abnormal. Therefore, clinically useful information is rarely gained from the HCG test in adult men.

Response to Gonadal-Steroid Hormone Antagonists and Inhibitors. Administration of either of the estrogen antagonists clomiphene citrate or tamoxiphen increases circulating gonadotropin and testosterone levels in healthy men by blocking the negative feedback effect of estradiol.[76] This is a dose and time-dependent effect, and several weeks of treatment are required before consistent changes occur. This approach is of limited clinical diagnostic usefulness and provides little additional information beyond that of basal hormone levels. Similarly, LH levels rise when testosterone production is blocked by steroidogenesis inhibitors such as ketoconazole.[77]

GnRH Test. Synthetic GnRH has been used extensively as a research probe. In general, the incremental rise in LH and FSH levels after GnRH administration is proportional to the basal hormone level. Thus peak gonadotropin levels are higher than normal in men with primary testicular failure. Patients with less severe testicular failure may have basal FSH levels within the range of normal, but an exaggerated response to GnRH. In patients with either pituitary or hypothalamic disease, the release of gonadotropins after stimulation with GnRH is usually reduced, but

may be normal. Thus the response to this test does not unequivocally distinguish between these two possibilities. In patients with GnRH deficiency and a normal pituitary gland, however, repeated administration with GnRH restores the deficient gonadotropin secretion.[78] Although repeated stimulation with GnRH may be useful in identifying those gonadotropin-deficient men who may be candidates for GnRH therapy, presently the test has little practical utility in the evaluation of most infertile men.

Testicular Biopsy. Histologic examination of testis tissue from infertile men almost always reveals abnormalities of the seminiferous tubules. These histologic findings provide little insight into the pathophysiology of infertility, however, and do not affect therapy. Therefore, routine testicular biopsy cannot presently be recommended. As newer biochemical analyses of testis tissue evolve, the procedure may prove more useful. In cases of azoospermia, it is helpful in delineating an obstructive from a proliferative etiology.

TREATMENT OF MALE INFERTILITY

The etiology and pathophysiology of most male infertility remains obscure, and consequently, treatments are generally unsatisfactory. Therefore, the diagnostic evaluation must attempt to identify those men with recognizable causes of infertility who may benefit from specific therapy. As described above, many endocrine and systemic disorders are associated with infertility and should be considered in all infertile men. An in-depth discussion of the treatment of each of these disorders exceeds the scope of this chapter, and interested readers are referred to a comprehensive text.[79]

Men with primary testicular failure and elevated serum FSH levels due to orchitis, Klinefelter's syndrome, cryptochidism, varicocele, or unknown causes, are not amenable to treatment for infertility. Azoospermia and severe oligospermia generally are associated findings, and additional diagnostic tests are unnecessary. Rare FSH-producing pituitary tumors must be excluded if suspected. The androgen deficiency of primary testicular failure is most practically treated with long-acting parenteral testosterone preparations.[80]

Gonadotropin Deficiency

Men with congenital or acquired gonadotropin deficiency require gonadotropins to stimulate spermatogenesis.[81,82] Most often, however, they are treated with testosterone until such time as fertility is desired. Therapy is then changed to HCG in doses of 1,500 to 2,000 IU one to three times weekly. Selected patients may produce sperm and impregnate their partners with HCG alone. It is likely that these subjects have some endogenous FSH secretion. Twelve to 18 months of treatment may be required before sperm begin to appear in the ejaculate. This is not surprising, because the production of sperm in healthy boys, based upon spermaturia, does not occur until several years after puberty has begun.[83] After approximately 1 year of HCG stimulation of Leydig cell function and increased intragonadal androgen production, FSH is added to the regimen. Most workers have used doses of 75 IU intramuscularly three times weekly, although lower doses may be effective. As the maturation of spermatogonia to mature sperm takes 72 days, several months of treatment are necessary before sperm are produced. Treatment should not be considered unsuccessful for at least 12 months with this regimen. Subjects with coexistent cryptorchidism, in spite of orchidopexy, respond poorly to therapy.

Patients with idiopathic hypogonadotropic hypogonadism (Kallmann's syndrome) may alternatively be treated with GnRH, as they have a defect in synthesis or release of GnRH, and otherwise normal pituitary and testicular function. An infusion pump is used to deliver pulses of GnRH into the subcutaneous tissue of the abdomen.[12,84] Doses of 2 to 8 μg/pulse every 90 to 120 minutes have been used to stimulate gonadotropin secretion. Serum testosterone levels generally rise into the normal range, and sperm begin to appear in the ejaculate 1 to 12 months after beginning treatment. As with HCG–HMG therapy, testis growth precedes the onset of complete spermatogenesis. The highest sperm counts are achieved in subjects whose pretreatment testis size is greater than 2.5 cm, suggesting that they have a partial gonadotropin deficiency. At present, no studies have prospectively compared the results of HCG-HMG with GnRH therapy. Patients can be taught to self-administer these medications, and compliance rates are high. Success rates, costs, and convenience of therapy ultimately determine which approach is preferable.

Varicocele-Associated Infertility

It remains a matter of controversy whether to recommend treatment for men with varicocele, because the results may not improve over those in untreated controls. Detachable balloons, stainless-steel coils, and other embolic and sclerosing materials can be placed in the internal spermatic vein by percutaneous catheterization.[85] This approach can be performed at less expense than surgical varicocelectomy and it does not require general anesthesia. Venography may also identify complex collaterals, as well as a right varicocele that might otherwise go undetected.

Idiopathic Oligospermia and Asthenospermia

Various medical therapies have been attempted in the management of idiopathic oligospermia. Although the literature contains many claims of success, most studies suffer from lack of appropriate control groups. In one study of 1,145 infertile couples,[86] pregnancy occurred in 191 (35%) of 548 untreated couples followed for 2 to 7 years. This included 75 (61%) of 122 men with sperm density of less than 20 million/mL and sperm motility of less than 40% on two occasions. These results mandate prospective studies with untreated control subjects in the evaluation of any treatment for male infertility, and indicate that such an approach is ethically permissible.

Probably the most frequently prescribed male fertility drugs are the estrogen antagonists clomiphene and tamoxifen. If given in sufficient doses, these drugs increase LH and FSH secretion by blocking the normal negative feedback inhibition of the hypothalamus and pituitary by estrogens.[76] The rationale is to stimulate spermatogenesis further by increasing the gonadotropin stimulation of the testes. The implied hypothesis (although thus far unproved) is that certain men are subtly deficient in gonadotropin secretion, resulting in infertility.

A second possibility is that testicular estrogens impair spermatogenesis directly, and that antiestrogens prevent this change. A pilot study with the aromatase inhibitor testolactone supported this hypothesis[87]; however, a subsequent randomized, placebo-controlled study did not confirm the findings.[88] Some authors reported improvement in sperm output with antiestrogens,[89] whereas others did not.[90] The issue is further clouded by the finding that pregnancy rates often are unrelated to changes in sperm output.[91] Randomized, prospective studies with these drugs demonstrated no significant effect on sperm output among groups of infertile men.[92] Additional investigation is needed to determine if there is a subpopulation of infertile men who will benefit from antiestrogen treatment. Hormonal therapy with HCG–HMG, GnRH and its agonistic analogs, or androgens is similarly ineffective and unwarranted.

Glucocorticoids have been used to alter the immune response in infertile men, particularly those in whom antisperm antibodies were identified. Due to lack of controlled studies, this approach remains unproved and can be dangerous. Short-term, high-dose glucocorticoids are safer than continuous treatment; however, 40 to 80 mg of prednisone for 10 days each month for 6 to 12 months produces clinical side effects. The difficulties in interpreting the effectiveness of glucocorticoid treatment in immune male infertility are underscored by a study in which 33% of 76 women whose husbands were treated with prednisolone for antisperm antibodies conceived over 9 months.[93] Antisperm antibody titers fell similarly in the pregnant and nonpregnant groups, and 11 of 25 women who eventually conceived were also treated for ovulatory dysfunction. There was no prospective control group. A double-blind, placebo-controlled study of methylprednisolone treatment of infertile men with sperm-associated immunoglobulins revealed a statistically greater decline in sperm-associated IgG in the steroid-treated group, but there was no effect on sperm density or motility, and no increase in the pregnancy rate, which was 10% over 3 months for the entire study population.[90]

The possible role in male infertility of chronic prostatitis of unknown etiology often leads to treatment of these men with antibiotics. In a carefully conducted multicenter study coordinated through the World Health Organization,[94] only 5.6% of 2,871 men evaluated for infertility fulfilled the criteria for male accessory gland infection. Of these, 34 couples in whom no other potential cause for infertiilty was found participated in a double-blind, placebo-controlled study of doxycycline.[95] Treatment averaged 5 months; there were two pregnancies in the doxycycline group and one in the placebo group. These data indicate that genital tract infection is uncommonly the only predisposing factor to male infertility, and further suggest that doxycycline is of limited use in these patients.

Accordingly, donor insemination is generally recommended when no treatable cause of male infertility is found. Additional approaches to the treatment of oligospermic men have focused on methods to treat abnormal sperm in vitro and to prepare an enriched fraction of more nearly normal sperm for intrauterine insemination,[96] gamete intrafallopian transfer,[97] and in-vitro fertilization.[98]

REFERENCES

1. Murphy DR, Torrano EF: Male fertility in 3620 childless couples. *Fertil Steril* 16:337, 1965.
2. Sharpe RM: Paracrine control of the testis. *Clin Endocrinol Metab* 5:185, 1986.
3. Wang C, Baker HWG, Burger HG, DeKretser DM, Hudson B: Hormonal studies in Klinefelter's syndrome. *Clin Endocrinol* 4:399, 1975.
4. Joseph A, Thomas IM: Cytogenetic investigations in 150 cases with complaints of sterility or primary amenorrhea. *Hum Genet* 61:105, 1982.
5. Retief AE: Cytogenetics and recombinant technology in male infertility. *Arch Androl* 17:119, 1986.
6. Lipshultz LI: Cryptorchidism in the subfertile male. *Fertil Steril* 27:609, 1976.
7. Nistal M, Paniagua R: Infertility in adult males with retractile testes. *Fertil Steril* 41:395, 1984.
8. Wolin LH: On the etiology of epididymitis. *J Urol* 105:531, 1971.
9. Lieblich JM, Rogol AD, White BJ, Rosen SW: Syndrome of anosmia with hypogonadotropic hypogonadism (Kallmann's syndrome). *Am J Med* 73:506, 1982.
10. Klingmuller D, Dewes W, Krahe T, Brecht G, Schweikert H-U: Magnetic resonance imaging of the brain in patients with anosmia and hypothalamic hypogonadism (Kallmann's syndrome). *J Clin Endocrinol Metab* 65:581, 1987.
11. Spratt DI, Carr DB, Merriam GR, et al: The spectrum of abnormal patterns of gonadotropin-releasing hormone secretion in men with idiopathic hypogonadotropic hypogonadism: Clinical and laboratory correlations. *J Clin Endocrinol Metab* 64:283, 1987.
12. Shargil AA: Treatment of idiopathic hypogonadotropic hypogonadism in men with luteinizing hormone-releasing hormone: A comparison of treatment with daily injections and with the pulsatile infusion pump. *Fertil Steril* 47:492, 1987.
13. Winters SJ, Troen P: Altered pulsatile secretion of luteinizing hormone in hypogonadal men with hyperprolactinemia. *Clin Endocrinol* 21:257, 1984.
14. Luton JP, Thieblot P, Valcke JC, Mahoudeau JA, Bricaire H: Reversible gonadotropin deficiency in male Cushing's disease. *J Clin Endocrinol Metab* 45:488, 1977.
15. Bonaccorsi AC, Adler I, Figueiredo JG: Male infertility due to congenital adrenal hyperplasia: Testicular biopsy findings, hormonal evaluation, and therapeutic results in three patients. *Fertil Steril* 47:664, 1987.
16. Ojeifo JO, Winters SJ, Troen P: Basal and adrenocorticotropic hormone-stimulated serum 17α-hydroxyprogesterone in men with idiopathic infertility. *Fertil Steril* 42:97, 1984.
17. Griffin JE, Wilson JD: The syndromes of androgen resistance. *N Engl J Med* 302:198, 1980.
18. Morrow AF, Gyorki S, Warne GL, et al: Variable androgen receptor levels in infertile men. *J Clin Endocrinol Metab* 64:1115, 1987.
19. Handelsman DJ: Hypothalamic–pituitary–gonadal dysfunction in renal failure, dialysis and renal transplantation. *Endocrinol Rev* 6:151, 1985.
20. Rojdmark S: Influence of short-term fasting on the pituitary–testicular axis in normal men. *Horm Res* 25:140, 1987.
21. Kussi T, Kostiainen E, Vartiainen E, et al: Acute effects of marathon running on levels of serum lipoproteins and androgenic hormones in healthy males. *Metabolism* 33:527, 1984.
22. Rogol AD, Veldhuis JD, Williams FA, Johnson ML: Pulsatile secretion of gonadotropins and prolactin in male marathon runners. *J Androl* 5:21, 1984.
23. MacConnie SE, Barkan A, Lampman RM, Schork MA, Beitins IZ: Decreased hypothalamic gonadotropin-releasing hormone secretion in male marathon runners. *N Engl J Med* 315:411, 1986.
24. Strauss RH, Lanese RR, Malarkey WB: Weight loss in amateur wrestlers and its effect on serum testosterone levels. *JAMA* 254:3337, 1985.
25. Ayers JWT, Komesu Y, Romani T, Ansbacher R: Anthropomorphic, hormonal and psychologic correlates of semen quality in endurance-trained male athletes. *Fertil Steril* 43:917, 1985.
26. Stanik S, Dornfeld LP, Maxwell MH, Viosca SP, Korenman SG: The effect of weight loss on reproductive hormones in obese men. *J Clin Endocrinol Metab* 53:828, 1981.
27. Kidd GS, Glass AR, Vigersky RA: The hypothalamic–pituitary–testicular axis in thyrotoxicosis. *J Clin Endocrinol Metab* 48:798, 1979.
28. Wortsman J, Rosner W, Dufau ML: Abnormal testicular function in men with primary hypothyroidism. *Am J Med* 82:207, 1987.
29. Davidson JM, Chen JJ, Crapo L, et al: Hormonal changes and sexual function in aging men. *J Clin Endocrinol Metab* 57:71, 1983.
30. Neaves WB, Johnson L, Porter JC, Parker CR Jr, Petty CS: Leydig cell numbers, daily sperm production, and serum gonadotropin levels in aging men. *J Clin Endocrinol Metab* 59:756, 1984.
31. Semple CG, Gray CE, Beastall GH: Male hypogonadism—A non-specific consequence of illness. *Q J Med* 64:601, 1987.
32. Boyden TW, Pamenter RW: Effects of ethanol on the male hypothalmic–pituitary–gonadal axis. *Endocrinol Rev* 4:389, 1983.
33. Kucheria K, Saxena R, Mohan D: Semen analysis in alcohol dependence syndrome. *Andrologia* 17:558, 1985.
34. Van Thiel DH, Gavaler JS, Sanghvi A: Recovery of sexual function in abstinent alcoholic men. *Gastroenterology* 84:677, 1982.
35. Brzek A: Alcohol and male fertility (preliminary report). *Andrologia* 19:32, 1987.
36. Gordon GG, Altman K, Southren AL, Rubin E, Lieber CS: Effect of alcohol (ethanol) administration on sex-hormone metabolism in normal men. *N Engl J Med* 295:793, 1976.
37. Whitehead ED, Leiter E: Genital abnormalities and abnormal semen analyses in male patients exposed to diethylstilbestrol in utero. *J Urol* 125:47, 1981.
38. Schilsky RL, Lewis BJ, Sherins RJ, Young RC: Gonadal dysfunction in patients receiving chemotherapy for cancer. *Ann Intern Med* 93:109, 1980.
39. Brauner, R, Czernichow P, Cramer P, Schaison G, Rappaport R: Leydig cell function in children after direct testicular irradiation for acute lymphoblastic leukemia. *N Engl J Med* 309:25, 1983.
40. Cosentino MJ, Chey WY, Takihara H, Cockett ATK: The effects of sulfasalazine on human male fertility potential and seminal prostaglan-

dins. *J Urol* 132:682, 1984.

41. Loriaux DL, Menard R, Taylor A, Pita JC Jr, Santen R: Spironolactone and endocrine dysfunction. *Ann Intern Med* 85:630, 1976.

42. Sonino N: The use of ketoconazole as inhibitor of steroid production. *N Engl J Med* 317:812, 1987.

43. Winters SJ, Banks JL, Loriaux DL: Cimetidine is an antiandrogen in the rat. *Gastroenterology* 76:504, 1979.

44. Schurmeyer T, Knuth UA, Belkien L, Nieschlag E: Reversible azoospermia induced by the anabolic steroid 19-nortestosterone. *Lancet* 1:417, 1984.

45. Ragni G, DeLauretis L, Gambaro V, et al: Semen evaluation in heroin and methadone addicts. *Acta Eur Fertil* 16:245, 1985.

46. Azizi F, Vagenakis AG, Longcope C, Ingbar SH, Braverman LE: Decreased serum testosterone concentration in male heroin and methadone addicts. *Steroids* 22:467, 1973.

47. Veldhuis JD, Rogol AD, Somojlik E, Ertel NH: Role of endogenous opiates in the expression of negative feedback actions of androgen and estrogen on pulsatile properties of luteinizing hormone secretion in man. *J Clin Invest* 74:47, 1984.

48. Dalterio SL, deRooij DG: Maternal cannabinoid exposure: Effects on spermatogenesis in male offspring. *Int J Androl* 9:250, 1986.

49. Handelsman DJ, Conway AJ, Boylan LM, Turtle JR: Testicular function in potential sperm donors: Effects of smoking and varicocele. *Int J Androl* 7:369, 1984.

50. Schrag SD, Dixon RL: Occupational exposures associated with male reproductive dysfunction. *Annu Rev Pharmacol Toxicol* 25:567, 1985.

51. Jequier AM, Holmes SC: Aetiological factors in the production of obstructive azoospermia. *Br J Urol* 56:540, 1984.

52. Handelsman DJ, Conway AJ, Boylan LM, Turtle JR: Young's syndrome: obstructive azoospermia and chronic sinopulmonary infections. *N Engl J Med* 310:3, 1984.

53. Afzelius BA, Eliasson R: Male and female infertility problems in the immotile-cilia syndrome. *Eur J Respir Dis* 64(suppl 127):144, 1983.

54. McCulloch DK, Campbell IW, Wu FC, Prescott RJ, Clarke BE: The prevalence of diabetic impotence. *Diabetologia* 18:279, 1980.

55. Murray FT, Wyss HU, Thomas RG, Spevack M, Glaros AG: Gonadal dysfunction in diabetic men with organic impotence. *J Clin Endocrinol Metab* 65:127, 1987.

56. Ver Voort SM: Infertility in spinal-cord injured male. *Urology* 29:157, 1987.

57. Hamer PM, Bain J: Ejaculatory incompetence and infertility. *Fertil Steril* 45:384 1986.

58. Nagao RR, Plymate SR, Berger RE, Perin EB, Paulsen CA: Comparison of gonadal function between fertile and infertile men with varicoceles. *Fertil Steril* 46:930, 1986.

59. Nilsson S, Edvinsson A, Nilsson B: Improvement of semen and pregnancy rate after ligation and division of the internal spermatic vein: Fact or fiction? *Br J Urol* 51:591, 1979.

60. Kass EJ, Chandra RS, Belman AB: Testicular histology in the adolescent with varicocele. *Pediatrics* 79:996, 1987.

61. Gump DW, Gibson M, Ashikaga T: Lack of association between genital mycoplasmas and infertility. *N Engl J Med* 310:937, 1984.

62. Berger RE, Smith D, Critchlow CW, et al: Improvement in the sperm penetration (hamster ova) assay (SPA) results after doxycycline treatment of infertile men. *J Androl* 4:126, 1983.

63. Desai S, Cohen MS, Khatamee M, Letier E: *Ureaplasma urealyticum (T. mycoplasma)* infection: Does it have a role in male infertility? *J Urol* 124:469, 1980.

64. Bronson R, Cooper G, Rosenfeld D: Sperm antibodies: Their role in infertility. *Fertil Steril* 42:171, 1984.

65. Fuchs EF, Alexander NJ: Immunologic considerations before and after vasovasostomy. *Fertil Steril* 40:497, 1983.

66. Zorgniotti AW, MacLeod J: Studies in temperature, human semen quality, and varicocele. *Fertil Steril* 24:853, 1973.

67. Zorgniotti AW, Cohen MS, Sealfon AI: Chronic scrotal hypothermia: results in 90 infertile couples. *J Urol* 135:944, 1985.

68. Morrow AF, Baker HW, Burger HG: Different testosterone and LH relationships in infertile men. *J Androl* 7:310, 1986.

69. Gross KM, Matsumoto AM, Southworth MB, Bremner WJ: Evidence for decreased luteinizing hormone-releasing hormone pulse frequency in men with selective elevations of follicle-stimulating hormone. *J Clin Endocrinol Metab* 60:197, 1985.

70. Mozaffarian GA, Higley M, Paulsen CA: Clinical studies in an adult male patient with "isolated follicle stimulating hormone (FSH) deficiency." *J Androl* 4:393, 1983.

71. Wang C, Dahl KD, Leung A, Chan SYW, Hsueh AJW: Serum bioactive follicle-stimulating hormone in men with idiopathic azoospermia and oligospermia. *J Clin Endocrinol Metab* 65:629, 1987.

72. Winters SJ, Troen P: A reexamination of pulsatile luteinizing hormone secretion in primary testicular failure. *J Clin Endocrinol Metab* 57:432, 1983.

73. Booth JD, Merriam GR, Clark RV, Loriaux DL, Sherins RJ: Evidence for Leydig cell dysfunction in infertile men with a selective increase in plasma follicle-stimulating hormone. *J Clin Endocrinol Metab* 64:1194, 1987.

74. Spitz IM, Zylber E, Cohen H, Almaliach U, Leroith D: Impaired prolactin response to thyrotropin-releasing hormone in isolated gonadotropin deficiency and exaggerated response in primary testicular failure. *J Clin Endocrinol Metab* 489:41, 1979.

75. Veldhuis JD, Sowers JR, Rogol AD, et al: Pathophysiology of male hypogonadism associated with endogenous hyperestrogenism: Evidence for dual defects in the gonadal axis. *N Engl J Med* 312:1371, 1985.

76. Winters SJ, Troen P: Evidence for a role of endogenous estrogen in the hypothalamic control of gonadotropin secretion in men. *J Clin Endocrinol Metab* 61:842, 1985.

77. Glass AR: Ketoconazole-induced stimulation of gonadotropin output in men: Basis for a potential test of gonadotropin reserve. *J Clin Endocrinol Metab* 63:1121, 1986.

78. Snyder PJ, Rudenstein RS, Gardner DF, Rothman JG: Repetitive infusion of gonadotropin-releasing hormone distinguishes hypothalamic from pituitary hypogonadism. *J Clin Endocrinol Metab* 48:864, 1979.

79. Santen RJ, Swerdloff RS (eds): *Male Reproductive Dysfunction: Diagnosis and Management of Hypogonadism, Infertility, and Impotence.* New York, Marcel Dekker, 1986.

80. Snyder PJ: Clinical use of androgens. *Annu Rev Med* 35:207, 1984.

81. Winters SJ, Troen P: Hypogonacotropic hypogonadism: Gonadotropin therapy, in Krieger DT, Bardin CW, Decker BC (eds): *Current Therapy in Endocrinology and Metabolism.* Toronto, BC Decker, 1985, pp 152–154.

82. Finkel DM, Phillips JL, Snyder PJ: Stimulation of spermatogenesis by gonadotropins in men with hypogonadotropic hypogonadism. *N Engl J Med* 313:651, 1985.

83. Nielsen CT, Skakkebaek NE, Richardson DW, et al: Onset of the release of spermatozoa (spermarche) in boys in relation to age, testicular growth, pubic hair and height. *J Clin Endocrinol Metab* 62:532, 1986.

84. Spratt DI, Findelstein JS, O'Dea LS, et al: Long-term administration of gonadotropin-releasing hormone in men with idiopathic hypogonadotropic hypogonadism. *Ann Intern Med* 105:848, 1986.

85. White RI Jr, Kaufman SL, Barth KH, et al: Occlusion of variococeles with detatchable balloons. *Radiology* 139:327, 1981.

86. Collins JA, Wrixon W, Janes LB, Wilson EH: Treatment-independent pregnancy among infertile couples. *N Engl J Med* 309:1201, 1983.

87. Vigersky RA, Glass AR: Effects of delta-1 testolactone on the pituitary–testicular axis in oligospermic men. *J Clin Endocrinol Metab* 52:897, 1981.

88. Clark RV, Sherins RJ: Clinical trail of testolactone for treatment of idiopathic male infertility (abstr). *J Androl* 4:31, 1983.

89. AinMelk Y, Belisle S, Carmel M, Jean-Pierre T: Tamoxifen citrate therapy in male infertility. *Fertil Steril* 48:113, 1987.

90. Paulson DF, Wacksman J, Hammond CB, Wiebe HR: Hypofertility and clomiphene citrate therapy. *Fertil Steril* 26:982, 1975.

91. Newton R, Schinfeld JS, Schiff I: Clomiphene treatment of infertile men: Failure of response with idiopathic oligospermia. *Fertil Steril* 34:399, 1980.

92. Ronnberg L: The effect of clomiphene citrate on different sperm parameters and serum hormone levels in preselected infertile men: A controlled double-blind cross-over study. *Int J Androl* 3:479, 1980.

93. Hendry WF, Treehuba K, Hughes L, et al: Cyclic prednisolone therapy for male infertility associated with autoantibodies to spermatozoa. *Fertil Steril* 45:249, 1986.

94. Hass GG Jr, Manganiello P: A double-blind, placebo-controlled study of the use of methylprednisone in infertile men with sperm-associated immunoglobulins. *Fertil Steril* 47:295, 1987.

95. Comhaire FH, Rowe PJ, Farley TMM: The effect of doxycycline in infertile couples with male accessory gland infection: A double-blind prospective study. *Int J Androl* 9:91, 1986.

96. Allen NA, Herbert CM, Maxson WS, et al: Intrauterine insemination: A critical review. *Fertil Steril* 44:569, 1985.

97. Asch RA, Balmaceda JP, Ellsworth LR, Wong PC: Preliminary experience with gamete intrafallopian transfer (GIFT). *Fertil Steril* 45:366, 1986.

98. Yovich J, Stonger J, Yovich J: The management of oligospermic infertility by in vitro fertilization. *Ann NY Acad Sci* 442:276, 1985.

CHAPTER 12

Surgical Management of Male Infertility

Sherman J. Silber

Surgical Management of Male Infertility

Diagnosis and Treatment of Obstructive Azoospermia	Ejaculatory Duct Obstruction
Vasectomy Reversal	Congenital Absence of Vas Deferens
Microsurgical Vasoepididymostomy	**Microsurgery for Undescended Testicle**
Evaluation of Obstruction Not Caused by Vasectomy	Rationale for Testicle Autotransplantation
Inguinal Disruption of Vas Deferens After Herniorrhaphy	Microsurgical Techniques
	Conclusions

DIAGNOSIS AND TREATMENT OF OBSTRUCTIVE AZOOSPERMIA

Vasectomy Reversal

Vasectomy is the most common cause of obstructive azoospermia. There are three major aspects to vasectomy reversal. The first concerns techniques for obtaining a reliable reanastomosis of the vas deferens. With modern microsurgery, accurate reanastomosis should be achievable in almost every case. The second aspect relates to the detrimental secondary effects of vasectomy, such as pressure-induced epididymal damage as a secondary result of vasectomy. The third aspect concerns microsurgically bypassing this secondary epididymal obstruction.

Microsurgical Approach. It is advisable to practice in animals before doing such surgery on humans.[1–12] For the best mucosal approximation in the human where lumina are of different diameter (because of chronic obstruction and increased pressure), I recommend a nonsplinted, two-layer approach (Fig. 12–1). A one-layer anastomosis provides poorer mucosal approximation when lumen diameters differ. A splint of any kind should never be used, and is only an

excuse for not being certain one has obtained a good anastomosis. It results in sperm leakage, inflammation, and more scarring.

It is not necessary to determine preoperatively what type of vasectomy was performed. Often a very large segment has been removed, and in the majority of cases that we have come across, the vasectomy has extended well into the convoluted portion. Such cases would have been considered impossible to correct with conventional techniques. With microsurgical techniques, they merely require a little more dissection, but essentially no change from a standard routine.

The preparation of the two ends of the vas deferens microscopic anastomosis is best performed with X 2½ loupe magnification. The healthy ends above and below the fibrosis are freed up several centimeters, and often more than that if a large gap has to be bridged. The more one frees up healthy tissue from surrounding attachments, the more easily the two ends will bridge any gap between them. As it is critical to have a tension-free anastomosis, no effort at anastomosis should be made until the ends above and below the obstruction have been adequately freed up. One generally need not fear devascularizing the vas deferens. The blood supply around the

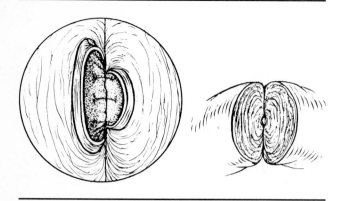

Figure 12–1. Diagrammatic representation of inner mucosal anastomosis of the small lumen on the abdominal side of the vas to the dilated lumen on the testicular side of the vasectomy site.

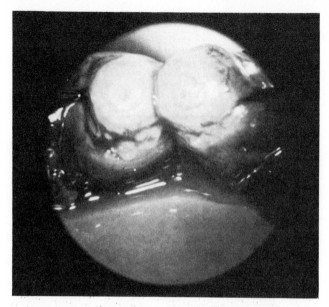

Figure 12–2. Luminal disparity before vas reanastomosis.

outer muscularis is quite extensive, and, contrary to conventional thinking, we have found that freeing the vas a good distance does nothing to injure the blood supply.

A microscope is necessary to make the operation easier and more accurate. Loupes can at best provide X 2½ to 4 magnification; to visualize the inner lumen of the vas deferens for easy and accurate placement of stitches requires 16 X magnification. Other advantages of the microscope are that the depth of focus is much clearer, the light is constantly supplied directly to the subject, and the instrument rests on a stand and thus is immobile. The operator can move his or her head or neck from time to time without in any way disturbing the steadiness of the view of the subject.

The fibrotic portion of the vas deferens is excised under the microscope until healthy lumen is reached. The testicular side lumen is generally noted to be dilated because of chronic high-pressure obstruction (Fig. 12–2). The abdominal side lumen will be extremely tiny by comparison. A tiny microcatheter is placed in the dilated end of the lumen on the testicular side of the vasectomy site, allowing sperm fluid to enter capillary action. This fluid is examined under a laboratory microscope for the presence or absence and characterization of sperm.

The information gained by microscopic characterization of sperm in the vas fluid allows extremely accurate prediction of success or failure after a properly performed vasovasostomy, and establishes the likelihood of secondary epididymal blockage. It is best not just to smear a slide on the cut end of the vas to obtain the fluid, as the specimen may dry quickly and give an inaccurate impression of the sperm content within the length of the obstructed side. If the fluid is very concentrated and mediocre microscope is used to examine the specimen, it is very easy to mistake densely packed, nonmotile sperm for

debris. The motility of sperm in the obstructed segment has no bearing on prognosis.

The inner mucosal anastomosis is performed under 16 to 25 X magnification. The object is to obtain as flawless as possible a mucosa-to-mucosa alignment despite the discrepancy in lumen diameter (Fig. 12–3). The surgeon places the first mucosal suture anteriorly, making sure that it includes the elastic layer directly next to the mucosa. By excluding as much muscularis as possible from this bite, a more precise approximation can be obtained. The suture is pulled through separately and then placed into the mucosa of the testicular side lumen. It is then pulled through, an instrument tie is performed, and the suture is cut. I recommend 10-0 nylon on a fine taper-cut needle (Sharpoint-Silber needle) for the inner mucosa.

After the first three mucosal sutures are placed anteriorly in such a fashion, the entire vasovasostomy clamp is rotated around 180 degrees, and what was the posterior wall of the vas is now in the anterior position. At this point it is easy to view the anterior row of sutures from the inside and inspect to see whether perfect mucosal alignment has been achieved. If large bites of muscle were included in these sutures, the edges do not come together properly and a muscle bridge is created between them. There should be no tearing or inaccuracy in the line-up of the mucosal margins. Finally, the outer muscularis is sutured separately. For the outer layer I recommend 9-0 nylon on a tougher taper-cut needle (Ethicon V-100-4).

Results. Semen analysis is obtained every month for the first 4 months, then at 8 months, 1 year, 1.5 years,

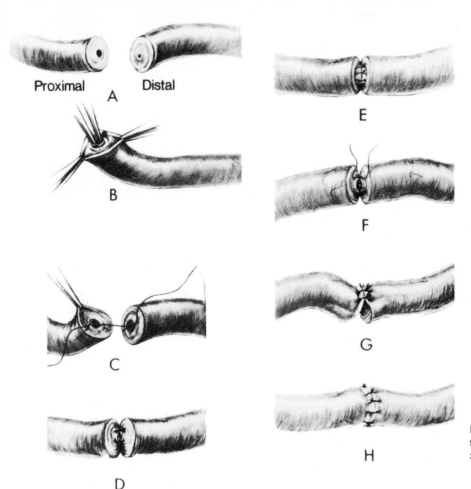

Figure 12–3. Steps of the microscopic two-layer vasal anastomosis. (From Silber.[13] Reproduced with permission.)

and 2 years postoperatively. The sperm count and quality tend to improve gradually with time. If the anastomosis is poor, however, the count may increase at first, but then eventually reduces to oligospermia or aspermia. If the patient is azoospermic 3 months or more after vasovasostomy, either the vas anastomosis or the epididymis is obstructed.

For patients who remain azoospermic, the interpretation of where the problem lies depends strictly upon the quality of sperm that was present in the vas fluid at the time of vasovasostomy. This findings indicates whether there is continuity in the epididymis (with fresh sperm continuing to come through and reach the vasectomy site), or whether a blockage in the epididymis prevents sperm from reaching the vas. If numerous long-tailed sperm are present in the fluid, the epididymal tubule is intact and the vasovasostomy should be successful.

From 1975 to 1978, over 400 patients subjected to this technique for vasovasostomy were carefully studied both preoperatively and postoperatively in an effort to determine the factors that affect recovery of fertility.[1] The overall pregnancy rate after 1.5 years of follow-up on the first 42 unselected patients was 71%. Five-year follow-up yielded an 82% pregnancy

rate. (The causes for the failures will become apparent below.) We now have performed over 1,800 such procedures, and results are similar throughout our long series. Very few women become pregnant before 6 months, and most do so between 8 and 16 months. An accurate assessment of pregnancy rate is not possible before a series has been followed for 3 years. Although some patients achieve normal sperm counts within the first month and impregnate their partners immediately, this is certainly the exception.

Most of the confusion in the literature on vasovasostomy stems from the lack of documentation of preoperative sperm quality in the vas fluid, inadequate postoperative semen analyses, sparse observations of the epididymal ductal system, and poor testis biopsy studies in vasectomized men. The group on whom we operated was studied carefully. Seminal fluid was sampled from the testicular side of the obstructed vas for each patient at the time of reanastomosis. The age of the patient, time since vasectomy, type of vasectomy, and area in which it was performed, were correlated to subsequent sperm count and pregnancy of the partner. Sperm counts were measured at monthly intervals after surgery for the first 4 months and then at intervals 4 months apart during the entire follow-up period. No patient was accepted for surgery who did not agree in advance to conform to this careful follow-up. The degree of dilatation of the vas lumen on the testicular side of the vasectomy site was measured in all patients. Appearance and quantity of vas fluid, as well as sperm morphology (electron and light microscopy), quantity, and motility were also recorded and correlated with postoperative results.

Sperm counts were arbitrarily considered as normal when there was a concentration of more than 10 million sperm/mL, 50% motility with good progression, and greater than 70% normal forms, according to the criteria of MacLeod and Gold.[14] It is recognized that lower sperm counts can be found in fertile men and higher counts in infertile men. The count does not have a dramatic effect on pregnancy rate unless it is below 10 million/cc. Even then, the distribution of sperm counts in patients with a patent vas postoperatively is not significantly different from that in control populations of fertile men.

A quantitatively meticulous testicle biopsy was performed in over 300 patients at the time of vasovasostomy and the findings were correlated with successful and unsuccessful postoperative results.[15] This was particularly important when there was no sperm in the vas fluid, and the patient remained azoospermic postoperatively despite a perfect anastomosis.

With this kind of careful investigation in patients subjected to as meticulous a microsurgical anastomosis as possible, physiologic data of greater reliability were obtainable. These data have led us to conclude that spermatogenesis is not significantly harmed by obstruction, and that failure to achieve fertility after an accurate vasovasostomy is caused by dilatation and then perforation of the epididymal duct with subsequent secondary epididymal obstruction.

We noted that the quality of sperm in the vas fluid appeared to be improved in patients who had minimal dilation of the testicular side lumen and in those who had a sperm granuloma at the site of the vasectomy. Fifty-nine (32%) of the first 184 vasa examined had an obvious sperm granuloma noted at the site of vasectomy. That is a much higher frequency than we have seen subsequently. This change is probably due to the increasing use of cautery for sealing the vas more effectively at the time of vasectomy. There were no particular symptoms of discomfort related to the sperm granuloma. The granuloma represented a continual leakage of sperm fluid at the vasectomy site (Fig. 12–4).

All of the men with sperm granuloma had abundant, morphologically normal sperm in the vas fluid. Even when the vasectomy had been performed over 10 years earlier, none had poor-quality sperm. The presence of a sperm granuloma assured a high quality of sperm in the vas fluid at the time of vasovasostomy.

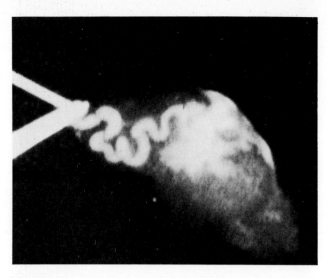

Figure 12–4. Vasogram of a sperm granuloma at the vasectomy site demonstrates continual sperm leakage into numerous diffuse channels from which seminal fluid can be reabsorbed.

The internal diameter of the testicular side lumen of the vas deferens was almost always 0.75 mm or less in vasa with sperm granuloma. In patients without sperm granuloma, it was usually 1 mm or greater. Thus, the presence of sperm granuloma was associated with less dilation of the vas on the testicular side of the obstruction. In addition, in patients who had unilateral granulomas, the sperm quality was always satisfactory on the side with the granuloma but was usually of poorer quality on the opposite side.

These data favored the postulate that failure to recover fertility after an accurate anatomic reconnection of the vas deferens is due to the local effects of high pressure created by the vasectomy. The presence of a sperm granuloma at the vasectomy site represents persistent and continual leakage of sperm, which alleviates the deleterious high intravasal and epididymal pressure that otherwise always occurs after vasectomy.

Effects of Vasectomy on the Testis and Epididymis. Despite the fact that vasectomy is one of the most frequently performed operations in the United States, a great deal of controversy has been generated in the scientific literature about its effects in humans.

Previous animal studies indicated that pressure changes induced by vasectomy could affect subsequent restoration of fertility even after accurate vas reanastomosis. If the problem was secondary ductal obstruction caused by rupture and sperm extravasation in the epididymis, more sophisticated microsurgery could restore fertility even in the least favorable cases. Although a clearly substantial pressure increase occurs in the epididymis after vasectomy, we found no discernible effect on spermatogenesis or

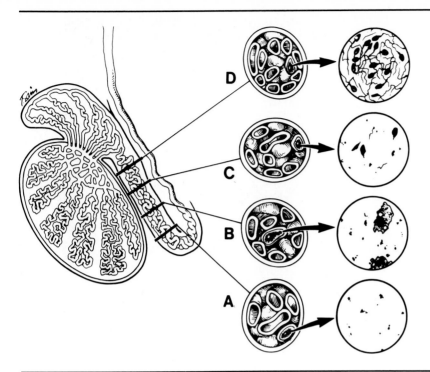

Figure 12–5. Stepwise transection of the epididymis, distal to proximal, in the course of determining the site of obstruction. **A.** No sperm or cells are seen in the epididymal fluid. **B.** Macrophages are visible, signifying that at least one site of epididymal perforation is near. **C.** Some sperm heads and debris are seen. **D.** The areas of obstruction are passed, as indicated by the multiplicity of normal sperm. Histologic sections between points C and D demonstrate epididymal inflammation, interstitial sperm granuloma, and tubular obstruction. (From Silber.[13] Reproduced with permission.)

testicular architecture. Since the testicle biopsy showed normal spermatogenesis in all patients who had no sperm in the vas fluid, we felt the problem had to be in the epididymis.

To resolve this matter, we explored patients who had azoospermia for at least 2 years after a patent vasovasostomy.[16] These patients, of course, had no sperm (or only sperm heads) in the vas fluid at the time of vasovasostomy. In 33 of the 39 such cases first explored, normal sperm were found in the epididymal fluid of the corpus epididymis despite absence of sperm in the vas fluid (Fig. 12–5). Epididymal histology distal to this site revealed extensive interstitial sperm granulomas resulting from rupture of the epididymal duct, similar to what Bedford observed in four other species.[17]

Once the epididymal rupture and subsequent blockage occur, the fluid that previously accumulated in the vas deferens is trapped there and isolated. The sperm in the fluid then eventually degenerate, the tails fall off, and then the heads finally degenerate into amorphous debris (Fig. 12–6). Thus the absence of sperm in the fluid just proximal to the vasectomy site indicates secondary epididymal blockage from epididymal ruptures caused by the pressure buildup that occurs after vasectomy. That is why the most accurate vasovasostomy cannot result in success if no sperm are present in the vas fluid. To treat such cases successfully requires bypassing the secondary blockage in the epididymis.[16,18–21]

The duration of time since vasectomy correlates with the likelihood of pressure-induced rupture of the epididymis in these patients, just as it did in

laboratory animal studies.[17] In humans, however, the time range is considerably expanded. Whenever reversal was performed within 1 year of vasectomy, high-quality sperm were always found in the vas fluid, and normal semen analyses were obtained after surgery.

There was no sudden period after which a blow-out could always be found. The risk of epididymal blow-out on each side gradually increased as an independent variable as the years progressed. The chances of finding no sperm in the vas fluid on either side at 10 years was 75%; the chances of finding no sperm on both sides at 10 years was about 50%. At 5 years after vasectomy, the chances of finding no sperm on one side was 25%, but the chances of finding no sperm on both sides was only 6%. In every patient in whom no sperm was found in the vas fluid, the testicle biopsy was normal. The absence of sperm was not caused by a disruption of spermatogenesis, but rather by epididymal ruptures and secondary blockage.

Patients who persist in having azoospermia or oligospermia and poor motility more than 1 year after vasovasostomy usually are found to have complete or partial blockage either at the vasovasostomy site or in the epididymis. Although this is usually clinically quite obvious, we developed a simplified quantitative testicle biopsy for cases that are uncertain.[15]

Quantitative Interpretation of Testicle Biopsy.
Testicle biopsy has been used by most clinicians in a nonquantitative fashion only. This has severely limited its usefulness and has led to many errors in its

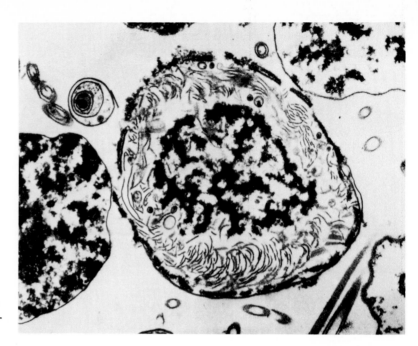

Figure 12–6. Degenerated sperm head in the vas fluid that, on light microscopy, showed only debris. (From Silber.[13] Reproduced with permission.)

interpretation.[22-25] A simplified quantitative evaluation of the testicle biopsy is very helpful for assessing male fertility. It is based on the normal histology and kinetics of spermatogenesis in the human.[26] Using radioactive tracers, it was determined that the rate of spermatogenesis in humans, or in any species, is constant, even when sperm production is reduced. Reduced production is always caused by lower numbers of sperm "on the assembly line," not diminished speed of production. Therefore the quantity of sperm being produced by the testicle at any given time is reflected by the testicle biopsy.

Using this principle, a method of quantitative interpretation of the testicle biopsy was developed.[27,28] Initial applications of the technique involved a small number of patients, and were limited to making a precise correlation with sperm count. Furthermore, the technique was elaborate and time consuming. In 1978 these same investigators counted all components of spermatogenesis and found a good correlation with sperm count.[29] The difficulty remained, however, that the method was time consuming, and very few fertility specialists had any inclination to put that much effort into photographing and analyzing every biopsy.

A simple method is available that can be performed in 10 to 15 minutes. Testicle biopsies of patients with both oligospermia and normal sperm counts were analyzed and found to be predictive of mean sperm count. Furthermore, comparing the results of quantitative testicle biopsy with the sperm count could document whether oligospermia was caused by a partially obstructed anastomosis or poor sperm transport, as opposed to simply deficient spermatogenesis.

Patients who are severely oligospermic after structured vasovasostomy become fertile after a microsurgical reanastomosis. Thus we know that obstruction in the ductal system can cause oligospermia and poor motility. In fact, most cases of poor sperm motility and low sperm count after vasectomy reversal have been found to be due to obstruction. When a patient's prior fertility is not known, or when documentation is necessary before embarking on a questionable case, a testicle biopsy should clarify whether or not blockage, or just poor spermatogenesis, is causing the poor semen quality.

The biopsy is performed with a careful "no touch" atraumatic technique under general anesthesia. The tunica albuginea is sharply incised with a scalpel. The protruding seminiferous tubules are excised with a wet, extremely sharp, microiris scissor, and then allowed to fall into Zenker's solution without being handled. Specimens are carefully fixed, cut in thin sections, and stained with hematoxylin and eosin. The technique of biopsy is important. If the specimen is handled roughly or fixed in formalin, it is difficult accurately to identify the cellular components of the seminiferous tubule.

The testicle biopsy is performed bilaterally and at least 10 seminiferous tubules are included in the count on each side. Only the mature spermatids (stages I, II, V, and VI) need be counted (Fig. 12–7); that is, the oval-shaped cells with dark, densely stained chromatin. Previous studies have shown that these cells have the greatest correlation with sperm count and are the easiest ones to recognize. All of the steps of spermatogenesis from spermatogonia though resting, leptotene, zygotene, and pachytene spermatocytes, and early spermatids, are excluded

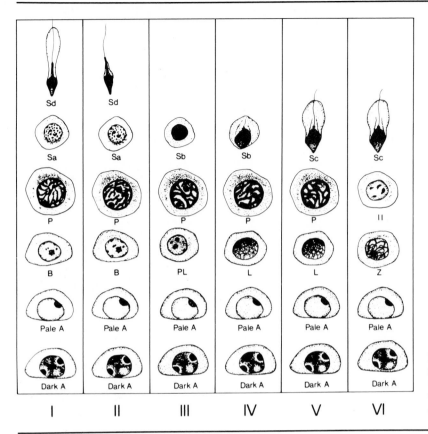

Figure 12–7. Six stages of human spermatogenesis. Mature spermatids are seen only in stages I, II, V, and VI. Note that they are the easiest cells to identify, and require very little time for quantification.

from consideration. The number of mature spermatids in a minimum of 20 tubules is summed and divided by the number of tubules.

Patients without obstruction with fewer than 10 million sperm/cc always have fewer than 20 mature spermatids per tubule. Those with over 20 million sperm/cc usually have greater than 20 mature spermatids per tubule. The number correlates very closely to the sperm count.

Using an expoential curve (Fig. 12–8), the number of mature spermatids per tubule can be used to predict the anticipated sperm count. In the absence of obstruction the correlation is remarkably close. For example, if the patient has 40 mature spermatids per tubule, the sperm count should be just under 60 million/cc; if there are 45 mature spermatids, the sperm count should be just over 85 million. The patient with a sperm count of only 3 million would be expected to have only 6 to 10 mature spermatids per tubule.

The postoperative sperm count of patients who undergo microscopic vasovasostomy or vasoepididymostomy correlates with their quantitative testicle biopsy. A constantly low count is usually caused by continuing obstruction. This can be determined objectively by comparing the mature spermatid count in the testicle biopsy to the sperm count in the semen.

For example, if the patient is simply not manufacturing many sperm, his count could be low without continuing obstruction. The semen usually have adequate motility because the low count does not reflect pathology, but rather a low rate of production.

Quantitative testicle biopsy can allow a firm diagnosis of obstruction prior to scrotal exploration that could otherwise require a great deal of guesswork as to the presence of epididymal blockage. In addition, it ensures that unwarranted medical therapy will not be haphazardly administered to patients who have obstruction.

Frequently patients undergo vasoepididymostomy inappropriately because the pathology report indicates normal spermatogenesis. The readings often are not quantitative, but rather qualitative impressions that tubules are filled with spermatocytes and some mature sperm. This has led to vasoepididymostomy in many men who do not have obstruction. If the biopsy shows thick tubules with large numbers of spermatocytes but only two or three mature spermatids per tubule, obstruction is not the cause of the patient's "azoospermia."

Some clinicians have attempted to use the serum follicle-stimulating hormone (FSH) level to monitor the amount of spermatogenesis: an elevated level in an azoospermic patient would supposedly indicate

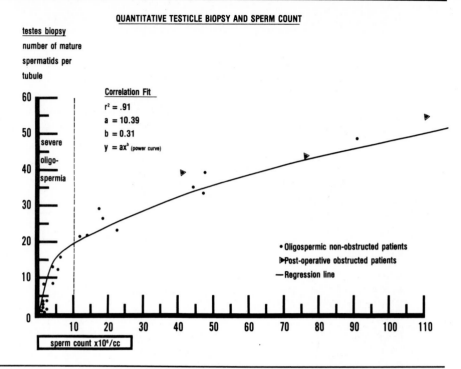

Figure 12–8. Graph demonstrates the relationship between the total number of mature spermatids per tubule on testis biopsy and the actual sperm count per cubic centimeter. This is an exponential relationship, as one would expect, as the testicle biopsy is two-dimensional. The sperm count relates to a volumetric function of the testicle. (From Silber and Rodriguez-Rigau.[15] Reproduced with permission.)

obstruction. Unfortunately, the correlation is very poor.[30] Patients with maturation arrest causing azoospermia have a normal FSH level. The level correlates most closely with the total number of spermatogonia and with the testicular volume, but not with the number of mature sperm. The feedback mechanism is not tuned finely enough for the serum

FSH level to reflect what the sperm count should be (B. Setchel, personal communication, 1980).

Ironically, it is the scattered mosaic arrangement of the various stages of spermatogenesis in the human seminiferous tubule (as opposed to the orderly wave moving across the tubule in most other species) that makes quantifying the human testicular

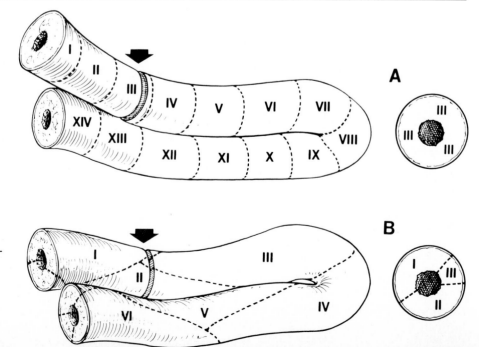

Figure 12–9. A. In most animals, spermatogenesis proceeds in an orderly wave across the seminiferous tubule from one stage to another. **B.** In humans, spermatogenesis has a mosaic, scattered arrangement that does not proceed in an orderly wave. (From Silber.[13] Reproduced with permission.)

formed by many urologists.[35] Although it was the best that could be performed in the 1950s, modern microsurgical facilities have rendered it obsolete, and these patients can now be given a much better prognosis with extremely extracting microsurgical procedures.

The microsurgical specific-tubule technique for vasoepididymostomy was described in 1978.[18-21] After the scrotal sac is entered, the tunica vaginalis is opened and the testis and epididymis are everted from the hydrocele sac. The dilated epididymal tubule is usually about 0.1 to 0.2 mm in diameter. The epididymal duct is extraordinarily delicate, with a wall thickness of about 30 μm. The conventional approach, in which a deep longitudinal incision is made into the outer epididymal tunic, reveals what looks like as many as 20 or 30 tiny tubules (Fig. 12–11). Without the benefit of microscopic observation, there is an illusion that sperm fluid is welling up from all of these tubules, but in truth the fluid is coming from only one of them. The other tubules are just blind loops disconnected from continuity with the testis by this incision. The ideal approach for reestablishing continuity of the ductal system is to

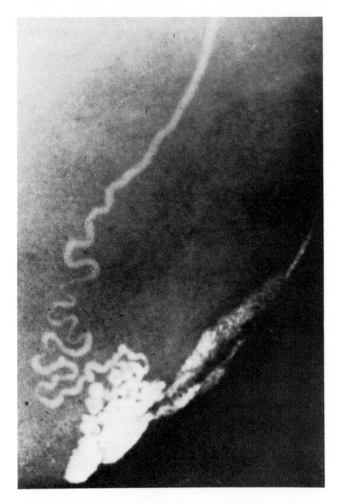

Figure 12–10. Retrograde vasogram of the vas deferens and epididymis shows that the epididymis is simply one long, intricately coiled tube that is continuous with the convoluted region of the vas.

biopsy so simple. In rats a cut through any particular seminiferous tubule shows only one particular stages (Fig. 12–9a). In humans, a cut through any area of the testicle reveals a scattered array of all the various stages of spermatogenesis (Fig. 12–9b). Thus, in humans it requires only 20 tubules for a good statistical sample of the total range of spermatogenesis in the entire testicle.

Microsurgical Vasoepididymostomy

Technique. The epididymis is a single, 20-foot-long, coiled tube with myriad intricate convolutions (Fig. 12–10). It is squeezed into 2-inch length like the pleats of an accordian. Because it is so tiny, even by microsurgical standards, the results with conventional surgery in repairing obstruction have been very poor.[31-34] The procedure used by Hanley and described by Hotchkiss formed the basis for the usual conventional vasoepididymostomy that is still per-

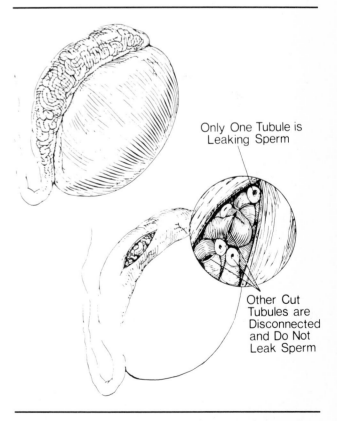

Only One Tubule is Leaking Sperm

Other Cut Tubules are Disconnected and Do Not Leak Sperm

Figure 12–11. In the first stage of a conventional approach to vasoepididymostomy the longitudinal slit is made in the tunic of the epididymis, with one epididymal tubule cut in so many different places that it looks like many cut tubules. Only one of those tubules is leaking sperm. (From Silber.[13] Reproduced with permission.)

anastomose (end-to-end) the inner lumen of the vas deferens specifically to the one epididymal tubule.

Originally, rather than making a conventional longitudinal incision, a *transverse* transection of the epididymis was made at the most distal point; that is, at the junction of the cauda and corpus epididymis (Fig. 12–12). With this approach one could slice off portions of the epididymis more and more proximally until sperm were recovered at the most distal possible level but proximal to the area of obstruction. I no longer transect the entire epididymis, and prefer a simpler, specific tubule approach that avoids epididymal dissection.

Under the operating microscope, 3 to 10 cut tubules are usually visible on the transected surface of the epididymis, and all are carefully examined for the efflux of sperm fluid. This cut surface of the epididymis is smeared on a slide, which is observed under a standard laboratory microscope or phase contrast microscope for the presence and quality of sperm as described above. Sometimes no fluid at all is observed, in which case transection must be continued proximally. The presence of fluid does not necessarily mean the presence of sperm, however. One must wait for the report on the fluid before

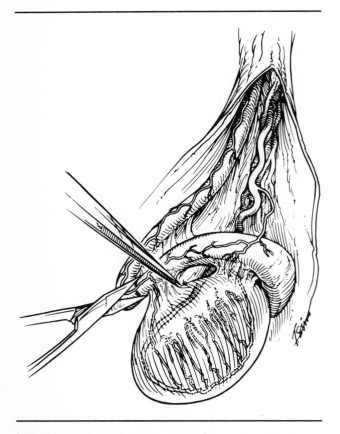

Figure 12–12. The epididymis is freed up without damaging the blood supply in preparation for a transverse sectioning before a specific tubule-to-tubule vasoepididymostomy. (From Silber.[13] Reproduced with permission.)

deciding whether to do the anastomosis at that point or to transect more proximally. The anastomosis is performed at the distal-most level where normal sperm are found in the epididymal fluid. This allows for the maximum possible length of epididymis.

The original technique is carried out as follows. For the first stitch the epididymis is held between the thumb and the forefinger, facing the microscope. A slight milking action may sometimes be necessary to promote a continual efflux of fluid in order to continue to see which is the correct tubule to anastomose. A 10-0 monofilament nylon on a V-75 taper-cut 75-μm needle is used for the inner layer, and a 9-0 nylon on V-100 vas cutting needle is used for the outer layer. The first suture is placed from the outside to the inside of the specific epididymal tubule that is leaking sperm fluid. Once the suture is placed, the epididymis is put into one jaw of the Silber vasovasostomy clamp and the vas is inserted into the other jaw. A blue piece of plastic is then placed underneath the epididymis and vas, which are held in the two jaws of the vasovasostomy clamp. From this point on, the anastomosis of the vas lumen to the epididymal tubule can be performed in a fashion somewhat similar to vasovasostomy (Figs. 12–13 and 12–14).

The first stitch is placed in the clamp before the epididymis because it is extremely difficult to locate the specific tubule leaking the fluid in any other way. The gentle milking action that the thumb and forefinger can provide is helpful in making sure that the fluid is continuing to flow from the tubule that is selected to suture. After the first suture is placed, the tubule is easily identified at all times.

An alternative technique, which yields equal results, is to open up the outer tunic and make a tiny cut into the epididymal tubule. The posterior muscle layer of the vas is then sutured to the posterior epididymal tunic. Subsequently, the inner mucosa of the vas is sutured end-to-side to the opening on the epididymal tubule.

Fertility After Vasoepididymostomy. What can be expected of sperm that have not progressed completely through the epididymis? It is well known that sperm from the cauda epididymis are mature and quite capable of fertilizing the ovum; however, it was formerly thought that a large percentage of sperm from the corpus epididymis were incapable of fertilization. Studies in animals revealed that sperm obtained from the head of the epididymis could not achieve maturity or directional motility, and thus could not achieve fertilization. We now know differently.

In the human, sperm from anywhere along the corpus epididymis that pass into the vas deferens and into the ejaculate can fertilize an ovum. If the anas-

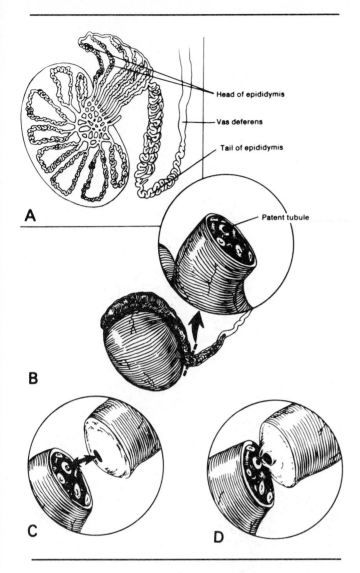

A

B

C   **D**

Head of epididymis

Vas deferens

Tail of epididymis

Patent tubule

Figure 12–13. Diagram of the specific tubule technique for vasoepididymostomy first described in 1978. (From Silber.[13] Reproduced with permission.)

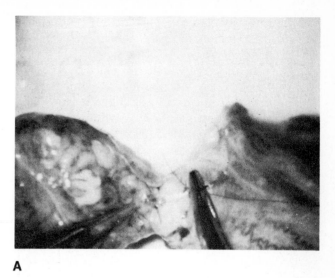

A

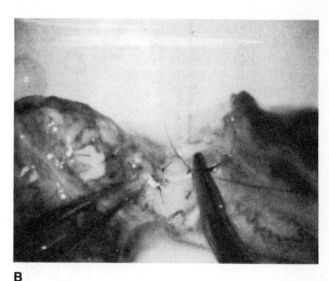

B

Figure 12–14. The final sutures are placed for an anastomosis of the vas lumen to the specific epididymal tubule. (From Silber.[13] Reproduced with permission.)

tomosis is successful anywhere within the corpus epididymis, pregnancy occurs in 73% of cases.[36–38] The prognosis is not as good when anastomosis is performed in the head of the epididymis in order to bypass the obstruction. Among such patients, we have attained pregnancy in 43%. Pregnancy has even resulted in several cases where the anastomosis had to be performed to the vasa efferentia, meaning the sperm never transited through any portion of the epididymis.

All of the animal data on sperm maturity in the epididymis come from studies in which sperm were sampled from an otherwise functioning epididymis that was intact along its entire length. The question of how well remaining segments of epididymal tubule and vas deferens would be able to promote sperm maturation in the physiologic context of vasoepididy-

mostomy could not be answered by any of the animal experiments that form the basis of our understanding of epididymal function.

For example, in the rabbit, spermatozoa were sampled from the seminiferous tubules, the ductuli efferentes, and various levels of the epididymis to determine their intrinsic motility and fertilizing capability.[39] Spermatozoa from the seminiferous tubules and ductuli efferentes showed only weak vibratory movements with no forward progress. Spermatozoa from the proximal head of the epididymis showed very irregular, erratic motility with no forward progression. Traversing the corpus epididymis, however, increasing numbers of spermatozoa began to show forward movement with proper longitudinal rotation as they progressed distally toward the cauda epididymis. Similar studies in the rabbit have been performed by others.[40,41]

In an effort to see whether or not the increase in maturity was merely a function of the time required for sperm to pass through the epididymis, or whether it was dependent on specific areas of the epididymis, various authors ligated different portions of the epididymis in rabbits and examined samples of the spermatozoa from each portion at intervals.[42-44] After interruption of sperm flow, epididymal spermatozoa that had been poorly motile in the caput region of the epididymis showed increased motility. Because of the pathologic nature of the chronic obstruction created by such an experimental model, however, all of these sperm once again lost their motility by 3 weeks. These researchers believed that it was possible for spermatozoa to mature at any level of the epididymal duct, but their experimental approach created such an abnormal environment that this hypothesis could not be tested adequately. Obstruction to the flow of spermatozoa within the epididymis has been shown clearly to result in stagnation of epididymal spermatozoa. Thus the increased time allowed for maturation in the experiment was counterbalanced by the abnormal obstructed environment.

Orgebin-Crist[45] first suggested that in humans, it was theoretically possible that sperm might be mature and be fertile after vasoepididymostomy even to proximal portions of the epididymis. The remaining epididymal tubule might undergo compensatory changes, or spermatozoa might have more time to mature after coming out of proximal regions of the epididymis than they would in the previously alluded to experimental models. Our results in humans with vasoepididymostomy for proximal epididymal obstruction indicate that sperm do not necessarily have to transit all or even part of the epididymis to mature sufficiently for fertilization. They only require sufficient time to mature and this can occur in the vas deferens as well as the epididymis. Yet it is clear nonetheless that the pregnancy rate is higher with corpus epididymis anastomosis than with caput anastomosis.

In most patients undergoing vasoepididymostomy, the most proximal obstruction is somewhat in the corpus region. We have seen no significant difference in pregnancy rates at any particular point along the corpus epididymis. In 78% of patients treated with this technique, a semen analysis reveals a sperm count of greater than 10 million/cc and adequate directional motility. About 60% of these patients impregnate their partners within 2 to 3 years. It is too early to know what the eventual pregnancy rate will be because it does seem that fertilizing capacity per monthly cycle of sexual exposure is somewhat less in these patients than the healthy population. Thus, it will take 5 years of follow-up before it can be stated with assurance how high the pregnancy rate will eventually be. Our impression, however, is that the results with vasoepididymostomy will parallel those with vasovasostomy.

Evaluation of Obstruction not Caused by Vasectomy

The diagnosis of obstruction should really be quite simple; however, it is sometimes approached in a confusing way that can lead to embarrassing situations, such as attempting to do a vasoepididymostomy on a patient who has no obstruction. Adherence to a few simple principles will avoid these difficulties and allow a proper preoperative decision to be made.

If a patient has a testicle biopsy that shows normal spermatogenesis, and if he is azoospermic, his infertility must be caused by obstruction. Everything else is superfluous. If in addition to these two criteria he also has a palpable vas deferens on physical examination, he is a candidate for surgical exploration and probable vasoepididymostomy. All other data are irrelevant.

Low semen volume (< 1.0 cc) may be due to ejaculatory duct obstruction. It can be managed by transurethral resection after vasography. Semen volume over 1.0 cc rules out ejaculatory duct obstruction, which in fact is quite rare.

A normal FSH level does not indicate obstruction. As previously mentioned, the serum FSH level correlates most closely with the total number of spermatogonia, and less well with the number of mature spermatids or the sperm count. The most likely diagnosis among patients with azoospermia and a normal serum FSH level is maturation arrest, not obstruction. The FSH is in the normal range because the total number of spermatogonia in these cases is normal. It is true that an elevated level usually means inadequate spermatogenesis, but even this axiom is not always true. Thus, semen volume and endocrine evaluations are not helpful in diagnosing obstruction.

A vasogram should be performed only as part of the operative procedure for correcting obstruction. It should not be used to make one diagnosis or to determine the need for surgery. Performing a vasogram as an isolated diagnostic procedure creates many problems. First, a scrotal exploration is not needed to ascertain that the vas is present; that should be easily discernible by physical examination. Second, unless performed as part of a careful microsurgical procedure, any injection or transection of the vas in performing a vasogram could result in obstruction where originally there was none. Third, the vasogram data are not necessary for preoperative planning. Most important, the test tells nothing about the epididymis, and can lead to a false positive diagnosis of obstruction as well as a false negative diagnosis of no obstruction. If a diagnosis of obstruction is certain, based on testicle biopsy and sperm count, the most logical time to perform is at the time of vasoepididymostomy, once the vas is transected, to make sure that the vas empties distally into the ejaculatory duct and prostatic urethra. It is not necessary to know this information ahead of time.

Many urologists consider that a vasogram can be used to make a diagnosis of epididymal obstruction. In fact, this is most decidedly not the case. Any retrograde injection of the vas deferens toward the epididymis can only result in potential damage to the epididymis. It cannot make a diagnosis of obstruction. Because the epididymis is a closed tubular system, the radiopaque fluid will come to a standstill somewhere in the epididymal duct, thus giving the illusion of obstruction. The point at which this happens depends strictly on the difference in pressure between the fluid in the tubule and the amount of exertion on the plunger of the syringe. What usually happens with forceful injection is that iatrogenic blow-outs are created, further complicating the patient's problem. Thus the only function of the vasogram at the time of microsurgical vasoepididymostomy is to make sure the distal vas empties properly into the ejaculatory duct.

Physical examination of the epididymis and testes, as well as history or lack of history of infection, can be very misleading as well. Testicles that produce a normal amount of sperm may be small, and those that produce no sperm (that have maturation arrest) may often be large. Historical data can be similarly confusing. At least half of our patients who were found to have epididymal obstruction from inflammatory causes gave no prior history of clinical epididymitis. We must assume that whatever caused their epididymal obstruction must have been subclinical.

In conclusion, most of the ancillary medical information that we routinely consider in fertility evaluations is irrelevant to the question of whether or not the patients have obstruction. The physical examination is only relevant in that if there is not palpable vas deferens (that is, congenital absence), no surgical anastomosis can be performed. These patients would require sperm aspiration combined with in-vitro fertilization of the partner. With that exception, the history and physical examination; serum FSH, luteinizing hormones, and testosterone levels; and vasography also are irrelevant to the diagnosis. All that are needed to determine the need for vasoepididymostomy are a palpable vas deferens on one or both sides, a testicle biopsy showing quanti-

tatively normal spermatogenesis, and a semen analysis showing azoospermia

Inguinal Disruption of Vas Deferens After Herniorrhaphy

We have encountered in routine evaluation of men with azoospermia the very unsettling discovery that bilateral inguinal herniorrhaphy, particularly in infancy, carries a high risk of causing iatrogenic obstruction of the vas deferens. Such patients generally complain of infertility in young adulthood. The semen analysis shows azoospermia, after which a testicular biopsy and a vasogram usually are performed. The vasogram reveals obstruction of the vas deferens near the external or internal inguinal ring on both sides, and the biopsy shows normal spermatogenesis. Such patients represent a major microsurgical challenge because an enormous segment of vas deferens has usually been removed throughout the inguinal canal together with the hernia sac, and the obstruction is of long duration (Fig. 12–15). One can usually expect to find either no vas deferens in the inguinal canal or some length of it missing, and enough must be freed up to bridge the gap. Furthermore, there is usually secondary epididymal blockage as well. This requires a vasoepididymostomy in which the blood supply to the intervening segment of vas must be preserved.

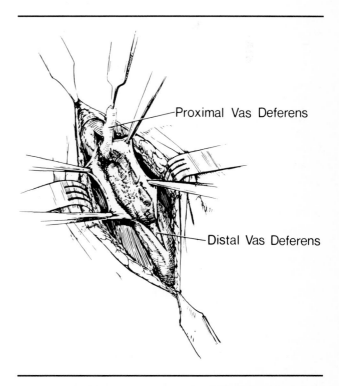

Figure 12–15. This figure demonstrates the problem encountered when attempting to anastomose a vas deferens that has been severed accidentally at the time of herniorrhaphy. (From Silber.[13] Reproduced with permission.)

My approach to the patient with azoospermia and a past history of bilateral inguinal herniorrhaphy is first to perform a testicle biopsy. If it is normal, for interruption of the vas deferens in the inguinal area a vasogram can be done operatively at the time of contemplated reconstruction.

Our findings should give some concern to pediatric surgeons who advocate bilateral inguinal herniorrhaphy for infants with unilaterally detected hernias based on the rationale that an undiscovered hernia probably exists on the other side and ought to be repaired also. When one considers that in some institutions as many as 15% of infant hernia sacs may be found to contain vas deferens, however, it follows that bilateral infant herniorrhaphy may conceivably sterilize as many as 2% of children. In addition, these unsettling figures argue strongly for using ocular loupes more routinely for certain pediatric procedures, including inguinal herniorrhaphy. The vas deferens is so incredibly tiny in the infant that it would be very easy for an excellent surgeon accidently to include it in the ligation of the sac at the internal ring.

Crossover Vasoepididymostomy. Frequently, inguinal disruption of the vas deferens is caused by herniorrhaphy on one side only, but the patient is still azoospermic because on the other side the testicle is atrophic. In such cases the extensive operation of inguinal vasovasostomy or inguinal vasoepididymostomy can be avoided by using a simple crossover procedure. On one side the inguinal vas deferens is completely intact, but no sperm are produced by the testicle on that side. On the other side the testicle is normal, but the inguinal vas deferens has been obstructed or destroyed by herniorrhaphy. It is far easier to make an opening in the median scrotal raphe and pull the vas from the healthy side through the raphe to the other side. Then either the scrotal vas deferens or the epididymis can be anastomosed in a crossover fashion to the inguinal vas from the opposite side (Fig. 12–16). These procedures are highly successful, and much easier both for the surgeon and the patient than trying to go though the area of the previous herniorrhaphy to bridge the gap of the missing vas deferens.

Ejaculatory Duct Obstruction

A rare cause of azoospermia is congenital obstruction of the ejaculatory duct. This diagnosis is made when the patient has a palpable vas deferens, azoospermia, and a normal testicle biopsy, in the presence of a low-volume semen with no fructose. A very low semen volume in a patient being assessed for epididymal obstruction should result in a high index of suspicion for ejaculatory duct obstruction. The vaso-

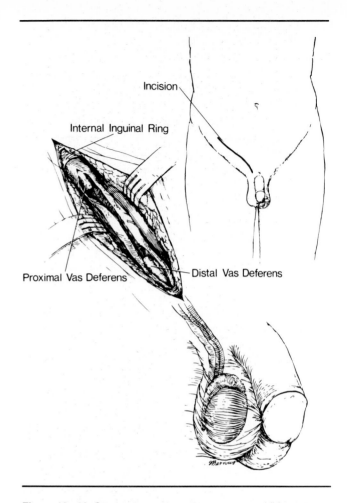

Figure 12–16. Crossover vasovasostomy or vasoepididymostomy. (From Silber.[13] Reproduced with permission.)

gram, which should always be performed routinely at the time of surgery, is the only definitive way to make this diagnosis.

If normal sperm are detected in the vas fluid and the vasogram shows ejaculatory duct obstruction, the patient is placed in lithotomy position and undergoes a transurethral resection of the ejaculatory duct orifice. If the patient has no sperm in the vas fluid, he may have already suffered a blow-out in the epididymis from this long-standing obstruction. In that event, a vasoepididymostomy is first performed and the incision closed before the patient is put in lithotomy position for transurethral resection of the ejaculatory duct.

A transurethral resection of the ejaculatory duct is not difficult for a competent resectionist to perform; however, unless one has had considerable experience with transurethral prostatectomy, it is best not to attempt this procedure.[46,47] First a resectoscope is inserted through the urethra and the prostatic fossa is inspected. A rectal sheath is used to allow an index finger in the rectum to palpate the posterior floor of the prostatic urethra. Using the finger as a guide, a hole is cut sharply into the floor of the prostatic urethra on either the right or the left side just proximal to the verumontanum but distal to the internal sphincter. Less experienced urologists have resected the "verumontanum" thinking that the ejaculatory duct empties there; it is simply the embryologic remnant of the Mullerian duct—the fetal uterus and upper vagina. The ejaculatory duct does not enter it.

It is important not to damage the internal sphincter so that the ejaculate will still go out the urethra rather than retrograde into the bladder. The external sphincter must not be damaged so as to prevent the complication of postoperative urinary incontinence. If the first tissue bite does not reveal the ejaculatory duct, one can continue to resect deeper. If it is truly a case of a blocked ejaculatory duct orifice, fairly soon after the first few bites one should come across a dramatically large, dilated opening with an equally dramatic efflux of translucent seminal fluid.

The semen volume and fructose level return to normal rapidly after this procedure. One of the ancillary benefits is that patients now have a reasonable volume of ejaculate. A normal sperm count with good motility returns within 3 to 8 months, and these patients are fertile. One problem is that they are more susceptible to the possibility of epididymitis because of urinary reflux up the vas deferens. The slightest hint of prostatitis or epididymitis should be treated aggressively with antibiotics. Adhering to this precaution, we have had good success treating this obstruction despite its rarity.

The diagnosis usually is not made definitively before surgery but becomes evident at the time vasography is performed while the patient is undergoing exploration for probable epididymal obstruction and low semen volume. One can be suspicious of ejaculatory duct obstruction when the patient has normal spermatogenesis on testicle biopsy, azoospermia, a palpable vas deferens, and low semen volume with absent fructose.

Congenital Absence of Vas Deferens

Congenital absence of the vas deferens is a rare condition with a poor prognosis for future fertility. The first successful use of sperm aspiration and in-vitro fertilization was reported in 2 couples.[48] The females underwent induction of follicular development using the gonadotropin-releasing hormone agonist leuprolide acetate (TAP Pharmaceuticals, Chicago) 1 mg/day intramuscularly; human follicle-stimulating hormone, 150 IU/day intramuscularly; and human menopausal gonadotropin, 150 IU/day

intramuscularly; from day 1 of the menstrual cycle until vaginal ultrasound examination and serum estradiol level revealed the presence of numerous preovulatory follicles. Human chorionic gonadotropin (HCG), 10,000 IU, was administered intramuscularly, and 36 hours later ultrasound-guided follicular aspiration was carried out transvaginally. Oocytes recovered were cultured at 37°C in an atmosphere of 5% carbon dioxide in air in tubes containing 1 mL Menezo's B2 medium supplemented with 15% heat-inactivated human fetal cord serum. The men underwent scrotal exploration immediately after oocyte aspiration in their wives. Under X 10-4 magnification with an operating microscope, a tiny incision was made with microscissors into the epididymal tunic to expose the tubules in the distal-most portion of the congenitally blind-ending epididymis. Sperm were aspirated with a #22 Medicut on a tuberculin syringe directly from the opening in the epididymal tubule. Great care was taken not to contaminate the specimen with blood, and precise hemostasis was achieved with microbiopolar forceps. The specimens were immediately diluted in HEPES-buffered medium, and a tiny portion examined for motility and quality of progression. If sperm motility was absent, another aspiration was made 0.5 cm more proximally. Sperm were obtained from successively more proximal regions until progressive motility was found. In both of these men sperm were not obtained until the most proximal portion of the caput epididymis was reached. Once the area of motile sperm was found, epididymal fluid was aspirated during a period of 10 to 15 minutes.

Sperm aspirated from the epididymis were washed in HEPES-buffered medium and centrifuged, and the resulting pellet resuspended in 100 μL of medium and incubated at 37°C for 1 hour. At the time of recovery, the total number of sperm was approximately 20 million, motility was less than 5%, and normal forms were only 20%. After wash and incubation the motility improved to 20%. Sperm remained motile in culture for 72 hours after recovery from the epididymis. Ten to 25 μL of the sperm resuspension was added to the culture tubes containing the oocytes and incubated for 12 to 15 hours.

In one patient, 28 oocytes were recovered at aspiration, resulting in 15 embryos, 5 of which were transferred to the fallopian tubes and the remaining frozen. Six embryos were generated from 24 oocytes recovered from the second patient, 5 of which were transferred to the fallopian tubes. The tubal embryo transfers were both performed 54 hours after the follicular aspiration.[49] After embryo transfer, the women received progesterone in oil, 25 mg/day intramuscularly. Both conceived as determined by increasing serum levels of β-HCG on days 14, 19, and 24 after tubal embryo transfer.

The fact that the first 2 couples in which this new treatment was attempted conceived, prompts us to believe that there is potentially desirable approach for achieving pregnancy in infertile couples with congenital absence of the vas.[50] Finally, and perhaps of importance scientifically, this is the first conclusive proof that sperm from the most proximal caput epididymis are capable of fertilizing the human oocyte in vitro, and casts doubt on the indispensable need for them to pass through the epididymis to achieve capacitation in the human.[51]

MICROSURGERY FOR UNDESCENDED TESTICLE

Rationale for Testicle Autotransplantation

Considerable discussion has taken place over how best to localize a nonpalpable cryptochid testis (spermatic venography, electromagnetic imaging scan, or spermatic arteriography), as well as over proper surgical management for the testis that is high and intraperitoneal.[52–57]

In our view, there is little need for controversy. We have found that laparoscopy is the simplest, safest, and most reliable method of localizing high intraabdominal testes.[58] For surgical management, the spermatic vessels must be divided for the testicle to be brought into the scrotum, but the collateral blood supply from the deferential artery is not reliable, and this procedure usually results in atrophy unless the spermatic vessels are revascularized.[55]

We originally reported on 7 patients with bilateral intraabdominal testes who underwent division of the spermatic vessels with microsurgical reanastomosis to the inferior epigastric vessels on one side, and on the other side simple division without reanastomosis.[59,60] On the side where revascularization of the spermatic vessels was performed, the testis retained its normal size and texture. On the other side, partial or complete testicular atrophy occurred.

The danger of unrecognized cancer in the intraabdominal testicle certainly provides one motive for placing such a testicle in the scrotum or possibly removing it.[61,62] It was generally assumed in previous years that the cryptorchid testicle suffered only loss of spermatogenic function; hormonal function was supposedly unaltered. Studies have demonstrated that the abdominal environment also affects the endocrine function of the testis, and results in premature loss of testosterone production. Cryp-

tochid patients have impaired intratesticular androgen production. An adult with untreated bilateral cryptochidism will have an elevated luteinizing hormone (LH) level, and will have premature loss of testosterone secretion.[54,58,63] Experimental studies in the rat demonstrated that when scrotal testes are transfered to the abdomen, there is an immediate and dramatic elevation in FSH corresponding to rapid deterioration of spermatogenesis.[64] Over a longer period of time, however, the LH levels begins to go up gradually also, indicating later loss of endocrine function of the cryptochid testes. The intraabdominal environment is detrimental not only to spermatogenesis, but to hormone production. It simply takes longer for this aspect of testicular function to deteriorate.

The question of whether transplanting these testes to the scrotum in a child will allow the development of fertility has been answered also. Evidence is overwhelming that making a testicle cryptochid diminishes spermatogenesis and that replacing the cryptochid testicle into the scrotum allows spermatogenesis to recover.[65–69] There are documented case reports of azoospermic adults (16 to 25 years of age) with bilateral simple cryptorchidism who after orchidopexy developed normal spermatogenesis and reasonable sperm counts.[70,71] Although these patients did not have intraabdominal testicles, the results support the idea that cryptorchid testes can make sperm if they are transferred to the scrotum. We now have very well-documented cases demonstrating that even intraabdominal testes will develop normal spermatogenesis after puberty if they are properly transferred to the scrotum without damaging the blood supply.[72]

What is the safest method for transferring the high intraperitoneal testis into the scrotum? The procedure of simply dividing the internal spermatic vessels was first recommended in 1903[73] and good results were reported.[74] Others, however, reported uniformly poor results with this operation.[75–77]

It was first demonstrated in 1963 that by dividing the internal spermatic vessels high up and not dissecting their attachment to the cord, it was sometimes possible to preserve collateral circulation by way of the deferential artery.[55] The spermatic vessels could be clamped first and the testicle biopsied to determine the adequacy of collateral blood flow. Almost half of the patients experienced some testicular atrophy, however, and in one third it was rather severe. Furthermore, the original diagrams demonstrate that this technique was most valuable in the management of the so-called long-looped vas, in which the testis is really located at the level of the internal inguinal ring and the vas loops down in the canal toward the external ring and then comes back to the testis at the internal ring. By avoiding dissection in the inguinal canal, the collateral circulation can be preserved. It should be noted that most of the cases these authors described did not involve severely high intraabdominal testes. Others have used the procedure for high intraperitoneal testes.[54,56,60] Favorable results are reported in the literature, but our observations leave no doubt that atrophy is caused by all groups employing this approach.

In our experience the deferential blood supply to the testicle cannot be relied on, and reports of good results of dividing the spermatic vessels without reanastomosis are very much overoptimistic. It was demonstrated in fresh autopsy dissections that the sum of the diameters of the deferential and cremasteric arteries was equal to the diameter of the testicular artery in only one third of cases, indicating that adequate functional collateral circulation to the testis is by no means universal.[69,78]

Microsurgical Techniques

Microvascular Scoville-Lewis, Schwartz, or Heifetz neurosurgical clips are placed on the deep inferior epigastric artery and both superficial and deep inferior epigastric veins inferiorly. These vessels are then

tied off superiorly. The inferior epigastric vessels are each divided and the lumina examined. The spermatic vessels are then brought into the area for anastomosis (Fig. 12–17).

For the microvascular anastomosis, 9-0 or 10-0 nylon on a BV-6 or BV-2 needle is ideal. Interrupted sutures are absolutely critical. Continuous suturing will result in a pursestring effect that will at best bunch, and at worst obstruct the anastomosis site. The interrupted sutures should be tied down and cut as one goes, rather than leaving them to be tied down at the end. With the latter, one will have an impossible puppet show, in which the spider-web-thin sutures become entangled with each other before even half of them have been placed. No attempt should be made to perform the arterial anastomosis until the spatulation has been performed, because the discrepancy between the lumina is otherwise too great.

The technique for the venous anastomosis is somewhat simpler. Since the vessel sizes here will generally match up very nicely, spatulation is not necessary. A standard anastomosis can be performed by placing two anterior stitches 120 degrees apart. Several sutures are placed between these two initial stay sutures, and the entire vessel is the rotated 180

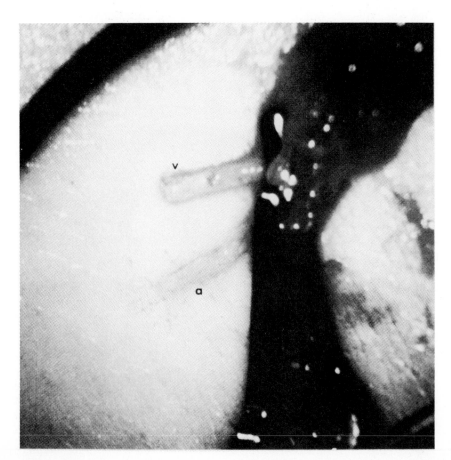

Figure 12–17. The divided spermatic vein (top) and artery (bottom).

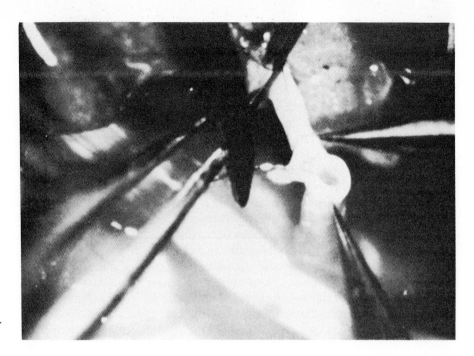

Figure 12–18. Venous anastomosis after the first 120 degrees have been sutured.

degrees so that the posterior 240 degrees that have not been sutured yet are facing anteriorly (Fig. 12–18). Another stay suture is placed halfway, dividing this into two 120-degree segments, each of which requires several sutures in between to complete the anastomosis (Fig. 12–19). After this, the clamps on the inferior epigastric vein and then the artery are removed. The testicle has now been completely revascularized; it can be placed into the

scrotal sac without any tension (Fig. 12–20). Adequacy of blood flow to the testis both intraoperatively and postoperatively is monitored with a Doppler probe.

In cases in which we reanastomosed the divided spermatic vessels on one side but relied on collateral circulation through the vas deferens on the other side, we have always wished that we had simply revascularized both sides.

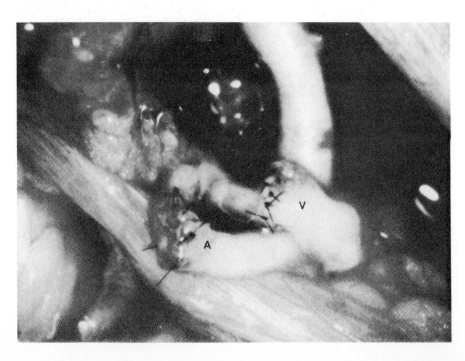

Figure 12–19. Completed arterial and venous anastomoses.

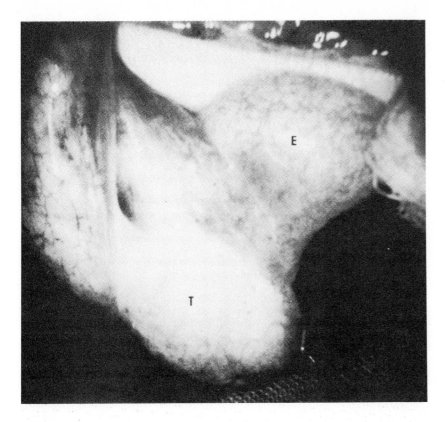

Figure 12–20. The blanched testicle before the vascular clamps are removed. It lies on the groin but is now free to be transferred to the scrotum.

CONCLUSIONS

Preoperative diagnosis and localization of the high intraabdominal testis is most reliably and easily accomplished by laparoscopy. These high testicles are best placed into the scrotum by dividing the spermatic vessels. Microsurgical reanastomosis to the inferior epigastric vessels is recommended to prevent partial or complete testicular atrophy, and to maximize the eventual prospect for fertility. Because we know that adults with bilateral cryptorchidism can recover fertility after the testes are placed in the scrotum, it is important not to compromise blood supply in the mistaken notion that these testicles are not very good anyway. There certainly is some hope for fertility if orchidopexy is performed with proper attention to blood supply.

REFERENCES

1. Silber SJ: Microscopic technique for reversal of vasectomy. *Surg Gynecol Obstet* 143:630, 1976.
2. Silber SJ: Perfect anatomical reconstruction of vas deferens with a new microscope surgical technique. *Fertil Steril* 28:72, 1977.
3. Silber SJ, Galle J, Friend D: Microscopic vasovasostomy and spermatogenesis. *J Urol* 117:299, 1977.
4. Silber SJ, Crudop J: Kidney transplantation in inbred rats. *Am J Surg* 125:551, 1973.
5. Silber SJ, Crudop J: A three kidney rat model. *Invest Urol* 11:466, 1974.
6. Silber SJ, Malvin RL: Compensatory and obligatory renal growth in rats. *Am J Physiol* 226:114, 1974.
7. Silber SJ: Growth of baby kidneys transplanted into adults. *Arch Surg* 111:75, 1976.
8. Silber SJ: Transplantation of rat kidneys with acute tubular necrosis into salt-loaded and normal recipients. *Surgery* 77:487, 1975.
9. Silber SJ: Successful autotransplantation of an intra-abdominal testicle to the scrotum using microvascular anastomosis. *J Urol* 115:452, 1976.
10. Silber SJ: Compensatory and obligatory renal growth in babies and adults. *Aust NZ J Surg* 44:421, 1974.
11. Silber SJ: Microscopic vasectomy reversal. *Fertil Steril* 28:1191, 1977.
12. Silber SJ: Vasectomy and vasectomy reversal. *Fertil Steril* 29:125, 1978.
13. Silber SJ: *Reproductive Microsurgery*. Baltimore, Williams & Wilkins, 1984.
14. MacLeod J, Gold RZ: The male factor in fertility and infertility. IV. Sperm morphology in fertile and infertile marriage. *Fertil Steril* 2:394, 1951.
15. Silber SJ, Rodriguez-Rigau LJ: Quantitative analysis of testicle biopsy: Determination of partial obstruction and prediction of sperm count after surgery for obstruction. *Fertil Steril* 36:480, 1981.
16. Silber SJ: Epididymal extravasation following vasectomy as a cause for failure of vasectomy reversal. *Fertil Steril* 31:309, 1979.
17. Bedford JM: Adaptation of the male reproductive tract and the rate of spermatozoa following vasectomy in the rabbit, rhesus monkey, hamster and rat. *Biol Reprod* 14:118, 1976.
18. Silber SJ: Microscopic vasoepididymostomy, specific microanastomosis to the epididymal tubule. *Fertil Steril* 30:565, 1978.
19. Silber SJ: Vasoepididymostomy to the head of the epididymis: Recovery of normal spermatozoa motility. *Fertil Steril* 34:149, 1980.
20. Silber SJ: Reversal of vasectomy in the treatment of male infertility. *J Androl* 1:261, 1980.
21. Silber SJ: Reversal of vasectomy in the treatment of male infertility: Role of microsurgery, vasoepididymostomy, and pressure-induced changes of vasectomy. *Urol Clin North Am* 8:53, 1981.
22. Charny CW: Testicular biopsy: Its value in male sterility. *JAMA* 115:1429, 1940.
23. Nelson WO: Interpretation of testicular biopsy. *JAMA* 151:1449, 1953.
24. Mannion RA, Cottrell TLC: Correlation between testicular biopsy and sperm count. *J Urol* 85:953, 1961.
25. Albert A: The mammalian testis, in Young WC (ed): *Sex and Secretions*, ed 3. Baltimore, Williams & Wilkins, 1961, vol 1, p 305.

26. Heller CG, Clermont Y: Kinetics of the germinal epithelium in man. *Recent Prog Horm Res* 20:545, 1964.

27. Steinberger E, Tjioe DY: A method for quantitative analysis of human seminiferous epithelium. *Fertil Steril* 19:960, 1968.

28. Tjioe DY, Steinberger E, Paulsen CA: A simple method for quantitative analysis of seminiferous epithelium in human testicular biopsies. *J Albert Einstein Med Center* 15:56, 1967.

29. Zuckerman Z, Rodriquez-Rigau LJ, Weiss DB, et al: Quantitative analysis of the seminiferous epithelium in human testicular biopsies, and the relation of spermatogenesis to sperm density. *Fertil Steril* 30:448, 1978.

30. DeKretser DM, Burger HG, Hudson B: The relationship between germinal cells and serum FSH levels in males with infertility. *J Clin Endocrinol Metab* 38:787, 1974.

31. Schoysman R: "Operative Treatment of Ductal Obstruction and/or Agenesis" Presented at the meeting of the American Fertility Society, Miami Beach, April 1977.

32. Schoysman R, Drouart JM: Progrès récents dans la chirurgie de la stérilité masculine et feminine. *Acta Clin Belg* 71:261, 1972.

33. Amelar RD, Dubin L: Commentary of epididymal vasostomy, vasovasostomy and testicular biopsy, in *Current Operative Urology*. New York, Harper & Row, 1975, pp 1181–1185.

34. Hanley HG: The surgery of male sub-fertility. *Ann R Coll Surg* 17:159, 1955.

35. Hotchkiss, RS: Surgical treatment of infertility in the male, in Campbell MF, Harrison HH (eds): *Urology*, ed 3. Philadelphia, Saunders, 1970, p 671.

36. Silber SJ: Pregnancy caused by sperm from vasa efferentia. *Fertil Steril*, in press. 49: xx, 1988.

37. Silber SJ: Results of specific tubule vasoepididymostomy: the role of epididymis in sperm maturation. *Human Reproduction*, Volume 4: xx, 1989.

38. Silber SJ: Apparent fertility of human sperm from the caput epididymis. *J Androl*, in press.

39. Gaddum P: Sperm maturation in the male reproductive tract: Development of motility. *Anat Rec* 161:47, 1969.

40. Bedford JM: Development of the fertilizing ability of spermatozoa in the epididymis of the rabbit. *J Exp Zool* 163:312, 1966.

41. Orgebin-Crist MC: Sperm maturation in rabbit epididymis. *Nature* 216:816, 1967.

42. Glover TD: Some aspects of function in the epididymis. Experimental occlusion of the epididymis in the rabbit. *Int J Fertil* 14:215, 1969.

43. Gaddum P, Glover TD: Some reactions of rabbit spermatozoa to ligation of the epididymis. *J Reprod Fertil* 9:119, 1965.

44. Paufler SK, Foote RH: Morphology, motility and fertility in spermatozoa recovered from different areas of ligated rabbit epididymis. *J Reprod Fertil* 17:125, 1968.

45. Orgebin-Crist MC: Studies of the function of the epididymis. *Biol Reprod* 1:155, 1969.

46. Silber SJ: *Transurethral Resection*. New York, Appleton-Century-Crofts, 1977.

47. Porch PP Jr: Aspermia owing to obstruction of distal ejaculatory duct and treatment by transurethral resection. *J Urol* 119:141, 1978.

48. Silber SJ, Asch R, Ord T, Borrero C, Balmaceda J: New treatment for infertility due to congenital absence of vas deferens. *Lancet* 2:850, 1987.

49. Devroey P, Braeckmans P, Smits, et al: Pregnancy after translaparoscopic zygote intrafallopian transfer in a patient with sperm antibodies. *Lancet* 1:1329, 1986.

50. Girgis SM, Etriby AN, Ibrahim AA, Kahil SA: Testicular biopsy and azoospermia. A review of the last ten years' experience in over 800 cases. *Fertil Steril* 20:467, 1969.

51. Orgebin-Crist MC: Studies of the function of the epididymis. *Biol Reprod* 1:155, 1969.

52. Levitt SB, Kogan SJ, Engel RM, et al: The impalpable testis: A rational approach to management. *J Urol* 120:515, 1978.

53. Weiss RM, Glickman MG, Lytton B: Clinical implications of gonadal venography in the management of the non-palpable undescended testis. *J Urol* 121:745.

54. Clatworthy NW, Hallenbaugh RS, Grossfeld JL: The long-louped vas orchidopexy for the high undescended testis. *Am Surg* 38:69, 1972.

55. Fowler R, Stephens FD: The role of testicular vascular anatomy in the salvage of high undescended testes, in Stephens FD (ed): *Congenital Malformations of the Rectum, Anus, and Genital Urinary Tract*. London, Livingstone, 1963, pp 306–320.

56. Gibbons MD, Cromie WJ, Duckett JW Jr: Management of the abdominal undescended testicle. *J Urol* 122:76, 1979.

57. Martin DC: The undescended testis: Evolving concepts in management. *Urol Dig* 1977.

58. Cohen R, Silber SJ: Laparoscopy for cryptorchidism. *J Urol* 124:928, 1980.

59. Silber SJ: The intra-abdominal testis: microvascular autotransplantaton. *J Urol* 125:329, 1981.

60. Silber SJ, Kelly J: Successful auto-transplantation of an intra-abdominal testis to the scrotum by microvascular technique. *J Urol* 115:452, 1976.

61. Campbell HE: Incidence of malignant growth of the undescended testicle: A critical and statistical study. *Arch Surg* 44:353, 1942.

62. Martin DC, Menck HR: The undescended testis: Management after puberty. *J Urol* 114:77, 1975.

63. Atkinson PM, Epstein MT, Rippon AE: Plasma gonadotropins and androgens in the surgically treated cryptorchid patient. *J Pediatr Surg* 10:27, 1975.

64. Altwein JE, Gittes RF: Effect of cryptorchidism and casteration on FSH and LH levels in the adult rat. *Invest Urol* 10:167, 1972.

65. Hadziselemovic F, Herzag B, Seguchi H: Surgical correction of cryptorchidism at two years: Electron microscopic and morphologic investigations. *J Pediatr Surg* 10:19, 1975.

66. Kiesewetter WB, Shull WR, Fetterman GH: Histologic changes in the testis following the anatomically successful orchidopexy. *J Pediatr Surg* 4:59, 1969.

67. Mengel W, et al: Studies on cryptorchidism: A comparison of histologic findings in the germinative epithelium before and after the second year of life. *J Pediatr Surg* 9:445, 1974.

68. Nelson WO: Mammalian spermatogenesis, effect of experimental cryptorchidism in the rat, and nondescent of the testis in man. *Recent Prog Horm Res* 6:29, 1951.

69. Sohval AR: Testicular dysgenesis as an etiologic factor in cryptorchidism. *J Urol* 72:693, 1954.

70. Britton BJ: Spermatogenesis following bilateral orchidopexy in adult life. *Br J Urol* 47:464, 1975.

71. Comhaire F, Derom F, Vermeulen L: The recovery of spermatogenesis in an azoospermic patient after operation for bilateral undescended testes at age of 25 years. *Int J Androl* 1:117, 1978.

72. Silber SJ: Recovery of spermatogenesis after testicle autotransplantation in an adult male. *Fertil Steril* 38:632, 1982.

73. Bevan AD: The surgical treatment of undescended testicle: A further contribution. *JAMA* 41:718, 1903.24.

74. Moschowitz AV: The anatomy and treatment of undescended testes, with special reference to the Bevan operation. *Ann Surg* 52:821, 1910.

75. Mixter EG: Undescended testicle: Operative treatment and end results. *Surg Gynecol Obstet* 39:275, 1924.

76. Wangenstein OH: Undescended testes: Experimental and clinical study. *Arch Surg* 14:653, 1927.

77. McCollum DW: Clinical study of spermatogenesis of undescended testicles. *Arch Surg* 31:290, 1935.

78. Silber SJ: Transplantation of human testis for anorchia. *Fertil Steril* 30:181, 1978.

CHAPTER 13

Assisted Reproductive Treatments for Oligospermia

Joel H. Batzofin, Larry I. Lipshultz

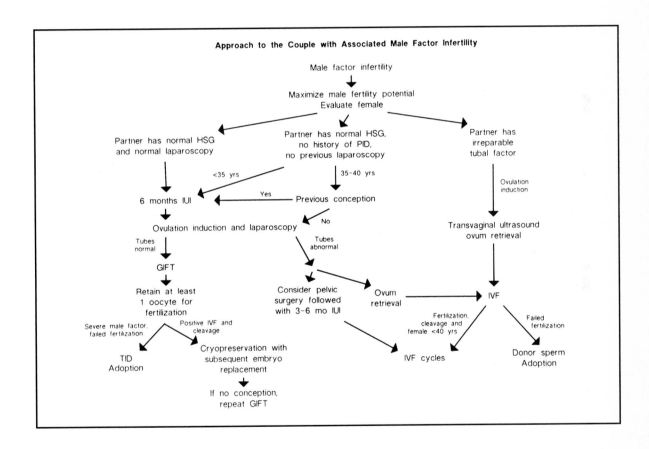

Since the mid-1970s there have been dramatic advances in our understanding of reproductive biology and in clinical applications of this knowledge. The coordinated efforts of basic scientists and clinicians have resulted in new therapeutic options for infertile and subfertile couples. It is generally agreed that infertility affects some 15 to 20% of couples who are attempting conception.[1] A thorough investigation of both partners shows the male factor to be the sole cause of the problem, or a significant contributing factor, in approximately 50% of couples with reproductive dysfunction. Several therapeutic treatments can be offered to infertile couples with an associated male factor problem.

A thorough history and physical examination are the initial steps in any infertility evaluation. Three semen analyses and determination of serum gonadotropin concentrations (i.e., luteinizing hormone, or LH, and follicle-stimulating hormone, or FSH), serum testosterone levels, and, when appropriate, serum prolactin levels are the primary laboratory tests. Three semen analyses are required because of the between-sample variability that is known to occur in certain individuals. The important semen characteristics and normal values are demonstrated in Table 13–1.[2]

After the semen analyses and the appropriate hormone tests, it can be determined whether the male values are completely normal, or whether an element of subfertility exists that necessitates additional testing and/or treatment. The two algorithms at the beginning of the chapter show the clinical approach we use after the initial basic evaluation.[3] All the steps outlined in the algorithms are directed toward maximizing fertility potential and may not ultimately be therapeutic in and of themselves. While some of the therapies may create a condition in which the male is capable of initiating a pregnancy spontaneously, many merely enhance fertility potential; consequently, the couple still requires additional treatment to initiate a pregnancy.

The initial diagnostic and therapeutic steps may halt or reverse a pathologic process that is detrimental to sperm production and/or function, but the patient remains relatively subfertile by virtue of persistent oligospermia, asthenospermia, or diminished fertilizing capacity of the spermatozoa. In such situations the clinician must resort to what are known as assisted reproductive treatments (ART). At present, these treatments include intrauterine insemination with processed spermatozoa (IUI), gamete intrafallopian transfer (GIFT), and in vitro fertilization with embryo transfer (IVF-ET).[4] Additional treatments such as transuterine tubal insemination (TUTI), direct intraperitoneal insemination (DIPI), and zygote intrafallopian transfer (ZIFT) are under investigation; if shown to be efficacious, these will be added to the assisted therapeutic options. There are three primary treatment options in terms of patient selection and results, as they specifically pertain to couples with an associated male factor. Prior to a discussion of the treatments per se, clarification of how and when we use the sperm-penetration assay is important, since we believe that when performed in an optimal fashion, this remains the most accurate test of sperm fertilizing capacity and also provides information useful in deciding on the best method of sperm processing for ART.

SPERM-PENETRATION ASSAY

Males with abnormalities of sperm production (oligospermia or asthenospermia) frequently have concomitant disorders of sperm function manifested as defective oocyte penetrability. Abnormalities in sperm function may also occur in males with normal bulk semen values (count, motility, and morphology). It is increasingly apparent that the functional competence of spermatozoa is not necessarily reflected by results obtained in the conventional semen analysis.[5] In efforts to analyze sperm competence, several laboratory tests have been developed and have received critical attention. Three of these are the zona-free hamster egg sperm-penetration assay (SPA), computer-assisted analysis of sperm movement, and measurement of sperm adenosine triphosphate (ATP) concentrations. Of these, only the SPA has had a significant impact of clinical management.

Species specificity of ovum fertilization is lost after enzymatic removal of the cumulus and zona pellucida from mouse, rat, and hamster ova. Heterologous combinations of spermatozoa and zona-free oocytes from guinea pig, mouse, rat, and hamster have demonstrated sperm chromatin decondensation within the egg cytoplasm, thus indicating that heterologous fusion had occurred.[6,7] Zona-free hamster oocytes demonstrate fusibility with spermatozoa from several species, including the human.[8,9]

It is known that gamete membrane fusion only occurs if the spermatozoa have been capacitated and have undergone the acrosome reaction[10,11]; therefore, fusion serves as a useful end point in determining the occurrence of these two phenomena. It has been demonstrated that heterologous fusion and the postfusion events of chromatin decondensation apparently do not differ from those in homologous fertilizations.[11–13] Consequently, the use of this heterologous system provides an excellent model for diagnostic evaluation of sperm function. Results from several laboratories indicate that the outcome of the SPA is highly correlated with results obtained in human IVF systems (Fig. 13–1). Furthermore, several different sperm-processing or sperm-enhancing procedures can be analyzed in the SPA, and the results

TABLE 13–1. SEMEN CHARACTERISTICS AND ACCEPTED NORMAL VALUES CHARACTERISTIC

Characteristic	Normal Values
Volume	1.5–5.0 ml
Color	Whitish gray
Liquefaction	Within 30 min
Density	20–200 million/ml
Motility	
Quantitative	>60%
Qualitative	Forward progression >2+ (scale 1 to 4)
Morphology	>60% normal
Clumping	Minimal
Leukocytes	<1 million/ml
Immature forms	1 million/ml

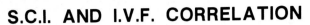

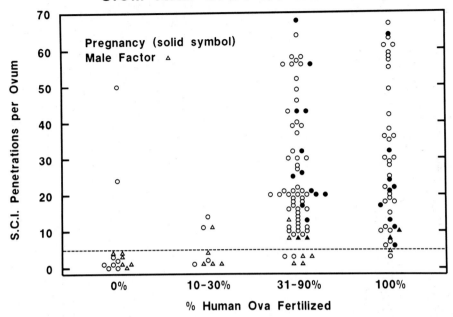

Figure 13–1. The correlation between results obtained in the sperm-penetration assay (SPA) and human IVF program (Baylor College of Medicine, Houston, TX). Sperm capacitation index (SCI) is an expression of the mean number of penetrations per ovum. The dotted line at five penetrations per ovum represents the sensitivity of this assay system, below which no pregnancies occurred in the 138 patients analyzed. Note the strong (but not perfect) correlation between results obtained in the SPA and ovum fertility rates in the human IVF program. (From Batzofin et al.[4] Reproduced with permission.)

can be compared with those obtained when the test is performed in the standard manner. In this way information regarding optimization of sperm function can be obtained and used in subsequent treatment cycles involving assisted reproductive treatments.

Factors that influence results of the SPA have been outlined by several authors.[11,14–16] Unfortunately, no consensus exists on the specific protocol used in the various laboratories, and consequently, valid comparison of results among the different centers frequently is not possible. It becomes extremely important, therefore, that for any given laboratory the test be reproducible and sensitive enough to avoid false negative results (failure to penetrate hamster oocytes but ability to penetrate human oocytes). Also results should correlate well with data obtained from the human IVF program.

There are several different methods for reporting results of SPA. In an optimized assay system, the sperm of pregnancy-proved donors will penetrate 100% of the ova at concentrations of 3 to 5 million sperm/ml. In addition, extensive polyspermy (often as high as 80 penetrations/ovum) will be detected. Since certain patients with infertility also achieve penetration scores of 100% but demonstrate no polyspermy, the results should be considered in terms of the degree of polyspermy, and not just the number of ova penetrated. The sperm capacitation index (SCI) is an expression of the mean number of penetrations per ovum. If the assay is sufficiently sensitive and reproducible, SPA data can be analyzed

and correlated with the IVF data, and a cut-off point can be established (e.g., five penetrations/ovum at a fixed concentration of motile sperm) above which the patient is considered fertile and below which the patient is considered subfertile (see Fig. 13–1). This information is helpful in patient counseling and assessment of the effect of sperm-enhancement procedures employed to improve gamete efficiency.

METHODS FOR SEPARATING SPERMATOZOA FROM SEMINAL PLASMA AND IMPROVING GAMETE EFFICIENCY

Several methods exist for separating motile spermatozoa from the male ejaculate. The most commonly used include direct swim-up separation, two-step washing with swim-up penetration, and Percoll discontinuous gradient-separation techniques (Table 13–2). These three methods have various advantages and disadvantages. For the most part, direct swim-up allows a highly motile fraction of sperm to be collected. The number of sperm recovered is significantly less than with the other two techniques, however. When increased numbers of abnormal and/or immature forms are present in the ejaculate or white blood cells and ejaculate debris concentrations are high, swim-up techniques provide a reasonable mechanism for isolating normal motile spermatozoa; however, the motile sperm may carry ejaculate debris into the swim-up suspension. The two-step washing

TABLE 13–2. SUMMARY OF THE USE OF SPERM-SEPARATING TECHNIQUES*

Semen Factor	Two-Step	Two-Step with Swim-Up	Percoll	Swim-Up
Oligospermia	+	++		+
Asthenospermia		+	++	+
Oligoasthenospermia		+		++
Increased abnormal spermatozoa			+	
Increased white blood cells and/or debris		+	++	+
Normal semen with abnormal penetration			++	+

*The method chosen for sperm processing will depend upon evaluation of both bulk semen values and sperm-fertilizing capacity determined by the SPA.

procedure provides the highest sperm recovery rate, but nonviable sperm and debris are collected as well. The two-step washing combined with sperm swim-up from the final sperm pellet yields a highly motile sperm fraction, with decreased debris, white cells, and nonviable forms.

Of these three methods, the two-step wash with swim-up is most frequently used. The Percoll gradient technique is used most commonly for males with normal sperm density and very low motility. Because ejaculates with increased concentrations of white blood cells or immature forms can benefit from Percoll separation, this is the method of choice to facilitate the collection of a highly motile sperm fraction.[17]

In essence, the goal of sperm processing is to select for a fraction of highly motile, morphologically normal sperm, as free as possible of white blood cells and other debris. In this way the most functional population of spermatozoa is collected. An equally important consideration is whether sperm-processing procedures are able to improve sperm function and penetrability when these mechanisms are defective.

The pathophysiologic basis of defective sperm function is highly complex. As noted previously, for successful ovum fertilization to occur, sperm must undergo capacitation and the acrosome reaction. For the most part, the specifics of these events are unclear. In efforts to determine whether sperm function can be enhanced by separation or coincubation techniques, several alternatives have been examined. The most commonly used methods are Percoll gradient separation and the addition of human follicular fluid to the culture medium. Our experience has shown that approximately 5 to 10% of males with abnormal SPAs improve after Percoll treatment, and that follicular fluid coincubation improves sperm-penetrating function in 40 to 50% of these patients.[18] Description of these methods has been published.[19] In addition, test-yolk buffer preparation has been extensively evaluated in the SPA system. Sensitivity of the assay was increased,[20] but clinical evaluation is pending.

Another aspect of sperm preparation under investigation is the effect of altering the sperm concentration at the time of oocyte insemination. It is likely that certain males have different subpopulations of spermatozoa in their ejaculate. Some spermatozoa are functionally competent while others are not. Increasing by a factor of 5 or 10 the number of sperm used for insemination increases the numbers of functionally competent sperm. Thus fertilization may occur with this higher sperm concentration when it is unlikely at a lower insemination concentration. The SPA serves as an extremely valuable assay for evaluating this phenomenon. Whether polyspermy rates would be increased in humans because of the higher concentrations of sperm used for the insemination is unknown.

Figure 13–2 summarizes clinical indications for SPA. With addition of the techniques described above to the standard SPA, the most effective method of improving sperm function can be identified prior to a couple's treatment cycle, and that particular method can be used in sperm penetration for IVF-ET, GIFT, or IUI.

ASSISTED REPRODUCTIVE TREATMENTS

After measures have been taken to maximize the fertility potential of the male, the couple frequently requires additional therapy by one of the assisted reproductive treatments involving IUI, IVF-ET, or GIFT. Choice of treatment is a complex decision involving a thorough work-up of both partners. If the female needs a laparoscopy, diagnostic and therapeutic steps may be combined (see flow diagram). Ideally, the treatment of choice is the one that carries the highest success rate and is the least invasive. To achieve these goals, decisions are based on three premises and guidelines.

First, the highest pregnancy rates occur when fertilization occurs in vivo rather than in vitro.[21] This implies that when clinically appropriate, IUI and/or GIFT would be preferred over IVF-ET. (At the present time, IVF-ET is the treatment of choice for couples in whom the female has irreparable damage to, or surgical absence of, fallopian tubes.) Second, for GIFT to be successful and without major risk of an ectopic pregnancy, fallopian tubes must be normal. A minor exception might include phimosis of the fimbriae with otherwise normal, patent tubes as demonstrated by hysterosalpingography and laparoscopy.

Finally, to document fertilization it may be necessary to perform routine GIFT procedures using some of the oocytes that are harvested, while retaining one or more oocytes in vitro.[22,23] The advent of cryopreservation techniques, offering the possibility

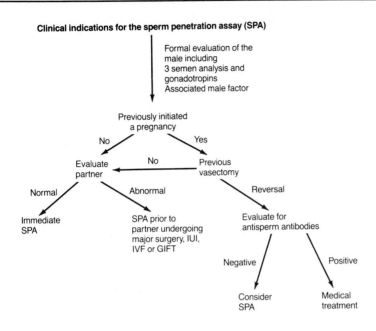

Figure 13–2. Clinical indications for the sperm penetration assay (SPA).

of subsequent transfer of frozen-thawed embryos, has circumvented some of the ethical dilemmas associated with this form of treatment and hence has greatly enhanced this option.

With these guidelines in mind, the clinician is able to formulate a comprehensive management plan for the couple with associated male factor infertility. Depending on the age and reproductive status of the female partner, diagnostic and therapeutic steps may be performed simultaneously. It is important to emphasize, however, that although this management plan can serve as a guideline, much remains to be learned about all of the assisted reproductive treatments. As new information becomes available, the clinical approach to infertile couples will require modification.

RESULTS

Intrauterine Insemination

In our clinic the criteria for patient selection for IUI as a treatment for male factor infertility included a semen analysis demonstrating oligospermia (fewer than 20 million/ml) and/or asthenospermia ($< 60\%$ motility), and/or an abnormal SPA on at least two occasions.[24] Complete evaluation of the females in this study revealed no evidence of compromising factors. In 201 treatment cycles involving 38 couples, the investigators reported 11 term pregnancies for a 5.5% pregnancy rate per treatment cycle. The overall pregnancy rate was 11 (29%) of 38. These data underscore the importance of an adequate therapeu-

tic trial in such couples. Most agree that there should be a period of 6 months with documented ovulation and accurately timed intrauterine insemination before the treatment is considered a failure and alternate therapy is considered.

In one study[25] pregnancy rates resulting from IUI were compared to those with timed intercourse for men with moderate and with severe semen defects. For the group with moderate semen defects ($10–40 \times 10^6$ sperm/ml, 30–44% motility, 30–40% normal forms), the pregnancy rate per IUI treatment cycle was 17 (8.8%) of 193 and for timed intercourse was 6 (4.5%) of 133 couples. This comparison demonstrated no statistically significant difference, and suggests that success in couples with moderate semen defects who are treated with IUI may be due to accurate timing of insemination rather than IUI per se. On the other hand, for patients with severe semen defects (counts $< 10 \times 10^6$ sperm/mL, motility $< 30\%$, morphology $< 30\%$ normal), pregnancy rates with IUI were significantly better (9/103 or 8.7%) than those resulting from timed intercourse alone (0/80). These data indicate that couples with severe semen defects benefit substantially from IUI. The improvement in pregnancy rates is most probably attributable to the fact that the insemination procedure bypasses some of the natural barriers of the female reproductive tract, principally, the cervix.

In Vitro Fertilization and Embryo Transfer

Figures 13–3 and 13–4 illustrates the results when 27 couples with severe male factor infertility ($< 3 \times 10^6$

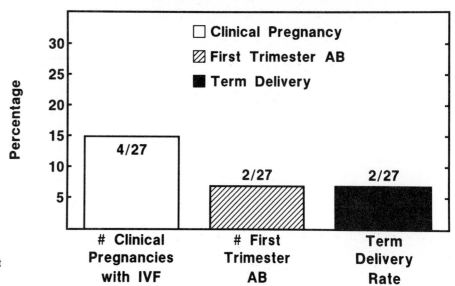

Figure 13–3. Pregnancy outcome after IVF with various sperm-preparation techniques for male infertility. (From Batzofin et al.[4] Reproduced with permission.)

total motile sperm/ejaculate), underwent treatment with IVF-ET. Fertilization of at least one oocyte occurred in 21 of 27 IVF cycles. The rate of fertilization of mature oocytes was significantly lower in the group with a male factor problem than in the one without it, which had an overall fertilization rate of 78%. In this series, the IVF treatment cycle yielded four clinical pregnancies, two of which aborted in the first trimester. Two patients had term deliveries that accounted for a 7 to 8% overall live birth rate per attempted IVF cycle. The overall pregnancy rate for this male factor subpopulation was lower than the overall term pregnancy rate for those without the male factor (15–20%). Other investigators noted the pregnancy rates in the two populations to be similar, and it has been suggested that partners of men with male factor as a group are more fertile than those of men without male factor infertility, and that this may result in similar pregnancy rates in both types of couples.[26,27]

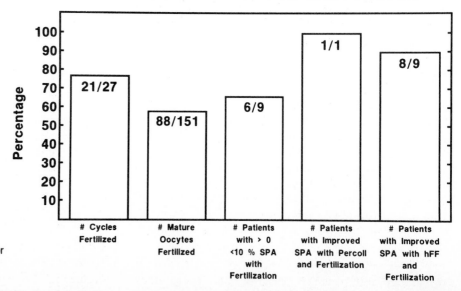

Figure 13–4. Fertilization outcome after IVF with various sperm-preparation techniques for male factor infertility (see text for discussion). (From Batzofin et al.[4] Reproduced with permission.)

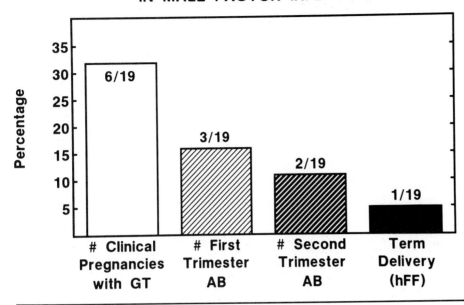

PREGNANCY OUTCOME WITH G.I.F.T. IN MALE FACTOR INFERTILITY

Figure 13–5. Pregnancy outcome with GIFT in male factor infertility. GT = gamete transfer = GIFT. (From Batzofin et al.[4] Reproduced with permission.)

GIFT

We reported on 19 cycles of GIFT in couples with male factor infertility identified by abnormal SPA.[19] Six of the 19 cycles resulted in pregnancies, but only one of these pregnancies went to term (Fig. 13–5). The term pregnancy occurred in an individual whose husband's sperm was coincubated with follicular fluid prior to GIFT. Two second-trimester losses were due to maternal factors without evidence of a genetic anomaly. The frequency of pregnancy wastage in this male factor GIFT population was unexpectedly higher than in those without male factor (22%). The specific reasons for the increased abortion rate are unknown at this time, but the limited size of this study population may be significant.

CONCLUSION

Accumulating data suggest that assisted reproductive treatments are useful for certain couples with male factor infertility. Selecting the specific treatment is a complex decision that can be made only after all factors for both members of a particular couple are evaluated. It is imperative that urologist, gynecologist, and reproductive biologist collaborate closely so that treatment can be tailored to the specific needs of each individual couple. If a fertilization abnormality is thought to be the cause of inability to conceive and the results of the SPA are inconclusive, in vivo testing may be recommended as outlined in Figure 13–4. For couples undergoing GIFT treatment cycles, this in-

volves retaining one or more of the harvested oocytes in vitro, with routine clinical transfer of the others. The retained oocytes can then be inseminated and observed for evidence of fertilization. In this way, the presence or absence of fertilization can be determined accurately. If failure of fertilization is documented in the face of superior-quality oocytes, the couple can be counseled to pursue other avenues, such as the use of donor insemination or adoption.

The role of the SPA in terms of its predictive value for ART remains somewhat unclear.[28,29] If the assay can be performed in a reliable, reproducible, and sensitive fashion, false positive and false negative results can be minimized or even eliminated. This can be of considerable assistance in patient counseling. In terms of analyzing the effects of sperm-processing procedures, the SPA seems to be an invaluable diagnostic aid, and as noted, the information thus obtained can be used clinically. In addition, the in vitro system, as well as newer tests of sperm function such as the hemi-zona assay,[30] will serve as extremely useful models with which to evaluate new therapeutic options as they become available. In particular, this will relate to newer methods of sperm-processing and sperm-enhancement procedures.

FUTURE CONSIDERATIONS

New information and therapeutic options have brought about significant advances in reproductive medicine, especially in the treatment of subfertile males. The IVF-ET, GIFT, and IUI methods have been applied with variable success. It is fair to say that we are still trying to understand the therapeutic applications of these treatment options. Much remains to be learned about the pathophysiologic mechanisms underlying disorders of male fertility; until these are better understood, much of the data we obtain from clinical investigations will be perplexing. It seems clear that adequate sperm production with normal bulk semen values is not necessarily associated with normal sperm-fertilizing capacity. Similarly, although disorders of sperm production are often associated with functional abnormalities, this is not always the case. Consequently, it is important to evaluate sperm function in any couple in whom the male has not previously initiated a pregnancy. At the present time, the most reliable means of assessing sperm function is the SPA. Investigations into the applications of computer-assisted semen analysis and other tests of sperm function are continuing.

The scientific and technologic advances relating to gamete accessibility and handling have reached a level of sophistication that has provided researchers with a unique opportunity to perform investigations and undertake therapeutic measures. For those individuals who suffer from defects of sperm function, several options exist now or will become available in the near future.

Methods to Improve Efficiency of Sperm

As noted earlier, sperm efficiency sometimes improves after the spermatozoa are processed with human follicular fluid, Percoll gradient separation, albumin gradients, swim-up procedures, or coincubation with test-yolk buffer or a variety of other sperm-capacitation media. Whether these methods improve sperm efficiency directly (by having an effect upon capacitation or the acrosome reaction) or indirectly (by changing the concentration of the motile fraction of sperm) is not clearly understood. Undoubtedly, additional methods of sperm processing will become available in the future, and improved understanding of underlying defects will increase the precision with which the different therapeutic options are applied.

In Vitro Management of Oocytes

Much of the initial work from IVF centers focused attention on in vitro handling of oocytes by methods such as enzymatic or mechanical removal of cumulus cells and prolonged incubation of immature oocytes prior to insemination. These studies demonstrated that laboratory handling of the oocyte is crucial to fertilization and early embryo development.[31] Studies pertaining to the optimization of the in vitro

handling of oocytes (and the early embryo) are continuing.

The importance of this aspect of reproductive treatments involving IVF-ET, GIFT, and IUI cannot be emphasized too strongly. In the future our understanding of these phenomena should improve still further. It is likely that a marginally subfertile male will not be able to fertilize oocytes under standard conditions, but if the oocytes (and the spermatozoa) are processed appropriately, fertilization will occur.

Zona Drilling

The zona pellucida of the oocyte represents a barrier to the passage of sperm. The enzymes released from the acrosomal cap during the acrosome reaction are necessary for the sperm to pass through the zona and subsequently to fuse with the vitellin membrane of the oocyte. For males with dysfunctional spermatozoa, acid drilling of the zona may allow passage of the sperm into the oocyte.[32] As yet, no pregnancy has been reported after these procedures, and research in this area continues.

Micromanipulation and Microinjection of Sperm

Micromanipulation and microinjection of sperm are the subjects of a great deal of interest and research. Processed spermatozoa can be placed in a micropipette of a micromanipulator and injected directly into the ooplasm, thereby bypassing the dysfunctional mechanisms of fertilization. At the present time these techniques are experimental, and concerns have been raised about possible genetic sequelae. Micromanipulation techniques will apply to several different aspects of reproductive medicine; however, it is anticipated that their major impact will be in the management of infertile males suffering from disorders of fertilization.

Miscellaneous

Several other options are being investigated and may have clinical application for subfertile males. Alloplastic spermatocele should be effective for males with congenital absence of, or damage to, the vas deferens, in whom microsurgery has either failed or is not feasible. The design of the spermatocele and the ability to maintain viable sperm in an artificial medium for a prolonged period may improve, so that the difficulties previously encountered with these techniques are overcome. Direct intraepididymal aspiration of sperm may become feasible for males with congenital absence of, or damage to, the epididymis and vas. As we understand more about sperm maturation and are able to provide a suitable in vitro environment in which the final stages of the process may occur, patients so affected may become candidates for treatment.

Although great strides have been made in the management of infertile males, much remains to be learned. Doubtless, as our knowledge increases, other options will become available for these patients. With the greater accessibility of the gametes and early embryos, and improved tissue culture techniques, the stage seems set for more sophisticated investigations into the mechanisms controlling reproductive processes. Molecular biologists and genetecists are making great progress in unraveling the genetic bases of many biologic phenomena, and will undoubtedly uncover the genetic mechanisms controlling capacitation and the acrosome reaction in healing individuals. The result will be that our understanding and ultimate therapy directed toward defects of these processes will continually improve.

REFERENCES

1. Hull MGR, Glazeuer CMA, Kelly NJ, et al: Population study of causes, treatment, and outcome of infertility. *Br Med J* 291:1693, 1985.
2. Overstreet JW, Katz DF: Semen analysis. *Urol Clin North Am* 441:449, 1987.
3. Lipshultz LI: Algorithms for the management of abnormal patterns by the semen analysis, in Lipshultz LI, Howards SS (eds): *Infertility in the Male*. London, Churchill Livingstone, 1983, p. 194.
4. Batzofin JH, Marrs RP, Serafini PC, Lipshultz LI: Assisted reproductive treatments for male factor infertility. *Probl Urol* 1:430, 1987.
5. Smith D, Rodriguez-Rigau LJ, Steinberger E: Relation between indices of semen analysis and pregnancy rate in infertile couples. *Fertil Steril* 28:1314, 1977.
6. Hanada A, Chang MC: Penetration of zona-free eggs by spermatozoa of different species. *Biol Reprod* 6:300, 1972.
7. Vanagimachi R: Penetration of guinea pig spermatozoa into hamster eggs in vitro. *J Reprod Fertil* 28:477, 1972.
8. Barros C, Leal J: In vitro fertilization and its use to study gamete interactions, in Hafez ESE, Semm K (eds): *In Vitro Fertilization and Embryo Transfer*. Lancaster, MTP Press, 1982, p. 37.
9. Yanagimachi R: Mechanisms of fertilization of mammals, in Mastrioianni L, Biggers JD (eds): *Fertilization and Embryonic Development In Vitro*. New York, Plenum Press, 1981, p. 81.
10. Moore HDM, Bedford JM: The interaction of mammalian gametes in the female, in Hartmen JF (ed): *Mechanism and Control of Animal Fertilization*. New York, Academic Press, 1983.
11. Overstreet JW, Yanagimachi R, Katz DF, et al: Penetration of human spermatozoa into the human zona pellicuda and zona-free hamster egg—a study of fertile donors and infertile patients. *Fertil Steril* 33:534, 1980.
12. Barros C, Gonzalez J, Herrera E, et al: Human sperm penetration into zona-free hamster oocyte as a test to evaluate the sperm fertilizing ability. *Andrologia* 11:197, 1979.
13. Rudak E, Jacobs PA, Yanagimachi R: Direct analysis of the chromosome constitution of human spermatozoa. *Nature* 274:911, 1978.
14. Johnson AR, Syms AJ, Lipshultz LI, et al: Conditions influencing human sperm capacitation and penetration of zona-free hamster ova. *Fertil Steril* 41:603, 1984.
15. Rogers BJ, Perrearlt S, Bentwood BJ, et al: Variability in the human-hamster ova in vitro assay for fertility evaluation. *Fertil Steril* 39:204, 1983.
16. Syms AJ, Johnson AR, Lipshultz LI, et al: Effect on aging and cold temperature storage of hamster ova as assessed in the sperm penetration assay. *Fertil Steril* 43:766, 1985.
17. Berger T, Marrs RP, Moyer D: Comparison of techniques for selection of motile spermatozoa. *Fertil Steril* 43:268, 1985.
18. Yee B, Cummings LM, Baxton P, Paulson RI, Marrs RP: Normalization of abnormal sperm penetration assays following treatment with human follicular fluid. Abstracts of the Pacific Coast Fertility Society, San Diego, 1986.
19. Marrs RP, Serafini PC, Kerin J, et al: Methods utilized to improve gamete efficiency. *NY Acad Sci*, in press.
20. Johnson AR, Lipshultz LI, Smith RG: Thermal shock (370) to spermatozoa stored at 40C optimizes capacitation. *J Urol* 133:74, 1985.
21. Kerin J, Serafini P, Quinn P, et al: The effect of maternal age on the pregnancy outcome of IVF and GT procedures. Presented at the 43rd annual meeting of the American Fertility Society, Reno, NV, September 1987.
22. Quigley MM, Sokoloski JE, Withers DM, et al: Simultaneous in vitro fertilization and gamete intrafallopian transfer (GIFT). *Fertil Steril* 47(5):797, 1987.
23. Braeckmans P, Devtocy P, Camus M, et al: Gamete intra-fallopian transfer: evaluation of 100 consecutive attempts. *Hum Reprod* 2:201, 1987.
24. Marrs RP, Quinn P, Brown J, et al: The use of intrauterine insemination for male factor infertility. Presented at the 43rd annual meeting of the American Fertility Society, Reno, NV, September 1987.
25. Kerin J, Quinn P: Washed intrauterine insemination in the treatment of oligospermic infertility semen. *Reprod Endocrinol* 5:23, 1987.
26. Hirsch I, Gibbons WE, Lipshultz LI, et al: In vitro fertilization in the couple with male factor infertility. *Fertil Steril* 45:659, 1986.
27. Cohen J, Edwards R, Fehilly C, et al: In vitro fertilization: A treatment for male infertility. *Fertil Steril* 43:422, 1985.
28. Margalioth EJ, Navot D, Laufer N, et al: Correlation between the zona-free hamster egg sperm penetration assay and human in vitro fertilization. *Fertil Steril* 45:665, 1986.
29. Belkien L, Bordt J, Freishchem CW, et al: Prognostic value of the heterologous ovum penetration test for human in vitro fertilization. *Int J Androl* 8:275, 1985.
30. Rosenwaks Z: In vitro fertilization: the state of the art. Plenary session presentation at the 43rd annual meeting of the American Fertility Society, Reno, NV, September 1987.
31. Marrs RP, Saito H, Yee B, Sata F, Brown J: Effect of variation of in vitro culture techniques upon oocyte fertilization and embryo development in human in vitro fertilization procedures. *Fertil Steril* 41:519, 1984.
32. Gordon JW: Plenary session presentation at the Fifth World Congress on In Vitro Fertilization, Norfolk, VA, April 1987.

CHAPTER 14

Therapeutic Insemination

Randall A. Loy, Machelle M. Seibel

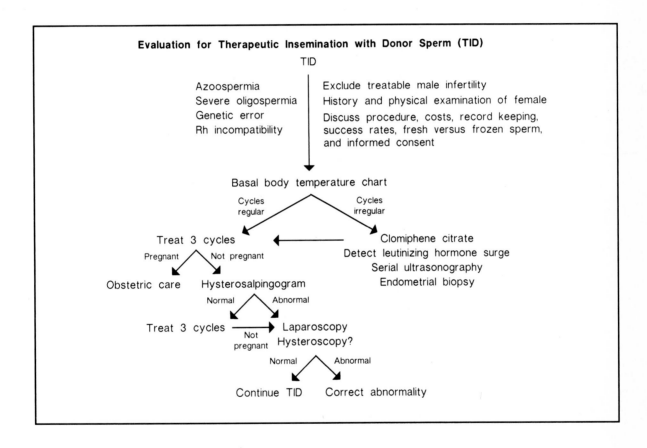

Evaluation for Therapeutic Insemination with Donor Sperm (TID)

Therapeutic insemination has evolved into one of the major treatment modalities of reproductive medicine. In the United States alone, an estimated 30,000 to 60,000 inseminations are performed each year, resulting in 6,000 to 10,000 live births.[1-3] The medicosocial reasons favoring the increasing practice of therapeutic insemination include a marked decrease in the number of adoptable children, later age for attempted conception, a greater number of single women interested in childrearing, wider public acceptance, and the recognition that effective treatment for the infertile male is wanting.

Male factor infertility is rarely appropriately treated with hormonal therapies and empirical medications are not efficacious. Some recent advances, adapted in part from in-vitro fertilization work, provide for laboratory preparation and treatment of subnormal semen and therapeutic insemination with selected populations of husband's sperm (TIH).[4] Although these in-vitro treatments may hold promise for the future, currently available evidence suggests that men with oligozoospermia (reduced number of spermatozoa), asthenospermia, (decreased sperm motility), or teratozoospermia (increased number of

199

spermatozoa with abnormal morphology) often have functional defects as well.[5] Therapeutic insemination by husband, however, has been used with good effect for other indications besides male infertility.

Most insemination procedures, therefore, involve the generally successful therapeutic insemination by donor (TID). The use of donor gametes evokes a number of ethical, legal, psychologic, and social questions, however, and their answers will affect the future directions of human insemination.

HISTORY

John Hunter (1728–1793) is credited with the first therapeutic insemination. Although probably best known for his methods of closing off an aneurysm,[6] Hunter was consulted by a London cloth merchant with hypospadias in the late 1770s. The husband was advised that his ejaculate could be collected in a warmed syringe and desposited into his wife's vagina. It is not certain whether Hunter performed the insemination himself or merely instructed the couple; however, a pregnancy did result.[7,8] Few subsequent cases of homologous insemination are reported in European medical literature until the mid-19th century. In New York City in 1866 J. Marion Sims performed 55 inseminations in 6 women, achieving 1 pregnancy. In each case Sims had as requisites for the procedure perfectly normal semen and an anatomic abnormality of the cervix.[9] He used the postcoital (Sims-Huhner) test in his studies, but the insemination success rate may have been low because he believed that ovulation was coincident with menstruation.

The first insemination by donor was performed by William Pancoast of Jefferson Medical College, Philadelphia, in 1884,[10] but the procedure received little attention in medical publications for more than 50 years until Sophia Kleegman in the United States[11,12] and Margaret Jackson in England[13] worked and wrote extensively on the subject, from the 1930s to the 1960s, and helped the public and medical profession better understand the procedure.

In 1953 Bunge and Sherman reported the first human pregnancies from the use of stored frozen semen,[14] ushering in a new era of infertility treatment. In the 1950s and 1960s the principal concerns regarding donor inseminations were its ethical, legal, and religious aspects. During this time the procedure gained general acceptance and clinically came of age.[15]

The 1970s saw a fourfold increase in demand for donor inseminations secondary to a dramatically changing social climate.[16] With the increased use of the method additional issues surfaced, especially relating to screening and selecting donors. In 1979 the results of a nationwide survey of physicians performing inseminations revealed that the screening of donors for both genetic and sexually transmitted diseases was inadequate. In the same year the American Fertility Society responded to these concerns and established guidelines for donor insemination.[17] Due to heightened awareness of the impact on reproductive medicine of acquired immunodeficiency syndrome (AIDS) and other sexually transmitted diseases, the American Fertility Society updated its guidelines and standards in 1986.[18]

THERAPEUTIC INSEMINATION—HUSBAND

If a nonspecific endoctrine deficiency, anatomic abnormality, or infection cannot be found as the cause of infertility, we prefer the use of therapeutic insemination with the husband's semen (TIH) to empiric endocrine therapy. The paucity of controlled, experimental designs in TIH studies make interpretation of published data difficult. The pregnancy rates achieved are approximately 18 to 20%, which are similar to the spontaneous pregnancy rates reported when oligospermia or poor motility is untreated. Because TIH involves insemination with the husband's semen it is not fraught with the same ethical, legal, and social questions as TID. The frustrated couple feels that something is finally being done. It is important for the couple to understand that, despite a wealth of studies, TIH remains an unproved treatment for male subfertility.[19]

Indications
The indications for homologous insemination may be divided into three major categories, as follows:

1. Demonstrated
   Anatomic defect(s) of the penis
   Retrograde ejaculation
   Ejaculatory or sexual dysfunction of either partner
   Anatomic defects of the vagina
2. Other
   Use of partner's semen after sterilization or death
   Sex selection, for gender or to avoid X-linked genetic diseases
3. Controversial
   Immunologic infertility
   Oligospermia, asthenospermia, or teratozoospermia
   Hostile cervical mucus
   Poor results of postcoital tests

The demonstrated indications are mostly anatomic and psychogenic, and the success rate should approach normal fecundity; no reliable data exist on pregnancy rates for controversial indications.[20] TIH is beneficial when normal coitus and ejaculation cannot take place due to an anatomic defect of the penis, retrograde ejaculation, ejaculatory or sexual dysfunction of either partner, or anatomic defect of the vagina or cervix. Insemination of whole ejaculates is of value in these instances.

In persons with the more controversial indications, the use of a split ejaculate may be beneficial. The first portion of the ejaculate contains the sperm-rich fraction and prostatic fluid. The seminal vesicles contribute most of the remaining ejaculate. The split-ejaculate method provides a specimen of high sperm density and motility. The ejaculate is collected by holding or taping two jars together with the first few drops collected in one jar and the remainder in the other. In 90% of instances the specimen in the first jar is superior, whereas in 5% that in the second jar is superior. In 5% no difference is found between the specimens, and in such instances this method is of no benefit.[21]

Intracervical Techniques

Several variations of TIH exist, and semen may be placed in the vagina, cervix, or uterus. Plastic cervical caps (oligospermia cup, Milex, Chicago) have been used to maintain semen–mucus interaction and to avoid the deleterious side effects of acidic vaginal secretions (Fig. 14–1a).[19] The total semen sample is placed into the cap, which is guided onto the cervix either along a speculum blade or without a speculum by palpation. An attached string protrudes from the vagina. Afterloading caps are also available, which are filled by a syringe through a hollow tube that protrudes from the vagina. The patient removes the cap 2 to 6 hours after the insemination. Because the cap forms suction with the cervix, the patient must reach into her vagina to dislodge it. It is removed easily by pulling on the string or tube, similar to removing a tampon. Patients should be warned that the sperm will rise into the uterus, but seminal plasma, mucus, and occasionally, tinges of blood will come out with the cap. The cap should be rinsed under warm running tap water without using soap, detergents, or antiseptics that could leach into the plastic and harm the sperm at future inseminations.

Inseminations are performed in our clinic in the immediate preovulatory period using fresh husband's semen less than 2 hours old. Speculums are stored on a heating pad to keep them warm; only warm water is used to lubricate them to avoid potential spermicidal effects of lubricants. After the cervix is exposed, packing forceps, Randall stone forceps, or nalsal polyp forceps are used to sample the endocervical mucus. Approximately 0.3 cc of semen is placed into the cervical canal through an acorn-tip cannula (Fig. 14–1b). The cannula is held in place for one minute to ensure adequate sperm–

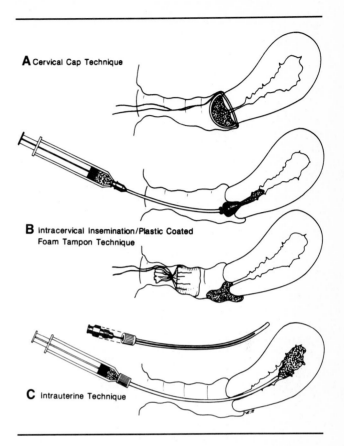

Figure 14–1. A. Plastic cervical cap. **B.** Acorn-tip catheter and syringe, and plastic-covered foam tampon. **C.** Shepard intrauterine catheter.

mucus interaction. By loosening the speculum, the excess semen is inseminated as a pool in the posterior vagina vault that covers the cervical os. The patient remains on the examining table for approximately 10 minutes, after which time a plastic-covered foam tampon (Fig. 14–1b) (Milex) is inserted, more to control leakage than as a fertility aid. The patient is asked to remove the tampon and dispose of it approximately 2 hours later.

Intrauterine Insemination

The condition for which intrauterine insemination (IUI) is most logically indicated is cervical factor due to the inability of sperm to penetrate cervical mucus and traverse the cervical canal.[22] The therapeutic value of IUI as treatment for oligospermia or asthenozoospermia remains inconclusive, largely because most previous studies have failed to control for the confounding variables.[23]

Sperm Preparation. Intrauterine insemination is now performed using various sperm preparations.[24–26] Whole, unwashed ejaculate should not be injected into the uterus, or severe pain or infection may follow. All sperm-preparation techniques attempt to remove prostaglandins and cellular debris from semen and to concentrate the population of highly motile, normal forms. In selecting the preparation method, the characteristics of the individual semen sample must be considered.

The simplest but least selective method of semen preparation is sperm washing. The liquified specimen is diluted with 7 to 10 mL of buffer and the sample is gently centrifuged at 270 to 300 g for 10 minutes. The resultant sperm pellet is resuspended in 0.5 mL buffer for IUI. Sperm washing does eliminate seminal fluid, but the cellular debris, abnormal sperm forms, and immotile sperm that remain are injected along with normal forms. No evidence exists however, that abnormal or immotile forms impair fertilization.

Sperm swim-up techniques prepare samples of highly motile sperm.[27] After one or two sperm washings by certrifugation to remove seminal plasma, the sperm migrate from the pellet into the overlaid diluent and are incubated at 37°C for 30 to 60 minutes. Thereafter, the sperm-rich supernatant containing only the most motile spermatozoa is removed for insemination. This may not be the method of choice for oligospermia, in that the total sperm number may be reduced to 10 to 30% of a fresh specimen,[25,26] and motile sperm are often incorporated into the pellet and unable to swim away.

Modifications of the swim-up technique for oligozoospermic samples include a single wash with lower centrifugation settings for shorter duration, performing swim-up without centrifugation,[28] and centrifuging spermatozoa against a ''soft cushion'' of iodized oil (rather than the centrifuge tube bottom) and then allowing swim-up.[29]

Another relatively common sperm preparation is the Percoll gradient system, which provides better recovery of motile spermatozoa than swim-up. A discontinuous gradient ranging from 30 to 95% Percoll is used, with the most motile sperm able to overcome the increasing concentration gradient. There is essentially a filtering effect, with the best sperm fractions collected after centrifugation.[30,31]

Two alternative methods less commonly employed are filtration through glass wool[32] and swim-up through albumin columns.[33] Both preparations reportedly concentrate viable spermatozoa but with considerable loss of sperm numbers.

Sperm Preparation with Antibiotics. Immunologically, the cervix is the first line of defense of the female genital tract and the site of most antibody activity.[34,35] When this natural barrier is bypassed, as in IUI, the risk of introducing microorganisms into the peritoneal cavity is increased.[36] The use of antibiotics in the media (streptomycin, 6,000 U/100 mL, and penicillin, 12,000 U/100 mL) has been shown to remove microorganisms from human semen when incorporated into sperm washing and swim-up preparations.[37]

Method of IUI. Inseminations are performed at the time of expected ovulation as predicted by basal body temperature graphs, radioimmunoassay (RIA) for luteinizing hormone (LH), or monoclonal antibody assay kits for urinary LH.[38] The importance of accurately timing the procedure with ovulation cannot be overemphasized because it bypasses the sperm reservoir function of the cervix. Spermatozoa from oligozoospermic males may be functionally suboptimal and their survival within the uterus may be compromised.

The 0.3 mL of prepared suspension (not whole ejaculate) is drawn into a tuberculin syringe and the syringe attached to a catheter. We prefer either a Shepard intrauterine catheter (Fig. 14–1c) (Cook Ob-Gyn, Spencer, IN) or a Tom Cat Catheter (Monoject Sherwood Medical, St. Louis, MO). The cervix is visualized using a speculum and the ectocervix is cleansed with a clean, dry, cotton ball. The catheter is then passed into the fundus and the suspension slowly injected. After the intrauterine catheter is removed the patient remains supine for approximately 10 minutes and is then free to leave with no restrictions on activity.

Complications of IUI

Several complications are possible when sperm are placed directly into the uterine cavity, such as vasomotor symptoms (from seminal plasma prostaglandins in the sperm preparation), pelvic infection, and development of antisperm antibodies. In our experience, severe uterine contractions and other vasomotor symptoms have been rare with washed or prepared samples. These reactions are far more likely to be seen with overzealous intracervical injection of aliquots of whole unprepared ejaculate.

The infection rate has been extremely low in our program and in the experience of others.[26] If either partner has a known pelvic infection, systemic antibiotics are administered prior to commencing IUI. Sperm washing and swim-up with antibiotics decreases the likelihood of infection,[37] even in the usual case of the overtly uninfected male partner. We do not, however, administer prophylactic systemic antibiotics with IUI.

The third possible complication is at present theoretical. Intrauterine insemination may increase exposure to sperm antigens and result in sensitization and antisperm antibody formation. For this reason, if pregnancy has not resulted within 4 to 6 IUI treatment cycles, other modalities should be considered, assuming absence of pelvic pathology. The risk of antibody formation may be increased with trauma associated with the insemination procedure itself,[22] allowing direct exposure of sperm antigens to the circulation.

Results of TIH

The interpretation of TIH results is hampered by the lack of controls and standards in generating and reporting these data. Some generalizations may be made on the efficacy of homologous insemination by dividing the published series into insemination type (nonintrauterine, intrauterine) and then according to the indication for the procedure.

Nonintrauterine TIH. Thirteen reports of nonintrauterine TIH for oligozoospermia published since 1960 were reviewed (Table 14–1).[19] Oligozoospermia was defined as a concentration of sperm less than 20 million/mL. In this series of 419 total couples the combined pregnancy rate was 16%.

Excluding two studies in which oligozoospermic whole ejaculates were inseminated intravaginally, the combined pregnancy rate for cervical insemination (intracervical injection or cervical cap using whole or split ejaculate) was approximately 17%. In this series of oligozoospermic couples, intracervical insemination using whole ejaculates of washed sperm yielded 6 pregnancies in 29 couples (21%)[39,40] and 8 in 37 couples (22%).[41] The spontaneous pregnancy rate in six series was 14% compared to 18% for treated couples.

Cervical factor infertility, defined in most TIH studies as poor results of postcoital tests, does not respond well to nonintrauterine TIH. Postcoital tests are difficult to quantify and the results may be "poor" on the basis of few progressively motile spermatozoa or poor quality of mucus. Six published trials involv-

TABLE 14–1. REPORTED RESULTS OF TIH FOR OLIGOZOOSPERMIA

Method	No. of Patients	Pregnant No. (%)
Split ejaculate	10	4 (40)
Cervical cap	14	5 (36)
Pooled frozen semen intravaginal	4	1 (25)
Intracervical, whole ejaculate	22	5 (23)
Split ejaculate	17	4 (23)
Intracervical, washed sperm	37	8 (22)
Pooled and frozen	155	27 (17)
Split ejaculate	7	1 (14)
Cervical cap	82	10 (12)
Split ejaculate	13	1 (8)
	34	2 (6)
Caffeine added to semen intravaginal, whole ejaculate	20	0 (0)

From Bunge and Sherman.[19] Reproduced with permission.

ing 192 couples reported a 12% pregnancy rate.[19] If two older reports involving several insemination methods[42,43] are excluded from this series of six works, 16 pregnancies were achieved in 55 couples, resulting in a 29% pregnancy rate.

Intrauterine TIH. A review[26] of IUI examined data for various forms of male infertility and noted a 25% pregnancy rate per couple. Another review of IUI in 261 couples with male factor infertility revealed a 17% pregnancy rate. If one combines the data from both of these reviews, the cumulative pregnancy rate per couple is 19%, differing little from the 17% with nonintrauterine insemination or the 14% background pregnancy rate reported by Nachtigall.[19] Results improve when intrauterine TIH is performed for cervical factor infertility.[4,24,26] The summarized results of three reviews reveal a combined pregnancy rate of 36% of 281 cases.

The role of IUI for immunologic infertility has not been elucidated fully. In the male with antisperm antibodies, current IUI preparation techniques may not prevent antibody binding from seminal or prostate fluids.[44] In the female, sperm antibodies may be present in the serum and diffuse into reproductive tract fluids or be synthesized by reproductive epithelia.[45] Intrauterine insemination bypasses the cervix, but the antigen–antibody reactions in the uterus, fallopian tubes, or fluid transudate cannot be eliminated.[22] Investigations involving IUI for immunologic infertility[46,47] have involved small numbers of patients, and results have been disappointing with a single exception[48] in which couples with either male or female serum sperm-agglutinating antibodies showed 25 and 40% pregnancy rates, respectively.

Idiopathic infertility may be an indication for IUI. In the majority of couples with unexplained infertility spontaneous pregnancies do tend to occur within 7 to 9 years, suggesting not infertility but reduced fertility.[49–51] An investigation of 36 couples diagnosed with unexplained infertility hypothesized that IUI with washed sperm would shorten the time interval for conception to occur.[52] Eight pregnancies (22% pregnancy rate) resulted during 117 treatment cycles, with a 6.8% pregnancy rate per cycle. This rate is statistically higher than anticipated from the spontaneous pregnancy rate during the 6 cycles of the study.

Ovulation induction with clomiphene citrate or human menopausal gonadotropins (HMG) may increase the effectiveness of IUI performed for oligoasthenozoospermia or unexplained infertility.[53] Among 49 couples with oligoasthenozoospermia who underwent superovulation, intrauterine inseminations were compared with intracervical inseminations.[54] Pregnancy occurred in seven patients having IUI (14.3%) and one with intracervical insemination

(2.0%). Untreated controls were not included. The conception rate may be increased after use of ovulation-induction agents by recruiting a greater number of oocytes for fertilization. In a controlled investigation of pharmacologic ovulation induction,[55] 17 infertile couples with either long-standing idiopathic or male-related infertility were studied after the administration of clomiphene citrate and purified follicle-stimulating hormone (FSH). Ten couples (58.8%) achieved pregnancy within 6 months of treatment; this was significantly higher than the rate obtained in 120 controls who underwent TIH either during normal cycles or after ovulation induction with clomiphene alone.

One review of IUI[26] found a mean of 3.3 cycles per conception, not unlike the experience of other investigations.[56-58] This review also reported 26% (25/96) spontaneous abortions among IUI-associated gestations. Two other studies reported spontaneous abortions of 50[59] and 12.5%[57] among TIH pregnancies. A relatively high rate of abortions is typical of an infertile population, and may reflect a combination of the early biochemical diagnosis of pregnancy, advanced maternal age, or fertilization with morphologically subnormal sperm, although other factors may play a role as well.

In summary, therapeutic insemination using husband's semen has various indications, some with demonstrated success and others more controversial. Male-related infertility is the most common reason that couples receive therapeutic insemination, but results are not high using either intracervical or intrauterine TIH. In fact, pregnancy rates with TIH have been little better than background pregnancy rates. Ovulation induction and IUI with homologouos sperm may hold some promise in oligoasthenozoospermia, but IUI seems best suited for anatomic or psychogenic abnormalities, or for cervical factor infertility. If no pregnancy is achieved after 4 to 6 timed cycles of TIH, other fertility treatment modalities should be considered.

TIH for Gender Selection

Historically, cultural and religious writings have suggested various manipulations of coital techniques to influence the sex of offspring. In 5th-century B.C. Greece, Anaxagoras proposed that males originated from the right testis and females from the left, and that to ensure a male heir one should tie off the left testicle.[60] Contemporary lay publications describe adjusting vaginal alkalinity or acidity and regulating the degree of penile penetration.[61] Two excellent recent reviews [62,63] of the "science" of human gender selection reveal that this body of literature is not scientific. Rather, it is both inconclusive and contradictory.

Although parents' preference for a child of a particular sex receives much discussion, approxi-

mately 200 sex-linked genetic diseases have been described,[64] representing definite medical reasons for gender selection. Among these diseases are various muscular dystrophies, hemophilia, and glucose-6-phosphate dehydrogenase deficiency. Most couples who desire an infant of a particular sex, however, do not seek medical consultation for genetic indications, but rather to complete their families according to their ideals of both number and gender of children.

In 1968 quinacrine mustard fluorescent staining provided a method to detect the human Y chromosome in nondividing nuclei.[65] Since that time numerous efforts to separate X and Y-bearing human spermatozoa have been made using gel filtration,[66] passage through mucus[67] or albumin,[68] electrophoresis,[69] and centrifugation techniques.[70,71] Two methods that have enjoyed the greatest success are the albumin gradient technique[68] for Y-sperm enrichment, and the sephadex G-50 gel chromatography approach for concentrating X-bearing sperm.[72] These methods have led to rates of approximately 75% male and female infants, respectively.[62] The procedures are time consuming and labor intensive, with recovery of approximately 10 to 15% of the initial motile sperm population by the former technique and 30 to 40% of the initial motile sperm by the latter. Patients who choose these techniques must be advised that results cannot be guaranteed. Fortunately, because the gender of choice occurs naturally in 50% of instances, no more than 50% of couples are disappointed.

THERAPEUTIC INSEMINATION—DONOR

Indications

Donor insemination has become a widely accepted form of treatment. A survey on the practice of donor insemination in the United States revealed that in over 95% of respondents' practices, the primary reason for therapeutic insemination by donor was infertility of the husband. The second most common reason was to avoid possible transmissions of genetic disease (especially Rh-factor incompatibility, cystic fibrosis, diabetes mellitus, hemophilia, Huntington's disease, muscular dystrophy, and Tay-Sachs disease), and third was for single women to have a biologic child.

The American Fertility Society's newest guidelines list the following indications for TID: irreversible azoospermia; sterility because of vasectomy, disease, or exposure to radiation or chemicals; oligospermia or seminal fluid abnormalities; a known hereditary or genetic disorder; noncorrectable ejaculatory dysfunction; and Rh incompatibility in the face of severe Rh isoimmunization.[18] Single women may also be candidates.[73] Social demography suggests movement away from the traditional two-parent family, with nearly half of all children living in a one-parent family before reaching age 18 years. One report proposed that programs refusing therapeutic insemination to single women may do so on an unfounded basis, for children in single-parent families have appropriate gender identity, gender role behavior, and sexual partner preference, and do not appear to be measureably psychologically damaged by the absence of a father.[74] Obviously, however, many legal, moral, regional, and even predjudicial factors must be considered to determine the appropriateness of TID for single women. Longer-term studies will also be required.

Psychologic Aspects of TID

Infertility is generally perceived by the couple as an enormous emotional strain. Surprise, denial, anger, isolation, guilt, and grief are confronted as they attempt to work through the problem.[75] When, after extensive investigation of infertility the couple is offered the option of donor insemination or adoption, the male often perceives himself to have "failed," and an identity crisis often follows.[76] Both sexual adequacy and concept of wholeness are challenged, and the couple is forced to confront the emotional trauma of personal loss. In light of a Western culture that emphasizes the concept of the "whole man," as well as familial and social expectations of the husband as father, the potential for feelings of guilt, anger, frustration, and despair clearly exists. If questions of sexual and personal inadequacy remain unresolved, martial strife and divorce may result.

The physician who pronounces the verdict of irreversible infertility bears a heavy responsibility to provide help in order to enable the couple to come through the painful process of adapting to a new form of identity.[76] Only after the partners have had an appropriate opportunity to work through the psychosocial dilemma should therapeutic insemination commence. Ethical and social questions often arise: Is it a sin? What will people think? Who should we tell? Will we be able to live with our sense of honesty if we do not tell? Does the resulting child deserve to know? What if the child is mentally or physically handicapped?

As the inseminations are performed, the woman may feel the intrusion of an unknown other into boundaries of self, a violation of "me" and "mine" potentially perceived as somewhere between a desired sexual experience and rape.[77] This can be prevented to some extent by telling the man that he is welcome to be present during the inseminations. Nevertheless, as many as one fourth of women in TID programs become anovulatory and experience decreased luteal function, which probably reflects the emotional impact on the menstrual cycle in these patients.[76,78]

It is of paramount importance that couples who select TID be encouraged to communicate openly with each other, to reflect introspectively, and to ventilate appropriately with psychiatrists, psychologists, or other counselors. The gynecologist must remain sensitive to the emotion-laden issues of TID, counsel patients about the questions likely to surface during treatment, and, when appropriate, refer the couple to a mental health professional.

Donor Selection and Screening

Donors for therapeutic insemination programs should ideally have proved fertility and excellent health, and be free of genetic abnormalities. The majority of donors tend to be students in the health sciences who are usually unmarried, middle-class, and white, 20 to 27 years of age, and who have been through a health and intelligence examination.[1] The use of younger donors reduces the risks of age-related hazards,[18] although in some instances older donors are used. Semen values judged as normal include volume of 2 mL or greater, greater than 60% motility (moving actively in purposeful direction), motility of 60 million/mL or greater, and 60% or more normal oval forms.[18]

A complete medical history should be obtained from each prospective donor. Careful questioning must be performed to exclude a history of hereditary, systemic, and mental diseases. A thorough sexual history should be obtained, and potential donors excluded if they have had any homosexual contact since 1978, if they have any other risk for AIDS such as a recent transfusion, or have recently had several sexual partners. Physical examination of the genitalia should optimally be performed by the physician group that performs the inseminations.

Many sexually transmitted organisms may be found in semen, and screening procedures to detect these agents have not been standardized.[79] Potential laboratory screening of prospective donors for sexually transmitted diseases (STDs) includes serologic tests for syphilis, serum hepatitis B surface antigen (HBsAg), urethral cultures for *Neisseria gonorrhoeae*, mycoplasma, and *Chlamydia trachomatis*, serum antibody tests for cytomegalovirus CMV, and serum screening for human immunodeficiency virus (HIV) antibodies. A suggested screening protocol for STDs[80] is as follows:

I. First visit
   A. Excluded by history
      1. Homosexual contact since 1978
      2. Parenteral drug abuse since 1978
      3. Hemophiliae
      4. From country with predominant heterosexual transmission of AIDS
      5. Sexual partner in AIDS risk group since 1978

6. More than one sexual partner within preceding 6 months
7. History of STD and related infections within preceding 6 months, including gonorrhea, nongonococcal urethritis, chlamydial infection, epididymitis, prostatitis, genital ulcer, syphilis, and hepatitis
8. Past history of genital herpes, genital warts, or chronic hepatitis, or prior exclusion from blood donation because of an infection
9. Current sexual partner with STD

B. If history negative, obtain CMV serology; if history positive, defer donation

II. Second visit (CMV serologic test negative)
A. Physical examination to exclude
1. Urethral discharge
2. Evidence of genital warts
3. Genital ulcers
B. If physical examination is negative, perform urethral culture for
1. N. gonorrhoeae
2. C. trachomatis
3. Optional
   a. Trichomonas vaginalis
   b. Ureaplasma urealyticum, Mycoplasma hominis, group B streptococci
C. Serology
1. HIV (AIDS virus)
2. HBsAg
3. Serologic test for syphilis (e.g., VDRL)
4. Optional: HSV-2
Accept donor if all results negative

III. Surveillance and follow-up
A. Exclude or discontinue donors: new acquisition of STD (e.g., genital warts, genital ulcers, urethritis)
B. New sexual partner: break in monogamy, break in abstinence
C. Rescreen donors at least every 6 months

A CMV-seronegative woman who receives semen containing CMV is at risk of transmitting the virus to the fetus and causing severe congenital infection. A CMV-positive woman may be susceptible to a heterologous strain of CMV. Therefore, it is maybe safest to use CMV-seronegative donors for all recipients, regardless of the recipient's serologic status.[80]

The human immunodeficiency virus was transmitted during therapeutic insemination to 4 of 8 patients who received semen from a single, asymptomatic, bisexual man.[81] Among the recipients of this donor, 4 had seroconversion from frozen semen stored for 1 to 4 months and none from semen stored for 16 to 17 months. Although other reports suggest that transmission of HIV by TID using fresh sperm is far less likely than predicted in the previous report,

every potential donor must initially be screened for HIV using an enzyme-linked immunosorbent assay (ELISA) for AIDS virus antibody. A positive assay should be confirmed by western blot analysis. If the results are positive, the potential donor should be excluded form the program; if they are negative the donor should be screened at least every 6 months. Because of the possibility that the patient or her partner could be HIV positive and could later suggest that the transmission occurred due to TID, we now routinely screen all patients for HIV prior to initiating therapy. Using these guidelines greatly reduces the potential risks associated with fresh semen. Because seroconversion can occur in the time interval between the screening of donors, however, the only way to ensure absolutely that donated semen is risk free is by using frozen sperm.[82] The potential donor should be screened for HIV prior to providing an initial specimen and again 60 to 90 days after donation. Interim semen samples should be used only if both results are negative. Tests for HBsAg, and urethral cultures for gonorrhea and chlamydia, should be repeated every 6 months.

Number of Pregnancies per Donor

A 1979 national survey of therapeutic insemination practice[1] revealed that most (77.1%) respondents had never used a donor for more than 6 pregnancies, whereas 5.7% had used a donor for 15 or more. The American Fertility Society recommended that the same donor not be used for more than 10 offspring,[73] although the limit could probably safely be placed somewhat higher.[4] With the wide geographic distribution of the 6,000 to 10,000 TID pregnancies per year,[1] the mobility of the American population, and the high frequency of matings across ethnic groups, unplanned consanguinity should occur exceedingly infrequently.[82] The risk of inbreeding increases, of course, as a single donor makes a large contribution to a fixed, local ethnic community.

Genetic Screening

Whether a complete chromosomal analysis should be performed on all prospective donors to exclude balanced translocations, inversions, or low-level aneuploidy remains controversial.[83] Although karyotyping each possible donor is not thought to be an absolute requirement, a detailed family history including specific inquiry about the physical and mental health of all first, second, and third-degree relatives is essential. Mediterranean races should ideally be tested for beta-thalassemia, Ashkenazi Jews for Tay-Sachs disease, blacks for sickle cell anemia and beta-thalassemia, and Asians for α-thalassemia. The donor and his family should also be free of multifactorial, chromosomal, and mendelian disorders.

Personality Screening

Physical matching of donors to husbands is attempted in nearly all TID programs; however, psychosocial characteristics are usually not matched and often not recorded.[1] Personality profiles in a group of 75 sperm donors were assessed using the Cattell 16PF test, and this population was quite distinct in some personality traits from the general community.[84] The donors were distinguished from the background community by features of intelligence, willingness to take risks, and boldness. The distinctions presumably reflect the donors' self-selection for the ability and desire to perform a task that is socially useful but not fully sanctioned. Donors who are in any way uncomfortable with TID, or who demonstrate qualities that to any extent alert the screening physician of a potential personality flaw, should simply not be used.

Evaluation of the Couple

When couples elect TID, it is helpful to have a standard presentation that overlooks none of the necessary information and details. The couple must be seen together at first to ensure that both partners are in agreement that TID is an acceptable form of treatment and that the decision is comfortable for them. It also conveys that they are being treated and that the man remains part of the process. Open dialogue with him must take place to ensure that he does not have a treatable cause for infertility. Because TID is often performed for oligospermia and not azoospermia, the options of TIH and in-vitro fertilization or gamete intrafallopian transfer should be raised if appropriate.

Once it is determined that TID will be employed, the couple should be told that thousands of children are born annually as a result of this procedure. A description of the technique should follow, including the method of timing the treatments, whether one or two inseminations per month will be used, and who other than the physician might be performing the inseminations (having several individuals perform the procedure increases the stress for some patients). Scheduling guidelines are also important; couples should be reassured that the physician has office hours on at least one weekend day in order to cover ovulation.

Couples should be told how donors are selected and who selects them. A discussion of fresh versus frozen sperm and their effectiveness follows. The discussion also should fully cover the potential costs, as most insurance companies do not cover TID. It is helpful for patients to be told anticipated time intervals for conception to occur. Finally, they should be informed as to how records are kept.

Evaluation of the female recipient involves a detailed medical and reproductive history and comprehensive physical examination. The American Fertility Society also recommends obtaining rubella titers (and rubella vaccination if antibody titers are not

TABLE 14-2. NEWER METHODS OF TIMING AND PREDICTING OVULATION

Product	Function	Time	Cost ($)	Manufacturer and Telephone Number
Thermometers				
Terumo	Digital BBT	60 sec	32.95	Terumo (301)398-8500
Cue	Oral sensor/vaginal probe measures changes in saliva, vaginal secretions	10 sec	300-700 rent 68/mo	Zetek (303)343-2122
Fertil-A-Chron	Computerized digital thermometer with memory	45 sec	95	Fertil-A-Chron (516)435-0913
Urine Test Kits				
First Response	1st morning urine, ovulation 12-24 hrs	30 min	30-40	Tambrands Inc (516)437-8800
Uvu Stick	Midafternoon urine, ovulation 24-36 hrs	30 min	60, 9 day 45, 6 day	Monoclonal Antibodies (800)227-8855
Quidel	Morning urine, repeat throughout day	35 min	30	Quidel (619)450-1533
Ramp	1st morning urine days 7,8,9 after LH surge to measure progesterone, quality of ovulation	5 min	115-140	Monoclonal Antibodies (800)227-8855
Clearplan	1st morning urine, ovulation 24-36 hrs (10-day test)	30 min	40-45	Unipath Ltd. (800)223-2329 In California (800)222-2329

present), a serologic test for syphilis, as well as serum testing for HBsAg, and HIV antibody (ELISA). Cultures for gonorrhoea and chlamydia should be taken from the cervix, and finally, antibody testing for CMV should be obtained. If the recipient is CMV seronegative, only CMV-negative donors should be used.

The timing of ovulation should be documented. Although several methods can be employed, including LH surge (radioimmunoassay or monoclonal home LH kit) (Table 14–2) with or without ultrasonographic monitoring of follicular maturation,[18] we prefer to use a basal body temperature (BBT) chart because it is inexpensive and reliable. Patients with irregular cycles should be administered clomiphene citrate in order to time insemination treatments better. Reproductive abnormalities detected during evaluation of the recipient should be fully explored and treated as necessary before beginning inseminations. Conversely, patients with a totally negative history and a perfectly regular cycle may be started almost at once with little or no evaluation.

Matching Donors and Recipients

Many clinics match donors to recipients by race, Rh factor, and unusual features of height and coloring. This can be achieved either by a detailed written physical charaterization or by taking a picture of each patient. The physical description or photograph should be placed in the patient's file. It should also be understood that although every effort will be made to match all desired characteristics, a donor is unlikely to represent a mirror image of the patient's partner.

Legal Aspects

The woman who undergoes TID should be informed of the indications, the nature of the procedure, the risks, and treatment alternatives.[85] Her partner's consent is required if he is to be legally recognized as the father and if he is to have the rights and responsibilities of parenthood. Currently, 29 states have statutes on the subject of donor insemination that make the consenting husband the legal father (Table 14–3). At least 12 states mandate that the executed consent be filed with a record-keeping body.

A donor consent form should be signed to affirm the medical, genetic, and sexual history, to maintain confidentiality, to define the terms of donor compensation (if any), to limit liability of the TID program, and to delineate the uses of the donor semen (Fig. 14–2).

Record-Keeping

The American Fertility Society's guidelines for donor insemination[18] suggest that permanent and confidential records, including the medical and genetic workup, be maintained and available on an anony-mous basis to the infertile couple, any resulting offspring, or both. Some state legislatures have proposed a more standardized medical record system for third-party reproduction, with recommendations for medical information disclosure similar to the above guidelines.[86] It is our practice to destroy all records after 1 year to ensure confidentiality and to prevent either the donor seeking out any resultant offspring or the reverse. Because only donors with a negative medical and genetic history are used, we feel that providing medical data about them is unnecessary. Furthermore, we believe that anonymity is one of the most important requisites of this procedure.

Techniques of TID

Insemination technique is as described for intracervical TIH. Approximately 0.3 cc of semen is placed just inside the external cervical os through a syringe–cannula. The excess semen flows into a vaginal pool. The speculum is loosened and the patient remains in a modified lithotomy position for approximately 10 minutes with the cervix in contact with the posterior vaginal seminal pool. A plastic-covered sponge tampon is inserted to prevent leakage, and the patient is released immediately thereafter. Studies suggest that time spent in lithotomy position after insemination, and the use of tampons, do not appear significantly to affect pregnancy outcome.[87]

Most physicians inseminate patients two times per cycle (61.4%), while others do so either three times (20.5%), or only once (17%). The success rates are independent of the number of times women are inseminated in a given cycle and the timing with which inseminations are spaced.[1] Others[88,89] support a schedule of two inseminations 2 days apart per treatment cycle as superior to a single insemination each month. The use of three or four inseminations did not measurably increase the success rate. Conception is more likely to occur when insemination is performed on or before the ovulatory day rather than after it.[90] This underscores the importance to the success of an insemination program of accurately predicting the day of ovulation.

When TID (or TIH) is to be employed in a gonadotropin-stimulated cycle, the timing of insemination is based on ultrasonographic monitoring of follicles, and measuring serum estradiol and LH values, similar to in-vitro fertilization. In the super-ovulated cycle, insemination should be within 12 to 24 hours after administration of human chorionic gonadotropin.[91]

If several inseminations are performed within a treatment cycle, the same donor should be used for each one. Although perhaps logistically more demanding, this decreases variables of uncertainty and allows for more straightforward record-keeping and

TABLE 14-3. SPERM DONATION LAWS BY STATE

State	Written Consent of Husband Required	Artificial Insemination Laws Make Consenting Husband the Legal Father	Donor is Not the Legal Father	Carriers of Venereal Disease or Genetic Defects Cannot Be Sperm Donors	Physician Required to File Information with State About TID	Provisions for Confidentiality
Alabama	X	X	X		X	X
Alaska	X	X				
Arizona						
Arkansas	X	X				
California	X	X	X		X	
Colorado	X	X	X		X	X
Connecticut	X	X	X		X	X
Delaware						
District of Columbia						
Florida	X	X				
Georgia		X				
Hawaii						
Idaho	X	X	X	X	X	X
Illinois	X	X	X			X
Indiana						
Iowa						
Kansas	X	X			X	X
Kentucky						
Louisiana	X	X				
Maine						
Maryland		X				
Massachusetts						
Michigan		X				
Minnesota	X	X	X		X	X
Mississippi						
Missouri						
Montana	X	X	X		X	X
Nebraska						
Nevada	X	X	X		X	X
New Hampshire						
New Jersey	X	X	X		X	X
New Mexico	X	X	X		X	X
New York	X	X		X(NYC)		
North Carolina	X	X				
North Dakota						
Ohio						
Oklahoma	X	X			X	X
Oregon	X	X	X	X	X	X
Pennsylvania						
Rhode Island						
South Carolina						
South Dakota						
Tennessee		X				
Texas	X	X	X			
Utah						
Vermont						
Virginia	X	X				
Washington	X	X	X		X	X
West Virginia						
Wisconsin	X	X	X		X	X
Wyoming	X	X	X		X	X

From Handelsman et al.[54] Reproduced with permission.

We_____and_____
authorize Dr._____and his/her designated associates and
assistants to perform one or more therapeutic insemination(s) on the women, with the sperm
obtained from an anonymous donor(s) for the purpose of achieving pregnancy.

We agree to rely on the judgment and discretion of the physicians to select an appropriate
donor(s), and we will never seek to identify the donor(s), nor will the donor(s) be advised of
the identity of either partner. We understand and agree that it cannot be guaranteed that
the same donor will be utilized for each insemination although every attempt will be made
to do so. We also understand that unless otherwise specified that frozen sperm will be used.

There is no guarantee that these inseminations will result in a pregnancy. Furthermore,
within the normal human population a certain percentage (approximately 3%) of children are
born with a physical or mental defect and that the occurrence of such defects is beyond the
control of physicians, and their associates and assistants do not assume responsibility for the
physical and mental characteristics of any child or children born as a result of donor
insemination. Therapeutic insemination carries with it a small risk of infection. Although
donors are regularly screened by blood tests and cultures, infections may occur that are
beyond the control of the physician.

Although therapeutic insemination places you at no more risk than the general population,
any pregnancy carries with it the possibility of spontaneous abortion (miscarriage), ectopic
pregnancy, or obstetric complications.

Signature of partners

_____

_____

Date of consent_____

Witnessed by_____

Date_____

I hereby certify that_____and_____,
known to me to be the individuals named herein, appeared before me and signed the above
consent to therapeutic insemination by donor.

Physician_____

Figure 14–2. Consent form for TID.   Date_____

interpretation of program results. Mixing donor semen with husband's semen is also to be discouraged as the husband's seminal fluid may cause agglutination of, or immobilize, donor spermatozoa.[92] In addition, sexual abstinence for 2 days prior to TID may lead to significantly improved fecundity, which is another reason not to mix semen.[93] Although semen mixing has been used to facilitate acceptance of TID by some couples,[94] it is both preferable and advisable to explore any emotional uncertainty in this area on the part of the couple prior to proceeding with donor insemination.

Results

Two distinct subpopulations of infertility are represented in any donor insemination program: women whose partners are azoospermic who have normal fecundity, and those whose partners are oligospermic who have subnormal fertility. The pregnancy rate in the former group is significantly higher (70%) than in the latter (48.8%). One must assume that this latter group is relatively hypofertile, because the women with high fertility have probably already been removed by spontaneous conception after prolonged exposure.[95] Alternatively, substances present in the seminal plasma or in the sperm of subfertile men may have initiated sperm antibody formation.

The success rate with TID has an approximate range of 40 to 85% and a mean of 70 to 75% (Table 14–4).[11,76,90,96–106] When reviewing success rates of insemination programs, there are several sources of variability: (1) differences in the methods of analysis; (2) differences in patient populations; and (3) differences in the technique used.[107] With respect to statistical methodology, studies that employ either life table analysis or the pregnancy rate (for all patients) per cycle of treatment are better than those that use the misleading method of distribution of conceptions by the number of cycles required for conception. The first two data analyses reflect the

TABLE 14–4. RESULTS OF TID USING FRESH SEMEN

Reference	No. of Patients (cycles)	Pregnancy Rate Crude/Corrected (%)	Mean Cycles to Conceive	Abortion (%)	Method
11	116	47/63	2.7	20	Cervical os
97	168	75	--	--	Cervical os/cap
98	219	52/65	3.8	11	Cervical os
99	129	47	3.0	14	Cervical cap
100	107	72/92	3.0	23	Cervical os
101	171	43/76	3.4	20	Cervical cap
102	168	81	3.5	4	Cervical os/cap
103	118	69	3.3	15	Cervical os
75	253(270)	85.2	3.3	16.5	Cervical os/cap
104	226(278)	58.6/82.4	4.9	10.7	Cervical cap
105	103(116)	80	2.3	12.8	Cervical os
106	330(404)	72.7/92.4	3.2	17.4	Cervical os/cap
89	80(90)	58	4.5/3.1	19	Cervical os
107	108(139)	54	5.5	16	Cervical os

Table constructed from Batzer and Corson.[91]

entire experience of the study group, whereas the last skews success rates and prognosis for conception by a certain cycle.[108]

The pattern of conceptions in the donor inseminations series above is remarkably similar in all studies. The majority of women who will become pregnant by TID do so by the end of the sixth cycle (Fig. 14–3). If the patient is entirely healthy (that is, negative results for all fertility tests) and her cycles are very regular, no initial evaluation may be needed. Patients with irregular cycles may require clomiphene citrate in order to schedule inseminations. After 3 months of therapy it is our practice to obtain a hysterosalpingogram. Women who do not conceive after 6 months of treatment should undergo further evaluation.[87] Diagnostic laparoscopy with chromopertubation may be performed. If a surgically correct-able factor is diagnosed and treated, an additional approximately 20% of TID patients may be expected to become pregnant using TID.[87,109] By the twelfth treatment cycle, 94% of TID pregnancies will be achieved.[89] For that reason, some authors have suggested that the most important factor in success with donor insemination is persistence.[93,103]

Fresh Versus Frozen Semen

Semen used for TID may be either fresh or frozen. Frozen semen has several distinct advantages. It may be stored until the presence of sexually transmitted diseases has been ruled out; matching of donors to recipients is easier, and donor logistics are potentially less complicated.[110] The cost of fresh and frozen sperm to the patient is generally comparable. Although several inseminations with the same donor are possible with frozen sperm, specimens often must be shipped by expensive overnight mail. In addition, frozen semen is less likely to result in pregnancy in a comparable period of time.

Pregnancy rates using fresh and frozen semen vary. A 73% success rate was reported using fresh semen as compared with 61% using preserved semen.[111] One group achieved a pregnancy rate of 37% with fresh semen and 20% when random fresh and frozen samples were used.[87] Others found that fresh samples were three times more effective than frozen ones in achieving a pregnancy.[93] In a comparative study in 381 randomly treated patients, the fecundability, or chance of becoming pregnant per cycle of exposure, was 18.9% with fresh and 5% with frozen semen.[112] One must recognize that in these studies, methods of biostatistical analysis, treatment, and populations varied. Nevertheless, the literature supports the general notion that the TID will result in

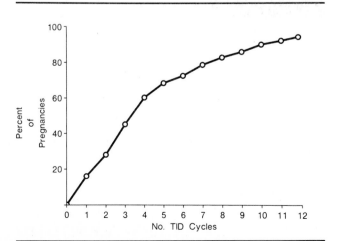

Figure 14–3. TID cumulative success rate.

pregnancy sooner with fresh than with frozen semen.[113]

Relationship of Age, Type of Infertility, and Gravidity to Success

Study population differences represent a major source of variability in published TID investigations; however, it is apparent that success is correlated with patient age, gynecologic abnormalities, and history of previous pregnancy. Advancing patient age has a deleterious effect upon fecundity and fertility (Figs. 14–4 and 14–5). Patients over age 35 have significantly lower rates of conception, require more insemination cycles per conception, and incur a higher frequency of spontaneous abortion.[107] Others [76,106,108,114] substantiate the finding that increasing maternal age is inversely correlated with successful conception. Except as a function of age itself, the duration of infertility probably does not significantly affect the pregnancy rate.[87]

Pelvic disease is a second important prognostic indicator of TID success.[87,106,108,115] The overall rate of success in those with gynecologic disorders other than anovulation (22%) is significantly lower than the rate (70%) in healthy women.[100] Patients not conceiving within 6 months should be strongly suspected of having pelvic adhesions.[109]

Ovulatory disturbances also coincide with a significantly lower pregnancy rate.[76] Approximately 1 in 4 previously ovulatory patients in a donor insemination program will develop secondary anovulation[116] and decreased luteal function.[76,78] It is our impression that this significant phenomenon is so frequent that patients should be warned that it is not

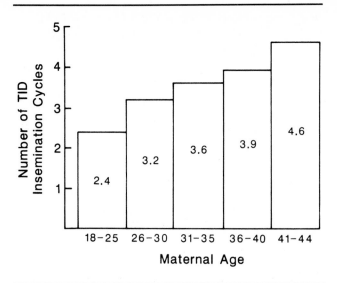

Figure 14–5. Number of cycles of artificial insemination with donor sperm required to conceive based on maternal age.

unusual and is most likely due to the stress associated with beginning TID. Usually the cycles become regular within a few months. Patients who require ovulation-induction therapy have decreased pregnancy rates and high rates of spontaneous abortion.

Patients with a history of a prior pregnancy have a higher TID success rate than those with no such history.[87] In a study of results of TID for first and subsequent pregnancies, the success rate was 54%, as opposed to 44% for patients who had never been pregnant.[117] This positive effect seems to be present whether the prior gestation ended in abortion, ectopic pregnancy, or viability.[106]

Discontinuation of Treatment

Patients with long-standing infertility, those of low socioeconomic status, and women whose husbands demonstrate apparent resistance to TID are significantly most likely to discontinue treatment.[76] Most insemination studies document a decreasing participation rate by couples as treatment periods extend; one report noted a dropout rate of approximately 40% at 3 months and nearly 75% after 6 months.[87] The most common reasons for discontinuing treatment are discouragement, relocation, adoption of a child, marital problems, and other infertility factors.[102,104] Discontinuation is the most common reason for TID failure.

Follow-Up of Pregnancies

Few longitudinal studies exist on the children produced from therapeutic insemination, due probably in large part to the constraints of data collection by questionnaire. It is well known that the obstetric

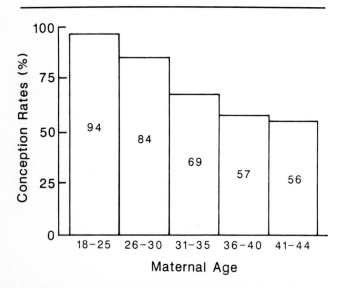

Figure 14–4. Conception rates versus maternal age.

histories closely parallel those of normal pregnancies, with comparable spontaneous abortion rates.[89]

One difference in the obstetric outcome is the possible predominance of male births with insemination. This phenomenon was first documented in 1941 by Seymour and Koerner,[118] who surveyed 30,000 physicians and obtained data on 9,489 women who had conceived with therapeutic insemination. Sixty-one percent (3,569 of 5,840) of successful TIH pregnancies were male infants, while TID accounted for 58% (2,107 of 3,649) male births. A review of nine TID studies[62] also noted a trend toward male offspring.

Above-average physical and mental development was noted in 133 children conceived through TID.[119] Medical students served as donors with semen cryopreserved. The mean intelligence quotient of those children was 112. Others have noted the excellent developmental progress of these children as well as the emotional strengths of the family.[120,121] These are extremely desired children, and the time devoted to them by somewhat more mature, stable parents in an atmosphere of love might well predispose toward better learning habits and thus higher achievement.[89]

Future Directions of Therapeutic Insemination

Therapeutic insemination will undoubtedly continue to evolve along the lines of its present development. The availability of rapid monoclonal antibody-type diagnostic tests for sexually transmitted diseases, including AID, should make the use of fresh semen safer. Procedures to wash and separate sperm developed by in-vitro fertilization laboratories will most likely be increasingly employed in IUI procedures using husband's sperm. These methods will allow for the use of less than optimal semen and perhaps overcome the defects of poor semen specimens. Should cryopreservation media and techniques be improved, frozen semen would gain widespread and instant increased usage. The use of a falloposcope, a flexible and directional fiberoptic scope less than 1 mm in diameter, for transuterine tubal insemination, is foreseen.[23] Other methods, now experimental, such as direct intraperitoneal insemination, may be an alternative for gamete intrafallopian transfer,[122] as may be superovulation with intrauterine insemination.[123]

SUMMARY

Therapeutic insemination has become a widespread and valuable tool in reproductive medicine. Insemination with husband's sperm has few indications for which the results are good, and traditional intracervical TIH for oligospermia, asthenospermia, or teratozoospermia should be viewed with caution. In-

stead, an aggressive approach to IUI with husband's semen appears more efficacious. Sperm washing and preparation with antibiotics, and possibly, superovulation in IUI, may yield higher success rates.

Therapeutic insemination by donor is generally successful and has as its primary indication male infertility. The emotional aspects of TID are pervasive, and educational and psychologic counseling should be part of the treatment protocol. Because of the stress involved, a number of patients develop secondary anovulation and luteal phase defects. Important, however, is the fact that almost all patients conceive as they continue in a TID program.

Donor selection should involve comprehensive screening, especially for genetic and sexually transmitted disease. Potential donors who are at risk for HIV infection by history must be excluded, and follow-up screening should be performed on all donors. Medical records that maintain confidentiality are to be kept on semen donors and TID couples, and state laws observed in reporting third-party pregnancies.

REFERENCES

1. Curie-Cohen M, Luttrell L, Shapiro S: Current practice of artificial insemination by donor in the United States. N Engl J Med 300:585, 1979.
2. Timmons MC, Rao KW, Sloan CS, Kirkman HN, Talbot LM: Genetic screening of donors for artificial insemination. Fertil Steril 35:451, 1981.
3. Stone SC: Complications and pitfalls of artificial insemination. Clin Obstet Gynecol 23:667, 1980.
4. Alexander NJ, Ackerman S: Therapeutic insemination. Obstet Gynecol Clin North Am, in press. 14:4 p. 905, 1988.
5. Mahadevan MM, Trounson AO: Influence of seminal characteristics on success rate of human IVF. Fertil Steril 42:400, 1984.
6. Lyons AS, Petrucelli RJ: Medicine: An Illustrated History. New York, Abrams, 1978, pp 481–482.
7. Siegler SL: Fertility in Women. Philadelphia, Lippincott, 1944, p 403.
8. Schellen AMCM: Artificial Insemination in the Human. Amsterdam, Elsevier, 1957, p 13.
9. Sims JM: Uterine Surgery. New York, William Wood, 1873, p 365.
10. Hard AD: Artificial impregnation. Med World 27:163, 1909.
11. Kleegman SJ: Therapeutic donor insemination. Fertil Steril 5:7, 1954.
12. Arny M, Quagliarello JR: History of artificial insemination: A tribute to Sophia Kleegman, M.D. Semin Reprod Endocrinol 5:1, 1987.
13. Jackson, MCN, Richardson DW: The use of fresh and frozen semen in human artificial insemination. J Biosoc Sci 9:251, 1977.
14. Bunge RG, Sherman JK: Fertilizing capacity of frozen human spermatozoa. Nature 172:767, 1953.
15. Peterson EP: Artificial insemination by donor—A new look. Fertil Steril 46:567, 1986.
16. Jacobsen E: Up 400%: Artificial insemination. Sexual Matters Today, Dec 6, 1976.
17. American Fertility Society: Guidelines for Donor Insemination 1979. Birmingham, AL, American Fertility Society, 1979.
18. American Fertility Society: New guidelines for the use of semen donor insemination: 1986. Fertil Steril 46(suppl):955, 1986.
19. Nachtigall RD: Indications, techniques and success rates for AIH. Semin Reprod Endocrinol 5:5, 1987.
20. American Fertility Society Artificial insemination—husband. Fertil Steril 46(suppl):34S, 1986.
21. Ericsson RJ, Langevin CH, Nishino M: Isolation of fractions rich in human Y sperm. Nature 246:421, 1973.
22. Moghissi KS: Some reflections on intrauterine insemination. Fertil Steril 46:13, 1986.
23. Kerin J, Quinn P: Washed intrauterine insemination in the treatment of oligospermic infertility. Semin Reprod Endocrinol 5(1):23, 1987.

24. Nachtigall RD, Faure N, Glass RH: Artificial insemination of husband's sperm. *Fertil Steril* 32:141, 1979.
25. Kerin JF, Peek J, Warnes GM, et al: Improved conception rate after intrauterine insemination of washed spermatozoa from men with poor quality semen. *Lancet* 1:533, 1984.
26. Allen NC, Herbert CM, Maxson WS, et al: Intrauterine insemination: A critical review. *Fertil Steril* 44:567, 1985.
27. Trounson AO, Moher LR, Wood C, Leeton JF: Effect of delayed insemination on in vitro fertilization, culture and transfer of human embryos. *J Reprod Fertil* 64:285, 1982.
28. Cohen J, Edwards R, Fehilly C, et al: In vitro fertilization: A treatment for male infertility. *Fertil Steril* 43:422, 1985.
29. Makler A, Morillo O, Huszar A, et al: Improved technique for separating motile spermatozoa from human semen. II. An atraumatic centrifugation method. *Int J Androl* 7:71, 1984.
30. Berger T, Marrs RP, Mayer DL: Comparison of techniques for selection of motile spermatozoa. *Fertil Steril* 43:268, 1985.
31. Hyne RV, Stojanoff A, Clarke GN, Lopata A, Johnston WIH: Pregnancy from in vitro fertilization of human eggs after separation of male spermatozoa by density gradient centrifugation. *Fertil Steril* 45:93, 1986.
32. Jeyendran RS, Perez-Pelaez M, Crabo BG: Concentration of viable spermatozoa for artificial insemination. *Fertil Steril* 45:132, 1986.
33. Glass RH, Ericsson RJ: Intrauterine insemination of isolated motile sperm. *Fertil Steril* 29:535, 1978.
34. Joyce D, Vassilopoulos D: Sperm–mucus interaction and artificial insemination. *Clin Obstet Gynaecol* 8:587, 1981.
35. Rebello R, Green FHY: A study of the secretory immune system of the female genital tract. *Br J Obstet Gynaecol* 82:812, 1975.
36. Stove SC, de la Maza LM, Peterson EM: Recovery of microorganisms from the pelvic cavity after intracervical or intrauterine artificial insemination. *Fertil Steril* 46:61, 1986.
37. Wong PC, Balmaceda JP, Blanco JD, Gibbs RS, Asch RH: Sperm washing and swim-up technique using antibiotics removes microbes from human semen. *Fertil Steril* 45:97, 1986.
38. Rodrick-Highberg G, Sapp L, Kasper K, Lakford J: Urinary LH test: Evaluation with clinical specimens. *Fertil Steril* 41:523, 1984.
39. Steiman RP, Taymor ML: AIH and its role in the management of infertility. *Fertil Steril* 28:146, 1977.
40. Taymor ML, Idriss WK: The role of AIH in male subfertility, in Emperaire JC, Audebert A (eds): *First International Symposium on Artificial Insemination Homologous and Male Subfertility.* Bordeaux, France, May 6–7, 1978.
41. Usherwood MMcD, Halim A, Evans PR: Artificial insemination (AIH) for sperm antibodies and oligospermia. *Br J Urol* 48:499, 1976.
42. Guttmacher AF: The role of artificial insemination in the treatment of human sterility. *Bull NY Acad Med* 19:573, 1943.
43. Mastroianni L Jr, Laberge JL, Rock J: Appraisal of the efficacy of artificial insemination with husband's sperm and evaluation of insemination technics. *Fertil Steril* 8:260, 1957.
44. Bronson R, Cooper G, Rosenfeld D: Sperm antibodies: Their role in infertility. *Fertil Steril* 42:171, 1984.
45. Moghissi KS: The function of the cervix in human reproduction. *Curr Probl Obstet Gynecol* 7:1, 1984.
46. Pepperell RJ, McBain JC: Unexplained infertility: A review. *Br J Obstet Gynaecol* 92:569, 1985.
47. Shulman S, Harlin B, Davis P, Reyniak JV: Immune infertility and new approaches to treatment. *Fertil Steril* 29:309, 1978.
48. Confino E, Friberg J, Dudkiewicz AB, Gleicher N: Intrauterine inseminations with washed human spermatozoa. *Fertil Steril* 46:55, 1986.
49. Lenton EA, Weston GA, Cooke ID: Long-term follow-up of the apparently normal couple with complaint of infertility. *Fertil Steril* 28:913, 1977.
50. Dor J, Homburg R, Rabau E: An evaluation of etiologic factors and therapy in 665 infertile couples. *Fertil Steril* 28:718, 1977.
51. Collins JA, Wrixon W, Javes LB, Wilson EH: Treatment-independent pregnancy among infertile couples. *N Engl J Med* 309: 1201, 1983.
52. Makler A: Washed intrauterine insemination in the treatment of idiopathic infertility. *Semin Reprod Endocrinol* 5:35, 1987.
53. Sher G, Knutzen VK, Stratton CJ, Montakhado MM, Allenson SG: In vitro sperm capacitation and transcervical intrauterine insemination for the treatment of refractory infertility: Phase I. *Fertil Steril* 41:260, 1984.
54. Canale D, Fioretti P: Pharmacologic induction of multiple follicular development improves the success rate of artificial insemination with husbands semen in couples with male-related or unexplained infertility. *Fertil Steril* 47:441, 1987.
55. Beck M, Beardsley L, Shelden R: A prospective study of intrauterine insemination of processed sperm from men with oligoasthenospermia in superovulated women. *Fertil Steril* 46:673, 1986.
56. Glezerman M, Bernstein D, Insler V: The cervical factor of infertility and intrauterine insemination. *Int J Fertil* 29:16, 1984.
57. Toffle RC, Nagel TC, Tagatz GE, et al: Intrauterine insemination: The University of Minnesota experience. *Fertil Steril* 43:743, 1985.
58. Huszar G, DeCherney A: The role of intrauterine insemination in the treatment of infertile couple: The Yale experience. *Semin Reprod Endocrinol* 5:11, 1987.
59. Moghissi KS, Gruber JS, Evans S, Yanez J: Homologous artificial insemination: A reappraisal. *Am J Obstet Gynecol* 129:909, 1977.
60. Parkes AS: Mythology of the human sex ratio. *Am Soc Animal Sci:* 38: 1971.
61. Glass RH: Sex preselection: Is it a possibility? *Contemp OB/GYN* 9:99, 1977.
62. Corson SL, Batzer FR: Human gender selection, *Semin Reprod Endocrinol* 5:81, 1987.
63. Batzofin JH: XY sperm separation for sex selection. *Urol Clin North Am* 14:609, 1987.
64. McKusick VA: X-linked phenotypes, in McKusic VA (ed): *Mendelian Inheritance in Man,* ed 5. Baltimore, Johns Hopkins University Press, 1978, p 705.
65. Casperson T, Farber S, Foley GE, et al: Chemical differentiation along metaphase chromosome. *Exp Cell Res* 49:219, 1968.
66. Quinlivan WLG, Preciado K, Long TL, Sullivan H: Separation of human X and Y spermatozoa by albumin gradients and sephadex chromatography. *Fertil Steril* 37:104, 1982.
67. Broer KH, Winkhaus I, Sombroek H, Kaiser R: Frequency of Y-chromatin-bearing spermatozoa in intracervical and intrauterine post coital tests. *Int J Fertil* 21:181, 1976.
68. Ericsson RJ, Langevin CN, Nishino M: Isolation of fractions rich in human Y sperm. *Nature* 246:421, 1973.
69. Sirai M, Matsuda S: Galvanic separation of X- and Y-bearing human spermatozoa. *Jpn J Fertil Steril* 37:104, 1982.
70. Rhode W, Portsmann T, Prehn S, Dorner G: Gravitational pattern of the Y-bearing sperm using Percoll density gradient centrifugation. *Fertil Steril* 40:661, 1983.
71. Kaneko S, Yamaguchi J, Kobayashi T, Iizuka R: Separation of human X- and Y-bearing sperm using Percoll density gradient centrifugation. *Fertil Steril* 40:661, 1983.
72. Steeno O, Adimoelja A, Steeno J: Separation of X- and Y-bearing spermatozoa using the sephadex-gel-filtration method. *Andrologica* 7:95, 1975.
73. American Fertility Society: Ethical considerations of the new reproductive technologies. Artificial insemination—donor. *Fertil Steril* 46:36S, 1986.
74. McGuire M, Alexander NJ: Artificial insemination of single women. *Fertil Steril* 43:182, 1985.
75. Seibel MM, Taymor ML: Emotional aspects of infertility. *Fertil Steril* 37:137, 1982.
76. Glezerman M: Two hundred and seventy cases of artificial donor insemination: Management and results. *Fertil Steril* 35:180, 1981.
77. Harvey B, Harvey A: How couples feel about donor insemination. *Contemp Obstet Gynecol* 49:93, 1977.
78. Vere MF, Joyce DN: Luteal function in patients seeking AID. *Br Med J* 6182:100, 1979.
79. Mascola L, Guinan ME: Screening to reduce transmission of sexually transmitted diseases in semen used for artificial insemination. *N Engl J Med* 314:1355, 1986.
80. Greenblatt RM, Handsfield HH, Sayers MH, Holmes KK: Screening therapeutic insemination donors for sexually transmitted diseases: Overview and recommendations. *Fertil Steril* 46:351, 1986.
81. Stewart GJ, Cunningham AL, Driscoll GL, et al: Transmission of human T-cell lymphotropic virus type III (HTLV-III) by artificial insemination by donor. *Lancet* 2:581, 1985.
82. Peterson EP, Alexander NJ, Moghissi KS: AID and AIDS—too close for comfort. *Fertil Steril* 49:209, 1988.
83. Verp MS: Genetic issues in artificial insemination by donor. *Semin Reprod Endocrinol* 5:59, 1987.
84. Handelsman DJ, Dunn SM, Conway AJ, Boylan LM, Jansen RPS: Psychological and attitudinal profiles in donors for artificial insemination. *Fertil Steril* 43:95, 1985.
85. Andrews LB: Ethical and legal aspects of in vitro fertilization and artificial insemination by donor. *Urol Clin North Am* 14:633, 1987.

86. Baylson MM: A medical advancement in search of a legal theory— artificial insemination by donor and the law. *Semin Reprod Endocrinol* 5:69, 1987.

87. Sulewski JM, Eisenberg F, Stenger VG: A longitudinal analysis of artificial insemination with donor semen. *Fertil Steril* 29:527, 1978.

88. Schoysman R, Schoysman-Deboeck A: Results of donor insemination with frozen semen: Sperm action. *Prog Reprod Biol* 1:252, 1976.

89. Behrman SJ: Artificial insemination. *Clin Obstet Gynecol* 22:245, 1979.

90. Meeks GR, McDonald J, Gookin K, Bates GW: Insemination with fresh donor semen. *Obstet Gynecol* 68:527, 1986.

91. Batzer FR, Corson SL: Inductions, techniques, success rates, and pregnancy outcome: New directions with donor insemination. *Semin Reprod Endocrinol* 5:45, 1987.

92. Quinlivan WLG, Sullivan H: The immunologic effects of husband's semen on donor spermatozoa during mixed insemination. *Fertil Steril* 28:448, 1977.

93. Quinlivan WLG: Therapeutic donor insemination: results and causes of nonfertilization. *Fertil Steril* 32:157, 1979.

94. Friedman S: Artificial insemination with donor semen mixed with semen of the infertile husband. *Fertil Steril* 33:125, 1980.

95. Emperaire JC, Gauzere-Saimireu E, Audebert AJM: Female fertility and donor insemination. *Fertil Steril* 37:90, 1982.

96. Behrman SJ: Artificial insemination. *Fertil Steril* 10:248, 1959.

97. Raboch J. Tomasek ZD: Therapeutic donor insemination—Results. *J Reprod Fertil* 14:421, 1967.

98. Strickler RC, Keller DW, Warren JC: Artificial insemination with fresh donor semen. *N Engl J Med* 293: 848, 1975.

99. Chong AP, Taymor ML: 16 years' experience with therapeutic donor insemination. *Fertil Steril* 26:791, 1975.

100. Dixon RE, Buttram VC Jr: Artificial insemination using donor semen: A review of 171 cases. *Fertil Steril* 27:130, 1976.

101. Koren Z, Lieberman R: 15 years' experience with artificial insemination. *Int J Fertil* 21: 119, 1976.

102. Corson SL: Factors affecting donor artificial insemination success rates. *Fertil Steril* 33:415, 1980.

103. Bergquist CA, Rock JA, MIller J, et al: Artificial insemination with fresh donor semen using the cervical cap technique: A review of 278 cases. *Obstet Gynecol* 60:195, 1982.

104. Aiman J: Factors affecting the success of donor insemination. *Fertil Steril* 37:94, 1982.

105. Virro MS, Shewchuk AB: Pregnancy outcome in 242 conceptions after artificial insemination with donor sperm and effects of maternal age on the prognosis for successful pregnancy. *Am J Obstet Gynecol* 148:518, 1984.

106. Yeh J, Seibel MM: Artificial insemination with donor sperm: A review of 108 patients. *Obstet Gynecol* 70:313, 1987.

107. Potter RG Jr: Artificial insemination by donors. *Fertil Steril* 9:37, 1958.

108. Albrecht BH, Cramer D, Schiff I: Factors influencing the success of artificial insemination. *Fertil Steril* 37:792, 1982.

109. Broekhuizen FK, Haning RV, Shapiro SS: Laparoscopic findings in twenty-five failures of artificial insemination. *Fertil Steril* 34:351, 1980.

110. Joyce D, Vassilopoulos D: Sperm–mucus interaction and artificial insemination. *Clin Obstet Gynaecol* 8:587, 1981.

111. Steinberger E, Smith KD: Artificial insemination with fresh or frozen semen. A comparative study. *JAMA* 223:778, 1973.

112. Richter MA, Haning RV Jr, Shapiro SS: Artificial donor insemination: Fresh versus frozen; the patient as her own control. *Fertil Steril* 41:277, 1984.

113. Sherman JK: Frozen semen: Efficiency in artificial insemination and advantage in testing for acquired immune deficiency syndrome. *Fertil Steril* 47:19, 1987.

114. Schwartz P, Mayanx MJ: Female fecundity as a function of age. *N Engl J Med* 306:404, 1982.

115. Friedman S: Artificial donor insemination with frozen human semen. *Fertil Steril* 28:1230, 1977.

116. Beck WW Jr: A critical look at the legal, ethical and technical aspects of artificial insemination. *Fertil Steril* 27:1, 1976.

117. David G, Czyglik F, Schwartz D, Mayaux JJ: Results of AID for a first and succeeding pregnancies, in David G, Price WS (eds): *Human Artificial Insemination and Semen Preservation*. New York, Plenum, 1980.

118. Seymour FI, Koerner A: Artificial insemination: present status in the United States as shown by a recent survey. *JAMA* 116:2747, 1971.

119. Mochimaru F, Sato H, Kobayashi T, Iizuka R: Physical and mental development of children born through AID, in David G, Price WS (eds): *Human Artificial Insemination and Semen Preservation*. New York, Plenum, 1980, pp 227–280.

120. Manuel CD, Czyba JC: Follow-up study on children born through AID, in David G, Price WS (eds): *Human Artificial Insemination and Semen Preservation*. New York, Plenum 1980, p 467.

121. Semenov G, Mises R, Bissery J: Attempt at follow up of children born through AID, in David G, Price WS (eds): *Human Artificial Insemination and Semen Preservation*. New York, Plenum, 1980, p 475.

122. Forrler A, Badoc E, Moreau L, et al: Direct intraperitoneal insemination: First results confirmed. *Lancet* 2:1468, 1986.

123. Dodson WC, Whitesides DB, Hughes CL Jr, Easley HA III, Haney AF: Superovulation with intrauterine insemination in the treatment of infertility: A possible alternative to gamete intrafallopian transfer and in vitro fertilization. *Fertil Steril* 48:441, 1987.

PART V

Specific Categories of Infertility

CHAPTER 15

Immunology

Richard A. Bronson

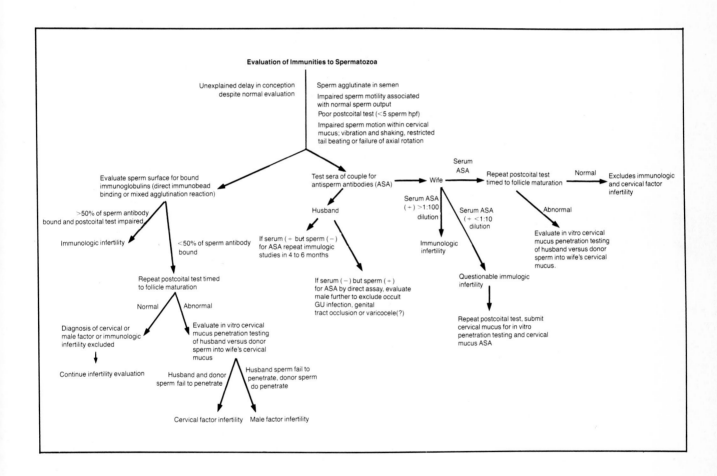

Since the end of the 19th century it has been known that animals immunized with sperm will produce antisperm antibodies. During the past decade, through the development of more specific tests and as a result of the acquisition of the ability to study fertilization *in vitro*, it has become clear that the spontaneous appearance of sperm-reactive antibodies in men or women can lead to impaired reproductive function.

IMMUNOGLOBULINS

Immunoglobulins are glycoproteins composed of a basic unit made up of four polypeptide chains (Fig. 15–1). One pair of chains is approximately twice the molecular weight of the other (designated heavy and light chain, respectively). The primary sequence of amino acids near the amino-terminal portion of the polypeptide (the variable region) is heterogeneous, while the carboxy-terminal portion contains a constant region. The antigen-combining site of the immunoglobulin molecule, which is formed by a small number of amino acids in the variable regions of the heavy and light chains, possesses a structural complementariness with a specific region of the antigen. Thus only restricted portions of antigen molecules, called determinants or epitopes, are recognized by the combining sites of individual antibodies.[1]

The five classes of immunoglobulin molecules found in humans are designated IgG, IgA, IgM, IgD, and IgE.[2] These are defined by structural differences in the constant regions of their heavy chains. They vary in molecular weight from 150,000 for IgG to 900,000 for IgM. Approximately 75% of the total serum immunoglobulin is IgG, of which four subclasses are known. In contrast, IgA is the predominant immunoglobulin in secretions. Secretory IgA is commonly composed of two IgA molecules. Two additional polypeptides, the J chain and the secretory component, are also present. The latter plays a role in the transport of IgA across mucosal surfaces. IgM makes up 10% of normal serum immunoglobulins and exists as a pentamer. IgD is normally present in only trace amounts, and its main function is not yet known. IgE binds with high affinity to mast cells and triggers the release of vasoactive substances in response to specific allergens, and is responsible for atopic symptoms.

The two large subclasses of lymphocytes are B cells and T cells. The T cells differentiate initially in the thymus, while B cells differentiate in fetal liver and spleen and adult bone marrow. The B cells synthesize surface antibody, which functions as an antigen receptor that is reactive with a single, specific

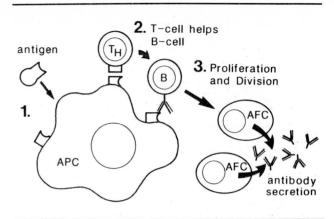

Figure 15–2. Overview of the immune response. 1. Antigen-presenting cells (APC) retain fragments of encountered antigens on their surface. 2. The surface antigen allows the surface receptors of T helper cells (TH) to recognize the antigen. The TH also help B cells (B) to recognize the antigen by their surface receptors (immunoglobulin). 3. The B cells are stimulated to proliferate and divide into antibody-forming cells (AFC), which secrete antibody.

epitope. Binding of a particular epitope to this receptor causes the B cells to proliferate and subsequently produce antibody. This process is augmented by interactions with T helper lymphocytes, which help B cells to produce immunoglobulins in two ways. B cells are activated by direct contact with T helper cells. During this process, new receptors are expressed on the B cell surface capable of binding growth and differentiation factors secreted by T helper cells.

Many antigens must first be processed by specific phagocytic cells (antigen processing cells or APC's) before they can be recognized by B cells; that is, bind to their receptors (Fig. 15–2). Macrophages, Langerhans cells, and dendritic cells have been documented to be capable of processing antigens. The exact molecular events by which native antigen is altered to a form recognized by T and B cells is unknown.

REGULATION OF IMMUNOGLOBULIN SECRETION IN THE REPRODUCTIVE TRACT

IgA is the major immunoglobulin present within external secretions. Large amounts are found in tears, saliva, colostrum, as well as respiratory, gastrointestinal and genitourinary tract secretions.

Secretory IgA is the product of two distinct cells: plasma cells and epithelial cells. IgA producing plasma cells are particularly prominent in the lamina propria of the gut, and salivary, lacrimal and lactating

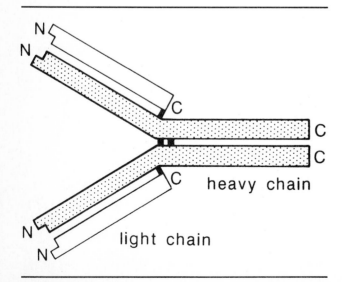

Figure 15–1. Basic structure of an immunoglobulin molecule.

mammary glands. Epithelial cells produce secretory component (SC), which acts as a regulatory transport protein.

Secretions of glands that are anatomically remote from the site of local immunization may also contain IgA antibodies to these antigens, and studies in several laboratory animals now suggest that there is a *common* mucosal immune system.

The sex steroids influence the total levels of IgA, IgG and secretory component in the reproductive tract secretions of ovariectomized rats. Administration of estradiol resulted in a decline in cervical and vaginal content of IgA, IgG, and secretory component.[3] Estradiol, in contrast, stimulated an increased tissue content of IgA in the uterus and also induced an increased production of secretory component. When administered with estradiol, progesterone blocked these responses. The opposing effect of estrogen on the secretion of immunoglobulins by the uterus and cervix demonstrates a different response of each compartment of the female reproductive tract to hormonal stimulus.

The regulation of secretion of IgG and IgA into the uterine lumen is complex. IgG is rapidly transferred, within 3 to 6 hours, from blood to the uterine lumen of ovariectomized rats treated with estrogen.[4] In contrast, IgA movement into the uterine lumen is gradual, requiring several days of hormone treatment. While IgG moves down a concentration gradient, IgA accumulation within the lumen is against such a gradient.

Sex steroids appears to act differently on IgA and IgG secretion in the rat uterus. Estradiol increases vascular permeability, which results in transudation of serum IgG into tissues and subsequently the uterine lumen.[5] In contrast, uterine IgA is synthesized locally by lymphocytes that migrate to the uterus in response to estradiol. IgA-producing lymphocytes, as part of the common mucosal system, are known to migrate into the rat genital tract during the estrus cycle in response to hormone treatment.[6] IgA plasma cells have been found in mouse endometrium in increased numbers at proestrus.[7]

The quantity of free secretory component is also increased by estradiol treatment in a pattern similar to that of IgA.[8] As this response is reduced by inhibitors of RNA synthesis, the estradiol regulation of secretory component appears to be mediated transcriptionally. Progesterone and testosterone administration is nearly without effect.

The coordinated increase in secretory component and IgA in the uterine lumen of ovariectomized rats treated with estradiol is consistent with the regulation of IgA transport across mucosal surfaces by secretory component. Secretory component production in the human reproductive tract is also under hormonal control. Secretory component levels are highest during the luteal phase and reduced significantly during the proliferative phase.[9]

The role of estradiol in regulating the presence of *specific* antibodies within the female reproductive tract has been studied.[10] Administration of estradiol to ovariectomized rats orally immunized with sheep red blood cells (sRBCs) results in an accumulation of anti-sRBC antibodies of both IgG and IgA classes in their uterine secretions. Vaginal antibody levels are also influenced by estradiol, but in contrast to the uterus, anti-sRBC IgA and IgG are present in vaginal secretions in the absence of hormonal stimulation and markedly inhibited in animals treated with estradiol.

The route of immunization influences local immunoglobulin secretion. While intraperitoneal and Peyer's patch immunization with sRBC stimulates specific anti-sRBC IgA antibodies in uterine and vaginal secretions, subcutaneous immunization results in a weak response in the reproductive tract.

The intragastric immunization of women with polio vaccine results in IgA antibodies in uterine and vaginal secretions.[11] It is interesting that studies of rats that received orally administered sperm demonstrated reduced fertility in association with antisperm antibody production.[12]

IMMUNOGLOBULINS PRESENT IN THE HUMAN REPRODUCTIVE TRACT

Vaginal fluid is a mixture of both transudate and cervical secretions. The average daily production of fluid from the vaginal wall ranges from 3 to 12 mL, varying in quantity throughout the menstrual cycle. Both IgG and IgA were detectable in secretions of the lateral vaginal wall of most women who had undergone hysterectomy; IgM, on the other hand, was rarely present.[13] Approximately 70% of the total IgA present is secretory, implying its local production. Specific antibodies have also been found in cervical and vaginal secretions after systemic and vaginal immunization. After vaginal application of a soluble antigen, antibodies to *Candida albicans* were induced in human volunteers.[14]

When levels of IgA and IgG in cervical mucus vary markedly throughout the cycle.[15] The early proliferative phase is characterized by high levels of IgG and IgA (100 to 300 and 20 to 70 mg%, respectively). These concentrations decrease markedly at midcycle to approximately 4 mg% for IgA and 10 mg% for IgG. Specific antibodies were observed in human cervical mucus against several microorganisms. Cyclic changes in specific antibody titer in cervical secretions were noted in monkeys experimentally immunized with T4 coliphage.[16]

Lymphocytes are scattered throughout the endometrial stroma of the human uterus, and IgG, IgA, and secretory component have been found by indirect immunofluorescence.[17,18] Little IgM staining was noted by this method. The immunoglobulin content of uterine secretions was measured by a blotting technique employed on surgical specimens.[19] IgG concentrations ranged from 250 to 280 mg%, IgA from 20 to 180 mg%, and IgM from 18 to 71 mg%. Small tissue cylinders were also obtained from fresh surgical specimens, and the release of immunoglobulin into agar gels was studied.[20] Preovulatory levels of diffusible IgA and IgG were significantly higher in the periovulatory phase of the cycle than during the early proliferative phase.

Immunoglobulin levels in human fallopian tubes have been studied by indirect immunofluorescence[21] and by cannulation.[22] Staining of IgA and IgG was documented along the basement membrane, and both immunoglobulin isotypes were present in specimens of human fallopian tube secretions.

The titers of specific antibodies were measured in oviductal secretions of rhesus monkeys immunized systemically or locally by intravaginal application of T4 coliphage.[23] After administration of human menopausal gonadotropin (HMG), a decrease in antibody titer occurred during follicular maturation parallel with an increase in serum estradiol. As the antibody titer fell lower than could be accounted for solely by an increase in the volume of secretion, it appears that estradiol regulates immunoglobulin production in the subhuman primate oviduct.

We compared the presence of antisperm antibodies in serum with that in vaginal secretions, uterotubal fluid, and peritoneal fluid (collected at laparoscopy). Immunoglobulins predominantly of the IgA class directed against specific regions of the sperm surface was found in uterotubal lavages but not in serum, thus indicating local production. In contrast, antisperm antibodies in peritoneal fluid were found to reflect those seen in plasma, consistent with their nature as transudates.[24]

These observations indicate that the mix of antibodies in each reproductive compartment varies throughout the menstrual cycle, and may not be a reflection of antibodies present in serum. These results highlight the difficulty in determining whether the presence of antisperm antibodies, detected in a serologic test, contributes to a delay in conception (see below).

EXPERIMENTAL INDUCTION OF INFERTILITY BY IMMUNIZATION WITH SPERMATOZOA

In 1932 Baskin[25] immunized women with large volumes of semen injected intramuscularly and found that they developed a humoral sperm-toxic factor (an antisperm antibody?) in their plasma. A delay in conception was also noted, despite repeated unprotected coitus.

In 1964 it was demonstrated that the specific induction of antisperm antibodies in mice resulted in diminished fertility.[26] Females with high titers of antisperm agglutinins showed a reduction in both litter size and total breeding performance over 6 months. The number of oviductal sperm was reduced after mating, while normal numbers of eggs were ovulated. The percentage of fertilized eggs in the oviducts 48 hours after coitus was diminished. In the same year, similar observations were made in mice immunized to sperm, although no association was noted between the degree of infertility and antisperm antibody titer.[27] Subsequently, however, a correlation was noted between titers and reproductive tract impairment.[28]

Immunization of female guinea pigs with homologous spermatozoa also results in reproductive impairment.[29] Autoantibodies induced in male guinea pigs also inhibit the acrosome reaction when added to a medium that supports in-vitro egg penetration, and reduced penetration of the zona pellucida by capacitated spermatozoa.[30,31]

Evidence exists that experimentally induced antisperm antibodies in rabbits have effects after fertilization. Embryo survival was impaired in situ after immunization with washed homologous spermatozoa. The development of blastocysts in vitro was inhibited in media containing uterine fluid from immunized animals.[32] Secretory IgA isolated from the uterine fluid of these animals inhibited blastocyst development. Bound antibodies were detected on the blastocyst by immunofluorescence. After absorption with spermatozoa, blastocysts expanded and hatched in culture normally, demonstrating that antisperm antibody is toxic to blastocysts.

Subsequently, immunizations were carried out with rabbit sperm plasma membrane solubilized with lithium idodosalicylate or the nonionic detergent NP40. Immunization with lithium idodosalicylate extracts resulted in failure of fertilization. Similar results were obtained in estrous rabbits artificially inseminated with sperm exposed in vitro to serum from similarly immunized animals.

In contrast, rabbits immunized with NP40 extract exhibited no impairment in fertilization, although the number of implantation sites was diminished. The uterine fluids of these rabbits contained immunoglobulins reactive with blastocysts. From these results it was concluded that antigens responsible for producing postfertilization infertility were extracted by the nonionic detergent from a subsurface site on spermatozoa.

Isoantibodies raised in mice against homologous sperm were also shown to cross-react with preimplantation embryos, resulting in failure of nidation.[28] Monoclonal antibodies raised against mouse spermatozoa impaired the development of preimplantation mouse embryos.[33] As these monoclonal antibodies react with a specific epitope derived from spermatozoa, such results suggest that the same antigenic determinant is expressed on the surface of the preimplantation embryo and spermatozoa.

ANTISPERM ANTIBODIES AND INFERTILITY

In 1955 Rumke and Hellinga[34] demonstrated that the presence of male autoantibodies to sperm was associated with unexplained infertility. Subsequently, a relationship was noted between the titer of circulating humoral antisperm antibodies and both the chance of and length of delay to conception.[35] Franklin and Dukes in the mid-1960s indicated that some women with failure to conceive possessed sperm agglutinins in their sera.[36] They raised the issue of whether these antisperm antibodies might play a role in the pathogenesis of human infertility.

Subsequent attempts to determine whether infertility in humans could have an immune basis have produced conflicting results (Table 15–1).[37] It is now apparent why these earlier investigations were unsuccessful. First, the extent of reproductive failure varies widely among individual animals sensitized to sperm. Furthermore, since antisperm antibodies may appear as either transudates from plasma or through direct local secretion by submucosal plasma cells, they may be present in plasma yet absent from the reproductive tract secretions or seminal plasma. Conversely, local immunity to sperm, demonstrable by antisperm antibody in the secretions of the reproductive tract, may be present despite the absence of humoral immunity. Finally, antisperm antibodies of IgA, IgG, or IgM isotype may be produced. Each of these immunoglobulins may have different potential to cause infertility.

Early work on the immune cause of infertility in humans was also hampered by reliance on agglutination techniques as the sole means of detecting sperm antibody. Bacterial contamination of semen[38] or the presence of β-globulins[39] can cause agglutination of spermatozoa in the absence of antisperm antibodies, especially with minimally diluted serum. Unfortunately, many of the early studies reporting the presence of antisperm antibodies were performed at low serum dilutions.[40]

NEW APPROACHES

It is now clear that antisperm humoral antibodies are not relevant to fertility unless they are present in the reproductive tract. The presence of immunoglobulins on sperm retrieved from the ejaculate is the most direct evidence of autoimmunity to sperm. This conclusion was corroborated in a study of ejaculates of nearly 2,000 men who had experienced a delay in conception.[41] The clinical indications for sperm antibody determination consisted of (1) spontaneous agglutination of sperm in semen; (2) poor sperm penetration of cervical mucus, despite "normal" semen analysis; (3) restricted sperm motion in cervical mucus, consisting of vibration, failure of longitudinal rotation, or sperm immobilization. Couples with idiopathic infertility were also screened when results of overnight postcoital tests, endometrial biopsy, and laparoscopy were normal.

Two hundred fifty-one (13.6%) of the 845 men tested were found to possess autoantibodies to sperm (the frequency for unselected infertile men is 8%).[42] In 20% of 856 matched semen and serum samples, humoral antibodies were detected in blood, *not* on sperm. As antisperm antibodies had not gained entry into the reproductive tract, they were not bound to the sperm surface, and their presence in serum would be expected to play no role in the couple's infertility. Conversely, the rate of negative serologic results not predictive of infertility was 14.1%. Here, spermatozoa were immunoglobulin bound, with no evidence of antisperm autoantibodies in serum. Their secretion was then purely local, in the male reproductive tract. Had only a serologic test for circulating humoral antisperm antibodies been relied on, a misleading result would have been obtained in approximately 35% of subjects.

Given these considerations, a number of investigators have developed techniques that allow the detection of immunoglobulins on the sperm surface. The radiolabeled antiglobulin assay uses radioiodonated xenogenic antibodies against human

TABLE 15–1. FREQUENCY OF IMMUNITY TO SPERMATOZOA IN WOMEN AS DETECTED BY MICROAGGLUTINATION TESTS PERFORMED IN DIFFERENT LABORATORIES

"Unexplained" Infertility (%)	Pregnant, Fertile, or "Organic" Infertility (%)
82/310 (26.4)	28/149 (18.7)
27/72 (37.5)	38/83 (45.8)
27/147 (18.4)	3/113 (2.7)
8/83 (24.2)	11/85 (12.9)
27/487 (5.5)	29/489 (5.9)
24/122 (19.7)	2/46 (4.4)
44/277 (15.9)	4/44 (9.1)
13/45 (29)	— —
90/216 (41.7)	10/50 (20)
9/40 (22.5)	3/80 (3.7)

(From Beer and Neaves.[37])

immunoglobulins.[43] This test is highly sensitive, due to use of a radiolabel, but does not allow assessment of individual spermatozoa.

The mixed agglutination reaction (MAR) uses human Rh-positive red blood cells sensitized by exposure to anti-Rh IgG.[44] When these sensitized cells are mixed with a drop of semen and a xenogenic antiglobulin (rabbit antihuman IgG), mixed agglutination of both cell types occurs if spermatozoa are antibody bound. This assay can be used to detect both antisperm IgG and IgA antibodies in a semi-quantitative way. Comparative studies between MAR and immunobead binding indicate a lower degree of sensitivity for the detection of IgA by MAR, however (H. Meinertz, R. A. Bronson, unpublished observations).

The sperm-panning test uses xenogenic antibodies raised against human immunoglobulins, which are then coated on microtiter wells.[45] Antibody-bound sperm bind to the wells. This assay is suitable for screening, but does not provide information for individual spermatozoa, nor does it allow the assessment of regional binding of immunoglobulins on the sperm surface (for example, head versus tail).

Immunobead binding uses polyacrylamide spheres to which rabbit antihuman antibodies are covalently linked.[46] These antibodies are isotype-specific, distinguishing IgG, IgA, and IgM. Spermatozoa are washed free of seminal fluid. A suspension of motile sperm is mixed with a drop of the immunobead suspension and observed under phase-contrast optics. As spermatozoa swim through the suspension, immunobeads adhere to the surface of spermatozoa that are immunoglobulin bound. The clustering of beads over different regions provides clinically useful information, such as the proportion of spermatozoa in an ejaculate that is coated with immunoglobulins over their surfaces (Fig. 15–3).

When the seminal fluid concentration of anti-sperm antibodies is high, agglutinates of sperm may appear that are large enough to form a grossly visible flocculation. In most instances agglutination is limited, and the majority of sperm remain motile. Immunobead binding has demonstrated that these motile sperm are also often antibody bound.

Spermatozoa that carry antibody over most of their surface may be completely motile in semen and are unable to enter the cervical mucus, as shown both on postcoital testing and in vitro (see below).[47–49]

Immunobead binding can be performed by both direct and indirect means. The indirect test is able to evaluate any biologic fluid by in vitro antibody transfer to antibody-free sperm. Spermatozoa that have been shown to be free of immunoglobulins by the direct assay can be exposed to serum, vaginal flushes, cervical mucus extracts, uterotubal lavage, follicular fluid, peritoneal fluid, or saliva, and then subjected to bead binding.

Immunobead binding is highly specific. The indirect assay also appears to be highly sensitive, compared with sperm agglutination and complement-dependent-immobilization assays.[50] This conclusion was reached after a multicenter, international study in which a large group of clinically defined sera were distributed as unknowns to participating laboratories under the auspices of the WHO Reference Bank for Reproductive Immunology (Tables 15–2 and 15–3).

Do those sperm-reactive antibodies remaining in seminal fluid reflect the cell-bound immunoglobulins present on the sperm surface? To answer this question, a comparison of sperm-bound versus sperm-free antibodies in the semen of 26 men with autoimmunity to sperm was carried out.[51] Spermatozoa were centrifuged from fresh ejaculates, washed, and analyzed by direct immunobead binding. Matched sperm-free seminal fluids were studied by the addition of antibody-free sperm from known fertile do-

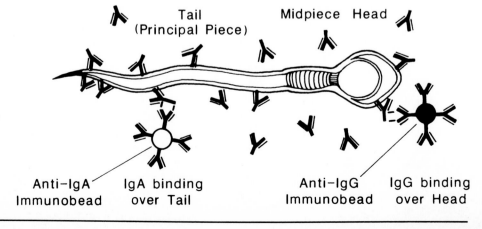

Figure 15–3. Schematic drawing of the immunobead test. Anti-IgA or anti-IgG covalently linked to polyacrylamide beads binds to IgA or IgG bound to the sperm surface. Quantification of antisperm antibody is by visualization of beads bound to the sperm surface.

Tail (Principal Piece)   Midpiece   Head

Anti-IgA Immunobead   IgA binding over Tail   Anti-IgG Immunobead   IgG binding over Head

TABLE 15-2. COMPARISON OF RESULTS BETWEEN IMMUNOBEAD BINDING AND GEL AGGLUTINATION TESTS IN 129 MALE SERA

Gel Agglutination Titer	Immunobead Binding Level			
	Negative	Low	Intermediate	High
Negative	73	25	6	3
4–8	1	0	0	2
16–32	1	0	1	7
≥64	0	0	0	10

(From Bronson et al.[50])

nors. After incubation in seminal fluid, the sperm were washed and reacted with immunobeads in an indirect assay (Fig. 15–4).

The diagnosis of autoimmunity to sperm would have been confirmed by analysis of the seminal fluid in 25 of 26 cases. In only 4 of the 26 ejaculates studied, however, was there no difference between sperm-bound and seminal fluid antisperm antibodies. In 85% of cases, neither the isotypes detected nor their regional binding specificities were reflective of those immunoglobulins detected on the sperm surface. Head-directed antibodies were absent from the seminal fluid in 12 cases (46%), but present on sperm. This finding is critical, as antibodies present over the sperm head could alter direct gamete interaction as well as impair sperm transport.

It is necessary to determine immunoglobulin isotype. IgA, IgG, and IgM antibodies are structurally different molecules that interact with complement in different ways and have different effects on spermatozoa.[52]

Immune Complement

The complement system consists of a cascade of more than 20 plasma proteins.[53] In association with IgM, IgG_1, or IgG_2, the final steps in the cascade lead to the generation of a membrane-attack complex (MAC) that is capable of creating a discontinuity in the plasma membrane, leading to cell lysis.[54] IgM antibodies are more efficient than IgG immunoglobulins in mediating hemolysis.[55,56] On the other hand, unaggregated IgA immunoglobulins do not interact with complement and thus cannot promote generation of the MAC.

The ability of antisperm antibodies of different isotypes to interact with complement, leading to sperm plasma membrane damage, has been studied.[57,58] Sera containing sperm head-directed IgAs had no effect on sperm motility or sperm ultrastructure in the presence of complement. In contrast, IgG antibody directed against the principal piece of the tail mediated complement-dependent immobilization. There is a direct correlation between the extent of immunoglobulin attachment along the sperm tail, as reflected by immunobead binding, and the degree of immobilization. In antibodies that bind solely to the sperm tail tip, no change in motility was noted. As the tail surface becomes immunoglobulin bound, however, spermatozoa rapidly lose motility in the presence of complement (Fig. 15–5). These results are quite similar to those previously noted in hemolytic dose-response curves. When red blood cells are sensitized with trinitrophenol (TNP), the number of hemolytic sites varies directly with the TNP antigen density as well as the concentration of anti-TNP IgG.[59] That is, both greater amounts of antigen on the red cell membrane as well as greater

TABLE 15-3. COMPARISON OF RESULTS (TITER) USING 4 METHODS OF DETECTING ANTISPERM ANTIBODY IN 14 MALE SERA ALL STRONGLY POSITIVE BY IMMUNOBEAD BINDING

Gel Agglutination (macro)	Tray Agglutination (micro)	Complement-Dependent Sperm Immobilization	Passive Hemagglutination
0	0	0	2
16	4	1	8
0	8	0	4
128	128	2	2
256	128	2	2
256	128	2	4
32	16	0	16
4	32	0	8
64	64	1	8
32	64	1	4
64	64	8	8
64	16	0	8
64	16	8	4
32	16	0	8

(From Bronson et al.[50])

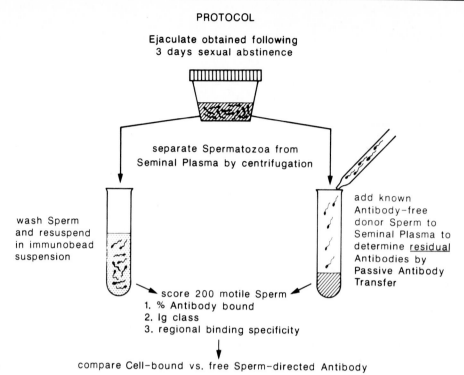

PROTOCOL

Ejaculate obtained following
3 days sexual abstinence

separate Spermatozoa from
Seminal Plasma by centrifugation

wash Sperm
and resuspend
in immunobead
suspension

add known
Antibody-free
donor Sperm to
Seminal Plasma to
determine <u>residual</u>
Antibodies by
Passive Antibody
Transfer

score 200 motile Sperm
1. % Antibody bound
2. Ig class
3. regional binding specificity

compare Cell-bound vs. free Sperm-directed Antibody

Figure 15–4. Immunobead protocol.

antibody concentration lead to an increased number of plasma membrane–lytic sites.

As seminal fluid contains complement inhibitors, spermatozoa of men with autoimmunity to sperm retain their viability in the ejaculate despite the presence of sperm-directed immunoglobulins on their sperm surface.[60] On entering the female reproductive tract, however, such sperm become liable to complement-mediated membrane damage.[61]

As anticipated from these studies, the Isojima test, a commonly used complement-dependent method of detecting immunity by sperm immobilization, would be expected to fail to detect sperm-directed immunoglobulins of the IgA class.[62]

Other Antibody Tests

Several enzyme-linked immunosorbant assays (ELI-SAs) have been developed to detect the presence of sperm-reactive antibodies in serum or semen, but dissatisfaction with this approach has increased. The presence of low-titer, naturally occurring antisperm antibodies is detectable by immunofluorescence in the majority of sera of men and women of all ages.[63,64] These antibodies are absorbed both by spermatozoa and testicular extracts, but not other tissues. Sera possessing antiacrosomal antibodies, when absorbed with lyophilized bacteria (*Escherichia coli*, and *Staphylococcus*, *Pseudomonas*, and *Klebsiella* species) as well *Candida albicans*, no longer react with sperm by indirect immunofluorescence. Of special importance, these sperm-reactive, naturally occur-

ring antibodies do not react with the surface of viable sperm in suspension, but only those after methanol fixation. Hence, these antibodies appear to be directed against subsurface antigens.

The high frequency of naturally occurring sperm-reactive antibodies poses a major problem of "immunologic background noise" for the ELISA. Thus the method of fixation of spermatozoa is critical in determining which antigens are "presented" to the test serum. Denaturation and loss of surface antigens might be expected to occur during fixation, and in addition, breakdown of the sperm plasma membrane may lead to exposure of intracellular antigens. Therefore this assay allows detection of antibodies that play no role in impaired reproduction.

The importance of distinguishing antibodies reactive with surface from those reactive with subsurface antigens was documented in a WHO-sponsored workshop on monoclonal antibodies raised against sperm antigens.[65] Given that unique the nature of monoclonal antibodies are directed against a single antigenic determinant, these reagents could be used as probes to test the premise that only antibodies reactive with the sperm surface alter sperm function. Of 49 monoclonal antibodies studied by immunobead testing, 27 exhibited reactivity with the living sperm surface. Thirty-six of these monoclonal antibodies were studied to determine their influence on the ability of motile spermatozoa to penetrate bovine cervical mucus in vitro. A correlation was found between the degree of reactivity of each monoclonal

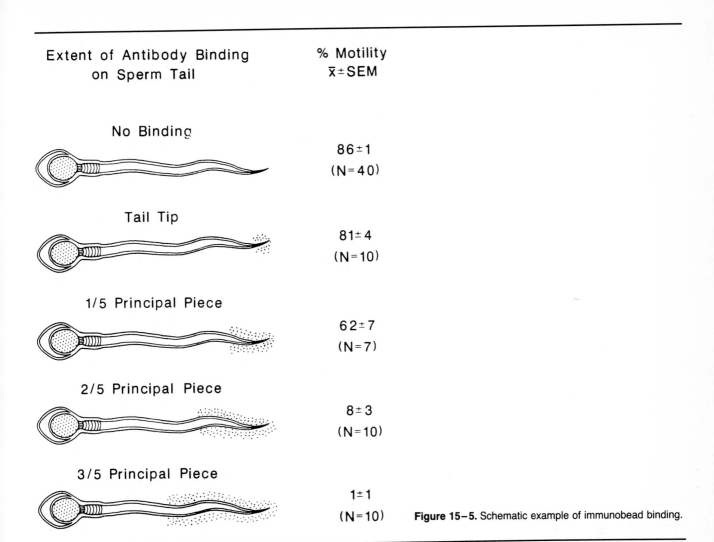

Extent of Antibody Binding on Sperm Tail	% Motility $\bar{x} \pm SEM$
No Binding	86±1 (N=40)
Tail Tip	81±4 (N=10)
1/5 Principal Piece	62±7 (N=7)
2/5 Principal Piece	8±3 (N=10)
3/5 Principal Piece	1±1 (N=10)

Figure 15–5. Schematic example of immunobead binding.

antibody with motile sperm and their subsequent ability to penetrate cervical mucus. Those antibodies directed against subsurface antigenic determinants failed to alter sperm cervical mucus penetration (Table 15–4).[66]

TABLE 15–4. RELATIONSHIP BETWEEN THE EXTENT OF BINDING OF MONOCLONAL ANTIBODY TO MOTILE SPERMATOZOA AND THEIR ABILITY TO PENETRATE A COLUMN OF BOVINE CERVICAL MUCUS IN VITRO

Mab Reactivity as Judged by % Sperm Binding Immunobeads*	Number of Samples	Location of Vanguard Spermatozoa (mm) x ± SD†
100%	11	17.5±6.2
50 < 100%	7	27.3±11.8
< 50%	6	33.0±11.7
None	12	37.4±5.8

*A population of nearly 100% motile spermatozoa obtained by swim-up were incubated with monoclonal antibody (Mab), then washed free of ascitic fluid or culture supernatant, and exposed to immunobeads.
† After 90 minutes' incubation at 37°C.
(From Bronson et al.[57] Reproduced with permission.)

When spermatozoa were fixed by different methods, a variation in the ability of an ELISA to detect sperm-reactive antibodies detected by immunobead binding also was documented. Typical methods of fixation were air-drying to wells, glutaraldehyde fixation, reaction with test serum while living, and freeze-thaw (Table 15–5).[67] No correlation was noted in the results of participating laboratories with the clinically defined sera provided by the WHO Reference Bank for Reproductive Immunology.[68] A correlation was found with results of indirect immunobead binding only when spermatozoa were first reacted with test serum and subsequently with enzyme-linked second antibody.

Antisperm Antibodies in Women

To gain an idea of the frequency of female immunity to sperm, a review of the indirect immunobead binding test results was carried out in 728 women who had experienced a delay in conception in association with an abnormal postcoital test. The husband's spermatozoa were first demonstrated to be free of antibodies and then were exposed to the wife's

TABLE 15–5. COMPARISON OF ANTISPERM ANTIBODIES DETECTED BY IMMUNOBEAD BINDING THEN TESTED BY ELISA USING DIFFERENT METHODS OF SPERM FIXATION

Patient Sera	Immunobead Binding Results			Sera Reacted First with Live Motile Sperm then Gluteraldehyde-fixed			Sera Reacted with Fresh Sperm Gluteraldehyde-fixed			Sera Reacted with Fresh Sperm Air-dried			Sera Reacted with Frozen Sperm Gluteraldehyde-fixed		
	IgG	A	M	IgG	A	M	IgG	A	M	IgG	A	M	IgG	A	M
R	+	+	−	+	+	−	+	−	+	+	+	+	+	+	+
M	+	+	+	+	+	+	+	−	+	+	−	+	+	−	+
Rm	+	+	−	+	+	−	+	−	−	−	−	−	−	−	−
E	+	+	−	+	+	−	+	+	+	+	−	+	+	−	+
B	+	+	−	+	+	−	+	+	+	+	−	+	+	−	+

The immunoglobulin classes of sperm-reactive antibodies detected by immunobead binding and ELISA were comparable only when live sperm were incubated in test serum *prior to fixation*, indicating that fixation of spermatozoa had altered their antigenicity. (From Bronson et al.[67])

serum. Three hundred ninety-nine (54.8%) of these women were totally free of detectable antisperm antibodies. A weakly positive result (more than 20%, but less than 50%, of sperm-binding immunobeads after serum exposure at 1:10 dilution) was noted in 27.5% of women, while 12.9% had intermediate levels of antisperm antibodies (immunobead-binding levels greater than 50% but less than 90%). Only 4.8% of the women (35 samples) possessed high levels of circulating antisperm antibodies, based on the observation that nearly all sperm were antibody bound after serum exposure at greater than 1:10 dilution.

The study of a large group of clinically defined sera supplied by the WHO Reference Bank for Reproductive Immunology provided insight into the nature of antisperm antibodies in women.[69] Low levels of antisperm antibody were found in 15.6 to 35% of sera from groups of known fertile females (low as defined by the previous immunobead-binding criteria). Levels were intermediate in 3 to 9% of these sera. In contrast, they were high in none of 57 sera (high was defined as 80% or more of spermatozoa-bound immunobeads after exposure to sera at 1:4 dilution). From these results it is apparent that the presence of antisperm antibodies in serum of a woman takes on clinical significance only if results of the test approach 100% at serum titers above 1:10.

Two provisos must be given in attempting to establish clinical guidelines for interpreting tests of antisperm antibodies in women. As noted above, the female immune system is capable of local secretion of immunoglobulins. Antisperm antibodies are present in vaginal–cervical secretions or solubilized cervical mucus in the absence of humoral antisperm antibodies in 3 to 10% of women. Hence, the need to study cervical mucus in the event of poor sperm survival despite negative serologic results for antisperm antibodies.[70] Finally, the presence of a low level immunity to sperm may be a marker that the cellular arm of the immune system has also been sensitized to spermatozoa; unfortunately, few studies have attempted to deal with this aspect of immune infertility.[71]

Evaluating the Poor Postcoital Test

Poor penetration and survival of sperm in cervical mucus may be associated with immunity to spermatozoa, although not invariably. The period of time during which spermatozoa may populate the female reproductive tract varies among women and indeed between cycles in the same woman. Absolute amounts of mucin present in human cervical mucus are similar throughout the reproductive cycle and only slightly elevated at midcycle.[72] Functional changes in the mucus viscoelasticity and penetrability to sperm appear to be due to an increased degree of hydration by transudated water, which is caused by alterations in the endocervical microvasculature in response to circulating estradiol.[73] The threshold of estradiol exposure at which mucus is formed by the mucus-secreting cells of the cervical crypts varies among women and may be influenced by cervicitis, prior in utero exposure to diethylstilbestrol, and prior surgery of the cervix. Depending on the set point of the hypothalamic–pituitary axis to positive feedback, the rapidity of rise of estradiol concentration prior to the initiation of the LH surge may vary. For this reason, cervical mucus production may be clinically manifest several days in advance of the surge, providing a wide window of opportunity for postcoital testing. Alternatively, abundant cervical mucus may become manifest only within the last possible hours in advance of the LH surge. In such instances, serial observation of mucus development in conjunction with basal body temperature and urinary LH monitoring may be necessary to time the postcoital test accurately.

The Zona-Free Hamster Egg-Penetration Test in the Study of Immune-Mediated Infertility

The significance of sperm-reactive antibodies detected by a particular method must be established by both clinical studies and by a demonstrable effect on sperm function. Antisperm antibodies have three potential mechanisms of action: (1) autoantibodies to spermatozoa in men may interfere with sperm production by the testis; (2) antibodies bound to the surface of spermatozoa, whether derived from the man or woman, may restrict the ability of sperm to penetrate or survive in cervical mucus; and (3) antibodies may hinder preparatory steps that lead to acquisition of egg-penetrating ability—capacitation, the acrosome reaction, and attachment to and penetration of the zona pellucida.

Determining the number of functionally active sperm in an ejaculate that are capable of penetrating eggs is an as yet unrealized goal of semen analysis. The same total number of sperm may be present in the ejaculates of two men, but with widely different values of semen volume, sperm concentration, and motility. Thus male fertility cannot be judged on the basis of those individual classic values, but only in the aggregate of the variables. In other words, male fertility must be judged as "population phenomenon."[74]

Spermatozoa retrived fresh from an ejaculate are unable to fertilize eggs placed in culture. The potential to acquire this ability develops as sperm pass through the epididymis. The proportion of spermatozoa capable of attaching to and penetrating the zona pellucida is highest for sperm that are recovered from regions of the epididymis most distal from the testis (cauda epididymis).[75,76]

The fertilizing ability of human sperm varies independent of motility, as shown by the sperm-penetration assay (SPA).[77] A wide range in the egg-penetrating ability of sperm was documented among known fertile men, despite insemination of zona-free hamster eggs with a constant number of motile sperm. These results are seen even when the most vigorously moving sperm are selected from an ejaculate by swim-up.

Several investigators have used the SPA to determine whether antisperm antibodies may alter sperm fertilizing potential. When capacitated spermatozoa were exposed to antisperm antibodies, penetration rates in the presence of sperm antibodies were 15% compared with 59% for control sera.[78] Six sera completely blocked penetration of zona-free hamster eggs, while 10 reduced the penetration rate substantially. The effect of plasma containing antisperm IgG added at the time of insemination of zona-free hamster eggs was studied.[79] Four of six positive samples significantly reduced sperm penetration.

In contrast, when spermatozoa were exposed to antisperm antibodies (without complement) prior to their capacitation, egg-penetration frequency was enhanced.[80] That the antibodies were directed against sperm head antigens that specifically promoted capacitation was determined by the observation that penetration rates declined after absorption with sperm. Subsequently, the authors showed that, in the presence of complement, complement-fixing, head-directed antibodies inhibited the ability of spermatozoa to penetrate zona-free hamster eggs without any evident change in motility (Table 15–6).[81]

In summary, several effects of antisperm antibodies on sperms' egg-penetrating ability have been observed under different experimental conditions. When sperm are preloaded with immunoglobulins (without complement) prior to capacitation, no impairment in egg-penetrating ability is evident. In this instance, a limited number of immunoglobulin molecules will bind to the sperm surface, either within

TABLE 15–6. EFFECT OF ANTISPERM ANTIBODIES IN THE PRESENCE OR ABSENCE OF COMPLEMENT ON ABILITY OF HUMAN SPERM TO PENETRATE ZONA-FREE HAMSTER EGGS

Immunoglobulin Class of Antisperm Antibody[†] Present in Test Serum	Complement* Present		Heat-inactivated Complement	
	% Eggs Penetrated (no. eggs Inseminated)	No. Penetrating Sperm/Inseminated Egg	% Eggs Penetrated (range) (no. eggs Inseminated)	No. Penetrating Sperm/Inseminated Egg
IgM	40.3 ± 14.8[‡] (60)	0.48 ± 0.14	73.4 ± 9.0 (51)	1.3 ± 0.19
IgG or A/G	54.6 ± 28.1 (95)	0.89 ± 0.55	76.1 ± 17.6 (97)	1.8 ± 0.67
IgA	93.8 ± 9.4 (80)	2.7 ± 1.7	87.6 ± 14.4 (58)	2.6 ± 2.0

*Guinea pig serum from a single animal was used as a source of complement.
[†]Antisperm antibodies directed solely against the sperm head postacrosomal and/or acrosomal regions as determined by immunobead binding.
[‡]Mean of % penetration for each serum ± SD.
Source: From reference 82. Reproduced by permission of MTP Press, Lancaster, England, Lobl T, Hafez ESE (eds): *Male Fertility and Its Regulation*, 1985. (From Lobl and Hafez (eds).[82] Reproduced with permission.)

the epididymis at the time of ejaculation when sperm and accessory gland secretions mix, or during their short-term intravaginal residence after coitus. In contrast, spermatozoa exposed to antisperm antibodies present in culture medium during capacitating incubation exhibit impaired egg-penetrating ability. Such conditions mimic those encountered by sperm in the reproductive tract of women sensitized to sperm. The mechanisms of these differences with respect to sperm capacitation and the acrosome reaction remain to be elucidated.

Effects of Antisperm Antibodies on Cervical Mucus-Penetrating Ability. The proportion of sperm that are antibody bound in the ejaculates of men with autoimmunity to sperm varies widely among individuals. For instance, 43 of 78 men with autoantibodies to sperm had ejaculates in which the vast majority of spermatozoa (81 to 100%) were antibody bound. In 16 of the 78 men, 50 to 80% of spermatozoa were antibody bound, and in the remaining 19 men this figure was less than 50%.

The amount of immunoglobulin bound to spermatozoa at the time of ejaculation depends on several factors: (1) the concentration of antisperm antibodies in male accessory gland secretions; (2) local production of antibodies compared with transudation from blood; (3) binding of antibodies to sperm in the epididymis before ejaculation versus that occurring when sperm mix with seminal fluid; (4) elapsed time since the last ejaculation; and (5) affinity antibody to the sperm surface.

Heterogeneity of antigen expression on spermatozoa in an ejaculate may also occur. Although it has been assumed that the variation in antibody binding reflected the limiting concentration of antibody in seminal fluid, this explanation has proved not to be adequate.[82] If antibody concentration were limiting in cases in which less than 100% of sperm are antibody bound, it would be expected that there would be no residual antibody remaining in the seminal fluid after centrifugation. On the contrary, it has been demonstrated that in some cases antibody-free sperm are detectable in the ejaculate, despite the presence of unbound antisperm antibody of similar immunoglobulin class and specificity remaining within the residual seminal fluid. Spermatozoa acquire glycoprotein surface coatings as they pass through the epididymis and at the time of ejaculation. Tissue-specific antigens are also secreted by the seminal vesicles at ejaculation.[83] Antigenic heterogeneity of ejaculate rabbit sperm plasma membrane was demonstrated in assays using monoclonal antibody directed against a specific sperm plasma membrane antigen.[84] Although all sperm obtained from the cauda epididymis expressed the antigen, a variable number of ejaculated sperm did not. These sperm placed in the uterus again possessed detectable surface antigen. This observation suggests that masking of surface antigens may occur in a nonuniform way during ejaculation.

Spermatozoa to which immunoglobulins are bound exhibit impaired ability to penetrate human cervical mucus.[47] This impairment results in part from an abnormal interaction between the Fc portion of sperm-bound IgA and IgG immunoglobulin and constituents of cervical mucus. Sperm bound by intact antibody become entrapped in cervical mucus, while sperm exposed to only Fab fragments show no reduction in mucus penetration.[48] Immunoglobulin-bound sperm treated with IgA_1 protease (which releases the Fc portion of the immunoglobulin molecule) displayed normal cervical mucus-penetrating ability. Antisperm IgA and IgG have both been shown to impair sperm motion within cervical mucus, although the former displays a greater degree of sperm entrapment than the latter.[49]

To determine whether the proportion of antibody-bound sperm in the ejaculate influences fertility, results of immunobead-binding tests on the ejaculate were compared with the number of motile sperm identified in cervical mucus at standard postcoital testing.[84] The total number of motile sperm in the ejaculate ranged from 42 to 638 million. When 100% of sperm were antibody bound, only rarely were more than 0 to 3 seen per high-power field. A small increase (often below 5 motile sperm/hpf) in the number of penetrating spermatozoa within cervical mucus was noted when binding levels were less than 100% but greater than 50%. Conversely, as immunobead-binding levels dropped under 50%, postcoital test results improved substantially. In several cases, 15 to 30 or 40 sperm per field were noted (Table 15–7).

The prognostic significance of the percentage of antibody-bound sperm in ejaculates was also determined by studying the pregnancy outcome of 108 couples in which the men had autoimmunity to sperm.[85] Immunobead-binding levels of less than 50% were associated with pregnancy rates of 43.3%, as observed retrospectively during a 2-year period when only the women were treated. When more than 50% of sperm were bound, the pregnancy rate was halved to 21.8% ($p < 0.05$) (Table 15–8).

Results were even more dramatic when the patient population was divided by clinical status. For couples in whom the presence of autoantibodies to sperm was the only abnormality in the fertility evaluation, pregnancy rates were 15.3% when more than 50% of sperm were bound, compared with 66.7% when less than 50% of sperm were antibody bound. Although only 35 couples were studied in this group, the difference was highly significant ($p < 0.005$).

TABLE 15–7. CORRELATION BETWEEN EXTENT OF AUTOIMMUNITY AND NUMBER OF MOTILE SPERMATOZOA IN CERVICAL MUCUS AT POSTCOITAL TESTING*

% Antibody-bound Sperm in Ejaculate Detected by Immunobead Binding	Total Number of Motile Sperm in Ejaculate × 10⁶	No. of Motile Sperm/hpf in Postcoital Cervical Mucus†
100%	42	0–3‡
	45	0–3
	69	0–1
	80	0–4
	82	0–4
	127	0
	157	0–8
	176	0–1
	345	0
	472	0
	638	7
> 50% but < 100%	15	15
	35	3
	45	2–7
	49	3
	49	0–1
	63	6–15
	67	4
	715	8
<50%	94	7
	118	15–40
	150	12
	153	15–26
	158	15–30

*Cervical mucus was examined within 48 hours preceding the thermal shift, 8 to 12 hours after coitus.

†Wives were free of sperm-directed antibodies.

‡Spermatozoa in cervical mucus are listed as the average observed or as a range in each hpf (× 400).

(From Bronson RA, Cooper GW, Rosenfeld DL: Complement-mediated effects of sperm head-directed human antibodies on the ability of human spermatozoa to penetrate zona-free hamster eggs. *Fertil Steril* 40:91, 1983. Reproduced with permission from the American Fertility Society.)

It is important to note that these results refer to spontaneous pregnancy rates in couples in which husbands manifested antisperm autoimmunity in the absence of treatment. The wide variation in pregnancy rates again emphasizes the need to document the proportion of sperm that are antibody bound. In addition, the fact that pregnancies do occur without treatment indicates the need for placebo-controlled studies to determine the efficiency of any treatments.

Sperm–Zona Interaction. To establish whether antisperm antibodies alter the ability of sperm to penetrate the egg vestments, aliquots of sperm from fertile men were exposed to sera containing antisperm antibodies reactive with the sperm head.[86] In addition, spermatozoa from the same ejaculate were exposed to the same panel of sera after absorption with spermatozoa. Nonviable human eggs were retrieved from surgical specimens of ovaries and exposed to these spermatozoa. The number of sperm bound to the zona pellucida was studied after their insemination in vitro and serial washing.

Samples that were antibody bound rarely yielded more than 5 sperm attached to the zona pellucida. That sperm-zona receptor sites were intact was documented by the second challenge with sperm incubated with absorbed sera; usually more than 100 sperm were attached to the zona surface. This was true for each of the sera studied. In two cases, although IgA antibodies were completely absorbed, IgG remained detectable on all sperm. Despite the presence of this residual IgG over the sperm head, sperm-zona binding increased markedly. These observations suggest that the isotype of antibody bound to the sperm head or the total immunoglobulin bound may be important in determining the degree of impairment of zona-penetrating ability.

To our surprise, each of these same sera containing antisperm antibodies promoted, rather than inhibited, the penetration of zona-free hamster eggs.

TABLE 15–8. PREGNANCY OUTCOME IN 198 COUPLES WHERE HUSBANDS MANIFESTED AUTOIMMUNITY TO SPERMATOZOA

Clinical Category	Proportion of Couples Pregnant		Level of Significance†
	More than 50% Sperm Antibody Bound*	Less Than 50% Sperm Antibody Bound*	
Normal men and women	4/26	6/9	0.005
Normal men and abnormal women	6/16	13/31	NS
Abnormal men and normal women	0/6	3/4	0.01
Abnormal men and women	2/7	1/9	NS
All groups	12/55	23/53	0.05

*As determined by immunobead binding of sperm washed free of seminal fluid.

†Chi-square analysis. NS = not significant.

(From Mettler et al.[65] Reproduced with permission.)

Hence, penetration frequencies for sperm incubated in antibody-negative sera were 76%, with 1.4 ± 0.27 sperm per penetrated egg. After exposure to antisperm antibody, nearly 100% of eggs were penetrated with 2 to 9 sperm per egg.

These results are important in indicating that the locus of impaired gamete interaction for men with autoantibodies to sperm is at the level of the zona pellucida and not at the egg surface. Whether all antisperm antibodies block zona penetration has not been determined. Indeed, these results also emphasize the need to identify the antigens to which sperm antibodies are directed. This is important, as the effects of antibody binding to the sperm surface depend upon their antigenic targets.

Antibodies directed against epitopes on or near the zona pellucida would be expected to block zona attachment. Antibodies to other antigens might have effects on oolemmal fusion, as well as on sperm cervical mucus transport. Indeed, this was the case in studies of the effects of different monoclonal antibodies on sperm function in different laboratory animals.[87,88] There is no currently satisfactory method to distinguish antisperm surface antibodies directed against fertilization-related antigens from those unrelated to fertilization.

In the future it should be possible to identify and purify specific antigens, which will substantially improve our diagnostic capabilities. The availability of such antigens will lead to specific enzyme-linked immunosorbant assays for each one, and determining the relative amounts of antibodies directed against different antigens should permit more specific diagnoses. The generation of polyclonal antisera to each antigen also might act as probes of the sperm surface during capacitation, allowing one to distinguish fertilization-related from unrelated antigens. Such sera may also allow the determination of shared antigenicity among sperm, fertilized eggs, and preimplantation embryos.

EFFECTS OF AUTOIMMUNITY TO SPERM ON SPERM PRODUCTION

Despite the presence of high levels of antisperm antibodies in the reproductive tract, the majority of men with this autoimmunity do not exhibit impairment of sperm production. Their sperm concentration in the ejaculate is similar to that of infertile men in the absence of such antibodies.

A blood–testis barrier exists between Sertoli cells as tight, junctional complexes and divides the seminiferous tubule into the basal and adlumenal compartments.[89] Naturally occurring orchitis in dark mink is associated with breakdown of these junctions, suggesting that the blood–testis barrier can become defective during seasonal regression of the testis.[90]

Experimental immunization of guinea pigs with testis extracts containing specific autoantigens has also been associated with the development of immune orchitis.[91] In humans, however, the question is unresolved as to whether autoimmunity to spermatozoa can impair spermatogenesis. After vasectomy, there is no evidence of the development of clinical orchitis.[92] In a single study, a man with prostatic cancer destined to undergo orchiectomy was immunized with spermatozoa and the testis subsequently examined for evidence of orchitis.[93] Only focal lesions were seen, suggesting that the antigens present on mature spermatozoa would not be expressed during the development of precursor sperm in the testis. Unfortunately, the cancer itself may have altered this individual's immune responsiveness to sperm antigens.

Spontaneously occurring sperm-reactive antibodies have been demonstrated in the serum of an infertile man with normal semen values that cross-reacted with intratesticular sperm in frozen, unfixed sections of human testis.[94] The presence of IgG deposits was shown on the seminiferous tubule wall, in germ cells, and in the interstitium of testis biopsy specimens from infertile patients.[95] Immunoelectron microscopy revealed immune complexes on the seminiferous tubule basement membrane in association with orchitis.[96] Antibodies induced experimentally against laminin (a basement membrane component) in rats were shown to alter Sertoli cell ultrastructure and spermatogenesis.[97]

Etiology of Immunity to Spermatozoa

At the onset of spermatogenesis in puberty, new antigens make their appearance on the sperm surface.[98] Because tolerance for self-antigens is established in the neonatal period, these antigens may be immunogenic. It has been theorized that sequestration by the blood–testis barrier of spermatozoa during spermatogenesis and subsequent spermiation in the lumen of the seminiferous tubule prevents the generation of autoantibodies to sperm. This concept, however, has been challenged, and the theory proposed that some testicular autoantigens are accessible to circulating antibodies and are immunogenic.[99]

Large number of lymphocytes ($\sim 1 \times 10^6$/cc) have been identified in the semen of healthy heterosexual men.[100] A population of intraepithelial suppressor T lymphocytes also was identified in the epididymis by immunoperoxidase staining with monoclonal probes to T cell surface antigens.[101] These T suppressor cells may play a role in preventing the development of autoimmunity to sperm.

Additional evidence suggests that the absence of autoimmunity to sperm may result from continuous active suppression by T suppressor cells. A diminished number of T suppressor cells relative to T helper cells was found in approximately one third of men with autoimmunity to sperm.[102]

Humoral antisperm antibodies are present in more than one half of men who have undergone vasectomy.[103] Several studies have documented that the chance of pregnancy is diminished in men who have undergone vasovasostomy, despite the presence of spermatozoa in the ejaculate in those in whom antisperm antibodies are detected within the reproductive tract.[104-106] Men with bilateral congenital absence of the vas deferens and seminal vesicles, as occurs in cystic fibrosis, have also been found to develop autoimmunity to sperm.[107] Both congenital and acquired obstruction to sperm egress may then play a role in the genesis of autoimmunity to sperm, perhaps by allowing entry of sperm antigens into the circulation. The question has been raised as to whether cryptic unilateral intratesticular or extratesticular obstruction could lead to antisperm antibody formation.[108] In fact, when mice undergo unilateral vas ligation these autoantibodies develop in association with diminished fertility.[109]

In 80 spontaneously infertile men in whom unilateral testicular obstruction was confirmed by exploratory scrototomy 40 had severe oligospermia, with sperm counts less than 5 million/mL, even though testicular biopsies showed adequate spermatogenesis and despite the presence of an unobstructed contralateral testis.[110] Seventy-five percent of these men had antisperm antibodies in their plasma. The most common sites of obstruction were the tail of the epididymis and the vas deferens. The author proposed that unsuspected unilateral disease might affect testicular sperm output through the development of an immune-mediated orchitis.

As mentioned earlier, naturally occurring orchitis leading to infertility occurs in the dark mink after seasonal regression of the testis.[90] An experimental immune orchitis that leads to aspermatogenesis was induced in guinea pigs after immunization with testis extracts.[91] It should be emphasized, however, that the majority of men from infertile couples with autoimmunity to sperm manifest no clinical evidence of orchitis or suppression of spermatogenesis. Indeed, it could be that those sperm antigens associated with autoimmunity to sperm in the majority of men do not appear in the testis during spermatogenesis but rather at some later stage of sperm maturation. Alterations in sperm surface moieties resulting from secretory products of the epididymis have been documented. Antisperm antibodies may also be directed against sperm-associated antigens that are surface-coating glycoproteins derived from secretions of the accessory glands at the time of ejaculation.[111] A tissue-specific antigen of ejaculation that binds to spermatozoa at the time of ejaculation and is secreted

by the seminal vesicles has been identified in the rat. We have noted, however, that epididymal sperm derived from men undergoing orchiectomy for prostatic malignancy exhibit an unaltered binding pattern of immunoglobulins to their surface compared with ejaculated sperm exposed to antisperm antibodies. This observation suggests that some sperm antigens to which antisperm autobodies are directed are expressed on epididymal sperm prior to ejaculation (R. A. Bronson, G.W. Cooper, unpublished observations).

It has also been hypothesized that during infection of the genital tract, macrophages and lymphocytes may encounter antigens on sperm to which the immune system is not tolerant. An increased frequency of antisperm antibodies was noted in men who were unresponsive to antibiotics who had repeatedly positive semen *Ureaplasma* cultures.[112] A subsequent study, however, did not corroborate this association.[113] Three hundred twenty-four semen specimens were tested for the presence of autoantibodies to sperm, leukospermia, and *Ureaplasma urealyticum*. Autoantibodies were detected on the sperm surface by immunobead binding in 46 of the ejaculates. Of those that were antibody positive, 10.9% cultured positive for *Ureaplasma* and 15.2% were found to have greater than 1 million polymorphonuclear leukocytes (PMNs)/cc. This compared with 28.4% positive results for antibody-negative ejaculates, in which 10.8% possessed more than 1 million PMNs/cc. It is hoped that additional evidence will determine whether acute or chronic genital tract infection can cause autoimmunity to sperm.

Experimental exposure of spermatozoa to the gastrointestinal tract results in the development of antisperm antibodies.[10,113] This has been demonstrated in mice orally immunized and rabbits rectally immunized with spermatozoa. A high frequency of antisperm antibodies also was documented in the sera of homosexual men.[114-116] The distribution of immunoglobulin isotypes of antisperm antibodies in these sera is different from that in heterosexual men from infertile couples.[114] While tail-directed antibody of the IgG class, and to a lesser extent IgA antibodies, predominate in the latter group, sperm head-directed IgMs are more frequently detected in the sera of homosexuals. Given the increasing evidence for the existence of a common mucosal immune system in humans, it is probable that lymphocytes in Peyer's patches or the colonic submucosa could become sensitized to spermatozoa, and then return to the male genital tract and locally secrete antisperm antibodies.

Etiology of Immunity to Sperm in Women

Although women are inoculated intravaginally with spermatozoa during coitus, this usually is not associated with the development of immunity to sperm. This observation is in contrast with the fact that the female reproductive tract of primates is not immunologically privileged, as demonstrated by the intravaginal inoculation of rhesus monkeys with T4 coliphage and a glycopolysaccharide of *Salmonella typhosa*.[16] The intravaginal inoculation of women with polio virus also leads to the formation of locally produced antiviral antibodies in the vaginal secretions.[11]

An immunoinhibitory substance has been detected and partially isolated from seminal plasma.[117] A relative lack of antigenicity was noted after epididymal mouse sperm were incubated in seminal fluid as opposed to saline.[118] Murine germ cells obtained from testicular suspensions and injected into syngeneic recipients yielded evidence of immunosuppression.[119] Although there has been some controversy as to the specificity of the immune modulation by seminal plasma, a broad spectrum of immunosuppressive effects on lymphocyte function in vitro has been documented.[120] These include blocking proliferation of T cells stimulated by mitogen, antigen, and allogeneic cells. Complement activity is also reduced by seminal plasma, possibly by several of protease inhibitors known to be present.[121]

Could nature provide the means through concomitant exposure at coitus to seminal fluid immunosuppressors, to prevent the development of immunity to sperm in women? Conversely, would a lack of immunosuppressive activity of seminal fluid lead to the development of antisperm antibodies? A pilot study was designed to answer these questions. The immunosuppressive activity of seminal plasma obtained from men in couples diagnosed to be free of antisperm antibodies was compared with that of men whose wives manifested high or low-level immunity to sperm.[122] Third-party peripheral blood lymphocytes were exposed to phytohemagglutinin, a mitogen that stimulates lymphoblast formation, in the presence of various dilutions of seminal fluid. Although a wide range in immunosuppressive activity of semen was noted between the two groups of men, no significant difference was seen between semen samples of husbands whose wives were highly sensitized to sperm versus those who were nonimmune.

REFERENCES

1. Goodman JW: Immunoglobulins' structure and function, in Stites DP, Stobo JD, Wells JV (eds): *Basic and Clinical Immunology*, ed 6. E. Norwalk, CT, Appleton & Lange, 1987, pp 27–36.
2. Nossal GV: The basic components of the immune system. *N Engl J Med* 316:132, 1987.
3. Wira CR, Sullivan DA: Sex steroid hormone regulation of IgA and IgG in rat uterine secretions. *Nature* 268:534, 1977.
4. Sullivan DA, Wira CR: Hormonal regulation of immunoglobulins in the rat uterus. Uterine response to multiple estradiol treatments. *Endocrinology* 114:650, 1984.
5. Sullivan DA, Wira CR: Hormonal regulation of immunoglobulins in rat uterus. Uterine response to a single estradiol treatment. *Endocrinology* 112:260, 1983.
6. Wira CR, Sullivan DA, Sandoe CP: Estrogen-mediated control of the secretory immune system in the uterus of the rat. *Ann NY Acad Sci* 409:534, 1983.
7. Parr MB, Parr EL: Immunochemical localization of immunoglobulins A, G, M in the mouse female genital tract. *J Reprod Fertil* 74:361, 1985.
8. Wira CR, Stern JE, Colby E: Estradiol regulation of secretory complement in the uterus of the rat: Evidence for involvement of RNA synthesis. *Immunology* 133:2624, 1984.
9. Sullivan DA, Richardson GS, MacLaughlin DJ, Wira CR: Variations in the levels of secretory component in human uterine fluid during the menstrual cycle. *J Steroid Biochem* 20:509, 1984.
10. Wira CR, Sandoe CP: Specific IgA and IgG antibodies in the secretions s of the female reproductive tract. Effects of immunization and estradiol on expression of this response in vivo. *J Immunol* 138:4159, 1987.
11. Ogra PL, Ogra SS: Local antibody response to polio vaccine in the human female genital tract. *J Immunol* 110:1307, 1973.
12. Allardyce RA: Effect of ingested sperm on fecundity in the rat. *J Exp Med* 159:1548, 1984.
13. Chodirker WB, Tomasi TB Jr: Gamma-globulin: quantitative relationships in human serum and nonvascular fluids. *Science* 142:1080, 1963.
14. Waldman RH, Cruz JM, Rowe DS: Intravaginal immunization of humans with *Candida albicans*. *J Immunol* 109:662, 1972.
15. Schumacher GFB: Humoral immune factors in the female reproductive tract and their changes during the cycle, in Dhindsa D, Schumacher GFB (eds): *Immunologic Aspects of Infertility and Fertility Regulation*. New York, Elsevier, 1980, pp 93–142.
16. Yang SL, Schumacher GFB: Immune response after vaginal application of antigens in the rhesus monkey. *Fertil Steril* 32:588, 1979.
17. Lippes J. Ogra SS, Tomasi TB Jr, Tourville OR: Immunohistological localization of G, A, M secretory piece and lactoferin in the female genital tract. *Contraception* 1:163, 1972.
18. Tourville DR, Ogra SS, Lippes J, Tomasi TB Jr: The human female reproductive tract. Immunohistological localizing of A, G, M secretory piece and lactoferin. *Am J Obstet Gynecol* 108:1102, 1970.
19. Schumacher GFB, Holt JA, Reale F: Approaches to the analysis of human endometrial secretion, in Baller FK, Schumacher GFB (eds): *Biology of the Fluids of the Female Genital Tract*. New York, Elsevier-North Holland, 1971.
20. Tauber PF: Biochemical components of the human endometrium, in Beller FK, Schumacher GFB (eds): *Biology of the Fluids of the Female Genital Tract*. New York, Elsevier-North Holland, 1971.
21. Lippes J, Enders RG, Pragay DA, Bartholomew WR: The collection and analysis of human fallopian tubal fluid. *Contraception* 5:85, 1972.
22. Lippes J: Applied physiology of the uterine tube. *Obstet Gynecol Annu* 4:119, 1975.
23. Schumacher GFB: Hormonal immune factors in the female reproductive tract and their changes during the cycle, in Dhindsa D, Schumacher GFB (eds): *Immunological Aspects of Infertility and Fertility Regulation*. New York, Elsevier, 1980, pp 93–142.
24. Bronson RA: Immunologic abnormalities of the female reproductive tract, in Gondos B, Riddick DH (eds): *Pathology of Infertility*. New York, Theime, 1987, pp 13–28.
25. Baskin MJ: Temporary sterilization by the injection of human spermatozoa: A preliminary report. *Am J Obstet Gynecol* 24:892, 1932.
26. McLaren A: Immunological control of fertility in female mice. *Nature* 201:583, 1964.
27. Edwards RG: Immunologic control of fertility in female mice. *Nature* 203:50, 1964.
28. Seki M, Mettler L: Influence of spermatozoal antibodies in the reproduction of mice. *Am J Reprod Immunol* 2:225, 1982.
29. Katsh S: Infertility in female guinea pigs induced by injection of homologous sperm. *Am J Obstet Gynecol* 78:276, 1959.
30. Tung KSK, Okada A, Yanagimachi R: Sperm autoantigens and fertilization. I. Effects of antisperm antibodies on rouleaux formation, viability and acrosome reaction of guinea pig sperm. *Biol Reprod* 23:877, 1980.
31. Yanagimachi R, Okada A, Tung KSK: Sperm autoantigens and fertilization. II. Effects of anti-guinea pig sperm antibodies on sperm-ovum interactions. *Biol Reprod* 24:512, 1981.
32. Menge AC, Peegel H, Riolo ML: Sperm factors responsible for immunologic induction of pre- and post-fertilization infertility in rabbits. *Biol Reprod* 20:93, 1979.

33. Lee CYG, Wong E, Zhang JH: Inhibitory effects of monoclonal sperm antibodies on the fertilization of mouse oocytes in vitro and in vivo. *J Reprod Immunol* 9:261, 1986.

34. Rumke PH, Hellinga G: Autoantibodies against spermatozoa in sterile men. *Am J Clin Pathol* 32:357, 1959.

35. Rumke P, Van Amstel N, Messa EN, Rezemar PD: Prognosis of fertility of men with sperm agglutinins in the serum. *Fertil Steril* 24:305, 1973.

36. Franklin RR, Dukes CD: Antispermatozoal antibody and unexplained infertility. *Am J Obstet Gynecol* 89:6, 1964.

37. Beer AE, Neaves WB: Antigenic status of semen from the viewpoints of the female and male. *Fertil Steril* 29:3, 1978.

38. Bell EB: An immune-type agglutination of mouse spermatozoa by *Pseudomonas maltophilia*. *J Reprod Fertil* 17:275, 1968.

39. Rose NR, Hjort T, Rumke P, Harper MJK, Vyazov O: Techniques for detection of iso- and auto-antibodies to human spermatozoa. *Clin Exp Immunol* 23:175, 1976.

40. Shulman S, Jackson H, Stone M: Antibodies to spermatozoa. V. Comparative studies of sperm-agglutinating activity in groups of infertile and fertile women. *Am J Obstet Gynecol* 123:139, 1975.

41. Pavia CS, Stites DP, Bronson RA: Reproductive immunology, in Stites DP, Stebo JD, Wells JV (eds): *Basic and Clinical Immunology*, ed 6. E. Norwalk, CT, Appleton & Lange, 1987, pp 609–613.

42. Clarke GN, Elliott PG, Smaila C: Detection of sperm antibodies in semen using the immunobead test. A study of 813 consecutive patterns. *Am J Reprod Immunol Microbiol* 7:61, 1985.

43. Haas GG, Cives DB, Schreiber AD: Immunologic infertility: Identification of patients with antisperm antibody. *N Engl J Med* 303:722, 1980.

44. Jager S, Kremer J, Van Slochteren-Draaisma T: A simple method of screening for antisperm antibodies in the human male. Detection of spermatozoal surface IgG with the direct mixed agglutination reaction carried out in untreated fresh human seman. *Int J Fertil* 23:12, 1978.

45. Hancock RJT, Farakis S: Detection of antibody-coated sperm by panning procedures. *J Immunol Methods* 66:149, 1984.

46. Bronson RA, Cooper GW, Rosenfeld DL: Membrane-bound sperm specific antibodies: Their role in infertility, in Vogel H, Jagiello G (eds): *Bioregulators in Reproduction*. New York, Academic Press, 1981, pp 526–527.

47. Bronson RA, Cooper GW, Rosenfeld DL: Auto-immunity to spermatozoa: effects on sperm penetration of cervical mucus as reflected by post coital testing. *Fertil Steril* 41:9, 1984.

48. Jager S, Kremer J. Kuiken J, et al: Induction of the shaking phenomenon by pretreatment of spermatozoa with sera containing antispermatozoal antibodies. *Fertil Steril* 36:784, 1981.

49. Bronson RA, Cooper GW, Rosenfeld DL, Gilbert JV, Plaut AG: The effect of IgA₁ protease on immunoglobulins bound to the sperm surface and sperm cervical mucus penetrating ability. *Fertil Steril* 47:985, 1987.

50. Bronson RA, Cooper G, Hjort T, et al: Antisperm antibodies, detected by agglutination, immobilization, microtoxicity and immunobead binding assays. *J Reprod Immunol* 8:279, 1985.

51. Bronson RA, Cooper GW, Rosenfeld DL: Seminal fluid antisperm antibodies do not reflect those present on the sperm surface. *Fertil Steril* 48:505, 1987.

52. Rapp HJ, Borsos T: *Molecular Basis of Complement*. New York, Appleton-Century-Crofts, 1970.

53. Cooper NR: The complement system, in Stites DP, Stobo JD, Wells JV (eds): *Basic and Clinical Immunology*, ed 6. E. Norwalk, CT, Appleton & Lange, 1987.

54. Fortin P, Babai F: Ultrastructural visualization of the membrane attack complex of the complement and its insertion in the glycocaly of the red cell using ruthinium red. Presented at the 6th international congress of immunology, Toronto, July 6–11, 1986.

55. Humphrey JH, Dourmashkin RR: Electron microscope studies of immune cell lysis, in Wolstenholme GEW, Knight J (eds): *CIBA Foundation Symposium on Complement*. Boston, Little, Brown, 1965, pp 175–189.

56. Colten HR, Borsos T, Rapp HJ: Titration of the first component of complement on a molecular basis: Suitability of IgM and unsuitability of IgG hemolysins as a sensitizer. *Immunochemistry* 6:461, 1969.

57. Bronson RA, Cooper GW, Rosenfeld DL: Correlation between regional specificity of antisperm antibodies to the spermatozoan surface and complement-mediated sperm immobilization. *Am J Reprod Immunol* 2:222, 1982.

58. Bronson RA, Cooper GW, Phillips D: Ultrastructural-physiologic correlates of human sperm egg penetrating ability. Presented at the 12th annual meeting of the American Society of Andrology, Denver, March 6–7, 1987.

12th annual meeting of the American Society of Andrology, Denver, March 6–7, 1987.

59. Kratz HJ, Borsos T, Isliker H: Mouse monoclonal antibodies and the red cell surface. II. Effect of hapten density on complement fixation and activation. *Mol Immunol* 22:229, 1985.

60. Brooks GF, Lammel CJ, Petersen BH, et al: Human seminal plasma inhibition of antibody complement-mediated killing and opsonization of *Neisseria gonorrhoeae* and other gram-negative organisms. *J Clin Invest* 67:1523, 1981.

61. Price RJ, Boettcher B: The presence of complement in human cervical mucus and its possible relevance to infertility in women with complement-dependent sperm immobilizing antibodies. *Fertil Steril* 32:61, 1979.

62. Isojima S, Tsuchiya K, Koyama K, Tanaka C: Further studies on sperm immobilizing antibody found in sera of unexplained cases of sterility in women. *Am J Obstet Gynecol* 112:199, 1972.

63. Tung KSK, Cooke WD Jr, McCarthy TA, Robitaille P: Human sperm antigens and antisperm antibodies. II. Age-related incidence of antisperm antibodies. *Clin Exp Immunol* 25:73, 1976.

64. Hjort T, Hansen RB: Immunofluorescent studies on human spermatozoa. I. The detection of different spermatozoal antibodies and their occurrence in normal and infertile women. *Clin Exp Immunol* 8:9, 1971.

65. Mettler L, Czuppon AB, Alexander N, et al: Antibodies to spermatozoa and seminal plasma antigens detected by various enzyme-linked immunosorbent (ELISA) assays. *J Reprod Immunol* 8:301, 1985.

66. Bronson RA, Cooper GW: Effects of sperm-reactive monoclonal antibodies on the cervical mucus penetrating ability of human spermatozoa. *Am J Immunol Microbiol* 14:59, 1987.

67. Bronson RA, Cooper GW, Witkin SS: Detection of spontaneously occurring sperm-directed antibodies in infertile couples by immunobead binding and enzyme-linked immunosorbent assay. *Ann NY Acad Sci* 438:504, 1984.

68. Hjort T, Johnson PM, Mori T: An overview of the WHO international multi-center study on antibodies to reproductive tract antigens in clinically defined sera. *J Reprod Immunol* 8:539, 1985.

69. Bronson RA, Cooper GW, Rosenfeld DL: Sperm antibodies: Their role in infertility. *Fertil Steril* 42:171, 1984.

70. Bronson RA, Cooper GW, Rosenfeld DL: Factors affecting the population of the female reproductive tract by spermatozoa: Their diagnosis and treatment. *Semin Reprod Endocrinol* 4:387, 1986.

71. McShane PM, Schiff I, Trentham MD: Cellular immunity to sperm in infertile women. *JAMA* 253:3555, 1985.

72. Wolf DP, Sokoloski J, Khan M, Litt M: Human cervical mucus. III. Isolation and characterization of rheologically active mucin. *Fertil Steril* 28:53, 1977.

73. Nicosia SV: Physiology of cervical mucus production. *Semin Reprod Endocrinol* 4:313, 1986.

74. Bronson RA: Sperm dysfunction: A new understanding of male infertility. *Sci Am*, in press.

75. Peterson RN, Hunt WP, Henry LH: Interaction of boar spermatozoa with porcine oocytes: Increase in proteins with high affinity for the zona pellucida during epididymal transit. *Gamete Res* 14:57, 1986.

76. Moore HDM, Hartman TD, Pryor JP: Development of oocyte-penetrating capacity of spermatozoa in the human epididymis. *Int J Androl* 6:310, 1983.

77. Rogers BJ: The sperm penetration assay: Its usefulness reevaluated. *Fertil Steril* 43:821, 1985.

78. Alexander NJ: Antibodies to human spermatozoa impede sperm penetration of cervical mucus and hamster eggs. *Fertil Steril* 41:433, 1984.

79. Haas GG Jr, Ansmanus M, Culp L, Tureck RW, Blasco L: The effect of immunoglobulin occurring on human sperm in vivo on the human sperm hamster ova penetration assay. *Am J Reprod Immunol* 7:109, 1985.

80. Bronson RA, Cooper GW, Rosenfeld DL: Ability of antibody-bound human sperm to penetrate zona-free hamster ova in vitro. *Fertil Steril* 36:778, 1981.

81. Bronson RA, Cooper GW, Rosenfeld DL: Complement-mediated effects of sperm head-directed human antibodies on the ability of human spermatozoa to penetrate zona-free hamster eggs. *Fertil Steril* 40:91, 1983.

82. Bronson R, Cooper G, Rosenfeld D: Reproductive effects of sperm surface antibodies, in Lobl T, Hafez ESE (eds): *Male Fertility and Its Regulation*. Boston, MTP Press, 1985, pp 417–436.

83. Dravland E, Josh MM: Sperm coating antigens secreted by the

epididymis and seminal vesicle of the rat. *Biol Reprod* 25:649: 1981.

84. Bronson RA, Cooper GW, Rosenfeld DL: Auto-immunity to spermatozoa: Effect on sperm penetration of cervical mucus as reflected by postcoital testing. *Fertil Steril* 41:609, 1984.

85. Ayvaliotis B, Bronson R, Cooper G, Rosenfeld D: Conception rates in couples where autoimmunity to sperm is detected. *Fertil Steril* 43:739, 1985.

86. Bronson RA, Cooper GW, Rosenfeld DL: Sperm-specific iso-antibodies and auto-antibodies inhibit the binding of human sperm to the human zona pellucida. *Fertil Steril* 38:724, 1982.

87. Saling PM, Irons G, Waibel R: Mouse sperm antigens that participate in fertilization. I. Inhibition of sperm fusion with egg plasma membrane using monoclonal antibodies. *Biol Reprod* 33:515, 1985.

88. Saling PM, Lakoski KA: Mouse sperm antigens that participate in fertilization. II. Inhibition of sperm penetration through zona pellucida using monoclonal antibodies. *Biol Reprod* 33:527, 1985.

89. Dym M, Caviacchia JC: Further observations on the blood–testis barrier in monkeys. *Biol Reprod* 17:390, 1977.

90. Tung KSK, Ellis L, Teuscher C, et al: The black mink *(Mustela vison)*. A natural model of immunologic male infertility. *J Exp Med* 154:1016, 1981.

91. Teuscher C, Wild GC, Tung KSK: Experimental allergic orchitis: The isolation and partial characterization of an aspermatogenic polypeptide (AP3) with an apparent sequential disease-inducing determinant(s). *J Immunol* 130:2683, 1983.

92. Massey FJ, Bernstein GS, Fallon WM, et al: Vasectomy and health. Results from a large cohort study. *JAMA* 252:1023, 1984.

93. Mancini RE, Andrada JA, Sarceni D, et al: Immunological and testicular response in a man sensitized with human testicular homogenate. *J Clin Endocrinol Metab* 25:859, 1965.

94. Haas GG Jr, D'Cruz G, DeBault LE: The distribution of HLA-ABC and Dr antigens in normal human testis. Presented at the 20th annual meeting of the Society for the Study of Reproduction, Urbana, IL, July 20–23, 1987.

95. Lehmann D, Temminck B, DaRugna D, et al: Role of immunological factors in male infertility. Immunohistochemical and serological evidence. *Lab Invest* 57:21, 1987.

96. Salomon F, Saremaslani P, Jakob M, Hedinger CF: Immunocomplex orchitis in infertile men: Immunoelectron microscopy of abnormal basement membrane structures. *Lab Invest* 47:555, 1982.

97. Lustig L, Doncel GF, Berenstein E, Denduchis B: Testis lesions, cellular and immune response induced in rats by immunization with laminin. *Am J Reprod Immunol Microbiol* 14:123, 1987.

98. O'Brien DA, Millett CF: Immunochemical identification of multiple cell surface antigens appearing during specific stages of mouse spermatogenesis. *Gamete Res* 13:199, 1986.

99. Tung KSK, Yule TD, Mahi-Brown CA, Listrom MD: Distribution of histopathology and Ia positive cells in actively induced and passively transferred experimental immune orchitis. *J Immunol* 138:752, 1987.

100. El-Demiry MIM, Hargreave TB, Busmittil A, et al: Lymphocytic sub-populations in the male genital tract. *Br J Urol* 57:769, 1985.

101. Ritchie AWS: Intraepithelial lymphocytes in the normal epididymis: A mechanism for tolerance to sperm auto-antigens? *Br J Urol* 56:79, 1984.

102. Witkin SS: Phenotypic characterization of seminal lymphocytes and their relations to sperm antibody production. Presented at the annual meeting of the American Fertility Society, Reno, NV, Sept 28–30, 1987.

103. Shulman S, Zappi E, Ahmed U, Davis J: Immunologic consequences of vasectomy. *Contraception* 5:269, 1972.

104. Linnet L, Hjort T, Fogh-Andersen D: Association between failure to impregnate after vasovasostomy and sperm agglutinins in semen. *Lancet* 1:117, 1981.

105. Alexander NJ: Antibody levels and immunologic infertility, in Isojima S, Billington WD (eds): *Reproductive Immunology*. New York, Elsevier, 1983, pp 207–214.

106. Wicklynd R, Alexander NJ: Vasovasostomy: Evaluation of success. *Urology* 13:532, 1979.

107. Girgis SM, Eklandroas EM, Iskander R, El-Dokhly R, Girgis RN: Sperm antibodies in serum and semen in men with bilateral congenital absence of the as deferens. *Arch Androl* 8:301, 1982.

108. Hendry WF: Surgery for testicular obstruction. *Recent Adv Urol/Androl* 4:313, 1987.

109. Kessler DL, Smith WD, Hamilton MS, Berger RE: Infertility in mice after unilateral vasectomy. *Fertil Steril* 43:308, 1985.

110. Hendry WF, Parslow JM, Stedronska J: Exploratory scrotomy in 168 azoospermic males. *Br J Urol* 55:785, 1983.

111. Isojima S, Kameda K, Tsuji Y, et al: Establishment and characterization of a human hybridoma secreting monoclonal antibody with high titers of sperm immobilizing and agglutinating activities against human seminal plasma. *J Reprod Immunol* 10:67, 1987.

112. Toth A, Lesser ML, Brooks C, Labriola D: Subsequent pregnancies among 161 couples treated for T-mycoplasma genital tract infection. *N Engl J Med* 308:505, 1983.

113. Bronson R, Cooper G, Rosenfeld D: Lack of correlation between seminal fluid ureaplasma status, leukospermia and auto-immunity to spermatozoa. Presented at the 30th annual meeting of the Society for Gynecologic Investigation, Washington, DC, March 17–20, 1983.

114. Bronson R, Cooper G, Rosenfeld D, et al: Comparison of antisperm antibodies in homosexual and infertile men with auto-immunity to spermatozoa. Presented at the 30th annual meeting of the Society for Gynecologic Investigation, Washington, DC, March 17–20, 1983.

115. Witkin SS, Sonnabend J: Immune response to spermatozoa in homosexual men. *Fertil Steril* 39:337, 1983.

116. Wolff H, Schill WB: Antisperm antibodies in infertile and homosexual men: Relationship to serologic and clinical findings. *Fertil Steril* 44:673, 1985.

117. Lord EM, Sensabaugh GF, Stites DP: Immunosuppressive activity of human seminal plasma. Inhibition of in vivo lymphocyte activation. *J Immunol* 118:1704, 1977.

118. Anderson DJ, Tarter TH: Immunosuppressive effects of mouse seminal plasma components in vivo and in vitro. *J Immunol* 128:535, 1982.

119. Hurtenbach U, Shearer GM: Germ cell induced immune suppression in mice: Effect of inoculation of syngenic spermatozoa on cell-mediated immune responses. *J Exp Med* 155:1719, 1982.

120. James K, Hargreave TB: Immunosuppression by seminal plasma and its possible clinical significance. *Immunol Today* 5:357, 1984.

121. Petersen BH, Lammel CJ, Stites DP, Brooks GF: Human seminal plasma inhibition of complement. *J Lab Clin Med* 96:582, 1980.

122. Bronson RA: Immunologic abnormalities of the female reproductive tract, in Gondos B, Riddick DH (eds): *Pathology of Infertility*. New York, Thieme, 1987, pp 13–28.

CHAPTER 16

Infections

Gilles R.G. Monif

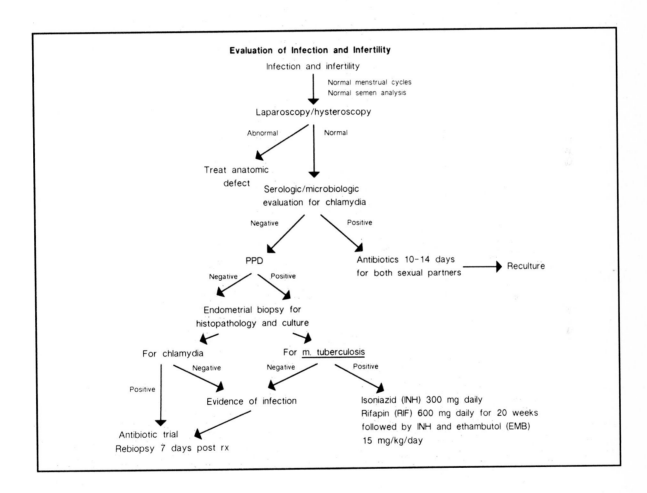

Evaluation of Infection and Infertility

Infection and infertility

Normal menstrual cycles
Normal semen analysis

Laparoscopy/hysteroscopy

Abnormal → Treat anatomic defect

Normal → Serologic/microbiologic evaluation for chlamydia

Negative → PPD

Positive → Antibiotics 10–14 days for both sexual partners → Reculture

PPD Negative / Positive → Endometrial biopsy for histopathology and culture

For chlamydia

For m. tuberculosis

Positive → Antibiotic trial Rebiopsy 7 days post rx

Negative → Evidence of infection

Negative

Positive → Isoniazid (INH) 300 mg daily
Rifapin (RIF) 600 mg daily for 20 weeks
followed by INH and ethambutol (EMB)
15 mg/kg/day

The quest for the microbiologic causation in infertility can be subdivided based on anatomic sites. Theoretically, microbiologic organisms can function at the cervical, endometrial, and fallopian tube levels and negatively affect fertilization or implantation.

FALLOPIAN TUBE INFERTILITY

Certain organisms, such as *Mycobacterium tuberculosis*, *Chlamydia trachomatis*, and *Neisseria gonorrhoeae*, by virtue of their replication, can alter fallopian tube structure and function.[1–3]

In the early 1970s, laparoscopic evaluation demonstrated a 12.8% frequency of tubal occlusion after a single episode of acute salpingitis; after two episodes the figure increased to 35.5%, and after three episodes, to 75%.[2] Reevaluation in 1980 of the effect on fallopian tube morbidity of expanded therapeutic techniques revealed frequency of tubal occlusion after one, two, and three episodes of acute salpingitis to be 11.4, 23.1, and 54.3%, respectively (Table 16–1.)[4]

TABLE 16–1. INCIDENCE OF TUBAL OCCLUSION DOCUMENTED BY LAPAROSCOPY FOLLOWING ONE, TWO, OR THREE EPISODES OF ACUTE SALPINGITIS

Number of Episodes of Acute Salpingitis	Am J Obstet Gynecol 121:707, 1975	Am J Obstet Gynecol 131:880, 1980
One	12.8%	11.4%
Two	35.5%	23.1%
Three	75 %	54.3%

Modified from Westrom.[9] Reproduced with permission.

The probability of secondary infertility is statistically linked to age, number of antecedent episodes of acute salpingitis, and severity of disease at the time of institution of appropriate antibiotic therapy (Tables 16–2 and 16–3). The frequency of infertility was reduced irrespective of the number of prior episodes of acute salpingitis in women aged 15 to 24 years, as opposed to those aged 25 to 34 years. The difference may reflect the increased prevalence of overt gonorrheal rather than chlamydial infection in the younger group. Women less than 25 years of age who previously had gonococcus-associated salpingitis had a significantly better fertility prognosis than those who previously had so-called nongonococcal salpingitis. Nongonococcal salpingitis usually has a chlamydial etiology or is a polymicrobial superinfection in which *N. gonorrhoeae* has autoeliminated.[5]

When the degree of the inflammatory reaction documented by laparoscopy is correlated with subsequent reproductive outcomes, a positive increased correlation can be demonstrated. Particularly with gonococcal disease, early effective antibiotic therapy gives the shortest value of erythrocyte sedimentation rate (ESR) half-time.[6] Little involuntary infertility occurs in patients who receive early antibiotic therapy and demonstrate a good therapeutic response.

Culdocentesis coupled with the application of sophisticated anaerobiology provided the opportunity to investigate what could be construed as both the front and the back of a conduit. With the information derived, it was possible to make a sophisticated guess as to what happened in the middle. The concept of polymicrobial superinfection of initial gonococcal salpingitis was developed from

TABLE 16–2. PERCENTAGE OF SECONDARY INFERTILITY POST-SALPINGITIS IN DIFFERENT AGE GROUPS

Number of Infections	Percent of Infertility Post-Salpingitis in Different Age Groups		
	15–24 yrs.	24–34 yrs.	Total
One	9.4	19.2	11.4
Two	20.9	31.0	23.1
Three or more	51.6	60.0	54.3

(Modified from Westrom.[4] Reproduced with permission.)

TABLE 16–3. CORRELATION BETWEEN MAGNITUDE OF INFLAMMATORY CHANGE AND SUBSEQUENT SECONDARY INFERTILITY FOLLOWING A SINGLE EPISODE OF SALPINGITIS

Magnitude of Inflammatory Change	Percent of Infertility Post-Salpingitis by Different Age Groups		
	15–24 yrs.	24–34 yrs.	Total
Mild	5.8	7.8	6.1
Moderately severe	10.8	22.0	13.4
Severe	27.3	40.0	30.0

(From Westrom.[4] Reproduced with permission.)

bacteriologic observations of the cul-de-sac.[7–10] *N. gonorrhoeae*, by virtue of its replication, sufficiently lowers the oxidation-reduction potential of the local microbiologic environment so as to initiate the anaerobic progression. This process is the principal mechanism by which a monomicrobial process becomes polymicrobial disease.[10,11]

As the progressive changes in the microbiologic environment select for the more microaerophilic organisms (class II anaerobes), *N. gonorrhoeae* undergoes autoelimination. This process occurs in the cul-de-sac and then sequentially in the fallopian tubes, endometrium, and endocervix. Ultimately, the gonococcus cannot be recovered from either end of the conduit. When nonrecovery of *N. gonorrhoeae* can be excluded because of technical problems (such as delayed plating, use of cold Thayer-Martin plates, or absence of initial ambient carbon dioxide), the absence of the gonococcus has come to imply either infection caused by *Chlamydia trachomatis* or advanced disease as a result of anaerobic superinfection of initial gonococcal salpingitis.

Based on therapeutic efficacy of single-drug therapy for acute salpingitis in terms of subgroups of patients with gonococcal salpingitis, determined by bacteriologic characterization of cul-de-sac aspirates, monomicrobial disease is relatively easy to treat with the new-generation tetracyclines.[5,11] These patients exhibit lysis of fever in 24 to 36 hours, marked amelioration of signs of peritoneal irritation and deep organ tenderness in 36 to 48 hours, and normal white blood cell count in 48 hours. Even when the initial white cell count is within normal limits, a significant decrease can be demonstrated in the first 48 hours of therapy.

The ability to achieve the anticipated therapeutic response observed for monomicrobial disease is significantly altered in patients with advanced polymicrobial superinfection. When *N. gonorrhoeae* is a constituent of a polymicrobial peritonitis, some patients develop what are called secondary febrile spikes. After initial reduction of temperature to below 37.6°C, there is a secondary elevation to 38°C or greater, which is sustained for a 4-hour period.[10,11]

Other patients fail to exhibit amelioration of physical findings and have a persistently elevated white blood cell count at 48 hours. The presence of a resistant anaerobic bacterial species in the cul-de-sac does not preclude duplication of the response of patients with monomicrobial disease, but when an altered therapeutic response is observed, invariably one or more class II or III anaerobic bacteria are present and are beyond the therapeutic efficacy of the drug used.

Once *N. gonorrhoeae* is no longer isolatable as a marker of the prevailing oxidation-reduction potential, the probability of reduplicating the anticipated therapeutic response seen monomicrobial disease drops precipitously.[11] In patients with polymicrobial peritonitis, this failure to respond varies between 40 to 60%, depending upon the criteria used to define therapeutic cure and whether *N. gonorrhoeae* can be concomitantly isolated from the cul-de-sac.

Once basement membrane destruction has been achieved by either anaerobic bacteria or *C. trachomatis*, the only resolution is healing by fibrosis, with its permanent alterations of fallopian tube function.

Chlamydia trachomatis is an obligate, intracellular, gram-negative organism that contains both RNA and DNA. Failure to supply the organism with essential growth factors can lead to a state of latency, which is recognized as a common state in the natural history of chlamydial infections. Women harboring the organism may be relatively or completely asymptomatic for months.

C. trachomatis has become the most common cause of sexually transmitted disease in many countries.[12] The frequency of isolation from the cervix of women with acute salpingitis is between 5 and 40%. In a limited series, the organism was recovered from the fallopian tubes or peritoneal exudates in up to 30% of patients with acute salpingitis. When one looks at the prevalence of *C trachomatis* in patients with prior salpingitis or infertility, the frequency of recovering the organism in asymptomatic patients is alarming.

In contrast to gonococcal salpingitis, chlamydial tubal infection appears to be a true chronic, active infection. Intracellular organisms may persist in the genital tissues for extremely long periods of time and continue to produce silent, progressive tubal damage unless treatment with appropriate antibiotics is instituted.[13-18] When infertile patients with chlamydial antibodies are evaluated at laparoscopy, frequently no history of an illness or procedure can be elicited to explain the presence of postinflammatory tubal damage.

Mycobacterium tuberculosis and *Coccidioides immitis*, among other organisms, are also fully capable of inducing permanent anatomic and functional sequelae, primarily by destroying the basement membrane.

The frequency of genital tuberculosis in infertile women ranges from 0.5 to 2.0% of all cases. A Mantoux intradermal skin test should be a standard part of every clinical evaluation of infertility. A positive reaction, which is induration more than 10 mm in diameter developing within 48 hours, should alert the physician to the possibility of genital tuberculosis. More important is a negative reaction, which in healthy patients effectively eliminates tuberculosis from diagnostic consideration.

ENDOMETRIAL–CERVICAL INFERTILITY OF INFECTIOUS ETIOLOGY

Gaps in our knowledge base have been inferred by the significant frequency of reproductive failures in patients without demonstrable evidence of endocrine dysfunction, hysterosalpingographic abnormalities, or any adverse finding in the postcoital test, and with normal menstrual cycles and partners with no abnormalities in semen analysis. Our frustration has caused us to seek out a possible causal relationship between infertility and a specific organism functioning at the endocervical level.

What has been the area of therapeutic controversy is whether or not a selected organism or flora existed, which is eradicated, would restore the potential for a successful pregnancy. The principal two organisms incriminated in the hypothesis that are thought to function at the cervical level are *Mycoplasma hominis* and *Ureaplasma urealyticum*.

The Mycoplasmas

Women with secondary infertility tend to have an elevated vaginal pH and complex microbiologic flora in which the anaerobic component is increased both quantitatively and qualitatively. *M hominis, U. urealyticum*, or both, can be isolated more frequently from such individuals than from matched controls. The fundamental question is whether either or both of these organisms can exert a negative cervical or endometrial influence on fertilization.[19-21]

The microbiologic hypothesis is based primarily on reports contending that initial isolation of mycoplasmas from the genital organs occurred more commonly in women with unexplained fertility than in matched controls, and the observation that frequently, after treatment of *Mycoplasma* infection, conception occurred.[18,21] Indirect support for the hypothesis was furnished by the inference that infection of the endometrial tissue by *M. hominis* may inhibit sperm migration by inducing changes in the ciliated cells lining the fallopian tubes in a manner similar to that described in *Mycoplasma pneumoniae* infections.

A somewhat better case has been made for *U. urealyticum* as a potentially correctable factor in secondary infertility.[22-27] At least one other study substantiated the report by Friberg of a higher frequency of *U. urealyticum* in a group of patients with unexplained infertility of at least 5 years' duration than in couples with proved fertility. A theoretical mechanism has been inferred from the observation that some strains of *U. urealyticum* isolated from infertile couples have been shown to be able to produce neuraminidase-like substances.[19] Neuraminidase can interfere with implantation and blastocyst development in mice. This blastocystotoxic effect has been postulated as an explanation for infertility and spontaneous abortions in patients infected with *U. urealyticum*.[21]

The problem with demographic studies has always been the appropriateness of the control group. The growth of *M. hominis* in the vagina is favored by pH shifts to the alkaline range. The organism achieves optimum growth of pH 7.4. *Ureaplasma urealyticum* prefers an environment somewhat acidic but relatively alkaline in comparison to the normal vaginal pH. Both organisms grow best in microaerophilic environments. When carefully controlled comparative studies are done, there is no difference in frequency of recovery of either *M. hominis* or *U. urealyticum*.[19,28] Any condition that elicits a local inflammatory response tends to enhance the probability of *Mycoplasma* colonization. The prevalence of the organism increases with pregnancy, abortion, and the development of with tubo-ovarian complexes.

In vitro studies have shown that *U. urealyticum* does not alter the physiologic characteristics of vaginal fluid or cervical mucus, sperm penetration, or sperm viability in cervical mucus. In well-controlled studies, eradication of *Mycoplasma* by doxycycline therapy is not associated with an improved conception rate.[28,29] It is the microbiologic environment that governs the presence or absence of these two organisms. At causal relationship between subclinical infection and secondary infertility for *Mycoplasma* is not tenable based on existing data.

MICROBIOLOGIC EVALUATION

Exclusion of a tubal pathogen is the key to the microbiologic evaluation of the infertile patient.

Mycobacterium tuberculosis

The diagnosis of genital tuberculosis may be established on the basis of the histopathologic features of a *premenstrual* endometrial biopsy or curettage fragments. Classically, one half of endometrial fragments are prepared for culture and guinea pig inoculation and the other half for histologic examination. Unfortunately, guinea pigs are not generally available, and

the regular culture media may have to be used. The diagnosis is generally established by the presence of characteristics granulomas in the material. Failure to demonstrate the acid-fast bacilli using Ziehl-Neelsen's technique does not invalidate the diagnosis except in the absence of evidence of delayed hypersensitivity (that is, a negative test using second-strength purified protein derivative, or PPD).

Occasionally, histologic examination of the endometrial tissue alone does not reveal the disease process, due to sampling errors or to noninvolvement of the endometrium when the fallopian tubes are the principal sites of infection. When a high index of suspicion exists, bacteriologic examination is important and should be done. Menstrual blood collected in a Tassette cup provides additional material for culture. One of the variables that is usually not controlled for is the point in the menstrual cycle in which the sample is taken. This influences the probability of organism recovery; for example, the progesterone phase is associated with diminished probability of recovery.

Hysterosalpingograms may reveal closed tubes with a tobacco-pouch deformity of the ampullary end, or a rigid pipestem pattern. In contrast to the morphologic changes in chronic salpingitis, the fimbriae are uninvolved. Some of the infected tubes demonstrate numerous fistulas.

Chlamydia trachomatis

Tissue culture is presently the gold standard for laboratory diagnosis of *C. trachomatis*. Although published methods are fairly standard, in practice many laboratories introduce variations that alter the sensitivity and specificity of the test.

Two major components are needed to culture for *C. trachomatis*: a cell-culture system and a method to identify inclusions growing in cell culture. The cell line of choice is McCoy. Alternatively, a particular strain of HeLa cells (HeLa 229) can be used, but this is usually restricted to research laboratories. Specimen material is centrifuged into the cells for 1 hour and then incubated for 2 to 3 days in medium containing cycloheximide. Incubation can take place in individual vials with coverslips at their base or on flat-bottomed wells in plastic microtiter plates. The choice between these methods is generally dictated by the number of specimens a laboratory has to process; the vial method is slightly more sensitive and less susceptible to cross-contamination, but is more time consuming and expensive.

Compared with other diagnostic tests for *C. trachomatis*, the major advantage of tissue culture is its specificity. With this method, the organism can be positively identified or saved for other marker studies such as immunotyping. It is clearly the method of choice for research studies. Determining its sensitivity and specificity has not been possible since it is the reference standard for other methods; however, it is estimated that culture has a sensitivity of 80 to 90% and a specificity of 100%.

Culture also has several disadvantages. The cost and complexity of laboratory requirements can be prohibitive. Specimens can be kept at 4°C for only up to 24 hours (preferably 12) before processing, or must be frozen at −70°C if they cannot be inoculated within 24 hours. They must be placed in specially prepared transport media. The cell monolayer may become contaminated with other bacteria or viruses, particularly in vaginal or rectal specimens.

Direct Smear Fluorescent Antibody Test. With this procedure, specimen material is obtained by swab and applied directly to a slide, which is fixed and then incubated with fluorescein-conjugated mono-clonal antibody before being examined under a fluorescence microscope. Total processing time is usually 30 to 40 minutes. Critical steps include (1) obtaining a satisfactory specimen and preparing a satisfactory smear (this can be checked before or after staining), (2) drying the specimen properly before fixing it, (3) using a high-quality fluorescence micro-scope, and (4) maintaining an experienced microsco-pist who can distinguish between elementary bodies and artifacts.

Compared with culture, the sensitivity of the direct smear test is greater than or equal to 90% in most published studies, and the specificity is greater than or equal to 98%. The positive predictive value of this test has ranged from approximately 80% (in populations with a *Chlamydia* prevalence of 10%) to 95% (in populations with a *Chlamydia* prevalence of 30%). Lower sensitivities and specificities are often encountered when specimens are less than optimal or when the individuals reading the slides are relatively inexperienced. In these instances, assessment of the proficiency of laboratory techniques is essential. This can be accomplished by comparing results with those obtained by a central reference laboratory that does proficiency testing.

The major advantages of the direct smear test are the uncomplicated transport and storage of speci-mens, rapid processing time compared with that required for other methods, high specificity, and the ability to check on the adequacy of specimen collec-tion (that is, cells on the slide). Disadvantages are the requirement of precise specimen collection, the need for high-quality fluorescence microscope equipment and an experienced microscopist, and the relatively labor-intensive nature of the process.

Enzyme Immunoassay. This test measures antigen–antibody reactions through an enzyme-linked immunoabsorbent assay (ELISA) and requires

a spectrophotometer. Processing time for specimens is approximately 4 hours. Questions continue to be raised about the reliability of ELISA for *C. trachomatis*. The sensitivity of the test has varied from 67 to 90%, specificity from 92 to 97%, and positive predictive value from 32 to 87%, depending on the population studied. Much of the observed disparity has been attributed to variable sensitivity of the tissue culture systems against which the ELISA has been com-pared.

The advantages of the ELISA are uncompli-cated transport and storage of specimens, the objec-tive method of measurement in the laboratory, which involves standard equipment and does not depend on a specially trained observer, and the ability to test large numbers of specimens at a time. The disadvantages are inability to check the adequacy of the specimen or to perform the test while the patient is waiting (although this is also true for the direct smear test if no fluorescence microscope is available).

Serology. Serologic diagnosis traditionally has re-lied on complement fixation (CF). Acute systemic infection produces a CF titer greater than 1:64, whereas infections limited to mucosal membranes produce a weak response. Microimmunofluores-cence is more sensitive and is preferentially used. To be indicative of infection, one must demon-strate a fourfold or greater rise in IgG antibody titer or the presence of IgM antibodies lasting for about 1 month.

Procedural Sequence

The microbiologic workup of the infertile patient starts with a PPD and serologic testing for *Chlamydia*. Smears or swabs to detect *C. trachomatis* must be obtained concomitantly. Once this information is received, endometrial biopsy is carried out for histo-logic analysis and possible culturing. If results of the PPD are positive, a portion of the biopsy or a second sample should be cultured for *M. tuberculosis*.

If a positive culture or serologic evidence of prior or current infection with *C. trachomatis* is identified, we advocate treating the patient with doxycycline, 100 mg twice a day for 14 days. If the patient has evidence of neither prior nor current infection with *M. tuberculosis* or *C. trachomatis*, but the endometrial biopsy exhibits evidence of a chronic inflammatory infiltrate, we rebiopsy the endometrium to obtain cultures for microbiologic processing. Given totally negative cultures, we most infrequently resort to a blind therapeutic challenge with a narrow-spectrum antibiotic and do another biopsy 14 days after ther-apy. For such a patient, we are functioning beyond the realm of our scientific knowledge.

SEMEN USED IN ARTIFICIAL INSEMINATION AS A VEHICLE FOR SEXUALLY TRANSMITTED PATHOGENS

Several viral agents are potentially transmissible through semen. It is possible that cytomegalovirus, the herpes simplex virus, and hepatitis B virus can all be transmitted through genital secretions.

Documentation of the dissemination of the acquired immunodeficiency syndrome (virus) through artificial insemination has changed the guidelines of the American Fertility Society. Potential semen donors are required first to give a detailed sexual history. Acceptable candidates should then be tested for antibodies to the cytomegaloviruses, and only men in whom the results are negative should undergo an examination, which includes urethral specimens, cultures for *N. gonorrhoeae* and *C. trachomatis*, and serologic tests for HIV, hepatitis B virus, and *Treponema pallidum* before donating sperm. Donors should ideally have negative results on two serologic tests for HIV 3 months apart, the second test being done 1 or 2 weeks before insemination. Moreover, the small possibility that such a donor might still be in the serologic window has argued for the use of frozen sperm obtained at the time of the first serologic surveillance, rather than the use of fresh sperm at the time of the second.

REFERENCES

1. Schachter J: Chlamydial infection. *N Engl J Med* 298:428, 1978.
2. Westrom L: Incidence: Effect of acute inflammatory disease on fertility. *Am J Obstet Gynecol* 121:707, 1975.
3. Trehanro JD, Ripa KT, March PA, et al: Antibodies to *Chlamydia trachomatis* in acute salpingitis. *Br J Vener Dis* 55:26, 1979.
4. Westrom L: Incidence, prevalence and trends of acute pelvic inflammatory disease and its consequences in industrialized countries. *Am J Obstet Gynecol* 138:880, 1980.
5. Monif GRG: Choice of antibiotics and length of therapy in the treatment of acute salpingitis. *Am J Med* 78(suppl 6B):188, 1985.
6. Viberg T: Acute inflammatory conditions of the uterine adnexa. *Acta Obstet Gynecol Scand* 38(suppl 4):1, 1964.
7. Chow AW, Malkasian KL, Marshall JR, et al: The bacteriology of acute pelvic inflammatory disease—Value of cul-de-sac cultures and relative importance of gonococci and other aerobic or anaerobic bacteria. *Am J Obstet Gynecol* 122:876, 1975.
8. Eschenbach DA, Buchanan TM, Pollock HM, et al: Polymicrobial etiology of acute pelvic inflammatory disease. *N Engl J Med* 293:166, 1975.
9. Monif GRG, Welkos SL, Baer H, Thompson RLJ: Cul-de-sac isolates from patients with endometritis/salpingitis/peritonitis and gonococcal endocervicitis. *Am J Obstet Gynecol* 126:158, 1976.
10. Monif GRG: Significance of polymicrobial superinfection in the therapy of gonococcal endometritis–salpingitis–peritonitis. *Obstet Gynecol* 55(suppl):1545, 1980.
11. Monif GRG: Clinical staging of acute bacterial salpingitis and its therapeutic ramification. *Am J Obstet Gynecol* 143:489, 1982.
12. Schachter J (ed): *Chlamydial Infections.* Proceedings of the 5th international symposium on human chlamydial infections, Lund, Sweden, June 15–19, 1982. Amsterdam, Elsevier, 1982.
13. Gump DW, Gibson M, Ashikawaga T: Infertile women and *Chlamydia trachomatis* infection, in March P-A, Holmes KK, Oriel JD, Piot P, Schachter J (eds): *Chlamydial Infections.* Proceedings of the 5th international symposium on human chlamydial infections, Lund, Sweden, June 15–19, 1982. Amsterdam, Elsevier, 1982.
14. Washington AE, Gove S, Schachter J, Sweet RL: Oral contraceptives, *Chlamydia trachomatis* infection, and pelvic inflammatory disease. A word of caution about protection. *JAMA* 253:2246, 1985.
15. Pummomen R, Terho P, Mikkanon V, et al: Chlamydia serology in infertile women by immunofluorescence. *Fertil Steril* 31:656, 1976.
16. Sweet RL: Chlamydia salpingitis and infertility. *Fertil Steril* 38:530, 1982.
17. Henry-Suchet J, Catalan F, Loffredo V, et al: *Chlamydia trachomatis* associated with chronic inflammation in abdominal specimens from women selected for tuboplasty. *Fertil Steril* 36:599, 1981.
18. Henry-Suchet J, Catalan F, Loffredo V, et al: *Chlamydia trachomatis* and mycoplasma research by laparoscopy in cases of pelvic inflammatory disease and in cases of tubal obstruction. *Am J Obstet Gynecol* 138:1022, 1980.
19. Friberg J: Mycoplasmas and ureaplasmas in infertility and abortion. *Fertil Steril* 33:351, 1980.
20. Bercovici B, Haas H, Sacks TH, Laufer A: Isolation of mycoplasma from the genital tract of women with reproductive failure, sterility or vaginitis. *Isr J Med Sci* 14:347, 1978.
21. Holmes KK: *Mycoplasma hominis*—A human pathogen. *Sex Transm Dis* 11:159, 1984.
22. Stray-Pedersen B: Femal genital colonization with *Ureaplasma urealyticum* and reproductive failure. *Obstet Gynecol Surv* 35:467, 1980.
23. Rehewy MS, Jaszczak S, Hafez ES, Thomas A, Brown WJ: *Ureaplasma urealyticum* (T-mycoplasma) in vaginal fluid and cervical mucus from fertile and infertile women. *Fertil Steril* 30:297, 1978.
24. Stray-Pedersen B, Eng J, Reikvam TM: Utero T-mycoplasma colonization in reproductive failure. *Am J Obstet Gynecol* 130:307, 1978.
25. Desai S, Cohen MS, Khatamee M, Lenter E: *Ureaplasma urealyticum* (T-mycoplasma) infection: Does it have a role in male infertility? *J Urol* 124:469, 1980.
26. Idriss WM, Patton WC, Taymor ML: On the etiologic role of *Ureaplasma urealyticum* (T-mycoplasma) infection in infertility. *Fertil Steril* 30:293, 1978.
27. Cassell GH, Brown MB, Younger JB, et al: Incidence of genital mycoplasmas in women at the time of diagnostic laparoscopy. *Yale J Biol Med* 56:557, 1983.
28. Nagata Y, Iwasaka T, Wada T: Mycoplasma infection and infertility. *Fertil Steril* 31:392, 1979.
29. Mathews CD, Clapp KH, Tansing JA, et al: T-mycoplasma genital infection: The effect of doxycyline therapy on human unexplained infertility. *Fertil Steril* 30:98, 1978.

CHAPTER 17

Genetics and Molecular Biology

William J. Butler, Paul G. McDonough

GENETIC CONTROL OF GAMETOGENESIS

Oogenesis

The primordial germ cells differentiate in the yolk sac entoderm and migrate to the genital ridge during the fourth week of embryonic development. Gonadal differentiation is induced as determined by the cytogenic sex of the germ cells. In the absence of testicular determinants, ovarian morphogenesis occurs. Although female development has been described as passive, ovarian determinants exist on both arms of the X chromosome, and privation of these determinants may lead to gonadal dysgenesis. The inactivation or lyonization of the X chromosome that occurs in most somatic cells[1] does not occur in germ cells, and two intact X chromosomes are required for ovarian development.[2]

The primordial oocytes undergo mitotic replication until approximately 20 weeks of gestational age, and shortly thereafter enter the first meiotic prophase. In the presence of two intact active X chromosomes, the primary oocytes are enveloped in a layer of granulosa cells and arrested in the dictyotene stage of the first meiotic prophase, where they stay until recruited for ovulation after puberty. In the absence of ovarian determinants (45, X0, or otherX chromosome deletions), the formation of this follicular mantle is incomplete and meiotic arrest doesnot occur. The primary oocytes complete meiosis and undergo atresia,[3] resulting in follicular depletion.

Female gametogenesis differs from male gametogenesis in the prolonged arrest of prophase of meiosis I, with the homologous chromosome pairs, already duplicated into sister chromatids, frozen in the synaptonemal complex with chiasmata indicating crossing over to exchange genetic material. Meiosis I is not completed until ovulation many years later, when it is accompanied by the development of the first polar body. Meiosis II is triggered by fertilization of the secondary oocyte, with formation of the mature ovum (female pronucleus) and second polar body. The long arrested prophase I renders the female more susceptible to genomic mutation with advancing age.

Spermatogenesis

Although the control of testicular differentiation by the Y chromosome has been apparent for many years, research has provided greater insight into this process. HY antigen, a cell surface antigen identified in male cells by serology and tissue transplantation, has been proposed to be the product of testicular-determining genes[4]; however, studies using recombinant DNA techniques have shown that the genes for testicular determination and HY antigen are distinct, although HY may have a role in spermatogenesis.[5,6] Deletion maps of the Y chromosome based on intersex persons now place testicular-determining genes on the short arm either just proximal to the tip[7] or more proximal and pericentric (Fig. 17–1).[8–10] The testicular determinants direct morphogenesis of the embryonic testis. Unlike in the embryonic ovary, minimal mitotic replication and no meiotic division of the spermatogonia occur, and therefore sperm have no prolonged meiotic arrest phase.

Meiotic division begins at puberty, and spermatogenesis exhibits several distinctive features compared to female gametogenesis. In meiosis I all chromosomes pair with their homologue to match genetic loci, but the male sex chromosome does not have a homologue. The short arms of male X and Y chromosomes pair and may undergo crossing over.[11] This raises the possibility that abnormal X–Y exchanges may result in clinical abnormalities of sexual differentiation, reproductive, or both. The male gametogenic cycle lasts 60 to 72 days; this continuous and rapid DNA turnover may make the male genome more vulnerable to single-point gene mutation, par-

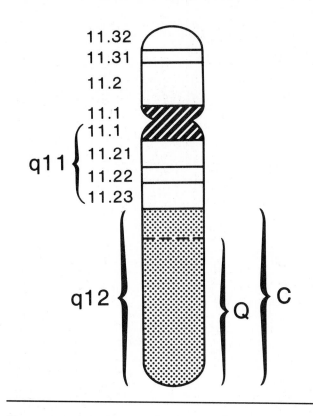

Schematic Y Chromosome

Figure 17–1. Map of Y chromosome with putative locations of testis-determinant genes (TDG) and HY antigen as determined by cytogenetic and molecular studies.

ticularly if there is compromise of DNA repair mechanisms as occurs with chronologic aging.

Pathophysiology of Gametogenesis and Fertilization

Absent or abnormal gametogenesis makes a significant contribution to the impairment of human fertility among affected individuals. The most basic identifiable problem occurs at the level of gamete production. Gonadal determinants on the sex chromosomes are required for gamete production, and loss of these determinants results in gonadal dysgenesis. Evaluation of patients with peripubertal amenorrhea (defined as primary amenorrhea or amenorrhea occurring within 6 months of menarche) revealed that 43% had hypergonadotropic hypogonadism; 63% of these patients had X chromosome privation with loss of ovarian determinants, resulting in follicular depletion and consequent amenorrhea and infertility.[12] Sex chromosomal aneuploidy is a much less likely etiology of adult-onset secondary amenorrhea.[13] The presence of excess active ovarian determinants in males also leads to infertility secondary to inhibited spermatogenesis, as seen in patients with 47,XXY Klinefelter's syndrome.[14] Abnormalities of testicular determinants are discussed below.

Chromosomal aneuploidy leading to the production of unbalanced gametes is an important cause of recurrent abortion,[15] but its role in infertility is only now being appreciated. The accepted frequency of spontaneous abortion of 10 to 15% of pregnancies has been challenged by data showing both a much higher conception rate than previously accepted and a much higher pregnancy loss rate. Late luteal urinary levels of human chorionic gonadotropin (HCG) were studied in women at risk for fertilization.[16] In 118 (60%) of 198 cycles studied, positive tests indicated early gestation, although only 51 cycles (26%) resulted in a clinical pregnancy. Fifty-seven percent of these pregnancies underwent early embryonic loss. In addition, 6 (12%) of 51 clinical pregnancies were early spontaneous abortions, giving a total pregnancy loss rate of 62%. These subjects were studied after cycle day 21, theoretically after implantation should have occurred. Any fertilized zygotes lost prior to implantation would not have been detected, so the actual number of pregnancies lost could exceed the documented 62%. Unrecognized early abortion may be a significant contributing factor in human infertility.

Early spontaneous abortions have been found to show a high frequency of aneuploidy.[17] These unbalanced zygotes may result from sporadic gametogenic errors, or from repetitive errors secondary to parental chromosome rearrangements or other mechanisms. In some cases the parental chromosome rearrangement may inhibit gametogenesis. Balanced chromosomal translocations account for 5.3% of infertile males,[18,19] which is 9 times the 0.6% frequency found in surveys of newborns.[20] Some male balanced translocation carriers are sterile secondary to the formation of long chromosome chains during meiosis I; it appears that this process interferes with inactivation of the X chromosome and thereby, spermatogenesis.[21] It is also possible that balanced translocation chromosomes may exert a remote effect to induce nondisjunction of other chromosome pairs and produce unbalanced gametes. To result in infertility, some selection process must be operative against either the unbalanced gametes or zygotes. Studies of sperm karyotypes using a zona-free hamster egg-penetration assay have shown that unbalanced sperm can penetrate an oocyte,[22] and this was confirmed by the finding of karyotypically abnormal embryos resulting from human in-vitro fertilization.[23] Zygote selection is probably the mechanism of prime importance in eliminating the products of unbalanced gametes. The known increase in aneuploidy with maternal age may also account for the observed increased frequency of early pregnancy loss and possibly infertility, in this age group, as zygote

selection against trisomy 21 fetuses can be demonstrated with 75% of these pregnancies lost prior to viability.

Recurrent aneuploidy not secondary to parental chromosomal anomalies is more difficult to demonstrate, but evidence is accumulating that various factors in gamete development can predispose to repetitive gametogenic errors and unbalanced conceptions or infertility (Table 17–1). These errors can occur in either the male or female in meiosis I or II. *Postnatal aging* is the term for the long arrest of oocytes in the dictyotene phase of meiosis I.

Oocytes are arrested in this late prophase I stage at approximately 24 weeks of fetal life and meiosis does not resume until the follicle is recruited for ovulation. Precocious terminalization of chiasmata may lead to premature disjunction of bivalents and resulting random malsegregation, forming unbalanced gametes. Aging may also affect the hypothalamic–pituitary axis such that in the older female, resumption of meiosis I leads to malsegregation (nondisjunction) and unbalanced gametes.[24] Older females do have a higher prevalence of both spontaneous abortion and aneuploid offspring, as well as compromised fertility. It has been shown that 70% of trisomy 21 infants result from errors in maternal meiosis I.[25]

Preovulatory aging refers to a prolongation of the follicular phase of the ovulatory cycle, interfering with normal completion of meiosis I. Studies have shown an increased frequency of abnormal zygotes when ovulation is experimentally delayed in animals.[26-28] An increased risk of aneuploidic abortion, particularly trisomy, was found in late ovulators.[17] The underlying mechanism may be spindle degeneration during intrafollicular aging.

Postovulatory aging refers to late fertilization of an ovulated oocyte. At ovulation the oocyte completes meiosis I and enters meiosis II, but does not complete meiosis II until after fertilization. Delayed fertilization therefore can predispose to errors in both meiosis II and fertilization. One group studied the outcome of conceptions that were probably caused by

TABLE 17–1. GAMETE AGING

	Postnatal	Preovulatory	Post Ovulatory
Time	Embryo → follicular recruitment	Follicular recruitment → ovulation	Ovulation → fertilization
Error	Meiosis I	Meiosis I	Meiosis II, fertilization
Result	Aneuploid gamete	Aneuploid gamete	Triploid zygote
Analogous male error	No	No	Yes

late fertilization as determined by basal body temperature, and found an increased rate of spontaneous abortion.[29] Karyotyping of zygotes resulting from fertilization of aged oocytes reveals increased frequency of triploidy, both from digyny (usually meiosis I error in oocyte) and dispermy.[30] Two thirds of all triploids are dispermic. The zona pellucida loses its integrity with aging and is less effective in blocking polyspermic penetration of the egg.[31,32] Dispermic triploids may undergo hydropic degeneration because of the diploid male genome, forming a partial mole.[33] Aging of sperm, in both the epididymis and female reproductive tract, has also been shown to increase the frequency of aneuploid zygotes.[34] As spermatogenesis is a continuous process and not subject to a period of meiotic arrest, however, older males would not be expected to be more likely to produce unbalanced gametes.

A unique feature of spermatogenesis that may result in impaired fertility is the process of X–Y interchange. Although meiotic pairing of X and Y does occur, the pair normally separates prematurely, probably to minimize genetic exchange.[11] Molecular studies of 46,XX males (clinical phenotype similar to Klinefelter's syndrome) show hybridization of DNA probes specific for Yp sequences.[35,36] This suggests that DNA from the paternal Y has been exchanged to the paternal X during spermatogenesis, and the presence of these testicular determinants in addition to a full complement of ovarian determinants in the offspring has resulted in male sexual development, but with impaired spermatogenesis causing sterility.

OTHER KNOWN GENETIC CAUSES OF INFERTILITY

Multifactorial Disorders

Müllerian aplasia (Rokitansky-Kuster-Hauser syndrome) has also been referred to as congenital absence of the vagina. In addition to aplasia of the upper vagina and cervix, usually only a rudimentary, nonfunctional uterus consisting of solid muscular cords is present.[37] These patients have primary amenorrhea but normal secondary sexual development. Less severe anomalies involving incomplete fusion or obstruction of the müllerian system can also occur. Family studies have shown a 2.7% prevalence of müllerian anomalies in first-degree female relatives of affected probands,[38] consistent with multifactorial inheritance, although inheritance by way of autosomal dominant or recessive genes with incomplete penetrance has also been proposed.[39] Aplasia and obstructive lesions result in infertility, while incomplete fusion (uterus didelphys, bicornis, or subseptus) can cause habitual abortion. Treatment consists of surgical correction, but in the case of müllerian

aplasia the only potential for fertility is oocyte aspiration and in-vitro fertilization, with the embryo to be carried by a surrogate. These patients should be evaluated for associated renal and vertebral anomalies.

Mendelian Disorders

Myotonic dystrophy is an autosomal dominant disorder characterized by progressive muscular dystrophy, myoclonus, cardiac involvement, and gonadal atrophy.[40,41] Linkage analysis using the blood group secretor locus mapped the gene to chromosome 19 between the centromere and q12.[42] Analysis by restriction fragment-length polymorphism is being used in an attempt to localize and identify the abnormal gene.[43]

Some cases of 46XX ovarian failure are inherited in an autosomal recessive fashion.[44] Genetic studies have been unsuccessful to date in determining the linkage of the defective gene. Other autosomal recessive diseases such as galactosemia and mucopolysaccharidoses are associated with ovarian failure, possibly secondary to gonadal infiltration by abnormal metabolites.[45] Deficiency of 17α-hydroxylase, a recessively inherited block in ovarian and adrenal steroidogenesis, causes high gonadotropin levels consistent with endocrine ovarian failure, and sexual infantilism.[46] Because of the inability to synthesize estrogen, the primordial follicles present in the ovaries cannot be induced to mature, which results in a functional agonadal state.

Congenital adrenal hyperplasia (CAH) results from an inherited block in adrenal steroidogenesis due to a deficiency of one of several enzymes necessary for cortisol biosynthesis.[47] Failure of cortisol negative feedback leads to increased production of adrenocorticotropic hormone (ACTH) from the pituitary and overproduction of androgenic steroid precursors. A deficiency of 21-hydroxylase accounts for 95% of cases. The classic form is genital ambiguity at birth in affected females.[48] The nonclassic or adult-onset form, resulting from a partial 21-hydroxylase deficiency, does not become apparent until puberty, with anovulation and signs of androgen excess.[49] Function of the hypothalamic–pituitary–ovarian axis is suppressed by the high levels of circulating steroid, resulting in anovulation in females[49] and poor spermatogenesis in males.[50] Congenital adrenal hyperplasia is inherited in autosomal recessive fashion, with the gene closely linked to the major histocompatibility complex (HLA) on chromosome 6.[51,52] Molecular analysis of this region has shown that the genetic defect involves the structural gene for cytochrome P450-21-hydroxylase.[53] Two copies of the gene are present on each chromosome, but one is a nonfunctional pseudogene.[54] Deletions of the active gene have been found in some cases of classic CAH,[55,56] but other classic and nonclassic cases are suspected to be secondary to as yet unidentified point mutations that affect gene transcription or messenger RNA (mRNA) processing. Treatment with glucocorticoid replacement lowers levels of ACTH and precursor steroids, relieving suppression of ovulation or spermatogenesis.[57]

In XY gonadal dysgenesis, or Swyer's syndrome, patients have sexual infantilism and gonadal dysgenesis; normal or tall stature differentiates this syndrome from X chromosome privation. Swyer's syndrome is inherited in an X-linked fashion.[58] Studies of HY antigen in these patients have proved to be equivocal, with conflicting results reported.[59-61] By using Y-specific DNA probes, microdeletions have been identified of the same DNA sequences that are present in 46,XX males.[9,10]

Testicular feminization, or complete androgen insensitivity, is due to absence or malfunction of the androgen receptor, which has been mapped to the X chromosome.[62] The molecular defects have yet to be defined, but genetic heterogeneity exists and could account for the variability of phenoytpic expression in incomplete forms.[63] These patients are sterile secondary to the presence of normal testes, which produce müllerian-inhibiting substance and therefore cause müllerian regression; breast development occurs under estrogen stimulation derived from peripheral conversion of androgens.

MOLECULAR GENETICS AND REPRODUCTIVE BIOLOGY

Advances in recombinant DNA technology have made it possible to identify molecular defects that can be examined without regard to gene expression. This approach has proved to be a powerful tool for investigating genes coding for hormones in the reproductive process. Gonadotropin-releasing hormone (GnRH) has been shown, by isolating and cloning the GnRH gene on the short arm of chromosome 8, to be derived from a large precursor molecule. The molecule contains an initial amino acid sequence, GnRH, and a subsequent larger peptide called gonadotropin- associated peptide (GAP) (Fig. 17–2).[64] Studies of GAP have shown it to have potent gonadotropin-secreting and prolactin-inhibiting activities,[65] suggesting that it may be a mediator of gonadotropin and prolactin release. Immunohistochemical studies have shown that both GnRH and GAP are expressed products of the GnRH gene in the hypothalamus.[66] The exact biologic function of GAP has yet to be determined, however. No molecular defects in the GnRH gene have been identified in humans with Kallmann's syndrome (isolated GnRH

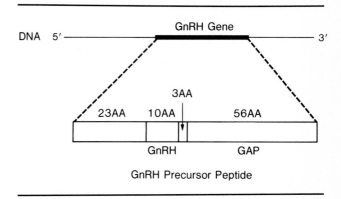

Figure 17–2. Diagrammatic representation of GnRH gene coding for GnRH and GAP.

deficiency), but deletion of the gene was reported in a hypogonadal mouse model.[67]

These glycoprotein hormones of the gonadotropin hormone family share a common α-subunit but have unique β-subunits that confer specific biologic activity (Table 17–2). The α-subunit gene has been isolated, sequenced, and localized to chromosome 6.[68,69] The gene for the β-subunit of follicle-stimulating hormone (FSH) is located on the short arm of chromosome 11, but has not been fully characterized.[70] The luteinizing hormone (LH) and human chorionic gonadotropin (HCG) β-subunits comprise a family of genes on chromosome 19q13. There is a single copy of the β-LH gene and seven copies of the β-HCG gene, not all of which are functional.[71,72] Structurally, these genes have been found to display 95% homology, showing that their structures are highly conserved and derived from a common ancestral gene.[73] This structural similarity probably accounts for the functional overlap and immunologic cross-reactivity of the respective peptides. The differences in the β-LH and β-HCG genes also are of functional significance. Different promoter regions allow for different physiologic regulation and tissue transcriptional specificity of the genes, and alteration of the translational stop signal in HCG adds additional glycosylation sites, resulting in a longer serum half-life.[74]

The α-subunit gene is expressed at a higher rate than each of the β-subunit genes, and although it does respond to regulatory factors, this constitutive synthesis indicates the α-subunit is not important in

TABLE 17–2. GONADOTROPIN GENES

	Alpha	LH	HCG	FSH
Chromosome	6	19q	19q	11p
Copy Number	1	1	7	?
Homologous	–	+	+	–

regulating the synthesis and biologic activity of these hormones.[75–77] Inhibition by estradiol of mRNA transcripts from both α and β genes has been demonstrated, showing that estrogen-negative feedback occurs at the level of either gene transcription or mRNA processing.[78] GnRH has been shown to increase mRNA transcription of both α and β-LH genes, suggesting gonadotropin regulation may act, at least in part, on alterations of gene expression.[79]

Characterization of the structure and expression of gonadotropin genes has proved to have direct clinical applications. Gonadotropin-secreting pituitary rumors are rare, but have been described as having unexpected endocrinologic effects, such as low gonadal steroid levels in the presence of high gonadotropin levels.[80–82] Some of these tumors secrete uncombined and therefore nonfunctional β-LH subunits.[83] Nonfunctioning pituitary tumors have been a diagnostic dilemma, but tumor mRNA analysis with specific DNA probes has demonstrated that most are derived from gonadotropin-producing cell types, with defects in mRNA translation or processing resulting in lack of detectable hormone secretion.[84]

It is possible to express cloned gonadotropin genes in in-vitro systems (Fig. 17–3). Such synthesis of glycoprotein hormones is more problematic than other hormones such as insulin and growth hormone because of the inability of bacterial systems to carry out glycosylation. Biologically active HCG, LH, and FSH have been produced in mammalian cells, however. This supply of such gonadotropins should provide large quantities of pure hormones for clinical use. In addition, this approach should provide an in-vitro system for studying genetic mutations and resultant functional derangements, with potential applications in the diagnosis and management of clinical disease.

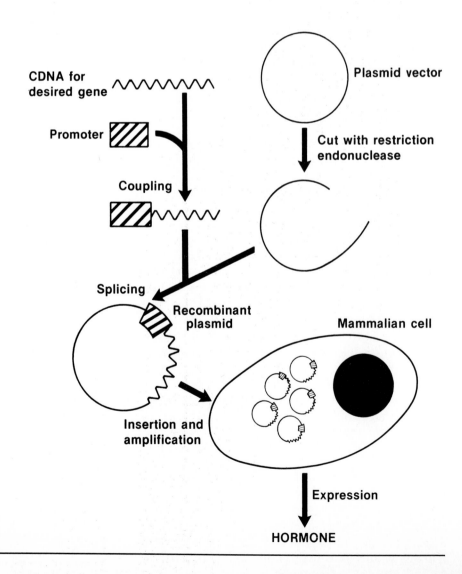

Figure 17–3. Molecular cloning and gene expression.

TABLE 17–3. INHIBIN GENE PRODUCTS

	Structure	Action of FSH
Inhibin A	α/βA	–
Inhibin B	α/βB	–
FRP	βA/βA	+
Activin	βA/βB	+

Molecular biologic techniques have proved to be critical in isolating and characterizing two long-sought hormones, inhibin and müllerian-inhibiting substance (MIS). It had been well documented that a peptide present in ovarian follicular fluid had FSH-suppressive effects, but biochemical attempts at isolation and characterization were not fruitful.[85] Recombinant DNA technology was used to isolate and sequence the genes for these hormones and to confirm that there are two forms of inhibin, A and B. Each is a heterodimer of a similar α-subunit and dissimilar β-subunit, βA or βB (Table 17–3).[86,87] It was also found that a dimer composed of inhibin β-subunits has FSH-releasing activity and has been called FSH-releasing peptide (FRP) or activin.[88,89] The exact biologic role of these hormones in regulating gonadotropins is under study. The β-subunit inhibin genes are closely homologous to the isolated gene for MIS.[90] At first MIS was thought to be produced only in the fetal testis, but it has now been shown to be synthesized in granulosa cells.[91] It is a homodimer that in the ovary may have a role inhibiting the breakdown of germinal vesicle and arresting oocyte maturation.[92] Recombinant MIS is being produced in cell culture and will be available for studies to determine its precise function and regulation.

REFERENCES

1. Migeon BR, Kennedy JB: Evidence for the inactivation of an X chromosome early in the development of the human female. *Am J Hum Genet* 27:233, 1975.
2. Gartler SM, Liskay RM, Gant M: Two functional X chromosomes on human fetal oocytes. *Exp Cell Res* 82:464, 1973.
3. Jirasek JE: Principles of reproductive embryology. IV. Development of the ovary, in Simpson JL (ed): *Disorders of Sexual Differentiation.* New York, Academic Press, 1976, p 75.
4. Wachtell SS: The genetics of intersexuality: Clinical and theoretic perspectives. *Obstet Gynecol* 54:671, 1979.
5. Goodfellow PJ, Darling SM, Thomas NS, Goodfellow PN: A pseudoautosomal gene in man. *Science* 234:740, 1986.
6. Burgoyne PS, Levy ER, McLaren A: Spermatogenic failure in male mice lacking HY antigen. *Nature* 320:170, 1986.
7. Page DC, De la Chapelle A: The parental origin of X chromosome in XX males determined using restriction fragment length polymorphisms. *Am J Hum Genet* 36:565, 1984.
8. Vergnaud G, Page DC, Simmler MC, et al: A deletion map of the human Y chromosome based on DNA hybridization. *Am J Hum Genet* 38:109, 1986.
9. Muller U, Doulon T, Schmid M, et al: Deletion mapping of the testis determining locus with DNA probes in 46,XX males and 46,XY and 46,X, dic (Y) females. *Nucleic Acids Res* 14:6489, 1986.
10. Disteche CM, Casanova M, Saal H, et al: Small deletions of the short arm of the Y chromosome in 46,XY females. *Proc Natl Acad Sci USA* 83:7841, 1986.
11. Ashley T: A re-examination of the case for homology between the X and Y chromosomes of mouse and man. *Hum Genet* 67:372, 1984.
12. Reindollar RH, Byrd JR, McDonough PG: Delayed sexual development: A study of 252 patients. *Am J Obstet Gyncol* 140:371, 1981.
13. Reindollar RH, Novak M, Tho SPT, McDonough PG: Adult-onset amenorrhea: A study of 262 patients. *Am J Obstet Gynecol* 155:531, 1986.
14. Simpson JL: Abnormal sexual differentiation in humans. *Annu Rev Genet* 16:193, 1982.
15. Tho SPT, Byrd JR, McDonough PG: Chromosome polymorphism in 110 couples with reproductive failure and subsequent pregnancy outcome. *Fertil Steril* 38:688, 1982.
16. Edmonds DK, Lindsay KS, Miller JF, Williamson E, Wood PT: Early embryonic mortality in women. *Fertil Steril* 38:447, 1982.
17. Boue J, Boue A, Lazar P: Retrospective and prospective epidemiological studies of 1500 karyotyped spontaneous human abortions. *Teratology* 12:11, 1975.
18. Tiepolo L, Zuffardi O, Fraccaro M, Giarola A: Chromosome abnormalities and male infertility, in Frajese G, Hafez ESE, Conti C, Fabbrini A (eds): *Oligozoospermia.* New York, Raven, 1981, p 233.
19. Hamerton JL, Canning N, Ray M, Smith S: A cytogenetic survey of 14,069 newborn infants. I. Incidence of chromosome abnormalities. *Clin Genet* 8:223, 1975.
20. Iselins L, Lindsten J: The 11q; 22q translocation, in Crosignani PG, Rubin BL, Fraccaro M (eds): *Genetic Control of Gamete Production and Function.* New York, Grune & Stratton, 1982, p 187.
21. Forejt J: Meiotic studies of translocations causing male sterility in the mouse. II. Double heterozygotes for robertsonian translocations. *Cytogenet Cell Genet* 23:163, 1979.
22. Rudak E, Jacobs PA, Yanigimachi R: Direct analysis of the chromosome constitution of human spermatozoa. *Nature* 274:911, 1978.
23. Rudak E, Dor J, Mashiach S, Nebel L, Goldman B: Chromosome analysis of multipronuclear human oocytes fertilized in vitro. *Fertil Steril* 41:538, 1984.
24. Brook JD, Gosden RG, Chandley AC: Maternal aging and aneupolid embryos—Evidence from the mouse that biological and not chronological age is the important influence. *Hum Genet* 66:41, 1984.
25. Hassold T, Chi D, Yamane JA: Parental origin of autosomal trisomies. *Ann Hum Genet* 48:129, 1984.
26. Witschi E, Laguens R: Chromosomal aberrations in embryos from overripe eggs. *Dev Biol* 7:605, 1963.
27. Mikamo K: Mechanism of nondisjunction of meiotic chromosomes and degeneration of maturation spindles in eggs affected by intrafollicular overripeness. *Experientia* 24:75, 1968.
28. Butcher RL, Fugo NW: Overripeness and mammalian ova. II. Delayed ovulation and chromosome anomalies. *Fertil Steril* 18:297, 1967.
29. Guerrero R, Rojas O: Spontaneous abortion and aging of human ova and spermatozoa. *N Engl J Med* 293:573, 1975.
30. Jacobs PA, Angell RR, Buchanan IM, et al: The origin of human triploids. *Ann Hum Genet* 42:49, 1978.
31. Adams CE, Chang MC: The effect of delayed mating on fertilization in the rabbit. *J Exp Zool* 151:155, 1962.
32. Szolollosi D: Mammalian eggs aging in the fallopian tubes, in Blandau RJ (ed): *Aging Gametes, Their Biology and Pathology.* International Symposium on Aging Gametes, Seattle, 1973. Basel, Karger, 1975, p 98.
33. Hunt PA, Jacobs PA, Szulman AE: Molar pregnancies and non-molar triploids—Results of a 7-year cytogenetic study. Presented at 34th annual meeting of the American Society of Human Genetics, Norfolk, Oct 1983.
34. Martin-Deleon PA, Boice ML: Sperm aging in the male and cytogenetic anomalies: An animal model. *Hum Genet* 62:70, 1982.
35. De la Chapelle A, Tippett PA, Wetterstrand G, Page D: Genetic evidence of X-Y interchange in a human XX male. *Nature* 307:172, 1984.
36. Guellean G, Casonova M, Bishop C, et al: Human XX males with Y single-copy DNA fragments. *Nature* 307:172, 1984.
37. Jones HW, Mermut S: Familial occurrence of congenital absence of the vagina. *Am J Obstet Gynecol* 114:1100, 1972.
38. Carson SA, Simpson JL, Malinak LR, et al: Heritable aspects of uterine anomalies. II. Genetic analysis of mullerian aplasia. *Fertil Steril* 40:86, 1983.
39. Shokeir MH: Aplasia of the mullerian system: Evidence for probable sex-limited autosomal dominant inheritance. *Birth Defects* 14(6c):147, 1978.

40. Hall JG: Disorders of connective tissue and skeletal dysplasia, in Schulman JD, Simpson JL (eds): *Genetic Disease in Pregnancy*. New York, Academic Press, 1981.

41. Clarke DG, Shapiro S, Monroe RG: Myotonia atrophica with testicular atrophy, urinary excretions of ICSH, androgens and 17-ketosteroids. *J Clin Endocrinol* 16:1235, 1956.

42. Renwick JH, Bundey SE, Ferguson-Smith MA, Izatt MM: Confirmation of linkage of the loci for myotonic dystrophy and ABH secretion. *J Med Genet* 8:407, 1971.

43. Bartlett RJ, Pericak-Vance MA, Yamaoka L, et al: A new probe for the diagnosis of myotonic muscular dystrophy. *Science* 235:1648, 1987.

44. Nazareth HRS, Farah LMS, Cunah AJB: Pure gonadal dysgenesis (type XX). Report of a family with four affected sibs. *Hum Genet* 37:117, 1977.

45. Kaufman FR, Kogut MD, Donnell GN, Goebelsman U, March C, Koch R: Hypergonadotropic hypogonadism in female patients with galactosemia. *N Engl J Med* 304:994, 1981.

46. Goldsmith O, Salomen DH, Horton R: Hypogonadism and mineralocorticoid excess. The 17-hydroxylase deficiency syndrome. *N Engl J Med* 277:673, 1967.

47. White PC, New MI, Dupont B: Congenital adrenal hyperplasia. Part I. *N Engl J Med* 316:1519, 1987.

48. Bongiovanni AM, Root AW: The adrenogenital syndrome. *N Engl J Med* 268:1283, 1963.

49. Kohn B, Levine LS, Pollack MS, et al: Late onset steroid 21-hydroxylase deficiency: A variant of classical congenital adrenal hyperplasia. *J Clin Endocrinol Metab* 55:817, 1982.

50. Wischusen J, Baker HWG, Hudson B: Reversible male infertility due to congenital adrenal hyperplasia. *Clin Endocrinol* 14:571, 1981.

51. Dupont B, Oberfield SE, Smithwick EM, Leli TD, Levine LS: Close genetic linkage between HLA and congenital adrenal hyperplasia (21-hydroxylase deficiency). *Lancet* 2:1390, 1977.

52. Levine LS, Zachmann M, New MI, et al: Genetic mapping of the 21-hydroxylase-deficiency gene within the HLA linkage group. *N Engl J Med* 299:911, 1978.

53. White PC, New MI, Dupont B: Congenital adrenal hyperplasia. Part II. *N Engl J Med* 316:1580, 1987.

54. Higoshi Y, Yoshioka H, Yamane M, Gotoh O, Fujii-Kuriyama Y: Complete nucleotide sequence of two steroid 21-hydroxylase genes tandemly arranged in human chromosome: A pseudogene and a genuine gene. *Proc Natl Acad Sci USA* 83:511, 1986.

55. Rumsby G, Carroll MC, Porter RR, Grant DB, Hjelm M: Deletion of the steroid 21-hydroxylase and complement C4 genes in congenital adrenal hyperplasia. *J Med Genet* 23:204, 1986.

56. Werkmeister JW, New MI, Dupont B, White PC: Frequent deletion and duplication of the steroid 21-hydroxylase genes. *Am J Hum Genet* 39:461, 1986.

57. Winter JSD: Current approaches to the treatment of congenital adrenal hyperplasia. *J Pediatr* 97:81, 1980.

58. Sternberg WH, Barclay DL, Kloepfer HW: Familial XY gonadal dysgenesis. *N Engl J Med* 278:695, 1968.

59. Gosh SN, Shah PN, Gharpure HM: Absence of H-Y antigen in XY females with dysgenetic gonads. *Nature* 276:180, 1978.

60. Moreira-Filho CA, Toledo SPA, Bagnoli VR, Frota-Pessoa O, Bisi H, Wajntal A: H-Y antigen in Swyer syndrome and the genetics of XY gonadal dysgenesis. *Hum Genet* 53:51, 1979.

61. Wachtel SS, Koo GC, De la Chapelle A, Kallio H, Heyman JM, Miller OJ: H-Y antigen in 46,XY gonadal dysgenesis. *Hum Genet* 54:25, 1980.

62. Migeon BR, Brown TR, Axelman J, Migeon CJ: Studies of the locus for androgen receptor: localization on the human X and evidence for homology with the TFM locus in the mouse. *Proc Natl Acad Sci USA* 78:6339, 1981.

63. Amrhein JA, Meyer WJ, Jones HW, Migeon CJ: Androgen insensitivity in man, evidence for genetic heterogeneity. *Proc Natl Acad Sci USA* 78:891, 1976.

64. Seeburg PH, Adelman JP: Characterization of the cDNA for precursor of human luteinizing hormone-releasing hormone. *Nature* 311:666, 1984.

65. Nikolics K, Mason AJ, Szonyi E, Ramachandran J, Seeburg PH: A prolactin-inhibiting factor within the precursor for human gonadotropin-releasing hormone. *Nature* 316:511, 1985.

66. Phillips HS, Nikolics K, Branton D, Seeburg PH: Immuno-cytochemical localization in rat brain of a prolactin release-inhibiting sequence of gonadotropin-releasing hormone. *Nature* 316:542, 1985.

67. Mason AJ, Hayflick JS, Zoeller RT, et al: A deletion truncating the gonadotropin-releasing hormone gene is responsible for hypogonadism in the hpg mouse. *Science* 234:1366, 1986.

68. Fiddes JC, Goodman HM: Isolation, cloning, and sequence analysis of the cDNA for the α-subunit of human chorionic gonadotropin. *Nature* 281:351, 1979.

69. Fiddes JC, Goodman HM: The gene encoding the common alpha subunit of the four human glycoprotein hormones. *J Mol Appl Genet* 1:3, 1981.

70. Fiddes JC, Talmadge K: Structure, expression and evolution of the genes for the human glycoprotein hormones. *Recent Prog Horm Res* 40:43, 1984.

71. Talmadge K, Boorstein WR, Fiddes JC: The human genome contains seven genes for the β-subunit of chorionic gonadotropin but only one gene for the β-subunit of luteinizing hormone. *DNA* 2:281, 1983.

72. Policastro PF, Daniels-McQueen SD, Carle G, Boime I: A map of the hCG β–hLH β gene cluster. *J Biol Chem* 261:5907, 1986.

73. Talmadge K, Vamvakopoulos NC, Fiddes JC: Evolution of the genes for the β subunits of human chorionic gonadotropin and luteinizing hormone. *Nature* 307:37, 1984.

74. Jameson JL, Lindell CM, Habener JF: Evolution of different transcriptional start sites in the human luteinizing hormone and chorionic gonadotropin beta subunit genes. *DNA* 5:277, 1986.

75. Corbani M, Counis R, Starzec A, Jutisz M: Effect of gonadectomy on pituitary levels of mRNA encoding gonadotropin subunits and secretion of luteinizing hormone. *Mol Cell Endocrinol* 35:83, 1983.

76. Nilson JH, Nejedlik MT, Virgin JB, Crowder ME, Nett TM: Expression of α-subunit and luteinizing hormone β genes in the ovine anterior pituitary. Estradiol supresses accumulation of mRNAs for both α-subunit and luteinizing hormone β. *J Biol Chem* 258:12087, 1983.

77. Laudelfeld T, Kepa J, Karsch F: Estradiol feedback effects on the α-subunit mRNA in the sheep pituitary gland: Correlation with serum and pituitary luteinizing hormone concentrations. *Proc Natl Acad Sci USA* 1:1322, 1984.

78. Gharib SD, Bowers SM, Need LR, Chin WW: Regulation of rat luteinizing hormone subunit messenger ribonucleic acids by gonadal steroid hormones. *J Clin Invest* 77:582, 1986.

79. Papavasiliou SS, Zmeili S, Khoury S, et al: Gonadotropin-releasing hormone differentially regulates expression of the genes for luteinizing hormone alpha and beta subunits in male rats. *Proc Natl Acad Sci USA* 83:4026, 1986.

80. Snyder PJ: Gonadotropin adenomas of the pituitary. *Endocr Rev* 6:552, 1985.

81. Whitaker MD, Prior JC, Scheithauer B, et al: Gonadotropin-secreting pituitary tumour: Report and review. *Clin Endocrinol* 22:43, 1985.

82. Beckers A, Stevenaert A, Mashiter K, Hennen G: Follicle-stimulating hormone-secreting pituitary adenomas. *J Clin Endocrinol Metab* 61:525, 1985.

83. Snyder PJ, Bashey JM, Kim SU, Chappel SC: Secretion of uncombined subunits of LH by gonadotropin cell adenomas. *J Clin Endocrinol Metab* 59:1169, 1984.

84. Jameson JL, Lindell CM, Habener JF, Ridgway EC: Expression of chorionic gonadotropin β-subunit like messenger ribonucleic acid in alpha-subunit secreting pituitary adenoma. *J Clin Endocrinol Metab* 62:1271, 1986.

85. Grady RR, Charlesworth MC, Schwartz NB: Characterization of the FSH-suppressing activity in follicular fluid, in Greep RO (ed): *Recent Progress in Hormone Research*. Proceedings of the 1981 Laurentian Hormone Conference. New York, Academic Press, 1981, vol 38, p 409.

86. Forage RG, Ring JM, Brown RW, et al: Cloning and sequence analysis of cDNA species coding for the two subunits of inhibin from bovine follicular fluid. *Proc Natl Acad Sci USA* 83:3091, 1986.

87. Mason AJ, Niall HD, Seeburg PH: Structure of two human ovarian inhibins. *Biochem Biophys Res Commun* 135:957, 1986.

88. Ling N, Ying S-Y, Ueno N, et al: Pituitary FSH is released by a heterodimer of the beta-subunits from the two forms of inhibin. *Nature* 321:779, 1986.

89. Vale W, Rivier J, Vaughn J, et al: Purification and characterization of an FSH-releasing protein from porcine ovarian follicular fluid. *Nature* 321:776, 1986.

90. Takahashi M, Hayashi M, Manganaro TF, Donahoe PK: The ontogeny of mullerian-inhibiting substance in granulosa cells of the bovine ovarian follicle. *Biol Reprod* 35:447, 1986.

91. Donahoe PK, Budzik GP, Trelstad R. Mullerian-inhibiting substance: An update, in Greep RO (ed): *Recent Progress in Hormone Research*. Proceedings of the 1981 Laurentian Hormone Conference. New York, Academic Press, 1981, vol 38, p 279.

92. Takahashi M, Koide SS, Donahoe PK: Mullerian-inhibiting substance as oocyte meiosis inhibitor. *Mol Cell Endocrinol* 47:225, 1986.

CHAPTER 18

Neurologic Considerations

Andrew G. Herzog

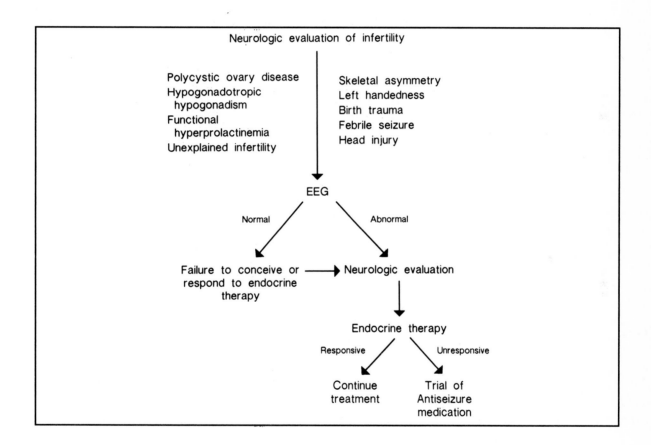

Some reproductive endocrine disorders that are common causes of infertility have been attributed to hypothalamic dysfunction. These include polycystic ovary syndrome (PCO), hypogonadotropic hypogonadism (HH), and functional hyperprolactinemia. Considerable animal experimental and clinical investigative evidence suggests that each of these conditions may be the result of altered secretion of gonadotropin-releasing hormone (GnRH) or abnormal dopamine activity in the hypothalamus. The demonstration of a primary etiology in the hypothal-

amus, however, is uncommon. It remains a possibility, therefore, that hypothalamic dysfunction in many cases may be secondary to extrahypothalamic influences. Indeed, the hypothalamus does not function in a vacuum in the brain. It is extensively and reciprocally interconnected with many cerebral and brain stem regions that modulate its activity. The epileptic involvement of temporal lobe structures may contribute to hypothalamic dysfunction, the development of reproductive endocrine disorders, and infertility.

NEUROANATOMY AND EPILEPSY

Epilepsy affects approximately 1% of the population in the United States. It can be divided into two types, generalized and partial. Primary generalized seizures originate synchronously from the entire cerebral cortical mantle and result in loss of consciousness and generalized tonic–clonic seizures. Secondary generalized seizures result from the generalization of partial seizures. About three fourths of adults with seizures have partial epilepsy,[1,2] that is, seizures that originate from a small portion of cerebral cortex. This region is known as a focus.

Medial temporal lobe structures, especially the amygdala and hippocampus, are highly epileptogenic and usually the sites of origin, or at least involvement, in partial epilepsy. These regions form part of the limbic system, where emotions are thought to be represented, and memory and learning take place. Activation of these regions with epileptic discharges can therefore lead to symptoms of heightened affect, including fear, anxiety, depression, and feelings of impending doom. Awareness may become intermittently impaired due to the episodic interference of continuous memory formation by epileptic discharges. Learning may be disrupted intermittently or become persistently impaired

Medial temporal lobe structures are heavily and reciprocally interconnected with other regions of the temporal lobe and with the insula. These areas of the brain elaborate preceptions of smell, taste, vision, and audition. Therefore, persons with epilepsy may experience auras of smells, tastes, sights, or sounds for which there are no environmental concomitants. Moreover, environmentally derived perceptions may be associated with exaggerated emotional and motivational significance by virtue of the heightened electrical activity in limbic structures. Deepened emotional state can lead to the development of persistently altered personality and behavior, commonly referred to as interictal features of temporal lobe epilepsy.[3] This syndrome is characterized by intense affect, depression, obsessions, paranoid ideation, circumstantiality, tangentiality, hyperreligiosity, hypergraphia, and altered sexuality or hyposexuality.

Medial temporal lobe structures are closely linked to the supplemental motor cortex and to the motor nucleus of the trigeminal nerve, regions of the brain that are responsible for motor activity such as deviation of the head and eyes, and mouthing and chewing movements. Medial temporal structures are also extensively interconnected with the orbital frontal cortex, rostral hypothalamus, dorsal motor nucleus of the vagus, and solitary nucleus. These are sites of motor and sensory autonomic nervous system representation. Therefore partial seizures are often associated with altered respiration, changes in cardiac rate, elevated blood pressure, enlargement of pupils, and even gooseflesh.

Finally, the medial temporal lobe structures have extensive, reciprocal, direct connections with hypothalamic regions that are involved in endocrine regulation. Transient endocrine changes commonly occur after seizures. Specifically, serum prolactin levels are significantly and markedly elevated during the first 15 minutes after a generalized[4] or partial[5] seizure. The levels gradually return to baseline over the subsequent hour. Levels of serum luteinizing hormone (LH) have also been observed to rise after generalized seizures and to return to baseline over a protracted 24-hour course.[6] Cortisol is another hormone that becomes dramatically elevated in the serum after generalized seizures.[4] This has also been shown to occur after simulated seizures.[4]

REPRODUCTIVE DYSFUNCTION AND EPILEPSY

Reproductive dysfunction is unusually common among individuals who have epilepsy.[7-9] Some observations suggest that they are more common with partial seizures of temporal lobe origin (temporal lobe epilepsy, or TLE) than with generalized or focal motor seizure disorders.[7] Studies that deal exclusively or predominantly with women who have TLE reveal that 14 to 20% have amenorrhea and that more than 50% overall have some form of menstrual dysfunction.[8,10,11] Fertility is reduced to 69% of the expected number of offspring.[12] Investigations of men who have TLE show that 49 to 71% have diminished potency or altered sexual interest.[13-18]

Elevated prolactin levels,[4-6] elevated[19-21] or elevated[24] or decreased[22,23] gonadotropin stimulation, decreased free testosterone (FT) levels,[25,26] and decreased 17-ketosteroid excretion[27] have all been shown to occur in the epileptic population. Two of these investigations in particular are noteworthy because they demonstrated reproductive endocrine abnormalities that correlated significantly with sexual dysfunction. Decreased urinary excretion of 17-ketosteroids, specifically androsterone and dehydroepiandrosterone (DHEA), was observed in epileptic men.[27] A positive correlation was found between the lowered excretion of androgens and reduced potency. It also was shown that epileptic men have reduced serum FT levels.[26] These concentrations were associated with higher serum gonadotropin and prolactin levels, and were significantly related to diminished sex drive.

Abnormalities in serum levels of gonadotropins and prolactin, and LH response to GnRH, suggest altered function of the hypothalamic–pituitary axis. Primary structural lesions at the level of the hypothalamus or pituitary, however, have not been evident by computerized tomography or clinical assessment and follow-up[8,9,22] Similarly, clinical evaluations and imaging studies of peripheral endocrine organs have not demonstrated structural lesions that provide an etiology for the findings.[8,9,22]

Abundant data suggest that altered function of temporal lobe structures, a factor common to all patients with TLE who have reproductive dysfunction, may contribute to reproductive and sexual changes. Temporal lobe epilepsy generally originates from or involves limbic portions of the temporal lobe.[28] Some of these limbic structures can be parcellated into anatomically distinct functional divisions that exert opposing modulator influences on the structure and function of reproductive organs.[29] A most notable example is the amygdala,[29] which is separated into corticomedial and basolateral divisions. Each has its largely separate outflow tract, the stria terminalis and ventral amygdalofugal pathway, respectively. Bilateral ablations of the basolateral portion of the amygdala in adult female deermice can induce anovulatory cycles and polycystic ovary changes.[30] Stimulation of the corticomedial amygdala in a number of mammalian species can induce ovulation and uterine contractions.[31,32] Transection of the stria terminalis blocks the ovulatory response, whereas a lesion of the ventral amygdalofugal pathway has no such effect.[32] Stimulation and ablation studies in rodents suggest that the corticomedial amygdala promotes sexual activity, while the basolateral amygdala inhibits it.[29,30] Bilateral amygdalectomy in adult male rats and cats results in marked degeneration of the testes.[33] Bilateral amygdalectomy in female monkeys induces amenorrhea and hypogonadal vaginal changes.[34] Temporal lobectomy in men and women with TLE is commonly associated with improved reproductive and sexual function, and less frequently with the development or exacerbation of reproductive and sexual dysfunction.[11,35,36]

Altered temporal lobe function may contribute to reproductive endocrine changes. Based on depth electrode recordings and video monitoring in human epileptic subjects, it was reported that prolactin elevation consistently follows seizures that produce intense, widespread, mesial temporal lobe limbic seizure discharges, and does not occur after seizures that do not involve these areas.[37] Electrical stimulation of the human amygdala, but not sham stimulation, has elicited significant elevations in serum prolactin levels.[38] With regard to gonadotropins, the amygdala has extensive, direct anatomic connections with the ventromedial and preoptic hypothalamic nuclei, which are involved in the regulation, production, and secretion of GnRH (Fig. 18–1).[39] Alterations

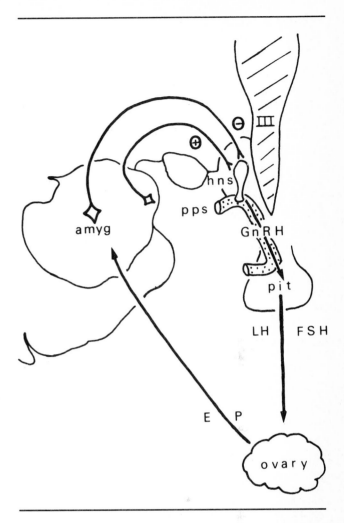

Figure 18–1. Cross-section of the anterior temporal lobe and diencephalon depicts direct projections from the two anatomically distinct functional divisions of the amygdala (amyg) to the same ventromedial hypothalamic neurons. The different influences of these projections on hypothalamic neurosecretory cells (hns) modulate pulsatile gonadotropin-releasing hormone (GnRH) secretion. Releasing hormones enter the pituitary portal system (pps), and regulate the pattern of luteinizing hormone (LH) and follicle-stimulating hormone (FSH) secretion by the pituitary (pit). These gonadotropins induce ovulation and stimulate production of estradiol (E) and progesterone (P). Gonadal steroids, in turn, bind to specific amygdaloid hormone receptors and influence neural activity, including epileptiform discharges.

in the physiologic frequency or concentration of pulsatile GnRH secretion can induce changes in serum LH and follice-stimulating hormone (FSH) that resemble patterns found in reproductive endocrine disorders such as PCO and HH.[40] Stimulation of the two major divisions of the amygdala or their outflow tracts can predictably and differentially affect the membrane potentials of the same ventromedial hypothalamic neurons.[41] Stimulation and ablation studies of the amygdala in conjunction with gonadotropin assays, moreover, have shown that the two functional divisions of the amygdala can produce eleva-

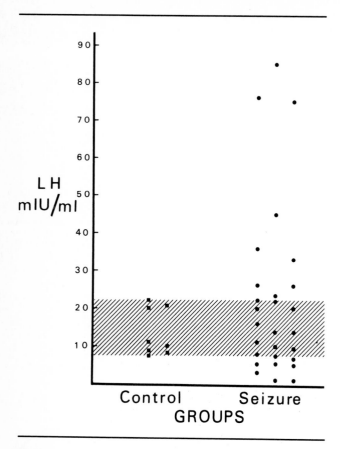

Figure 18–2. This graph shows the much broader range of base-line LH serum levels as measured during the early follicular phase among 28 women with partial seizures of temporal lobe origin, in comparison to 8 age-matched, healthy controls. This finding is consistent with the concept that involvement of the limbic system with epileptiform discharges may disrupt normal limbic modulation of hypothalamic regulation of pituitary gonadotropin secretion. (From Herzog et al.[9] Reproduced with permission.)

tions or reductions in pituitary and serum LH levels.[30]

Consistent with these animal data is the finding that women with TLE have a range of early follicular-phase serum LH levels that extends well above and below normal control values (Fig. 18–2).[8] This has led to the hypothesis that involvement of temporal lobe limbic structures with seizure discharges may disrupt normal limbic modulation of hypothalamic regulation of pituitary secretion and promote the development of reproductive endocrine disorders (Fig. 18–3).

NEUROLOGIC CONSIDERATIONS OF MALE REPRODUCTIVE DYSFUNCTION

Reproductive endocrine abnormalities in men with TLE have been ascribed to the use of antiseizure medications. Changes were demonstrated in the levels of both adrenal and gonadal steroids during 21

days of carbamazepine administration in healthy men.[42] Levels of serum sex hormone-binding globu-lin (SHBG) increased; levels of testosterone, FT, DHEA sulfate (DHEAS), and androsterone declined. All but DHEAS returned to baseline levels by the end of the treatment period.

Levels of serum testosterone and SHBG were elevated in epileptic men undergoing long-term anti-convulsant therapy.[43] The authors postulated that despite normal pituitary and testicular regulatory function, anticonvulsant-induced increases in SHBG synthesis and secretion may result in elevated serum total testosterone (TT) levels but decreased FT con-centration, which may contribute to diminished sex-ual activity. Elevated levels of SHBG and TT, and diminished levels of FT were confirmed in epileptic men receiving extended anticonvulsant medica-tions.[26] No consistent correlations were noted be-tween serum hormone levels and dosages, however. Neuroendocrine dysfunction was demonstrated among untreated as well as treated men and women with TLE.[22] It is unlikely, therefore, that all of the reproductive endocrine abnormalities associated with TLE were attributable to medications.

Low serum testosterone and elevated gonado-tropin and prolactin levels were demonstrated in epileptic men.[44] Data suggested an inverse relation-ship between serum testosterone levels and the ages of the subjects. No relationship was noted between reproductive hormone level and antiseizure medica-tion dosage. These investigators questioned why clinical hyposexuality was reported to be more com-mon with TLE than with primary generalized sei-zures if it were related to drug use.

In our own investigation,[9] 11 of 20 men with TLE had diminished sexual interest or potency. Nine of these 11 had reproductive endocrine disorders, in-cluding features of HH in 5, functional hyperprolac-tinemia in 2, and hypergonadotropic hypogonadism in 2. Among these 9 were 4 patients in whom the relationship of reproductive endocrine abnormal-ities to antiseizure medication was not apparent because either they had no history of such therapy or reproductive symptoms preceded the use of these agents.

Reproductive endocrine disorders may favor the development of TLE in men. Brain wave abnormali-ties, including temporal lobe epileptiform discharges, may occur with greater than expected frequency among men with these disorders.[45] Medial temporal lobe structures bind sex steroids, including testos-terone.[46] Animal experimental data suggest that testosterone raises electroshock seizure threshold and orchiectomy lowers it.[47] Serum levels of FT are usually decreased in the reproductive endocrine disorders that are associated with TLE in men,[2,25,26] and may therefore favor the occurrence of epilepti-form activity.

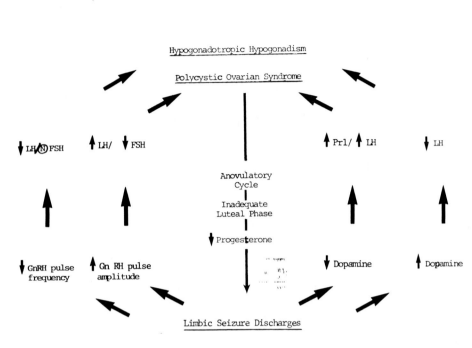

Figure 18–3. Shown are possible mechanisms by which limbic seizure discharges may promote reproductive endocrine disorders, and how abnormal reproductive hormone levels may influence epilepsy. It is based on a hypothesis that involvement of limbic structures with epileptiform discharges may disrupt normal limbic modulatory influences on hypothalamic secretion of GnRH. Altered frequency or amplitude of GnRH secretion may lead to patterns of pituitary secretion of LH and FSH, which are found in hypogonadotropic hypogonadism and PCO syndrome. Kindled limbic seizures alter brain dopamine levels. Hypothalamic dopamine exerts an inhibitory effect on pituitary LH and prolactin (Prl) secretion. Abnormal brain dopamine levels may alter pituitary gonadotropin and prolactin secretion, and promote the development of reproductive endocrine disorders. Reproductive endocrine disorders that are associated with partial seizures of temporal lobe origin are characterized by anovulatory cycles and diminished progesterone secretion. An elevated serum estrogen:progesterone ratio may promote the development of seizure discharges in the brain. (From Herzog et al.[9] Reproduced with permission.)

NEUROLOGIC CONSIDERATIONS OF FEMALE REPRODUCTIVE DYSFUNCTION

In an investigation of 50 women with clinical and electroencephalographic features of TLE, 19 had reproductive endocrine disorders: PCO in 10, HH in 6, premature menopause in 2, and functional hyperprolactinemia in 1. The occurrence of PCO (20%) and of HH (12%) was significantly greater that the estimated frequencies in the general female population. The data in our investigations confirmed that antiseizure medication use is associated with diminished free: total testosterone ratios.[8,9] Furthermore, they demonstrated for the first time in an epileptic population an association between antiseizure medication and markedly diminished DHEAS serum levels.[8,48]

Analysis of the female data, however, did not show a statistically significant relationship overall between the occurrence of menstrual disorders and the use of antiseizure medications. Some individual endocrine syndromes also did not appear to be related to those agents. Six of the 10 women with TLE and PCO, for example, did not take antiseizure medication; nor did those who had hyperprolactinemia. Both of the women with premature menopause took these agents, but the amenorrhea preceded the

institution of therapy in one. One of the 6 women who had HH did not take antiseizure medication, and 2 of the 6 who did had had irregular menses since menarche, which preceded the institution of therapy. Furthermore, no relationship was found between any of the endocrine syndromes and the type or serum level of antiseizure medication. It is unlikely, therefore, that the reproductive endocrine disorders can be attributed entirely to drug effects.

Central dopaminergic mechanism may also contribute to the relationship between TLE and reproductive endocrine disorders (see Fig. 18–3). Bromocriptine[49] and dopamine[50] lessen LH[49] and prolactin[50] secretion by the pituitary, and are thought to act in the lateral palisade zone of the median eminence to inhibit GnRH secretion.[51] Clinical studies of PCO syndrome reveal exaggerated suppression of LH levels with dopamine infusion[52,53] and supranormal elevation of prolactin levels in response to haloperidol.[54] These features and elevated baseline levels of LH and prolactin suggest a decreased level of dopamine activity in the hypothalamus of women with PCO syndrome.

The opposite has been proposed to explain HH. In the absence of hypothyroidism and structural lesions of the pituitary and peripheral endocrine glands, no organic origin is usually demonstrated to explain the low gonadotropin levels in HH. The amenorrhea is generally attributed to a functional derangement of the hypothalamic–pituitary axis, especially excessive dopaminergic tone in the tubero-infundibular region of the hypothalamus.[55] Altered dopamine and homovanillic acid concentrations in the brains of animals with kindled amygdaloid seizures[56] and in the spinal fluid of patients with TLE[57] suggest a relationship between TLE and brain dopamine metabolism. There is reason to consider, therefore, that epileptic discharges in medial temporal limbic structures may influence reproductive endocrine function by modulating dopamine as well as GnRH levels in the hypothalamus.

Neural innervation of the gonads provides another potential mechanism by which altered brain function may induce reproductive and endocrine changes (Fig. 18–4). This possibility, however, has remained largely unexplored. It has been demonstrated that bilateral ovariectomy is followed by unilateral right-sided reduction in hypothalamic GnRH content, while unilateral ovariectomy on either side produces an ipsilateral increase in hypothalamic GnRH content.[58] These findings cannot readily be explained by endocrine factors alone.

The ovary is innervated both by sympathetic noradrenergic fibers originating from neurons in the intermediolateral cell column of the spinal cord, and by parasympathetic cholinergic fibers from the dorsal motor nucleus of the vagus. In rodent models, unilateral ovariectomy is generally associated with contralateral compensatory ovarian hypertrophy. Unilateral ovariectomy in association with 6-hydroxydopamine application to the remaining ovary results in decreased compensatory ovarian hypertrophy.[59] This has been attributed to blockage of noradrenergic neural transmission. Unilateral ovariectomy in association with bilateral vagotomy also results in diminished compensatory ovarian hypertrophy, as well as in diminished elevation of serum LH and FSH levels and a prolonged estrus cycle.[60]

The amygdala has direct efferent projections to both the dorsal motor nucleus of the vagus[61] and the dorsomedial and lateral regions of the hypothalamus.[61] The latter regulate sympathetic response through direct projections to the neurons of the intermediolateral cell column of the spinal cord.[62] Temporolimbic stimulation in adrenalectomized and hypophysectomized rats has been shown to increase or decrease estradiol and progesterone concentrations in the contralateral ovarian vein at 105 to 120 minutes, while ovarian blood flow remains unchanged.[63] Thus there is reason to investigate the possibility that involvement of medial temporal lobe structures with epileptiform discharges may disrupt normal limbic neural as well as neuroendocrine modulation of gonadal structure and function. The reverse may also be true. Sensory vagal fibers from

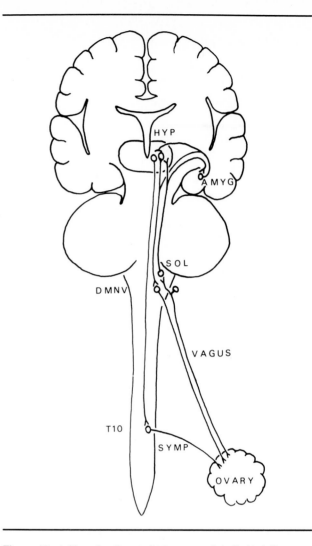

Figure 18–4. Neural pathways that may mediate limbic influences on gonadal structure and function. The amygdala (AMYG) has direct fiber projections to the dorsomedial and lateral regions of the hypothalamus (HYP). These regions are connected directly to the preganglionic sympathetic neurons in the intermediolateral cell column of the thoracolumbar spinal cord, from which originate sympathetic nerve fibers to the gonads. The amygdala also has direct and indirect projections to the dorsal motor nucleus of the vagus (DMNV), from which originate vagal fibers to the gonads. Afferent vagal fibers from the gonads project to the solitary nucleus in the medulla (SDL). The solitary nucleus has direct projections to the amygdala as well as to the hypothalamus.

the gonads terminate in the solitary nucleus of the medulla. The solitary nucleus is directly and extensively connected to the amygdala.[64] The amygdala shows sensitive, short-latency electrophysiologic responses to vagal stimulation.[65] Therefore sensory input from pelvic reproductive structures may exert modulatory influences on limbic discharges.

Reproductive endocrine disorders may favor the development of TLE in women (see Fig. 18–3). Medial temporal lobe limbic structures bind hormones[46,66] and show sensitive electrophysiologic changes in response to hormonal influence.[67] Animal experimental and human clinical data suggest that estrogen promotes interictal epileptiform brain wave activity and can precipitate clinical seizures.[47,58] The antiestrogen clomiphene citrate has been shown significantly to lessen both kainic acid-induced seizures in rats[69] and seizure frequency in epileptic women with reproductive endocrine disorders.[70] Progesterone also lessens the probability of interictal epileptiform activity[71] and has benefited some patients with epilepsy.[72-74] The anovulatory cycles in PCO and HH, therefore, may expose temporal lobe limbic structures to a constant estrogen effect without the normal progesterone elevation in the luteal phase, and thereby heighten interictal epileptiform activity. In this regard, 56.5% of women with anovulatory cycles or amenorrhea were found to have electroencephalographic (EEG) abnormalities, including some with focal paroxysmal epileptogenic discharges.[75] Treatment with clomiphene citrate restored EEG findings to normal in 54% of them. There was, moreover, an association between correction of the EEG and ovulation and pregnancy. Thus the hormonal changes associated with anovulatory cycles may favor the development of EEG abnormalities.

PRENATAL FACTORS, TLE, AND REPRODUCTIVE ENDOCRINE DISORDERS

Another possibility to consider is that the association between TLE and some reproductive endocrine disorders may represent the parallel effects of prenatal factors that are common to the development of both the brain and the reproductive system. Both categories of disorders have a tendency to be familial. A genetically determined susceptibility to TLE was suggested by its greater than expected occurrence in first-order relatives.[76] Sex-linked dominant transmission[77] and autosomal dominant inheritance with variable expression[78] have been proposed to explain the high familial occurrence of PCO. Comparable studies of HH are not available. Premature menopause is reported to be familial,[79,80] and was attributed in 4 women members of one family to an interstitial deletion of the long arm of the X chromosome.[81] Autosomal dominant transmission with variable penetrance was proposed to explain the high familial frequency of HH in men.[82] Hypergonadotropic hypogonadism in disorders of gonadal differentiation is commonly associated with autosomal or sex chromosomal anomalies.[83] The possible contribution of hereditary traits or genetic linkage to the parallel development of both TLE and reproductive endocrine disorders warrants further investigation.

In addition, data suggest that TLE and reproductive endocrine disorders may promote their mutual development. Specifically, involvement of limbic structures with epileptiform discharges may disrupt the normal modulation of reproductive endocrine function, and reproductive endocrine disorders may adversely affect neural activity in limbic structures and thereby lead to TLE. Critical evaluation of these hypotheses by further research is required to obtain a better understanding of the interactions between hormones and seizure activity in the pathogenesis and treatment of both conditions.

Men and women with partial seizures may have a wide array of symptoms and findings. In the most obvious cases, seizures occur in clearly definable episodes and disrupt consciousness, memory, and continuing activities. In more subtle forms, symptoms blend in with regular activities and perceptions, and are more difficult for the patient and physician alike to diagnose. In such cases, many years may pass without recognition that the symptoms may be the manifestations of a potentially treatable, neuropathologic process that may also contribute to infertility. Therefore the gynecologist and endocrinologist should obtain an EEG in patients who have reproductive or reproductive endocrine disorders that have neither a clearly definable primary etiology in the reproductive or endocrine system nor adequate response to therapy.

The EEG studies are especially important if patients have emotional, behavioral, learning, perceptual, or autonomic manifestations that are consistent with a diagnosis of TLE. Suspicion should also be raised if there is evidence of left-handedness or skeletal asymmetry to suggest anomalous brain development or brain injury early in life. Other predisposing factors for brain wave abnormalities include a history of birth difficulty, febrile seizure, or significant head injury with loss of consciousness or memory. The majority of patients with partial seizures of temporal lobe origin have paroxysmal epileptiform activity or at least slowing of brain waves in temporal derivatives of the EEG. If results of the regular EEG are negative, there is an additional 10% yield of positive findings in EEG tests carried out while the patient is asleep, especially with the use of nasopharyngeal or sphenoidal leads.

Some evidence exists that return of brain wave function to normal may be associated with increased fertility. As noted earlier, results of the EEG were abnormal in the majority of one series of infertile women, and correction of the EEG was associated with ovulation and pregnancy.[75] The anticonvulsant phenytoin was used to treat 80 infertile women with inadequate luteal phase and EEG abnormalities.[84] A 45% pregnancy rate was observed within 4 months of the onset of therapy.

We used antiseizure medications to treat 5

women with newly diagnosed partial seizures and a 5 to 7-year history of unsuccessfully treated infertility in association with PCO syndrome. Three of the 5 women became pregnant within 3 months. Two of these continued using antiseizure medication to term. The third tapered and discontinued the medication after learning of her pregnancy. All 3 delivered apparently healthy, full-term babies. Finally, in several surgical series of unilateral temporal lobectomy for intractable epilepsy, improved seizure control was associated with normalization of reproductive function, restored fertility, and improved sexual behavior.[15–17,35,85]

Further investigations are required to establish the precise role of brain wave therapy in the treatment of infertility. Thorough neurologic and EEG evaluations of potential extrahypothalamic influences on reproductive and endocrine function, however, should be considered in all infertile men and women who do not have a clearly definable primary etiology identified in the reproductive or endocrine system.

REFERENCES

1. Plan for Nationwide Action on Epilepsy. DHEW publication (NIH) 78-311. Washington, DC, Department of Health, Education, and Welfare, 1978, vol 2.
2. Schomer DL: Current concepts in neurology: Partial epilepsy. N Engl J Med 309:356, 1983.
3. Bear D, Fedio P: Quantitative analysis of interictal behavior in temporal lobe epilepsy. Arch Neurol 34:457, 1976.
4. Abbott RI, Browning MCK, Davidson DLW: Serum prolactin and cortisol concentrations after grand mal seizures. J Neural Neurosurg Psychiatry 43:163, 1980.
5. Pritchard PB III, Wannamaker BB, Sagel J, et al: Endocrine function following complex seizures. Ann Neurol 14:27, 1983.
6. Dana-Haeri J, Trimble MR, Oxley J: Prolactin and gonadotropin change following generalized and partial seizures. J Neurol Neurosurg Psychiatry 46:331, 1983.
7. Gastaut H, Collomb H: Étude du comportement sexuel chez les épileptiques psychomoteurs. Ann Med Psychol 112:657, 1954.
8. Herzog AG, Seibel MM, Schomer DL, Vaitukaitis JL, Geschwind N: Reproductive endocrine disorders in women with partial seizures of temporal lobe origin. Arch Neurol 43:341, 1986.
9. Herzog AG, Seibel MM, Schomer DL, Vaitukaitis JL, Geschwind N: Reproductive endocrine disorders in men with partial seizures of temporal lobe origin. Arch Neurol 43:347, 1986.
10. Jensen I, Vaernet K: Temporal lobe epilepsy: Follow-up investigation of 74 temporal lobe resected patients. Acta Neurochir 37:173, 1977.
11. Trampuz V, Dimitrijevic M, Kryanovski J: Ulga epilepsije u patogenezi disfunkeije ovarija. Neuropsihijatrija 23:179, 1975.
12. Dansky LV, Andermann E, Andermann F: Marriage and fertility in epileptic patients. Epilepsia 21:261, 1980.
13. Hierons R, Saunders M: Impotence in patients with temporal lobe lesions. Lancet 2:761, 1966.
14. Kolarsky A, Freund K, Machek J, et al: Association with early temporal lobe damage. Arch Gen Psychiatry 17:735, 1967.
15. Taylor DC: Sexual behavior and temporal lobe epilepsy. Arch Neurol 21:510, 1969.
16. Blumer D: Changes of sexual behavior related to temporal lobe disorders in man. J Sex Res 6:173, 1970.
17. Jensen I, Larsen JK: Mental aspects of temporal lobe epilepsy. J Neurol Neurosurg Psychiatry 42:256, 1979.
18. Shukla GD, Srivastava ON, Katiyar BC: Sexual disturbances in temporal lobe epilepsy: A controlled study. Br J Psychiatry 134:288, 1979.
19. Toone, BK, Wheeler M, Fenwick PBC: Sex hormone changes in epileptics. Clin Endocrinol (Oxf) 12:391, 1980.
20. Hoffmann J, Kahlert T: Veraenderungen von sexual Hormonen bei maennlichen Epilepsie-Patienten unter Langzeittherapie. Nervenarzt 52:715, 1981.
21. Rodin E, Subramanian MG, Gilroy J: Investigation of sex hormones in male epileptic patients. Epilepsia 6:690, 1984.
22. Herzog AC, Russell V, Vaitukaitis JL, et al: Neuroendocrine dysfunction in temporal lobe epilepsy. Arch Neurol 39:133, 1982.
23. Murialdo G, Manni R, DeMaria A, et al: Luteinizing hormones pulsatile secretion and pituitary response to gonadotropin-releasing hormone and to thyrotropin-releasing hormone in male epileptic subjects on chronic phenobarbital treatment. J Endocrinol Invest 10:27, 1987.
24. Dana-Haeri J, Oxley J, Richens A: Pituitary responsiveness to gonadotropin-releasing and thyrotrophin-releasing hormones in epileptic patients receiving carbamazepine or phenytoin. Clin Endocrinol (Oxf) 20:163, 1984.
25. Dana-Haeri J, Oxley J, Richens E: Reduction of free testosterone by antiepileptic drugs. Br Med J 284:85, 1982.
26. Toone BK, Wheeler M, Nanjee M, et al: Sex hormones, sexual activity and plasma anticonvulsant levels in male epileptics. J Neurol Neurosurg Psychiatry 46:824, 1983.
27. Christiansen P, Deigaard J, Lund M: Potens, fertilitet of konshormonudskillelse hos yngre manglige epilepsilidende. Ugeskr Laeger 137:2402, 1975.
28. Falconer MA, Serafetinides EA, Corsellis JAN: Etiology and pathogenesis of temporal lobe epilepsy. Arch Neurol 10:233, 1964.
29. Kaada B: Stimulation and regional ablation of the amygdaloid complex with reference to functional representations, in Eleftheriou BE (ed): The Neurobiology of the Amygdala. New York, Plenum, 1972, pp 205–281.
30. Zolovick AJ: Effects of lesions and electrical stimulation of the amygdala on hypothalamic-hypophyseal regulation, in Eleftheriou BE (ed): The Neurobiology of the Amygdala. New York, Plenum, 1972, pp 745–762.
31. Koikegami H, Yamada T, Usui K: Stimulation of the amygdaloid nuclei and periamygdaloid cortex with special reference to its effects on uterine movements and ovulation. Folia Psychiatr Neurol Jpn 8:7, 1954.
32. Velasco ME, Taleisnik S: Release of gonadotropins induced by amygdaloid stimulation in the rat. Endocrinology 84:132, 1960.
33. Yamada, T, Greer MA: The effect of bilateral ablation of the amygdala on endocrine function in the rat. Endocrinology 66:565, 1960.
34. Erickson LB, Wada JA: Effects of lesions in the temporal lobe and rhinencephalon on reproductive function in adult female rhesus monkeys. Fertil Steril 21:434, 1970.
35. Savard RJ, Walker E: Changes in social functioning after surgical treatment for temporal lobe epilepsy. Social Work 10:87, 1965.
36. Taylor DC, Falconer MA: Clinical socioeconomic and psychological adjustment after temporal lobectomy for epilepsy. Br J Psychiatry 114:124, 1968.
37. Sperling MR, Pritchard PB, Engle J Jr, Daniel C, Sagel J: Prolactin in partial epilepsy: An indicator of limbic seizures. Ann Neurol 20:716, 1986.
38. Parra A, Velasco M, Cervantes C et al: Plasma prolactin increase following electric stimulation of the amygdala in humans. Nueroendocrinol 31:60, 1980.
39. Renaud LP: Influence of amygdala stimulation on the activity of identified tuberoinfundibular neurons in the rat hypothalamus. J Physiol 260:237, 1976.
40. Knobil E: The neuroendocrine control of the menstrual cycle. Recent Prog Horm Res 36:53, 1980.
41. Dreifuss JJ, Murphy JT, Gloor P: Contrasting effects of two identified amygdaloid efferent pathways on single hypothalamic neurons. J Nuerophysiol 31:237, 1986.
42. Connell JM, Rapeport WG, Beastall GH, Brodie MJ: Changes in circulating androgens during short-term carbamazepine therapy. Br J Clin Pharmacol 17:347, 1984.
43. Barragry JM, Makin HLJ, Trafford DJH, et al: Effect of anticonvulsants on plasma testosterone and sex hormone-binding globulin levels. J Neurol Psychiatry 41:913, 1978.
44. Rodin E, Subramanian MG, Gilroy J: Investigation of sex hormones in male epileptic patients. Epilepsia 25:690, 1984.
45. Spark R, Wills C, Royal H: Hypogonadism, hyperprolactinemia, and temporal lobe epilepsy in hyposexual men. Lancet 1:413, 1984.
46. Stumpf WE: Steroid-concentrating neurons in the amygdala, in Eleftheriou BE (ed): The Neurobiology of the Amygdala. New York, Plenum, 1972, pp 763–774.
47. Longo LPS, Saldana LEG: Hormones and their influence in epilepsy. Acta Neurol Latinoam 12:29, 1969.
48. Levesque LA, Herzog AG, Seibel MM: The effect of phenytoin and

carbamazepine on serum dehydroepiandrosterone sulfate in men and women who have partial seizures with temporal lobe involvement. *J Clin Endocrinol Metab* 63:243, 1986.

49. Lachelin GCL, Leblanc H, Yen SSC: The inhibitory effect of dopamine agonists on LH release in women. *J Clin Endocrinol Metabol* 44:728, 1977.

50. Leblanc H, Lachelin GCL, Abu-Fadil S et al: Effects of dopamine infusion on pituitary hormone secretion in humans. *J Clin Endocrinol* 43:668, 1976.

51. McNeill TH, Sladek JR: Fluorescenceimmunocytochemistry: Simultaneous localization of catecholamines and gonadotropin- releasing hormone. *Science* 200:72, 1978.

52. Pehrson J, Vaitukaitis JD: Altered dopaminergic control of gonadotropin and prolactin secretion in polycystic ovary syndrome. Annual Meeting of the Endocrine Society, Cincinnati, June 17, 1981.

53. Quigley MF, Rakoff JF, Yen SSC: Increased luteinizing hormone sensitivity to dopamine inhibition in polycystic ovary syndrome. *J Clin Endocrinol Metab.* 52:231, 1981.

54. Falashchi P, del Pozo E, Rocco A et al: Prolactin release in polycystic ovary. *Obstet Gynecol* 55:579, 1980.

55. Rakoff JS, Rigg LA, Yen SSC: The impairment of progesterone-induced pituitary release of prolactin and gonadotropin in patients with hypothalamic chronic anovulation. *Am J Obstet Gynecol* 130:807, 1978.

56. Sato M, Nakashima T: Kindling: Secondary epileptogenesis, sleep and catecholamines. *Can J Neurol Sci* 2:439, 1975.

57. Papeschi R, Molina-Negro P, Sourkes TL, et al: The concentration of homovanillic and 5-hydroxyindoleacetic acid in ventricular and lumbar CSF. *Neurology* 22:1151, 1972.

58. Gerendai I, Rotstejn WH, Marchetti B, et al: Unilateral ovariectomy-induced luteinizing hormone-releasing hormone content changes in the two halves of the mediobasal hypothalamus. *Neurosci Lett* 9:333, 1978.

59. Gerendai I, Marchetti B, Maugeri S, Amico-Roxas M, Scapagnini U: Prevention of compensatory ovarian hypertrophy by local treatment of the ovary with 6-OHDA. *Neuroendocrinology* 27:272, 1978.

60. Burden HW, Lawrence IE: The effect of denervation on compensatory ovarian hypertrophy. *Neuroendocrinology* 23:368, 1977.

61. Price JL, Armaral DG: An autoradiographic study of the projections of the central nucleus of the monkey amygdala. *Neuroscience* 1:124, 1981.

62. Saper CB, Loewy AD, Swanson LW, Cowan WM: Direct hypothalamo-autonomic connections. *Brain Res* 117:305, 1976.

63. Kawakami M, Kubo K, Vemura T, Nagase H, Hayashi R: Involvement of ovarian innervation in steroid secretion. *Endocrinology* 109:136, 1981.

64. Ricardo JA, Koh ET: Anatomical evidence of direct projections from the nucleus of the solitary tract to the hypothalamus, amygdala, and other forebrain structures in the rat. *Brain Res* 153:1, 1978.

65. Dell P, Olson R: Projections secondaires mesencéphaliques, diencéphaliques et amygdaliennes désafferences viscérales vagales. *C R Soc Biol* 145:1088, 1951.

66. Pfaff DW, Keiner M: Estradiol-concentrating cells in the rat amygdala as part of a limbic–hypothalamic hormone-sensitive system, in Eleftheriou BE (ed): *The Neurobiology of the Amygdala*. New York, Plenum, 1972, pp 775–792.

67. Sawyer CH: Functions of the amygdala related to the feedback actions of gonadal steroid hormones, in Eleftheriou BE (ed): *The Neurobiology of the Amygdala*. New York, Plenum, 1972, pp 745–762.

68. Logothetis J, Harner R, Morrell F, et al: The role of estrogens in catamenial exacerbation of epilepsy. *Neurology* 9:352, 1958.

69. Nicoletti F, Speciale C, Sortino MA, et al: Comparative effects of estradiol benzoate, the antiestrogen clomiphene citrate, and the progestin medroxyprogesterone acetate on kainic acid-induced seizures in males and female rats. *Epilepsia* 26:252, 1985.

70. Herzog AG: Clomiphene therapy in epileptic women with menstrual disorders. *Neurology* 38:432, 1988.

71. Backstrom T, Zetterlund B, Blum S, Romano M: Effects of IV progesterone infusions on the epileptic discharge frequency in women with partial epilepsy. *Acta Neurol Scand* 69:240, 1984.

72. Zimmerman AW, Holden KR, Reiter EO, et al: Medroxyprogesterone acetate in the treatment of seizures associated with menstruation. *J Pediatr* 83:959, 1973.

73. Mattson RH, Cramer JA, Caldwell BV, Siconolfi BC: Treatment of seizures with medroxyprogesterone acetate: Preliminary report. *Neurology* 34:1255, 1984.

74. Herzog AG: Intermittent progesterone therapy and frequency of complex partial seizures in women with menstrual disorders. *Neurology* 36:1607, 1986.

75. Sharf M, Sharf B, Bental E, et al: The electroencephalogram in the investigation of anovulation and its treatment by clomiphene. *Lancet* 1:750, 1969.

76. Andermann E: Multifactorial inheritance of generalized and focal epilepsy, in Anderson VE, Hauser WA, Penry JK, et al (eds): *Genetic Basis of the Epilepsies*. New York, Raven, 1982, pp 355–374.

77. Givens JR: Hirsutism and hyperandrogenism. *Adv Intern Med* 21:221, 1976.

78. Jaffee WL, Vaitukaitis JL: Polycystic ovarian syndrome, in Vaitukaitis JL (ed): *Clinical Reproductive Neuroendocrinology*. New York, Elsevier, 1982, pp 207–230.

79. Coulam CB, Stringfellow S, Hoefnagel D: Evidence for a genetic factor in the etiology of premature ovarian failure. *Fertil Steril* 40:693, 1983.

80. Mattison DR, Evans MI, Schwimmer WB, et al: Familial premature ovarian failure. *Am J Hum Genet* 36:134, 1984.

81. Krauss CM, Turksoy RN, Atkins L, et al: Familial premature ovarian failure due to an interstitial deletion of the long arm of the X chromosome. *N Engl J Med* 317:125, 1987.

82. Santen RJ, Paulsen CA: Hypogonadotropic eunuchoidism. I. Clinical study of the mode of inheritance. *J Clin Endocrinol* 36:47, 1973.

83. Grumbach MD, Conte FA: Disorders of sex differentiation, in Williams RH (ed): *Textbook of Endocrinology*. Philadelphia, Saunders, 1981, pp 423–514.

84. Gautray JP, Jolivet A, Goldenberg F, et al: Clinical investigation of the menstrual cycle. II. Neuroendocrine investigation and therapy of the inadequate luteal phase. *Fertil Steril* 29:275, 1978.

85. Cogen PH, Antunes JL, Correll JW: Reproductive function in temporal lobe epilepsy: The effect of temporal lobectomy. *Surg Neurol* 12:243, 1979.

CHAPTER 19

Unexplained Infertility

John Collins

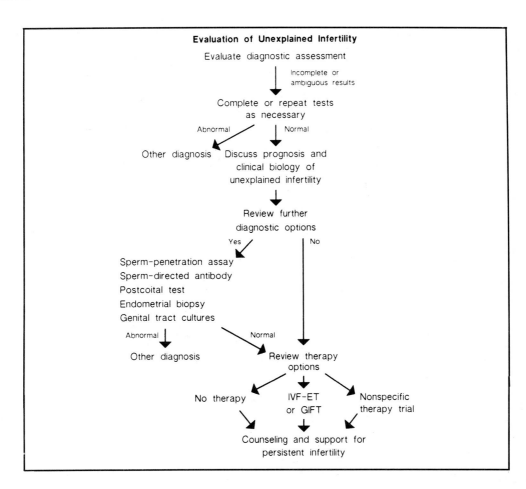

Evaluation of Unexplained Infertility

Evaluate diagnostic assessment

↓ Incomplete or ambiguous results

Complete or repeat tests as necessary

Abnormal ← | → Normal

Other diagnosis ← Discuss prognosis and clinical biology of unexplained infertility

↓

Review further diagnostic options

Yes ↙ | No ↓

Sperm-penetration assay
Sperm-directed antibody
Postcoital test
Endometrial biopsy
Genital tract cultures

Abnormal ↓ | Normal ↘

Other diagnosis → Review therapy options

↓

No therapy / IVF-ET or GIFT / Nonspecific therapy trial

→ Counseling and support for persistent infertility

Although knowledge of the integral requirements for fertilization and the establishment of pregnancy is expanding rapidly, the clinical assessment of infertility is limited in its ability to evaluate gamete preparation, endocrine regulation, genital tract adaptations, and other prerequisites of successful conception. Among the components of the reproductive process that have been clarified to date, numerous possible errors remain inaccessible to clinical assessment; moreover, much remains to be discovered about human reproduction, and some of the gaps in this knowledge may represent as yet undetectable causes of infertility. Thus unexplained infertility stems in part from shortcomings in the ability to evaluate fully the countless prerequisites for conception, both male and female.

Before 1900 virtually all cases of infertility were unexplained because of the lack of clinical tests. Innovations between 1900 and 1940, however, made possible significant improvements in the diagnosis of tubal, seminal, and ovulatory causes. Rubin's[1] report on oxygen insufflation as a test of tubal patency in 1920 made possible the diagnosis of tubal disease without resorting to diagnostic laparotomy, which had been the previous standard method. Within 1 year Rubin predicted a shift to carbon dioxide as the insufflation medium, thus instituting a diagnostic test that survives to the present era in some countries.[2,3]

In 1928 Macomber and Sanders[4] reported pregnancy results among a group of infertile men who were the subjects of the first study in which spermatozoa were methodically counted. The orderly counting of living sperm in the ejaculate and the associated pregnancy results defined a new understanding of male reproduction factors in which not only azoospermia but also oligospermia were found to cause infertility; these authors proposed a normal cutoff at 60 million sperm/mL.

By the late 1930s, understanding of the endometrial and basal temperature responses to progesterone in the luteal phase clarified ovulatory causes of infertility, which had depended previously on a history of amenorrhea.[5,6] Notwithstanding these advances, a relatively large proportion of infertility remained unexplained after the deployment of the state-of-the-art investigation methods in 1960.[7] In a thoughtful discussion, Southam[7] considered whether this represented a "misfortune due to the laws of chance, or a limitation in our knowledge."

Although diagnosis has improved vastly since 1960, clinical experience and the literature confirm that unexplained infertility remains a problem almost a century after the beginning of the modern era.

Numerous publications highlight the dilemma, including articles of clinical opinion, literature reviews, and descriptive studies. Several of the latter report on the results of investigations and provide data on the pregnancy rate outcomes for such couples; this chapter relies mainly on the aggregate clinical experience from these descriptive studies to guide clinical action.

PREVALENCE AND PROGNOSIS OF UNEXPLAINED INFERTILITY

For many reasons, the prevalence of unexplained infertility as reported in the literature is variable; the proportion of couples whose infertility has no apparent cause ranges from 0 to 31%. Table 19–1 shows an apparent reduction in the extent of the condition during the period covered by these reports. This trend may be attributable to concurrent improvements in diagnostic protocols; the observed trend disappears, however, when the two studies with highest and lowest percentages are excluded from the aggregate results.

With respect to prognosis, the outcome of interest for couples with unexplained infertility is pregnancy, an event that may occur months or years after the initial consultation. Although survival analysis is preferable for estimating event rates during follow-

TABLE 19–1. COMPARISON OF REPORTS ON UNEXPLAINED INFERTILITY

Decade of Report	Number of Couples	Unexplained Infertility (%)	Lower/Upper 95% Confidence Limit
1950s	134	13.0	7/19[8]
	658	5.0	3/7[9]
	1437	31.0	29/33[10]
Subtotal	2229		
Mean		22.2	
1960–79	644	22.0	19/25[11]
	500	13.0	10/16[12]
	512	18.0	15/21[13]
Subtotal	1656		
Mean		18.0	
1980s	1020	0.0	[14]
	196	18.0	13/23[15]
	291	7.0	4/10[16]
	400	24.0	20/28[17]
	141	11.0	6/16[18]
	493	26.0	22/30[19]
	1297	13.0	11/15[20]
	708	24.0	21/27[21]
Subtotal	4546		
Mean		13.9	
Total	8431		
Mean		16.9	

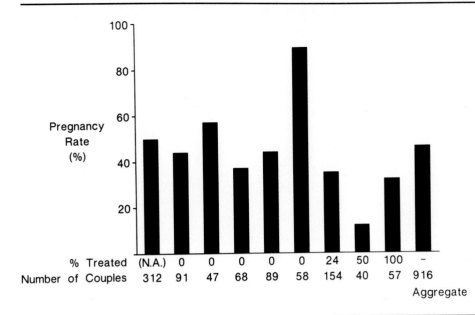

Figure 19–1. Pregnancy rates and treatment rates among reported groups of couples with unexplained infertility.

up, the majority of studies report simple pregnancy rates (pregnancies observed/total number of couples registered) and do not take into account losses to follow-up and varying lengths of observation. Simple pregnancy rates serve as an approximate estimator of the outcome because the denominator includes couples who have been lost to follow-up, among whom the outcome is unknown. The reported rates range from 22 to 57% (Fig. 19–1); in general, they are 5 to 10% lower than cumulative rates, which make use of life tables to account for losses and withdrawals.[30]

The prognosis for couples with unexplained infertility appears to depend upon the chance that some undiscoverable defect may be corrected with the passage of time.[31] In some cases, the defect is severe and the probability of correction approaches zero; such couples remain infertile, thus contributing to the poor prognosis among those with a longer duration of infertility. The effect of this distributional factor on the prognosis is shown in Table 19–2, together with the effect of a history of a previous pregnancy in the partnership (secondary infertility).

TABLE 19–2. EFFECT OF PREGNANCY HISTORY AND DURATION OF INFERTILITY ON THE PROGNOSIS WITH UNEXPLAINED INFERTILITY

Diagnosis: Unexplained Infertility (no. of couples)	Cumulative Pregnancy Rate (%) (95% Confidence Limits)	
	12 Months	36 Months
Primary infertility		
Duration <36 months (131)	40 ± 9	62 ± 14
Duration ≤36 months (89)	13 ± 8	40 ± 19
Secondary infertility (47) (both duration groups)	46 ± 16	65 ± 19

Adapted from Collins et al.[32]

Cumulative pregnancy rates for couples with unexplained infertility 1 year and 3 years after their first visit, even in the group with the worst prognosis, are 13 and 40%, respectively.

PROBLEMS IN DEFINING UNEXPLAINED INFERTILITY

The optimum assessment of the infertile couple depends upon an orderly evaluation of the fertile potential of both partners. An extensive set of diagnostic tests is available to complement the clinical history and physical findings, including assessment of seminal fluid and the properties and functions of sperm cells, ovulatory functions, and genital tract integrity, and detection of associated disorders such as infectious diseases. Additional tests that are required in specific cases to search for the underlying cause of infertility-associated disorders such as azoospermia, amenorrhea, and hyperprolactinemia are discussed in other chapters of this text; such investigations are not applicable among couples with unexplained infertility who have no apparent abnormality.

In practice, numerous factors influence the extent of the diagnostic investigation, such as the duration of infertility, travel time, and the wishes of the couple. Thus it is not surprising that the extent of diagnostic testing that is required before the label of unexplained infertility may be applied is the subject of much debate.[33,34] As a result, our understanding of this condition is hampered by variability in the diagnostic protocols that contribute to the published clinical experience. The tests stipulated for defining unexplained infertility in several reports in the literature are shown in Table 19–3.

TABLE 19–3. DIAGNOSTIC TESTS REQUIRED TO HAVE NORMAL RESULTS IN REPORTED STUDIES OF UNEXPLAINED INFERTILITY

Semen Analysis	Ovulation Confirmation*	Hysterosalpingogram	Laparoscopy	Postcoital Test	Sperm Antibody
Yes	EB	Yes	Yes	Yes	No[23]
Yes	BBT	Yes	No	Yes	No[26]
Yes	NA	Yes	No	No	Yes[29]
Yes	BBT	Yes	No	No	No[22]
Yes	P4	Yes	Yes	Yes	No[28]
Yes	EB	Yes	No	No	No[7]
Yes	P4	No	Yes	No	No[24]
Yes	EB	Yes	Yes	Yes	No[27]
Yes	P4	Yes	Yes	Yes	No[35]
Yes	P4	Yes	Yes	Yes	No[36]

*EB = endometrial biopsy; BBT = basal body temperature shift; P4 = midluteal progesterone concentration; NA = not available.

Laparoscopy was not a uniform requirement, even in recent publications, provided that tubal patency had been evaluated by hysterosalpingography. Also, postcoital tests and the evaluation of sperm-directed antibody were not included in some of these investigations; decision making on whether to include these and other procedures in clinical protocols is discussed below.

An additional problem lies in the inconsistency of clinical findings: some apparent causes of infertility are subject to change over a period of time; also, reproductive defects may have different potency in a given partnership. As a result, an individual clinician's previous experience is likely to influence the meaning of a diagnostic test result, and the debate on protocols will undoubtedly continue. A widely accepted minimum assessment, expressed in current terms, includes evaluation of the ejaculate for its content of normal, progressively motile spermatozoa; a properly timed endometrial biopsy or estimate of the concentration of progesterone in peripheral blood during the middle week of the luteal phase; and evaluation of the female genital tract, including tubal patency, by laparoscopy.[37]

A second problem in defining unexplained infertility lies in the use of different cutoffs for the normal range of semen analysis variables and progesterone concentration. When different standards are applied, two otherwise similar groups of subjects would appear to include disparate percentages of couples with unexplained infertility. Selecting cutoffs for diagnostic tests is a trade-off between better sensitivity (high sperm density cutoff values include more abnormal results in the infertile group) and better specificity (low cutoff values exclude more fertile men from the infertile group). Continuing with this example, values of 5, 10, 20, 40, and 60 million sperm/mL have been suggested as the threshold for subfertile sperm density.[38–42] Different criteria also exist for motility and morphology of sperm.[43–46] The number of different standards is due in part to the lack of an absolute association between semen analysis results and pregnancy rates; thus there is an overlap in results recorded among fertile and infertile groups.[47]

As noted above, when different cutoff values are chosen, the sensitivity and specificity of a diagnostic test mutually fluctuate; plotting the sensitivity and specificity throughout the range of possible cutoffs creates a receiver-operating characteristics (ROC) curve that can be used to access the predictive value of the test.[48] The ROC curves for semen analysis variables reveal that, with respect to the prediction of pregnancy, there is little to choose among the various cutoffs proposed in the literature.[49] Thus selection of a specific cutoff value by consensus would have a minimal effect on the clinical interpretation of the test, and could lead to wider agreement with respect to the definition of unexplained infertility.

A third problem among many that bedevil the definition of unexplained infertility is the extent of reproductive pathology that is undetectable by even the most comprehensive assessment available. In the male, for example, no combination of available tests can provide a complete profile of sperms' fertilizing ability.[50] Such a profile would incorporate the ability to penetrate cervical mucus, undergo capacitation, and negotiate the uterotubal junction. The ability of sperm to undergo the acrosome reaction, penetrate the zona pellucida, and attach to the oocyte plasma membrane can be assessed only in part by in-vitro penetration and fertilization tests. Thus, although it is possible to enumerate normal, progressively motile sperm in the ejaculate and to characterize further some aspects of sperm function through in-vitro testing, other essential sperm cell properties and functions may elude assessment.[50]

Similar limitations hamper the complete assessment of reproductive potential in the female. Although ovulation can be assumed to occur when there is evidence of progesterone secretion from the corpus luteum, it is not possible on a regular basis to observe ovulation, or to recover an ovum from the female genital tract to confirm the fact.[51] Also, the clinical test of tubal patency, in which contrast medium is passively transmitted through the fallopian tubes, does not assess characteristics of bidirectional tubal motility that could be essential for fertilization and embryo transport.[52] Furthermore, the hormonal assessment of luteal function and the study of endometrial histology may not reveal possible important deficiencies in the vascular, biochemical, and immunologic preparation of the endometrium that is essential for attachment and implantation of the developing embryo.[53–55]

In addition to the difficulties inherent in different protocols, various cutoffs, and the limited scope of the diagnostic assessment, several other problems of definition complicate the understanding of unexplained infertility. For example, different definitions of "normal" are reported for categoric test results such as endometrial biopsy.[56–60] Also, when couples conceive prior to having a test such as a laparoscopy, to what category should they be allocated? The choice here is a trade-off between uncertainty and overselection; excluding such couples increases the certainty of correct diagnosis, but decreases the degree to which the selected sample represents infertile couples in general. It is evident that the orderly study of unexplained infertility will require much discussion leading to a consensus on the arbitrary decisions

that will be needed to refine the definition of this clinical state.

Potential Explanations

Although unexplained infertility may in part represent flaws in diagnostic assessment, other possible explanations have been considered. Several authors have proposed that a proportion of otherwise healthy couples appear to be infertile by chance alone.[7,27,29,31] In any population, excluding totally sterile couples, a small proportion of so-called normal couples with low fecundity will fail to conceive and will appear to be infertile.[31] Because the definition of infertility is arbitrarily set at no conception in 1 year of unprotected intercourse, those who do not conceive within that time will be assigned to the apparently infertile group. Provided their diagnostic test results are not falsely abnormal, these couples would be included in the unexplained group after diagnostic assessment.

Although their fecundity is relatively low, such couples should have an excellent long-term prognosis; after 1 year, theoretically over 50% will conceive within the next year.[31] If these couples are more likely to conceive before the infertility becomes long standing, they may be expected to be overrepresented among groups with a shorter duration of infertility. Data from the Canadian Infertility Therapy Evaluation Study are useful in exploring this matter.[61] Recruitment began in this collaborative study of more than 2,000 infertile couples in 1984, and a standardized diagnostic assessment protocol was used. The proportion of unexplained infertility is

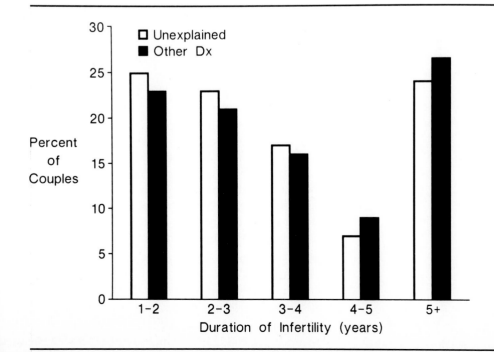

Figure 19–2. Distribution of the duration of infertility among 454 couples with unexplained infertility and 1471 couples with other diagnoses enrolled in the Canadian Infertility Therapy evaluation study.[38]

not significantly associated with the duration of infertility (χ^2, 4 $df = 1.98$; $p = 0.74$) (Fig. 19–2). The small observed excess in the short-duration groups does not suggest that random delays in conception account in a major way for the category of unexplained infertility. It follows that the condition includes a substantial proportion of couples with real but unobservable defects that lead to prolonged infertility.

The search for reproductive defects that might contribute to unexplained infertility has generated extensive clinical research literature. The reports can be broadly classified into two groups: those that explore the boundaries of known infertility factors, and those in which fertility implications arise in the course of investigations not primarily focused on infertility. In the first and larger group, abnormal follicular development, elevation of peritoneal fluid prostanoid concentration, and low endometrial uptake of progesterone have been observed in couples with otherwise unexplained subfertility.[62–65] Significantly high titers of autoantibodies to zona pellucida have been observed also among patients with unexplained infertility, as compared with those who had a known cause of infertility and their healthy counterparts.[66,67] Transitory, relatively mild hyperprolactinemia and euprolactinemic galactorrhea may be associated with otherwise unexplained infertility, leading to impaired fertilization or implantation, while not interfering with follicular maturation, ovulation, or corpus luteum function.[68,69]

The findings of such studies are not always immediately applicable in practice. For example, mycoplasma cells were demonstrated to be capable of attaching to human spermatozoa, leading to gross alterations in sperm cell morphology[70]; the presence of mycoplasma cells does not appear, however, to alter the number of motile sperm or hamper their ability to fertilize eggs.[71] In another example, the ability of spermatozoa to reach the site of fertilization was assessed as a potential cause of otherwise unexplained infertility by laparoscopic sperm recovery from the peritoneal fluid. Among some patients, spermatozoa failed to reach the site of fertilization, an observation that was unrelated to any of the conventional criteria of semen quality.[72] This potentially useful diagnostic test involves time-consuming peritoneal fluid preparation and tedious scanning for sperm cells that limit its clinical usefulness.

Investigations in the immunology of early pregnancy exemplify studies not primarily directed to infertility that may nevertheless be relevant to understanding some cases of unexplained infertility. Both decidual and embryonic factors appear to intervene in the process by which maternal rejection of the implanting blastocyst is prevented.[55,73] The local secretion of factors by the embryo combines with hormonal secretions from the corpus luteum to prepare the endometrium for implantation. Rejection of the implanting embryo by cytotoxic maternal T cells appears to be suppressed by a population of non-T suppressor cells in the decidua.[73] Further research in this area may reveal the existence of recurring deficiencies in the preparation for implantation that could lead to infertility.

Thus unexplained infertility may represent in part random delays in conception among normal couples; also, an array of as yet undiscovered defects in fertilization and implantation exists that could be the subject of continuing research to develop a more comprehensive understanding of infertility. Research designs to investigate the potential causes are burdened by the lack of consensus on the definition, and by the need to show that any observed abnormality, if it is to explain infertility, must be recurring or continuous. Meticulous designs with control group observations are needed to distinguish between random events and aberrations that may be important in the origin of infertility.

MAKING DECISIONS ON DIAGNOSTIC TESTS

Couples with unexplained infertility are under constant pressure to reexplore the problem. Other infertile couples, well-meaning relatives, and the media only too freely offer ideas for new tests and treatment. Should tests with previously normal results be repeated? Will new tests lead to conception? The best available answers to these questions lie in the ability of diagnostic tests to predict conception.

In clinical decision making, the value of tests lies in their ability to predict a specific outcome[74]; the diagnostic process for infertility specifically evaluates the probability of conception by searching for disorders that are known to be associated with impaired fertility. Usually the discovery of such disorders is followed by treatment, which, if successful, masks the prediction. For unexplained infertility, however, no specific treatment is known, and test results have a more direct relationship to outcome. The existence of different criteria for the assessment of infertility is thought-provoking, and the process is complicated further because couples with long-standing unexplained infertility may expect to participate in the decisions. A reasonable standard for guidance in deciding on further testing is the effect of a specific assessment on the probability of pregnancy.

Which Additional Tests Should be Performed?

Beyond the minimum assessment of semen analysis, confirmation of luteinization, and laparoscopy with its attendant procedures, what further diagnostic tests are reasonable? From the numerous ones available, which choice or choices will be useful for the individual couple? An approach that may help to answer these questions is discussed in this section with three diagnostic tests as examples: the postcoital test, a well-defined, traditional assessment; the sperm-directed antibody (SDA), another traditional test for which new methods are available; and the human sperm-hamster oocyte-penetration test (SPA), a more recent evaluation of certain sperm cell functions. The discussion focuses not on the methodology, but on the application of diagnostic principles reflected in the predictive value of a given test result.

Postcoital Test. Few clinicians question that disorders of cervical function may lead to infertility. The cervix appears to serve both a filtering and a storage function, and thus contributes to maintaining a supply of live spermatozoa for a period of 3 to 5 days after deposition.[75] It is debatable, however, whether the postcoital test is capable of detecting disorders in cervical function. Cervical mucus characteristics, when judged at midcycle, seem uniformly good to excellent.[76,77] Thus scoring tends to reveal uniformly high-quality cervical mucus when the test is timed correctly in association with ovulation. Postcoital tests also enumerate the motile sperm in the mucus, and the results appear to correlate with total motile sperm counts in the ejaculate,[78] with impaired penetration of zona-free hamster egg plasma membranes,[79] and with lower conception rates among infertile couples.[78,80-85]

The results of postcoital tests appear to be predictive of pregnancy in several studies in which the 95% confidence intervals for the pregnancy rate associated with normal results are significantly superior (Fig. 19–3). The difference between the preg-

nancy rates with normal or abnormal results seems greater when the best result is selected from a series of tests[80] and when couples with oligospermia and other disorders are excluded.[83] On the other hand, the kappa statistic (which expresses the extent of agreement beyond chance and usually takes a numeric value between 0 and 1) suggests that postcoital test findings are only weakly linked with observed pregnancy rates; also, the results are less persuasive with larger sample sizes, which may be more representative of unselected clinical practices; furthermore, the correlation with sperm count results may account in part for the observed predictions of postcoital test results. As well, the predictive power of the postcoital test is gained at the expense of a high prevalence of abnormal results: in the studies in Figure 19–3, 43 to 60% of results were abnormal by the cutoff criterion of 5 sperm per high-power field. Although studies of unexplained infertility should include postcoital testing in order to improve our understanding of infertility, because of its low discriminatory power, in clinical practice the test may be indicated only as an elective choice for couples who understand its limitations.

Sperm-Directed Antibody Test. Immunity to spermatozoa may cause infertility through several mechanisms, including reduced sperm motility, agglutination, and complete immobilization.[86] Sperm-associated antibodies may be evaluated by conventional assays based on the observation of an antibody function such as agglutination or immobilization of sperm. Techniques that make use of an intermediate marker such as immunobeads enable the identification of specific immunoglobulin types on the sperm

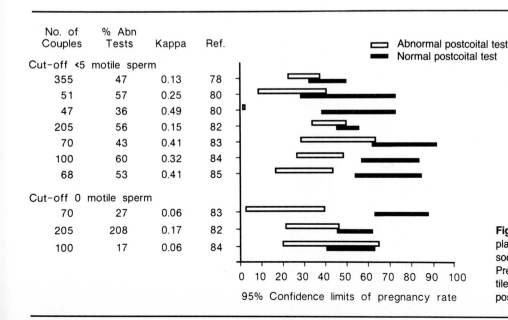

No. of Couples	% Abn Tests	Kappa	Ref.
Cut-off <5 motile sperm			
355	47	0.13	78
51	57	0.25	80
47	36	0.49	80
205	56	0.15	82
70	43	0.41	83
100	60	0.32	84
68	53	0.41	85
Cut-off 0 motile sperm			
70	27	0.06	83
205	208	0.17	82
100	17	0.06	84

☐ Abnormal postcoital test
■ Normal postcoital test

0 10 20 30 40 50 60 70 80 90 100
95% Confidence limits of pregnancy rate

Figure 19–3. The proportion of unexplained infertility is not significantly associated with the duration of infertility. Pregnancy rates among studies of infertile couples with normal and abnormal postcoital tests.

surface, and in seminal plasma, cervical mucus, and either partner's serum.[87] Although a single assay method has not yet been selected as superior to all others, several techniques for identifying immunoglobulins show highly correlated results.[88-92] The prevalence of abnormal antibody titers appears to be higher in both male and female infertile partners than among fertile individuals, and the difference is especially notable among couples with unexplained infertility.[93,94,88]

The degree of correlation among the methods appears to justify grouping together the results of studies that also report the occurrence of pregnancy during follow-up. Follow-up without specific immune therapy reveals that pregnancy rates generally are lower with antibody detected either on the sperm surface or in the male's serum (Fig. 19–4); the agreement between antibody presence and conception failure as reflected in the kappa values is not, however, strong. In studies that focus on antibody assessment among infertile female partners, the results are more variable and the kappa values are generally lower. In five of the eight reports on

antibody presence in the female's serum or cervical mucus, the pregnancy rates were not significantly different for those with normal and abnormal antibody assay results.

It has been suggested that antibodies may be a relative rather than an absolute impediment to fertilization; thus further research is needed to clarify the specific role of sperm-directed antibodies in the origins of infertility.[86,88] Clinical studies of antibody influence continue in many centers, and comprehensive studies of unexplained infertility should include this factor among those tested. In other infertility management settings, unless there is a specific indication for this test, such as obstruction or infection of the male ductal system, its routine use does not appear to offer decisive predictive information.

Sperm-Penetration Assay. Last among these examples of additional diagnostic tests that may be considered for an infertile couple is the SPA, or human sperm-hamster oocyte-penetration test. The hamster is one of the few species in which the oocyte depends entirely on the zona reaction to block polyspermy;

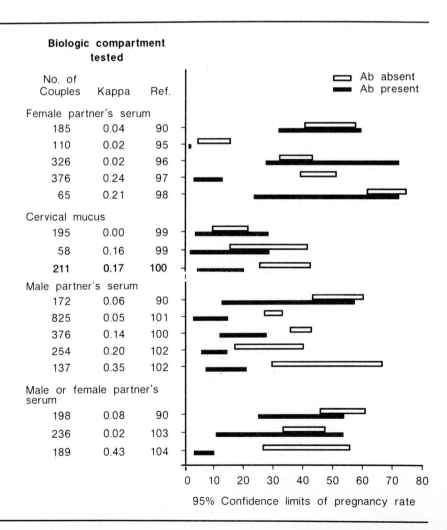

Figure 19–4. Sperm directed antibody (Ab) assay results, agreement statistics, and pregnancy rates among studies of infertile couples.

when the zona is removed, the hamster oocyte is vulnerable to both polyspermy and to cross-species fertilization.[105] The SPA model of fertilization yields information about the ability of sperm to acrosome-react, fuse with plasma membranes, and undergo nuclear decondensation. The test is thus a versatile research tool for evaluating correlations among seminal variables.[105,106] During the 1980s the methodology for this assay has been carefully refined, and the results have been compared with in-vitro fertilization (IVF) of human oocytes.[106,107]

The SPA test has potential as a clinical predictor of IVF, although comparing studies is complicated by the use of different cutoffs for normal results. The association varies from outstanding in some reports to unmeasurable in others.[108,109] Moreover, the pregnancy rates that follow successful IVF do not appear to reflect SPA performance[108,109]; one report included three patients who scored zero on the SPA yet initiated a pregnancy through IVF and embryo transfer.[109]

On the other hand, SPA results seem to correlate with in-vitro pregnancy rates during the follow-up of couples in whom no known female factors cause infertility. Pregnancy rates were lower with an abnormal SPA result (10 to 20%) than with a normal result (40 to 50%).[24,110] This correlation may reflect sperm functions other than the ability to penetrate egg-enveloping structures; also, the correlation with in-vivo conception may be independent of conventional semen values (Table 19–4). Under some conditions, then, the SPA may reflect a combination of sperm survival and fertilizing capacity; only the latter is important in IVF, for which a freshly prepared specimen is needed, while both attributes are required for in-vivo fertilization and pregnancy.[50] Poor performance on a sperm-penetration assay may not be a contraindication to IVF; rather, because the test predicts a lower probability of conception in vivo, an abnormal result is a possible reason for referral to an IVF and embryo transfer (IVF-ET) program.

Although it is not possible to review every diagnostic test for infertility, these examples illustrate the value of certain assays according to the degree to which their results revise the probability of pregnancy. Although the diagnosis of infertility-associated pathology can be made with certainty in some conditions, for couples with unexplained infertility, considerable uncertainty remains about the value and need for specific tests. Focusing on the predictive value may help to reduce the extent of this uncertainty.

Should Test with Previously Normal Results be Repeated?

When faced with persistent unexplained infertility, the possibility of new disease and the desire to ascertain current status are powerful stimulants to repeat tests the results of which previously were reported as normal. The major components of semen analysis (sperm density, progressive motility, and morphology) are subject to considerable observer variability[111] and also to inherent variability within the individual.[112–114] Because of this, during the initial workup it is important to repeat the test as often as necessary to establish a true range. Therefore, provided that the results are within the normal range, it is not clinically useful to repeat the semen analysis unless a new exposure factor arises. If results of the initial workup are unavailable, incomplete, or outdated, a new series of tests is necessary to establish the current range.

No studies report on the findings of a repeat laparoscopy during the otherwise uneventful follow-up of infertility. When searching for an explanation for long-standing infertility, however, an as yet undetectable cause seems far more likely to be the case than a clinically "silent" change in the status of a previously normal pelvis. When laparoscopy has been performed after 2 to 3 years of infertility, and the pelvis has been described reliably as normal, the probability of new pathology after another year or two is likely to be very low. Thus it should be repeated only if doubt exists about earlier findings or there has been a substantial change in the clinical risk of endometriosis, tubal disease, or other infertility-associated pathology.

Clinical biology can render certain types of repeated tests unnecessary. One common question concerns whether or not ovulation is occurring regularly; when the menstrual intervals are 25 to 35 days, there is 95% confidence that ovulation, as documented by luteinization, is occurring.[58,115] Useful also for couples who despair of the frenzied activity that takes place around midcycle is the information available from laboratory studies on the longevity of sperm in the cervix; sperm appear to survive for 3 to 5 days after deposition.[75] Among couples with normal intercourse patterns, lack of sperm availability at the time of ovulation is unlikely to be the case of prolonged unexplained infertility.

TABLE 19–4. TOTAL MOTILE SPERM COUNT, RESULTS OF HUMAN-HAMSTER OOCYTE-PENETRATION TESTS, AND CONCEPTION AMONG 177 INFERTILE COUPLES*

Total Motile Sperm Count Ejaculate	Sperm-Penetration Rates (%)	Conception	Number of Couples	Pregnancy Rate (%)
<5 million	<10	0	12	0
	≥10	1	5	20
≥5 million	<10	4	69	6
	≥10	18	91	20
All count groups	<10	4	81	5
	≥10	19	96	20

*Mean duration of follow-up 10.2±3.1 (SD) months.

It is important to repeat tests when previous results are ambiguous. Biologic variability, recall errors on the part of referring physicians, and occasional slips in the laboratory all contribute to confusing results. The chart for each couple should include copies of operative notes, and actual laboratory reports regardless of where the investigations took place. When the evidence is ambiguous, the couple may be invited to choose between accepting the ambiguity or undergoing confirmatory assessments.

MANAGEMENT OF UNEXPLAINED INFERTILITY

The Role of Treatment

Medical practice is both more successful and more satisfying when rational, effective therapy is available to correct specific defects and lead to a desirable outcome. Couples with unexplained infertility present a special dilemma, because although they have no specific defect, and although they may intellectually appreciate the importance of a rationale for treatment, many feel compelled to take some action. If the published data are representative, a large proportion of these couples continue to be childless (see Fig.19–2); for many, no viable alternative such as adoption exists. Thus it is important to explore the available clinical data to help them choose among the treatment options.

In the absence of a specific cause that could be corrected, any treatment effects in these couples might be expected to be randomly distributed; thus the proportion receiving treatment does not appear to influence observed pregnancy rates (Fig. 19–1). From the subset of couples with unexplained infertility who continue under observation in the Canadian Infertility Therapy Evaluation Study, preliminary data stratified by duration of infertility and treatment are shown in Figure 19–5.[61] In each duration category, approximately 30% of couples received treatment (defined as some form of standard infertility therapy, not including diet, vitamins, and other nonspecific therapy). There are no appreciable differences in pregnancy rates between couples who received treatment and those who did not. This study did not include randomized allocation, however, and the results may have been influenced by various kinds of bias related to treatment decisions.

More specific studies of treatment among couples with unexplained infertility have been reported.[116] Among those with superior designs, three randomized trials of bromocriptine compared with placebo revealed no measurable difference in observed pregnancy rates.[117-119] In a study in which allocation to groups was not randomized, a superior

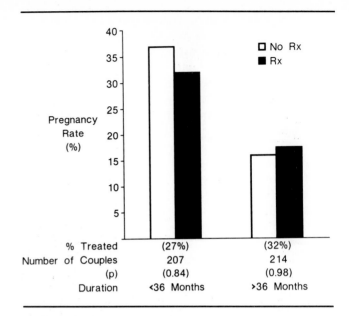

Figure 19–5. Duration of infertility treatment and pregnancy among couples with unexplained infertility enrolled in the Canadian Infertility Evaluation Study.[38]

pregnancy rate was associated with patients receiving bromocriptine therapy (with or without clomiphene) compared with pyridoxine-treated controls, in whom unexplained infertility was associated with expressible galactorrhea.[69] The latter results are promising, as they incorporate follicular and periovulatory administration of bromocriptine during a phase of the cycle when thyrotropin-releasing hormone responses may be exaggerated in some couples.[120] Nevertheless, studies that compare results after patients have selected themselves into specific therapy groups may be subject to unrecognized biases. For example, although the differences were not significant, the pyridoxine-treated subjects in this study were older, had a longer duration of infertility, and had lower pretreatment prolactin levels than the bromocriptine-treated group.[69]

Many reports of therapy rely on the prolonged duration of unexplained infertility as a control. In theory, even after a prolonged duration, some couples may be considered to be normal, and predictable spontaneous rates of cure have been published.[31] This spontaneous cure rate may explain why the extent of treatment-independent pregnancy among couples with unexplained infertility may be as high as 90%.[27,121,122] Spontaneous cure cannot be isolated from treatment-related pregnancy in single-arm studies, nor is the rate of spontaneous cure predictable in any given sample. For example, in one report on human menopausal gonadotropin treatment in women with 2 to 9 years' duration of infertility, 3 pregnancies occurred among 6 women within 1 or 2 treatment cycles.[123] In a second study of several different protocols of gonadotropin administration, there were no conceptions in 50 cycles.[124] Among 11 women with 2 to 4 years' duration of unexplained infertility (who had been treated with clomiphene for up to 13 cycles and with human menopausal gonadotropin for up to 6 cycles), 3 pregnancies were observed after 1 or 2 cycles of treatment with 20 μg of gonadotropin-releasing hormone administered in 90-minute pulses.[125] Evidently, trials are required to evaluate the results of such therapy to increase follicle recruitment in this heterogeneous clinical state. Direct intraperitoneal insemination of approximately 3 million motile washed sperm was associated with 3 continuing pregnancies among 10 couples with unexplained or cervical infertility lasting 2 to 9 years.[126] In part because intraperitoneal instillation may enhance the immunologic response to spermatozoa antigens, a controlled trial is suggested to evaluate the role of this procedure.[126,127]

Because of the potential for harmful as well as beneficial results from empiric treatment, the concept of a therapeutic trial is useful when a couple considers treatment that has unknown value. If by random chance the treatment were to restore normal fecundity, 75% or more of couples would conceive within 6 months and 87% within 9 months,[31] and a longer trial of empiric therapy may be unwarranted. Although the prognosis for unexplained infertility is superior to that in other clinical diagnoses, after 3 years the expected pregnancy rates fall below 50%; thus couples in whom the condition persists are more likely to experience continuing infertility than success.

In-Vitro Techniques

The management outlined above is unsatisfactory because it has no rational basis and a uniform response to any treatment cannot be expected in view of the many possible causes of unexplained infertility. Several types of in-vitro techniques may, however, be considered for these couples. These include inducing ovulation associated with ultrasound timing of intrauterine insemination of prepared spermatozoa, IVF-ET, ovum donation, and gamete intrafallopian transfer (GIFT). After the initial success with IVF, the technique and various modifications were adapted to provide the above list of therapies for couples with unexplained infertility as well as other infertility diagnoses.

Although initially promising,[128] intrauterine insemination techniques have not always been associated with rewarding pregnancy rates among couples with unexplained infertility.[129] They appear to be applicable mainly among couples waiting for IVF-ET programs. The procedure involving transfer of a fertilized ovum recovered from a donor is a special development that has not been widely adopted[130]; IVF-ET and GIFT are more commonly employed.

Lower fertilization rates were initially reported in vitro for couples with unexplained infertility, in comparison with those with bilateral tubal obstruction.[131] In a summary of reports from several centers, however, fertilization rates in unexplained infertility ranged from 55 to 85% of those noted in patients with tubal disease.[132] More recently, the rate was 96% among 25 couples with unexplained infertility undergoing IVF-ET after failed intrauterine insemination.[129] Regardless of fertilization rates, pregnancy rates with IVF-ET appear to be equivalent for unexplained infertility and anatomic factors.[132–134] Reported pregnancy rates for unexplained infertility range from 7 to 25% of cycles in which an embryo was transferred.[132] The GIFT procedure, in which mature oocytes and prepared spermatozoa are deposited in the ampullary portion of one or both fallopian tubes, has been associated with promising early results,[135,136] with pregnancy rates as high as 31% reported.[137]

The spontaneous cure rate of unexplained infertility remains a problem in interpreting pregnancy rates after IVF-ET and GIFT.[133] Treatment-independent pregnancies were reported after unsuccessful IVF-ET among couples with apparent tubal dysfunction and other infertility diagnoses.[138–140] Spontaneous cure among couples with unexplained infertility does not, however, fully explain such results; only 4 of the 18 treatment-independent pregnancies observed in follow-up after failed IVF-ET in 245 couples occurred in the group with unexplained infertility.[140]

Counseling

For many couples with persistent infertility, regardless of their diagnosis, IVF-ET or GIFT is a last resort. The waiting list for successful programs is long, and couples can be enrolled or registered at an early stage in their infertility history. Pregnancy while on the waiting list is not uncommon, but couples who complete such programs without success have a real need for continuing support and counseling.

Although psychologic factors may contribute to the etiology of unexplained infertility, the anxiety and stress observed among these couples appear to be a consequence rather than a cause of the condition.[141] Couples respond in different ways to continuing childlessness, to the procedures used in infertility investigation and treatment, and to the apparent failure of management when childlessness persists.[142,143] It is important to have an understanding of the possible sources of anxiety and stress among all infertile couples; in particular among those with unexplained infertility, it is essential to appreciate the extent to which uncertainty about the diagnosis and prognosis may aggravate their feelings. Such couples frequently change physicians during the course of management; this may reflect dissatisfaction, not with the treatment plan, but with the attitude of the physician or other members of the clinical team. To offset misunderstandings, conventional counseling can be an important service.[144] It is provided in many IVF-ET programs, and many hospital-based infertility clinics have ready access to knowledgeable counseling by social workers and interested psychiatrists. For each couple, the type of support needed can be individualized and an appropriate program found.

After diagnosis and treatment are completed, counseling should recognize serious negative emotional and social effects of infertility, which have been observed 2 years after medical and surgical therapy.[143] In addition to the standard techniques, it may be important at this time to ensure that infertility management, such as recommendations for coital timing, does not interfere with a normal sexual relationship.[145]

Although such specific attention may be important for some couples, virtually all those with persistent infertility require extended discussions with clinical personnel. For these to be effective, it is essential that a detailed discussion of biologic and clinical information about infertility be presented in a straightforward fashion. The prognosis for pregnancy is the chief interest, and so it is prudent to ensure that couples understand as clearly as possible what their prognosis may be, making use of data from the literature where possible. This review leads naturally to questions about the biology of reproduction, and couples should be provided with information that is tailored to their needs and their preexisting knowledge. For those with unexplained infertility in particular, this should include an unvarnished description of the limitations of the diagnostic assessment, and the potential for undiscoverable defects that may be factors leading to infertility.

REFERENCES

1. Rubin IC: The nonoperative determination of patency of fallopian tubes. *JAMA* 75:661, 1920.
2. Rubin IC: Subphrenic pneumoperitoneum: Produced by intrauterine insufflation of oxygen as a test of patency of the fallopian tubes in sterility and in allied gynecological conditions. *Am J Roentgenol* 8:120, 1921.
3. World Health Organization: Comparative trial of tubal insufflation, hysterosalpingography, and laparoscopy with dye hydrotubation for assessment of tubal patency. *Fertil Steril* 46:1101, 1986.
4. Macomber D, Sanders MB: The spermatozoa count: Its value in the diagnosis, prognosis and treatment of sterility. *N Engl J Med* 200:981, 1928.
5. Rubinstein BB: The relation of cyclic changes in human vaginal smears to body temperatures and basal metabolic rate. *Am J Physiol* 119:635, 1937.
6. Rock J, Bartlett M: Biopsy studies of human endometrium: Criteria of dating and information about amenorrhea, menorrhagia and time of ovulation. *JAMA* 108:2022, 1937.
7. Southam AL: What to do with the "normal" infertile couple. *Fertil Steril* 11:543, 1960.

8. Frank R: A clinical study of 240 infertile couples. *Am J Obstet Gynecol* 60:645, 1950.
9. Johansson CJ: Clinical studies on sterile couples with special reference to the diagnosis, etiology and prognosis of infertility. *Acta Obstet Gynecol Scand* 36:1, 1957.
10. Southam AL, Buxton CL: Factors influencing reproductive potential. *Fertil Steril* 8:25, 1957.
11. Newton J, Craig S, Joyce D: The changing pattern of a comprehensive infertility clinic. *J Biosoc Sci* 6:477, 1974.
12. Raymont A, Arronet BH, Arrata WSM: Review of 500 cases of infertility. *Int J Fertil* 14:141, 1969.
13. Dor J, Homburg R, Rabau E: An evaluation of etiologic factors and therapy in 665 infertile couples. *Fertil Steril* 28:718, 1977.
14. Harrison RF: Pregnancy successes in the infertile couples. *Int J Fertil* 25:81, 1980.
15. Serenson SS: Infertility factors. *Acta Obstet Gynecol Scand* 59:513, 1980.
16. Thomas AK, Forrest MS: Infertility: A review of 291 infertile couples over eight years. *Fertil Steril* 34:106, 1980.
17. West CP, Templeton AA, Lees MM: The diagnostic classification and prognosis of 400 infertile couples. *Infertility* 5:127, 1982.
18. Verkauf BS: The incidence and outcome of single-factor, multifactorial, and unexplained infertility. *Am J Obstet Gynecol* 147:175, 1983.
19. Kliger BE: Evaluation, therapy, and outcome in 493 infertile couples. *Fertil Steril* 41:40, 1984.
20. Collins JA, Rand CA, Wilson EH, Wrixon W: The better prognosis in secondary infertility is associated with a higher proportion of ovulation disorders. *Fertil Steril* 45:611, 1986.
21. Hull MGR, Glazener CMA, Kelly NJ, et al: Population study of causes, treatment and outcome of infertility. *Br Med J* 291:1693, 1985.
22. Lenton EA, Weston GA, Cooke ID: Long-term follow-up of the apparently normal couples with a complaint of infertility. *Fertil Steril* 28:913, 1977.
23. Rousseau S, Lord J, Lepage Y, Van Campenhout J: The expectancy of pregnancy for "normal" infertile couples. *Fertil Steril* 40:768, 1983.
24. Aitken RJ, Best FSM, Warner P, Templeton A: A prospective study of the relationship between semen quality and fertility in cases of unexplained infertility. *J Androl* 5:297, 1984.
25. Collins JA, Gwatkin RB, Bissessar HK, et al: The predictive value of semen analysis and sperm function assays. Presented at the annual meeting of the Canadian Fertility and Andrology Society, Val David, Quebec, Oct 1987.
26. Barnea ER, Holford TR, McInnes DRA: Long-term prognosis of infertile couples with normal basic investigations: life-table analysis. *Obstet Gynecol* 66:24, 1985.
27. Collins JA, Wrixon W, Janes LB, Wilson EH: Treatment-independent pregnancy among infertile couples. *N Engl J Med* 309:1201, 1983.
28. van Dijk JG, Frolich M, Brand EC, van Hall EV: The "treatment" of unexplained infertility with danazol. *Fertil Steril* 31:481, 1979.
29. Koninckx PR, Muyldermans M, Brosens IA: Unexplained infertility: "Leuven" considerations. *Eur J Obstet Gynecol Reprod Biol* 18:403, 1984.
30. Lamb EJ, Cruz AL: Data collection and analysis in an infertility practice. *Fertil Steril* 23:310, 1972.
31. Leridon H, Spira A: Problems in measuring the effectiveness of infertility therapy. *Fertil Steril* 41:580, 1984.
32. Collins JA, So Y, Wilson EH, Wrixon W, Casper RF: Clinical factors affecting pregnancy rates among infertile couples. *Can Med Assoc J* 130:269, 1984.
33. Templeton AA, Penney GC: The incidence, characteristics, and prognosis of patients whose infertility is unexplained. *Fertil Steril* 37:175, 1982.
34. Blackwell RE: Patients with unexplained infertility. *Fertil Steril* 38:261, 1982.
35. Haxton MJ, Black WP: The aetiology of infertility in 1162 investigated couples. *Clin Exp Obstet Gynecol* 14:75, 1987.
36. Trimbos-Kemper GCM, Trimbos JB, van Hall EV: Pregnancy rates after laparoscopy for infertility. *Eur J Obstet Gynecol Reprod Biol* 18:127, 1984.
37. Taylor PJ, Gomel V: Endoscopy in the infertile patient, in Gomel V, Taylor PJ, Yuzpe AA, Rioux JE (eds): *Laparoscopy and Hysteroscopy in Gynecologic Practice*. Chicago, Year Book, 1986, pp 75–94.
38. Bostofte E, Serup J, Rebbe H: Relation between sperm count and semen volume and pregnancies obtained during a twenty-year follow-up. *Int J Androl* 5:167, 1982.
39. Zuckerman Z, Rodriguez-Rigau LJ, Smith KD, Steinberger E: Frequency distribution of sperm counts in fertile and infertile males. *Fertil Steril* 28:1310, 1977.

40. MacLeod J, Gold RZ: The male factor in fertility and infertility. II. Spermatozoon counts in 1000 men of known fertility and in 1000 cases of infertile marriage. *J Urol* 66:436, 1951.

41. Aafjes JH, Van der Vijver JCM, Burgman FW, Schenck PE: Double-blind crossover treatment with mesterolone and placebo of subfertile oligospermic men. Value of testicular biopsy. *Andrologia* 15(T):531, 1983.

42. Smith D, Rodriguez-Rigau LJ, Steinberger E: Relation between indices of semen analysis and pregnancy rate in infertile couples. *Fertil Steril* 28:1314, 1977.

43. Amelar RD, Dubin L, Schoenfeld C: Sperm motility. *Fertil Steril* 34:197, 1980.

44. Bostofte E, Serup J, Rebbe H: Relation between number of immobile spermatozoa and pregnancies obtained during a twenty-year follow-up period. *Andrologia* 16:136, 1984.

45. Fredriccson B, Sennerstam R: Morphology of live seminal and postcoital cervical spermatozoa and its bearing on human fertility. *Acta Obstet Gynecol Scand* 63:329, 1984.

46. Bostofte E, Serup J, Rebbe H: The clinical value of morphology rating of spermatozoa. *Int J Fertil* 30:31, 1985.

47. Hargreave TB, Elton RA: Fecundability rates from an infertile male population. *Br J Urol* 31:71, 1981.

48. Hanley JA, McNeil BJ: The meaning and use of the area under the ROC curve. *Radiology* 143:29, 1982.

49. Peng HQ, Collins JA, Wilson EH, Wrixon W: Receiver-operating characteristics curves for semen analysis variables: Methods for evaluating diagnostic tests for male gamete function. *Gamete Res* 17:229, 1987.

50. Aitken RJ, Clarkson JS, Irvine DS, Richardson DW: Contribution of defective sperm function to infertility. *Acta Eur Fertil* 16:273, 1985.

51. Jeffcoate SL: Use of rapid hormone assays in the prediction of ovulation, in Jeffcoate SL (ed): *Ovulation: Methods for Its Prediction and Detection.* New York, Wiley, 1983, pp 67–83.

52. Jansen RPS: Endocrine response in the Fallopian tube. *Endocr Rev* 5:525, 1984.

53. Kennedy TG: Prostaglandins and uterine sensitization for the decidual cell reaction. *Ann NY Acad Sci* 476:43, 1986.

54. Moulton BC, Koenig BB: Biochemical responses of the luminal epithelium and uterine sensitization. *Ann NY Acad Sci* 476:95, 1986.

55. Lala PK, Kearns M, Parkar RS, Scodras J, Johnson S: Immunological role of the cellular constituents of the decidua in the maintenance of semiallogeneic pregnancy. *Ann NY Acad Sci* 476:183, 1986.

56. Noyes RW: The underdeveloped secretory endometrium. *Am J Obstet Gynecol* 77:929, 1959.

57. Moszkowski E, Woodruff SD, Jones GES: The inadequate luteal phase. *Am J Obstet Gynecol* 83:363, 1972.

58. Rosefeld DL, Garcia CR: A comparison of endometrial histology with simultaneous plasma progesterone determinations in infertile women. *Fertil Steril* 27:1256, 1976.

59. Daly DC, Walters CA, Soto-Albors CE, Riddick DH: Endometrial biopsy during treatment of luteal phase defects is predictive of outcome. *Fertil Steril* 40:305, 1983.

60. Balasch J, Vanrell JA, Marquez M, Gonzalez-Merlo J: Endometrial biopsy inadvertently taken in the cycle of conception. *Int J Gynecol Obstet* 44:699, 1984.

61. Collins JA and the coinvestigators of the Canadian Infertility Therapy Evaluation Study: A comparison of pregnancy rates among treated and untreated infertile couples. Presented at 43rd annual meeting of the Society of Obstetricians and Gynecologists of Canada, Ottawa, June 1987.

62. Lewinthal D, Furman A, Blankstein J, et al: Subtle abnormalities in follicular development and hormonal profile in women with unexplained infertility. *Fertil Steril* 46:833, 1986.

63. Ylikorkala O, Koskimies A, Laatkainen T, Tenhunen A, Viinikka L: Peritoneal fluid prostaglandins in endometriosis, tubal disorders and unexplained infertility. *Obstet Gynecol* 63:616, 1984.

64. Drake TS, O'Brien WF, Ramwell PW: Peritoneal fluid prostanoids in unexplained infertility. *Am J Obstet Gynecol* 147:63, 1983.

65. Maynard PV, Baker PN, Symonds EM, et al: Nuclear progesterone uptake by endometrial tissue in cases of subfertility. *Lancet* 2:310, 1983.

66. Bousquet D, St-Jacques S, Roberts KD, Chapdelaine A, Bleau G: Zona pellucida antibodies in a group of women with idiopathic infertility. *Am J Reprod Immunol* 2:73, 1982.

67. Singh J, Mhaskar AM: Enzyme-linked immunosorbent determination of autoantibodies to zona pellucida as a possible cause of infertility in women. *J Immunol Methods* 79:133, 1985.

68. Ben-David M, Schenker JG: Transient hyperprolactinemia: A correctable cause of idiopathic female infertility. *J Clin Endocrinol Metab* 57:442, 1983.

69. DeVane GW, Guzick DS: Bromocriptine therapy in normoprolactinemic women with unexplained infertility and galactorrhea. *Fertil Steril* 46:1026, 1986.

70. Busolo F, Zanchetta R, Bertoloni G: Mycoplasmic localization patterns on spermatozoa for infertile men. *Fertil Steril* 41:412, 1984.

71. Hill AC, Tucker MJ, Whittingham DG, Craft I: Mycoplasmas and in vitro fertilization. *Fertil Steril* 47:652, 1987.

72. Templeton A, Aitken J, Mortimer D, Best F: Sperm function in patients with unexplained infertility. *Br J Obstet Gynaecol* 89:550, 1982.

73. Daya S, Clark DA, Devlin C, Jarrell J: Preliminary characterization of two types of suppressor cells in the human uterus. *Fertil Steril* 44:781, 1985.

74. Schecter MT, Sheps SB: Diagnostic testing revisited: Pathways through uncertainty. *Can Med Assoc J* 132:755, 1985.

75. Gould JE, Overstreet JW, Hanson FW: Assessment of human sperm function after recovery from the female reproductive tract. *Biol Reprod* 31:888, 1984.

76. Pandya IJ, Mortimer D, Sawers RS: A standard approach for evaluating the penetration of human spermatozoa into cervical mucus in vitro. *Fertil Steril* 45:357, 1986.

77. Schats R, Aitken RJ, Templeton AA, et al: The role of cervical mucus–semen interaction in infertility of unknown aetiology. *Br J Obstet Gynaecol* 91:371, 1984.

78. Collins JA, Ying S, Wilson EH, Wrixon W, Casper RF: The postcoital test as a predictor of pregnancy among 355 infertile couples. *Fertil Steril* 41:703, 1984.

79. Soules MR, Moore DE, Spadoni LR, et al: The relationship between the postcoital test and the sperm penetration assay. *Fertil Steril* 38:384, 1982.

80. Hamilton CJCM, Evers JLH, deHaan J: Ultrasound increases the prognostic value of the postcoital test. *Gynecol Obstet Invest* 21:80, 1986.

81. Harrison RF: The diagnostic and therapeutic potential of the postcoital test. *Fertil Steril* 31:71, 1981.

82. Jette NR, Glass RH: Prognostic value of the postcoital test. *Fertil Steril* 23:29, 1972.

83. Hull MGR, Savage PE, Bromham DR: Prognostic value of the postcoital test: prospective study based on time-specific conception rates. *Br J Obstet Gynaecol* 89:299, 1982.

84. Samberg I, Martin-Du-Pan R, Bourrit B: The value of the postcoital test according to etiology and outcome of infertility. *Acta Eur Fertil* 16:147, 1985.

85. Santomauro AG, Sciarra JJ, Varma AO: Clinical investigation of the role of semen analysis and postcoital tests in the evaluation of male infertility. *Fertil Steril* 23:245, 1972.

86. Bronson R, Cooper G, Rosenfeld D: Sperm antibodies: Their role in infertility. *Fertil Steril* 42:171, 1984.

87. Haas GG: Clarifying antibody-mediated infertility. *Am J Reprod Immunol Microbiol* 7:148, 1985.

88. Hjort T, Johnson PM, Mori T: An overview of the WHO international multi-centre study on antibodies to reproductive tract antigens in clinically defined sera. *J Reprod Immunol* 8:359, 1985.

89. Meinertz H, Hjort T: Detection of autoimmunity to sperm: Mixed antiglobulin reaction (MAR) test or sperm agglutination? A study of 537 men from infertile couples. *Fertil Steril* 46:86, 1986.

90. Adeghe JHA, Cohen J, Sawers SR: Relationship between local and systemic autoantibodies to sperm, and evaluation of immunobead test for sperm surface antibodies. *Acta Eur Fertil* 17:99, 1986.

91. Francavilla F, Catignani P, Romano R, et al: Immunological screening of a male population with infertility marriages. *Andrologia* 16:578, 1984.

92. Jennings MG, McGowan MP, Baker HWG: Immunoglobulins on human sperm: Validation of a screening test for sperm autoimmunity. *Clin Reprod Fertil* 3:335, 1985.

93. Clarke GN, Elliott PJ, Smaila C: Detection of sperm antibodies in sperm using the immunobead test: A survey of 813 consecutive patients. *Am J Reprod Immunol* 7:118, 1985.

94. Hargreave TB: Incidence of serum agglutinating and immobilizing sperm antibodies in infertile couples. *Int J Fertil* 17:90, 1982.

95. Blumenfeld Z, Gershon H, Makler A, Stoler J, Brandes JM: Detection of antisperm antibodies: A cytotoxicity immobilization test. *Int J Fertil* 31:207, 1986.

96. Ingerslev HJ, Ingerslev M: Clinical findings in infertile women with circulating antibodies against spermatozoa. *Fertil Steril* 33:514, 1980.

97. Portuondo JA, Echanojaurigui AD, Irala JP, Calonge J: Triple evaluation of tubal patency. *Int J Fertil* 25:307, 1980.

98. Rumke P, Renckens CNM, Bezemer PD, van Amstel N: Prognosis of fertility in women with unexplained infertility and sperm agglutinins in the sperm. *Fertil Steril* 42:561, 1984.

99. Chen C, Jones WR: Application of a sperm microimmobilization test to cervical mucus in the investigation of immunologic infertility. *Fertil Steril* 35:542, 1981.

100. Menge AC, Medley NE, Mangione CM, Deitrich JW: The incidence and influence of antisperm antibodies in infertile human couples on sperm–cervical mucus interactions and subsequent fertility. *Fertil Steril* 38:439, 1982.

101. Baker HWG, Clarke GN, Hudson B, et al: Treatment of sperm autoimmunity in men. *Clin Reprod Fertil* 2:55, 1983.

102. Rumke PH, van Amstel N, Messer EN, Bezemer PD: Prognosis of fertility of men with sperm agglutinins in the serum. *Fertil Steril* 25:393, 1974.

103. Hanafiah MJ, Epstein JA, Sobrero AJ: Sperm-agglutinating antibodies in 236 infertile couples. *Fertil Steril* 23:493, 1972.

104. Mathur S, Williamson HO, Baker ME, et al: Sperm motility on postcoital testing correlates with male autoimmunity to sperm. *Fertil Steril* 41:81, 1984.

105. Yanagimachi R, Yanagimachi H, Rogers BJ: The use of zona-free animal ova as a test system for the assessment of the fertilizing capacity of human spermatozoa. *Biol Reprod* 15:471, 1976.

106. Rogers J: The sperm penetration assay: Its usefulness reevaluated. *Fertil Steril* 43:821, 1985.

107. Aitken RJ: The zona-free hamster egg penetration test, in Hargreave TB (ed): *Male Infertility*. New York, Springer-Verlag, 1983, p 75.

108. Margalioth EJ, Navot D, Laufer N, et al: Correlation between the zona-free hamster egg sperm penetration assay and human in vitro fertilization. *Fertil Steril* 45:665, 1986.

109. Kuzan FB, Dixon LL, Muller CH, Soules MR, Zarutskie PW: Human sperm penetration assay as an indicator of sperm function in human vitro fertilization. *Fertil Steril* 48:282, 1987.

110. Sutherland PD, Matson PL, Moore HDM, et al: Clinical evaluation of the heterologous oocyte penetration (HOP) test. *Br J Urol* 57:233, 1985.

111. Jequier AM, Ukombe EB: Errors inherent in the performance of a routine semen analysis. *Br J Urol* 55:434, 1983.

112. Baker HWG, Burger HG, de Kretser DM, et al: Factors affecting the variability of semen analysis results in infertile men. *Int J Androl* 4:609, 1981.

113. Sherins RJ, Brightwell D, Sternthal PM: Longitudinal analysis of semen of fertile and infertile men, in Troen P, Nankin HR (eds): *The Testis in Normal and Infertile Men*. New York, Raven, 1977, p 473.

114. Tjoa WS, Smolensky MH, Hsi BP, et al: Circannual rhythm in human sperm count revealed by serially independent sampling. *Fertil Steril* 38:454, 1982.

115. Orrell KGS, Wrixon W, Irwin AC: The clinical prediction of ovulation. *Nova Scotia Med Bull* 59:119, 1980.

116. Pepperell RJ, McBain JC: Unexplained infertility: A review. *Br J Obstet Gynaecol* 92:569, 1985.

117. Wright CS, Steele SJ, Jacobs HS: Value of bromocriptine in unexplained primary infertility: A double-blind controlled trial. *Br Med J* 1:1037, 1979.

118. Harrison RF, O'Moore RR, McSweeney J: Idiopathic infertility: A trial of bromocriptine versue placebo. *J Irish Med Assoc* 72:479, 1979.

119. McBain JC, Pepperell RJ: Use of bromocriptine in unexplained infertility. *Clin Reprod Fertil* 1:145, 1982.

120. Archer DF: Prolactin response to thyrotropin-releasing hormone in women with infertility and/or randomly elevated serum prolactin levels. *Fertil Steril* 47:559, 1987.

121. Bernstein D, Levin S, Amsterdam E, Insler V: Is conception in infertile couples treatment related? A survey of 309 pregnancies. *Int J Fertil* 24:65, 1979.

122. Grant A: The spontaneous cure rate of various infertility factors or post hoc and propter hoc. *Aust NZ J Obstet Gynaecol* 9:224, 1969.

123. Wang CF, Gemzell C: Pregnancy following treatment with human gonadotrophins in primary unexplained infertility. *Acta Obstet Gynecol Scan* 58:141, 1979.

124. Lenton EA, Harper R, Smith SK, Khatchikian MA, Corda A: Administration of FSH to regularly cycling women. Presented at the annual conference of the Society for the Study of Fertility, Reading, England, July 11–13, 1984.

125. Bohnet HG: Unexplained infertility and its treatment with intermittent GnRH application. *J Steroid Bichem* 23:863, 1985.

126. Forrler A, Dellenbach P, Nisand I, et al: Direct intraperitoneal insemination in unexplained and cervical infertility. *Lancet* 1:916, 1986.

127. Studd J, Lim-Howe D, Dooley M, Savvas M: Direct intraperitoneal insemination. *Lancet* 1:326, 1987.

128. Sher G, Knutzen VK, Stratton CJ, Montokhaol MM, Allenson SG: In vitro sperm capacitation and transcervical intrauterine insemination for the treatment of refractory infertility: Phase I. *Fertil Steril* 41:260, 1984.

129. Hewitt J, Cohen J, Krishnaswamy V, et al: Treatment of idiopathic infertility, cervical mucus hostility, and male infertility: Artificial insemination with husband's semen or in vitro fertilization? *Fertil Steril* 44:350, 1985.

130. Buster JE, Bustillo M, Thorneycroft IH, et al: Non-surgical transfer of in vivo fertilized donated ova to five infertile women: Report of two pregnancies. Lancet 1:816, 1983.

131. Mahadevan MM, Trounson AO, Leeton JF: The relationship of tubal blockage, infertility of unknown cause, suspected male infertility, and endometriosis to success of in vitro fertilization and embryo transfer. *Fertil Steril* 40:755, 1983.

132. Navot D, Schenker JG: The role of in vitro fertilization in unexplained and immunological infertility. *Congr Gynecol Obstet* 14:160, 1985.

133. Leeton J, Mahadevan M, Trounson A, Wood C: Unexplained infertility and the possibilities of management with in vitro fertilization and embryo transfer. *Aust NZ J Obstet Gynaecol* 23:131, 1984.

134. Fishel SB, Edwards RG: Essentials of fertilization, in Edwards RG, Purdy JM (eds): *Human Conception in Vitro*. London, Academic Press, 1982, pp 157–179.

135. Guastella G, Comparetto G, Gullo D, et al: Gamete intra-fallopian transfer (GIFT): A new technique for the treatment of unexplained infertility. *Acta Eur Fertil* 16:311, 1985.

136. Asch RH, Balmaceda JP, Ellsworth LR, Wong PC: Preliminary experiences with gamete intrafallopian transfer (GIFT). *Fertil Steril* 45:366, 1986.

137. Asch RH, Balmaceda JP, Ellsworth LR, et al: Gamete intrafallopian transfer (GIFT). Experiences with an individualized induction of follicular development regime and mini-laparotomy. Presented at the 33rd annual meeting of the Society for Gynecologic Investigation, Toronto, March 19–22, 1986.

138. Jarrell J, Gwatkin R, Lumsden B, et al: An in vitro fertilization and embryo transfer pilot study: Treatment-dependent and treatment-independent pregnancies. *Am J Obstet Gynecol* 154:231, 1986.

139. Ben-Rafael Z, Mashiach S, Dor J, Rudak E, Goldman B: Treatment-independent pregnancy after in vitro fertilization and embryo transfer trial. *Fertil Steril* 45:564, 1986.

140. Haney AF, Hughes CL Jr, Whitesides DB, Dodson WC: Treatment-independent, treatment-associated, and pregnancies after additional therapy in a program of in vitro fertilization and embryo transfer. *Fertil Steril* 47:634, 1987.

141. Seibel MM, Taymor ML: Emotional aspects of infertility. *Fertil Steril* 37:137, 1982.

142. Mahlstedt PP: The psychological component of infertility. *Fertil Steril* 43:335, 1985.

143. Lalos A, Lalos O, Jacobsson L, von Schoultz B: The psychological impact of infertility two years after completed surgical treatment. *Acta Obstet Gynecol Scand* 64:599, 1985.

144. Rosenfeld DL, Mitchell E: Treating the emotional aspects of infertility: Counseling services in an infertility clinic. *Am J Obstet Gynecol* 135:177, 1979.

145. Lalos A, Lalos O, Jacobson L, von Schoultz B: Psychological reactions to the medical investigation and surgical treatment of infertility. *Gynecol Obstet Invest* 20:209, 1985.

CHAPTER 20

Recurrent Pregnancy Loss

W. Page Faulk, Carolyn B. Coulam, and John A. McIntyre

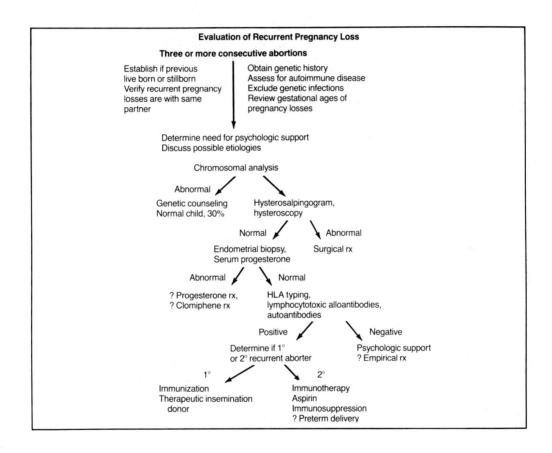

Spontaneous abortion is the expression of products of conception prior to 20 weeks' gestation. Its etiologies have been reported as being chromosomal, infectious, hormonal, and anatomic.[1-4] Therefore, the term *spontaneous abortion* is neither a diagnosis nor a disease, but rather a description of an event that occurs as a result of a disease or diseases. Spontaneous abortion can occur sporadically or recurrently within individuals. The sporadic variety occurs in 1 of 6 pregnancies[5-7] and accounts for 93% of pregnancy failures.[8] The recurrent type has been defined as 3 or more consecutive pregnancy losses and has been described as a syndrome.[9] Its prevalence is approximately 1% of reproducing couples and it accounts for about 7% of recognizable fetal losses.[10,11]

Although sporadic spontaneous abortions are assumed to be due to identifiable karyotypic abnormalities,[12] the prevalence of abnormal chromosome analyses among recurrent abortions is low[1-4] Although the range of prevalence rates for causes of recurrent spontaneous abortion have varied widely in the studies reported,[1-4] our estimates are chromosomal 6%, infectious 0%, hormonal 29%, anatomic 10%, and immunologic 40%.[1] The roles of anatomic defects[1] and hormonal deficiencies[13] have been questioned, and the role of infection seriously doubted,[1] however, leaving the principal causes to be chromosomal abnormalities and immunologic factors.

DIAGNOSIS

A difficulty in making a diagnosis of recurrent spontaneous abortion results from observations that not all pregnancy losses are clinically evident.[5-7,14-16] Eighty-five percent of all reproductive wastage occurs prior to clinical awareness.[17-19] These results suggest that a large proportion of women who experience recurrent pregnancy losses would complain of infertility rather than of miscarriages. Nonetheless, a significant number of women have clinical histories documenting early pregnancy losses.

Recurrent spontaneous abortions are classified as primary or secondary. The term *primary* is applied to women who have had 3 or more consecutive spontaneous abortions and no pregnancies continuing beyond the 20th week of gestation while mating with the same partner.[20] This condition occurs in 1 of 144 pregnancies and accounts for 6% of pregnancy failures.[8] It affects approximately 26,000 women in the United States.

Secondary recurrent spontaneous abortion refers to women who have had 3 spontaneous abortions after a live birth or stillbirth while mating with the same partner.[20] It occurs in 1 of 500 pregnancies and accounts for 1.5% of pregnancy failures.[8] Approximately 7,400 women in the United States can be said to be afflicted with this condition.

The diagnosis of the cause of recurrent spontaneous abortion cannot be made from history alone. The investigation includes chromosome analysis of both partners, hysteroscopy or hysterosalpingography, luteal phase evaluation with measurement of serum progesterone level and endometrial biopsy, and immunologic tests. Less than half of the couples will have a diagnosis after these tests have been performed[1-4] (Tables 20-1 and 20-2). Immunologic

TABLE 20-1. EVALUATION OF COUPLES EXPERIENCING RECURRENT PREGNANCY LOSS

Chromosome Analysis
Hysteroscopy/hysterosalpingogram
Endometrial biopsy, serum progesterone
HLA typing
Lymphocytotoxic antibodies
Phospholipid antibodies
Lupus anticoagulant
Antinuclear antibodies
Mixed lymphocyte culture

TABLE 20-2. PREVALENCE OF DIAGNOSIS IN 225 COUPLES WITH RECURRENT PREGNANCY LOSS

Diagnosis	Prevalence
Genetic causes	6%
Anatomic defects	1%
Hormonal deficiency	1%
Immunologic causes	67%
Unexplained	25%

testing of these couples yields results suggestive of an underlying immunologic problem in about half of them.[1] Such tests include HLA typing, lymphocytotoxic antibodies, mixed lymphocyte culture reactions, and autoantibodies.

HLA Typing

Before differences were discovered between primary and secondary aborters, early studies of HLA types reported increased sharing of the major histocompatibility complex (MHC) antigens of these couples compared with normally reproducing couples.[21,22] These early reports were confirmed[23-28] and denied[29-34] with about equal frequency, until the populations being investigated were subgrouped as primary and secondary aborters.[35-38] This grouping indicated that antigen sharing between partners in the secondary group was not significantly different from that of normal couples,[35,37,38] but those in the primary group differed both from secondary aborting[35,37] and normally fertile couples.[28,36,37]

The significance of shared MHC antigens between partners in recurrent spontaneous abortions is not clear.[39] However, reproduction has been found to be better in couples who share fewer HLA antigens compared with those who share 2 or more.[40] Indeed, indexes such as number of children and interchild intervals seem to vary as a function of the degree of HLA sharing among Hutterite couples who do not practice contraception.[41]

One interpretation of the role of MHC antigens in human reproduction is that it is the HLA markers that are important; their association with trophoblast antigens is important to generate maternal immunologic protection of trophoblast,[42] and compatibility between mother and blastocyst results in failure of such recognition.[20,43] Thus shared HLA may be an index of shared trophoblast antigens.[44] This interpretation has yet to be proved.

Lymphocytic Antibodies

Primary recurrent spontaneous aborters rarely have antibodies to their partners' lymphocytes,[38] yet such antibodies are commonly identified in women who experience secondary abortion.[20,38] These antibodies are broadly reactive with lymphocytes from many different donors,[45] and they are removed by absorption with trophoblast membranes[46] or with tissues that express trophoblast-lymphocyte cross-reactive (TLX) antigens, such as platelets.[47]

Lymphocytotoxic antibodies in sera of secondary aborters are broadly reactive, and they are not anti-HLA.[46] By definition, the antibodies are anti-TLX because they are differentially absorbed from sera with either trophoblast or lymphocytes. Serologic studies with rabbit anti-TLX sera indicate that TLX antigens are restricted to a few serologic groups,[48] possibly only 3.[49] This may explain why pregnancy-associated lymphocytotoxic antibodies were found to have such broad specificities.[50] These authors also found few serologic groups, and interpreted this to mean the antibodies had public specificities for class I antigens of the MHC. Human syncytiotrophoblast at the maternal–fetal interface do not express MHC class I antigens.[46]

It is often diagnostically useful to identify lymphocytotoxic antibodies,[20] but these antibodies are not identified in sera of all women with clinical histories of secondary abortion.[51] If present, they strengthen the clinical diagnosis.[52] In addition, they usually are considered to be a contraindication to the use of leukocyte immunotherapy.[53] There are also practical reasons to expect that patients with lymphocytotoxic antibodies could respond adversely to immunotherapy with leukocytes.

Different tests for lymphocytotoxic antibodies can produce different results on the same sample. For example, complement-fixation assays only detect complement-fixing antibodies. Complement-independent assays, such as antibody-dependent cellular cytotoxicity, are sometimes positive when complement-fixation assays are negative, and vice versa.[20,38] In addition, lymphocytotoxic antibodies in secondary aborters are sometimes present with inhibitors that disallow complement fixation.[54] This problem usually can be overcome if the lymphocytes are washed free of the patient's serum after incubation. This step removes the inhibitors and allows complement fixation to proceed.[55] A similar inhibitor has been identified in a complement-independent assay.[56]

Mixed Lymphocyte Culture Reactions

Mixed lymphocyte cultures (MLC) are used as invitro models of allogeneic recognition reactions. In the laboratory they are performed by using maternal lymphocytes as responder cells and irradiated paternal lymphocytes as stimulator cells. In third-party nonpregnant sera, maternal lymphocytes should respond to stimulation by paternal lymphocytes by proliferating at a comparable rate to that obtained by stimulation with third-party lymphocytes.[57] Lym-

phocytes from couples with primary abortion sometimes have depressed stimulation indexes compared with those from fertile couples.[20,36] Such hyperactivity often cannot be correlated with the HLA-D locus-related antigens that are thought to be responsible for T cell stimulation by B cells, although primary aborting couples frequently share these antigens.[36,37] This defect in allogeneic recognition response is compatible with the idea that primary aborters fail to recognize adequately and mount protective immunologic responses to trophoblast antigens,[42] particularly to trophoblast antigens represented on lymphocytes.[48]

Another finding in MLC reactions that can be useful in evaluation is the absence from the blood of primary aborters of factors that block maternal lymphocyte responses to paternal lymphocytes.[57] Such factors are usually present in the blood of normally reproducing women during pregnancy,[58] and the blockade that they produce is specific for paternal lymphocytes.[59] Blocking factors have been eluted from normal placentas and immunologically shown to be maternal IgG.[60] Present evidence indicates that the blocking factors in maternal blood are also immunoglobulins.[61]

Lymphocytes of secondary aborters produce normal stimulation indexes in MLC reactions with paternal or third-party stimulator cells when the reactions are done in the presence of nonpregnant control sera. Thus, there is no lack of paternal cellular allogeneic recognition, as can be observed with lymphocytes of some primary aborters. When the MLC reaction is done in the presence of sera from pregnant or nonpregnant secondary aborters, however, it is blocked regardless of the source of the stimulator cells.[20] In other words, secondary aborters produce blocking factors, but these factors are present in nonpregnant blood, and they block stimulation by third-party as well as by paternal lymphocytes.[62] This is similar to an experimental observation that rabbit antibodies to a group of human trophoblast antigens are inhibitory for MLC reactions.[63] The rabbit produces its antibody in response to trophoblast immunization; it is thought that secondary aborters produces their antibody for the same reason.

Autoantibodies

The study of autoantibodies is an emerging area in pregnancy research. If antibodies exist in maternal blood as a consequence of allogeneic stimulation during pregnancy, they are not autoantibodies unless they existed before the pregnancy. There has been little agreement on the effect of pregnancy on the production of autoantibodies. In a study of 136 women, none of whom had a known autoimmune disorder, the frequency of autoantibody detection was not significantly different between the pregnant and nonpregnant groups.[64] These results do not support an idea that pregnancy has an effect on the induction or suppression of autoantibody production. Several well-studied pregnancy-associated antibodies obviously are not autoimmune, such as maternal antibodies to fetal erythrocytes or platelets, and allotypic antigens on immunoglobulin heavy and light chains.[65]

Although no clear increase in autoantibodies occurs in normal pregnancy,[64] an increase has been reported in abnormal pregnancies,[65] some of which have been described as phospholipid antibodies.[66] A phospholipid antibody often found in patients with systemic lupus erythematosus has been referred to as lupus anticoagulant.[67] Lupus anticoagulant is also present in spontaneous aborters who do not have systemic lupus erythematosus.[68-71] Pregnant patients with circulating lupus anticoagulant have a syndrome much like that seen in secondary aborters with lymphocytotoxic alloantibodies, inasmuch as they produce cold-reactive lymphocytotoxic antibodies that can be absorbed with HLA-negative trophoblast membranes.[72] These women often abort after the 20th week of gestation.

Anticardiolipin is another phospholipid autoantibody not uncommonly identified in patients who suffer repeated spontaneous abortions.[73,74] Antinuclear antibodies have also been reported in these women.[3] Cross-reactivity between phospholipid membrane antigens and nuclear antigens has been reported.[75,76] Many unanswered questions remain regarding the nature of autoantibodies directed toward phospholipids. For example, there is scant information about whether such antibodies were produced during the pregnancy or if they were present before the patient became pregnant. Nonetheless, the presence of maternal antibodies to phospholipids is of obvious clinical importance in the management of high-risk patients.

PATHOPHYSIOLOGY

The pathophysiology of spontaneous abortions is not known. Immunologic mechanisms may not be involved in sporadic abortions, whereas in many recurrent abortions they seem to be a factor.[20,23,26,36,38,42,46,51,53,57,62,72] The clinical and immunologic differences between primary and secondary aborters suggest that these conditions involve different immunopathologic processes.[20] The evidence in primary aborters is drawn from negative findings, the only positive finding being the occurrence of HLA antigen sharing between the patient and her partner. When the woman has another partner, she often bears normal children.[77] This is in striking contrast with secondary aborters, who continue to abort with other men. In other words, the problem in primary abortion seems to be mate-specific and that in secondary abortion seems to be patient-specific.[77]

This observation suggests that the defect in primary recurrent spontaneous abortion is inability of the women to recognize and mount immunologically protecting responses to a specific paternally transmitted allogeneic trophoblast antigen, perhaps due to compatibility between genes that code for trophoblast antigens.[42] The genetic compatibility argument is frequently supported by pointing out that miscarriage often can be prevented in primary aborters by immunizing them with the partner's[78,79] or third-party[23,80] lymphocytes.

Immunogenetics

Some insight into the immunologic and genetic roles in the pathophysiology of recurrent spontaneous abortion has been obtained from studies of CBA × DBA mice.[81-83] In this combination the $H-2^k$ female mated with the $H-2^d$ male experiences a fetal resorption rate of about 35%. The resorption rate falls to about 8% if the female is immunized with lymphocytes from a third-party donor, but does not significantly change if she is immunized with paternal cells. Continued immunization of multigravid, multiparous mice is associated with a high percentage of late-onset fetal resorptions, regardless of whether the mothers receive paternal or nonpaternal leukocytes.[84] This gives cause to ask if continued immunotherapy could convert a primary to a secondary aborter. Epidemiologic evidence suggests that such conversions can occur in the natural history of primary abortion.[77]

Further studies of the CBA × DBA mouse model have shown that passively transferred sera from third-party immunized females to pregnant mice produces inhibition of fetal resorptions,[85] and a similarly beneficial result has been obtained with the use of antiidiotypic sera.[86] Autoantiidiotypic antibodies to anti-HLA receptors also have been demonstrated in normal human pregnancy.[87] These findings indicate that maternal autoantiidiotypic responses may be central in building an immunologic understanding of normal and abnormal pregnancies.

Immunochemical data from normal human pregnancies have been used to build a model of how maternal autoantiidiotypic responses form a pathophysiologic basis for primary and secondary recurrent spontaneous abortions.[88] This model suggests that if a primary aborter is genetically compatible for trophoblast antigens with her partner, she fails to produce antibody (Ab_1) to trophoblast antigen and thus fails to produce autoantiidiotypic antibody (Ab_2). In the absence of Ab_2, maternal allogeneic rejection reactions are not down-regulated,[89] and innate killer cell response can reject the blastocyst.

Similarly, if a secondary aborter is a poor autoantiidiotype producer and produces Ab_1 but not Ab_2, her cytotoxic Ab_1 could be transported into the placenta and fetus (Fig. 20–1).

Phospholipid Antibodies

Attention has been drawn to a possible role for antibodies to phospholipids in certain recurrent spontaneous abortions.[68–71] Some of these (such as lupus anticoagulants) have the paradoxic effect of prolonging partial thromboplastin times in the laboratory while being clinically associated with thrombotic disease.[90] They interfere with the phospholipid component of the prothrombin–convertase macromolecular complex,[91] and they are thought to block prostacycline release from endothelium and increase thromboxane release from platelets in vivo.[92] The placentas of some women with antibodies to phospholipids and histories of recurrent spontaneous abortions are reported to have infarcts that have been deemed to be etiologically related to the abortion.[69,73,93]

Hemostasis and Fibrinolysis

Pregnancy is the quintessential allogeneic relationship. Surgically created allogeneic relationships, such as renal transplantations, cause the activation of coagulation and fibrinolysis.[94] This is explained in part by reports that products of allogeneically activated lymphocytes and macrophages cause endothelial cells to present tissue factor.[95] This activates factor VII, which activates factor X to begin the assembly of prothrombin convertase.[96] The allogeneic relationship of human pregnancy also initiates clotting and fibrinolysis.[97,98]

Certain clotting factors are abnormal in normal pregnancies,[99,100] and these abnormalities are further exaggerated in abnormal pregnancies.[98–101] Some fibrinolytic enzymes and enzyme inhibitors also undergo significant changes during pregnancy.[102] Immunohistologic studies have shown both coagulation and fibrinolysis products in chorionic villi,[103–105] as well as evidence of accelerated coagulation in abnormal placentas.[106] The pathophysiologic basis of these observations may relate to the finding that antibodies to endothelium as well as products of allogeneic recognition reactions can change the normally thromboresistant endothelium into a thrombogenic surface.[107]

IgE

Heterologous antisera to IgE inhibit allogeneic recognition reactions in vitro,[108] and some patients with preeclamptic toxemia produce IgE autoantibodies to smooth muscle.[109] Eosinophils are associated with IgE and graft rejection, and they collaborate with IgE in the elaboration of type I immunopathologic reactions. Major basic protein (MBP) is a product of eosinophils that mediates these reactions.[110] Of interest, MBP also is found in a subset of cytotrophoblast in human placentas.[111] Longitudinal studies of maternal blood throughout pregnancy show that trophoblasts apparently release their MBP before delivery.[112,113] This raises the intriguing possibility that IgE-mediated MBP could be involved in the pathophysiology of spontaneous abortions.

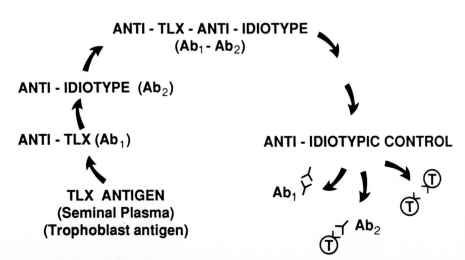

CONTROL CIRCUIT IN HUMAN PREGNANCY
(TLX/Anti - TLX/Anti - anti - TLX)

ANTI - TLX - ANTI - IDIOTYPE
(Ab_1 - Ab_2)

ANTI - IDIOTYPE (Ab_2)

ANTI - TLX (Ab_1)

TLX ANTIGEN
(Seminal Plasma)
(Trophoblast antigen)

ANTI - IDIOTYPIC CONTROL

Ab_1

Ab_2

Figure 20–1. Schematic representation of the network hypothesis for normal control of immunologic responses. The first antibody produced (Ab_1) is to inoculated antigen. The second (Ab_2) is usually to an epitope in the hypervariable region of Ab_1. These responses circulate as immune complexes (Ab_1–Ab_2). The Ab_2 binding site is also represented on T cells, which operate to control subsequent cellular responses to antigen. Both humoral and cellular responses are thus controlled through mediations of the network hypothesis.

TREATMENT

Therapy should be directed toward the cause of recurrent pregnancy loss. In addition to the tests mentioned above, phospholipid antibodies, antinuclear antibodies, and lupus anticoagulant or activated partial thromboplastin time should be obtained.

Anatomic Defects

Müllerian duct anomalies have been thought to be causal in recurrent spontaneous abortions. Reports show a marked improvement in fetal salvage rates after metroplasty (Table 20–3). When the outcome in patients undergoing metroplasty was compared with women with the same uterine abnormality and not having surgery, however, the live birth rates were the same (Table 20–4). This study analyzed the reproductive outcome of 140 patients with uterine anomalies.[1] Twenty-one patients underwent metroplasty, and 119 did not. Seventeen of the nonsurgical patients were matched with the surgical patients by age, chief complaint at the time of diagnosis, gravidity, and type of anomaly, and these women served as matched controls. The remaining 102 nonsurgical patients did not have significant clinical problems and served as additional controls.

Follow-up data were available after the diagnosis of uterine anomaly for 20 of the surgical patients, 17 of the nonsurgical matched controls, and 52 of the other controls. The percentages of patients with living children after the diagnosis of uterine anomaly were 71 and 80% for each of the nonsurgical groups, compared with 70% for those who underwent metroplasty. Although fetal salvage rates improved markedly after metroplasty, outcome was similar to that of the controls for whom surgery was deferred.

Observations with the hysteroscope have provided evidence that uterine adhesions represent an effect rather than a cause of multiple pregnancy losses.[114] Just as the efficacy of metroplasty in the treatment of multiple pregnancy loss is being questioned, so too is the role of these anatomic defects as a cause.

Two additional anatomic defects also deserve mention. A small, T-shaped uterus identified by hysterosalpingogram suggests in-utero exposure to diethylstilbestrol. The hypoplastic uterine corpus is associated with recurrent spontaneous abortions and

TABLE 20–3. REPRODUCTIVE PERFORMANCE BEFORE AND AFTER METROPLASTY

Patients	Before	After
Total	21	10
Pregnant	20 (95%)	17 (85%)
With living children	0 (0%)	14 (70%)

TABLE 20–4. OBSTETRIC OUTCOME WITH AND WITHOUT METROPLASTY AFTER THE DIAGNOSIS OF UTERINE ANOMALY WAS MADE

Patients	Surgical	Nonsurgical Matched	Controls Other
Total	20	17	52
Pregnant	17 (85%)	17 (100%)	49 (94%)
With living children	14 (70%)	12 (71%)	42 (80%)

premature labor. No treatment exists for this problem. A history of recurrent second trimester pregnancy losses preceded by painless cervical effacement and dilatation is a typical history of an incompetent cervix. Treatment involves placing a McDonald or Shirodkar cervical cerclage during the second trimester of the subsequent pregnancy.

Hormonal Deficiencies

The role of progesterone deficiency in recurrent spontaneous abortion has been investigated in two areas. The first was an attempt to implicate low pregnanediol levels in pregnancy. Results in women who were treated with exogenous progesterone were no different from those in patients who received placebo.[115,116] The second approach was to diagnose the insufficient effect of progesterone on the endometrium during the luteal phase of the menstrual cycle, and to initiate treatment with exogenous hormones a few days after ovulation. To date, these studies have not been controlled to determine whether correcting the luteal phase defect prior to the missed menstrual period is of value in recurrent spontaneous aborters who are diagnosed as having an inadequate luteal phase.

The existence of luteal phase defects has been a subject of considerable debate. Most of the controversy results from inconsistencies in diagnosis based on an endometrial biopsy. The prevalence of diagnosis of luteal phase defect among couples with recurrent pregnancy loss falls from 32% when the dating of the endometrial biopsy is compared with the onset of the next menstrual period, to 1% when interpretation of the endometrial biopsy is referenced to ovulation documented by ultrasonic examination[117] (Fig. 20–2). These data call into question the existence of luteal phase defect as a significant clinical entity. They furthermore question the role of endometrial biopsies in the evaluation of these patients.[117]

Genetic Causes

The relative frequency of chromosomal abnormalities among spontaneous abortions is shown in Table 20–5. Although almost one half of all spontaneous abortions occurring during the first trimester have an abnormal karyotype, only 6% of recurrent abortions

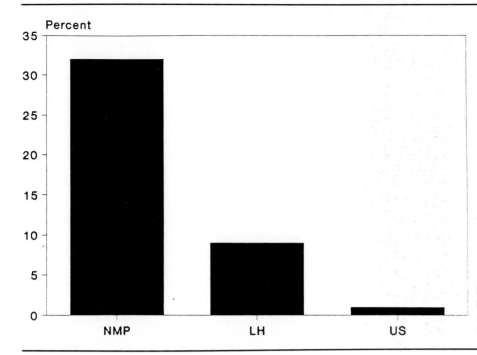

Figure 20–2. Prevalence of diagnosis of luteal phase defect based on onset of next menstrual period (NMP), urinary luteinizing hormone surge (LH), and ultrasound (US).

do. Moreover, the types of chromosomal abnormalilties observed in recurrent abortions are different from those seen in sporadic abortions (Table 20–6). Another difference is that trisomies and monosomy for X chromosome are the most frequent chromosomal abnormalities in all first-trimester abortions, and robertsonian translocations usually are seen in recurrent abortions.[118]

At the time of initial visit, pedigree analysis and chromosomal studies of peripheral blood in both parents will identify known genetic factors. There presently is no available treatment either for a detected parental chromosomal translocation, or for a multifactorial genetic disorder that is operative in the production of abortions, with or without fetal malformations. Therapeutically speaking, the chance of a full-term living child is in the range of 20 to 30% depending on the specific translocation or genetic disorder. Cytogenetic studies of chorionic villi and amniotic fluid, ultrasonography, and α-fetoprotein levels are indicated in future pregnancies for these patients.

Immunologic Causes

Reports in 1981 generated interest in the possibility that immunotherapy might prevent primary recurrent spontaneous abortions.[25,44] Therapy is based on the concept that successful pregnancy requires maternal allogeneic recognition.[42] Such recognition results in the production of blocking antibodies, suppressor cells, and autoantiidiotypic responses.[88] It also results in the release of interleukin-1, which down-regulates endothelial thrombomodulin and up-regulates tissue factor.[119] The presentation of tissue factor activates factor VII, which in turn activates the clotting system by the extrinsic pathway.[96] Such responses to the implanting blastocyst could provide the deposition of fibrin, which secures the implantation site.[97,120] Stimulating allogeneic recognition or modulating response to allogeneic recognition by affecting its immunologic or hematologic amplification systems would be expected to result in successful immunotherapy for those who have an immunologic cause of recurrent pregnancy loss. Several such regimens have been introduced. As with all forms of

TABLE 20–5. CHROMOSOMAL ABNORMALITIES IN SPONTANEOUS ABORTION

Abortion	Total Number	Karyotype Normal	Abnormal
First trimester	131	72 (54%)	59 (46%)
Second trimester	259	221 (85%)	38 (15%)
Recurrent	51	48 (94%)	3 (6%)

TABLE 20–6. TYPES OF CHROMOSOMAL ABNORMALITIES IN SPONTANEOUS ABORTIONS

Sporadic		Recurrent	
Trisomies	46%	Translocations	83%
45, X	31%	Inversions	10%
Triplody	13%		
Other	10%	Other	7%

treatment, the benefits of immunotherapy must be weighed against its risks.

More complications in untreated pregnancies that progress beyond 28 weeks' gestation occur in women with a history of recurrent miscarriage[121] than in women without such a history. In a study of 97 mothers who gave birth to 118 babies, 72 had had a viable first pregnancy before experiencing 3 or more miscarriages. This group had an increase in small-for-gestational-age (SGA) infants, preterm births, and perinatal mortality rates.[121] Others also reported an increase in preterm delivery,[122,123] SGA infants,[124] and congenital anomalies[123] among offspring of secondary aborters.

Specific Therapeutic Approaches

Primary Recurrent Spontaneous Aborters. Women who have been evaluated and found to be negative for known causes of primary recurrent spontaneous abortions, and who lack humoral or cellular evidence of alloantigen recognition for their partners' lymphocytes, have been immunized with leukocytes from either their partners or third-party donors. The intravenous route has been used for both third-party and partner immunizations, and the intradermal route for inoculation with partner leukocytes. All methods of treatment have resulted in a viable birth rate of 70 to 80%.[11,59,78-80,125]

It is perplexing that immunizations with paternal and third-party donor lymphocytes produce similar results, because a rationale for the use of the latter is to stimulate maternal response that would not be forthcoming without immunization, because of genetic incompatibilities between partners. This concept is supported by results of studies with CBA × DBA mice, in which third-party cells protect and paternal cells do not.[81,82] A possible immunogenetic interpretation is that humans are sufficiently outbred to produce cross-reactive autoantiidiotypic responses, but among inbred mice such responses would not be expected to cross-react. In clinical practice there are also examples of primary aborters who fail with immunizations of paternal cells and subsequently succeed with immunizations of third-party lymphocytes,[126] but these findings are probably extensions of the observation that such women often experience a successful pregnancy after changing mates.[11] For this reason, therapeutic insemination with donor sperm may be offered as an empiric form of treatment.

The safety of leukocyte transfusions remains controversial. The association of acquired immunodeficiency syndrome with transfusion of blood products has complicated the use of this therapy. Other considerations include risks of maternal sensitization to leukocyte, erythrocyte, or platelet antigens; perin-atal host-versus-graft disease; and transfusion-related risks including infections. Severe intrauterine growth retardation has been reported in several women after intradermal immunization with paternal leukocytes,[79] but this has not been the experience of other investigators.

Alternative approaches to inducing the necessary maternal immunologic responses are being evaluated. One study uses isolated trophoblast microvillous membranes and another employs seminal plasma. Both of these materials contain trophoblast antigens such as TLX.[127] These approaches have the advantage of lacking intact cells and nuclear material. If they are effective, they have the potential of offering couples suffering from primary recurrent spontaneous abortion a safer option for treatment.

Secondary Recurrent Spontaneous Aborters. Secondary aborters do not receive leukocyte immunizations, but no agreement exists about how these patients should be treated. Twice-daily subcutaneous injections of heparin, 500 U, have been used successfully to prevent secondary abortions.[20] Rationale for this therapy is drawn from laboratory studies of sera from these women before and after solid-phase heparin absorption.[128,129] These investigations revealed significant decreases in lymphocytotoxic antibody activity after heparin absorption.[54,55]

A link between the morbidity of infants of secondary aborters and the tendency of these women to miscarry has been suggested.[130] This arises from the observation that in human placentation, nonvillous trophoblast invades the maternal decidua and infiltrates the spiral arteries, thereby increasing blood flow through these arteries to supply the growing conceptus.[131] This process has been shown to be defective in some women who abort,[130] as well as in those whose pregnancies result in SGA infants.[132] The defective placentation may provide an explanation for the risk of pregnancy failure throughout intrauterine life. This may be relevant for the late pregnancy losses manifest by secondary aborters.

Antiphospholipid antibodies are associated with autoimmune conditions characterized by vascular abnormalities.[67] Individuals in whom these antibodies are observed have adverse pregnancy outcomes, including maternal thrombosis, severe preeclampsia, and early and late fetal death.[68-74] Because the vascular lesions and the range of pregnancy outcomes are similar to those observed in secondary abortions, a role for hemostasis and fibrinolysis in the pathophysiology of recurrent pregnancy loss has been postulated. There are very few published cases of viable infants delivered of untreated women who were clearly documented to have lupus anticoagulant activity prior to or early in pregnancy.

Preterm delivery is one approach to managing

pregnancies complicated by circulatory anticoagulants,[133,134] but this is usually preceded by attempts to decrease antibody titers to phospholipids by immunosuppression. Experience has accumulated with the use of prednisone,[68,69,135,136] and more refractory patients have been given azathioprine or cyclophosphamide.[68] Aspirin is given concomitantly with immunosuppression. This is done to inhibit thromboxane synthetase with the expectation of reducing the threat of small-vessel thrombosis.[137] No studies with aspirin or immunosupressive agents have been controlled, and the results are descriptive. Definition of the efficacy of the various treatments awaits results of randomized clinical trials.

Risks of Immunotherapy. The risks to the fetus in primary aborters is by definition 100% loss. No published data have described pregnancy outcome among women who experienced 3 or more spontaneous abortions and then produced a viable infant without treatment. In one series describing 45 infants born to women after intravenous immunization with third-party leukocytes, 7 preterm births, 3 infants with congenital anomalies, and 6 SGA infants were reported.[138] Whether the increase of preterm births and congenital anomalies observed in this study can be compared with the pregnancy outcomes reported in secondary aborters is questionable, because primary and secondary abortion seem to be distinct clinical entities with different etiologies. Information describing perinatal and pediatric follow-up of children of treated primary aborters shows that complications are fewer than those expected from untreated secondary aborters,[121] but more than those expected from normally reproducing couples.[138] Clearly, controlled investigation with better experimentally and clinically defined objectives is required before objective judgments can be drawn as to optimal therapeutic procedures.

SUMMARY

In the past, a cause of recurrent pregnancy loss could be found in only a few couples. Advances in the understanding of the pathophysiology of this problem have diminished the numbers of unexplained recurrent pregnancy losses, and have limited the known causes to genetic and immunologic etiologies. With the availability of more diagnostic tools, the prevalence of pregnancy loss will continue to decrease, thus allowing treatment to be focused more specifically on the cause.

Although it is beyond the scope of this chapter to discuss in detail the emotional component of recurrent pregnancy loss, it must be remembered that this event takes an enormous emotional toll on couples,

and in some ways is even more devastating and anxiety provoking than failing to conceive at all.[139] It is hoped that specific therapy based on pathogenesis rather than empiricism will lead to successful treatment for this very frustrating clinical problem.

REFERENCES

1. Coulam CB: Unexplained recurrent pregnancy loss: epilogue. *Clin Obstet Gynecol* 29:999, 1986.
2. Tho PT, Byrd JR, McDonough PG: Etiologies and subsequent reproductive performance of 100 couples with recurrent abortion. *Fertil Steril* 32:389, 1979.
3. Harger JH, Archer DF, Marchese SG, Muracca-Clemmens M, Garver KL: Etiology of recurrent pregnancy losses and outcome of subsequent pregnancies. *Obstet Gynecol* 62:574, 1983.
4. Stray-Pedersen B, Stray-Pedersen S: Etiologic factors and subsequent reproductive performance in 195 couples with a prior history of habitual abortion. *Am J Obstet Gynecol* 148:140, 1984.
5. Miller JF, Williamson E, Glue J, et al: Fetal loss after implantation: A prospective study. *Lancet* 2:554, 1980.
6. Edmonds DK, Lindsay KS, Miller JF, Williamson E, Wood PJ: Early embryonic mortality in women. *Fertil Steril* 38:447, 1982.
7. Whittaker PG, Taylor A, Lind T: Unsuspected pregnancy loss in healthy women. *Lancet* 1:1126, 1983.
8. Roman E: Fetal loss rates and their relation to pregnancy order. *J Epidemiol Commun Health* 38:29, 1984.
9. Strobino BR, Kline J, Shrout P, et al: Recurrent spontaneous abortion: Definition of a syndrome, in Porter IH, Hook EB (eds): *Embryonic and Fetal Death*. New York, Academic Press, 1980, p 315.
10. Malpas P: A study of abortion sequences. *Br J Obstet Gynaecol* 45:932, 1938.
11. Stray-Pedersen B, Peterson JO, Omland T: Estimations of the incidences of toxoplasma infections among pregnant women from different areas in Norway. *Scand J Infect Dis* 11: 247, 1979.
12. Hassold T, Chen N, Funkhouser J, et al: A cytogenetic study of 1000 spontaneous abortions. *Ann Hum Genet* 44:151, 1980.
13. Lloyd R, Coulam CB: Recurrent spontaneous abortion: Frequency of diagnosis of luteal phase defect. *Am J Reprod Immunol Microbiol* 16:103, 1988.
14. Block SK: Occult pregnancy. *Obstet Gynecol* 48:365, 1986.
15. Braunstein GD, Karow WG, Gentry WD, Wade ME: Subclinical spontaneous abortion. *Obstet Gynecol* 50(suppl): 41s, 1977.
16. Chartier M, Roger M, Barrat J, Michelon B: Measurement of plasma human chorionic gonadotropin (hCG) and βhCG activities in the late luteal phase: Evidence of the occurrence of spontaneous menstrual abortions in infertile women. *Fertil Steril* 31:134, 1979.
17. French FE, Bierman JM: Probabilities of fetal mortality. *Public Health Rep* 77:835, 1962.
18. Poland BJ, Miller JR, Harris M, Livingston J: Spontaneous abortion. A study of 1961 women and their conceptuses. *Acta Obstet Gynecol Scand* 102(suppl):1, 1981.
19. Leridan H: *Human Fertility: The Basic Components.* Chicago, University of Chicago Press, 1977.
20. McIntyre JA, Faulk WP, Nichols-Johnson VR, Taylor CF: Immunological testing and immunotherapy is recurrent spontaneous abortion. *Obstet Gynecol* 67:169, 1986.
21. Komlos L, Zamir R, Joshua H, Halbrecht I: Common HLA antigens in couples with repeated abortions. *Clin Immunol Immunopathol* 7:330, 1977.
22. Gerencer M, Drazancic A, Kovacic I, Tomaskovic Z, Kastelan A: HLA antigen studies in women with recurrent gestational disorders. *Fertil Steril* 31:401, 1979.
23. Unander AM, Olding LB: Habitual abortion: Parental sharing of HLA antigens, absence of maternal blocking antibody, and suppression of maternal lymphocytes. *Am J Reprod Immunol Microbiol* 4:171, 1983.
24. Schacter B, Muir A, Gyves M, Taskin M: HLA-A,B compatibility in parents of offspring with neural tube defects or couples expressing involuntary fetal wasteage. *Lancet* 1:796, 1979.
25. Beer AE, Quebbeman JF, Ayers JW, Haines RF: Major histocompatibility complex antigens, maternal and paternal immune responses and chronic habitual abortions in humans. *Am J Obstet Gynecol* 141:987, 1981.

26. Gill TE: Immunogenetics of spontaneous abortions in humans. *Transplantation* 35:1, 1983.
27. Thomas ML, Harger JH, Wagener DK, Rabin BS, Gill TJ: HLA sharing the spontaneous abortion in humans. *Am J Obstet Gynecol* 151:1053, 1983.
28. McIntyre JA, Faulk WP: HLA and the generation of diversity in human pregnancy, in Klopper A, Eastbourne W (eds): *Immunology of Human Placental Proteins*. Philadelphia, Saunders, 1982.
29. Jeannet M, Bischof P, Bourrit B, Vuagnat P: Sharing of HLA antigens in fertile, subfertile and infertile couples. *Transplant Proc* 17:903, 1985.
30. Lauritsen JG, Jorgensen K, Kissmeyer-Nielsen F: Significance of HLA and blood-group incompatibility in spontaneous abortion. *Clin Genet* 9:575, 1976.
31. MacQueen JM, Sanfilippo FP: The effect of parental HLA compatibility on the expression of paternal haplotypes in offspring. *Hum Immunol* 11:155, 1984.
32. Rocklin RE, Kitzmiller JL, Garvoy MR: Maternal-fetal relation. II. Further characterization of immunologic blocking factor that develops during pregnancy. *Clin Immunol Immunopathol* 22:305, 1982.
33. Caudle MR, Rote NS, Scott JR, DeWitt C, Barney MF: Histocompatibility in couples with recurrent spontaneous abortion and normal fertility. *Fertil Steril* 39:793, 1983.
34. Mowbray JF, Gibbings CR, Sidgwick AS, Ruszkiewicz M, Beard RW: Effects of transfusion in women with recurrent spontaneous abortion. *Transplant Proc* 15:896, 1983.
35. McIntyre JA, Faulk WP: Histocompatibility and recurrent abortion. *Fertil Steril* 41:653, 1984.
36. McIntyre JA, Faulk WP: Recurrent spontaneous abortion in human pregnancy: Results of immunogenetical, cellular and humoral studies. *Am J Reprod Immunol Microbiol* 4:165, 1983.
37. Coulam CB, Moore SB, O'Fallon WM: Association between major histocompatibility antigen and reproductive performance. *Am J Reprod Immunol Microbiol* 14:54, 1987.
38. McIntyre JA, McConnachie PR, Taylor CS, Faulk WP: Clinical, immunologic and genetic definitions of primary and secondary recurrent spontaneous abortion. *Fertil Steril* 42:849, 1984.
39. Johnson PM, Chia KV, Risk JM: Immunological question marks in recurrent spontaneous abortion, in Clark DA, Croy BA (eds): *Reproductive Immunology*. Amsterdam, Elsevier, 1986, p 239.
40. Ober CL, Matin AO, Simpson JL, et al: Shared HLA antigen's and reproductive performance among Hutterites. *Am J Hum Genet* 5:994, 1983.
41. Ober C, Hauck WW, Kostyu DD, et al: Adverse effects of HLA-DR antigen sharing on fertility: A cohort study in a human isolate. *Fertil Steril* 44:227, 1985.
42. Faulk WP, McIntyre JA: Trophoblast survival. *Transplantation* 32:1, 1981.
43. Faulk WP, Temple A, Lovins R, Smith NC: Antigens of human trophoblast: A working hypothesis for their role in normal and abnormal pregnancies. *Proc Natl Acad Sci USA* 75:1947, 1978.
44. Taylor C, Faulk WP: Prevention of recurrent abortions with leukocyte transfusions. *Lancet* 2:68, 1981.
45. Torry DS, McIntyre JA, Faulk WP, McConnachie PR: Characterization of maternal trophoblast–lymphocyte cross-reactive (TLX) immunity. *Trophoblast Res* 2:173, 1986.
46. Faulk WP, McIntyre JA: Immunological studies of human trophoblast: Markers, subsets and functions. *Immunol Rev* 75:139, 1983.
47. Kajino T, Faulk WP, McIntyre JA: Antigens of human trophoblast: Trophoblast–lymphocyte cross-reactive antigens on platelets. *Am J Reprod Immunol Microbiol* 14:70, 1987.
48. McIntyre JA, Faulk WP: Allotypic trophoblast lymphocyte cross-reactive (TLX) cell surface antigens. *Hum Immunol* 4:27, 1982.
49. McIntyre JA, Faulk WP, Verhulst SJ, Colliver J: Human trophoblast lymphocyte cross-reactive (TLX) antigens define a new alloantigen system. *Science* 22:1135, 1983.
50. Konoeda Y, Terasaki P, Wakisaka A, Park MS, Mickey MR: Public determinants of HLA indicated by pregnancy antibodies. *J Immunol* 41:253, 1986.
51. McConnachie PR, McIntyre JA: Maternal antipaternal immunity in couples predisposed to repeated pregnancy loss. *Am J Reprod Immunol* 5:145, 1984.
52. Denegri JF, Altin M, McConnachie PR, et al: Immunotherapy of primary immunological aborters: Rationale for the use of pooled cryopreserved purified normal peripheral blood mononuclear cells. *Am J Reprod Immunol Microbiol* 12:65, 1986.

53. Mowbray JF: Genetic and immunological factors in human recurrent abortion. *Am J Reprod Immunol Microbiol* 15:138, 1987.
54. McIntyre JA, Faulk WP: Antibody responses in secondary aborting women: Effect of inhibitors in blood. *Am J Reprod Immunol Microbiol* 9:113, 1985.
55. Torry DS, McIntyre JA, Faulk WP, McConnachie PR: Inhibitors of complement-mediated cytotoxicity in normal and secondary aborter sera. *Am J Reprod Immunol Microbiol* 10:53, 1986.
56. Faulk WP, Torry D, McIntyre JA: Effects of serum versus plasma on agglutination of antibody-coated indicator cells by human rheumatoid factor. *Clin Immunol Immunopathol* 46:169, 1988.
57. McIntyre JA, Faulk WP: A cell-mediated immune defect in recurrent spontaneous abortion. *Trophoblast Res* 1:315, 1983.
58. Rocklin R, Kitzmiller J, Carpenter B, Garovoy MR, David JR: Maternal-fetal relation: Absence of an immunologic blocking factor from the serum of women with chronic abortions. *N Engl J Med* 295:1209, 1976.
59. Takakuwa K, Kanazawa K, Takeuchi S: Production of blocking antibodies by vaccination with husband lymphocytes in unexplained recurrent aborters—The role in successful pregnancy. *Am J Reprod Immunol* 10:1, 1986.
60. Faulk WP, Jeannet M, Creighton WD, Carbonara A: Immunological studies of immunoglobulins on trophoblastic basement membranes. *J Clin Invest* 54: 1011, 1974.
61. Sargent IL, Redman CWG: Maternal cell-mediated immunity to the fetus in human pregnancy. *J Reprod Immunol* 7:95, 1985.
62. McIntyre JA, Faulk WP: Trophoblast antigens in normal and abnormal human pregnancy. *Clin Obstet Gynecol* 29:976, 1986.
63. McIntyre JA, Faulk WP: Antigens of human trophoblast: Effects of heterologous anti-trophoblast sera on lymphocyte responses in vitro. *J Exp Med* 149:824, 1979.
64. Patton PE, Coulam CB, Bergstralh E: The prevalence of autoantibodies in pregnant and nonpregnant women. *Am J Obstet Gynecol* 157:1345, 1987.
65. Faulk WP, van Loghem E, Stickler GB: Maternal antibody to fetal light chain (Inv) antigens. *Am J Med* 56:393, 1974.
66. Cowchock S, Dehoratius RD, Wapner RJ, Jackson LG: Subclinical autoimmune disease and unexplained abortion. *Am J Obstet Gynecol* 50:367, 1984.
67. Hughes GRV: Autoantibodies in lupus and its variants: Experience in 1000 patients. *Br Med J* 289:339, 1984.
68. Lubbe WF, Liggins GC: Lupus anticoagulant and pregnancy. *Am J Obstet Gynecol* 153:322, 1985.
69. Branch DW, Scott JR, Kochenour NR, Hershgold E: Obstetric complications associated with the lupus anticoagulant. *N Engl J Med* 313:1322, 1985.
70. Feinstein DI: Lupus anticoagulant, thrombosis and fetal loss. *N Engl J Med* 313:348, 1985.
71. Harris EN, Chan JKH, Asherson RA, et al: Thrombosis, recurrent fetal loss, and thrombocytopenia. *Arch Intern Med* 146:2153, 1986.
72. Bresnihan B, Grigor RR, Oliver M, et al: Immunological mechanism for spontaneous abortion in systemic lupus erythematosus. *Lancet* 2:1205, 1977.
73. Lockshin MD, Druzin ML, Goer S, et al: Antibody to cardiolipin as a predictor of fetal distress or death in pregnant patients with systemic lupus erythematosus. *N Engl J Med* 313:152, 1985.
74. Unander M, Norberg R, Hahn L, Arfors L: Anticardiolipin antibodies and complement in ninety-nine women with habitual abortion. *Am J Obstet Gynecol* 156:114, 1987.
75. Hughes, GRV, Harris EN, Gharavi AE: The anticardiolipin syndrome. *J Rheumatology* 13:486, 1986.
76. Shoenfeld Y, et al: Polyspecificity of monoclonal lupus autoantibodies produced by human–human hybridomas. *N Engl J Med* 308:414, 1983.
77. Coulam CB, McIntyre JA, Faulk WP: Reproductive performance in women with repeated pregnancy losses and multiple partners. *Am J Reprod Immunol Microbiol* 12:10, 1986.
78. Mowbray J, Gribbings C, Liddell H, et al: Controlled trial of treatment of recurrent spontaneous abortion by immunization with paternal cells. *Lancet* 1:941, 1985.
79. Beer AE: New horizons in the diagnosis, evaluation and therapy of recurrent spontaneous abortion. *Clin Obstet Gynecol* 13:115, 1986.
80. Taylor CG, Faulk WP, McIntyre JA: Prevention of recurrent spontaneous abortions by leukocyte transfusions. *J R Soc Med* 78:623, 1985.
81. Chaouat G, Kiger N, Wegmann TG: Vaccination against spontaneous abortion in mice. *J Reprod Immunol* 5:389, 1983.
82. Kiger N, Chaouat G, Kolb JP, Wegmann TG, Guenet JL: Immunoge-

netic studies of spontaneous abortion in mice. Pre-immunization of females with allogeneic cells. *J Immunol* 134:2966, 1985.

83. Clark DA, Chaput A, Tutton D: Active suppression of host versus graft reaction in pregnant mice. VII. Spontaneous abortion of allogeneic CBA/JX DBA/2 fetuses in the uterus of CBA/J mice correlates with deficient non-T suppressor cell activity. *J Immunol* 136:1668, 1986.

84. Chavez DJ, McIntyre JA, Colliver J, Faulk WP: Allogeneic matings and immunization have different effects in nulliparous and multiparous mice. *J Immunol* 139:85, 1987.

85. Chaouat G, Kolb JP, Kiger N, Stanislawski M, Wegmann T: Immunologic consequences of vaccination against abortion in mice. *J Immunol* 134:1594, 1985.

86. Chaouat G, Lanker D: Vaccination against spontaneous abortion in mice: Protection against spontaneous abortion by preimmunization with an antiidiotypic antibody. *Am J Reprod Immunol Microbiol* 16:146, 1988.

87. Suciu-Foca N, Reed E, Rohowsky C, Kung P, King DW: Antiidiotypic antibodies to anti-HLA receptors induced by pregnancy. *Proc Natl Acad Sci USA* 80:830, 1983.

88. Faulk WP, McIntyre JA: Role of anti-TLX antibody in human pregnancy, in Clark DA, Croy BA (eds): *Reproductive Immunology.* Amsterdam, Elsevier, 1986, p 106.

89. Suciu-Foca N, Reemtsma K, King DW: The significance of the idiotypic anti-idiotypic network in humans. *Transplant Proc* 18:230, 1986.

90. Colaco CB, Elkon KB: The lupus anticoagulant. *Arthritis Rheum* 28:67, 1985.

91. Pengo V, Thiagarajan P, Shapiro SS, Heine MJ: Immunological specificity and mechanism of action of IgG lupus anticoagulants. *Blood* 70:69, 1987.

92. Elias M, Eldor A: Thromboembolism in patients with the "lupus"-type circulating anticoagulant. *Arch Intern Med* 144: 510, 1984.

93. De Wolf F, Carreras, LO, Moerman P, et al: Decidual vasculopathy and extensive placental infarction in a patient with repeated thromboembolic accidents, recurrent fetal loss, and a lupus anticoagulant. *Am J Obstet Gynecol* 142:829, 1982.

94. Faulk WP, Gargiulo P, McIntyre JA, Bang NU: Hemostasis and fibrinolysis in renal transplantation. *Semin Hemostas Thromb* In press.

95. Helin H, Edgington TS: A distinct "slow" cellular pathway involving soluble mediators for the T cell-instructed induction of monocyte tissue factor activity in an allogeneic immune response. *J Immunol* 132:2457, 1984.

96. Nemerson Y: Tissue factor and hemostasis. *Blood* 71:1, 1988.

97. Faulk WP: Hemostasis and fibrinolysis in human normal placentae: Possible role in early pregnancy failure, in Beard RW, Sharp F (eds): *Early Pregnancy Loss: Mechanisms and Treatment.* Ashton-under-Lyne, Lancastershire, Peacock Press, 1988, p 193.

98. Saleh AA, Bottoms SF, Welch RA, et al: Preeclampsia, delivery, and the hemostatic system. *Am J Obstet Gynecol* 157:331, 1987.

99. Pritchard JA, Cunningham FG, Mason RA: Coagulation changes in eclampsia: their frequency and pathogenesis. *Am J Obstet Gynecol* 124:855, 1976.

100. Von Hugo R, Graeff H: Thrombohemorrhagic complications in the obstetric patient, in Coleman R, Hirsh J, Marder V, Salzman E (eds): *Hemostasis and Thrombosis*, ed 2. Philadelphia, Lippincott, 1987, p 926.

101. Pekonen F, Rasi V, Ammala M, Viinikka L, Ylikorkala O: Platelet function and coagulation in normal and preeclamptic pregnancy. *Thromb Res* 43:553, 1986.

102. Kruithof E, Tran-Thang C, Gudinchet A, et al: Fibrinolysis in pregnancy: A study of plasminogen activator inhibitors. *Blood* 69:460, 1987.

103. Johnson PM, Faulk WP: Immunological studies of human placentae: Identification and distribution of proteins in immature chorionic villi. *Immunology* 34:1027, 1978.

104. Faulk WP, Johnson PM: Immunological studies of human placentae: Identification and distribution of proteins in mature chorionic villi. *Clin Exp Immunol* 27:365, 1977.

105. Hsi BL, Faulk WP, Yeh CJG, McIntyre JA: Immunohistology of clotting factor V in human extraembryonic membranes. *Placenta* 8:529, 1987.

106. Matter L, Faulk WP: Fibrinogen degradation products and factor VIII consumption in normal pregnancy and preeclampsia: Role of the placenta, in Bonner J, McGillivray I, Symonds M (eds): *Pregnancy Hypertension.* Lancaster, MTP, 1978, p 357.

107. Schorer AE, Kaplan ME, Rao GHR, Moldow CF: Interleukin 1 stimulates endothelial cell tissue factor production and expression by a prostaglandin-independent mechanism. *Thromb Haemost* 56:256, 1986.

108. Faulk WP, McIntyre JA: Immunological aspects of the materno–fetal

109. Alanen A: Serum IgE and smooth muscle antibodies in pre-eclampsia. *Acta Obstet Gynecol Scand* 63:581, 1984.

110. Gleich G, Loagering DA, Frigas E, et al: Major basic protein of the eosinophil granule: Physiocochemical properties, localization, and function, in Mahmoud AAF, Austen RF (eds): *The Eosinophil in Health and Disease.* New York, Grune & Stratton, 1980, p 79.

111. Maddox DE, Kephart GM, Coulam CB, et al: Localization of a molecule immunochemically similar to eosinophil major basic protein in human placenta. *J Exp Med* 160:29, 1984.

112. Wasmoen TL, Coulam CB, Leiferman KM, Gleich G: Increase of plasma eosinophil major basic protein levels late in pregnancy predicts onset of labor. *Proc Natl Acad Sci USA* 84:3029, 1987.

113. Coulam CB, Wasmoen T, Creasy R, Suteri P, Gleich GD: Major basic protein as a predictor of preterm labor: A preliminary report. *Am J Obstet Gynecol* 156:790, 1987.

114. Shaffer W: Role of uterine adhesions in the cause of multiple pregnancy losses. *Clin Obstet Gynecol* 29:912, 1986.

115. Goldzieher JW: Double-blind trial for a progestin in habitual abortion. *JAMA* 188:651, 1964.

116. Klopper A, Macnaughton MC: Hormones in recurrent abortion. *Br J Obstet Gynaecol* 72:1022, 1965.

117. Lloyd R, Coulam CB: Role of endometrial biopsy in diagnosing luteal phase defect. *Fertil Steril* Suppl:S57, 1988.

118. Durald GW, Michels VV: Recurrent miscarriages: Cytogenetic causes and genetic counseling of affected families. *Clin Obstet Gynecol* 29:865, 1986.

119. Esmon CT: The regulation of natural anticoagulant pathways. *Science* 235:1348, 1987.

120. Boyd JD, Hamilton WJ: *The Human Placenta.* Cambridge, Heffer, 1970, p 275.

121. Reginald PW, Beard RW, Chapple J, et al: Outcome of pregnancies progressing beyond 28 weeks gestation in women with a history of recurrent miscarriage. *Br J Obstet Gynaecol* 94:643, 1987.

122. Funderburk SJ, Guthrie D, Meldrum D: Suboptimal pregnancy with prior abortions and premature births. *Am J Obstet Gynecol* 126:55, 1976.

123. Schoenbaum SC, Monson RR, Stubblefield PG, Dorny PD, Ryan K: Outcome of the delivery following induced and spontaneous delivery. *Am J Obstet Gynecol* 136:19, 1980.

124. Alberman E, Roman E, Pharoah POD, Chamberlain C: Birthweights before and after spontaneous abortions. *Br J Obstet Gynaecol* 87:275, 1980.

125. Unander AM, Lindholm A: Transfusions of leukocyte-rich erythrocytes: A successful treatment in selected cases of habitual abortion. *Am J Obstet Gynecol* 154:516, 1986.

126. Beer AE, Quebbeman JF, Xiaoyu Z: Nonpaternal leukocyte immunization in women previously immunized with paternal leukocytes: Immune responses and subsequent pregnancy outcome, in Clark DA, Croy BA (eds): *Reproductive Immunology.* Amsterdam, Elsevier, 1986, p 261.

127. Kajino T, Torry DS, McIntyre JA, Faulk WP: Trophoblast antigens in human seminal plasma. *Am J Reprod Immunol Microbiol* 17:91, 1988.

128. McIntyre JA, McConnachie PR, Faulk WP: Characterization of maternal antipaternal antibodies in secondary aborting women. *Contrib Gynecol Obstet* 14:131, 1985.

129. McConnachie PR, Denegri JR, Lower FE, Torry DS, McIntyre JA: Differences in immunoglobulin subclasses between dye exclusion and 51Cr release complement-dependent lymphocytotoxicity assay. *Transplantation* 42:212, 1986.

130. Robertson WB, Brosens I, Landells W: Abnormal placentation. *Obstet Gynecol Annu* 14:421, 1985.

131. Pijnenborg R, Dixon G, Robertson WB, Brosens I: Trophoblastic invasion of human decidua from 8–18 weeks of pregnancy. *Placenta* 1:3, 1980.

132. Brosens I, Robertson WB, Dickson HG: The physiological response to the vessels of the placental bed to normal pregnancy. *J Pathol Bacteriol* 93:569, 1967.

133. Nilsson IM, Astedt B, Hedner U, Berizin D: Intrauterine death and circulating anticoagulant. *Acta Med Scand* 197:153, 1975.

134. Soulier RP, Boffa MC: Avortements a repetition, thromboses et anticoagulant circulant antithromboplastine. *Nouv Presse Med* 9:244, 1980.

135. Lubbe WF, Butler WS, Palmer SJ, Liggins GC: Fetal survival after prednisone suppression of maternal lupus-anticoagulant. *Lancet* 1:1361,

1983.

136. Lubbe WF, Butler WS, Palmer SJ, Liggins GC: Lupus anticoagulant in pregnancy. *Br J Obstet Gynaecol* 91:357, 1984.

137. Patrignani P, Filabozzi P, Patrono C: Selective cumulative inhibition of platelet thromboxane production by low-dose aspirin in healthy subjects. *J Clin Invest* 69:1366, 1982.

138. MacLachlan NA, Wilson JK, Apps P, et al: Outcome of infants born following maternal immunization to prevent primary recurrent spontaneous abortions.

139. Seibel MM, Taymor ML: Emotional aspects of infertility. *Fertil Steril* 37:127, 1982.

PART VI
Ultrasound

CHAPTER 21
Ultrasound in Infertility

Colin R. McArdle

Ultrasound in Infertility

Male Factor Infertility
    Normal Testes
    Varicocele
    Small Testes
    Testicular Tumor
Female Infertility Factors
    Normal Uterus and Ovaries
    Fibroids
    Uterine Anomalies
    Endometriosis
    Tubal Conditions
    Cervical Factors
    Ovulatory Factors
    Normal Cycle
    Endometrial Changes

Monitoring Therapy
    Artificial Insemination
    Ovulation Induction
    Other Monitoring Techniques
Complications of Ovulation Induction
    Ovarian Hyperstimulation
    Multiple Pregnancies
    Oocyte Retrieval Using
      Ultrasonic Guidance
Monitoring Pregnancy
    Early Pregnancy
    Ectopic Pregnancy

In 1978 Hackeloer first described the ultrasonic development of the maturing follicle in the normal menstrual cycle.[1] Ten years later follicular development and oocyte harvesting by ultrasound are commonplace. Further developments in the diagnosis and treatment of both male and female infertility will no doubt occur in the next 10 years. By then, much of the material discussed in this chapter will be considered outdated. One constant, however, will remain: The ultrasound picture demonstrates faithfully, according to certain physical principles, exactly what is being scanned. It is never wrong; only the interpretation can be wrong. The better the anatomy can be demonstrated, the more probable a correct interpretation will be made. For this reason it is essential that the persons interpreting the scans be both knowledgeable about ultrasound and committed to expanding their knowledge.

Similarly, the ultrasound equipment used should be of high quality. For the investigation of infertility, two probes should be considered essential, a sector scanner for transabdominal scanning and a vaginal probe. Although a straight linear array is good for evaluating the pregnant uterus once it has extended out of the pelvis, it is less appropriate for viewing the pelvis.

According to the American Institute of Ultrasound in Medicine, no confirmed biologic effects on patients or instrument operators caused by exposure at intensities typical of present diagnostic ultrasound instruments have ever been reported. Although the possibility exists that such effects may be identified in the future, current data indicate that the benefits to patients of the prudent use of the procedure outweigh the risks, if any, that may be present.[2] The NIH consensus report came to generally similar conclusions, suggesting that ultrasound examinations of pregnant women should not be performed on a routine basis but rather when suggested clinical indications are present.[3]

MALE FACTOR INFERTILITY

A male factor is present in 30 to 40% of infertile couples. In the majority of instances, ultrasound of the testis is unrevealing; however in certain cases, the procedure is warranted to confirm or rule out diagnosis or suspicion of some structural abnormality.

Normal Testes
The normal testis measures between 3 and 5 cm in length and 2 and 3 cm in diameter. It has a uniformly heterogeneous echo texture (Fig. 21–1). Occasion-

ally, the septa that extend from the mediastinum testis and divide the testis into the lobuli testis may produce an echogenic linear pattern. It is characteristic and easily recognized. Occasional small densities with posterior shadowing are seen within the substances of the testes. These probably represent phleboliths and are not of pathologic significance. The epididymis lies posterolateral to the testis. It consists of a head superiorly, a body, and a tail. It is generally between 6 and 8 mm thick and should not be greater than 10 mm in diameter. Small amounts of fluid in the tunica vaginalis (hydrocele) are normal.

Varicocele
In varicocele the veins of the pampiniform plexus are tortuous and distended.[4] Although it is stated that the left side is involved in 98% of cases,[5] the frequency of ultrasonographically demonstrable varioceles on the right is probably considerably higher than 2%. Ultrasound examination, preferably performed using a high-resolution, near-focused transducer, reveals serpiginous tubular structures within the epididymis (Fig. 21–2). The adjacent testis should show a normal, uniformly heterogeneous echo pattern. Further distention of these veins may be demonstrated by having the patient stand or perform a Valsalva's maneuver.

Small Testes
Mumps orchitis with subsequent testicular atrophy, Klinefelter's syndrome, and infantile testis syndrome are all causes of small testes and infertility.[5] Sono-

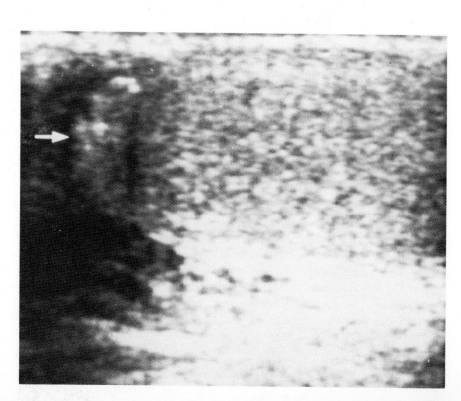

Figure 21–1. Longitudinal scan shows the homogeneous pattern of the testis. Superior to the testis lies the epididymis (arrow).

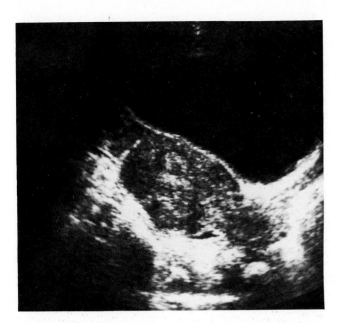

Figure 21–5. Longitudinal scan of a fibroid uterus. The uterus is enlarged and irregular, and has an inhomogeneous echo texture. Note that each individual fibroid is not well delineated.

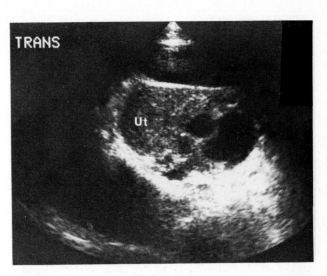

Figure 21–7. Endometriosis is evident on this transverse scan of the pelvis. Several cystic areas are adjacent to the uterus. Those containing low-level echoes are characteristic of endometriomas.

eral low-level echoes caused by the bloody fluid they contain. The enhanced through-transmission and well-defined back wall confirm their cystic nature (Fig. 21–7). The size and number of the endometriomas should be recorded so that response to medical therapy can be assessed.

Tubal Conditions

Although a sonographic method of determining tubal patency has been described, hysterosalpinography remains the best method for determining the presence of tubal obstruction. Normal fallopian tubes cannot be visualized by ultrasound. The changes associated with acute or chronic inflammatory disease, often a cause of infertility, frequently are

detectable, however. A hydrosalpinx appears as a clear, cystic area of varying shape. More frequently there is generalized thickening of the adnexae often associated with small, somewhat amorphous collections of fluid (Fig. 21–8). Transvaginal sonography offers a more detailed examination of the adnexal region and in many cases allows visualization of the fallopian tubes when inflamed.

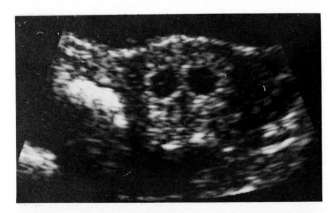

Figure 21–6. Transverse scan of a pregnant bicornuate uterus. Two small gestational sacs can be seen in the separate uterine cavities. In the nonpregnant state, the cavities may be more difficult to visualize.

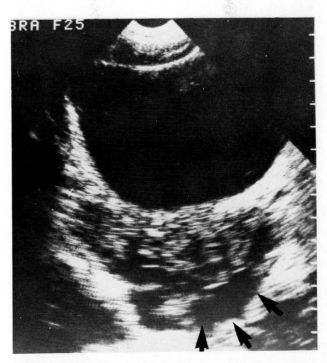

Figure 21–8. Transverse scan of the pelvis. The somewhat poorly defined, fluid-filled areas posterior to the uterus in the left adnexa (arrows) are typical of hydrosalpinx.

Cervical Factors

No generally accepted role for ultrasound has been found for diagnosing cervical factors that cause infertility. Because vaginal sonography allows such good demonstration of the cervix, cervical canal, and uterine vessels, some role for this technique may be uncovered.

Ovulatory Factors

Ultrasound has a significant role in the treatment of anovulation. With two exceptions, however, it is much less useful in determining the causative factors of anovulation or oligoovulation. The two areas in which ultrasound may assist in diagnosis are polycystic ovary disease (PCO) and the luteinized unruptured follicle syndrome (LUF).

Polycystic Ovary Disease. The diagnosis of PCO can be established by the characteristic hormonal profile coupled with obesity, hirsutism, and infertility, and confirmed by ovarian biopsy. It may also be suggested by certain ultrasonic features. In about 71% of patients witch hormonally defined PCO,

ovarian enlargement is seen (> 6 cm^3).[11] The ovaries typically become spherical rather than ellipsoid.

In addition, several discrete cysts, less than 1 cm in diameter, situated around the periphery may be seen (Fig. 21–9). These represent the immature, atretic follicles typical of this disease. When using the standard transabdominal transvesical scanning technique, these small cysts can be seen in about 50% of patients with PCO. In the remainder they are too small to identify separately, and the ovaries then appear large and relatively sonolucent. The enhanced resolution that endovaginal sonography provides allows these smaller cysts to be visualized, and makes the diagnosis of PCO easier. Nevertheless, approximately 29% of patients have no ovarian enlargement. These variances probably reflect the broad spectrum of clinical features typical of the disease.

Luteinized Unruptured Follicle Syndrome. As the name implies, LUF is a condition in which the follicle fails to rupture within the ovulatory interval of 38 hours after the luteinizing hormone (LH) surge. The luteinized unruptured follicle is easily demonstrated

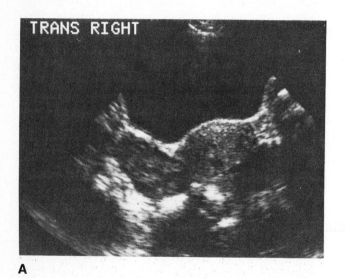

A

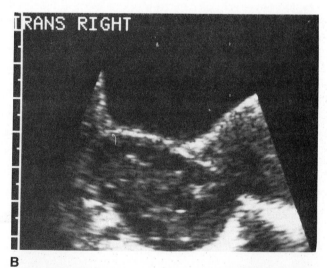

B

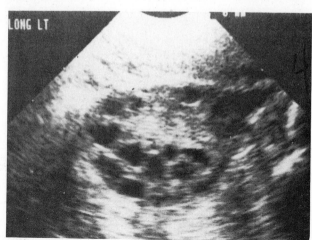

C

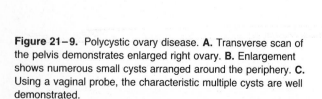

Figure 21–9. Polycystic ovary disease. **A.** Transverse scan of the pelvis demonstrates enlarged right ovary. **B.** Enlargement shows numerous small cysts arranged around the periphery. **C.** Using a vaginal probe, the characteristic multiple cysts are well demonstrated.

on ultrasound. Therefore, any dominant follicle that persists 48 hours beyond the LH peak is abnormal and may be taken as evidence of LUF.

Normal Cycle

Follicular development and ovulation during the normal menstrual cycle have been elegantly demonstrated by serial ultrasound examination.[13] The hormonal changes that occur during these cycles determine the sequence of events that can be observed in both the ovaries and the uterus. Without a thorough understanding of the hormonal changes during the menstrual cycle, interpretation of any ultrasonographic findings will inevitably be incomplete and often inadequate.

In the early follicular phase of the menstrual cycle, a cohort of developing follicles is recruited from the pool of nonproliferating primordial follicles present within the ovaries.[14] The initiation of follicular development is a continuous process. The vast majority of these primordial follicles never develop beyond the early preantral phase and undergo spontaneous regression. These follicles are not detectable by ultrasound. Some, however, under the influence of follicle-stimulating hormone (FSH), do develop, and the granulosa cells contained within these antral follicles start to produce estrogen. When they have reached around 5 mm, they may be detected ultrasonically. From this group will be selected a single dominant follicle,[15] at about day 8 when it is around 8 to 10 mm. While the other follicles undergo atresia or developmental arrest, the dominant follicle continues to grow at a rate of approximately 2 mm a day (Fig. 21–10). In 5 to 11% of normal cycles 2 dominant follicles develop, but always on opposite ovaries.[14] The dominant follicle continues to grow until ovulation occurs, generally when the mean diameter of the follicle is between 20 and 24 mm. There is such

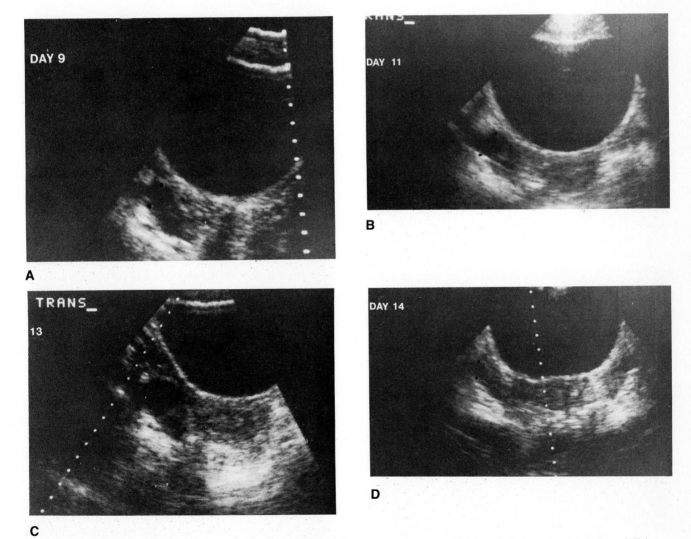

Figure 21–10. Normal follicular development. **A.** Transverse scan of the right ovary on the 9th day of the cycle demonstrates a follicle measuring 14 mm. **B.** Two days later the follicle measures 19 mm. **C.** Two days later the follicle measures 23 mm and the ovary 47 mm. **D.** One day later ovulation has occurred and the follicle is reduced in size.

variation in the maximum preovulatory diameter, however, that the size of the follicle has not proved particularly useful for predicting ovulation. During the later stages of development, a cumulus oophorus may be seen (Fig. 21–11), and this may be regarded as a sign of maturity.[13]

Other signs of follicle maturity and impending ovulation have been documented.[16] Crenellation of the lining of the follicle and decreased reflectivity around it indicate that ovulation will occur within 6 to 10 hours. These signs reflect the changes in and around the follicle that occur after the LH surge has begun. They are probably not seen frequently enough and are too operator dependent to be useful on a routine basis.

Ovulation occurs about 36 to 38 hours after the serum LH surge begins (Fig. 21–12). Because detection of the LH surge in urine is somewhat delayed, ovulation will occur approximately 24 hours after a positive urine assay is found. The process of ovulation was observed ultrasonically.[17] There was some variation among patients, but all showed a decrease in size of the follicle either occurring rapidly or over a period of 30 minutes, followed by the development of a corpus hemorrhagicum soon after. It is interesting to note that these authors did not observe either crenellation of the lining of the follicle or decreased reflectivity around the follicle. Evidence of ovulation can be seen in about 90% of normal cycles.[18] These changes are described as the follicle disappearing completely, becoming smaller and irregular in shape, and filling with low-level echoes as the corpus hemorrhagicum forms. In the absence of pregnancy, this corpus luteum lasts for 14 days, at which time it rapidly regresses and menstruation occurs. On ultra-

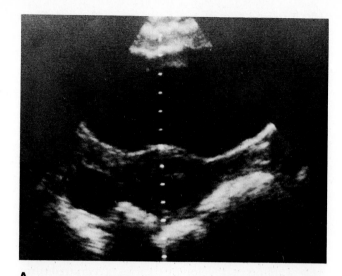

A

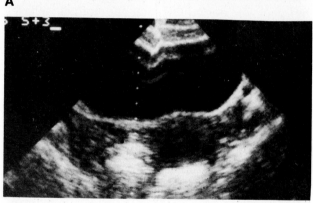

B

Figure 21–12. A. Transverse scan shows a preovulatory follicle on the right ovary. **B.** After ovulation the follicle is no longer seen.

sound, a corpus luteum typically appears as a cyst with well-defined walls and low-level internal echoes reflecting its hemorrhagic contents. Through most of the normal cycle, from the development of the follicle to the disappearance of the corpus luteum at menstruation, a cystic structure is present on one or the other ovary. For this reason, care must be taken not to interpret a cyst seen on ultrasound examination erroneously as evidence of pathology, because more commonly it is a normal finding in most premenopausal women.

Endometrial Changes

After menstruation, in the early proliferative phase the endometrial cavity is seen as a thin, continuous line. As the proliferative phase continues the endometrium thickens (Fig. 21–13), while the continuous endometrial line becomes less and less pronounced. At the time of ovulation the total endometrial thickness is between 8 and 14 mm.[19] After ovulation, a small, hypoechoic, ringlike structure with a central echogenic line appears. This is considered to be

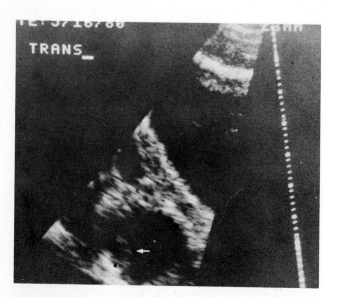

Figure 21–11. Longitudinal scan of a mature follicle shows the presence of a cumulus (arrow). Although a good sign of maturity, it is not reliably seen.

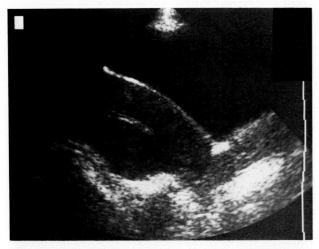

A

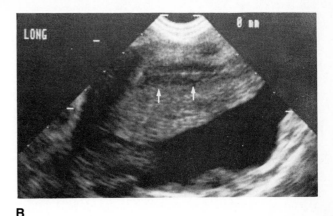

B

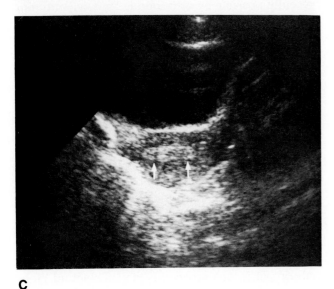

C

Figure 21–13. Endometrial changes. **A.** In the early proliferative phase the endometrium is a thin, echogenic line. **B.** In the large proliferative phase (vaginal probe) the thickened endometrium (arrows) is hypoechoic. A central, thin echogenic line is still present. **C.** In the secretory phase, the endometrium is thickened in the cul-de-sac (arrows).

strong evidence that ovulation has occurred. A similar appearance may be seen in association with ectopic pregnancy. In the secretory phase, the endometrium continues to thicken until menstruation occurs.

MONITORING THERAPY

Artificial Insemination

In patients with irregular cycles, monitoring follicular development and endometrial thickness may be of considerable help in timing of insemination. Once the dominant follicle achieves a diameter of 18 mm, ultrasound examinations may be performed daily. Insemination should be performed on the day ultrasound criteria of ovulation are demonstrated.

Ovulation Induction

Oligoovulation or anovulation is present in approximately 20% of infertile couples. Except in patients with ovarian failure, ovulation can be induced successfully in most cases. The aim is to induce the development of one or more follicles and continue their growth to maturity and ovulation. Typically, the drugs used are clomiphene citrate and human menopausal gonadotropin (HMG).[20] Urinary FSH is also used. Gonadotropin-releasing hormone has been given on a limited basis.[21]

Ultrasound monitoring allows the number and size of developing follicles to be observed easily. The likelihood of multiple gestations and the complications of ovulation induction such as ovarian hyperstimulation can be predicted. Because repeated ultrasound examinations are both costly and time consuming for patients, follicular development is not monitored in all instances, as, for example, when clomiphene citrate is administered. The chances of large numbers of follicles developing when this drug is employed is small, because the development of more than two dominant follicles is uncommon.[19]

When gonadotropins are the induction agents,

ultrasound monitoring is advised.[22] An initial scan of the pelvis is performed prior to initiating therapy to establish the presence of any ovarian or uterine pathology. Even if all subsequent monitoring is to be performed with a vaginal transducer, it is recommended that the standard, full-bladder, transabdominal scan be performed initially. This technique allows the whole pelvis to be well visualized. The vaginal transducer has only limited field of view, and any pathology that lies more than 6 or 7 cm from the transducer may not be resolved.

Ultrasound monitoring of the ovaries is normally started on the 5th day after the beginning of HMG administration. By this time the developing follicles are around 10 mm in diameter. If several follicles are present, they may be compressed, giving a cartwheel appearance (Fig. 21–14). Although many advocate measuring the follicles in all three dimensions, in practice this often proves to be very painstaking to perform and frequently confusing to interpret, particularly when large numbers of follicles are present. A single mean diameter for each follicle averaged from only two dimensions is usually all that is necessary. This may be obtained with the ovary in either the longitudinal or transverse projection, but the same projection must be repeated in all subsequent scans.

As previously stated, follicles grow approximately 2 mm a day. Between 18 and 23 mm is regarded as an optimal size for mature follicles; however, they may vary considerably in size, particularly in cycles induced with HMG. For this reason, in patients with oligoovulation or anovulation, the diameter of the largest follicle is commonly used as a guide for oocyte maturity. If the largest follicle has reached a size of 18 mm, ovulation will be initiated by the administration of human chorionic gonadotropin (HCG).

In patients undergoing in-vitro fertilization (IVF), it is necessary to develop a larger number of follicles so that more than one or two ova can be harvested. Various protocols may be used, but all are designed to develop many more follicles than would be desirable in women with oligoovulation or anovulation.[23] The optimum size is again between 18 and 23 mm, but it is unlikely that all follicles develop at the same rate. Mature ova may be obtained from follicles between 12 and 34 mm, although 15 and 23 mm are more typical diameters. The gynecologist must therefore attempt to develop many follicles in this range while avoiding a spontaneous LH surge. When oocytes are harvested under ultrasound guidance, it should be remembered that puncturing a follicle larger than 20 mm is considerably easier than puncturing one of 12 mm.

Accurate prediction of an LH surge is not presently possible by ultrasound. Thus when timing oocyte harvesting, the ultrasound findings must not be used in isolation. Other values such as serum estradiol (E_2) and LH levels should also be monitored. If the patient has had previous induced cycles, these should also be reviewed, as cyclic patterns frequently emerge and can assist in timing oocyte retrieval.

Other Monitoring Techniques

The timing of HCG administration is critical: too early and the oocytes may undergo atresia or fail to provide mature eggs; too late and the oocytes may be overmature. In addition, in many patients, a spontaneous LH surge may occur, causing considerable difficulty in correctly timing oocyte retrieval. Because the size of the follicle does not always correlate with maturity, it is not surprising that ultrasound alone has not been completely successful for estimating maturity.[24] For this reason, most programs monitor E_2 levels at the same time as performing ultrasound examinations.[25] In the normal cycle there is a reasonable correlation between the E_2 level and mean follicular diameter.[13,26] In the presence of numerous follicles, the correlation is poor.[27] Claims of a significant correlation between E_2 and mean follicular volume in these patients[28] do not appear to be valid. Generally, when the E_2 level is between 1,000 and 2,000 pg/mL the follicles are mature. Because a satisfactory E_2 level may be produced by a few mature follicles or a larger number of smaller immature follicles, the combination of ultrasound findings and measurement of E_2 level allows for better patient management. As the E_2 level rises, there is an increasing frequency of ovarian hyperstimulation (OHS) syndrome.[29] The gynecologist must therefore attempt to balance the need for many mature follicles with the likelihood of OHS if the E_2 level rises too high.

In most circumstances follicular development does not require further monitoring after HCG ad-

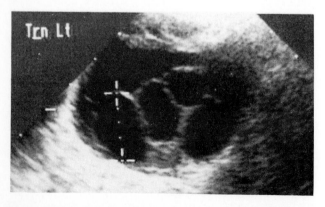

Figure 21–14. Multiple follicles are seen adjacent to one another, giving a cartwheel appearance. Measurement of each follicle should be the mean of both diameters.

ministration. The follicles usually grow between 2 and 4 mm in the 36 hours prior to ovulation. If evidence of ovulation is required, another ultrasound 2 days after HCG administration is recommended to search for the signs such as decrease or disappearance in the size or number of follicles, and fluid in the cul-de-sac. In addition, if cystic enlargement of the ovaries occurs, this indicates the development of OHS and may be taken as evidence of ovulation. This rarely occurs in any but induced cycles. Conversely, in the absence of ultrasound evidence of ovulation, a second dose of HCG may be administered.

COMPLICATIONS OF OVULATION INDUCTION

Ovarian Hyperstimulation

Ovarian hyperstimulation is characterized by cystic enlargement of the ovaries after ovulation. In its severest form, the OHS syndrome, massive cystic enlargement of the ovaries, ascites, pleural effusions, and hemoconcentration occur (Fig. 21–15). This degree of severity is uncommon. Other forms of OHS

(severe, moderate, and mild) characterized by ovarian enlargement (< 9, < 7, and < 5 cm, respectively) without evidence of ascites, effusion, or hemoconcentration are common, being demonstrated in 44% of ovulation inductions.[30]

A definite correlation exists between the development of OHS and the number of follicles present at ovulation[31] and also the E_2 level. The greater the number of follicles and the higher the E_2 level, the more likely OHS will occur. Because typically a larger number of follicles and higher E_2 levels are present in patients having IVF, some degree of OHS is present in almost all patients. In fact, the term *controlled ovarian hyperstimulation* is often used to describe ovulation induction for IVF. Withholding HCG will not necessarily prevent ovulation and subsequent OHS, because spontaneous LH surges do occasionally occur. The symptoms and signs of OHS start developing soon after ovulation and are worst at around 8 to 10 days. In the absence of pregnancy the symptoms diminish over a period of 10 days (Fig. 21–16). If the patient becomes pregnant, ovarian enlargement may persist for many weeks.[30]

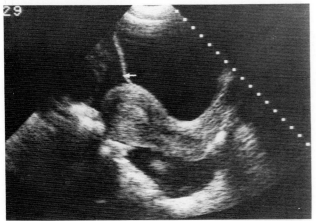

A

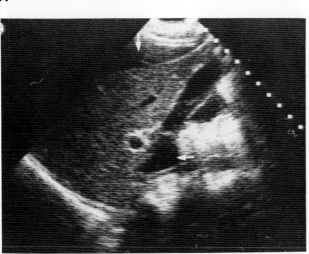

C

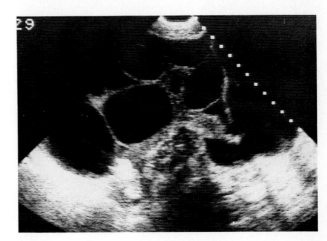

B

Figure 21–15. Ovarian hyperstimulation syndrome. **A.** Longitudinal scan shows fluid in the cul-de-sac and above the fundus (arrow). **B.** Longitudinal scan through right ovary, which is massively enlarged with numerous follicular and luteal cysts. **C.** Longitudinal scan of the liver shows free ascitic fluid (arrow) around the liver.

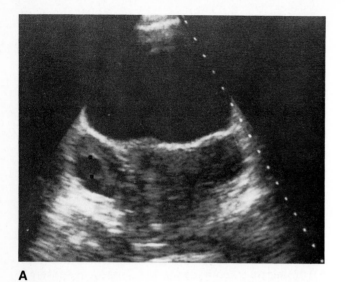

A

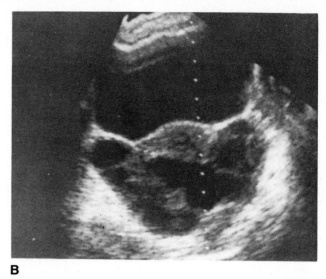

B

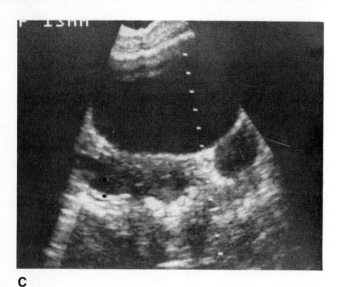

C

Figure 21–16. Ovarian hyperstimulation. **A.** Preovulatory scan shows numerous developing follicles on both ovaries. **B.** Ten days after ovulation, bilateral cystic enlargement of both ovaries has occurred. **C.** Ten days later both ovaries have returned to near normal size. The patient did not become pregnant.

Multiple Pregnancies

Although it is ideal if only 1 or 2 follicles develop in patients who require ovulation induction, numerous follicles develop in the majority of women.[32] This does increase the probability of multiple gestations, but these actually occur in only about 20% of instances. Therefore the presence of many follicles should not preclude the administration of HCG. When 3 or more preovulatory follicles are detected, however, careful discussion with the couple prior to administering HCG is essential.

Oocyte Retrieval Using Ultrasonic Guidance

Three methods of ultrasound-guided oocyte retrieval have been reported: transabdominal–transvesicle, transuretheral–transversicle, and transvaginal. The first reports used a transabdominal–transvesical approach.[33,34] Although a satisfactory rate of oocyte recovery has been achieved with this technique, it is not widely used in the United States because of the considerable discomfort to the patient. A perurethral–transvesical approach has had wider application.[35] This technique can be accomplished without significant discomfort in a sedated patient (Fig. 21–17). The oocyte recovery rate is comparable to that with laparoscopic retrieval, and a slightly higher pregnancy rate has been observed (C. R. McArdle, M. M. Seibel, unpublished data, 1987). In the transvaginal, ultrasonically guided, follicle-puncture method the needle is guided using a standard transabdominal technique, scanning the vagina and ovaries through a full bladder.[36]

The advent of the intravaginal probe with biopsy attachment has made it possible to harvest oocytes using the transvaginal approach (Fig. 21–18).[37] The same advantages that apply to the use of the vaginal transducer in assessing follicular growth apply to oocyte harvesting. Because of the proximity of the transducer to the ovaries, a high-frequency, high-

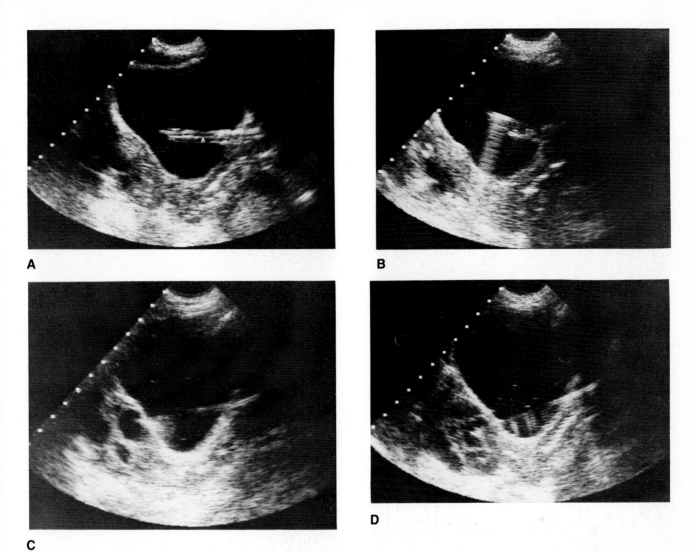

Figure 21–17. Oocyte retrieval per urethra (longitudinal scans). After a Foley catheter has filled the bladder with Ringer's lactate solution, (**A**) a needle is introduced into the bladder by placing its tip into the tip of the catheter. **B.** The needle is unhooked from the Foley catheter. **C.** The tip of the needle is aligned with a follicle. **D.** The needle is pushed into the follicle and the oocyte is retrieved.

definition transducer can be used, ensuring excellent visualization of the follicles. Better control of all aspects of oocyte retrieval is possible with this over other ultrasound guidance methods. Furthermore, it can be performed by a single operator instead of requiring both a radiologist and a gynecologist. This procedure is regarded as the method of choice for the majority of patients.

In many patients with extensive tubal disease and adhesions, however, the ovaries may not be equally accessible to all approaches. An ovary that lies high within the pelvis is more likely to be accessible to the perurethral than the transvaginal approach. Similarly, an ovary lying behind the uterus or low within the cul-de-sac can be approached only through the vagina. Some competency in more than one method of oocyte retrieval is therefore recommended in order to accommodate all patients.

In cycles in which gamete intrafallopian transfer (GIFT) is employed, ultrasound is generally used only to assist ovulation induction. Laparoscopy is used to retrieve oocytes and place them into the fallopian tubes; however, reports of doing this under ultrasound guidance using a specially designed catheter have been published.[38]

MONITORING PREGNANCY

Early Pregnancy
During the earliest phases of embryologic life, before a chorionic cavity has formed, the embryo is not detectable by ultrasound. This chorionic cavity forms at around 30 to 34 days after the last menstruation, when it rapidly becomes detectable by ultrasound. Using a vaginal transducer, a clearly defined gestational sac usually can be detected by 32 days. No yolk sac or fetal parts can be seen, and a gestational sac may be confused with a decidual cast. By 35 days, using a vaginal transducer, a yolk sac can be seen

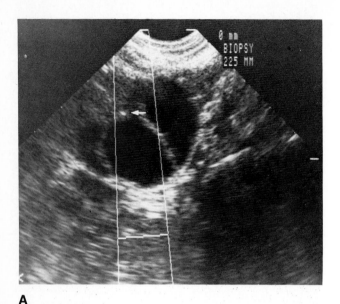

A

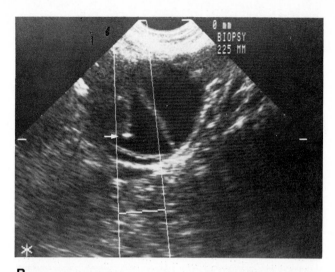

B

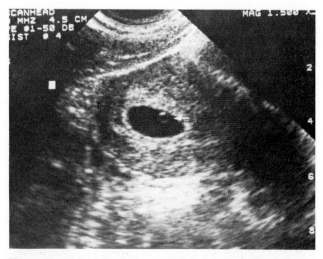

Figure 21–18. Transvaginal oocyte retrieval. **A.** The tip of the needle (arrow) is seen prior to aspiration of a follicle. **B.** The needle is advanced into the follicle. **C.** The follicle has been aspirated. It will be flushed several times or until the oocyte is seen. The tip of needle is seen (arrow).

C

within the gestational sac. This proves conclusively the presence of an intrauterine pregnancy. The gestational sac grows around 1 mm a day[39]; if the standard sector scanner is used, it is usually not easily visible until day 35, and the yolk sac generally is not seen until day 40 (Fig. 21–19). By this time or soon after, a fetal pole may be detected with the vaginal probe. From these data, it can be seen that an intrauterine pregnancy cannot be detected for at least 16 days from conception, or 30 days after the last menstruation (Table 21–1). Unless a yolk sac can be detected, the presence of an intrauterine pregnancy cannot be determined absolutely. The gestational sac without a yolk sac or fetal pole detectable may be confused with a decidual cast, a point of confusion when an ectopic pregnancy is suspected.

Attempts have been made to distinguish between a gestational sac and a decidual cast, often referred to as a pseudogestational sac or pseudosac of pregnancy.[40,41] When implantation of the blastocyst

Figure 21–19. Longitudinal scan of the uterus reveals a yolk sac (arrow) within a gestational sac. This is absolute proof that this sac represents an intrauterine pregnancy. A double decidual sac sign is also seen on the fundal and posterior aspects of the gestational sac.

TABLE 21–1. AFFIRMATION OF INTRAUTERINE PREGNANCY

Day After Last Menstrual Period	β-HCG 2nd IS (mIU/ml)	Ultrasound Findings
23	—	Positive
32	±500	Gestational sac
35	±1,800	Yolk sac, gestational sac
40	>5,000	Fetal pole, yolk sac
45	>10,000	Embryo, fetal pole

occurs at around the 6th day after conception, it does so into one or another wall of the endometrium. As the embryo develops and the chorionic sac appears, it tends to lie in an eccentric position within the uterine cavity, surrounded by markedly thickened endometrium. This position forms the basis of what is termed the intradecidual sign[42] (Fig. 21–20a and b), which is claimed to be both highly sensitive and specific for the diagnosis of intrauterine pregnancy.[40] Conversely, a decidual cast or pseudosac is a centrally located, sac-shaped lucency, with the endometrium of the uterine wall of similar thickness on both sides of the sac (Fig. 21–20c and d). These are the findings whether the transvaginal or transabdominal transducer is used.

Another sign that may be helpful in confirming the presence of pregnancy when neither yolk sac nor fetal pole is detectable is the ultrasonographic demonstration of line of separation between the decidua parietalis and the decidua capsularis (Fig. 21–20e and f). This is represented as a lucent line between the two echogenic lines caused by the two decidual layers. This sandwich is what is called the double decidual sac sign,[41] which is again good evidence of an intrauterine rather than an ectopic pregnancy.

Even when one or another of these signs is present, if an ectopic gestation is suspected it is prudent to repeat the ultrasound examination in 5 to 7 days to confirm the presence of a yolk sac or fetal pole within the gestational sac, thus proving beyond doubt the existence of an intrauterine pregnancy.

Ectopic Pregnancy

The prevalence of ectopic pregnancy has risen threefold since 1970, and although the associated mortality has dropped during this period, it remains a leading cause of maternal death.[42] Many of the causes that predispose to infertility, such as endometriosis and pelvic inflammatory disease, also predispose to the development of tubal pregnancy.

To exclude an ectopic pregnancy, three questions must be answered: (1) is the patient pregnant?; (2) is it an intrauterine pregnancy?; and (3) is there evidence of an ectopic gestation?

Is the Patient Pregnant?   In the absence of a positive pregnancy test, all but chronic ectopic pregnancies can be excluded. The radioimmunoassay for β-HCG either in the blood or the urine is both highly sensitive and specific. It may be detected on the 9th day after conception (day 23 after last menstruation). This is approximately 9 days before a gestational sac can be seen sonographically with a vaginal probe. If results of the qualitative test are positive, the patient is pregnant. Blood β-HCG should then be measured quantitatively. Two standards are commonly used for β-HCG assay results, the second international standard (2nd IS) and the international reference preparation (IRP).[43] Roughly 100 mIU/mL 2nd IS approximates 200 mIU/mL IRP. It is very important to know which standard a laboratory is using when trying to correlate sonographic appearances with quantitative β-HCG results. Even when the reference units are the same, some variation among laboratories is often present. Although there is a very small false negative rate for the detection of β-HCG at the lowest levels, for practical purposes, negative results of a pregnancy test properly performed exclude the diagnosis of acute ectopic pregnancy.

The quantitative level of β-HCG level can be useful in distinguishing between intrauterine and ectopic pregnancy. Typically, the latter is associated with lower values for dates than a corresponding intrauterine pregnancy.[44] Using a transabdominal technique, an intrauterine gestational sac should be visible sonographically in all patients in whom the HCG level is greater than 1800 m IU/mL 2nd IS.[45] A sac may be detected at levels much below this, but not reliably. If a vaginal transducer is used, an intrauterine sac can be detected at levels as low as 500 IU/mL.[46] Failure to demonstrate an intrauterine pregnancy at these levels strongly suggests an ectopic gestation.

When a diagnosis cannot be established with certainty, serial quantitative measurements of β-HCG can be performed with advantage. A normal intrauterine pregnancy has an HCG doubling rate of approximately 2 days, whereas in a patient with either an ectopic pregnancy or early abortion, the level will show either a subnormal increase or a decline.

Is It an Intrauterine Pregnancy?   While a single elevated HCG level confirms the presence of pregnancy, it does not adequately distinguish between a normal intrauterine or ectopic pregnancy, or spontaneous abortion, particularly if the patient's dates are not totally reliable. In most instances, ectopic pregnancy can be excluded with complete certainty by the ultrasonographic demonstration of a viable intrauterine pregnancy. This can be done by demonstrating a fetal pole with fetal cardiac activity or a yolk sac.

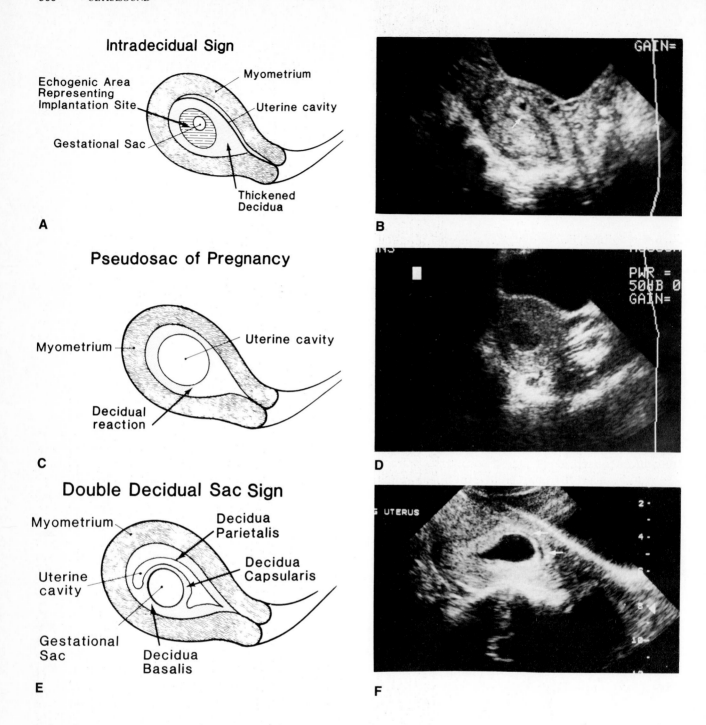

Figure 21–20. A. Illustration of the intradecidual sign. The small gestational sac lies eccentrically to the endometrial cavity. The thickened decidua surrounds the sac. **B.** The gestational sac is seen lying superiorly to the echogenic line (arrows) of the endometrial cavity. **C.** Decidual cast (pseudogestational sac or pseudosac of pregnancy). The central position of the fluid collection and the limited endometrial echoes around the sac are characteristic of a decidual cast. **D.** Decidual cast (pseudogestgational sac). A hyperechoic area is present within the uterine cavity. The limited decidual reaction and the absence of an eccentric position of the sac suggest that this is a decidual cast. This patient had an ectopic pregnancy. **E.** Double decidual sac sign (DDSS). The separation between the decidua parietalis and the decidua capsularis forms a lucent line on ultrasound and forms the basis of this sign. **F.** A lucent line is seen around part of the gestational sac (arrows).

Except in the very rare instance of concurrent intrauterine and extrauterine pregnancy,[47] ectopic gestation can be excluded in these circumstances.

Using the standard transabdominal technique, a fetal pole or yolk sac is evident by week 6 after the last menstrual period. Using a vaginal probe, the fetus or

yolk sac can generally be resolved by day 32 to 35 from the last menstruation. Demonstration of a sac within the uterus without demonstrating fetus or a yolk sac is also good evidence of an intrauterine pregnancy if certain criteria are met. If the sac demonstrates the double decidual sac sign (DDSS) or

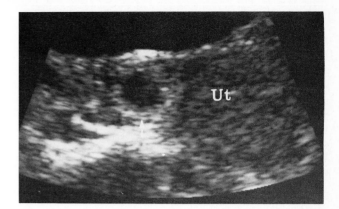

Figure 21–21. Ectopic pregnancy. Transverse scan through the pelvis. An extrauterine sac is seen in the right adnexa (arrow). The body of the uterus is adjacent (Ut).

the intradecidual sign (described earlier in the "Early Pregnancy" section), an intrauterine pregnancy may be called with confidence. If results of the patient's pregnancy test are positive but no intrauterine pregnancy can be demonstrated, the pregnancy is too early to be detected by ultrasound, the patient has aborted, or an ectopic gestation is present.

Is There Evidence of an Ectopic Gestation? When an ectopic pregnancy is suspected and no intrauterine pregnancy is demonstrated, about 43% of patients have an ectopic pregnancy.[43] The presence of any of the signs of ectopic pregnancy greatly improves the accuracy of this diagnosis. On occasion, a viable fetus can be seen within the adnexa, but this is only demonstrated in about 5% of cases with standard techniques (Fig. 21–21).[40] It will probably be higher when vaginal probes are used. In these cases, an ectopic pregnancy may be diagnosed with total confidence. If either a mass or free fluid is detected in

the pelvis, an ectopic pregnancy is present in 71% of patients (Fig. 21–22). In all cases, a search for free fluid in the abdomen should be conducted particularly around the liver, for occasionally the blood from a bleeding ectopic gestation collects in this region and is not detected within the pelvis.

When neither an intrauterine pregnancy nor signs of an ectopic pregnancy are seen, the differential diagnosis remains as before: an intrauterine pregnancy too early to see, an abortion, or an ectopic pregnancy. Unfortunately, approximately 20% of women with an ectopic pregnancy demonstrate neither adnexal mass nor pelvic fluid. The physician must therefore determine on clinical grounds what to do next. Three alternatives are reasonable: (1) an immediate laparoscopy, if suspicion for ectopic pregnancy is high; (2) when the most likely diagnosis is early abortion, dilation and curettage to determine whether chorionic villi are present; and (3) a repeat ultrasound in 4 to 5 days, and serial estimates of the β-HCG levels.

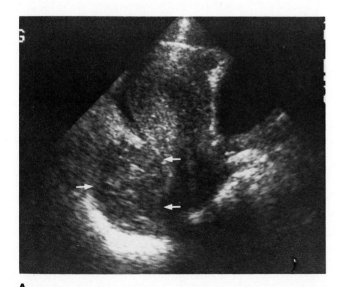

A

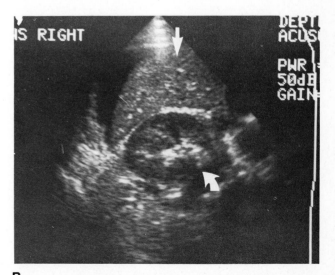

B

Figure 21–22. Ectopic pregnancy. **A.** No intrauterine sac is present. Some fluid is present around the uterus and a mass representing thrombus is present in the cul-de-sac (arrows). **B.** Fluid is demonstrated around the liver (straight arrow) and kidney (curved arrow). All signs suggest ruptured ectopic pregnancy.

REFERENCES

1. Hackeloer BJ: Ultrasonic demonstration of follicular development. *Lancet* 1:941, 1978.
2. American Institute of Ultrasound in Medicine: *Safety Considerations for Diagnostic Ultrasound Equipment.* Bethesda, AIUM, 1985.
3. National Institutes of Health: Diagnostic ultrasound imaging in pregnancy. Publication no. 84-667. Bethesda, NIH, 1984.
4. Rifkin MD, Foy PM, Kurtz AB, Pasto ME, Goldberg BB: The role of diagnostic ultrasonography in varicocele evaluation. *J Ultrasound Med* 2:271, 1983.
5. Mostof FK: Testes, scrotum and penis, in Anderson WAD, Kissure JM (eds): *Pathology.* St. Louis, CV Mosby, 1977, p 1013.
6. Hricak M., Hoddick WK: Scrotal ultrasound, in Hricak M (ed): *Genitourinary Ultrasound.* New York, Churchill Livingstone, 1986, pp 219–240.
7. Dubin TS, Amelar RD: Etiologic factors in 1294 consecutive cases of male infertility. *Fertil Steril* 22:469, 1971.
8. Giorlandino C, Gleicher N, Nanni C, et al: The sonographic picture of endometrium in spontaneous and induced cycles. *Fertil Steril* 47:508, 1987.
9. McArdle CR, Berezin A: Ultrasound demonstration of uterus subseptus. *J Clin Ultrasound* 8:139, 1980.
10. Friedman H, Vogelzang RL, Mendelson EB, Neiman HL, Cohen M: Endometriosis detection by ultrasound with laparascopic correlation. *Radiology* 157:217, 1985.
11. Hann LE, Hall DA, McArdle CR, Seibel MM: Polycystic ovarian disease: Sonographic spectrum. *Radiology* 150:531, 1984.
12. Luikkonen S, Koskimies AL, Tenhunen A, Ylostalo P: Diagnosis of luteinized unruptured follicle (LUF) syndrome by ultrasound. *Fertil Steril* 41:26, 1984.
13. Hackeloer BJ, Fleming R, Robinson MP, Adam AH, Coutts JR: Correlation of ultrasonic and endocrinologic assessment of human follicular development. *Am J Obstet Gynecol* 135:122, 1979.
14. Ritchie WG: Ultrasound in the evaluation of normal and induced ovulation. *Fertil Steril* 43:167, 1985.
15. Hodgen GD: The dominant ovarian follicle. *Fertil Steril* 38:281, 1982.
16. Picker RH, Smith DH, Tucker MM, Saunders DM: Ultrasonic signs of imminent ovulation. *J Clin Ultrasound* 11:1, 1983.
17. O'Herlihy C, de Crespigny L, Robinson HP: Monitoring ovarian follicular development with real time ultrasound. *Br J Obstet Gynaecol* 87:613, 1980.
18. Queenan JT, O'Brien GD, Bains LM, et al: Ultrasound scanning of the ovaries to detect ovulation. *Fertil Steril* 34:105, 1980.
19. Ritchie WG: Sonographic evaluation of normal and induced ovulation. *Radiology* 161:1, 1986.
20. Seibel MM, McArdle CR, Thompson IE, Berger MJ, Taymor ML: The role of ultrasound in ovulation induction: A critical appraisal. *Fertil Steril* 36:573, 1981.
21. Zacur HA: Ovulation induction with gonadotropin-releasing hormone. *Fertil Steril* 44:435, 1985.
22. McArdle CR, Seibel MM, Weinstein F, et al: Induction of ovulation monitored by ultrasound. *Radiology* 148:809, 1983.
23. Seibel MM: A new era in reproductive technology: In vitro fertilization, gamete intra fallopian transfer and donated gametes and embryos. *N Engl J Med* 318:828, 1988.
24. Buttery B, Trouson A, McMaster R, Wood C: Evaluation of diagnostic ultrasound as a parameter of follicular development in an in vitro fertilization program. *Fertil Steril* 39:458, 1983.
25. Bryce RL, Shuter B, Sinosich MJ, et al: The value of ultrasound, gonadotropin, and estradiol measurements for precise ovulation prediction. *Fertil Steril* 37:42, 1982.
26. Kerin JF, Edmonds DK, Warnes GM, et al: Morphological and functional relationships of graafian follicle growth to ovulation in women using ultrasonic, laparoscopic and biochemical measurements. *Br J Obstet Gynaecol* 88:81, 1981.
27. Mantzavinos T, Garcia JE, Jones HW: Ultrasound measurement of ovarian follicles stimulated by human gonadotropins for oocyte retrieval and in vitro fertilization. *Fertil Steril* 40:461, 1983.
28. Marrs RP, Vargyas JM, March CM: Correlation of ultrasonic and endocrinologic measurements in human menopausal gonadotropin therapy. *Am J Obstet Gynecol* 145:417, 1983.
29. Schenker JG, Weinstein D: Ovarian hyperstimulation syndrome: A current survey. *Fertil Steril* 30:255, 1978.
30. McArdle CR, Seibel MM, Hann LE, Weinstein F, Taymor ML: The diagnosis of ovarian hyperstimulation (OHS): The impact of ultrasound. *Fertil Steril* 39:464, 1983.
31. Blankstein J, Shalev J, Saadon T, et al: Ovarian hyperstimulation syndrome: Prediction by number and size of preovulatory follicles. *Fertil Steril* 47:597, 1987.
32. Sallan HN, Marinho AO, Collins WP, Rodeck CH, Campbell S: Monitoring gonadotropin therapy by real time ultrasonic scanning of ovarian follicles. *Br J Obstet Gynaecol* 89:155, 1982.
33. Lenz S, Lauritsen JG: Ultrasonically guided percutaneous aspiration of human follicles under local anesthesia: A new method of collecting oocytes for in vitro fertilization. *Fertil Steril* 38:673, 1982.
34. Lewin A, Laufer N, Rabinowitz R, et al: Ultrasonically guided oocyte collection under local anesthesia: The first choice method for in vitro fertilization—A comparative study with laparoscopy. *Fertil Steril* 46:257, 1986.
35. Parsons J, Riddle A, Booker M, et al: Oocyte retrieval for in vitro fertilization by ultrasonically guided needle aspiration via the urethra. *Lancet* 1:1076, 1985.
36. Dellenbach P, Nisand I, Moneau L, et al: Transvaginal sonographically controlled follicle puncture for oocyte retrieval. *Fertil Steril* 44:656, 1985.
37. Russel J, DeCherney AH, Hobbins J: A new transvaginal probe and biopsy guide for oocyte retrieval. *Fertil Steril* 47:656, 1985.
38. Jansen RP, Anderson JC: Catheterisation of the fallopian tubes from the vagina. *Lancet* 2:309, 1987.
39. Bernard KG, Cooperberg PL: Sonographic differentiation between blighted ovum and early viable pregnancy. *AJR* 144:597, 1985.
40. Yeh H, Goodman JD, Carr L, Rabinovitz JG: Intradecidual sign: A US criterion for early intrauterine pregnancy. *Radiology* 161:463, 1986.
41. Bradley WA, Fiske CE, Filly RA: The double decidual sac sign of early pregnancy: Use in exclusion of ectopic pregnancy. *Radiology* 143:223, 1982.
42. Weinstein L, Morris MB, Dotters D, Christian CD: Ectopic pregnancy—A new surgical epidemic. *Obstet Gynecol* 61:698, 1983.
43. Filly RA: Ectopic pregnancy: The role of sonography. *Radiology* 163:661, 1987.
44. Nyberg DA, Filly RA, Duarte DLD, Laing FC, Mahoney BS: Abnormal pregnancy: Early diagnosis by US and serum chorionic gonadotropin levels. *Radiology* 158:393, 1986.
45. Nyberg DA, Filly RA, Mahoney BS, et al: Early gestation: Correlation of HCG levels and sonographic identification. *AJR* 144:951, 1985.
46. Timor-Tritsch IE, Shraga R, Thaler I: Review of transvaginal ultrasonography: A description with clinical application. *Ultrasound Q* 6:1, 1988.
47. Hann LE, Bachman DB, McArdle CR: Co-existent intrauterine and ectopic pregnancy: A re-evaluation. *Radiology* 152:151, 1984.

PART VII

Hormonal Treatment of Female Infertility

CHAPTER 22

Ovulation Initiation: Clomiphene Citrate

Eli Y. Adashi

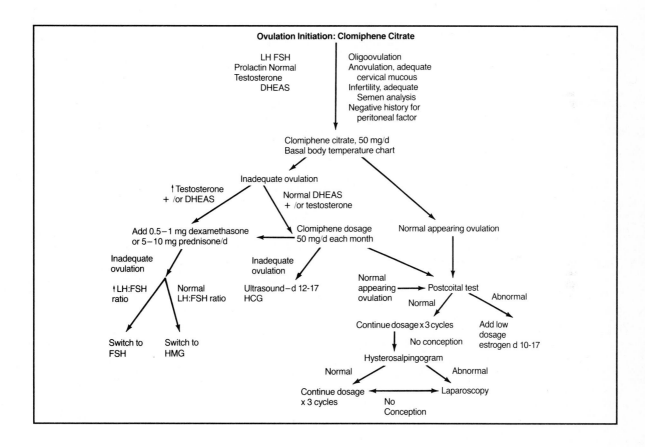

Synthesized in 1956, clomiphene citrate was first used in clinical trials as early as 1960 (Fig. 22–1). These efforts were followed in short sequence by the appearance of the first published report describing the successful use of the drug in inducing ovulation in humans.[2] Specifically, clomiphene citrate (still known as MRL/41) was shown to effect ovulation in 28 of 36 women with chronic anovulation; subsequent confirmatory reports followed.[3-11] An investi-

gational new drug application having been filed in 1962, approval for widespread clinical use was ultimately granted by the Food and Drug Administration (FDA) in 1967 with the stipulation that the total dosage consumed per cycle not exceed 750 mg. At this time, the original William S. Merrell Company patent rights[12] have expired, leading to the introduction of preparations listed under brand names other than Clomid, such as Serophene, a product of Serono

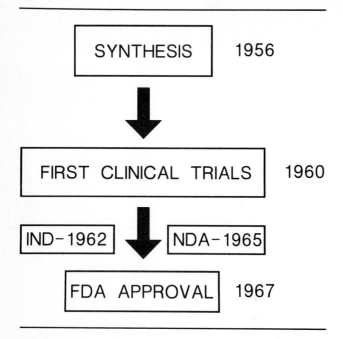

SYNTHESIS 1956

FIRST CLINICAL TRIALS 1960

IND-1962 NDA-1965

FDA APPROVAL 1967

Figure 22–1. Developmental landmarks of clomiphene citrate. IND = investigational new drug application; NDA = new drug application.

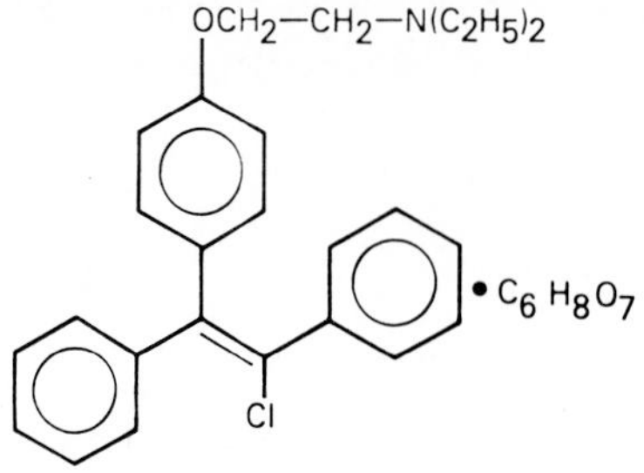

OCH₂-CH₂-N(C₂H₅)₂

• C₆H₈O₇

Cl

2-[p-(2-chloro-1,2-diphenylvinyl) phenoxy] triethylamine dihydrogen citrate

Figure 22–2. Structural formula of clomiphene citrate.

Laboratories (Randolph, MA). By most accounts, the efficacy of the various brands of clomiphene citrate appears comparable.

PHARMACOLOGY

Clomiphene citrate is a triphenylchloroethylene derivative in which the 4 hydrogen atoms of the ethylene core have been substituted with 3 phenyl rings and a chloride anion, respectively (Fig. 22–2). One of the 3 phenyl rings bears an aminoalkoxy $(OCH_2\text{-}CH_2\text{-}N[C_2K_5]_2)$ side chain, the significance of which to clomiphene citrate's action remains uncertain. The dihydrogen citrate moiety $(C_6H_8O_7)$ ac-

counts for the fact that commercially available preparations in clinical use represent the dihydrogen citrate salt form of clomiphene proper. Clomiphene citrate is available as a racemic mixture of two stereochemical isomers referred to as the trans (62%) and cis (38%) isomers, respectively (Fig. 22–3). In certain parts of the world the drug is available in its cis form as a 10-mg tablet, which is reportedly equipotent with the 50-mg tablet sold in the United States. Limited experience suggests that the clinical utility of clomiphene citrate may indeed be due to its cis isomer.[13,14] It remains uncertain, however, whether cis clomiphene citrate is more effective than clomiphene citrate proper in terms of ovulation and conception rates.[15–18]

A nonsteroidal estrogen, clomiphene citrate is capable of interacting with estrogen receptor-binding proteins not unlike native estrogens.[19] The nature of the interaction may differ from that of the naturally occurring ligand. Specifically, the drug is known for its propensity to prolong nuclear receptor occupancy.[20–22] Indeed, it may occupy nuclear receptor sites for weeks at a time, as compared with native estrogens capable of clearing the cell within 24 hours. Of significance, clomiphene does not display proges-

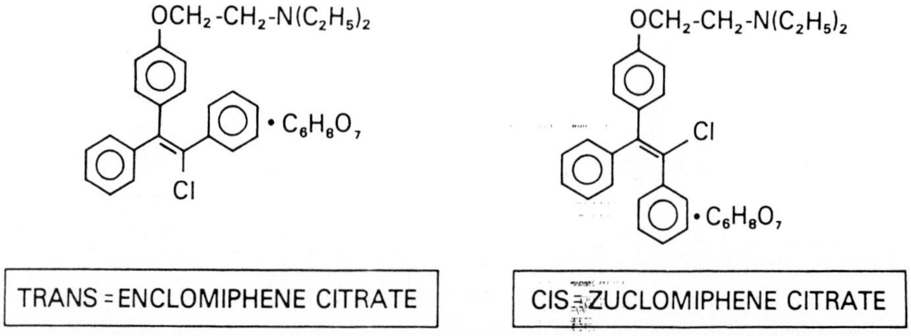

OCH₂-CH₂-N(C₂H₅)₂

• C₆H₈O₇

Cl

OCH₂-CH₂-N(C₂H₅)₂

Cl

• C₆H₈O₇

Figure 22–3. Sterochemical isomers of clomiphene citrate.

TRANS = ENCLOMIPHENE CITRATE

CIS = ZUCLOMIPHENE CITRATE

tational, corticotropic, androgenic, or antiandrogenic properties.

Studies with ^{14}C-labeled clomiphene citrate in humans disclosed that it is readily absorbed and that it is excreted primarily in the feces.[23-25] Computations based on a half-life estimate of 5 days suggest finite residual drug concentrations until and possibly beyond midcycle. The role of the residual at midcycle in the ovulatory agenda remains uncertain.[26]

ADMINISTRATION

Indications

The primary indication for the use of clomiphene citrate is normotropic (or inappropriate) gonadotropic, normoprolactinemic, anovulatory infertility.[27-29] Eligible patients are likely to be afflicted with a chronic anovulatory disorder often dating back to puberty. They are also likely to be well estrogenized as assessed by progestin-induced withdrawal bleeding, the circulating levels of estrone and extradiol-17β, and the occasional finding of abnormal endometrial growth such as cystic hyperplasia. Of significance, it is the adequate estrogen milieu of eligible patients that resulted in the suggestion that clomiphene citrate may initiate ovulation by virtue of its antiestrogenic property. In contrast, initiation of ovulation with this compound is generally unsuccessful in hypogonadotropic (estrogen-poor) women, although an empirical trial may be in order.[30-32] Although hyperprolactinemic chronic anovulation may respond to the agent,[33] such patients should be managed with a dopamine receptor agonist such as bromocriptine. Furthermore, empirical use of clomiphene in normally ovulating women to "enhance fertility" is not warranted.

Contraindications

Pregnancy. The inadvertent administration of clomiphene citrate during pregnancy might occur under unmonitored circumstances wherein absence of a period after a clomiphene cycle may be taken to mean an apparent treatment failure. Thus, the old clinical dictum of no period, no clomiphene citrate appears to be just as timely now as it was when the drug was originally formulated. Increased physician awareness, basal body temperature charting, and pregnancy testing should minimize if not eliminate the drug's use during early pregnancy.

Liver Dysfunction. Liver disease or a history of liver dysfunction is generally viewed as a contraindication to the use of clomiphene citrate. Because the drug is metabolized, if only in part when administered in the

setting of suboptimal liver function, its effects may prove unmanageable and even harmful.

Ovarian Cysts. Because clomiphene citrate is capable of stimulating follicular growth, further enlargement of a preexisting ovarian cyst may prove potentially harmful,[34,35] such as in the rare occurrence of massive ovarian enlargement.[36] Instead, allowances must be made for the ovary to return to normal size either spontaneously over time or with the use of combination oral contraceptives.

Vision Symptoms. Withholding clomiphene citrate on the basis of its causing vision symptoms is a precautionary measure for which little scientific support exists. Discontinuation appears warranted if such symptoms do occur, however, because the use of the agent is elective and because unforeseen ophthalmologic sequelae may thus be avoided.

Monitoring

The use of clomiphene citrate generally does not require intense monitoring. Basal body temperature charting as an adjunctive measure is recommended, however, given its low cost, simplicity, and harmlessness. Other monitoring options might also be considered.

Steroidogenic Monitoring. The so-called triple 7 regimen is based on the anticipation that the successful initiation of ovulation with clomiphene citrate is marked by unique alterations in serum levels of estradiol-17β and progesterone.[37] Specifically, documentation is sought for a preovulatory estradiol-17β rise and a subsequent rise in luteal progesterone level.[38,39] By timing the various hormonal determinations relative to the last oral dose of clomiphene, the triple 7 regimen can be employed whether clomiphene is administered for 5, 7, or 10 days.

The protocol used at the University of Maryland calls for determining the circulating levels of estradiol-17β 7 days after the last clomiphene tablet (Fig. 22-4). Accordingly, monitoring for estradiol-17β occurs well within the projected window of ovulation, that is, 5 to 10 days after the last oral dose. Using this approach, a preovulatory estradiol-17β rise is commonly detected assuming successful follicular recruitment, selection, and assertion of dominance. Progesterone sampling is generally carried out 7 days later—that is, 14 days after the last oral dose of clomiphene citrate—thereby optimizing the detection of a possible luteal rise. A follow-up office visit is scheduled 7 days later, 21 days after the last clomiphene tablet.

Although this regimen involves two hormonal determinations in the course of a cycle, useful

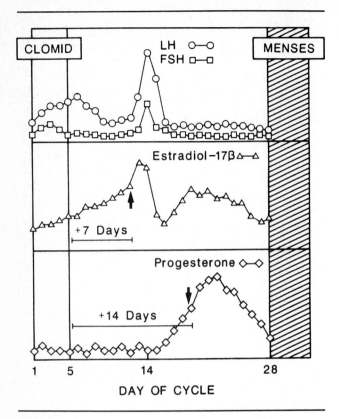

Figure 22–4. Hormonal monitoring of clomiphene-initiated ovulation.

TABLE 22–1. DOSE EFFECTS OF CLOMIPHENE CITRATE

Dose (mg)	Ovulatory Rate (%)	Conception Rate (%)
50	52.1	52.8
100	21.9	20.7
150	12.3	9.8
200	6.9	8.8
250	4.9	6.2

From Gysler et al.[44] Reproduced with permission.

information may be derived under circumstances characterized by apparent lack of response, for example, when basal body temperature charting remains inconclusive or in the face of an apparent treatment failure. Under these circumstances, hormonal monitoring yields indispensible information relative to the occurrence of ovulation or the lack thereof.

Sonographic Monitoring of Follicular Development. Now widely available, ultrasound may be employed independent of or concurrently with hormonal monitoring.[40,41] Best results may be anticipated by combining several monitoring modalities.

Establishing the Dosage

The recommended starting dosage is 50 mg daily for a total of 5 days. Although an unequivocal relationship between dose level and multiple gestation has not been demonstrated, it is likely that such correlation does exist. It is thus suggested that use be made of the lowest dose of clomiphene citrate consistent with successful outcome. Therapy may be initiated at any time in the absence of recent uterine bleeding, and in patients with chronic anovulation, treatment may be started at any time. Indeed, uterine bleeding, either spontaneous or induced, is not imperative

prior to initiating ovulation. More commonly, treatment is started on or about the 5th day of the cycle after progestin-induced bleeding or spontaneous dysfunctional uterine bleeding, although an earlier starting date is perfectly acceptable.

The simplest protocols call for graded incremental therapy when the subsequent cycle dosage proves ineffective in inducing ovulation. Such decisions can and should be made immediately after the treatment cycle in question. In the absence of ovulation, new treatment courses may begin as early as 30 days after initiation of the previous cycle. Lack of response to 200 or 250 mg daily for 5 days suggests that a change of course is in order; however, the vast majority of pregnancies occur at dosages of 150 mg daily or less (Table 22–1).

Once an ovulatory dosage is obtained, additional modification is neither advantageous nor required. Instead, a 4 to 6-month effort at conception is indicated prior to any further intervention. This is due to the finding that most clomiphene-citrate-associated conceptions[44] are anticipated within the first 6 ovulatory cycles (Table 22–2). Intercourse every other day for 1 week beginning 4 days after the last day of clomiphene administration ensures optimal timing for conception.

TABLE 22–2. CLOMIPHENE CITRATE-RELATED CONCEPTIONS: EFFECT OF DURATION OF TREATMENT

Ovulatory Cycle	Cumulative Conceptions (%)
1	51.8
2	76.7
3	84.5
4	91.2
5	95.4
≥6	100.0

From Gysler et al.[44] Reproduced with permission.

OVULATION FAILURE

Total Lack of Response

Total lack of response refers to the absence of follicular development and the consequent lack of ovulation (Fig. 22–5). Under these circumstances, consideration might be given to increasing the duration of clomiphene therapy.[45–47] Indeed, it has long been recognized that prolonged administration of relatively low doses may succeed where shorter-term high-dose regimens have failed. Although the mechanism(s) underlying this phenomenon remain uncertain, it is tempting to speculate that this form of therapy results in more persistent and seemingly more efficient increments in release of pituitary gonadotropins with consequent ovarian stimulation.

In addition, consideration may be given to dexamethasone supplementation.[48–55] The mechanism(s) underlying the ability of dexamethasone to synergize with clomiphene citrate are unknown, but it is abundantly clear that these two agents may promote ovulation initiation, particularly in the face of elevated dehydroepiandrosterone sulfate. It remains unknown whether dexamethasone lowers the circulating levels of adrenal androgens (which might otherwise inhibit folliculogenesis or aromatase activ-

ity), or whether glucocorticoids may synergize with clomiphene citrate at the level of the hypothalamus— that is, participate in the release of hypothalamic gonadotropin-releasing hormone (GnRH).[56]

Partial Lack of Response

Clomiphene-citrate-associated ovulation failure need not be complete. The drug may bring about follicular maturation and progressive increments in serum estradiol-17β (Fig. 22–6). Despite a seemingly adequate preovulatory rise in estradiol-17β, however, ovulation may fail to occur for reasons that remain largely unknown. Although ovulation, and obviously conception, will not occur, the apparent lack of a midcycle gonadotropin surge can be bypassed by the exogenous administration of human chorionic gonadotropin (HCG).

It is anticipated that hormonal monitoring and follicle ultrasound measurements will precisely identify those patients in whom clomiphene results in follicular maturation but not ovulation, and who are candidates for HCG administration. Failure to use these adjunctive modalities may result in the administration of HCG either unnecessarily or at a suboptimal time.

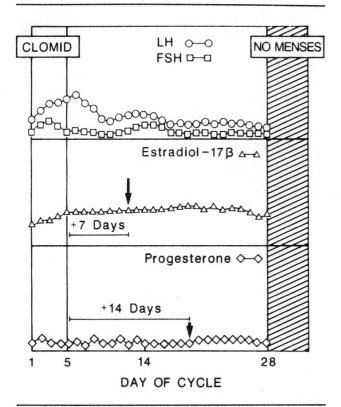

Figure 22–5. Anovulatory response to clomiphene.

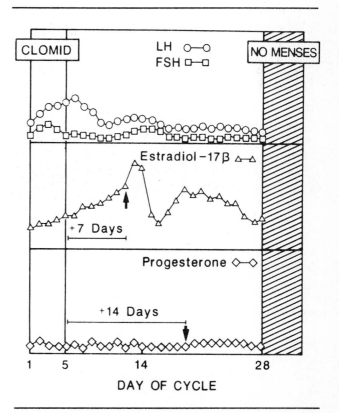

Figure 22–6. Anovulatory response to clomiphene despite pre-ovulatory rise in estradiol.

CONCEPTION FAILURE

Failure to conceive refers to the lack of conception in the face of an apparent ovulatory pattern. This requires that clomiphene-citrate-associated luteal phase dysfunction be ruled out.[57-59] In addition, other possible concurrent infertility factors (for example, male or tuboperitoneal) must be evaluated. If not properly evaluated before-hand.

Although the possible adverse effect of clomiphene on the cervical mucus deserves further consideration, the existence or significance of this complication remains a matter of debate.[44,60-66] Repeating the postcoital test after each successive dosage increment should obviate any deleterious effects of the drug on cervical mucus.

OVULATION AND CONCEPTION RATES

Whereas approximately 80% of well-selected patients treated with clomiphene can be expected to ovulate, only about 40% will ultimately conceive.[67,68] This apparent discrepancy may be more apparent than real, and may well involve other causes of infertility or loss to follow up. Indeed, conception rates approaching 90% have been reported[42,43] in the absence of other infertility factors. In addition, using life table analysis to correct for loss to follow-up, one group demonstrated that the conception rate per ovulatory cycle is the same in clomiphene cycles as it is for spontaneously encountered cycles.[69] Moreover, the pregnancy rate in 70 patients ovulating for 3 cycles was 55.7%, comparable to that observed in the population at large.[70] Finally, another report further documents that in otherwise healthy patients, the monthly conception rate in clomiphene-intitiated cycles does not differ from that expected in women who discontinued diaphragm contraception.[71] Taken together, these findings suggest that pregnancy rates in clomiphene-citrate-initiated ovulation may approach that of spontaneously occurring cycles, provided therapy is sustained for the required length of time.

ADVERSE EFFECTS

Multiple Pregnancies

Multiple gestation[72,73] is likely due to the ability of clomiphene citrate to stimulate a pronounced rise in the circulating levels of pituitary gonadotropins. This phenomenon was stressed by the finding that the mean early follicular levels of follicle-stimulating hormone (FSH) and luteinizing hormone (LH) were significantly higher in women given the drug than those in untreated controls.[74] Representing primarily an increase in pulse frequency, this relatively acute burst of gonadotropins may well support the growth of numerous follicles. Consequently, the relative increase in the frequency of multiple gestation associated with clomiphene therapy is likely to be accounted for by multiple ovulation rather than zygotic cleavage. Rates established in earlier reports have ranged from 6.25 to 12.3%.[73,75,76]

Hot Flushes

Reportedly occuring in up to 11% of patients, clomiphene-citrate-associated hot flushes are rarely severe and clearly reversible.[77] Although the cellular mechanism(s) involved are unknown, the antiestrogenic properties of clomiphene may well be involved. According to this view, the clomiphene-associated hot flush, like its menopausal counterpart, is causally linked to net effective estrogenic deprivation. Inasmuch as the menopausal hot flush is a central neuroendocrine phenomenon, that associated with clomiphene is likely to represent a similar, if not identical situation.

Vision Symptoms

Vision symptoms with clomiphene therapy occur at an estimated rate of less than 2%.[73] Described as "blurring," or spots or flashes (scintillating scotomata), such symptoms have been correlated with a high total dose. The underlying mechanism(s) have not been established, but this side effect is considered self-limited.

Although measured visual acuity has not generally been affected, it can be severely (albeit reversibly) diminished in exceptional circumstances. As a matter of prudence, patients having any vision symptoms should discontinue treatment, and consideration must be given to other modes of initiating ovulation.

Toxicity and Birth Defects

Clomiphene in LH-free medium and in concentrations that exceed the dosages used to induce ovulation is capable of inducing meiotic-like changes in follicle-enclosed mouse oocytes.[78] At higher concentrations, degenerative changes are noted in a high proportion of oocytes. Clomiphene itself, and not changes in follicular fluid steroid levels, is believed to be responsible. One study[79] observed abnormal karyotypes in nearly 50% of oocytes obtained from infertile women undergoing preovulatory oocyte retrieval after clomiphene stimulation. Whether this was true of fertile women not taking clomiphene was not addressed. Clomiphene has been found to increase the interval of time required for oocytes to reach metaphase I compared to oocytes obtained from natural cycles. Furthermore, the interval of time required for metaphase I oocytes to achieve metaphase II is statistically significantly shortened for clomiphene cycles (2.4 hours for clomiphene citrate versus 10 hours for natural cycles).[80] Although it has been suggested that clomiphene does increase the frequency of chromosomal anomalies in spontaneous abortions and recurrent molar pregnancies,[81,82] there is no evidence that it increases the prevalence of congenital malformations among live births.[83]

SUMMARY

Clomiphene citrate remains one of the most widely prescribed medications in the treatment of infertility. It is indicated for a wide range of ovulatory dysfunctions. Women who ovulate normally or who have hyperprolactinemia should not receive the drug. These two relative contraindications notwithstanding, clomiphene citrate remains a safe, effective, reasonably inexpensive method of treating infertility due to disorders of ovulation.

REFERENCES

1. Palopoli FP, Feil VJ, Allen RE, Holtkamp DE, Richardson A Jr: Substituted aminoalkoxytriarylhaloethylenes. J Med Chem 10:84, 1967.
2. Greenblatt RB, Barfield WE, Jungck EC, Ray AW: Induction of ovulation with MRL/41. JAMA 178:101, 1961.
3. Charles D: M.R.L. 41 in the treatment of secondary amenorrhea and endometrial hyperplasia. Lancet 2:278, 1962.
4. Greenblatt BR, Roy S, Mahesh VB, Barfield WE, Jungck EC: Induction of ovulation. Am J Obstet Gynecol 84:900, 1962.
5. Roy S, Greenblatt RB, Mahesh VB, Jungck EC: Clomiphene citrate: Further observations on its use in induction of ovulation in the human and on its mode of action. Fertil Steril 14:575, 1963.
6. Whitelaw MJ, Grams LR, Stamm WJ: Clomiphene citrate: Its uses and observations on its probable action. Am J Obstet Gynecol 90:355, 1964.
7. Puebla RA, Greenblatt RB: Clomiphene citrate in the management of anovulatory uterine bleeding. J Clin Endocrinol 24:863, 1964.
8. Kistner R: Further observations on the effects of clomiphene citrate in anovulatory females. Am J Obstet Gynecol 92:380, 1965.
9. Lamb EJ, Guderian AM: Clinical effects of clomiphene in anovulation. Obstet Gynecol 28:505, 1966.
10. Jones GS, Moraes-Ruehsen MD: Clomiphene citrate for improvement for ovarian function. Am J Obstet Gynecol 99:814, 1967.
11. MacGregor AH, Johnson JE, Bunde CA: Further clinical experience with clomiphene citrate, Fertil Steril 19:616, 1968.
12. Allen RE, Palopoli FP, Schumann EL, VanCampan MG Jr: U.S. Patent Office. 2:914, 561, 1959.
13. Charles D, Klein T, Lunn SF, Loraine JA: Clinical and endocrinological studies with the isomeric components of clomiphene citrate. J Obstet Gynaecol Br Commonw 76:1100, 1969.
14. Pandya G, Cohen MR: The effect of cis-isomer of clomiphene citrate (cisclomiphene) on cervical mucus and vaginal cytology, J Reprod Med 8:133, 1972.
15. MacLeod SC, Mitton DM, Parker AS, Tupper WRC: Experience with induction of ovulation. Am J Obstet Gynecol 108:814, 1970.
16. Murthy YS, Parekh MC, Arronet GH: Experience with clomiphene and cisclomiphene. Int J Fertil 16:66, 1971.
17. Van Campenhout J. Borreman E, Hyman A, et al: Induction of ovulation with cis clomiphene. Am J Obstet Gynecol 115:321, 1973.
18. Connaughton JF Jr, Garcia CR, Wallach EE: Induction of ovulation with cisclomiphene and a placebo. Obstet Gynecol 43:697, 1974.
19. Clark JH, Markaverich, BM: The agonistic-antagonistic properties of clomiphene: review. Pharmacol Ther 15:467, 1982.
20. Clark JH, Peck EJ Jr: Oestrogen receptors and antagonism of steroid hormone action. Nature 251:446, 1974.
21. Clark JH, Peck EJ Jr: Estrogen-receptor binding: Relationship to estrogen-induced responses. J Toxicol Environ Health 1:561, 1976.
22. Adashi EY, Hsueh AJW, Yen SSC: Alterations induced by clomiphene in the concentrations of oestrogen receptors in the uterus, pituitary gland and hypothalamus of female rats. J. Endocrinol 87:383, 1980.
23. Schreiber E, Johnson JE, Plotz EJ, Wiener M: Studies with ^{14}C labeled clomiphene citrate. Clin Res 14:287, 1966.
24. Holtkamp DE, Staples RE, Greslin JG, Davis RH: Pharmacodynamics of clomiphene in animals. Excerpta Med Int Congr Ser 133:68, 1966.
25. Clomiphene citrate (Clomid), the William S. Merrell Company. Clin Pharmacol Ther 8:891, 1967.
26. Terakawa N, Shimizu I, Tsutsumi H, Aono T, Matsumoto K: A possible role of clomiphene citrate in the control of pre-ovulatory LH surge during induction of ovulation. Acta Endocrinol 190:58, 1985.
27. Goldfarb AF, Crawford R: Polycystic ovarian disease, clomiphene and multiple pregnancies. Obstet Gynecol 34:307, 1969.
28. Yen SSC, Vela P, Ryan KJ: Effect of clomiphene citrate in polycystic ovary syndrome: Relationship between serum gonadotropin and corpus luteum function. J Clin Endocrinol 31:7, 1970.
29. Lunenfeld B, Insler V: Classification of amenorrhoeic states and their treatment by ovulation induction. Clin Endocrinol 3:223, 1974.
30. Spellacy WN, Cohen WD: Clomiphene treatment of prolonged secondary amenorrhea associated with pituitary gonadotropin deficiency. Am J Obstet Gynecol 97:943, 1967.
31. Marshall JC, Fraser TR: Amenorrhea in anorexia nervosa: Assessment and treatment with clomiphene citrate. Br Med J 4:590, 1971.
32. Garcia-Flores RF, Vazquez-Mendez J: Progressive dosages of clomiphene in hypothalamic anovulation. Fertil Steril 42:543, 1984.
33. Greenblatt RB, Faucher G, Mahesh VB, et al: Ovulation and pregnancy in the Chiari–Frommel syndrome. Report of 10 cases. Fertil Steril 17:742, 1966.
34. Roland M: Problems of ovulation induction with clomiphene citrate with report of a case of ovarian hyperstimulation. Obstet Gynecol 33:55, 1970.
35. Scommegna A, Lash SR: Ovarian overstimulation, massive ascites and singleton pregnancy after clomiphene. JAMA 207:753, 1969.
36. Southam AL, Janovski NA: Massive ovarian hyperstimulation with clomiphene citrate. JAMA 181:443, 1962.
37. Swyer GIM, Radwanska E, McGarrigle HHG: Plasma oestradiol and progesterone estimation for the monitoring of induction of ovulation with clomiphene and chorionic gonadotropin. Br J Obstet Gynaecol 82:794, 1975.
38. Fritz MA, Speroff L: The endocrinology of the menstrual cycle: the interaction of folliculogenesis and neuroendocrine mechanisms. Fertil Steril 38:509, 1982.
39. Fritz MA, Speroff L: Current concepts of the endocrine characteristics of normal menstrual function: The key to diagnosis and management of menstrual disorders. Clin Obstet Gynecol 26:647, 1983.
40. O'Herlihy C, de Crespigny LJC, Robinson HP: Monitoring ovarian follicular development with real-time ultrasound. Br J Obstet Gynaecol 87:613, 1980.
41. O'Herlihy C, Pepperell RJ, Robinson HP: Ultrasound timing of human chorionic gonadotropin administration in clomiphene stimulated cycles. Obstet Gynecol 59:40, 1982.
42. Rust LA, Israel R, Mishell DR Jr: An individualized graduated therapeutic regimen for clomiphene citrate. Am J Obstet Gynecol 120:785, 1974.
43. Drake TS, Tredway DR, Buchanan GC: Continued clinical experience with an increasing dosage regimen of clomiphene citrate administration. Fertil Steril 30:274, 1978.
44. Gysler M, March CM, Mishell DR Jr, Bailey EJ: A decade's experience with an individualized clomiphene treatment regimen including its effect on the postcoital test. Fertil Steril 37:161, 1982.
45. Adams R, Mishell DR Jr, Israel R: Treatment of refractory anovulation with increased dosage and prolonged duration of cyclic clomiphene citrate. Obstet Gynecol 39:562, 1972.
46. Lobo RA, Granger LR, Davajan V, Mishell DR JR: An extended regimen of clomiphene citrate in women unresponsive to standard therapy. Fertil Steril 27:762, 1982.
47. O'Herlihy C, Pepperell RJ, Brown JB, et al: Incremental clomiphene therapy: A new method for treating persistent anovulation. Obstet Gynecol 58:535,1981.
48. Chang RJ, Abraham GE: Effect of dexamethasone and clomiphene citrate on peripheral steroid levels and ovarian function in a hirsute amenorrheic patient. Fertil Steril 27:640, 1972.

49. Lobo RA, Paul W, March CM, Granger L, Kletzky OA: Clomiphene and dexamethasone in women unresponsive to clomiphene alone. *Obstet Gynecol* 60:497, 1982.

50. Check JH, Rakoff AE, Roy BK: Induction of ovulation with combined glucocorticoid and clomiphene citrate therapy in a minimally hirsute woman. *J Reprod Med* 19:159, 1977.

51. Lisse K: Combined and clomiphene–dexamethasone therapy in cases with resistance to clomiphene. *Zentrabl Gynakol* 102:645, 1980.

52. Higashiyama S, Yasuda J, Otubo K, Ikada H: Ovulation induction with prednisolone-clomiphene therapy in clomiphene failure. *Jpn J Fertil Steril* 26:1, 1981.

53. Diamant YZ, Evron S: Induction of ovulation by combined clomiphene citrate and dexamethasone treatment in clomiphene citrate nonresponders. *Eur J Obstet Gynaecol Reprod Biol* 11:335, 1981.

54. Daly DC, Walters CA, Soto-Albors CE, Tohan N, Riddick DH: A randomized study of dexamethasone in ovulation induction with clomiphene citrate. *Fertil Steril* 41:844, 1984.

55. Hoffman D, Lobo RA: Serum dehydroepiandrosterone sulfate and the use of clomiphene citrate in anovulatory women. *Fertil Steril* 43:196, 1985.

56. Miyake A, Tasaka K, Sakumoto T, Nagahara Y, Aono T: Hydrocortisone elicits the effect of clomiphene citrate on luteinizing hormone-releasing hormone in vitro. *Acta Endocrinol* 107:145, 1984.

57. Van Hall EV, Mastboom JL: Luteal phase insufficiency in patients treated with clomiphene. *Am J Obstet Gynecol* 103:165, 1969.

58. Jones GS, Maffezzoli RD, Strott CA, et al: Pathophysiology of reproductive failure after clomiphene-induced ovulation. *Am J Obstet Gynecol* 108:847, 1970.

59. Garcia J, Jones SG, Wentz AC: The use of clomiphene citrate. *Fertil Steril* 28:707, 1977.

60. Riley GM, Evans TN: Effects of clomiphene citrate on anovulatory ovarian function. *Am J Obstet Gynecol* 89:97, 1964.

61. Eichenbrenner I, Insler V, Serr DM, Salomy M, Faktor J: The effect of clomiphene on vaginal cytology and cervical mucus. *Harefuah* 78:171, 1970.

62. Graff G: Suppression of cervical mucus during clomiphene therapy. *Fertil Steril* 22:209, 1971.

63. Sharf M, Groff M, Kuzminski T: Quinestrol therapy in hypomucorrhea due to clomiphene. *Am J Obstet Gynecol* 110:423,1971.

64. Taubert H-D, Dericks-Tan JSE: High doses of estrogens do not interfere with the ovulation-inducing effect of clomiphene citrate. *Fertil Steril* 27:375,1976.

65. Van der Merwe JV: The effect of clomiphene and conjugated estrogens on cervical mucus. *S Afr Med J* 60:347, 1981.

66. Maxson WS, Pittaway DE, Herbert CM, Garner CH, Colston-Wentz A: Antiestrogenic effect of clomiphene citrate: Correlation with serum estradiol concentrations. *Fertil Steril* 42:356, 1984.

67. Whitelaw MJ, Kalman CG, Grams LR: The significance of the high ovulation rate versus the low pregnancy rate with Clomid. *Am J Obstet Gynecol* 107:865, 1970.

68. Hancock KW, Oakey RE: The low incidence of pregnancy following clomiphene therapy. *Int J Fertil* 18:49, 1973.

69. Lamb EJ, Colliflower WW, Williams JW: Endometrial histology and conception rates after clomiphene. *Obstet Gynecol* 39:389, 1972.

70. Gorlitsky GA, Kase NG, Speroff L: Ovulation and pregnancy rates with clomiphene citrate. *Obstet Gynecol* 51:265, 1978.

71. Hammond MG, Halme JK, Talbert LM: Factors affecting the pregnancy rate in clomiphene citrate induction of ovulation. *Obstet Gynecol* 62:196, 1983.

72. Kistner RW: The infertile woman. *J Nurs* 73:1937, 1973.

73. Asch RH, Greenblatt RB: Update on the safety and efficacy of clomiphene citrate as a therapeutic agent. *J Reprod Med* 17:175, 1976.

74. Ross GT, Cargille CM, Lipsett MB, et al: Pituitary and gonadal hormones in women during spontaneous and induced ovulatory cycles. *Recent Prog Horm Res* 26:1, 1970.

75. Atlay RD, Pennington GW: The use of clomiphene citrate and pituitary gonadotropin in successive pregnancies: the Sheffield quadruplets. *Am J Obstet Gynecol* 109:402, 1971.

76. Aiken RA: An account of the "Birmingham sextuplets." *J Obstet Gynaecol Br Commonw* 76:684, 1969.

77. Jones GS, De Moraes-Ruehsen M: Induction of ovulation with human gonadotropins and with clomiphene. *Fertil Steril* 16:461, 1965.

78. Laufer N, Pratt BM, DeCherney AH, et al: The in vivo-in vitro effects of clomiphene citrate on ovulation, fertilization and development of cultured mouse oocytes. *Am J Obstet Gynecol* 147:633, 1983.

79. Wramsby H, Fredga K, Liedholm P: Chromosome analysis of human oocytes recovered from preovulatory follicles in stimulated cycles. *N Engl J Med* 316:121, 1987.

80. Seibel MM, Smith DM: The effect of clomiphene citrate on human preovulatory oocyte maturation in vivo. *J In Vitro Fert* 6:3, 1989.

81. Boue JG, Boue A: Increased frequency of chromosomal anomalies in abortions after induced ovulation. *Lancet* 1:679, 1973.

82. Mor-Joseph S, Anteby SO, Granat M, Brzezinski A, Evron S: Recurrent molar pregnancies associated with clomiphene citrate and human menopausal gonadotropins. *Am J Obstet Gynecol* 151:1095, 1985.

83. Harlap S: Ovulation induction and congenital malformations. *Lancet* 2:961, 1976.

CHAPTER 23

Ovulation Induction: HMG

Bruno Lunenfeld, Eitan Lunenfeld

HISTORICAL PERSPECTIVES

One of the most far-reaching discoveries ever made in reproductive biology was that the male and female reproductive systems are under the functional control of the anterior hypophysis. Crowe and associates[1] demonstrated in 1909 that partial hypophysectomy in the adult dog provoked atrophy of the reproductive organs and prevented sexual development in juvenile animals. It took nearly 20 years to obtain firm evidence that the male and female reproductive systems were under the functional control of the pituitary gland. This was based on the demonstration that implantation of anterior pituitary glands evoked rapid development of sexual puberty in immature animals[2]; hypophysectomized immature male and female animals failed to mature sexually[3]; and in the adult hypophysectomized animal, sexual characteristics regressed rapidly.

Shortly afterward the three gonadotropic factors were discovered. Follicle-stimulating hormone (FSH), as its name indicates, is primarily responsible for follicular recruitment, selection, growth, and ripening. Luteinizing hormone (LH) is responsible for the final maturation of the FSH-stimulated follicles, ovulation, and transformation of the follicular remnants into functional corpora lutea. Human chorionic gonadotropin (HCG), the hormone secreted by the trophoblastic cells, has biologic actions similar to those of LH.

These hormones, in the past obtained from pregnant mares' serum (PMS) and animal pituitaries, have been used clinically to induce ovulation. Gonadotropins of animal origin are no longer used for this purpose because humans rapidly produce antibodies to nonprimate gonadotropins that neutralize their clinical effects. The antibodies formed tend to be specific for the preparations injected and do not affect the action of gonadotropins obtained from other sources. In 1954 it was demonstrated that kaolin extracts from pooled menopausal urine contained FSH and LH activity in comparable amounts.[4] These extracts prevented atrophy of Leydig cells and retained complete spermatogenesis in hypophysectomized rats. Based on these findings the authors predicted that such extracts could open up interesting therapeutic possibilities. In 1957 the same group demonstrated that these extracts were capable of inducing follicular growth and promotion of corpora lutea in hypophysectomized rats.[5] The recognition of the therapeutic potential of human gonadotropins stimulated the search for suitable sources for their extraction. Most investigators were purifying gonadotropins from menopausal urine (HMG); however, a Stockholm group obtained them by processing human pituitaries (HPG).

One pituitary contains as much FSH as 2 to 5 L of postmenopausal urine. A suitable product was obtained by single-fraction purification with ammonium sulfate or ethanol. Ovulation was successfully induced with HPG followed by HCG.[6]

The scarcity of postmortem pituitary glands required for the production of HPG eliminates the possibility of their widescale use, however. For this reason, attention was directed by pharmaceutical companies (Serono, Randolph, MA, and Organon, West Orange, NJ) to prepare purified extracts from menopausal urine for clinical use. The initial urinary extract was prepared by the kaolin–acetone method, purified first by ammonium acetate ethanol and then by permutit chromatography. This preparation is a potent ovarian stimulant in the human.[7] Three pregnancies resulted after 16 courses of treatment in 10 women.[8] Since that time, over 8,000 patients have been treated for more than 22,000 cycles, resulting in 3,120 pregnancies (Table 23–1).[9]

CHEMISTRY, CLEARANCE, AND PHYSIOLOGY

Since the 1960s the major elements of the mechanisms of action, control, and regulation of secretion of gonadotropins have been elucidated, and the structure of the hormones has been determined. Gonadotropins are glycoproteins with a molecular weight around 30,000 daltons and consisting of about 20% carbohydrate. The carbohydrate moieties in their molecules are fucose, manose, galactose, acetyl glucosamine, and N-acetyl neuraminic acid.[10] The sialic acid content varies widely among the glycoprotein hormones, from 20 residues in HCG and 5 in FSH to only 1 or 2 in LH. These differences are largely responsible for the variations in the isoelectric points of gonadotropins. The carbohydrate moieties are complex. They may be branched or straight chains, and they contain sialic acid as an important constituent, particularly at the ends of the chains.

Different sialic acid content also accounts for both the variation in molecular weight of the hormone isolated from various sources and the differences in biologic activity determined by in-vivo assays. The higher the sialic acid content, the longer the biologic half-life. Thus the increased amount of carbohydrate in HCG is responsible for the fact that its half-life is significantly longer than that of LH or FSH. Whereas the β-subunit of LH contains only one carbohydrate group, the β-subunit of HCG contains six. The function of these carbohydrate groups is not fully known, except that removing the terminal neuraminic acid (sialic acid) residues drastically shortens the half-lives of the circulating hormones in blood. For this reason, desialylated preparations of human LH, HCG, and FSH show considerably reduced biologic activity in vivo, but retain activity in

TABLE 23–1. INDUCTION OF OVULATION WITH HMG-HCG: RESULTS OF 15 TRIALS

	No. of Patients	No. of Cycles	No. (%) of Pregnancies
	756	1585	224 (33.0)
	1056	4008	552 (52.3)
	134	438	31 (23.1)
	101	343	62 (61.4)
	77	322	43 (55.8)
	228	463	101 (44.3)
	62	225	26 (41.9)
	1190	2798	334 (28.1)
	1107	3646	424 (38.3)
	442	1098	118 (26.7)
	320	?	163 (50.9)
	232	655	136 (58.6)
	40	159	33 (82.5)
	2166	6096	523 (24.2)
	95	320	72 (75.8)
Totals	8008	22,156	3120 (39.9)

From Lunenfeld et al.[9] Reproduced with permission.

either specific in-vitro biologic assays employing membrane receptors or isolated target cells. Therefore, attempting to measure these hormones by immunoassay or by in-vitro bioassay does not express their actual bioactivity in vivo. Deglycosylated hormones in vitro can act as competitive antagonists of the actions of the intact hormone on cyclic adenosine monophosphate production and to a lesser extent on steroid hormone biosynthesis.

The gonadotropic hormones consist of two hydrophobic, noncovalently associated α and β-subunits. The three-dimensional structure of each subunit is maintained by internally cross-linked disulfide bonds. Gonadotropic hormones can be disassociated into the individual subunits by denaturing agents (10 M urea at pH 4.5 or 1 M propionic acid).[11] The pure subunits possess limited biologic activity, but the activity is regenerated by allowing the two subunits to recombine. All of the gonadotropins as well as thyroid-stimulating hormone (TSH) share a common α-subunit of 92 amino acid residues in the same sequence, containing five disulfide bonds as well as two carbohydrate moieties at positions 52 and 78. The β-subunits of FSH, LH, and HCG are unique to each hormone and confer their biologic specificity; they have amino acid chains of variable lengths (116 to 147 amino acid residues) and contain six disulfide bonds. In the β-subunits of HCG, two branched-chain moieties are attached to asparagine at positions 13 and 30. Smaller, linear sugar groups are attached by o-serine linkage to serines within the unique HCG COOH-terminal peptide at residues 121, 127, 132, and 138. Highly purified FSH isolated from human pituitaries has a specific activity of 10,000 IU/mg, while FSH recovered from urine of postmenopausal women contains 1,255 IU/mg, and highly purified HCG has a specific activity of 11,000 to 13,500 IU/mg.

Methodologies that have allowed analysis of the genes and gene products showed that the two subunits of the gonadotropic hormones are translated from separate messenger RNAs[12] and both are synthesized as precursors. This is followed by cleavage of the signal peptide leader sequence by the signal peptidase. The nascent polypeptide α and β-subunits are then glycosylated by en bloc attachment of high-manose complex type oligosaccharides to two aspargine residues of each subunit. Excess manose and glucose residues are trimmed from the intermediates (Fig. 23–1). Thereafter, peripheral monosaccharides N-acetyl glucosamine, galactose, and N-acetyl neuraminic acid are attached sequentially to complete the oligosaccharide structures. The α and β-subunits then combine noncovalently in a two-step reaction to form the biologically active glycoproteins.[13]

Integrated genetics cloned the genes for HCG, LH, and FSH. Producing these glycoproteins by recombinant DNA technology has, however, met with a considerable number of obstacles. Insertion of the gene and expressing it in *Escherichia coli* produced polypeptides devoid of the carbohydrate chains. Expressing it in yeast yielded excess glycosylation. Thus efforts were made to express the gene in mammalian cells.

Initial results seem promising. It is expected that by the 1990s, recombinant DNA technology will produce sufficient amounts of gonadotropins in mammalian cells for clinical use.

Information regarding metabolism of gonadotropic hormones is scarce. It has been shown that purified preparations of human FSH, LH, and HCG injected intravenously into humans have serum half-lives (as determined by bioassays) of 180 to 240 minutes, 42 to 60 minutes, and 6 to 8 hours,

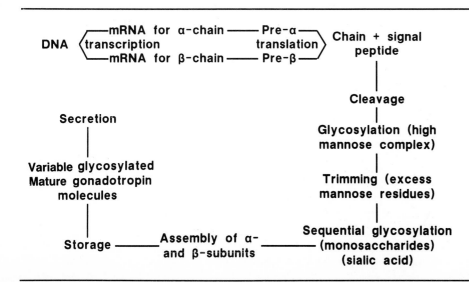

Figure 23–1. Schematic presentation of the main steps of gonadotropin production in the gonadotrope.

respectively. The half-lives of the α and β-subunits of LH were found to be only 16 minutes. The higher carbohydrate content of HCG (10%) is responsible for its significantly longer half-life than that of human FSH (5%) and LH (2%). Due to rapid hepatic clearance, removal of sialic acid from HCG reduces its half-life to minutes and results in correspondingly low biologic activity in vivo.

The mean metabolic clearance rate (MCR) of FSH in women has been determined to be 14 mL/minute; it has not been determined in men. The MCR of LH is 25 to 30 mL/minute in women regardless of ovulatory state, and is almost 50% higher in healthy men. The disappearance curves for both hormones are multiexponential, indicating distribution in more than three mathematical compartments. In premenopausal women, daily production rates of LH are 500 to 1,000 IU, with a marked preovulatory rise, whereas rates in postmenopausal women are 3,000 to 4,000 IU daily. These values indicate that the pituitary content of LH (and probably of FSH) is turned over once or twice daily, and that rapid biosynthesis of gonadotropins must be necessary to maintain the normal levels of pituitary storage and secretion. Only 3 to 10% of the daily production of FSH and LH is excreted in the urine in a biologically active form; however, the rate of urinary gonadotropin secretion may be used to reflect both physiologic and pathologic conditions. The recovery of exogenous gonadotropins in the urine of fertile and infertile subjects is 10 to 20% of the administered hormone. Urinary excretion of gonadotropins accounts for only 5% of the MCR. The MCR of HMG in hypogonadotropic subjects is 0.4 to 1.7 mL/minute.

FOLLICULAR DEVELOPMENT

Early studies based on animal experiments suggested that follicular development up to the antrum stage was gonadotropin independent.[14,15] In gonadotropin-deprived prepubertal mice, follicular development can proceed; however, it is markedly altered and retarded.[16] In women, it was suggested that it may take 10 weeks for a primordial follicle (oocyte surrounded by a single layer of granulosa cells) to develop into an antral follicle capable of gonadotropic responsiveness.[17] Final growth, maturation, and ovulation then occur within 2 weeks under optimal stimulation of FSH and LH, and normal ovarian response. Whereas several hundred primordial follicles initiate growth, no more than 20 precursor follicles are likely to be present at the beginning of the menstrual cycle.[18] All the other follicles degenerate at early stages of development. About 20 remain, and under physiologic conditions, some are selected for

further growth and development. Only one matures, reaches dominance, and ovulates. The others undergo atresia or luteinization (Fig. 23–2).

As follicles enter the gonadotropin-sensitive phase, it becomes apparent that a specific frequency and amplitude of gonadotropin-releasing hormone (GnRH) pulses are necessary to assure the proper milieu to accomplish this process.[19] FSH almost exclusively binds to membrane receptors on the granulosa cells, induces their multiplication, and stimulates biochemical processes such as aromatase activity, while LH stimulates thecal cell development and androgen production. The aromatase system converts androgens, diffusing into the granulosa cell layer to estrogens. Together with estrogens, FSH induces synthesis of FSH and LH receptors on the granulosa cells, leading to increased sensitivity of the growing follicle to gonadotropins.

On the other hand, LH, or LH-mediated androgens, inhibits the synthesis of both FSH and LH receptors, and thus is thought to play a major role in degeneration or atresia. Exogenous gonadotropin stimulation, specifically FSH, can save follicles from degeneration and permit multiple ovulation.[20] Disturbances in the pulsatile pattern of GnRH secretion or improper gonadotropin stimulation deranges follicular development, which may result in anovulation. The severity of this may range from hypoestrogenic amenorrhea to regular cycles with only subtle

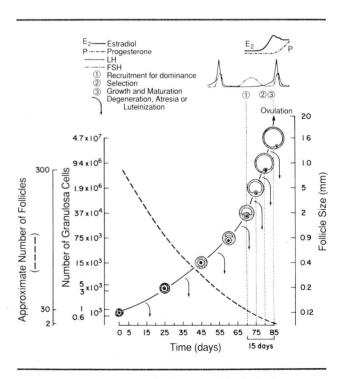

Figure 23–2. Recruitment, growth, and degeneration trajectory of primordial follicles.

abnormalities in follicular development and hormonal profiles in women with unexplained infertility.[21]

SELECTION OF PATIENTS FOR FIRST AND SECOND-LINE GONADOTROPIN THERAPY

The possibilities for classifying anovulatory patients are virtually unlimited, depending on the clinical laboratory facilities available and the purpose to be served. Every classification may be valuable as long as acceptable, measurable, and well-defined variables are used, and a reasonable compromise is achieved among accuracy, effort, and cost. The guidelines are based on up-to-date scientific information and technical advances. They are therapeutically oriented to gonadotropins whether as first or second-line therapy.

Hypothalamic–Pituitary Insufficiency
The etiology of amenorrhea in women who fail to have withdrawal vaginal bleeding after progesterone challenge may be due to target unresponsiveness or hypothalamic–pituitary insufficiency. Bleeding after cyclic estrogen–progesterone administration eliminates the diagnosis of uterine causes such as congenital abnormalities or severe uterine adhesion such as Asherman's syndrome. A low or normal FSH and LH level rules out ovarian failure and points to pituitary insufficiency.

All women with pituitary insufficiency benefit from HMG–HCG therapy. When using pulsatile GnRH, it is necessary to differentiate between hypothalamic insufficiency and pituitary failure. Patients with pituitary failure cannot respond to pulsatile GnRH (Fig. 23–3).

Hypothalamic Dysfunction with Normal Prolactin and Androgen Levels
Failure to ovulate in nonandrogenized, normoprolactinemic women secondary to chronic hypothalamic dysfunction is probably the most common cause of menstrual disorders. Patients in this category also have a variety of symptoms that may range from luteal phase defects to amenorrhea. This form of amenorrhea usually responds to progesterone challenge with vaginal bleeding.

Stress, alterations in body weight, and excessive athletic activity can result in chronic hypothalamic anovulation. If change in lifestyle does not restore ovulation, clomiphene citrate should be considered first. Only in women who fail to ovulate with doses of

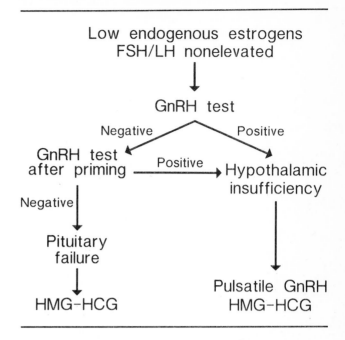

Figure 23–3. Algorithm for the differential diagnosis of amenorrhea in patients with low endogenous estrogens.

up to 150 mg/day for 5 days, or who do not conceive despite suggestive ovulation for 3 to 6 cycles, should HMG–HCG therapy be initiated.

Iatrogenically Induced Cervical Factor
When a patient with hypothalamic dysfunction with normal prolactin and androgen levels appears to respond well to treatment with clomiphene but fails to conceive, a postcoital test should be repeated. Should serial determinations of the cervical score[22] and well-timed postcoital tests reveal persistently poor cervical mucus with predominately immotile spermatozoa, a deleterious effect of clomiphene on the cervical mucus should be taken into consideration (Fig. 23–4).

Clomiphene citrate, acting as an antiestrogen, may severely depress the vaginal epithelium and, to a lesser degree, the endocervical crypts. Because clomiphene therapy results in multifollicular development, the elevated estrogen levels usually override this effect. In some cases, however, the antiestrogenic effect results in thick, tenacious mucus, which may prevent conception by hindering sperm migration through the cervical canal. The discrepancy between the ovulation rate and the conception rate after clomiphene therapy may in some cases be due to the suppressive effect of the drug on the uterine cervix. The use of estrogens in combination with clomiphene as a means of improving the quality of the cervical mucus remains a controversial issue. Low

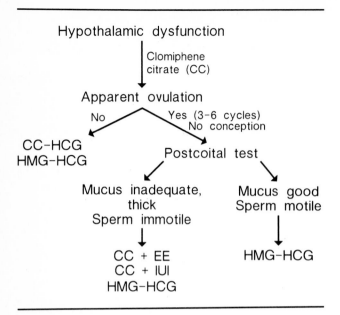

Figure 23–4. Iatrogenic cervical factor in patients with hypothalamic dysfunction treated with clomiphene citrate (CC).

dosages of synthetic estrogens such as ethinyl estradiol, 20 μg, or conjugated estrogens such as Premarin (Ayerst Laboratories, New York, NY), 0.3 mg daily on cycle days 10 to 17, are typical.

If the penetration of the cervical mucus by spermatozoa does not improve after treatment with estrogens in combination with clomiphene, artificial intrauterine insemination with the partner's sperm may be attempted. Therapy with HMG–HCG may also serve as a second-line therapy in such patients, as it induces ovulation without deleterious effect on the cervical mucus.

Premature Luteinization

Premature luteinization is a specific category of anovulation. It is frequently unrecognized, or misdiagnosed as unexplained infertility, luteal phase defect, or luteinized unruptured follicle (LUF) syndrome. It occurs if there is an untimely LH surge in response to rising estrogen at a time when the follicle is still immature. It can only be diagnosed if an LH

peak is detected in the presence of immature follicles as seen by ultrasonography. It can be speculated that this entity represents an exaggerated sensitivity of the pituitary to the rising levels of estrogen, resulting in an LH surge. This assumption may explain the failure of clomiphene citrate or HMG to restore ovulation in these women. Since both of these agents cause multiple follicular development with exaggerated estrogen responses, a premature LH peak is even more likely to occur. A rational therapeutic approach is to abolish the estrogen-evoked positive feedback mechanism. This can be effectively accomplished by the use of a potent GnRH agonist.[23]

Thus anovulation due to recurrent premature luteinization requires a triphasic therapeutic approach. A GnRH agonist is administered until the positive feedback is abolished (2 to 7 weeks). Thereafter, HMG is given in conjunction with the agonist until at least 1 follicle reaches maturation as judged by ultrasonography and estrogen levels. Then HCG is administered to induce ovulation (Fig. 23–5).

Hypothalamic–Pituitary Dysfunction Associated with Hyperandrogenism

The androgenized anovulatory patient typically has a past or present history of acne, seborrhea, and hirsutism that may or may not be associated with obesity. Elevated androgen production may arise from the ovaries, the adrenal cortex, or both. Accurately determining the predominant source assists in choosing the correct treatment to restore ovulation. Figure 23–6 illustrates such an approach.

An androgenized patient with normal or elevated testosterone levels who also has normal levels of dehydroepiandrosterone sulfate should be suspected as having polycystic ovary disease. An elevated LH:FSH ratio (greater than 3) is an additional characteristic feature of this entity. High-resolution ultrasound imaging of the pelvis provides anatomic confirmation of this diagnosis. Peripheral cysts of 4 to 6 mm average diameter and an echo-dense central stroma are typically observed. This corresponds well with the macroscopic appearance of the cut surface of the polycystic ovary. In patients with polycystic

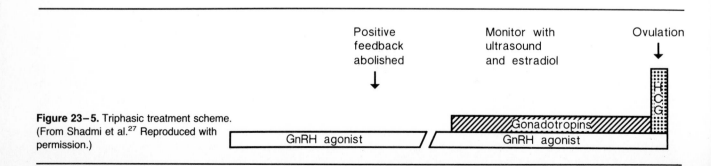

Figure 23–5. Triphasic treatment scheme. (From Shadmi et al.[27] Reproduced with permission.)

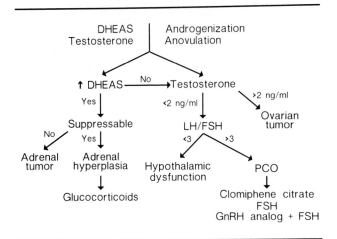

Figure 23–6. Algorithm for the differential diagnosis of androgenized women.

ovary disease, chronic increased LH secretion continuously stimulates the proliferation of stromal and thecal cells, and increases production of intraovarian and intrafollicular androgens. Intrafollicular androgens are associated with follicular atresia, probably through inhibition of both FSH and LH receptors. This mechanism fits the hormonal pattern and morphologic appearance described above.

Chronically elevated LH secretion may have manifold etiologies, however. It may be initiated through increased androstenedione–testosterone production from either an ovarian or adrenal source. Its peripheral conversion to estrone/estradiol, primarily in adipose tissue, enhances LH secretion. The relationship of obesity with this disease is unequivocal and its impact on the clinical expression of the syndrome most important; however, a hypothalamic–pituitary disorder as its origin cannot be excluded. The first-line treatment, regardless of etiology, is clomiphene citrate. This agent increases gonadotropin secretion and, despite an even further increase in LH levels in some women, allows selection, growth, and maturation of a single follicle. In other patients clomiphene citrate causes many follicles to grow and results in hyperstimulation. In those with an inappropriate response to clomiphene, gonadotropin therapy, preferably a purified FSH preparation, should be used to attempt to override the FSH:LH imbalance. In some cases FSH is capable of interrupting the self-perpetuating biochemical cycle of polycystic ovary disease.[24–26]

In women in whom both of these types of therapy fail, a more rational approach may be indicated. Long-term administration of GnRH analogs (GnRHa) has been shown to be effective in down-regulating pituitary gonadotropin secretion.[27] These agents were used successfully in conjunction with gonadotropins in 8 women with the syndrome who

had previously failed to conceive with exogenous gonadotropin therapy alone.[28] During GnRHa therapy, gonadotropin secretion diminishes and the FSH:LH imbalance is corrected within 3 to 4 weeks.[9,27] When this stage has been reached, treatment with HMG is initiated. Figure 23–7 illustrates this approach in a patient in whom other therapeutic regimens had failed and who conceived after this kind of triphasic therapy.

Empiric Use of HMG in Presumably Ovulating Women

Although the use of HMG–HCG in anovulatory women is widely accepted and of definite value, the applicability of these agents in ovulatory women such as those with unexplained infertility or luteal phase defect, and for mucus production in patients with a cervical factor, is not without controversy. The potential exists for ovarian hyperstimulation and multiple gestation. In contrast to these risks is the realization that in these women, empiric use of HMG is associated with a pregnancy rate of approximately 12%.[29] Although still low, this rate was significantly higher than those in corresponding control groups, and not dissimilar from rates achieved with in-vitro fertilization. Others, however, found pregnancy rates of 14% among untreated women with unexplained infertility.[30] Therefore, the empiric use of HMG remains of uncertain value.

PRINCIPLES OF OVULATION INDUCTION

To induce ovulation, FSH is necessary in the early phase of the cycle to recruit and select follicles. For growth and maturation, both FSH and LH are necessary. In cases of in-vitro fertilization where the aim is to obtain many oocytes, increased gonadotropin stimulation should theoretically commence during the early recruitment phase. To induce ovulation in vivo, the aim is the development of 1 or 2 mature follicles, and gonadotropin stimulation should be delayed until the selection phase (see Fig. 23–2).

Most gonadotropin preparations used for therapeutic purposes contain both FSH and LH in various proportions. It has been shown that administration of HMG or purified FSH can override the normal mechanism of ovarian follicular selection. It was demonstrated that in normogonadotropic patients, administration of HMG on day 2 produced significantly more follicles than administration from day 9.[31] Apparently, the earlier that FSH administration is started during the cycle (prior to the selection phase), the more follicles are recruited.

Although the timing and FSH content of the HMG preparation determine the number of follicles

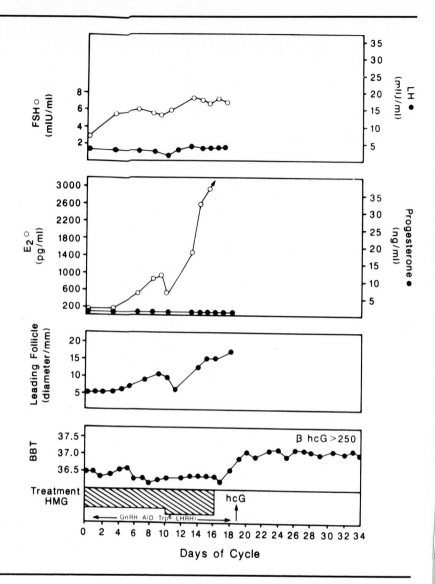

Figure 23–7. Profile of women who conceived after triphasic therapy. (From Shadmi et al.[27] Reproduced with permission.)

recruited and selected, the LH content determines the steroidogenic pattern. Final maturation of the follicles is brought about by the combination of FSH and LH. This stage takes between 4 and 6 days and is expressed by a steady geometric increment of estrogens, as well as a daily increase of follicular diameter of about 1.5 to 2 mm/day. Ovulation is induced by administration of LH or LH-like material (HCG) when one or two follicles have reached a diameter of 16 mm or more and serum estradiol levels are ideally between 450 and 900 pg/mL. When estradiol levels are above 2,000 pg/mL or 3 or more preovulatory follicles are present, HCG should be withheld.

MONITORING GONADOTROPIN THERAPY

By monitoring ovulation induction, one can assess the gonadotropin dose that is effective in evoking an ovarian response, the length of time required for

follicular maturation, and the appropriate time to trigger ovulation with HCG. Furthermore, it should help to prevent hyperstimulation, or at least to detect it as early as possible. Ideally, for these purposes a combination of ultrasonography to assess the number and size of growing follicles, and measurement of estrogen level to indicate functional integrity, should be used.[32] As the levels of estrogens reflect the total estrogen secretion of all functional follicular structures, however, a baseline ultrasonography prior to initiating gonadotropin administration is useful in all instances and crucial in women who received ovulation-induction therapy in the previous cycle. Endogenous estrogen production affects several cervical values, which can be assessed by a point scoring system (the cervical score).[22] The score shows a reasonably good correlation with rising estrogen levels and is a particularly useful guide in establishing the effective daily dosage of gonadotropins.

The initial dosage of FSH is usually 75 to 150

IU/day (1 to 2 ampules of Pergonal). If no rise in estrogen occurs within 5 days (as determined by cervical score or measuring the level) and no alarming clinical signs are noted, the daily dosage is increased by 1 to 2 ampules. Treatment is continued at the higher dosage for 4 to 6 days, the growth and maturation phase. This phase is monitored by ultrasonography to determine the number and size of follicles, and by estrogen level measurement to determine their functional capacity.[32,33] The effective dosage is one that causes a significant and steady estrogen rise. With this method of monitoring ovulation induction, two ultrasonographies and estrogen determinations usually are sufficient. Increases in estrogen levels greater than 100% a day are excessive. If this occurs, the dosage should be reduced by 1 ampule. If the estrogen level does not rise steadily, the daily dosage is again increased by 1 to 2 ampules for 4 to 6 days. If the estrogen rise is steady and not excessive, the same dosage is continued until the level is between 450 and 900 pg/mL and 1 or 2 follicles have reached a diameter of 16 mm or greater. At that stage, ovulation is triggered by the administration of 5,000 to 10,000 IU of HCG.

In the past, when more than 2 large follicles were present or when estradiol levels were excessive, HCG administration was withheld and the treatment cycle aborted. This was done to prevent multiple gestations or hyperstimulation. In centers where in-vitro fertilization (IVF) and embryo freezing are available, cycles resulting in multiple follicular development could be salvaged using follicular reduction.[34] This technique involves aspirating excessive follicles after HCG administration. The excessive eggs are fertilized and cryopreserved, and the remaining follicles are allowed to ovulate in vivo. Should the patient not conceive in this specific cycle, the cryopreserved embryos are transferred in subsequent cycles. The use of this technique should reduce multiple gestations and hyperstimulation to a minimum.

RESULTS OF TREATMENT

The efficacy of HMG–HCG treatment reported below was determined retrospectively by life table analysis from a data base. Pregnancy was related to both the primary etiology of the infertility disturbance and the age of the patient.

The pregnancy rate with HMG–HCG therapy in amenorrheic patients with hypothalamic–pituitary insufficiency or failure is very high. Of 279 patients in our series, 82% conceived.[9] The cumulative pregnancy rate is significantly affected by age, however. In patients under age 35 years it was over 95% after 6 treatment cycles, and in patients above 35 years it was only 60%.[9]

The pregnancy rates in amenorrheic, oligoovula-

tory, or anovulatory patients with clomiphene citrate therapy was 55%. Patients above age 35 years have a very poor chance to become pregnant.

Rates in women with polycystic ovary disease are difficult to estimate, because the diagnosis of this entity has been ill defined. In 827 patients treated with clomiphene citrate, 76% ovulated but only 33% conceived within 6 months.[35] In those with clomiphene-resistant disease, treatment with HMG resulted in a 58% conception rate after an average of 2.4 treatment cycles.[36] A multicenter study was conducted using purified FSH (Metrodin, Serono Laboratories) in patients who failed to conceive after various therapies. This clinical trial achieved a pregnancy rate of 30%. The average length of therapy was 2.4 cycles per patient. Since the introduction of long-term administration of GnRH analogs, promising reports with a triphasic treatment regimen have appeared in the literature. Although there is no doubt about its effectiveness, it cannot be quantifed because the numbers are too small.

Results in the treatment of LUF syndrome, infertility due to untimely LH surge, and unexplained infertility have been disappointing. The introduction of purified FSH and GnRHa may change the poor prognosis for these patients. Theoretically, these medications alone or combined with IVF and embryo transfer, or with gamete intrafallopian transfer, seem to be promising. Again it is too early to quantify results as the number of patients treated is too small.

True success rates are concealed in the number of live births. A review of 1,346 miscarriages after HMG therapy showed an abortion rate of 21.5%.[9] There was no significant difference in the rate with respect to diagnostic groups; however, it was significantly higher in the first conception cycle than in the second or third. This was independent of whether the second conception occurred spontaneously (13%) or whether it followed induction of ovulation with HMG–HCG (12.8%).

Short-Term Safety
No consistent drug-related adverse effects have been reported with gonadotropin therapy. Most of the adverse reactions noted with HMG–HCG are due to ovarian responsiveness and sensitivity to the amount administered. As most of the treatment protocols aim to induce multifollicular development, the main complications are hyperstimulation, multiple pregnancy, and obstetric and postnatal complications due to multiple gestation.

Hyperstimulation. Mild hyperstimulation (Table 23–2) ranges between 31 and 60% in different large series. Severe hyperstimulation ranges between 0.25 and 1.8% and has been declining with the use of serum estradiol and sonography. With correct moni-

TABLE 23–2. CLASSIFICATION OF HYPERSTIMULATION

Laboratory and Clinical Findings	Adverse Reaction					
	Mild				Severe	
	1		2		3	
	1	2	3	4	5	6
Excessive steriod production	+	+	+	+	+	+
Ovarian enlargement		+	+	+	+	+
Abdominal discomfort		+	+	+	+	+
Palpable ovarian cysts		?	+	+	+	+
Abdominal distention			+	+	+	+
Nausea			+	+	+	+
Vomiting				+	+	+
Diarrhea				?	+	+
Ascites					+	+
Hydrothorax						+
Severe hemoconcentration						+
Thromboembolic phenomena						?

From Lunenfeld et al.[9] Reproduced with permission.

toring, the rate of severe hyperstimulation should not surpass 0.25%.

Multiple Gestations. The overall multiple pregnancy rate is about 26%. Of these, 74% are twins. Using ultrasonic monitoring, it is possible to prevent or at least decrease the occurrence of multiple pregnancies; however, every such attempt has significantly reduced the overall pregnancy rate. The increased conception rate with multifollicular development and transfer of more than 1 embryo has been well demonstrated in IVF programs.

The course of gestation appears to be normal. Analysis of the mode of delivery showed a high frequency of interventions, breech extractions, vacuum extractions, forceps deliveries, and cesarean sections. The high prevalence of obstetric interventions may be explained by a high rate of multiple pregnancies, primiparity ratios, and psychologic factors involved in delivering a "premium child" in patients with long-standing infertility.

Sex Ratios. The sex ratio (M:F) of single births was 1.06 (54% boys) and of twins 0.72 (42% boys).[9] The number of triplets was too small to analyze. One group reported 32 males and 50 females in the single births (39%), with a twin M:F ratio of 0.78.[37] In another series, the rate of male children in single pregnancies was 51.8%,[38] but in twins and triplets it was 53.8 and 66.7%, respectively. The normal secondary sex ratio at 28 weeks' gestation is considered to be 106 males to 100 females.[39,40] This higher number of males probably reflects the interplay between the primary sex ratio and sex differences in early prenatal mortality. It is known that the number

of males decreases with an increasing number of children at birth. This is regarded as being due to the better survival of female offspring rather than a relative loss of males.[41,42]

The sex ratios were 1.043 for twins, 1.007 for triplets, and 0.940 for quadruplets.[42] The high frequencies of females in our twin series, and of males in twins and triplets in two other series,[38] were probably due to the rather small numbers involved. By combining all three series, one approaches the expected sex ratios, indicating clearly the importance of sufficiently large numbers in order to estimate similarity or divergence in the figures.

Congenital Malformations. Until 1970 major malformations were reported in 4 of 122 infants born.[43] During the years 1970 to 1972 no major malformations occurred among the 87 infants examined in the neonatal period. Another report on 157 infants born after gonadotropin therapy revealed 4 infants classified as having major malformations and 11 with various minor malformations.[37] Preliminary data on 66 infants born as a result of HMG–HCG treatment after 28 weeks' gestation revealed 2 with a major malformation and 5 with minor malformations (15.21 and 75.8/1,000 live births, respectively).[44] This frequency did not differ significantly from the 10.3 major and 72.4 minor malformations per 1,000 live births reported for the population as a whole. The frequency of congenital malformations in healthy populations has been reported to be 12.7 per 1,000 live births after 28 weeks' gestation, with a range of 3.1 to 22.5.[45,46] This increases to 23.1 per 1,000, which is manifested by 5 years. A congenital malformation rate of 3% was observed in the neonatal period, with twice as many occurring in twin births, most of which were monozygotic.[47] The clinical evidence does not indicate that babies born after HMG–HCG ovulation induction are at any greater risk of malformation than the population as a whole.

The postnatal development of the children born did not deviate from acceptable norms. Of 26 daughters,[48] including 5 pairs of twins, of amenorrheic women who conceived before 1969, 22 (84.6%) reported regular menses, usually associated with pelvic pain (95%). One girl had oligomenorrhea (interval 35 to 45 days), and two experienced menarche 2 and 4 months previously. Only in one girl had menarche not yet occurred. The mean age at menarche was 12.3 years (range 10 to 14 years), which was slightly lower than the mean age of 12.6 years in the general female populations of children born in Israel[49] and the United States.[50] The mean weight and height of the girls was similar to the 50th percentile values of the healthy population of the same ages born in Israel.[47] Examination of medical histories did not disclose any special data except the usual childhood diseases. In all cases psychomotor and mental development was normal.

It can be concluded that the girls investigated are developing normally, both physically and mentally, and have normal secondary sex characteristics. A functional hypothalamic–pituitary–ovarian–uterine axis is evidenced by the appearance of menarche followed by normal regular cycles. This observation is of special importance in the girls whose mothers had pituitary failure or insufficiency, indicating that the disease is not necessarily hereditary. Although the number of postpubertal girls investigated so far is too small to reach final conclusions, we believe that the group studied was of sufficient size to reassure clinicians, the treated mothers, and their offspring that no serious defect in pubertal development is expected to occur as the result of treatment.

Long-Term Safety

Nulliparity has been a consistently reported risk factor for carcinoma of the breast and endometrium.[51–55] Among the 1,438 functionally infertile patients in our series,[9] the rate of hormone-associated tumors was 1.5 times the expected rate. For carcinoma of the breast it was 1.4 times higher and for endometrial cancers 8.0 times higher. In an attempt to assess whether risk factors could be linked to different etiologies in this heterogeneous group, these infertile patients were analyzed according to three types: (1) amenorrheic patients with low endogenous estrogens and gonadotropins (141 patients); (2) infertile women displaying both estrogens and postovulatory progesterone whose infertility was due to mechanical infertility, male factor, or unexplained infertility (712 patients); and (3) amenorrheic or anovulatory women displaying endogenous estrogens, but lacking or having less than normal postovulatory progesterone levels (992 patients).

In the first group, the observed hormone-associated cancer rate was lower than expected for all sites. Not a single case of breast, endometrial, or other hormone-associated cancer was detected (although 1.68 were expected) in patients of this group independent of whether or not HMG–HCG therapy was followed by pregnancy.

In the women in the second group, no increased risk for hormone-associated cancer was observed. In the third group the observed rates of uterine and breast cancer were 10.3 and 1.8 times greater than expected, respectively.

For 187 women with functional infertility who were treated with HMG–HCG, no record of conception exists. In this group, 3 breast cancers were observed compared to 1.1 expected. This figure is 2.83 times greater than the expected rate in a matched population. Furthermore, 2 cases of endometrial cancer were found, whereas only 0.07 were expected.

This figure is 28.6 times the expected rate. In contrast, among the 198 women who conceived between 1965 and 1975 after induction of ovulation with HMG–HCG, not a single case of breast or endometrial cancer was observed. Our investigation indicates that women treated with HMG–HCG are not at increased risk for cancer.

Because the number of women receiving each specific treatment was small, the statistical power to detect minor effects of treatment was low; however, a large cancer risk would certainly have been detected. It seems from the results presented that, of the infertile patients, only anovulatory women with unopposed estrogens are at increased risk for uterine and breast cancer. Induction of ovulation with HMG–HCG followed by conception seems to reduce the risk. The interpretation of these results must be tempered by the fact that the majority of these women have not yet entered the natural cancer age. We have learned from carcinogenic agents such as irradiation that the effects of exposure are most evident when the population reaches that age, and so we will have to wait another 10 to 15 years for a conclusive answer.

Gonadotropins as ovulation-inducing drugs, if administered to properly selected patients, in correct dosages, and with effective monitoring of treatment, are relatively safe for both patients and offspring. It can be concluded that anovulatory patients have a 60 to 80% chance of delivering a healthy baby. For infertility due to mechanical factors, microsurgery and IVF procedures have changed the once-grim prognosis. The chances of conception vary from 60 to 70% for tubal anastamosis or adhesiolysis, to 20 to 30% for neosalpingostomy[56] and 10 to 20% for IVF,[57] and are still significantly smaller than for infertility due to endocrine factors.

REFERENCES

1. Crowe SJ, Cushing H, Homans J, cited by Lunenfeld B, Donini P: Historic aspects of gonadotrophins, in Greenblat RB (ed): *Ovulation*. Toronto, Lippincott, 1966, pp 105–115.
2. Zondek B, Ascheim S: Das Hormon des Hypophysenvorderlappens: Testobject zum Nachweis des Hormons. *Klin Wochenschr* 6:248, 1927.
3. Smith PE, Engle ET: Experimental evidence regarding role of anterior pituitary in development and regulation of genital system. *Am J Anat* 40:159, 1927.
4. Borth R, Lunenfeld B, de Watteville H: Activité gonadotrope d'un extrait d'urines de femmes en ménopause. *Experientia* 10:266, 1954.
5. Borth R, Lunenfeld B, Riotton G, et al: Activité gonadotrope d'un extrait des femmes en ménopause (2e communication). *Experientia* 13:115, 1957.
6. Gemzell CA, Diczfalusy E, Tillinger G: Clinical effect of human pituitary follicle-stimulating hormone (FSH). *J Clin Endocrinol Metab* 18:1333, 1958.
7. Borth R, Lunenfeld B, Menzi A: Pharmacologic and clinical effects of a gonadotropin preparation from human postmenopausal urine, in Albert A, Thomas MC (eds): *Human Pituitary Gonadotropins*. Springfield, IL, Charles C Thomas, 1961, p 255.
8. Lunenfeld B, Sulimovici S, Rabau E, et al: L'induction de l'ovulation dans les amenorrhees hypophysaires par un traitement combiné de gonadotrophines urinaires ménopausiques et de gonadotrophines chorioniques. *Compt Rend Soc Fr Gynecol* 5:287, 1962.

9. Lunenfeld B, Blankenstein J, Ron E, et al: Short and long term survey of patients treated with HMG/HCG and follow-up of offspring, in Genazziani AR, Volpe A, Faechinettle (eds): *Proceedings of the First International Congress on Gynecological Endocrinology*. Lancashire, Parthenon, 1987, p 459.

10. Butt WR, Kennedy JF: Structure–activity relationships of protein and polypeptide hormones, in Margoulis M, Greenwood FC (eds): *Protein and Polypeptide Hormones*. Amsterdam, Excerpta Medica, 1971, p 115.

11. De la Llosa P, Jutisz M: Protein and polypeptide hormones, in Margoulis M (ed): Amsterdam, Excerpta Medica, 1969, p 229.

12. Fiddes JC, Goodman HM: Isolation, cloning and sequence analysis of the cDNA for the alpha-subunit of human chorionic gonadotropin. *Nature* 281:351, 1979.

13. Hussa RO: Biosynthesis of human chorionic gonadotropin. *Endocr Rev* 1:268, 1980.

14. Greep RP: Histology, histochemistry and ultrastructure of adult ovary, in Grady HG, Smith DE (eds): *The Ovary*. Baltimore, William & Wilkins, 1963, p 48.

15. Hertz R: Pituitary independence of the prepubertal development of the ovary of the rat and rabbit and its pertinence of hypoovarianism in women, in Grady HG, Smith DE (eds): *The Ovary*. Baltimore, Williams & Wilkins, 1963, p 48.

16. Lunenfeld B, Eshkol A: Immunology of follicle-stimulating hormone and luteinizing hormone. *Vitam Horm* 27:131, 1970.

17. Gougeon A: Origin and growth of the preovulatory follicle(s) in spontaneous and stimulated cycles, in Testart J, Frydman R (eds): *Human In Vitro Fertilization*. INSERM symposium no 24. New York, Elsevier, 1985, p 3.

18. Baker TG: Oogenesis and ovulation, in Austin CR, Short RV (eds): *Germ Cells and Fertilization in Mammals*. Cambridge, Cambridge University Press, 1982, vol 1, p 17.

19. Wildt L, Hausler A, Marshall G, et al: Frequency and amplitude of gonadotropin-releasing hormone stimulation and gonadotropin secretion in the rhesus monkey. *Endocrinology* 109:376, 1981.

20. diZerega GS, Turner CK, Stouffer RL, et al: Suppression of follicle-stimulating hormone dependent folliculogenesis during the primate ovarian cycle. *J Clin Endocrinol Metab* 52:451, 1981.

21. Lewinthal D, Furman A, Blankstein G, et al: Subtle abnormalities in follicular development and hormonal profile in women with unexplained infertility. *Fertil Steril* 46:833, 1986.

22. Insler V, Melmed H, Eichenbrenner J, et al: The cervical score—A simple semiquantitative method for monitoring the menstrual cycle. *J Gynecol Obstet* 10:223, 1972.

23. Lunenfeld E, Potashnik J, Insler V: Combined GnRH agonist and gonadotropin therapy in patients who failed to respond to previous ovulation-inducing therapy. *Isr Fertil Soc* 1986.

24. Flamigni C, Venturoli S, Paradisi R, et al: Human urinary follicle-stimulating hormone in infertile women with polycystic ovaries. *J Reprod Med* 30:184, 1985.

25. Claman P, Seibel MM: Purified human follicle-stimulating hormone for ovulation induction: A critical review. *Semin Reprod Endocrinol* 4:227, 1986.

26. Seibel MM, Kamrava MM, McCardle C, Taymor ML: Treatment of polycystic ovary disease with chronic low-dose follicle-stimulating hormone: Biochemical changes and ultrasound correlation. *Int J Fertil* 29:39, 1984.

27. Shadmi AL, Lunenfeld B, Bahari C, et al: Abolishment of the positive feedback mechanism: A criterion for temporary medical hypophysectomy by LH-RH agonist. *Gynecol Endocrinol* 1:1, 1987.

28. Fleming R, Haxton MJ, Hamilton MPR, et al: Successful treatment of infertile women with oligomenorrhoea using a combination of an LH–RH agonist and exogenous gonadotrophins. *Br J Obstet Gynaecol* 92:369, 1985.

29. Welmer SL, Polan ML, Graebe TA, Barnea E, DeCherney AH: The use of empiric Pergonal therapy in patients with infertility of unknown origin. Presented at the 41st meeting of the American Fertility Society, Chicago, Sept 1985.

30. Nachtegall RD: Indications, techniques and success rates for AIH. *Semin Reprod Endocrinol* 5:15, 1987.

31. Blankstein J, Saadon T, Mashiach S, et al: The effect of human menopausal gonodotropins on ovarian follicular selection in women. *J IVF/ET* 1:100, 1984.

32. Seibel MM, McArdle C, Thompson IE, et al: The role of ultrasound in ovulation induction: A critical appraisal. *Fertil Steril* 36:573, 1981.

33. McCardle CR, Seibel MM, Weinstein F, et al: Induction of ovulation monitored by ultrasound. *Radiology* 148:809, 1983.

34. Belaisch-Allart J: L'aspiration ovocytaire: une conduite possible devant l'hyperstimulation. *Horm Reprod Metab* 4:95, 1987.

35. MacGregor AH, Johnson JE, Bunde CA: Further clinical experience with clomiphene citrate. *Fertil Steril* 19:616, 1968.

36. Kemmann E, Tavakoli F, Shelden RM, et al: Induction of ovulation with menotropins in women with polycystic ovary syndrome. *Am J Obstet Gynecol* 141:58, 1981.

37. Caspi E, Ronen J, Schreyer P, et al: Pregnancy and infant outcome after gonadotropin therapy. *Br J Obstet Gynaecol* 83:967, 1976.

38. Bettendorf G, Braendle W, Sprotte CH, et al: Overall results of gonadotropin therapy, in Insler V, Bettendorf G (eds): *Advances in Diagnosis and Treatment of Infertility*. New York, Elsevier-North Holland, 1981, p 21.

39. Tricomi V, Serr DM, Solish G: The ratio of male and female embryos as determined by the sex chromatin. *Am J Obstet Gynecol* 75:504, 1960.

40. Serr DM, Ismajovich B: Determination of the primary sex ratio for human abortions. *Am J Obstet Gynecol* 87:63, 1963.

41. Benirshke K, Kim CK: Multiple pregnancy. *N Engl J Med* 288:1276, 1973.

42. Nichols JB: Statistics of births in the USA, 1915–1948. *Am J Obstet Gynecol* 64:376, 1952.

43. Hack M, Lunenfeld B: The influence of hormone induction of ovulation on the fetus and newborn. *Pediatr Adolesc Endocrinol* 5:191.

44. Harlap S: Ovulation induction and congenital malformations. *Lancet* 2:961, 1976.

45. Stevenson AC, Johnson HA, Stewart PMI, et al: Congenital malformations: A report of a study of a series of consecutive births in two centers. *Bull WHO* 34(suppl):9, 1966.

46. McKeown J: Malformations in a population observed for five years, in *Foundations Symposium on Congenital Malformations*. London, Churchill, 1960, p 2.

47. Hendricks CH: Twinning in relation to birth weight mortality and congenital malformations. *Obstet Gynecol* 27:47, 1966.

48. Ben-Rafael Z, Blankstein J, Sack J, et al: Menarche and puberty in daughters of amenorrheic women. *JAMA* 250:3202, 1983.

49. Leiba S, Lunenfeld B, Sheba C: Comparative study of growth and development of immigrant children from Morocco, Iran and India and of Israeli-born children. *Harefuah* 70:1, 1966.

50. Zacharias L, Wurtman RJ, Schatzoff M: Sexual maturation in contemporary American girls. *Am J Obstet Gynecol* 108:833, 1970.

51. Ron E, Lunenfeld B, Menczer J, Serr D, Katz L: Cancer incidence in a cohort of infertile women. *Am J Epidemiol* 122:516, 1985.

52. Kelsey JL: A review of the epidemiology of human breast cancer. *Epidemiol Rev* 1:74, 1979.

53. Brinton LA, Hoover R, Fraumeni JF Jr: Reproductive factors in the aetiology of breast cancer. *Br J Cancer* 47:757, 1983.

54. Kelsey JL, LiVolsi VA, Holford TR, et al: A case-control study of endometrial cancer. *Am J Epidemiol* 116:333, 1982.

55. LaVecchia C, Franceschi S, Decarli A, Gallus G, Tognoni G: Risk factors for endometrial cancer at different ages. *J Natl Cancer Inst* 3:667, 1984.

56. Diamond MP: Surgical aspects of infertility, in Sciarra JJ (ed): *Gynecology and Obstetrics*. 1988.

57. Seibel MM: A new era in reproductive technology: In vitro fertilization, gamete intrafallopian tube transfer and donated gametes and embryos. *N Engl J Med* 318:828, 1988.

CHAPTER 24

Ovulation Induction: FSH

Machelle M. Seibel

Ovulation Induction: FSH

Structure and Pharmacology
Physiology
Clinical Studies
    Hypothalmic Amenorrhea
    Polycystic Ovary Disease
       Low-dose Protocols Without HCG
       Intermediate-Dose Protocols Without HCG
       FSH with HCG as "Surrogate" LH Surge
    U-FSH for In-Vitro Fertilization

Ovarian function was first shown to be dependent on pituitary gonadotropins in the 1920s.[1,2] Pregnant mare serum gonadotropin was soon isolated, extracted,[3] and used successfully[4] for ovulation induction. Unfortunately, its high antigenicity precluded widespread clinical use.[5]

Subsequently, extracts of human pituitary gonadotropins, containing both follicle-stimulating hormone (FSH) and luteinizing hormone (LH), were administered successfully,[6] but limited availability restricted their use. By the early 1960s gonadotropins were being extracted from the urine of menopausal women, providing a plentiful source of this substance.[7] The ensuing clinical trials by Lunenfeld and colleagues[8] in 1962 resulted in the successful induction of ovulation and pregnancy using human postmenopausal gonadotropins (HMG, Pergonal, Serono Laboratories, Randolph, MA) in combination with human chorionic gonadotropin (HCG).

Unfortunately, with only cervical mucus ferning and pelvic examination available to follow patients, ovarian hyperstimulation often resulted.[9,10] The introduction of estrogen monitoring[11] and ultrasonography[12] added safety as well as effectiveness in achieving a high pregnancy rate without complications.

Donini and associates[7,13] at Serono Laboratories used anti-HCG antibodies to cause absorption of LH onto gel columns, and eluted out highly purified FSH extracts from HMG. This purified urinary extract (U-FSH, Metrodin, Serono Laboratories) was not made available for clinical investigation until the late 1970s. Prior to that time, so-called pure FSH pituitary extracts were simply crude ammonium sulfate precipitates of anterior pituitary tissue[14,15] that contained significant amounts of LH as contaminant. With the development of gel filtration techniques,[15] limited quantities of highly purified FSH pituitary extracts were also made available for clinical investigations by the National Pituitary Agency of the National Institutes of Health. Approximately 70 mg of LH and 20 mg of FSH can be obtained from 1,000 human glands.

STRUCTURE AND PHARMACOLOGY

Follicle-stimulating hormone is an acidic glycoprotein with an approximate molecular weight of 33,000. The discovery of the subunit nature of anterior pituitary hormones provided the breakthrough for establishing the primary structure of many glycoprotein hormones, including FSH, LH, and HCG (Table 24–1). Human FSH is composed of two subunits, a hormone-nonspecific α-subunit and a hormone-specific β-subunit. The α-subunit consists of 89 amino acids with 2 carbohydrate moieties attached to asparagine at positions 49 and 75. The β-subunit has a variable chain length of between 108 and 115 amino acids with 2 carbohydrate residues attached to asparagine at positions 7 and 24. In total, human FSH contains approximately 27% carbohydrate and 73% protein. The carbohydrate moieties consist of sialic acid, galactose, mannose, and glucosamine, with small amounts of galactosamine and fucose.[15] The gene structures for both subunits are known, and a single gene type apparently is responsible for coding all α and β-subunits within a species.[16]

Several species of FSH are found in the pituitary gland and serum.[17,18] These forms differ most significantly in their sialic acid residues, which occupy the terminal positions of the carbohydrate residues. The degree of sialic acid incorporation affects the molecule's acidity, receptor-binding affinity, and most important, its half-life[19] and biologic activity.[17]

A sustained estrogenic milieu causes the pituitary to secrete FSH with a lower sialic acid content.[17,18,20] Thus, men and postmenopausal women secrete FSH with a high sialic acid content and a longer half-life and less biologic activity than the less acidic forms present in menstruating women and in estrogen-treated men.[18,21]

Little information is available on serum half-lives of FSH, although based on radioimmunoassay there seem to be fast and slow components in the disappearance rates of FSH glycoproteins.[22,23] After hypophysectomy in 5 postmenopausal women,[22] disappearance rate half-lives of fast and slow components of endogenous FSH were 4 and 70 hours, respectively.[22] Others reported that infusions of less acidic pituitary FSH extracts have shorter half-lives of 3 and 50 hours.[23] The metabolic clearance rate of FSH is approximately 14 mL/minute.

Reported measurements of "units" of pituitary and menopausal urinary extracts of FSH might be equivalent in that they are routinely based on a 1953 ovarian weight augmentation bioassay[24] using the second international reference preparation HMG as standard. This gross bioassay measurement, however, may not be equivalent to the in-vivo biologic effect of FSH on granulosa cell aromatase activity in which clinicians are most interested. Preliminary unpublished data from our laboratory suggest that they are not. The use of different standards has resulted in a wide range of values for FSH measured in different laboratories; however, the profile of FSH throughout the menstrual cycle and in other physiologic changes is identical. Furthermore, when the biologic and immunologic properties of LH and FSH were studied in three commercially available urinary gonadotropin preparations and in the first international standard preparation of human urinary gonadotropins before and after fractionation by isoelectrofocusing (IEF),[25] significant differences were found in the IEF profiles of both bioactive and immunoreactive LH and FSH, and in the biologic: immunologic ratios of the preparations studied. These differences seem to be due to the purification procedures employed. Differences in the in-vivo potencies, circulating half-lives, and clinical responses suggest that not only

TABLE 24–1. PRIMARY STRUCTURE OF LH, FSH, AND HCG

	Molecular Weight	Amino Acids	Carbo-hydrates	Sialic Acid Residues	Half-life in Circulation
LH	28,000			1–2	≅ 50 min
α		89	2		
β		115	2		
FSH	33,000			5	≅ 3–4 hrs
α		89	2		
β		115	2		
HCG	38,000			20	≅ 6–8 hrs
α		89	2		
β		145	6		

different preparations, but also different batches of the same preparation, may yield quite variable results.

PHYSIOLOGY

Briefly, the role of FSH in folliculogenesis is as follows. Early in the normal menstrual cycle a large cohort of follicles starts to develop. During the transition of granulosa cell autodifferentiation from squamous to cuboidal shapes, FSH receptors appear. The absolute number of FSH receptors per granulosa cell does not increase beyond this early stage of follicle growth. Elevated FSH levels are thought to play a significant role in recruiting the cohort of follicles. With advancement of follicular development to the late secondary and early tertiary stage, receptors for estradiol, progesterone, testosterone, and glucocorticoids appear. From this point on, however, further development requires FSH.

For reasons that are not totally clear, a single follicle is selected that dominates the rest of the cohort. This dominant follicle is enriched with FSH receptors, which allow it to grow despite declining FSH levels. FSH crosses the basal lamina and binds to granulosa cell membrane FSH receptors. These receptors rapidly destabilize after solubilization with detergents, making them very difficult to purify and study.[26] FSH activates adenylate cyclase, which results in the synthesis of the intracellular second messenger cyclic adenosine 3',5'-monophosphate (cAMP)[27] The cAMP binds to a regulatory protein subunit of protein kinase, resulting in the phosphorylation of regulatory proteins. Estrogen amplifies FSH action by enhancing the formation of FSH-stimulated cAMP and cAMP-dependent protein kinase. In this fashion, granulosa cells are capable of a maximal response to a minimal concentration of follicular fluid FSH; however, FSH is only detectable in follicular fluid when the androgen:estrogen ratio is above 1. Therefore, in conditions such as polycystic ovary disease in which androgen levels predominate, exposure of the granulosa cells to FSH is markedly reduced.

The developing follicle secretes, among other things, low levels of estrogen and inhibin, further reducing pituitary FSH output. Under the influence of LH, the ovarian stroma produces androgens, which the dominant follicle uses as a precursor for estrogens. In a time and dose-dependent manner, FSH is also responsible for the induction of aromatase enzyme and LH receptors.[28] These androgens also serve to suppress additional follicular development, causing atresia of the previously synchronous cohort of follicles.[28,29] When a critical level of estrogen (principally estradiol) is reached, the pituitary gland

paradoxically responds with a gonadotropin surge. The rise of LH triggers follicle rupture.[30] The simultaneous rise of FSH is responsible for expansion of the cumulus.[31] An FSH-releasing substance has been identified in porcine follicular fluid.[32,33] It is a heterodimeric protein composed of the two β-subunits of inhibins A and B, linked by interchain disulfide bonds. It has been suggested that this substance be called activin. Activin acts independently of the gonadotropin-releasing hormone (GnRH) receptor and increases stored as well as released FSH. The role of this substance in humans remains to be determined.

In disordered menstrual cycles, the dynamic interactive chain of events among hypothalamus, pituitary, and ovary is disturbed. In hypothalamic anovulation there is a relative deficiency of both FSH and LH. In polycystic ovary disease (PCO) the production of LH relative to FSH is overabundant. A high LH:FSH ratio results in the production of more androgens from ovarian stroma than can be aromatized to estradiol by an immature cohort of developing follicles. These "excess" ovarian androgens, in concert with adrenal androgens, are partially aromatized to weak estrogens in adipose tissues, which further inhibits the pituitary from increasing its FSH output (Fig. 24–1).[34] This self-perpetuating cycle leads to the clinical picture of the obese, hirsute, anovulatory patient with PCO.

Purified FSH is less effective in hypothalamic anovulation, because both LH and FSH are deficient.

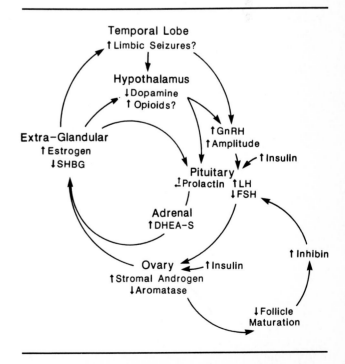

Figure 24–1. Self-perpetuating cycle of hormonal imbalance observed in polycystic ovary disease.

In contrast, the relative deficiency of FSH in PCO provides a rationale for interrupting the self-perpetuating cycle in a physiologically sound manner.

CLINICAL STUDIES

FSH for Ovulation Induction in Hypothalamic Amenorrhea

The role of HMG in ovulation induction in patients with hypothalamic amenorrhea has been clearly established.[8] Purified FSH preparations do not appear useful in severe disease, as some LH activity (endogenous or exogenous) is critical for stromal production of androgenic precursors that are aromatized into estrogens by granulosa cells under the influence of FSH.[28]

It has been shown in animal as well as human studies that LH is required for follicular development.[34-39] The level of endogenous gonadotropins separates the response of anovulatory patients into two distinct groups. In those with low endogenous gonadotropins, pure pituitary FSH preparations are totally ineffective in stimulating follicular estrogen production. The same or a lower dose of FSH given with LH in the form of HMG results in a good follicular response, however.

In contrast, anovulatory patients with endogenous gonadotropins demonstrate an adequate response to pure pituitary FSH. When endogenous LH:FSH ratios are high, addition of LH in the form of HMG tends to increase the frequency of ovarian overstimulation.[36]

One primate study suggested that LH is unimportant for follicular development.[40] The investigators "turned off" endogenous LH production using a gonadotropin-releasing hormone analog that may itself have an LH effect on the ovary.[41] The suggestion that LH is unnecessary for human follicular development was also raised based on ovulatory responses to U-FSH-HCG; however, the investigators failed to divide patients into those with or without endogenous gonadotropins.[42] Suffice to say, the overwhelming weight of the evidence suggests strongly that either endogenous or exogenous LH must be available for pure FSH to induce ovulation optimally.

FSH for Ovulation Induction in Polycystic Ovary Disease

Urinary FSH became approved for clinical use in the United States in November 1986 for use in clomiphene-resistant patients with PCO. High endogenous levels of LH suggest that the additional LH in HMG is unnecessary for folliculogenesis in PCO and in fact may be detrimental. In-vitro studies performed on granulosa cells obtained from polycystic ovarian follicles demonstrated that the polycystic ovary is not inherently defective but rather does not receive sufficient exposure to FSH. Granulosa cells from PCO follicles have the same potential ability to aromatize androstenedione into estrogens as granulosa cells from "normal" follicles, if FSH is added to the culture medium[43] (Fig. 24-2). This observation provided the necessary impetus to use purified FSH in PCO to interrupt the self-perpetuating cycle of chronic anovulation by providing the specific hormone that is deficient. It was further hoped that purified FSH would reduce the hyperstimulation and multiple pregnancy rate observed when these patients are treated with HMG, which contains an equal amount of FSH and LH.[35,44,45]

To date, clinical studies using purified FSH in PCO can be divided into several groups. Earlier studies were dependent on pituitary preparations.[35,36,44,46,47] Some used HCG as an ovulatory trigger[35,36,44,47] and some did not.[46,48] Postmenopausal urinary extracts of FSH (U-FSH) have also been studied in PCO. As with pituitary FSH, these studies were performed both with [49-52] and without HCG[52-54] as an ovulatory trigger. Dosages used and duration of therapy also varied from study to study (Table 24-2).

Low-Dose Protocols Without HCG

Polycystic ovary disease is a state of chronic hormonal imbalance. In contrast to hypothalamic amenorrhea, however, the hypothalamus–pituitary–ovarian axis is intact. The pathophysiology of PCO results in inappropriate secretion of gonadotropins, resulting in a relative deficiency of FSH. The goal of protocols is to supply exogenously the deficient FSH over an extended time interval in order to allow for the endogenous correction of the hormonal imbalance. Patients with PCO respond to appropriate estradiol levels with an endogenous LH surge (Fig. 24-3a).[34,36] Similarly, granulosa cells obtained from these patients are capable of aromatizing androgens to estrogens if exposed to adequate levels of FSH.[28] For these reasons, long-term low dosages (40 to 150 IU/day) of pure FSH without HCG were investigated.

These clinical trials unequivocally substantiated that patients with PCO have an intact HPO axis. Interruption of the self-perpetuating cycle with FSH induced an endogenous LH surge, ovulation, and conception without HCG as an ovulatory trigger. Furthermore, no more than 2 preovulatory follicles were seen to develop, thus reducing the potential risk of multiple births (Table 24-3). Reasonable pregnancy rates were achieved with no complications (see Table 24-2).[46,47,53,54] Unfortunately, because daily intramuscular injections of U-FSH are occasionally required for more than 30 days to induce ovulation, low-dose protocols are impractical.

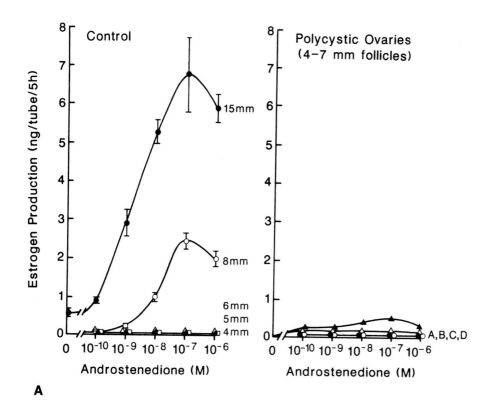

A

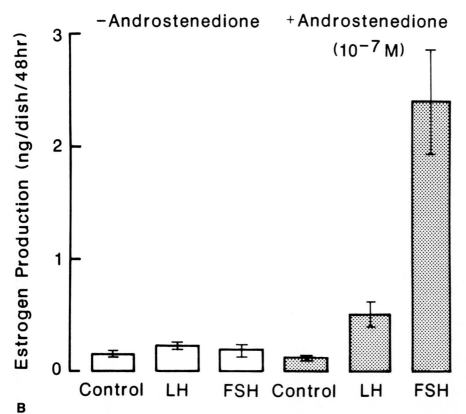

B

Figure 24–2. A. Neither granulosa cells from small control follicles nor small PCO follicles have acquired aromatase, whereas larger control follicles have acquired the aromatase enzyme. **B.** Granulosa cells isolated from 4 to 6-mm follicles of healthy women and those with polycystic ovaries are capable of converting an androgen precursor (androstenedione) into estrogen in the presence of FSH due to the induction of the aromatase enzyme. (From Erickson et al.[43] Reproduced with permission.)

TABLE 24–2. STUDIES REPORTING THE USE OF PURIFIED FSH PREPARATIONS FOR THE TREATMENT OF ANOVULATION

FSH Source	No. of Patients	No. of Cycles	Daily Dose*	HCG	Ovarian Enlargements	Ovulations	Pregnancies	Reference
Polycystic ovary disease								
Pituitary	4	5	Intermediate	Yes	2	?	?	35
Pituitary	10	18	Low	Yes	5	14	2	44
Pituitary	4	10	Intermediate	Yes	2	6	1	48
Pituitary	2	2	Low	No	0	2	2	46
Pituitary	5	6	Low	No	0	4	3	47
Urinary	21	25	Intermediate	Yes	10	22	8	50
Urinary	4	8	Intermediate	Yes	0	8	3	52
Urinary	18	43	High Intermediate	Yes	9	39	9	51
Urinary	10	11	Low	No	0	5	1	54
Urinary	10	28	Intermediate	No	8	9	3	52
Urinary†	8	8	Low	Yes	5	6	2	57
Undefined diagnosis of anovulation								
Urinary	18	38	Intermediate	Yes	9	?	?	56
Urinary	15	16	Intermediate	Yes	0	16	4	42

*FSH (IU/day); low = 40–150; intermediate =75–225; high intermediate = 150–375.
†Administered intravenously.
From Claman and Seibel.[53] Reproduced with permission.

Intermediate-Dose Protocols Without HCG

Intermediate doses (75 to 225 IU/day) of U-FSH were subsequently employed to reduce both the number of injections and the duration of treatment. It was hoped that an endogenous LH surge would occur and HCG would not be necessary after a shortened interval of treatment. Spontaneous LH surges occurred in less than half the cycles, however, despite adequate preovulatory estrogen levels (Fig. 24–3b). Of those women who did have an endogenous LH surge and ovulate, many had short luteal phases.[51]

The reduced luteal phase length appeared to be due to a blunted LH surge. These findings suggest that intermediate dosages of FSH, like HMG, are capable of stimulating developing follicles to secrete an "LH surge-inhibiting factor."[55] Nevertheless, a direct effect of FSH on LH release cannot be entirely excluded. The fact that ovulation occurred in less than half the cycles despite the development of preovulatory follicles and preovulatory estradiol levels reduced the clinical usefulness of the intermediate dosage of U-FSH without HCG. If intermediate dosages of shorter duration were to be consistently effective, an ovulatory trigger of HCG appeared necessary.

In contrast to low-dose regimens, ovarian hyperstimulation does occur with intermediate doses of FSH without HCG in cycles that are not carefully monitored. Two studies[51,56] reported significant symptoms of abdominal pain, ascites, and multiple pregnancy when estrogen assays were performed retrospectively. When estrogen levels were run prospectively in conjunction with pelvic ultrasound, no significant sequelae developed.

FSH with HCG as "Surrogate" LH Surge

The lack of consistent ovulation using intermediate-dose U-FSH with HCG for patients with PCO led to preliminary studies using HCG as an ovulatory trigger with prospective monitoring using both rapid estradiol and ultrasonography. Eight of 8 treatment cycles were ovulatory, with 3 pregnancies and no hyperstimulation[52] (Table 24–4). When dosages above 225 IU of FSH daily are used in conjunction with HCG, the rate of ovarian overstimulation rises greatly.[50] A review of the world literature suggests that if ovulation does not occur after 3 ampules (225 IU) of FSH daily administered for 2 weeks, it will not occur with higher dosages administered over a longer interval of time. A proposed protocol is shown in Figure 24–4.

I generally begin a new patient on day 4 to 6 of a spontaneous or induced cycle with 1 ampule admin-

TABLE 24–3. SERUM ESTROGEN LEVELS AND FOLLICLE SIZE AND NUMBER ON DAY OF PRESUMED OVULATION

Estradiol (pg/ml)	No. of Follicles (mm)			Largest Follicle (mm)	Outcome
	≥15	10–14	<10		
360	–	–	–	–	+β–Subunits
1120	1	0	2	30	+β–Subunits
4260	1	1	3	20	+β–Subunits
1375	1	0	1	30	Ovulation
138	0	0	5	7	Nonovulation
264	0	1	1	10	Nonovulation

From Seibel et al.[48] Reproduced with permission.

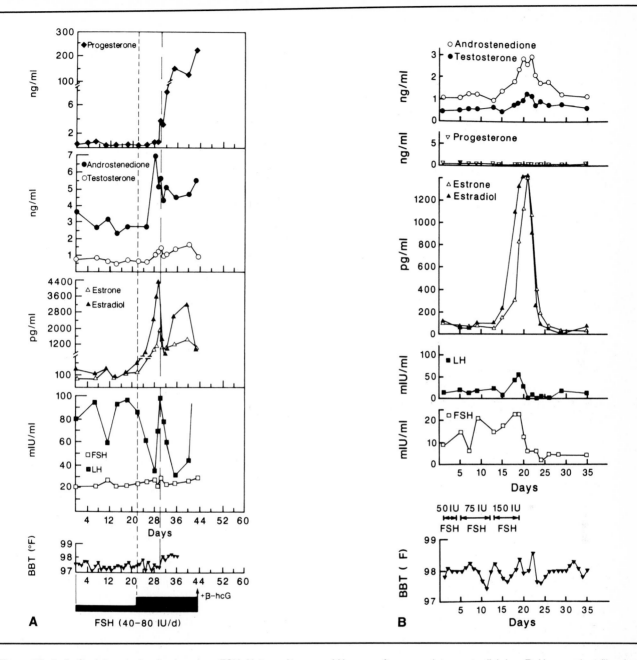

Figure 24–3. A. Ovulatory cycle after low-dose FSH. Note endogenous LH surge after preovulatory estradiol rise. **B.** Hormonal profile of a patient receiving U-FSH demonstrates an anovulatory cycle. Notice that despite the preovulatory rise in E₂, the LH rise is blunted and luteal phase progesterone levels are anovulatory.

istered daily for 6 days. On day 7 of treatment a pelvic ultrasound is performed and serum estradiol level is measured. If the largest follicle is smaller than 10 mm and the serum estradiol is below 200 pg/mL, the daily dosage is increased by 1 ampule for 3 days; otherwise the current dosage is maintained. A repeat ultrasound and estradiol is obtained on treatment day 10. The dosage of FSH is increased by 1 ampule daily if the largest follicle is less than 13 mm and the estradiol level is below 300 pg/mL. If the desired follicular development does not occur the cycle is discontinued and the next treatment cycle is initiated with 2

ampules daily for 6 days and the same general guidelines followed.

When the lead follicle becomes 15 mm in diameter, daily ultrasounds and serum estradiol determinations are obtained, and 5,000 IU of HCG is administered when the lead follicle achieves a diameter of 17 mm or more and serum estradiol levels exceed 350 pg/mL. However, if more than 3 follicles are larger than 17 mm or the serum estradiol is above 1,800 pg/mL, the HCG is withheld. In instances where serum estradiol levels are sufficient but follicle diameter is 15 or 16 mm, FSH may be withheld and

TABLE 24–4. U-FSH WITH AND WITHOUT HCG IN PCO

	HCG	No HCG
Patients	4	10
Cycles	8	28
Ovulations	8 (100%)	9 (32%)*
Pregnancies	3 (38%)	3 (11%)†
Ovarian enlargement	0	8 (28%)

*Percentage of cycles = 0.0008.
†Not significant, Fisher's exact test.
From Claman et al.[52] Reproduced with permission.

the patient "coasted" for 24 hours. A serum estradiol and pelvic ultrasound are repeated the next day and HCG administered that afternoon. Patients who require more than 14 days of treatment or more than 3 ampules daily are unlikely to respond to this form of treatment.

In a separate protocol, we compared the administration of a short course of UFSH (5 ± 1 days) which is similar to clomiphene to the protocol described above (11 ± 4 days). Despite comparable estradiol levels (short = 887 pg/mL vs long = 856 pg/mL) and numbers of preovulatory follicles (short = 2.0 vs long

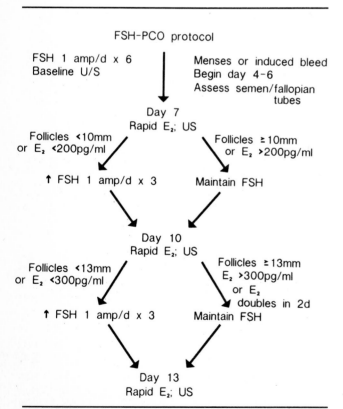

Figure 24–4. Proposed protocol for ovulation induction in PCO using purified FSH.

= 1.7), no pregnancies occurred in the short protocol group. These data further suggest that effective follicleogenesis in PCO requires longer than 6 days of UFSH to simulate the normal physiology for oocyte maturation.

One group of authors administered urinary FSH intravenously to patients with PCO using a pulsatile infusion pump.[57] Eight patients were administered 75 to 112.5 IU daily. A pulse interval of 120 minutes was used to infuse 6.7 IU/pulse. Human chorionic gonadotropin was used to trigger ovulation. All patients developed 4 or more follicles and 4 patients developed between 7 and 15. Five of 8 patients developed ovarian overstimulation; in 1 woman it was severe, with ascites and altered coagulation values. There was 1 triplet and 1 quadruplet pregnancy. Although innovative, in my opinion, the intravenous administration of FSH has no role in the treatment of ovulatory disorders associated with PCO. It is possible, however, that it may prove useful in women who respond poorly to ovulation-induction protocols for in-vitro fertilization.

Controlled, prospective studies comparing U-FSH and HMG are necessary to determine which drug is more effective for ovulation induction in PCO. Preliminary data suggest that ovulation and pregnancy rates are comparable,[49–51,54]; however, U-FSH appears to result in fewer complications if cycles are monitored prospectively with estrogens and pelvic ultrasound examinations. Further refinement of dosage and duration will no doubt only enhance the effectiveness and safety of U-FSH for the treatment of anovulation in patients with PCO.

U-FSH for In-Vitro Fertilization

Successful in-vitro fertilization (IVF) and embryo transfer is positively correlated with the number of oocytes retrieved and the number of embryos transferred.[58] For this reason, many IVF centers have begun incorporating U-FSH into their treatment protocols for controlled ovarian hyperstimulation.[59] Studies on intact monkeys have shown U-FSH capable of recruiting several follicles with infrequent spontaneous LH surges.[55] Although this is a potentially undesirable outcome for ovulation induction in PCO, an absent LH surge is highly desirable for IVF centers, which must precisely document the onset of the LH surge or time of HCG administration in order to plan oocyte retrieval.

Administering U-FSH for IVF also poses a theoretical concern. Unlike patients with hypothalamic amenorrhea who respond poorly to purified FSH, patients undergoing IVF have normal levels of circulating endogenous LH. Therefore, the addition of exogenous LH could result in enhanced androgen production and follicle atresia. To address this concern, 28 ovulatory cycles were studied prospectively

TABLE 24–5. PERIPHERAL SEX STEROID VALUES IN OVULATORY MENSTRUAL CYCLES AUGMENTED WITH REGIMENS OF PURE UFSH AND HMG

Treatment	$E_2\ \bar{x}\ \Delta$	$P\ \bar{x}\ \Delta$	$T\ \bar{x}\ \Delta$	$\Delta_4\ \bar{x}\ \Delta$
CI–HMG (n= 7)	698.2 (NS)	0.14 (NS)	0.24 (NS)	2.25 (p Δ0.05)
CI–UFSH (n = 13)	638.5 (NS)	0.43 (NS)	0.07 (NS)	0.45
UFSH (n= 8)	55.8 (NS)	0.19 (NS)	0.11 (NS)	0.17

CI = Clomiphene.
From reference 60. Reproduced with permission.

and randomly treated with clomiphene citrate, 50 to 100 mg/day for 5 days and HMG, 225 IU/day for 3 days; clomiphene citrate and U-FSH: or U-FSH alone. Peripheral levels of androstenedione were significantly decreased by the use of U-FSH alone or in sequence with clomiphene citrate.[60] Mean serum estradiol levels were not statistically different (Table 24–5). This study suggests that U-FSH is less androgenic than human menopausal gonadotropins for ovulation induction in IVF cycles. Furthermore, ovulation induction with HMG compared to U-FSH results in a significant increase in follicular fluid androgen levels.[61] Both of these findings suggest that U-FSH may improve oocyte quality and, indirectly, pregnancy rates achieved by IVF.

Clinical trials with U-FSH alone have in fact resulted in a tendency to larger number of oocytes retrieved, embryos transferred, and pregnancies achieved compared with HMG regimens.[62–65] When U-FSH is compared with extra HMG for augmenting treatment during follicular recruitment (cycle days 3, 4, and possibly 5), more mature oocytes are retrieved, higher numbers of embryos are transferred, and pregnancy rates are increased significantly.[62,66,67] Other groups have not found an advantage of U-FSH alone over HMG,[68–70] and in fact a higher frequency of short luteal phase lengths in U-FSH-stimulated cycles was reported.[65] Furthermore, one report suggested that U-FSH may be associated with an increased prevalence of empty follicle syndrome.[71] All of the empty follicles occurred in patients with unexplained infertility, however, and could represent an entity that existed prior to entering IVF. More work is necessary to determine the specific advantages of purified FSH for IVF.

REFERENCES

1. Zondek B, Aschheim S: Des Hormon des Hypophysenvorderlappens. *Klin Wochenschr* 6:248, 1927.
2. Smith PE, Engle ET: Experimental evidence regarding the role of anterior pituitary in the development and regulation of the genital system. *Am J Anat* 40:159, 1927.
3. Cole HH, Hart GH: The potency of blood serum of mares in progressive stages of pregnancy in effecting the sexual maturation of immature rats. *Am J Physiol* 93:57, 1930.
4. Hamblem EC, David CD: Treatment of hypoovarianism by the sequential and cyclic administration of equine and chorionic gonadotropins. *Am J Obstet Gynecol* 50:137, 1945.
5. Buxton CL: The pitfalls of clinical research. *J Clin Endocrinol Metab* 13:231, 1953.
6. Gemzell CA, Diczfalusy E, Tillinger KG: Clinical effect of human pituitary follicle stimulating hormone. *J Clin Endocrinol Metab* 18:1333, 1958.
7. Donini P, Puzzuoli D, Montezeniola R: Purification of gonadotropins from human menopause urine. *Acta Endocrinol* (Copenh) 45:321, 1964.
8. Lunenfeld B, Sulimovici S, Rabau E, Eshkol A: L'induction de l'ovulation dans les amenorrhoea hypophysaires par un traitement combiné de gonadotrophines urinaires ménopausiques et de gonadotrophines chorionique. *C R Soc Fr Gynecol* 35:346, 1962.
9. Taymor ML, Sturgis SH, Lieberman BL, Goldstein DP: Induction of ovulation with human postmenopausal gonadotropin. I. Case selection and results of therapy. *Fertil Steril* 17:731, 1966.
10. Taymor ML, Sturgis SH: Induction of ovulation with human postmenopausal gonadotropin. II. Probable causes of overstimulation. *Fertil Steril* 17:736, 1966.
11. Karam K,Taymor ML, Berger KJ: Estrogen monitoring and the prevention of ovarian overstimulation during gonadotropin therapy. *Am J Obstet Gynecol* 115:L972, 1973.
12. McArdle C, Seibel M, Hann LE, et al: The diagnosis of ovarian hyperstimulation (OHS). The impact of ultrasound. *Fertil Steril* 39:464, 1983.
13. Donini P, Puzzuoli D, D'Alessio I, et al: Purification and separation of FSH and LH from human postmenopausal gonadotropin. II. Preparation of biological apparently pure FSH by selective binding of the LH with an anti-HCG serum and subsequent chromatography. *Acta Endocrinol* 52:169, 1966.
14. Parlow AF, Wilhelm AE, Reichert LE Jr: Further studies on the fractionation of human pituitary glands. *Endocrinology* 77:1126, 1965.
15. Saxena BB, Rathnam P: The structure and function of follicle stimulating hormone, in McKerns K (ed): *Structure and Function of the Gonadotropins.* New York, Plenum, 1978, p 183.
16. Fiddes JC, Goodman HM: The gene encoding the common alpha subunit of the four human glycoprotein hormones. *J Molec Appl Genet* 1:3, 1981.
17. Miller C, Ulloa-Aguirre A, Hyland L, Chappel S: Pituitary follicle stimulating hormone form. *Fertil Steril* 40:242, 1983
18. Wide L: Male and female forms of human follicle stimulating hormone in serum. *Fertil Steril* 55:682, 1982.
19. Morell AG, Gregoriadis G, Sheinberg IH, et al: The role of sialic acid in determining the survival of glycoproteins in the circulation. *J Biol Chem* 246:1461, 1971.
20. Galle PC, Ulloa-Aguirre A, Chappel SC: Effects of oestradiaol, phenobarbitone and luteinizing hormone releasing hormone upon the isoelectric profile of pituitary follicle stimulating hormone in ovariectomized hamsters. *J Endocrinol* 99:31, 1983.
21. Wide L, Wide M: Higher plasma disappearance rate in the mouse for pituitary follicle stimulating hormone of young women compared to that of men and elderly women. *J Clin Endocrinol Metab* 58:426, 1984.
22. Yen SSC, Llerena LA, Pearson OH, Littell AS: Disappearance rates of endogenous follicle stimulating hormone in serum following surgical hypophysectomy in man. *J Clin Endocrinol* 30:325, 1970.
23. Kjeld JM, Harsoulis P, Kuku SF, et al: Infusions of hFSH and hLH in normal men. I. Kinetics of human follicle stimulating hormone. *Acta Endocrinol* 81:225, 1976.
24. Steelman SS, Pohley FH: Assay of the follicle stimulating hormone based on the augmentation with human chorionic gonadotropin. *Endocrinology* 53:604, 1953.
25. Harlin J, Khan SA, Diczfalusy E: Molecular composition of luteinizing hormone and follicle-stimulating hormone in commercial gonadotropin preparations. *Fertil Steril* 46:1055, 1986.
26. Dattatreyamurty E, Schneyer A, Reichert LE: Solubilization of functional and stable follitropin receptors from light membranes of bovine calf testes. *J Biol Chem* 261:13104, 1986.
27. Richards JS, Sengal N, Tash JS: Changes in content and cAMP-dependent phosphorylation of specific proteins in granulosa cells of preantral and preovulatory ovarian follicles and in corpora lutea. *J Biol Chem* 258:5227, 1983.
28. Erickson GF, Magoffin DA, Dyer CA, Hofeditz C: The ovarian androgen producing cells: A review of structure/function relationships. *Endocrinol Rev* 6:371, 1985.

29. Hodgen GD: The dominant ovarian follicle. *Fertil Steril* 38:281, 1982.

30. Seibel MM, Smith DM, Levesque L, Borten M. Taymor ML: The temporal relationship between the luteinizing hormone surge and human oocyte maturation. *Am J Obstet Gynecol* 142:568, 1982.

31. Eppig JJ: FSH stimulates hyaluronic acid synthesis by oocyte–cummulus cell complexes from mouse preovulatory follicles. *Nature* 281:483, 1979.

32. Ling N, Shao-Yao Y, Ueno N et al: Pituitary FSH is released by a heterodiner of the β subunits from the two forms of inhibin. *Nature* 321:779, 1986.

33. Vale W, Rivier J, Vaughan J, et al: Purification and characterization of an FSH releasing protein from porcine ovarian follicular fluid. *Nature* 321:776, 1986.

34. Seibel MM: Toward understanding the pathophysiology and treatment of polycystic ovary disease. *Semin Reprod Endocrinol* 2:297, 1984.

35. Berger MJ, Taymor ML, Karam K, Nudemberg F: The relative roles of exogenous and endogenous follicle stimulating hormone (FSH) and luteinizing hormone (LH) in human follicular maturation and ovulation induction. *Fertil Steril* 23:783, 1972.

36. Taymor ML, Berger MJ, Thompson IE, Karam KS: Hormonal factors in human ovulation. *Am J Obstet Gynecol* 114:445, 1972.

37. Jewelewicz R, Warren M, Dyrenfurth I, Vande Wiele RL: Physiological studies with purified human pituitary FSH (HP-FSH). *J Clin Endocrinol Metab* 32:688, 1971.

38. Jacobson A, Marshall JR: Ovulatory response rate with human menopausal gonadotropins of varying FSH-LH ratios. *Fertil Steril* 20:171, 1969.

39. Berger MJ, Taymor ML: The role of LH in human follicular maturation and function. *Am J Obstet Gynecol* 111:708, 1971.

40. Kenigsberg D, Littman BA, Williams RF, Hodgen GD: Medical hypophysectomy. II. Variability of ovarian response to gonadotropin therapy. *Fertil Steril* 42:116, 1984.

41. Bramley TA, Menzies GS, Baird DT: Specific binding of gonadotropin-releasing hormone and an agonist to human corpus luteum homogenates: Characterization, properties, and luteal phase levels. *J Clin Endocrinol Metab* 61:834, 1985.

42. Hoffman DI, Lobo RA, Campeau JD, et al: Ovulation induction in clomiphene-resistant anovulatory women: Differential follicular response to purified urinary follicle-stimulating hormone (FSH) versus purified FSH and luteinizing hormone. *J Clin Endocrinol Metab* 60:922, 1985.

43. Erickson GF, Hsueh AJW, Quigley ME, Rebr RW, Yen SSC: Functional studies of aromatase activity in human granulosa cells from normal and polycystic ovaries. *J Clin Endocrinol Metab* 49:514, 1979.

44. Raj SG, Berger MJ, Grimes EM, Taymor ML: The use of gonadotropins for the induction of ovulation in women with polycystic ovarian disease. *Fertil Steril* 28:1280, 1979.

45. Wang CF, Gemzell C: The use of human gonadotropins for the induction of ovulation in women with polycystic ovarian disease. *Fertil Steril* 33:479, 1980.

46. Kamrava MM, Seibel MM, Berger MJ, et al: Reversal of persistent anovulation in polycystic ovarian disease by administration of chronic low-dose follicle-stimulating hormone. *Fertil Steril* 37:520, 1982.

47. Schoemaker J, Colston-Wentz A, Jones GS, et al: Stimulation of follicular growth with "pure" FSH in patients with anovulation and elevated LH levels. *Obstet Gynecol* 51:270, 1978.

48. Seibel MM, Kamrava MM, McArdle C, Taymor ML: Treatment of polycystic ovary disease with chronic low-dose follicle-stimulating hormone: biochemical changes and ultrasound correlation. *Int J Fertil* 29:39, 1984.

49. Venturoli S, Paradisi R, Fabbri R, et al: Comparison between human urinary follicle-stimulating hormone and human menopausal gonadotropin treatment in polycystic ovary. *Obstet Gynecol* 63:6, 1984.

50. Flamigni C, Venturoli S, Paradisi R, et al: Use of human urinary follicle-stimulating hormone in infertile women with polycystic ovaries. *J Reprod Med* 30:184, 1985.

51. Garcea N, Campo S, Panetta V, et al: Induction of ovulation with purified urinary follicle-stimulating hormone in patients with polycystic ovarian syndrome. *Am J Obstet Gynecol* 151:635, 1985.

52. Claman P, Seibel MM, McArdle C, Berger MJ, Taymor ML: Comparison of intermediate-dose purified urinary follicle stimulating hormone with and without HCG for ovulation induction in polycystic ovarian disease. *Fertil Steril* 46:518, 1986.

53. Claman P, Seibel MM: Purified human follicle-stimulating hormone for ovulation induction: A critical review. *Semin Reprod Endocrinol* 4 (3):277, 1986.

54. Seibel MM, McArdle C, Smith D, Taymor ML: Ovulation induction in polycystic ovary syndrome with urinary follicle-stimulating hormone or human menopausal gonadotropin. *Fertil Steril* 43:703, 1985.

55. Schenken RS, Hodgen GD: Follicle-stimulating hormone blocks estrogen-positive feedback during the early follicular phase in monkeys. *Fertil Steril* 45:556, 1986.

56. Check JH, Chung-Hsiu W, Gocial B, Adelson HG: Severe ovarian hyperstimulation syndrome from treatment with urinary follicle-stimulating hormone. Two cases. *Fertil Steril* 43:317, 1985.

57. Lanzone A, Fulghesu AM, Conte M, et al: Induction of ovulation by intermittent intravenous purified follicle-stimulating hormone in polycystic ovary disease. *Fertil Steril* 48:1058, 1987.

58. Seibel MM: A new era of reproductive technology: In vitro fertilization, gamete intrafallopian transfer, and donated gametes and embryos. *N Engl J Med* 318:828, 1988.

59. Navot D, Rosenwaks Z: The use of follicle-stimulating hormone for controlled ovarian hyperstimulation in in vitro fertilization. *J IVF/ET* 5:3, 1988.

60. Oskowitz SP, Seibel MM, Taymor ML: Comparative effects on sex steroids of pure urinary follicle-stimulating hormone and human menopausal gonadotropins in clomiphene-primed ovulatory cycles. Presented at the 41st annual meeting of the American Fertility Society, Chicago, Sept 27–Oct 2, 1985.

61. Polan ML, Daniele A, Russell JB, DeCherney AF: Ovulation induction with human menopausal gonadotropin compared to human urinary follicle-stimulating hormone results in a significant shift in follicular fluid androgen levels without discernible differences in granulosa–luteal cell function. *J Clin Endocrinol Metab* 63:1284, 1986.

62. Jones GS, Acosta AA, Garcia JE, et al: The effect of follicle-stimulating hormone without additional luteinizing hormone on follicular stimulation and oocyte development in normal ovulatory women. *Fertil Steril* 43:696, 1985.

63. Russell JM, Polan ML, DeCherney AH: The use of pure follicle-stimulating hormone for ovulation induction in normal ovulatory women in an in vitro fertilization program. *Fertil Steril* 45:829, 1986.

64. Scoccia B, Blumenthal P, Wagner C, et al: Comparison of human urinary follicle stimulating hormone and human menopausal gonadotropins for ovarian stimulation in an in vitro fertilization program. *Fertil Steril* 48:446, 1987.

65. Belaisch-Allart J: Pure FSH for ovulation stimulation in an IVF and ET programme. Presented at the 4th world conference on in vitro fertilization, Melbourne, Nov 18–22, 1985.

66. Muasher SJ, Garcia JE, Rosenwaks Z: The combination of follicle stimulating hormone and human menopausal gonadotropin for the induction of multiple follicular maturation for in vitro fertilization. *Fertil Steril* 44:62, 1985.

67. Crosignani PG, Lombroso GC, Caccamo A, et al: Ovarian stimulation with human gonadotropins: Doubling of pregnancy rate with combined Metrodin and Pergonal. Presented at the 4th world conference on in vitro fertilization, Melbourne, Nov 18–22, 1985.

68. Willemsen ENP, Goverde H, Bastiaans LA, et al: HMG versus FSH in follicular maturation. A prospective randomized study in in vitro fertilization in human and in an animal model. Presented at the 4th world conference on in vitro fertilization, Melbourne, Nov 18–22, 1985.

69. Ronnberg L, Martikainen H, Puistola U: Comparison of ovarian response to HMG and pure FSH in an in vitro fertilization program. Presented at the 4th world conference on in vitro fertilization, Melbourne, Nov 18–22, 1985.

70. Brodie BL, Hill GA, Herbert CM et al: Human menopausal gonadotropins and pure FSH compared in a program for in vitro fertilization and embryo transfer. Presented at the 5th world congress on in vitro fertilization, Norfolk, April 5–10, 1987.

71. Ashkenazi J, Feldberg D, Shelef M, Dicker D, Goldman JA: Empty follicle syndrome: An entity in the etiology of infertility of unknown origin, or a phenomenon associated with purified follicle-stimulating hormone therapy? *Fertil Steril* 48:152, 1987.

CHAPTER 25

Ovulation Induction: GnRH

Paul Claman, Machelle M. Seibel

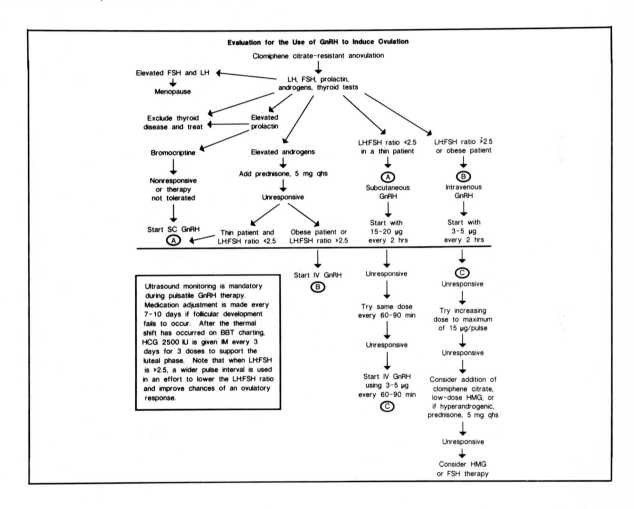

Evaluation for the Use of GnRH to Induce Ovulation

Clomiphene citrate and bromocriptine are widely used in the treatment of various types of anovulation. A high percentage of patients respond, complications are rare, and there is little need for involved endocrine or ultrasound monitoring. Substantial numbers of women fail to ovulate with these medications, however. Until 1980, human menopausal gonadotropin (HMG) was the only alternative treatment for these refractory patients. When the pulsatile nature of gonadotropin-releasing hormone (GnRH) release became appreciated,[1] the clinical application of this medication followed almost immediately.

Gonadotropin-releasing hormone is also referred to as luteinizing hormone-releasing hormone (LH-RH), luteinizing hormone-releasing factor (LRF), luteinizing hormone–follicle-stimulating hormone (LH–FSH)-releasing factor, luliberin, and gonadoliberin. It was first proposed in 1937 by Harris,[2] who hypothesized the release of a hypothalamic factor into the portal system, which in turn stimulated the release of trophic hormones from the pituitary. In 1960 Campbell, McCann, and co-workers found that crude hypothalamic extracts stimulated LH release from the pituitary[3,4]; however, more than a decade elapsed

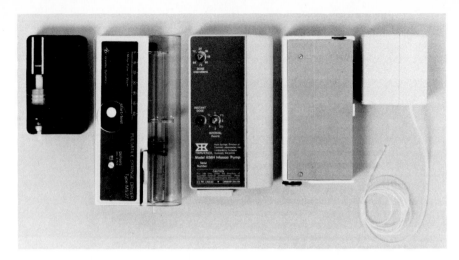

Figure 25–1. Various available pumps are, from left to right: Zyklomat (Ferring GmbH, Keil, FRG), Mill Hill (modified by Blows, Mill, Hill, UK), Travenol Autosyringe AS6H (Autosyringe, Hooksett, NH), Graseby MS27 (Graseby Medical), and the NIMR (General Purpose, Nordisk, Gentofte, Denmark). (From Chambers et al.[38] Reproduced with permission.)

before the structure of this substance was characterized independently.[5-8]

Soon after its isolation, GnRH was employed with great enthusiasm as a possible tool for the investigation of hypothalamic–pituitary–ovarian physiology, a role that although important, has never fully materialized.[9-14] Due to lack of understanding of the pulsatile nature of this substance, however, early efforts to induce ovulation were not encouraging. Initially, GnRH was used with mixed results to induce an LH surge or to augment clomiphene citrate or HMG therapy.[15-26] Later attempts at ovulation induction employed GnRH alone, with dosages ranging from 5 µg to 3 mg/day in up to 3 divided doses given subcutaneously, intravenously, or intramuscularly. Ovulation and pregnancy rates were disappointing and much lower than those observed with HMG.[27-37]

Experiments performed in GnRH deficient primates with lesions of the arcuate nucleus clearly demonstrated that replacement GnRH administered in a pulsatile manner was capable of simulating the release of LH and FSH typical of a natural cycle.[1] The availability of portable pulsatile infusion pumps[38] (Fig. 25–1) for GnRH provided the necessary technology for clinicians to apply primate reproductive physiology to the treatment of certain types of human ovulatory disorders.[39]

PHYSIOLOGY OF GnRH

Location and Biochemistry

Gonadotropin-releasing hormone is a decapeptide whose structural formula is identical in all species studied to date (Fig. 25–2).[7] Although it has been found in human placenta,[40] breast milk,[41] ovary,[42] and rat pancreas,[43] its most important source relevant to the control of gonadotropin secretion is in the medial basal hypothalamus, primarily the arcuate

nucleus (Fig. 25–3). Disconnecting the medial basal hypothalamus from the remainder of the central nervous system does not abolish regular secretion of GnRH. Destruction of the arcuate nucleus does abolish pituitary gonadotropin secretion, however, suggesting that the arcuate nucleus is the primary hypothalamic source of GnRH secretion.[1]

The hormone is a neurohumeral agent originating from a high- molecular-weight precursor that has been found in human placenta and hypothalamus using recombinant DNA technology. As predicted from cloned nucleotide sequences, this GnRH precursor comprises the decapeptide preceded by a signal sequence of 23 amino acids (AA) and followed by a GLY-LYS-ARG sequence necessary for enzymatic processing and carboxy-terminal amidation of GnRH. A sequence of 56 AA occupies the carboxy-terminal region of the precurser and constitutes the GnRH-associated peptide (GAP) (Fig. 25–4), which appears to be a potent inhibitor of prolactin secretion.[44,45]

Pharmacology

The serum half-life of GnRH is 2 to 8 minutes.[46-49] When a large bolus of GnRH is administered intravenously, LH and FSH are observed in the blood within 5 minutes. Peak levels of LH are noted by 25 minutes and of FSH by 45 minutes after injection. Basal gonadotropin levels are again observed several hours later. If GnRH is given as a constant infusion, a biphasic response is observed. Gonadotropins initially peak at 30 minutes, and then plateau. A second rise is observed at approximately 230 minutes. Subsequently, gonadotropin levels decay due to downregulation of the pituitary gonadotropes. This biphasic response is thought to demonstrate GnRH's effect on two functional pools of gonadotropins. The first is a secretory pool, which is ready for immediate release as demonstrated by the initial gonadotropin surge after 30 minutes of constant GnRH infusion. The second is a reserve pool. Here, gonadotropins are

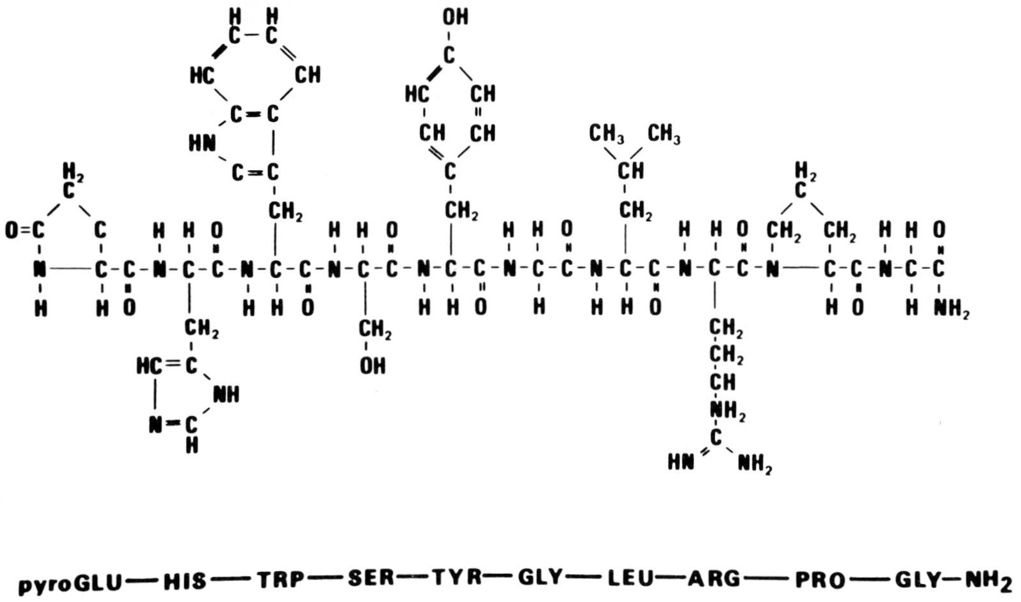

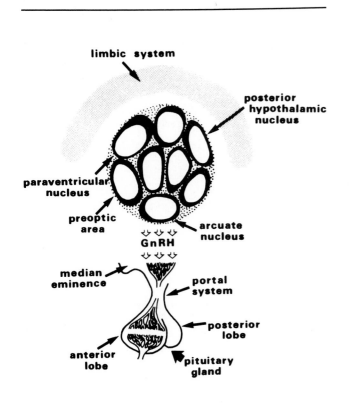

Figure 25–2. Structural formula of GnRH. (From Blankstein et al.[39] Reproduced with permission.)

pyroGLU—HIS—TRP—SER—TYR—GLY—LEU—ARG—PRO—GLY—NH₂

Figure 25–3. Modulated by the central nervous system, GnRH is secreted primarily into the portal circulation by the arcuate nucleus. It is then carried to the gonadotroph cell in the anterior pituitary, where it stimulates the synthesis, storage, and release of FSH and LH. (From Blankstein et al.[39] Reproduced with permission.)

synthesized, stored, and ultimately transferred to the secretory pool under the influence of GnRH, accounting for the second LH and FSH rise observed during a constant infusion of the releasing hormone (Fig. 25–5).[50]

It is thought that GnRH activates the gonadotrope cell by way of a second messenger. After binding of the hormone to the cell membrane, a cyclase system is activated, producing either cyclic adenosine 3′,5′-monophosphate (cAMP) or, as some data suggest, cyclic guanosine 3′,5′-monophosphate (cGMP).[51,52] Gonadotropin secretion is dependent on movement of calcium ion, with an associated redistribution of calmodulin (the cellular calcium cation receptor). Calmodulin has been shown to move from the cytosol to the plasma membranes of pituitary cells after GnRH administration, with an associated rise in LH.[53,54] Repeated pulses of GnRH probably either stimulate an increase in the number of receptors or modulate postreceptor calcium-dependent mechanisms on the pituitary gonadotrope. This is thought to account for the mechanism of GnRH self-priming, or so-called up-regulation. Constant infusions of GnRH down-regulate by depleting receptors (or desensitize postreceptor response).

Analogs of GnRH with higher potency and longer half-lives than the parent peptide have been developed by substituting or omitting certain amino acids from the decapeptide. When administered intermittently, these agonists/antagonists (Fig. 25–6) act as if a constant GnRH infusion were being given. Down-regulation ensues, with a profound reduction

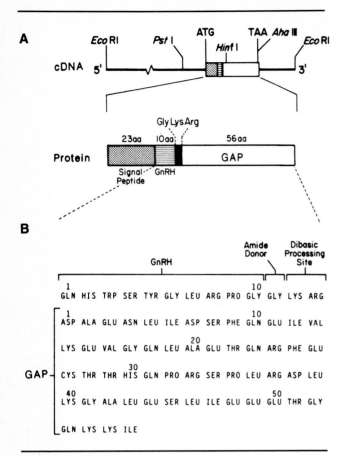

A

B

Figure 25–4. Structure and encoded amino acid sequence of human placental cDNA for prepro-GnRH.[45] **A.** Partial-restriction endonuclease map. The coding region is located between the initiation codon for protein synthesis ATG and the termination codon TAA. Schematic representation of the encoded protein identifies the three domains of signal peptide, GnRH, and GAP with the respective sizes in amino acid (aa) residues. **B.** Amino acid sequences of GnRH and GAP with an enzymatic processing site separating the two moieties. Numbers refer to the respective positions within GnRH (1–10) or GAP (1–56). (From Seeberg et al.[45] Reproduced with permission.)

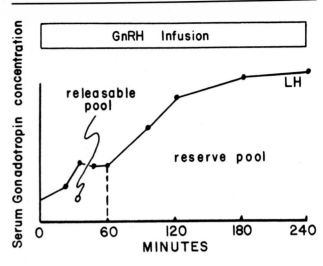

Figure 25–5. Gonadotropin responses to the continuous intravenous infusion of GnRH. (From Keye.[50] Reproduced with permission.)

in gonadotropin secretion. Iatrogenic induction of a hypogonadal state with GnRH analogs appears useful in the treatment of steroid-hormone-dependent disorders such as precocious puberty, endometriosis, uterine fibroids, prostate disease, and hyperandrogenic states. Furthermore, by blocking endogenous gonadotropin secretion, especially the LH surge, these analogs appear helpful in improving the predictability of ovarian response to HMG therapy, especially among clomiphene-resistant patients with polycystic ovary disease (PCO) and in superovulation regimens for in-vitro fertilization.[55,55a]

Secretion

Gonadotropin-releasing hormone is cleaved from its precursor and secreted primarily by cells located

	D-Trp[6]	Leuprolide	Buserelin	Nafarelin	GNRH		ANTAGONISTS	
		AGONISTS						
1	—	—	—	—	pyro-Glu	N-Ac-D-Na(2)	Ac-Δ²-Pro	NAc-D-p-Cl-Phe
2					His	D-pCl-Phe	p-F-D-Phe	NAc-D-p-Cl-Phe
3					Trp	D-trp	D-Trp	D-Trp
4					Ser			
5					Tyr			
6	D-Trp	D-Leu	D-Ser(tBu)	D-Nal(2)	Gly	D-hArg(Et₂)	D-Trp	D-Phe
7					Leu			
8					Arg			
9					Pro			
10		NHEt	NHEt		Gly-NH₂	D-Ala		D-Ala

Figure 25–6. Structure of GnRH decapeptide, and sites of substitutions in some of its agonistic and antagonistic analogs. (From Andreyko et al.[55] Reproduced with permission.)

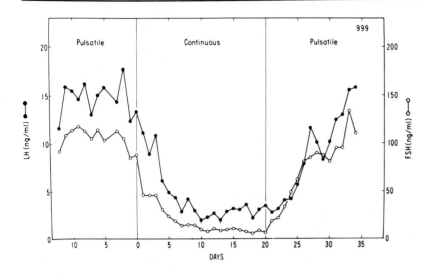

Figure 25–7. When GnRH is administered by continuous infusion to a hypothalamic-lesioned rhesus monkey, desensitization and down-regulation of the GnRH receptor take place. This leads to marked reduction of both LH and FSH. (From Belchetz et al.[56] Reproduced with permission.)

within the arcuate nucleus. These cells share characteristics of both neuronal and endocrine gland cells. They respond to steroid hormones as well as to neurotransmitters such as catecholamines and endogenous opiates. The releasing hormone and its precurser are synthesized on ribosomes, packaged into granules by the Golgi apparatus, and transported down the axon for storage and secretion primarily into the portal vessels of the pituitary stalk. It is these GnRH fibers of the tuberoinfundibular tract that govern gonadotropin secretion.

Physiologic studies have shown that gonadotropin response to GnRH is strikingly dependent on the mode of administration and the surrounding hormonal milieu. In the primate, intermittent pulsed administration of this peptide results in a sustained release of FSH and LH, whereas continuous infusion results in inhibition of both gonadotropins (Fig. 25–7). In addition, ovarian products (steroids and protein hormones) can modulate gonadotropin secretion, resulting in the cyclic hormonal changes observed during a normal menstrual cycle even if GnRH is administered at a set pulse frequency.[1]

GnRH Physiology in the Normal Menstrual Cycle

Endogenous GnRH is difficult to measure directly due to its very short half-life, the fact that it is secreted into the pituitary portal circulation, and the possibility that peripheral levels do not reflect portal values. Therefore our understanding of its physiology has been facilitated by animal experiments demonstrating that observed peripheral blood LH pulses accurately reflect a preceding bolus of hypothalamic GnRH secreted into the portal circulation (Fig. 25–8).[57] These data support the notion that hypotha-

lamic GnRH activity may be inferred by the study of pituitary LH pulses in peripheral blood.[58]

Studies of the normal menstrual cycle conducted in this manner have shown that GnRH is regulated by neurotransmitters such as catecholamines and endogenous opiates. Norepinephrine appears to stimulate hypothalamic GnRH secretion by way of

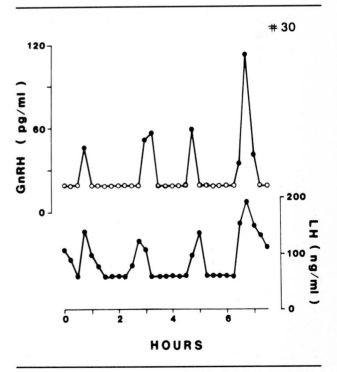

Figure 25–8. Pulsatile release of GnRH and LH in an ovariectomized monkey. (From Van Vugt et al.[57] Reproduced with permission.)

α-adrenergic receptors.[59,60] Conversely, dopamine and endorphins are major inhibitors of GnRH release.[61-63] These neurotransmitters are in turn regulated by ovarian hormones. In this fashion, GnRH pulse frequency and amplitude are further modulated throughout the menstrual cycle.[58]

Changes in the frequency and amplitude of GnRH pulsations have different effects on LH and FSH secretion. Increasing the amplitude is associated with an increase in the ratio of LH:FSH secretion. Shortening the pulse frequency from 180 to 60 minutes also increases this ratio (Figs. 25–9 and 25–10),[1,64] and widening the pulse frequency reduces the ratio. Further shortening of the pulse interval leads to down-regulation, with a decrease in both gonadotropins (Fig. 25–7). During the menstrual cycle the pulse frequency increases from every 90 minutes in the early follicular phase to every 60 minutes in the late follicular phase. The midcycle surge is associated with very rapid LH pulses occur-

ring at least every 45 minutes, followed by a luteal phase slowing observed to occur every 3 to 4 hours.[58]

The physiologic significance of these alterations in GnRH frequency throughout the normal menstrual cycle is unclear. Normal menstrual cycles can be induced in GnRH-deficient women[65] or rhesus monkeys[1] by pulsatile administration of GnRH at an unvarying dose or frequency (Fig. 25–11). Convincing data in GnRH-deficient rhesus monkeys and humans show that the cyclic patterns of gonadotropins seen throughout the menstrual cycle can be regarded as resulting from the negative and positive feedback effects of ovarian hormones on pituitary function.[1] Furthermore, imposing a rapid (follicular phase) gonadotropin secretory pattern in healthy women during the luteal phase with exogenous GnRH has no discernible effects on the corpus luteum or on follicular development in the subsequent cycle.[66] These clinical findings suggest that although an optimal GnRH pulse frequency may

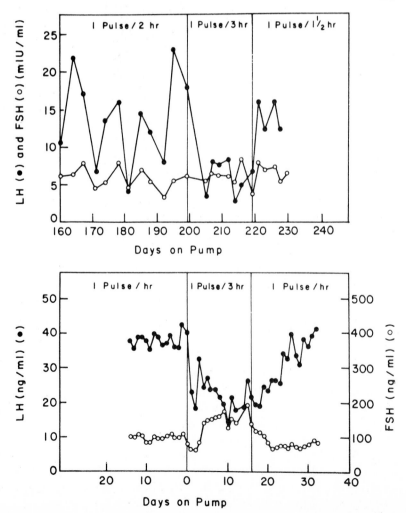

Figure 25–9. Top. Serum FSH and LH values during administration of GnRH at different intervals to a woman with Kallmann's syndrome (GnRH deficiency). Widening the pulse interval from 2 to 3 hours while maintaining the same 20-μg pulse resulted in reduction of LH levels; FSH levels did not change. Serum LH increased when the pulse interval was reduced to 90 minutes. **Bottom.** Response to a changing pulse frequency in primates. (From Seibel et al.[64] Reproduced with permission.)

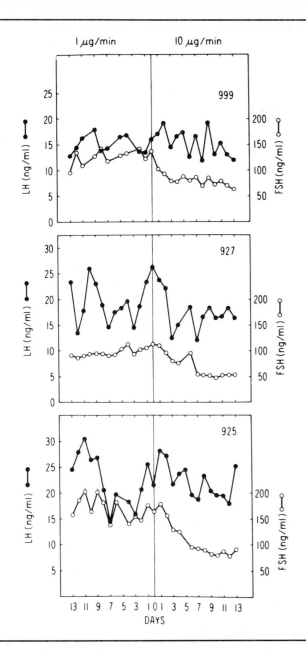

Figure 25–10. Increasing the GnRH dose given intravenously to a GnRH-deficient rhesus monkey every 60 minutes causes a marked increase in the LH:FSH ratio. (From Knobil.[1] Reproduced with permission.)

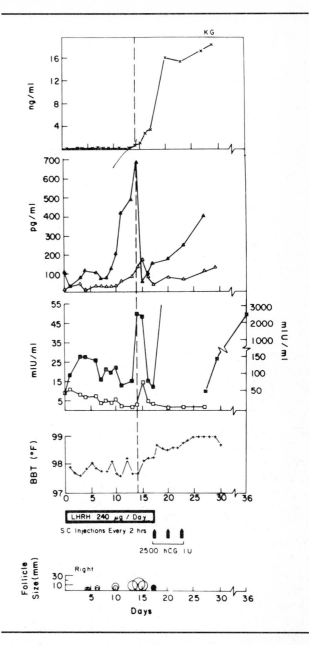

Figure 25–11. A patient with hypothalamic amenorrhea ovulates and becomes pregnant during the subcutaneous administration of GnRH, 20 μg every 2 hours. After ovulation, the luteal phase is supported with human chorionic gonadotropin (HCG), 2,500 IU intramuscularly every 3 days for 3 doses. Composite drawing shows daily levels of luteinizing hormone (LH), follicle-stimulating hormone (FSH), estrone (E_1), estradiol (E_2), progesterone (P), basal body temperature (BBT), and follicular development as observed on ultrasound examinations. X = P; black triangle = E_2; white triangle = E_1; black square = LH; white square = FSH; asterisk = β-HCG. (From Seibel et al.[65] Reproduced with permission.)

occur normally, a wide range of variations can be tolerated.

For clinical applications, the dose and pulse frequency must be established within certain limits, although there is substantial flexibility in this system (Tables 25–1 and 25–2). Successful induction of ovulation and pregnancy have been established in patients with hypothalamic anovulation using intravenous GnRH, self-administered every 2 hours during waking hours only.[67] There seems to be a frequency window (60 to 120 minutes in humans and primates) within which GnRH can be given at a fixed frequency, with normal gonadotropin stimulation, follicular development, release of an LH surge, ovulation, and development of a healthy corpus luteum.

TABLE 25–1. SUBCUTANEOUS GnRH IN WOMEN WITH HYPOTHALAMIC INSUFFICIENCY

Reference	Dose (μg)	Frequency (min)	Patients	Cycles	Ovulations (pts/cycles)	Pregnancies/ Abortions
82	20	120	10	16	10/15	4/1
83	19	90	19	?	17/55	12/3
84	2–20	90–180	5	14	0	0
85	5–10	120–180	2	3	0	0
	2–20	60–240	3	8	2/2	0*
86	10–25	90	25	83	25/80	25/8
87	5–15	90	14	36	14/30	13/2
88	50–200/day	60–120	14	?	10/?	6/?
89	2.5–15	90	4	9	4/9	4/?
90	5–20	90	?	21	/13	4/?
91	1–40	60–90	14	50	5/15	2/1
92	50–100 ng/kg	90	7	16	6/15	3/?

*GnRH given only during daytime.

PATHOPHYSIOLOGY OF OVULATORY DISORDERS

Studies modulating GnRH pulses have led to a better understanding of many ovulatory disorders. Inadequate or infrequent doses of GnRH given to women with hypothalamic amenorrhea result in cycles with luteal phase deficiency (Fig. 25–12).[68,69] Higher doses or more rapid pulses lead to an increased LH:FSH ratio[1,64,70,71] and hyperandrogenism[72] characteristic of PCO.[73] Very rapid pulsing of low-dose GnRH during the follicular phase in healthy women induces

TABLE 25–2. INTRAVENOUS GnRH IN WOMEN WITH HYPOTHALAMIC INSUFFICIENCY

Reference	Dose (μg)	Frequency (min)	Patients	Cycles	Ovulations (pts/cycles)	Pregnancies/ Abortions
93	2.5–20	90	33	143	33/143	38/9
94	1–5	96–120	8	23	8/20	7/3
95	12	96	49	?	/58	12/?
	12	180	4	?	/4	2/?
96	12	96	25	?	22/28	7
97	20	90	27	40	22/32	11/3
68	25 ng/kg	60	7	10	/8	2(only 5 infertile pts)
	100 ng/kg	60	12	20	12/20	6(only 7 infertile pts)
98	2.5–5	70–90	26	79	/77	26
84	2–20	90–180	10	25	6/10	2
99	4–15	64–128	22	45	/28	6(only 23 cycles for infertility therapy)
100	5	90	18	?	/39	9/4
101	1.2–10	90	14	24	13/23	7/2
91	10–15	60–90	9	23	3/3	1/1
86	10–25	90	3	6	3/6	3
67	10	120*	16	34	16/34	11
102	5	120	8	15	6/12	4
103	100	120*	?	8	5	0
	20	120*	?	20	17	5
	20	96	?	3	3	1
	10	90	?	2	1	0
104	5–10	90	20	88	74	25/6

*Daytime only.

25 ng/kg

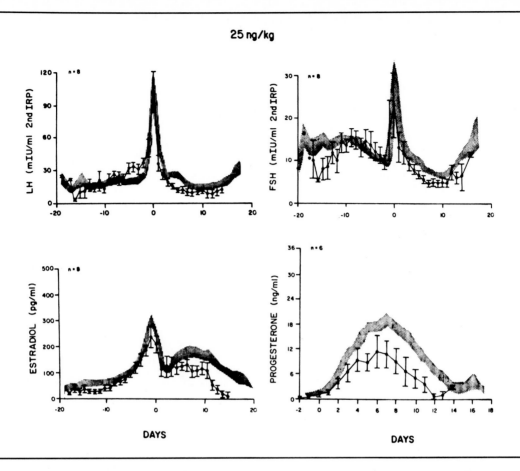

Figure 25–12. Patients with hypothalamic amenorrhea (solid line) treated with aa suboptimal dose of intravenous GnRH every 60 minutes demonstrate lower levels of follicular phase gonadotropins and luteal phase progesterone compared to healthy menstruating women (hatched area). (From Santoro et al.[68] Reproduced with permission.)

a deficient luteal phase.[74] High doses given every 60 to 90 minutes may lead to frank ovarian hyperstimulation and multiple pregnancy (Fig. 25–13 and Table 25–3).

Indirect evidence obtained in studies of LH pulses in patients with hypothalamic amenorrhea,[75] luteal phase defects,[76] and PCO[73,77,78] also supports the hypothesis that these disorders may be due either to deficient or exaggerated GnRH secretion.[58,79] Most forms of ovulatory dysfunction may thus be viewed as a spectrum of abnormalities in the hypothalamic GnRH pulse generator. Pulse abnormalities may be modulated further by catecholamines, corticotropin-releasing factor (CRF), and opioid secretion from higher central nervous system centers. Increasing dopaminergic tone with bromocriptine decreases the LH:FSH ratio in PCO.[73] Opioid administration in healthy menstruating women reduces gonadotropin secretion.[63] Conversely, patients with hypothalamic amenorrhea treated with opioid blockers such as naloxone or naltrexone demonstrate increased gonadotropin secretion. Patients with hypothalamic

amenorrha have responded to opioid blockers with ovulatory menses.[63,80] Animal studies have demonstrated that CRF is secreted by the brain during stress and that it inhibits GnRH secretion into the hypophyseal portal circulation. The result is blunting of LH pulsation. When a CRF antagonist is administered during stress, the blunted LH pulsatility is reversed.[81] All of these studies emphasize the concept that regulating GnRH pulse frequency and amplitude greatly affects the maintenance of a normal menstrual cycle.

ADMINISTRATION OF PULSATILE GnRH

Route of Administration

Significant controversy has arisen over the relative merits of intravenous versus subcutaneous administration of GnRH. Although some authors have reported discouraging results using the latter, patients with hypothalamic insufficiency treated with ade-

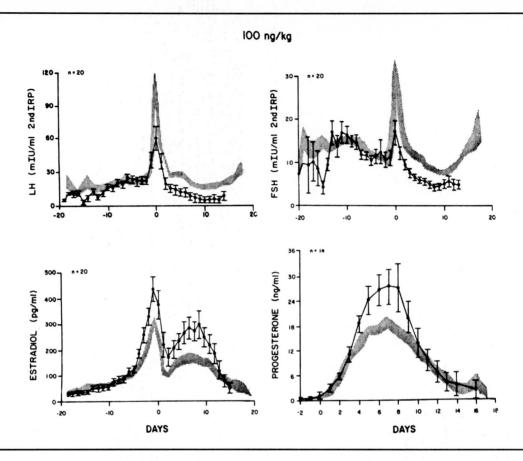

Figure 25–13. Patients with hypothalamic amenorrhea (solid line) treated with a supraphysiologic dose of intravenous GnRH every 60 minutes have evidence of overstimulation, with a high LH:FSH ratio early in the cycle and higher estradiol and progesterone levels in the luteal phase compared to healthy menstruating women (hatched area). (From Santoro et al.[68] Reproduced with permission.)

TABLE 25–3. MULTIPLE PREGNANCIES WITH GnRH

Reference	Route	Dose (μg)	Frequency (min)	Diagnosis	Outcome
118	IV	18	90	HI	Quadruplets
119	IV	15–20	90	HI	Triplets
120	IV	8	90	HI	Hyperstimulation
98	IV	2.5,5,14	90	HI	Twins (3 sets)
121	IV	5	60	PCO	Triplets
90	IV	2.5–20	90	HI	Triplets, twins (2 sets)
Saffan, Seibel, unpublished data	IV	4.5	90	PCO	Quadruplets, born at 36 weeks, 3 surviving
122	SC	10–25	90	HI	Triplets
123	SC	20	90	HI	Twins (3 sacs)

A review of several series revealed 3(4.6%) of 72 SC cycles (various doses and frequencies) and 8(5.7%) of 140 IV cycles (doses 2.5–20 μg, frequency q 90 min) ending in multiple pregnancies.[124]
HI = hypothalamic insufficiency; PCO = polycystic ovary disease.

TABLE 25–4. ADMINISTRATION OF GnRH IN WOMEN WITH POLYCYSTIC OVARY SYNDROME

Reference	Route	Dose (μg)	Frequency (min)	Pts.	Cycles	Ovulations (pts/cycles)	Pregnancies	Comments
105	IV	10–20	90	15	42	10/29	8	
99	IV	8	90–128	8	18	/9	2	7/8 ovulations and all pregnancies with a 128-min frequency
106	IV	5–20	90	26	74	21/41	3	
108	IV	20	90	13	20	/2	4 (2 miscarriages)	
109	IV	5–40	60–120	11	85	9/74	5 (3 pts., also 2 miscarriages)	
100	IV	5	90	4	?	/16	0	
101	IV	1–40	90–153	10	17	6/19	1	
98	IV	2.5–5	60–120	5	14	2/7	1	
110	IV	1.2–2.2	90	3	5	2/4	0	
111	IV	15	90	?	26	/11	4 (4 miscarriages)	(all 11 PCO pregnancies in 8 women)
	SC	15	90	?	41	/16	7 (2 miscarriages)	
112	IV	15	90	4	7	/3	0	
	SC	15	90	8	17	/2	1	
82	SC	5–20	120	3	5	1/2	0	Ovulations all with 8.5 μ dose

quate pulse doses and intervals demonstrate little difference in ovulation and pregnancy rates between the routes (Tables 25–1 and 25–2).[67,68,82–104] Ovulation rates of well over 90% are observed in hypothalamic insufficiency, and most patients become pregnant within 6 months with subcutaneous GnRH therapy. Although the doses required for subcutaneous administration are greater than those for intravenous administration, the former has significant advantages over the latter route. First, it is better tolerated. Patients can be instructed to change their own fine-gauge catheter, and the need to maintain a long-term intravenous line with its attendant risks of infection are obviated. Second, chemical thrombophlebitis and infectious complications, although rare, are less common than with the intravenous route. Also, the presence of a significant heart murmur is a contraindication to intravenous GnRH due to the theoretical risk of subacute bacterial endocarditis. Finally, intravenous catheters occasionally pull out or clot. This problem can be prevented in part by mixing in heparin, 1,000 IU/mL diluent. Should the economic benefits of a lower daily dose become important or a patient be unresponsive to subcutaneous treatment, the intravenous route can be used.

For patients with PCO, however, subcutaneous administration seems to be less efficacious than intravenous administration (Table 25–4).[82,98–101, 105–112] An even lower response to subcutaneous treatment can be anticipated in obese patients.[91,99,113]

Therefore we suggest using the intravenous route from the outset in these less responsive women.

Although nasal administration of GnRH has been used to treat hypogonadotropic hypogonadism in males, its use in treating ovulatory disorders has yet to be assessed. The 200-μg dose required every 2 hours makes this route impractical.[114]

Several pulsatile infusion devices are available.[38] We have found the Travenol Autosyringe (model AS6H, Travenol Autosyringe, Hooksett, NH) both practical and versatile. It is relatively small, weighing only 400 g, and allows for adjustment of pulse interval and bolus volumes. A drug-concentration chart makes calculating and adjusting the dosage simple and efficient (Table 25–5). After the powdered GnRH is dissolved in diluent, it can be left in solution for over a month without concern for deterioration of biologic efficacy.[115]

Our approach is to administer a combined oral contraceptive for 7 to 10 days to induce withdrawal bleeding, which serves as a useful reference point from which to begin treatment. When menstruation follows an ovulation-induction cycle, this step is disregarded. We ask the patient to keep a basal body temperature (BBT) chart and start the GnRH pump within 7 days of the first day of flow. Ultrasound examination of ovarian response is used for follicle tracking once or twice weekly until a 15-mm follicle is observed. Where available, the transvaginal ultrasound transducer is ideal for observing follicle growth. At this time it is helpful to perform an ultrasound examination daily until it reveals evidence of ovulation and a thermal shift is observed on BBT.[116,117] Ultrasound monitoring is necessary to decrease the risk of ovarian overstimulation and multiple pregnancy.[90,98,118–124] It also is helpful in adjusting the GnRH dosage in hyporesponders.[82] Thus it is incorrect to assume patients receiving pulsatile GnRH do not require monitoring.

The GnRH is administered through a 1.2-cm, 27-gauge needle (24″ set, no. 3M8472P; 42″ set, no. 3M8463P, Travenol) inserted into the subcutaneous fatty tissue of the lower abdomen or upper arm. The attached microtubing leads to the pump device, which can be worn on a belt or under clothing secured by an elastic strap. When using the subcutaneous route, we start with a dosage of 15 to 20 µg every 2 hours. Some patients appear to respond better to a 90-minute pulse interval; however, since most adverse experience with multiple pregnancies have been reported with this interval, we reserve it for poor responders (see Table 25–3). Depending on the ovarian response determined by ultrasound monitoring, it is occasionally necessary to alter the dosage or pulse interval. This should be considered only after 7 days of stimulation without demonstrable follicular development. Ovulation should occur by 21 days of treatment, although in most instances no more than 14 days are required.

More than 90% of patients with hypothalamic amenorrhea or oligoovulation respond well to GnRH given as described (Fig. 25–14). Some nonresponders respond to intravenous GnRH. To prevent clotting when using this route, heparin, 1,000 IU, is added to each cc of diluent along with the medication. A 5-cc syringe (no. 1M8474, Travenol) is used in the Travenol AS6H pump. The medication is delivered through a 21-gauge intravenous catheter placed in a comfortable place in the cephalic vein of the distal

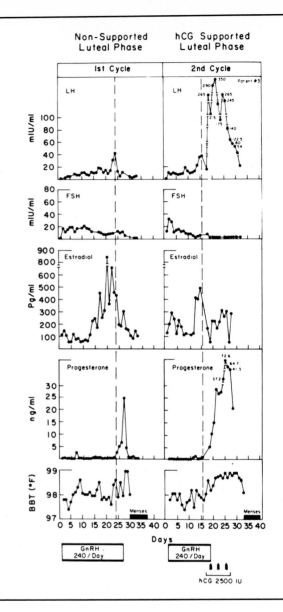

Figure 25–14. Hormone levels and temperature variations in a patient with hypothalamic amenorrhea treated with pulsatile GnRH. Note the shortened luteal phase in the left panel when human chorionic gonadotropin was withheld. (From Weinstein et al.[125] Reproduced with permission.)

TABLE 25–5. GnRH CONCENTRATIONS

Pulse Volume (µl)	Final dilutions (µg/ml)					
	100	200	250	300	400	500
	Actual per pulse dose (µg/ml)					
12	1.2	2.4	3	3.6	4.8	6
24	2.4	4.8	6	7.2	9.6	12
36	3.6	7.2	9	10.8	14.4	18
48	4.8	9.6	12	14.4	19.2	24
60	6.0	12.0	15	18.0	24.0	30
72	7.2	14.4	18	21.6	28.8	36
84	8.4	16.8	21	25.2	33.3	42

GnRH (Factrel, Ayerst Labs, New York), available in 500 and 100 µg ampules, is diluted with the accompanying diluent. We use a dilution of 250 µg/ml in a 5 cc syringe to fit the Travenol Auto Syringe model AS6H. Heparin, 1000 IU, is added to each cc of diluent for intravenous use.

forearm so that it can be hidden under long-sleeved clothing. The catheter is then connected to the pump by microtubing (60″ length, no. 3M8511, Travenol). It has been suggested that intravenous dosages be adjusted based on the severity of the hypothalamic insufficiency.[90,116] In our experience and after reviewing the wide range of effective dosages (See Table 25–2), we feel it best to start most patients on a dosage of 3-µg every 90 minutes and increase it as needed up to a maximum of 15 µg per dose. Multiple pregnancies have generally been reported with dosages of 5 µg and greater. Furthermore, it has been well documented that hyperphysiologic responses are observed at dosages of 4 to 5 μg (75 ng/kg).[68]

Of note, after an unsuccessful trial of subcutaneous GnRH, before administering intravenous GnRH we have had some success in giving clomiphene citrate. After the pituitary is primed with the subcutaneous hormone, these patients with hypothalamic amenorrhea who were previously resistent to clomiphene may go on to respond to the agent.

After follicles mature with GnRH, an endogenous LH surge occurs that initiates ovulation. The quality of the LH surge is often not sufficient to provide adequate luteal phase support, however. Therefore, after ovulation (documented by the thermal shift on the BBT chart combined with a change in cervical mucus and disappearance of the dominant follicle), medication must be continued.[125] This can be accomplished either by continuing the pulsatile GnRH or discontinuing it and administering progesterone or human chorionic gonadotropin (HCG). We have found it most convenient and cost-effective to administer HCG, 2,500 IU intramuscularly, beginning the day after ovulation and every 3rd day thereafter for a total of 3 doses.

Risks

One often-discussed advantage of pulsatile GnRH therapy over human menopausal gonadotropin (HMG) therapy for anovulation is a low rate of multiple pregnancies. On reviewing a series of over 200 treatment cycles using the intravenous or subcutaneous route at various pulse doses and intervals, it is noted that multiple pregnancy does occur about 5% of the time.[124] We have not, however, found a single report of a multiple pregnancy using our regimen of 20 μg subcutaneously every 120 minutes in women with oligoanovulation due to hypothalamic insufficiency (see Table 25–3).

Allergic reactions and even anaphylaxis with the development of anti-GnRH antibodies have been documented in patients receiving long-term GnRH.[126,127] These patients may become refractory to the treatment.[128] Furthermore, the presence of anti-GnRH antibody may contribute to the slightly higher than expected miscarriage rate of about 20% that occurs in GnRH-induced pregnancies.[124,129]

PATIENT SELECTION FOR PULSATILE GnRH TREATMENT

Since its introduction as a ovulation-inducing agent, pulsatile GnRH has been used to treat a wide variety of ovulatory dysfunctions. Proper evaluation of the etiology of anovulation is essential prior to initiating therapy in order to ensure that GnRH is the optimal ovulation-inducing agent. A good history and physical examination in conjunction with measuring serum levels of LH, FSH, androgens, and prolactin usually are sufficient to suggest the etiology.

Hypothalamic Amenorrhea or Insufficiency

Patients with hypothalamic amenorrhea or insufficiency who are anovulatory are ideally suited for ovulation induction with GnRH. These are the same patients who traditionally have been treated with human menopausal gonadotropins. Typical histories include substantial weight loss, anorexia nervosa, excessive exercise, or significant physical or psychologic stress. Serum levels of LH, FSH, and prolactin are usually in the normal to low normal range. Primary amenorrhea in association with anosmia and undetectable levels of LH and FSH should suggest a congenital absence of GnRH production (Kallmann's syndrome). Patients with a pituitary stalk transection do not respond to pulsatile GnRH and require HMG therapy.

When administered at an appropriate dosage and pulse interval, GnRH effectively restores normal ovulatory function and fertility in over 90% of women treated. Excellent response rates are observed for both the subcutaneous and intravenous routes. As shown in Tables 25–1 and 25–2, wide ranges of dosages and dose intervals have been used successfully. When administered intravenously at 60-minute intervals, the ideal dose appears to be between 25 and 100 ng/kg.[68] An effective alternative is a 90-minute interval with doses between 2 and 10 μg.

We prefer the subcutaneous route of administration for women with hypothalamic amenorrhea. Excellent response rates can be obtained, with lower potential risks and easier patient management. The vast majority of these patients respond well to a standard 20-μg dose given every 120 minutes.[82]

Efforts should first be made to correct underlying contributory factors, such as reducing excessive exercise, improving the diet, or gaining weight. Patients with hypothalamic amenorrhea associated with weight loss ovulate well with GnRH treatment, but have a higher risk of intrauterine growth retardation if a pregnancy begins when they are significantly underweight. For this reason, it is best to bring these patients closer to their ideal body weight before considering GnRH treatment.[111] Where indicated, patients with hypothalamic amenorrhea should have appropriate radiologic studies of the pituitary area to exclude mass lesions.

Polycystic Ovary Disease

One of the most common causes of chronic anovulation is PCO. Oligoamenorrhea, acne, obesity, and hirsutism in association with an inappropriately high LH:FSH ratio are classically associated with this disease. Although the majority of patients respond to clomiphene citrate, 15 to 20% do not. In these women, alternative methods of inducing ovulation have been the use of HMG and extracts of purified FSH.[130] These drugs work directly on the ovaries and bypass pituitary control of follicular recruitment. For this reason, HMG and purified FSH must be administered carefully to prevent complications. Despite diligent monitoring with serum estrogen levels and ovarian ultrasound, ovarian hyperstimulation and multiple pregnancy can occur in 20 to 30% of women.

The finding of high LH:FSH ratios suggests that this syndrome may at least in part be due to excessive hypothalamic GnRH secretion[73,77-79] and is not exclusively a primary ovarian defect.[131] It had been hoped that manipulation of the pulse frequency and amplitude of exogenously administered GnRH might reset or restore the correct or optimal GnRH signal to the pituitary gland. In practice, however, results have not been all that encouraging.

Investigators report ovulation rates of about 50% per treatment cycle, as opposed to more than 90% observed in patients with hypothalamic insufficiency. It has been noted by some that ovulation and pregnancy rates using GnRH in this group of patients are similar to those with HMG, albeit with fewer complications.[132] Among patients with PCO, the subcutaneous route has a much lower response rate than the intravenous route. Although higher ovulation and pregnancy rates might be anticipated by using a wider pulse interval[99] (such as every 120 minutes) to lower the LH:FSH ratio (see Table 25–4 and Fig. 25–9), clinical experience has not borne this out. Perhaps this is because in these patients, in contrast to GnRH-deficient women, their own GnRH secretion continues to function in parallel with the administered medication.

It has been suggested that patients with PCO who have high baseline LH:FSH ratios are unlikely to respond to pulsatile GnRH, compared to hyperandrogenic anovulatory women with normal LH:FSH ratios.[133] Of interest, we observed a marked increase of both LH and prolactin levels in unresponsive normoprolactinemic patients with PCO who were unresponsive to GnRH therapy.[82] It appears that at least in some patients, exogenous GnRH may override or correct the abnormal hypothalamic GnRH pulses that occur in PCO. The addition of clomiphene citrate, glucocorticoids, or low-dose HMG may increase GnRH responsiveness in otherwise resistant patients.[106,107,107a]

Hyperprolactinemia

The first series of women successfully treated with pulsatile GnRH included a patient with hyperprolactinemic amenorrhea.[134] Good data support the use of GnRH in hyperprolactinemic patients in whom bromocriptine is not effective.[134-137] Uncorrected hyperprolactinemia does not appear to interfere with ovulation and pregnancy rates when these women are treated with GnRH[134-137] or HMG.[138] All hyperprolactinemic patients should have appropriate radiologic examination of the sella turcica and measurement of serum TSH levels to exclude either a pituitary adenoma or hypothyroidism, both of which can cause hyperprolactinemia.

Luteal Phase Deficiency

Luteal phase inadequacy is believed to be a cause of recurrent miscarriage and infertility. Pulse studies of LH throughout the luteal phase have demonstrated aberrant frequencies among these patients.[76] Furthermore, inadequate GnRH replacement in hypothalamic amenorrhea leads to ovulatory cycles with an inadequate luteal phase (see Fig. 25–12).[68,69] Therefore, luteal phase inadequacy could theoretically be due to inadequate GnRH and could respond to exogenous pulsatile GnRH. Preliminary data support the possible application of GnRH therapy in some of these women.[98,139,140] Because there are simpler means to correct this disorder and only preliminary data exist on the possible efficacy of this treatment, however, it should be reserved for women refractory to the more established treatments for the insufficient luteal phase.

Deficient Cervical Mucus

The use of pulsatile GnRH to treat patients with poor cervical mucus production has been suggested.[141] Until further experience is gained, this treatment application should be considered experimental.

Superovulation for In-Vitro Fertilization and Embryo Transfer

Controlled ovarian hyperstimulation is a necessary step to induce ovulation for in-vitro fertilization (IVF). Because ovarian hyperstimulation and multiple pregnancies have been observed as adverse effects of GnRH ovulation induction, it has been hoped that higher doses of the drug could be used to induce multiple follicular growth in IVF-ET programs. Although there are reports of pulsatile GnRH used for this purpose, we have not found a consistent superovulation response in patients undergoing IVF even when high doses are used. Furthermore, in contrast to menopausal gonadotropins, patients treated with GnRH demonstrate an exaggerated LH pulse amplitude, making it difficult to determine with certainty either the presence or the initiation of the LH surge. Therefore other treatment protocols appear highly preferable to GnRH for controlled ovarian hyperstimulation associated with IVF.[142-145]

REFERENCES

1. Knobil E: The neuroendocrine control of the menstrual cycle. *Recent Prog Horm Res* 36:53, 1980.
2. Harris GW: The pituitary stalk and ovulation, in Vilee CA (ed): *Control of Ovulation.* New York, Pergamon, 1961, p 56.
3. Campbell HJ, Feuer G, Garcia J, Harris GW: The infusion of brain extracts into the anterior pituitary gland and the secretion of gonadotrophic hormones. *J Physiol* 157:30P, 1961.
4. McCann SM, Talesnik S, Friedman H: LH-releasing activity in hypothalamic extracts. *Proc Soc Exp Biol Med* 104:432, 1960.
5. Matsuo H, Baba Y, Nair RMG, Arimura A, Schally AV: Structure of the porcine LH and FSH releasing factor. 1. The proposed amino acid sequence. *Biochem Biophys Res Commun* 43:1334, 1971.
6. Burgus R, Butcher M, Ling N, Guillemin R: Structure moleculaire du facteur hypothalamique (LRF) d'origina ovine controlant la secretion de l'hormone gonadotrope hypophysaire de luteinisation (LH). *Seances Acad Sci (III)* 273:1611, 1971.
7. Schally AV: Aspects of hypothalamic regulation of the pituitary gland: Its implications for the control of reproductive processes. *Science* 202:18, 1978.
8. Guillemin R: Peptides in the brain: The new endocrinology of the neuron. *Science* 202:390, 1978.
9. Taymor ML: The use of luteinizing hormone-releasing hormone in gynecologic endocrinology. *Fertil Steril* 25:992, 1974.
10. Grimes EM, Thompson IE, Taymor ML: The sequence of pituitary responses to synthetic luteinizing hormone-releasing hormone (LH-RH) throughout the normal menstrual cycle. *Acta Endocrinol* 79:625, 1975.
11. Feore JC, Taymor ML: The relationship between the pituitary response to luteinizing hormone-releasing hormone and the ovulatory response to clomiphene citrate. *Fertil Steril* 27:1240, 1976.
12. Mortimer RH, Fleischer N, Lev-Gur M, et al: Correlation between integrated LH and FSH levels and the response to luteinizing hormone-releasing factor (LRF). *J Clin Endocrinol Metab* 43:1240, 1976.
13. Reiter EO, Root AW, Duckett GE: The response of pituitary gonadotrope to a constant infusion of luteinizing hormone-releasing hormone (LHRH) in normal prepubertal and pubertal children and in children with abnormalities of sexual development. *J Clin Endocrinol Metab* 43:400, 1976.
14. Wentz AC, Andersen RN: Response to repetitive luteinizing hormone-releasing hormone stimulation in hypothalamic and pituitary disease. *Am J Obstet Gynecol* 138:364, 1980.
15. Kastin AJ, Zarate A, Midgley AR, et al: Ovulation confirmed by pregnancy after infusion of porcine LHRH. *J Clin Endocrinol Metab* 33:980, 1971.
16. Grimes EM, Taymor ML, Thompson IE: Induction of timed ovulation with synthetic luteinizing hormone-releasing hormone in women undergoing insemination therapy. 1. Effect of a single parenteral administration at mid-cycle. *Fertil Steril* 26:277, 1975.
17. Acosta AA, Buttram VC, Malinak LR, et al: The use of synthetic luteinizing hormone-releasing hormone in induction of ovulation. *Fertil Steril* 26:1173, 1975.
18. Huang KE: The induction of ovulation in amenorrheic patients with synthetic luteinizing hormone-releasing hormone: The significance of pituitary responsiveness. *Fertil Steril* 27:65, 1976.
19. Huang KE: Use of synthetic luteinizing hormone-releasing hormone in induction of ovulation in amenorrheic patients. *Fertil Steril* 26:796, 1975.
20. Keller PJ: Induction of ovulation by synthetic luteinizing hormone-releasing factor in infertile women. *Lancet* 2:570, 1972.
21. Breckwoldt M, Czygan PJ, Lehman F, Bettendorf G: Synthetic LH-RH as a therapeutic agent. *Acta Endocrinol* 75:209, 1974.
22. Crosignani PG, Trojsi L, Attansio A, et al: Hormonal profiles in anovulatory patients treated with gonadotropins and synthetic luteinizing hormone-releasing hormone. *Obstet Gynecol* 46:15, 1975.
23. Maia H Jr, Barbosa I, Maia H, et al: Induction of ovulation with clomiphene citrate followed by LH-RH in women. *Int J Gynaecol Obstet* 21:1, 1983.
24. Nakano R, Katayama K, Mizuno T, Tojo S: Induction of ovulation with synthetic luteinizing hormone-releasing hormone. *Fertil Steril* 24:471, 1974.
25. Phansey SA, Barnes MA, Williamson HO, et al: Combined use of clomiphene and intranasal luteinizing hormone-releasing hormone for induction of ovulation in chronically anovulatory women. *Fertil Steril* 34:446, 1980.
26. Kotsuji F, Kitaguchi M, Okamura Y, Tojo S: Luteinizing hormone-releasing hormone (LH-RH) treatment for inducing clomiphene response in anovulatory patients with hypogonadotropic hypogonadism. *Asia Oceania J Obstet Gynaecol* 8:139, 1982.
27. Akande EO, Carr PJ, Dutton A, et al: Effect of synthetic gonadotropin-releasing hormone in secondary amenorrhea. *Lancet* 2:112, 1972.
28. Casas PRF, Badano AR, Aparicio N, et al: Luteinizing hormone-releasing hormone in the treatment of anovulatory infertility. *Fertil Steril* 26:549, 1975.
29. Hammond CB, Wiebe RH, Haney A, Yancy SG: Ovulation induction with luteinizing hormone-releasing hormone in amenorrheic infertile women. *Am J Obstet Gynecol* 135:924, 1979.
30. Hanker JP, Bohnet HG, Leyendecker G, Schneider HPG: LH-RH therapy in functional amenorrhea based on clinical subclassification. *Int J Fertil* 25:222, 1980.
31. Henderson SR, Bonnar J, Moore A, MacKinnon PCB: Luteinizing hormone-releasing hormone for induction of follicular maturation and ovulation in women with infertility and amenorrhea. *Fertil Steril* 27:621, 1976.
32. Keller PJ: Treatment of anovulation with synthetic LH-RH. *Am J Obstet Gynecol* 116:698, 1973.
33. Nillus SJ, Fries H, Wide L: Successful induction of follicular maturation and ovulation by prolonged treatment with LH-releasing hormone in women with anorexia nervosa. *Am J Obstet Gynecol* 122:921, 1975.
34. Rabin D, MacNeil LW: Long-term therapy with luteinizing hormone-releasing hormone in isolated gonadotropin deficiency: Failure of therapeutic response. *J Clin Endocrinol Metab* 52:557, 1981.
35. Zanartu J, Dabancens A, Kastin AJ, Schally AV: Effect of synthetic hypothalamic gonadotropin-releasing hormone (FSH/LH-RH) in anovulatory sterility. *Fertil Steril* 25:160, 1974.
36. Zarate A, Canales ES, Schally AV, et al: Successful induction of ovulation with synthetic luteinizing hormone-releasing hormone in anovulatory infertility. *Fertil Steril* 23:672, 1972.
37. Zarate A, Canales ES, Soria J, et al: Further observations on the therapy of anovulatory infertility with synthetic luteinizing hormone-releasing hormone. *Fertil Steril* 25:3, 1974.
38. Chambers GR, Sutherland IA, White S, Mason P, Jacobs HS: A new generation of pulsatile infusion devices. *Ups J Med Sci* 89:91, 1984.
39. Blankstein J, Mashiach S, Lunenfeld B: *Ovulation Induction and In Vitro Fertilization.* Chicago, Year Book, 1986.
40. Khodr GS, Siler-Khodr TM: Placental luteinizing hormone-releasing factor and its synthesis. *Science* 307:315, 1980.
41. Gonzalez ER: Does breast milk unleash gonadotropins? *JAMA* 244:634, 1980.
42. Popkin R, Bromley TA, Currie A, et al: Specific binding of LHRH to human luteal tissue. *Biochem Biophys Res Commun* 114:750, 1983.
43. Seppala M, Wahlstrom T, Leppaluoto G: Luteinizing hormone-releasing factor (LRF)-like immunoreactivity in rat pancreatic islet cell. *Life Sci* 25:1489, 1979.
44. Nikolics K, Mason AJ, Szonyi E, et al: A prolactin-inhibiting factor within the precursor for human gonadotropin-releasing hormone. *Nature* 316:511, 1985.
45. Seeberg PH, Adelman JP: Characterization of cDNA for precursor of human luteinizing hormone-releasing hormone. *Nature* 311:666, 1984.
46. Jeffcoate SL, Greenwood RH, Holland DT: Blood and urine clearance of luteinizing hormone-releasing hormone in man measured by radioimmunoassay. *J Endocrinol* 60:305, 1974.
47. Pimstone B, Epstein S, Hamilton SM, LeRoith D, Hendricks S: Metabolic clearance and plasma half-disappearance time of exogenous gonadotropin-releasing hormone in normal subjects and in patients with liver disease and chronic renal failure. *J Clin Endocrinol Metab* 44:356, 1977.
48. Arimura A, Kastin AJ, Gonzales-Barcena D, et al: Disappearance of LH-releasing hormone in man as determined by radioimmunoassay. *Clin Endocrinol* 3:421, 1974.
49. Miyachi Y, Mecklenburg RS, Hansen JW, Lipsett MG: Metabolism of ^{125}I-luteinizing hormone-releasing hormone. *J Clin Endocrinol Metab* 37:63, 1973.
50. Keye WR Jr: Regulation of pituitary response to gonadotropin-releasing hormone, in Sciarra JJ (ed): *Gynecology and Obstetrics.* New York, Harper & Row, 1987, vol 5.
51. Naor Z, Leifer AM, Catt KJ: Calcium-dependent actions of GnRH on pituitary 3',5'c-GMP production and gonadotropin release. *Endocrinology* 107:1438, 1980.

52. Snyder G, Naor Z, Fawcett CP, et al: Gonadotropin release and cyclic nucleotides—Evidence for LHRH-induced elevation of 3',5'c-GMP levels in gonadotropins. *Endocrinology* 107:1627, 1980.

53. Borges JLC, Scott D, Kaiser DL, et al: Ca^{++} dependence of gonadotropin-releasing hormone-stimulated luteinizing hormone secretion: In vitro studies using continuously perfused dispersed rat anterior pituitary cells. *Endocrinology* 113:557, 1983.

54. Conn PM, Chafouleas JG, Rogers D, et al: Gonadotropin-releasing hormone stimulates calmodulin redistribution in rat pituitary cells. *Nature* 292:264, 1981.

55. Adreyko JL, Marshall LA, Dumesic DA, Jaffe RB: Therapeutic uses of gonadotropin-releasing hormone analogs. *Obstet Gynecol Surv* 42:1, 1987.

55a. Claman P, Bayer S, Garner P, Berger E, Seibel MM: Human menopausal gonadotropin or purified follicle stimulating hormone induction of ovulation in polycystic ovarian syndrome after down regulation with a gonadotropin releasing hormone analogue. 44th annual meeting of The American Fertility Society, Atlanta, Georgia, Oct 8–13, 1988.

56. Belchetz PE, Plant TM, Nakai Y, Keogh EJ, Knobil E: Hypophyseal responses to continuous and intermittent delivery of hypothalamic gonadotropin-releasing hormone. *Science* 202:631, 1978.

57. Van Vugt DA, Diefenbach WD, Alston IE, Ferin M: Gonadotropin-releasing hormone pulses in third ventricular cerebrospinal fluid of ovariectomized rhesus monkeys: Correlation with luteinizing hormone pulses. *Endocrinology* 117:1150, 1985.

58. Crowley WF Jr, Filicori M, Spratt DI, Santoro NF: The physiology of gonadotropin-releasing hormone (GnRH) secretion in men and women. *Recent Prog Horm Res* 41:473, 1985.

59. Negro-Vilar A, Advis JP, Ojeda SR, et al: Pulsatile luteinizing hormone (LH) patterns in ovariectomized rats: Involvement of norepinephrine and dopamine in the release of LH-RH and LH. *Endocrinology* 111: 932, 1982.

60. Ojeda SR, Negro-Vilar A, McCann SM: Evidence for involvement of alpha-andrenergic receptors in norepinephrine-induced prostaglandin E$_2$ and luteinizing hormone-releasing hormone release from the median eminence. *Endocrinology* 110:409, 1982.

61. Fritz MA, Speroff L: The endocrinology of the menstrual cycle: The interaction of the folliculogenesis and neuroendocrine mechanisms. *Fertil Steril* 38:509, 1982.

62. Vijayan OE, McCann SM: The effects of systemic administration of dopamine and apomorphine on plasma LH and prolactin concentration in conscious rates. *Neuroendocrinology* 25:221, 1978.

63. Ferin M, Van Vugt D, Wardlaw S: The hypothalamic control of the menstrual cycle and the role of endogenous opioid peptides. *Recent Prog Horm Res* 40:441, 1984.

64. Seibel MM, Claman P, Oskowitz SP, McCardle C, Weinstein FG: Events surrounding the initiation of puberty with long-term subcutaneous pulsatile gonadotropin-releasing hormone in a female patient with Kallmann's syndrome. *J Clin Endocrinol Metab* 61:575, 1985.

65. Seibel MM, Kamrava M, McArdle C, Taymor ML: Ovulation induction and conception using subcutaneous pulsatile luteinizing hormone-releasing hormone. *Obstet Gynecol* 61:292, 1983.

66. Soules MR, Steiner RA, Clifton DK, Bremner WJ: The effects of inducing a follicular phase gonadotropin secretory pattern in normal women during the luteal phase. *Fertil Steril* 47:45, 1987.

67. Corenblum B, Mackin J, Taylor P: Ovulation induction and pregnancy in women with hypothalamic amenorrhea treated with intermittent GnRH. *R Reprod Med* 30:736, 1985.

68. Santoro N, Wierman ME, Filicori M, Waldstreicher J, Crowley WF Jr: Intravenous administration of pulsatile gonadotropin-releasing hormone in hypothalamic amenorrhea: Effects of dosage. *J Clin Endocrinol Metab* 62:109, 1986.

69. Hutchinson JS, Zeleznik AJ: Effects of varying gonadotropin pulse frequency on corpus luteum function and lifespan during the menstrual cycle of rhesus monkey. Abstract 613. Presented at the 67th annual meeting of the Endocrine Society, Baltimore, June 19–21, 1985.

70. Wildt L, Hausler A, Marshall G, et al: Frequency and amplitude of gonadotropin-releasing hormone stimulation and gonadotropin secretion in the rhesus monkey. *Endocrinology* 109:376, 1981.

71. Gross KM, Matsumoto AM, Bremner WJ: Differential control of luteinizing hormone and follicle-stimulating hormone secretion by luteinizing hormone-releasing hormone pulse frequency in man. *J Clin Endocrinol Metab* 64:675, 1987.

72. Soules MR, Clifton DK, Steiner RA, Cohen NL, Bremner WJ: Gonado-

tropin-releasing hormone-induced changes in testosterone secretion in normal women. *Fertil Steril* 48:423, 1987.

73. Seibel MM: Toward understanding the pathophysiology and treatment of polycystic ovary disease. *Semin Reprod Endocrinol* 2:297, 1984.

74. Clifton DK, Soules MR, Steiner RA: Neuroendocrine regulation of pulsatile gonadotropin-releasing hormone secretion, in Coelingh Bennink HJT, Dogterom AA, Lappohn RE, Rolland R, Schoemaker J (eds): *Pulsatile GnRH 1985.* Proceedings of the 3rd Ferring Symposium, Noordwijk, The Netherlands, Sept 11–13, 1985. Haarlem, The Netherlands, Ferring, 1986, p 19.

75. Marshall JC, Kelch RP: Gonadotropin-releasing hormone: Role of pulsatile secretion in the regulation of reproduction. *N Engl J Med* 315:1459, 1986.

76. Soules MR, Steiner RA, Clifton DK, Bremner WJ: Abnormal patterns of pulsatile luteinizing hormone in women with luteal phase deficiency. *Obstet Gynecol* 63:626, 1984.

77. Rebar RW, Judd HL, Yen SSC, et al: Characterization of the inappropriate gonadotropin secretion in polycystic ovarian syndrome. *J Clin Invest* 57:1320, 1976.

78. Waldstreicher J, Santoro NF, Hall JE, Filicori M, Crowley WF Jr: Hyperfunction of the hypothalamic–pituitary axis in women with polycystic ovarian disease: Indirect evidence for partial gonadotrope desensitization. *J Clin Endocrinol Metab* 66:165, 1988.

79. Santoro N, Crowley WF Jr: Disorder of endogenous GnRH secretion: Hypogonadotropic hypogonadism, polycystic ovarian disease, inadequate luteal phase, in Coelingh Bennink HJT, Dogterom AA, Lappohn RE, Rolland R, Schoemaker J (eds): *Pulsatile GnRH 1985.* Proceedings of the 3rd Ferring Symposium, Noordwijk, The Netherlands, Sept 11–13, 1985. Haarlem, The Netherlands, Ferring, 1986, p 51.

80. Wildt L, Leyendecker G: Induction of ovulation by the chronic administration of naltrexone in hypothalamic amenorrhea. *J Clin Endocrinol Metab* 64:1334, 1987.

81. Rivera C, Rivier J, Vale W: Stress-induced inhibition of reproductive functions: Role of endogenous corticotropin-releasing factor. *Science* 231:603, 1986.

82. Saffan D, Seibel MM: Ovulation induction with subcutaneous pulsatile gonadotropin-releasing hormone in various ovulatory disorders. *Fertil Steril* 45:475, 1986.

83. Skarin G, Nillius SJ, Wide L: Pulsatile subcutaneous luteinizing hormone-releasing hormone treatment of anovulatory infertility. Abstract 2630. Presented at the 7th International Congress of Endocrinology, Quebec City, Quebec, 1984. Excerpta Medica, International Congress series 652. Amsterdam, Elsevier, 1984.

84. Loucopoulos A, Ferin M, Van der Wiele RL, et al: Pulsatile administration of GnRH for induction of ovulation. *Am J Obstet Gynecol* 148:895, 1984.

85. Reid RL, Sauerbrei E: Evaluation of techniques for induction of ovulation in outpatients employing pulsatile gonadotropin-releasing hormone. *Am J Obstet Gynecol* 148:648, 1984.

86. Jacobs HS, Adams J, Franks S, et al: Induction of ovulation with luteinizing hormone-releasing hormone: Problems, indications and contraindications. *J Steroid Biochem* 20:A36, 1984.

87. Hurley DM, Brian R, Outch K, et al: Induction of ovulation and fertility in amenorrheic women by pulsatile low-dose gonadotropin-releasing hormone. *N Engl J Med* 310:1069, 1984.

88. Keogh, EJ, Carote C, Meakin J, et al: Clinical application of pulsatile GnRH. Abstract 1166. Presented at the 7th International Congress of Endocrinology, Quebec City, Quebec, 1984. Excerpta Medica, International Congress series 652, Amsterdam, Elsevier, 1984.

89. Woodhouse NJY, Niles N, Othman HO: Hypothalamic hypogonadism: Induction of ovulation—Pregnancy by subcutaneous pulsatile injections of GnRH. *Horm Res* 20:172, 1984.

90. Leyendecker G, Wildt L: Pulsatile administration of gonadotropin-releasing hormone in hypothalamic amenorrhea. *Ups J Med Sci* 89:19, 1984.

91. Molloy BG, Hancock KW, Glass MR: Ovulation induction in clomiphene nonresponsive patients: The place of pulsatile gonadotropin-releasing hormone in clinical practice. *Fertil Steril* 43:26, 1985.

92. Soules MR, Southworth MB, Norton ME, Bremner WJ: Ovulation induction with pulsatile gonadotropin-releasing hormone: A study of the subcutaneous route of administration. *Fertil Steril* 46:578, 1986.

93. Leyendecker G, Wildt L: Induction of ovulation with pulsatile administration of gonadotropin-releasing hormone in hypothalamic amenorrhea. *J Steroid Biochem* 20:1382, 1984.

94. Miller DS, Reid RL, Cetel NS, Rebar RW, Yen SSC: Pulsatile adminis-

tration of low-dose gonadotropin-releasing hormone: Ovulation and pregnancy in women with hypothalamic amenorrhea. *JAMA* 250:2937, 1983.

95. Hanker JP, Nieschlag L, Schneider HPG: Pulsatile LH-RH substitution in hypothalamic amenorrhea. Abstract 972. Presented at the 7th International Congress of Endocrinology, Quebec City, Quebec, 1984. Excerpta Medica, International Congress series 652. Amsterdam, Elsevier, 1984.

96. Hanker JP, Schneider HPG: Induction of ovulation by pulsatile GnRH in hypothalamic amenorrhea, in Coelingh Bennink HJT, Dogterom AA, Lappohn RE, Rolland R, Schoemaker J (eds): *Pulsatile GnRH 1985*. Proceedings of the 3rd Ferring Symposium, Noordwijk, The Netherlands, Sept 11–13, 1985. Haarlem, The Netherlands, Ferring, 1986, p 115.

97. Berg D, Mickan H, Michael S, et al: Ovulation and pregnancy after pulsatile administration of gonadotropin-releasing hormone. *Arch Gynaekol* 233:205, 1983.

98. Jansen RPS, Handelsman DJ, Boyland LM, et al: Pulsatile intravenous GnRH for ovulation induction in infertile women. 1. Safety and effectiveness with outpatient therapy. *Fertil Steril* 48:33, 1987.

99. Bringer J, Hedon B, Jaffiol C, et al: Influence of the frequency of gonadotropin-releasing hormone (GnRH) administration on ovulatory responses in women with anovulation. *Fertil Steril* 44:42, 1985.

100. Rolland R, Lorijn RHN, Willemsen WNP: Chronic intermittent administration of GnRH in infertile women with different cycle abnormalities. *J Steroid Biochem* 20:1402, 1984.

101. Schriock ED, Jaffe RB: Induction of ovulation with gonadotropin-releasing hormone. *Obstet Gynecol Surv* 41:414, 1986.

102. Malo JW, Bezdicek B, Campbell E, Pavelka DA, Covato T: Ovulation induction with pulsatile intravenous GnRH. *J Reprod Med* 30:902, 1985.

103. Schoemaker J, Simons AHM, Burger CW, Delemarre HA, Van Kessel H: Induction of ovulation with LH/FSH releasing hormone (LHRH), in Roland R, Van Hall EV, Hillier SG, McNatty P, Schoemaker J (eds): *Follicular Maturation and Ovulation*. Amsterdam, Excerpta Medica, 1982, p 373.

104. Willemsen WNP, Rolland RHW, Lorijn RHN, Franssen AMHW: Results of GnRH therapy in anovulatory infertile women, in Coelingh Bennink HJT, Dogterom AA, Lappohn RE, Rolland R, Schoemaker J (eds): *Pulsatile GnRH 1985*. Proceedings of the 3rd Ferring Symposium, Noordwijk, The Netherlands, Sept 11–13, 1985. Haarlem, The Netherlands, Ferring, 1986, p 139.

105. Coelingh Bennink HJT, Weber HW, Alsbach GPJ, Thijssen JHH: Induction of ovulation by pulsatile intravenous administration of GnRH in polycystic *Ovarian Disease*. Abstract 344. Presented at the 7th International Congress of Endocrinology, Quebec City, Quebec, 1984. Excerpta Medica, International Congress series 652. Amsterdam, Elsevier, 1984.

106. Berg FD, Hinrichsen H, Mickan: Administration of gonadotropin-releasing hormone in hyperandrogenic women with anovulation, in Coelingh Bennink HJT, Dogterom AA, Lappohn RE, Rolland R, Schoemaker J (eds): *Pulsatile GnRH 1985*. Proceedings of the 3rd Ferring Symposium, Noordwijk, The Netherlands, Sept 11–13, 1985. Haarlem, The Netherlands, Ferring, 1986, p 155.

107. Corenblum B, Taylor PJ: Augmentation of gonadotropin-releasing hormone induced follicular growth with exogenous gonadotropins. *Fertil Steril* 48:954, 1987.

107a. Eshel A, Abdulwahid NA, Armar NA, Adams JA, Jacobs HS: Pulsatile LH-RH therapy in women with polycystic ovary syndrome. *Fertil Steril* 49:956, 1988.

108. Birkhauser MH, Huber PR: Pathophysiological aspects and clinical results of ovulation induction by pulsatile intravenous administration of GnRH in polycystic ovary syndrome (PCOS), in Coelingh Bennink HJT, Dogterom AA, Lappohn RE, Rolland R, Schoemaker J (eds): *Pulsatile GnRH 1985*. Proceedings of the 3rd Ferring Symposium, Noordwijk, The Netherlands, Sept 11–13, 1985. Haarlem, The Netherlands, Ferring, 1986, p 161.

109. Burger CW, Korsen TJM, Hompes PGA, Schoemaker J: PCO-like disease: To pulse or not to pulse, that is the question, in Coelingh Bennink HJT, Dogterom AA, Lappohn RE, Rolland R, Schoemaker J (eds): *Pulsatile GnRH 1985*. Proceedings of the 3rd Ferring Symposium, Noordwijk, The Netherlands, Sept 11–13, 1985. Haarlem, The Netherlands, Ferring, 1986, p 181.

110. Ory SJ, London SN, Tyrey L, Hammond CB: Ovulation induction with pulsatile gonadotropin-releasing hormone administration in patients with polycystic ovarian syndrome. *Fertil Steril* 43:20, 1985.

111. Adams J, Polsam DW, Abdulwahid N, et al: Multifollicular ovaries: Clinical and endocrine features and response to pulsatile gonadotropin-releasing hormone. *Lancet* 2:1375, 1985.

112. Tucker M, Adams J, Mason WP, et al: Multiple cystic ovatian disease—A new classification. Abstract 2657. Presented at the 7th International Congress of Endocrinology, Quebec City, Quebec, 1984. Excerpta Medica, International Congress series 652. Amsterdam, Elsevier, 1984.

113. Lyles R, Elkind-Hirsch E, Goldzieher JW, Besch PK: Plasma gonadotropin-releasing hormone profiles after intravenous and subcutaneous bolus injection in thin and obese women. *Obstet Gynecol* 71:44, 1988.

114. Klingmuller D, Meschi M, Schweikert HU: Successful intranasal administration of LH-RH in men with hypogonadotropic hypogonadism. *J Steroid Biochem* 20:1395, 1984.

115. Hahn PM, Van Vugt DA, Reid RL: The stability of synthetic gonadotropin-releasing hormone in solution. *Fertil Steril* 48:155, 1987.

116. Leyendecker G, Wildt L: Induction of ovulation with chronic intermittent (pulsatile) administration of GnRH in women with hypothalamic amenorrhea. *J Reprod Fertil* 69:397, 1983.

117. Seibel MM, McArdle CR, Thompson IE, et al: The role of ultrasound in ovulation induction: A critical appraisal. *Fertil Steril* 36:573, 1981.

118. Heineman MJ, Bouckaert PXJM, Schellekens LA: A quadruplet pregnancy following ovulation induction with pulsatile luteinizing hormone-releasing hormone. *Fertil Steril* 42:300, 1984.

119. Bogchelman P, Lappohn RE, Janssens J: Triplet pregnancy after administration of gonadotropin-releasing hormone. *Lancet* 2:45, 1982.

120. Geisthovel F, Peters F, Breckwoldt M, Freiburg FRG: Ovarian hyperstimulation due to long-term pulsatile intravenous gonadotropin-releasing hormone treatment. *Arch Gynecol* 236:255, 1985.

121. Filicori M, Michelacci L, Ferrari P, et al: Triplet pregnancy after low-dose pulsatile gonadotropin-releasing hormone in polycystic ovarian disease. *Am J Obstet Gynecol* 155:768, 1986.

122. Mason P, Adams J, Morris OV, et al: Induction of ovulation with pulsatile luteinizing hormone-releasing hormone. *Br Med J* 288:181, 1984.

123. Skarin G, Nillius SJ, Wide L: Pulsatile subcutaneous low-dose gonadotropin-releasing hormone treatment of anovulatory infertility. *Fertil Steril* 40:454, 1983.

124. Jansen RPS: Ovulation induction with pulsatile GnRH, in Thomsen K, Ludwig H (eds): *Gynecology and Obstetrics: Proceedings of the 11th World Congress of Gynecology and Obstetrics*, Berlin, 1985. Heidelberg, Springer-Verlag, 1986, p 842.

125. Weinstein FG, Seibel MM, Taymor ML: Ovulation induction with subcutaneous pulsatile gonadotropin-releasing hormone: Role of supplemental human chorionic gonadotropin in the luteal phase. *Fertil Steril* 41:546, 1984.

126. Claman P, Elkind-Hirsch K, Oskowitz SP, Seibel MM: Urticaria associated with antigonadotropin-releasing hormone antibody in a female Kallmann's syndrome patient being treated with long-term pulsatile gonadotropin-releasing hormone. *Obstet Gynecol* 69:503, 1987.

127. MacLeod TL, Eisen A, Sussman GL: Anaphylactic reaction to synthetic luteinizing hormone-releasing hormone. *Fertil Steril* 48:500, 1987.

128. Meakin JL, Keogh EJ, Martin CE: Human anti-luteinizing hormone-releasing hormone antibodies in patients treated with synthetic luteinizing hormone-releasing hormone. *Fertil Steril* 43:811, 1985.

129. Das C, Gupta SK, Talwar GP: Pregnancy interfering action of LHRH and anti-LHRH. *J Steriod Biochem* 23:803, 1986.

130. Claman P, Seibel MM: Purified human follicle-stimulating hormone for ovulation induction: A critical review. *Semin Reprod Endocrinol* 4:277, 1986.

131. Erickson GF, Hsueh AJW, Quigley ME, Rebar RW, Yen SSC: Functional studies of aromatase activity in human granulosa cells from normal and polycystic ovaries. *J Clin Endocrinol Metab* 49:514, 1979.

132. Bringer J, Hedon B, Gibert F, et al: Treatment of anovulation by HMG or GnRH: Contribution of a cross-over randomized study to a rational management of PCO, in Coelingh Bennink HJT, Dogterom AA, Lappohn RE, Rolland R, Schoemaker J (eds): *Pulsatile GnRH 1985*. Proceedings of the 3rd Ferring Symposium, Noordwijk, The Netherlands, Sept 11–13, 1985. Haarlem, The Netherlands, Ferring, 1986, p 171.

133. Jansen RPS, Handelsman DJ, Boyland LM, et al: Pulsatile intravenous gonadotropin-releasing hormone for ovulation induction in infertile women. II. Analysis of follicular and luteal phase responses. *Fertil Steril* 48:39, 1987.

134. Leyendecker G, Struve T, Plotz EJ: Induction of ovulation with chronic

intermittent (pulsatile) administration of LH-RH in women with hypothalamic and hyperprolactinemic amenorrhea. *Arch Gynecol* 229:177, 1980.

135. Bergh T, Skarin G, Nillius SJ, Wide L: Pulsatile treatment with gonadotropin-releasing hormone (GnRH) in hyperprolactinemic women, in Coelingh Bennink HJT, Dogterom AA, Lappohn RE, Rolland R, Schoemaker J (eds): *Pulsatile GnRH 1985.* Proceedings of the 3rd Ferring Symposium, Noordwijk, The Netherlands, Sept 11–13, 1985. Haarlem, The Netherlands, Ferring, 1986, p 103.

136. Franks S, Mason HD, Sagle M, et al: Hypothalamic disorders in hyperprolactinaemia: The place of GnRH treatment, in Ludwig H, Thomsen K (eds): *Gynecology and Obstetrics:* Proceedings of the 11th World Congress of Gynecology and Obstetrics, Berlin, 1985. Springer-Verlag, 1986, p 829.

137. Morris DV, Abdulwahid NA, Armar A, Jacobs HS: The response of patients with organic hypothalamic–pituitary disease to pulsatile gonadotropin-releasing hormone therapy. *Fertil Steril* 47:54, 1987.

138. Fairne D, Dor J, Lupovici N, Lunenfeld B, Mashiach S: Conception rate after gonadotropin therapy in hyperprolactinemia and normoprolactinemia. *Obstet Gynecol* 65:658, 1985.

139. Lorijn RHN, Rolland R: Induction of ovulation with pulsatile LH-RH in infertile women. *Ups J Med Sci* 89:47, 1984.

140. Loucopoulos A, Ferin M: The treatment of luteal phase defects with pulsatile infusion of gonadotropin-releasing hormone. *Fertil Steril* 48:933, 1987.

141. Loucopoulos A, Ferin M, Van der Wiele RL: Cervical mucus-related infertility treated by pulsatile administration of gonadotropin-releasing hormone. *Fertil Steril* 41:139, 1984.

142. Shaw RW, Ndukwe G, Imoedemhe D, Burford G, Chan R: Stimulation of multiple follicular growth for in vitro fertilization by administration of pulsatile luteinizing hormone-releasing hormone during the midfollicular phase. *Fertil Steril* 46:135, 1986.

143. Jones GS, Muasher S, Acosta AA, Rosenwaks Z: The use of GnRH in an in vitro fertilization program, in Coelingh Bennink HJT, Dogterom AA, Lappohn RE, Rolland R, Schoemaker J (eds): *Pulsatile GnRH 1985.* Proceedings of the 3rd Ferring Symposium, Noordwijk, The Netherlands, Sept 11–13, 1985. Haarlem, The Netherlands, Ferring, 1986, p 199.

144. Liu JH, Durfee R, Muse K, Yen SSC: Induction of multiple ovulation by pulsatile administration of gonadotropin-releasing hormone. *Fertil Steril* 40:18, 1983.

145. Seibel MM: A new era in reproductive technology: In vitro fertilization, gamete intrafallopian tube transfer and donated gametes and embryos. *N Engl J Med* 318:828, 1988.

CHAPTER 26

Treatment of Infertility Using Bromocriptine Mesylate

Eugene Katz, Eli Y. Adashi

Treatment of Infertility Using Bromocriptine Mesylate

History
Pharmacology
Mechanism of Action
Adverse Effects
Therapeutic Indications
   Prolactin-Producing Pituitary

Adenomas
Idiopathic Hyperprolactinemia
Polycystic Ovary Syndrome
Idiopathic Infertility
Luteal Phase Dysfunction
Summary

The identification of human prolactin as a distinct lactogenic hormone and its isolation are relatively recent events.[1] The development of a specific radioimmunoassay for prolactin heralded an era in which the physiology of prolactin secretion by the pituitary gland and its hypothalamic control became better understood.[2] In addition, elevated levels of circulating prolactin were found to be associated with several clinical entities of reproductive pertinence.[3]

HISTORY

Bromocriptine (2-bromo-α-ergocriptine) (Fig. 26–1) is a semisynthetic product derived from a family of ergot alkaloids or ergopeptines. Ergot itself is the product of the fungus *Claviceps purpura* that grows on edible grains, mainly rye.[4] Descriptions of the noxious effects of ergot poisoning can be found as early as 600 B.C. on an Assyrian tablet. Much later, in the Middle Ages, the disease caused by the ingestion of the fungus was named Holy Fire, or St. Anthony's fire, after the saint at whose shrine relief was said to be obtained. Indeed, at that location, pilgrims received contamination-free grain. The symptoms of poisoning consisted of gangrene of the limbs as a result of intense vasoconstriction. Although poison-

ing was also accompanied by abortion, the use of ergot as an uterotonic agent preceded its identification as the cause of St. Anthony's fire. In addition, infants of poisoned women died because of lack of breast milk.[5]

The use of bromocriptine mesylate (hereafter, referred to as bromocriptine) as an agent capable of lowering the circulating levels of prolactin was sparked by the discovery that ergot alkaloids inhibited endometrial decidualization in the rat,[6] an effect that could be reversed by the administration of progesterone or prolactin.[7] Due to the lack of radiometric methods for the measurement of prolactin, however, two bioassays were used, both of which were based on the inhibition of the luteotropic action of prolactin in the rat. The specific end points under study were the interruption of leukocyte dominance in vaginal smears of pseudopregnant rats and the inhibition of ovum implantation in inseminated rats. The suppression of lactation constituted an additional bioassay.[8,9]

Using this approach, bromocriptine was selected in 1967 for further development as a therapeutic agent[8] and introduced for clinical testing in 1969.[10] The drug was ultimately approved for clinical use in the United States in 1979. To date, approved indications are for the treatment of hyperprolactinemic

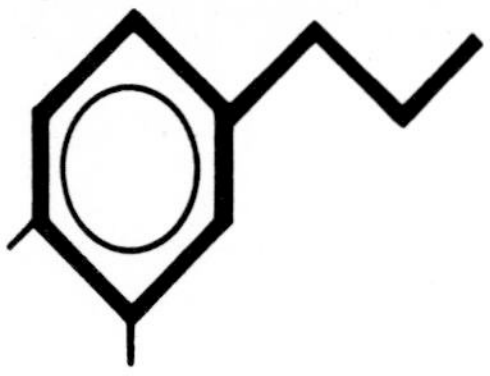

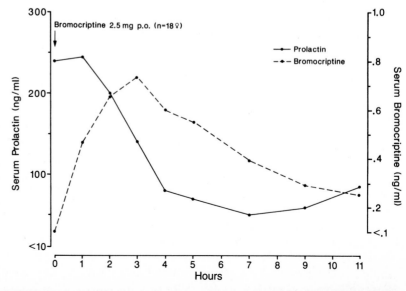

Dopamine

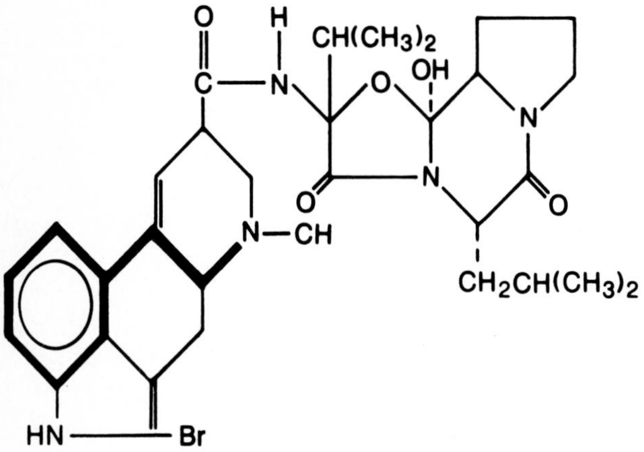

Bromocriptine

Figure 26–1. Structural formulas of dopamine and bromocriptine.

disorders including prolactin-producing pituitary tumors, and the inhibition of physiologic postpartum lactation, acromegaly, and Parkinson's disease. The drug is also used for a variety of other endocrine and nonendocrine conditions.[10]

PHARMACOLOGY

After an oral dose of bromocriptine, 28% of the drug is absorbed. Of that fraction, 94% is metabolized after the first passage through the liver.[11,12] Thus between 90 and 98% of the absorbed drug is excreted in the bile and feces, and the remainder is excreted in the urine.[10,13] After a single oral dose of 2.5 mg, drug levels tend to peak at 3 hours, falling with a half-life of 3.3 hours.[14] As expected, the drug is still detectable in serum 11 hours after the initial dose (Fig. 26–2). As a result, the circulating levels of prolactin decline by 40% at a time when peak concentrations of bromocriptine have been reached. The peak effect is observed 7 hours after the initial dose. Of significance, there appears to be no difference in the pharmacokinetics of bromocriptine among responders and nonresponders. Rather, differences in sensitivity to the drug seem to be at play.[14]

Attempts to administer bromocriptine vaginally have also proved successful.[15] Given in this fashion, its circulating levels display a continuous rise over a period of 8 hours, accompanied by a decrease in serum prolactin levels.

Although a long-acting form of bromocriptine has been developed for intramuscular injection, it is not as yet available for widespread clinical use.[16] In this case, the drug is incorporated into polylactic acid microspheres and suspended in a dextran-containing vehicle prior to injection. Maximum serum levels are reached about 2 hours after injection, followed by slow clearance with a half-life of 16 days. A 50-mg dose of injectable, long-acting bromocriptine inhibits prolactin secretion for 4 to 11 weeks. Side effects—nausea and vomiting—last only 1 hour to 2 days.[17,18] Limited clinical experience suggests the

Figure 26–2. Serum levels of bromocriptine and prolactin after oral bromocriptine, 2.5 mg. (Modified from Thorner MO, Schran HF, et al: A broad spectrum of prolactin suppression by bromocriptine in hyperprolactinemic women: a study of serum prolactin and bromocriptine levels after acute and chronic administration of bromocriptine. *J Clin Endocrinol Metab* 50(b): 1026, 1986.[14] ©1986, the Endocrine Society. Reproduced with permission.)

utility of this preparation in the treatment of prolactin-producing pituitary adenomas and in inhibiting puerperal lactation.[19] Other ergot derivatives have been evaluated in the search for a preparation with fewer side effects; however, bromocriptine continues to be the most widely used of these substances.[20,21]

The initial 2.5-mg dose is generally given at bedtime, thereby minimizing the possibility of orthostatic hypotension (discussed later). Additional increments are provided with meals and increased in a stepwise fashion every 4 to 7 days to avoid unpleasant side effects. Optimal dosing is determined by the return of circulating levels of prolactin to normal. Dosages above 20 mg/day are seldom needed in the treatment of prolactin-producing pituitary tumors.[22] Indeed, dosages as low as 1.25 mg/day are in many instances sufficient to normalize serum prolactin levels in cases of idiopathic hyperprolactinemia.[23,24]

MECHANISM OF ACTION

The secretion of pituitary prolactin is known to be under tonic inhibitory control by hypothalamic dopamine.[25] The latter neurotransmitter is secreted by the tuberoinfundibular neurons and released at the level of the median eminence into the long portal vessels, which convey it to the anterior pituitary.[8] The consequent binding of dopamine to its lactotrope receptors results in the inhibition of cyclic adenosine 3',5'-monophosphate (cAMP) and calcium-dependent prolactin release.[26,27] That bromocriptine may exert a direct effect at the pituitary level is evident from its ability to compete with dopamine for binding to isolated bovine anterior pituitary membranes.[28] In addition, bromocriptine inhibits the secretion of prolactin by isolated rat pituitary glands[29] and reduces the serum levels of prolactin in hypophysectomized rats bearing a heterotopic pituitary.[30] Significantly, it inhibits the release of prolactin not only at the level of the lactotrope but also at the level of the tuberoinfundibular neurons in the hypothalamus. Indeed, bromocriptine reduces dopamine turnover in the tuberoinfundibular neurons of the lactating rat, thereby increasing the hypothalamic content of this neurotransmitter.[31] In addition to reducing prolactin secretion (an exocytotic event), bromocriptine has been shown to inhibit lactotrope proliferation.[32,33]

ADVERSE EFFECTS

Some unwanted reactions to bromocriptine appear to be associated with the initiation of therapy, while others appear to be the result of long-term administration. Initially, bromocriptine may induce nausea, vomiting, postural hypotension, headaches, and na-

sal stuffiness. These effects are transient and can be minimized by administering the drug at bedtime, by avoiding large dosage increments, and by providing the drug in conjunction with meals. Bromocriptine may produce alcohol intolerance and gastrointestinal bleeding. Very high doses (as prescribed in Parkinson's disease) may result in cold-induced digital vasospasm (not ergotism), erythromelalgia, hallucinations, delusions, dementia, and depression.[8] To date, there is no evidence of long-term harmful effects on hepatic, renal, or hematologic functions. An exhaustive review of the rare and almost all reversible side effects can be found elsewhere.[34]

An important issue in patients receiving bromocriptine for infertility is its teratogenic potential. The medication does indeed cross the placenta and has been shown to lower fetal serum levels of prolactin.[35,36] However, analysis of the outcome of more than 2,000 pregnancies in which embryos and fetuses of all gestational ages were exposed to bromocriptine did not reveal an increase in the frequency of congenital anomalies or of spontaneous abortions.[34] In addition, reports of more than 350 children born of mothers receiving bromocriptine during pregnancy, some for more than 30 weeks of continuous exposure, and followed for up to 9 years, confirm the safety of the drug.[34,37-39]

These facts notwithstanding, it is suggested that, in the absence of overriding indications, bromocriptine be discontinued in the immediate postovulatory phase and that its administration during pregnancy be avoided whenever possible. This note of caution is prompted by the recognition that its teratogenic potential has not as yet been exhaustively evaluated. Indeed, it would be difficult to rule out at this time the possibility of subtle neurologic damage inflicted by the agent during gestation, particularly in reference to organizing dopaminergic nerve systems. Although no evidence exists to support such a possibility, it appears reasonable to minimize gestational exposure and thereby the possibility of as yet uncovered adverse consequences.[37,40]

THERAPEUTIC INDICATIONS

Prolactin-Producing Pituitary Adenomas

In 1975 bromocriptine was used successfully for the first time in the treatment of two patients with large prolactin-producing pituitary tumors.[41] Successful normalization of visual fields was reported in 1978,[42] the same year in which the first radiographic documentation of tumor regression was presented.[43,44] The drug's inhibitory effect on the growth of pituitary tumors in experimental animals was, in fact, discovered early in its development.[45-47] Used at much higher concentrations than those employed in women, bromocriptine also proved inhibitory to DNA synthesis by cultured lymphocytes and proliferation of cultured pituitary cells.[48-50]

The mechanism by which bromocriptine reduces the size of human prolactin-producing pituitary tumors has been elucidated. This is an important issue, for if the drug's effect were a consequence solely of a reduction in size of individual tumor cells—that is, merely cytostatic—its benefit would be restricted to the time during which it is administered. On the other hand, if bromocriptine had a cytocidal effect, a greater and perhaps a more permanent effect could be expected. In fact, both mechanisms seem to be at play. Indeed, bromocriptine has been shown to produce necrotic changes in tumoral pituitary tissue of certain patients.[51] These findings were later extended in studies comparing untreated patients with prolactin-producing pituitary adenomas with those receiving bromocriptine for 2 weeks and those who after 2 weeks of taking the drug discontinued therapy 1 week prior to surgery.[52] The tumors treated with bromocriptine displayed necrotic changes and fibrosis, as well as a reduction in size of individual tumor cells and an increase in the amount of stromal tissue. In contrast, patients who discontinued bromocriptine prior to surgery developed areas of regrowth of tumor cells. It has therefore been proposed that these tumors may contain two populations of cells. While most cells may respond to bromocriptine with cytostasis, others undergo necrosis. Conceivably, it is the first group of cells that is responsible for the regrowth of the tumor (see below).

Only a reduction in cell size but little in the way of a tumoricidal effect of bromocriptine was observed in 5 patients with prolactin-producing pituitary tumors.[53] Similar results were reported by others.[54,55] Specifically, the reduction in cell size was mostly apparent in the cytoplasm, perhaps due to the destruction of the prolactin-producing apparatus—the rough endoplasmic reticulum and the Golgi complex. Some cells showed an increase in the number of secretory granules, perhaps as a consequence of an unequal dopaminergic effect on the synthesis and release of prolactin. It was significant, however, that all studies revealed regrowth of pituitary tumor cells as soon as 1 week after discontinuation of therapy.[52,53,55,56]

Taken together, the literature extensively supports the ability of bromocriptine to reduce the size of prolactin-producing pituitary tumors to return the serum prolactin level to normal and thus restore reproductive cyclicity, and to correct the visual defects or palsies of the third and fourth nerves that occur secondary to compression of adjacent cranial structures.

Macroadenomas. Theoretically, macroadenomas, defined as prolactin-producing pituitary tumors that exceed 10 mm in diameter, can be managed with radiotherapy, surgery, dopaminergic agents, or combinations thereof. Radiotherapy has not been widely employed in the United States, given the slow rate of response as well as the potential development of secondary panhypopituitarism. Similarly, significant concerns persist with respect to the utility of the transsphenoidal approach for removing these adenomas.[57] Although capable of effecting immediate (albeit transient) resolution in up to 60% of cases[58-63] with relatively low morbidity and mortality, this procedure is associated with an unacceptable recurrence rate that can reach 91% (Table 26–1).[63] Consequently, this therapy is not curative, strongly suggesting that the more conservative, although equally noncurative, medical approach may be superior.

More than 300 cases of macroprolactinomas treated with bromocriptine have been reported. Most of those published after 1980 are summarized in Table 26–2. The drug effectively reduces the size of the macroadenomas in 33 to 100% of patients, including those with suprasellar extension. Although serum prolactin values appear to reach normal levels in 50 to 100% of patients, a significant but not necessarily complete decrease in circulating levels of the hormone is observed in practically all bona fide cases.[64-77] The significance of this finding lies in the observation that the reduction in the size of the tumor, and the improved oculomotor, sensorial, and pituitary endocrine function, are associated with a reduction, although not necessarily to normal, of hyperprolactinemia. Conversely, although reduced tumor size is always preceded by diminished prolactin release, a lower serum prolactin level does not assure subsequent reduction in size. The positive effects of the drug are the result of either the elimination of the mass effect on the hypothalamic–pituitary system or the correction of the putative underlying hypothalamic dysfunction (dopamine deficiency).[78,79] Although the effect of bromocriptine is dramatic, regrowth can occur with discontinuation of the drug.[66,67,71,74,76,80-84]

In summary, bromocriptine constitutes the initial treatment of choice for all macroprolactinomas, particularly in view of the limitations and potential complications of alternative forms of therapy.

During pregnancy, symptomatic macroadenomas respond dramatically to bromocriptine.[84-89] Specifically, prolactin levels are lowered in both maternal and cord blood, while levels in the amniotic fluid (presumably of decidual origin not subject to dopaminergic control) remain normal.[87] The drug does not alter maternal serum levels of progesterone, testosterone, or estradiol during early pregnancy.[88]

TABLE 26–1. RESULTS OF SURGICAL TREATMENT OF PROLACTINOMAS

Reference	N	Remission of Hyper–PRL	%	Microadenomas Recurrence N(%)	N	Remission of Hyper–PRL	%	Microadenomas Recurrence N(%)
58	40	37	92.5	0 (at least 1 follow-up visit)	60	37	62	1(2.7)
					27 extrasellar	10	37	1(4)
59	54	39	72 (88% if preop PRL 100 ng/dl)	NR	46	16	35	NR
					17 diffuse	8	47	
					29 invasive	8	29	
60	61	46	75	NR	8	4	50	NR
61	50	37	54	NR	48	9	19	NR
					27 expansive	9	33	
					21 invasive	0	0	
62	28	24	85	12(50)	16	5	47	4(80)
63		13	NR	4(31) (3–9 mo)	NR		10	NR	9(91) (× 26 mo)

NR = not reported

Microadenomas.   The therapeutic options for microadenomas, which are prolactin-producing tumors of less than 10 mm in diameter, include medical treatment with bromocriptine, surgery, or observation alone. Transsphenodial resection of these tumors has been reported to lead to the immediate correction of hyperprolactinemia in 55 to 92% of cases (see Table 26–1).[57–62] The morbidity associated with surgery, however, although low, is certainly higher than that associated with bromocriptine alone.[57] Even in experienced hands, recurrence rates can reach 50%.[61,62] Furthermore, occasionally microprolactinomas cannot be found at surgery.

Bromocriptine represents a highly effective, noninvasive alternative to surgery. It also may be preferred because microprolactinomas, as is discussed below, left untreated display a slow rate of progression. In general, bromocriptine reduces prolactin levels in 94 to 100% of patients, although not always to within the normal range (Table 26–3).[90–93] Even such apparently incomplete response is in most cases adequate to bring about the return of ovulation and fertility. It is conceivable that some of the immunoreactive prolactin represents a nonbioactive form.[94]

Although pregnancy is generally perceived as a negative influence on prolactin-producing pituitary tumors, it may in fact exert a therapeutic effect on microadenomas. Thus, in a group of 58 hyperprolactinemic women of whom 39 had abnormal tomograms, assessed before and after a bromocriptine-induced pregnancy, prolactin levels were reduced by more than half in 20 patients after pregnancy.[95]

Levels decreased even further in 15 women who became pregnant a second time. Although persistent remission of hyperprolactinemia was reported in 22% of 36 patients with microprolactinoma after discontinuation of treatment with bromocriptine, other investigators reported that only seldom do the hormone levels remain normal after the medication is withdrawn.[96]

In selecting the appropriate treatment, particularly when fertility is not a consideration, it is important to take into account that the natural history of the disease is not completely understood. Obviously, all macroadenomas were at one time microadenomas; however, it is not known what proportion of smaller tumors progress into macroadenomas. In 120 autopsies performed in an unselected group of men and women between ages 16 and 91 years who had no clinically apparent pituitary disease, 27% of the pituitaries were found to harbor a microadenoma; 41% of these tumors stained for prolactin. No sex difference could be noted, and the age distribution of patients with microadenoma did not differ from that in the autopsy group.[97] The fact that microadenomas are so prevalent while invasive macrodenomas are seldom seen suggests that prolactinomas are in most cases nonprogressive.

In addition, 43 patients with hyperprolactinemia, of whom 28 had a tomographic (CT) scan consistent with the presence of a pituitary tumor, were followed untreated, with prolactin levels measured biannually and CT scans every 9 to 24 months for 3 to 20 years.[98] In 3 patients, the levels returned to normal. Further-

TABLE 26–2. RESULTS OF BROMOCRIPTINE THERAPY FOR MACROADENOMAS

Reference	No. of Patients	No. of Patients with PRL Reduced	Patients with Reduced Tumor Size N (%)	Comments
64.65	2	2 (1 to normal)	2 (100)	Rapid regrowth of tumor upon discontinuation of bromocriptine, and reduction after reinstitution of therapy.
66	8	8	8 (100)	5 patients who discontinued BCR had elevation of PRL of less than 40% of initial levels.
67	10	10 (8 to normal)	9 (90)	8 patients previously treated with surgery or radiotherapy.
68	18	18 (7 to normal)	11 (61)	All patients had extra-sellar extension of tumor, 2 had been previously treated with surgery and radiotherapy.
69	4 11 nonsecretory tumors 5 nonprolactin-secreting tumors	4 (100)9 (82)	4 (100)	All with extrasellar extension.
70	19	19	10 (53)	All patients received BCR prior to surgery. Those who received BCR did significantly better after surgery.
71	12	12 (10 to normal)	4 (33)	2 patients with suprasellar extension.
72	15	15 (14 to normal)	10 (67)	6 patients with suprasellar extension. Hyperprolactinemia redeveloped in 14 patients after discontinuation of therapy.
73	6	6 (3 to normal)	4 (67)	
74	27	27 (18 to normal)	27 (100)	All had extrasellar extension.
75	38	37 (30 to normal)	29 (76)	4 patients received lisuride instead of BCR.
76	12	12 (10 to normal)	12 (100)	
77	24	23 (15 to normal)	23 (96)	All with extrasellar extension 8 patients had been previously treated with surgery.

more, visual fields remained normal in all patients, and only 2 showed progression of the tumor. Similarly, 25 patients with prolactin levels of at least 50 ng/mL for at least 2 years were followed for an average of 11.3 years without treatment.[99] Although conventional sella tomograms have serious limitations,[100] this radiologic examination remained unchanged or improved in 24 patients; 21 had lower prolactin levels at reevaluation. In view of these findings, simple observation without treatment appears an acceptable management option when symptoms are not intolerable and fertility is not being sought. One possible exception to this rule, however, is the hyperprolactinemic hypoestrogenic patient, the management of whom is discussed below.

It is worthwhile to note that follicle-stimulating hormone-producing tumors[101,102] and other nonprolactin and nonfunctioning pituitary tumors may sometimes respond to bromocriptine.[69,103,104]

Idiopathic Hyperprolactinemia

The term *idiopathic hyperprolactinemia* is used in reference to hyperprolactinemic patients who have no radiologically demonstrable pituitary tumor. In these

TABLE 26–3. EFFECT OF BROMOCRIPTINE ADMINISTRATION ON PATIENTS WITH MICROADENOMA AND HYPERPROLACTINEMIC PATIENTS WITHOUT EVIDENCE OF ADENOMA

| Reference | Microadenoma | | | No Evidence of Microadenoma | | |
	No. of Patients	Reduction of PRL N(%)	Normalization of Menses N(%)	No. of Patients	Reduction of PRL N(%)	Normalization of Menses N(%)
90	19	19(100) [14 to normal]	19(100)	21	21(100)	21(100)
91	35	31(89)	33(94)	23	22(96)	23(100)
92	36	36(100) [8 to normal]				
93	17	16(94)	15/16(94)			

*35 patients received metergoline and 23 received bromocriptine; both were equally effective.

patients bromocriptine is highly effective in correcting the hyperprolactinemia (See Table 26–3).[90,91] Expectant management also is an acceptable option in most but not all cases.

A decrease in bone density was reported to occur in hyperprolactinemic women.[105,106] Although the lack of estrogen probably contributes to the bone loss, by itself it may not fully account for the development of osteoporosis. Rather, prolactin may affect bone economy either directly or indirectly. In some but not all in vitro studies, prolactin induced the formation of 1,25-dihydroxyvitamin D_3.[107,108] It also was reported to increase bone calcium mobilization in rats.[109] In addition, calcitonin administration lowers prolactin levels in humans,[110] an effect in which the central dopaminergic system may be involved.[111] Indeed, patients with Parkinson's disease who are treated with L-dopa have a high bone mineral content.[112] Because correction of hyperprolactinemia restores bone density,[113,114] patients who choose not to be treated must be counseled as to the effects of high levels of prolactin on bone density.

Polycystic Ovary Syndrome

Hyperprolactinemia was observed at one point in 20 to 40% of patients with polycystic ovary syndrome (PCO).[115] Although the mechanism(s) underlying this association remain uncertain, this phenomenon suggests the existence of a decrease in central dopaminergic activity.[116–118] It is on these tentative grounds that bromocriptine has been proposed as an alternative therapeutic modality in the management of PCO, its addition being viewed in the context of dopamine replacement therapy. The accuracy of this prediction appears to be supported by the agent's ability to correct some of the endocrine dysfunctions associated with PCO, namely, the inappropriate release of luteinizing hormone (LH)[119–128] and the attendant hyperandrogenism. Although additional studies are clearly necessary, it has been generally presumed that the ability of bromocriptine to diminish the overall LH release represents an inhibitory effect of dopamine at the level of arcuate gonadotropin-releasing hormone (GnRH) neurons. In any event, as only a fraction of patients with PCO have hyperprolactinemia, it is possible that the elevated LH is a consequence of an entirely different phenomenon, namely, the associated hyperestrogenic milieu.[116,124,125]

The ability of bromocriptine to improve the PCO-associated hyperandrogenism may well represent two distinct mechanisms of action. For one, bromocriptine's action in lowering LH release may be accompanied by diminishing stimulation of the ovarian androgen-producing theca-interstitial cells.[117] In addition however, the agent may diminish adrenal androgen production, which may[126–129] or may not[130] be subject to positive control by prolactin.

Few studies have addressed the treatment of PCO with bromocriptine, and most of them are uncontrolled (Table 26–4).[123,131–134] This is of utmost importance, because it was reported that 35 to 45% of patients have occasional ovulatory cycles prior to or while receiving bromocriptine.[134] The same reservation exists with respect to studies on the effectiveness of the agent in normoprolactinemic anovulatory patients without the clinical or laboratory characteristics of PCO (Table 26–5).[125,135–139] In this connection, nocturnal levels of prolactin, as well as peak levels of the hormone after metoclopramide stimulation test, were analyzed in a group of normoprolactinemic, chronically anovulatory patients receiving bromocriptine either alone or in combination with clomiphene citrate if they failed to ovulate with the

TABLE 26–4. TREATMENT OF CLASSIC POLYCYSTIC OVARY DISEASE WITH BROMOCRIPTINE

Reference	Patients	Treatment	Results	Comments
121	20 normoprolactinemic	BCR 7.5 mg	12 patients resumed menses	Uncontrolled study.
131	7 normoprolactinemic	BCR 2.5–5.0 mg	3 patients ovulated (4 cycles)	Uncontrolled study, all clomiphene failures.
132	Total 37 21 normoprolactinemic 16 normoprolactinemic	BCR 5.0 mg	Total 31 "markedly improved menses"; 19 "markedly improved menses" 12 "markedly improved menses"	Uncontrolled study.
133	55 normoprolactinemic	BCR 2.5–5.0 mg 28 pts Placebo; 27 pts	12 regular ovulation (53%) (NS)	Double-blind controlled study.
134	23 (3 with moderate hyperprolactinemia)	BCR 5.0 mg	7 ovulatory patients (30%) (31 of 91 cycles) 8 occasional ovulatory cycles	All clomiphene failures. 35–45% of patients had occasional ovulation with or prior to BCR therapy.

NS = not significant.

single-drug therapy.[139] The patients who ovulated with bromocriptine alone had higher nocturnal and peak postmetoclopramide prolactin levels, suggesting that latent or nocturnal hyperprolactinemia was responsible for their anovulation.

In conclusion, controlled studies fail to show that bromocriptine alone may be beneficial in anovulatory women with or without PCO. Although a subgroup of normoprolactinemic anovulatory patients may be particularly responsive to the drug, their characteristics have yet to be defined.

Idiopathic Infertility

In 1977 a cumulative 63% pregnancy rate was reported after 10 months of bromocriptine therapy in 40 ovulatory, normoprolactinemic (but infertile)

women.[140] Unfortunately, no control group was studied, thereby invalidating any conclusion. Indeed, subsequent data derived from controlled studies showed no benefit from the drug for idiopathic infertility.

A controlled crossover study administered bromocriptine or placebo to 50 patients with unexplained infertility for 3 months.[141] If no pregnancy occurred, the patients were crossed over for an additional 3 months. The group was subsequently followed for a total of 12 months. The overall pregnancy rate was 36%. Ten patients became pregnant without specific therapy, 5 before and 5 after treatment. Four became pregnant while taking bromocriptine and 4 while taking placebo, demonstrating no benefit from the medication. When bromocriptine was administered for 6 months to 47 patients with unexplained infertil-

TABLE 26–5. BROMOCRIPTINE THERAPY FOR CHRONIC ANOVULATION

Reference	Patients	Treatment	Results	Comments
125	21 normoprolactinemic	BCR 2.5 mg	15 ovulatory	Uncontrolled study.
135	30 normoprolactinemic, normohypogonadotropic amenorrhea	BCR 5.0 mg 17 patients Placebo 13 patients	2 normal menses (12%) (NS) 4 normal menses (31%) (NS)	
136	38 normoprolactinemic anovulatory	BCR 2.5 mg days 5–26 Cyclophenyl 600 mg days 5–12	30 patients conceived within 3 cycles	Uncontrolled study.
137	37 anovulatory 20 hyperprolactinemic 17 normoprolactinemic	BCR 5.0 mg	18 patients ovulated 17 ovulated 1 ovulated	BCR not effective for normoprolactinemic anovulation.
138	15 patients: 12 ovulatory with clomiphene, 3 resistant to clomiphene	BCR 5.0 mg for 6 mo	14 ovulated 13 pregnancies	Uncontrolled study.
139	34 normoprolactinemic	BCR 10 mg	13 ovulatory	Patients ovulatory with BCR have higher peak nocturnal and higher peak post-metoclopramide test levels of prolactin before treatment.

NS = not significant.

ity, the cumulative pregnancy rate was similar to that of a matched control group.[142]

Others studied prolactin levels throughout the cycle in a group of 48 patients with unexplained infertility and a control group of 28 fertile women.[143] The control group showed an insignificant midcycle rise and a midluteal phase elevation of serum prolactin level; however, 45 (94%) of the infertile women displayed a significant but transient midcycle elevation of prolactin. Although 18 (40%) of these 45 women displayed no other prolactin peak, the remaining 27 had a late luteal phase elevation as well. When bromocriptine was then given to the infertile group at dosages sufficient to suppress any elevation of prolactin, 18 (40%) of 45 patients conceived within 3 months of treatment. The lack of a treatment control group in the study conspires against assigning bromocriptine a role in the restoration of fertility. Moreover, the role of possible transient hyperprolactinemia is questionable. Indeed, the effects of prolactin on hypothalamic and ovarian function are preceded by a latency period.[144]

Luteal Phase Dysfunction

A discussion of the role of prolactin in the function of the corpus luteum of several species can be found elsewhere.[145] Briefly, prolactin is essential in forming and maintaining the corpus luteum in rodents. In rhesus monkeys, a minimal concentration also may be necessary for adequate luteogenesis.[146] Early luteal hypophysectomy in this species does not affect luteal function, however. [147]

In hypophysectomized women, ovulation induction with exogenous gonadotropins and human chronic gonadotropin (HCG) results in the formation of a normal corpus luteum despite the absence of prolactin. On the other hand, in-vitro lutenized human granulosa cells require prolactin for maximum production of progesterone. However, the presence of high prolactin levels results in reduced progesterone production.[148] In women, bromocriptine-induced hypoprolactinemia as well as metoclopramide-induced hyperprolactinemia (initiated early in the menstrual cycle) have been reported to reduce progesterone production by the corpus luteum and the binding of LH to the structure.[149,150] Corpus luteum function remains unaffected when hyperprolactinemia is induced once the corpus luteum is formed, suggesting that the excess prolactin exerts its deleterious effects on the developing follicle. Some studies showed that bromocriptine prolongs the luteal phase,[150,151] while one showed an increased area under the basal body temperature curve but slightly shortened luteal phases.[152] In the latter study, the patients were normoprolactinemic and the luteal phase defects were diagnosed purely on the basis of shortened secretory phases. Some studies

have failed to demonstrate either suboptimal midluteal serum progesterone levels in hyperprolactinemic patients, or elevated circulating prolactin in patients with suboptimal midluteal levels.[153]

In conclusion, although correcting hyperprolactinemia with bromocriptine may improve folliculogenesis and thereby assist in correcting a luteal phase defect, there is no evidence that normoprolactinemic women with a luteal phase defect may benefit from the drug. Indeed, some evidence appears to support a deleterious effect of bromocriptine-induced hypoprolactinemia on luteal cell function.

SUMMARY

The development of bromocriptine mesylate and its introduction as a therapeutic option in disorders of reproductive endocrinology represented a cornerstone in the study of the physiology of prolactin secretion in normal and pathologic conditions. Its use in inhibiting postpartum lactation is widespread. In addition, it constitutes the first line treatment for prolactin-producing pituitary adenomas. However, the literature does not seem to support the use of bromocriptine in polycystic ovary syndrome, idiopathic infertility, and normoprolactinemic luteal phase defect.

REFERENCES

1. Hwang P, Guyda H, Friesen HG: Purification of human prolactin. *J Biol Chem* 247:1955, 1972.
2. Hwang P, Guyda H, Friesen H: A radioimmunoassay for human prolactin. *Proc Natl Acad Sci USA* 68:1902, 1971.
3. Frank S, Murray MF, Jequier AM: Incidence and significance of hyperprolactinemia in women with amenorrhea. *Clin Endocrinol* 4:597, 1975.
4. Rall TW, Schleifer LS: Oxytocin, prostaglandins, ergot alkaloids, and other drugs; tocolytic agents, in Gilman AG, Goodman LS, Rall TW, Murad M (eds): *The Pharmacological Basis of Therapeutics.* New York, Macmillian, 1985, pp 482–483, 937–938.
5. Barbieri RL, Ryan KJ: Bromocriptine endocrine pharmacology and therapeutic applications. *Fertil Steril* 39:727, 1983.
6. Shelesnyak MC: Ergotoxine inhibition of deciduoma formation and its reversal by progesterone. *Am J Physiol* 179: 3a02, 1954.
7. Shelesnyak MC: Maintenance of gestation in ergotoxine-treated pregnant rats by exogenous prolactin. *Acta Endocrinol* 27:99, 1958.
8. Thorner MO, Fluckiger E, Calne DB: *Bromocriptine. A Clinical and Pharmacological Review.* New York, Raven, 1980, pp 5–18, 143–153.
9. Fluckiger E, Wagner H: 2-Br-alpha-ergokryptin: Beeinflussung von Fertilität und Laktation bei der Ratte. *Experientia* 24:1130, 1968.
10. Vance ML, Evans WS, Thorner MO: Bromocriptine. *Ann Intern Med* 100:78, 1984.
11. Aellig WH, Nuesch E: Comparative pharmokinetic investigations with tritium-labelled ergot alkaloids after oral and intravenous administration in man. *Int J Pharm* 15:606, 1977.
12. Schran HF, Bhuta SI, Schwartz HJ, Thorner MO: The pharmacokinetics of bromocriptine in man, in Goldstein M, Calde DB, Lieberman A, Thorner MO (eds): *Ergot Compounds and Brain Function: Neuroendocrine and Neuropsychiatric Aspects.* New York, Raven, 1980, pp 125–139.
13. Kiechel JR: Pharmacocinetique et metabolisme des dérives de l'ergot. *J Pharmacol* [Paris] 10:533, 1980.
14. Thorner MO, Schran HF, Evans WS, Rogol AD, Morris JL, Macleod RM: A broad spectrum of prolactin suppression by bromocriptine in hyperprolactinemic women: A study of serum prolactin and bro-

mocriptine levels after acute and chronic administration of bromocriptine. *J Clin Endocrinol Metab* 50:1026, 1980.

15. Katz E, Schran HF, Adashi EY: Successful treatment of a prolactin-producing pituitary macroadenoma with intravaginal bromocriptine mesylate: A novel approach to intolerance of oral therapy. *Obstet Gynecol* 73:517, 1989.

16. Del Pozo E, Schluter K, Nuesch E, Rosenthalem J, Kemp L: Pharmacokinetics of a long-acting bromocriptine preparation (Parlodel LA) and its effects on release of prolactin and growth hormone. *Eur J Clin Pharmacol* 29:615, 1986.

17. Benker G, Gieshoff B, Freundlieb O, et al: Parenteral bromocriptine in the treatment of hormonally active pituitary tumors. *Clin Endocrinol* 24:505, 1986.

18. Montiru M, Pagani G, Gianola D, et al: Long-acting suppression of prolactin secretion and rapid shrinkage of prolactinomas after a long-acting, injectable form of bromocriptine. *J Clin Endorinol Metab* 63:266, 1987.

19. Peters F, del Pozo E, Coriti A, Breckwoldt M: Inhibition of lactation by a long-acting bromocriptine. *Obstet Gynecol* 67:82, 1986.

20. Crosignani PG, Ferrari C, Liuzzi A, et al: Treatment of hyperprolactinemic states with different drugs: A study with bromocriptine, metergoline, and lisuride. *Fertil Steril* 37:61, 1982.

21. Borges JLC, Schran HF, Evans WS, et al: Mesulergine, a new dopamine agonist: Effects on anterior pituitary function and kinetics. *Clin Pharmacol Ther* 36:696, 1984.

22. Borenstein R, Kessler L, Ben-David M: Prolactin resistance to bromocriptine treatment: A case report. *Int J Fertil* 26:287, 1981.

23. De Bernal M, de Villamizar M: Restoration of ovarian function by low nocturnal single daily doses of bromocriptine in patients with the galactorrhea-amenorrhea syndrome. *Fertil Steril* 37:392, 1982.

24. Soto-Albors CE, Daly DC, Walters CA, Ying YK, Riddick DH: Titrating the dose of bromocriptine when treating hyperprolactinemic infertile women. *Fertil Steril* 43:485, 1985.

25. Leong DA, Frawley LS, Neill JD: Neuroendocrine control of prolactin secretion. *Annu Rev Physiol* 45:109, 1983

26. Schettini G, Cronin MJ, Macleod RM: Adenosine 3′5′-monophosphate (cAMP) and calcium-calmodulin interrelation in the control of prolactin secretion: Evidence for dopamine inhibitor of cAMP accumulation and prolactin release after calcium mobilization. *Endocrinology* 1112:1801, 1980.

27. Nagasawa H, Yanai R, Flueckiger E: Counteraction by 2-Br-alpha-ergocryptine of pituitary prolactin release promoted by dibutyrila-denosine-3′,5′-monophosphate, in Pasteels JL, Robyn C (eds): *Human Prolactin.* Amsterdam, Excerpta Medica, 1973, p. 313.

28. Calabro MA, Macleod RM: Binding of dopamine to bovine anterior pituitary gland membranes. *Neurondocrinology* 25:32, 1978.

29. Pasteels JL, Danguy A, Frerotte M, Ectors F: Inhibitor de la secretion de prolactive par l'ergocornine et la 2-Br-α-ergocryptine: action directe sur l'hypophyse en culture. *Ann Endocrinol* [Paris] 32:188, 1971.

30. Mueller EE, Cocchi D, Panerai AE, et al: Pituitary hormones and ergot alkaloids. *Pharmacology* 1:63, 1978.

31. Hokfelt T, Fuxe K: Effects of prolactin and ergot alkaloids on the tuberoinfundibular dopamine neurons. *Neuroendocrinology* 9:100, 1972.

32. Lloyd HM, Jacobi JM, Meares JD: DNA synthesis and depletion of prolactin in the pituitary gland of the male rat. *J Endocrinol* 77:129, 1978.

33. Lloyd HM, Meares JD, Jacobi J: Effects of oestrogen and bromocriptine on in vivo secretion and mitosis in prolactin cells. *Nature* 255:497, 1975.

34. Weil C: The safety of bromocriptine in long-term use: A review of the literature. *Curr Med Res Opin* 10:25, 1986.

35. Andersen A, Pedersen H, Westergard J, Schioler V, Arends J: Normal and abnormal prolactin levels during human pregnancy: Lack of influence on fetoplacental endocrine function. *Acta Obstet Gynecol Scand* 63:145, 1984.

36. Bigazzi M, Ronga R, Lancranjan I, et al: A pregnancy in an acromegalic woman during bromocriptine treatment: Effects on growth hormone and prolactin in the maternal, fetal, and amniotic fluid compartments. *J Clin Endocrinol Metab* 48:9, 1979.

37. Raymond JP, Goldstein E, Konopka P, Leleu MF, Merceron RE, Loria Y: Follow-up of children born of bromocriptine-treated mothers. *Horm Res* 22:239, 1985.

38. Turkalj I, Braun P, Krupp P: Surveillance of bromocriptine in pregnancy. *JAMA* 247;1589, 1982.

39. Kurachi K, Aono T, Koike K, et al: A follow-up survey of infants born to mothers treated with bromocriptine. *Sanka Fujinka* 50:126, 1978.

40. Polatti F, Bolis PF, Ravagni-Probizer MF, Baruffini A, Cavalleri A:

Treatment of hyperprolactinemic amenorrhea by intermittent administration of bromocriptine (CB 154). *Am J Obstet Gynecol* 131:792, 1978.

41. Corenblum B, Webster BR, Mortimer CB, Ezrin C: Possible antitumor effect of 2-bromo-ergocryptine (CB-154 Sandoz) in 2 patients with large prolactin-secreting pituitary adenomas [abstr]. *Clin Res* 23:614A, 1975.

42. Vaidya R, Aloorkar SD, Rege NR, et al: Normalization of visual fields following bromocriptine treatment in hyperprolactinemic patients with visual field constriction. *Fertil Steril* 29:632, 1978.

43. Ezrin C, Kovacs K, Horvath E: Hyerprolactinemia: Morphologic and clinical considerations. *Med Clin North Am* 62:393, 1978.

44. Sobrinho LG, Nunes MCP, Santos MA, Mauricio JC: Radiological evidence for regression of prolactinomas and treatment with bromocriptine. *Lancet* 2:257, 1978.

45. Quadri SK, Lu KH, Meites J: Ergot-induced inhibition of pituitary tumor growth in rats. *Science* 176:417, 1972.

46. MacLeod RM, Lehmeyer JE: Suppression of pituitary tumor growth and function by ergot alkaloids. *Cancer Res* 33:849, 1973.

47. Stepien H, Wolaniuk A, Pawlikowski M: Effects of pimozide and bromocriptine on anterior pituitary cell proliferation. *J Neural Transm* 42:239, 1978.

48. Petrini GO: Antiproliperative properties of bromocriptine (CB-154) on human cells: A further rationale for medical management of pituitary macroadenomas. *Int J Clin Pharm Res* 3:279, 1983.

49. Melmed S: Bromocriptine inhibits colony formation by rat pituitary tumor cells in a double-layered agar clonogenic assay. *Endocrinology* 109:2258, 1981.

50. Prysor-Jones RA, Jenkins JS: Effects of bromocriptine on DNA synthesis, growth and hormone secretion of spontaneous pituitary tumors in the rat. *J Endocrinol* 88:463, 1981.

51. Gem M, Uozumi T, Ohta M, et al: Necrotic changes in prolactinomas after long-term administration of bromocriptine. *J Clin Endocrinol Metab* 59:463, 1984.

52. Mori H, Mori S, Saitoh Y, et al: Effects of bromocriptine on prolactin-secreting pituitary adenomas. Effects of reduction in tumor size evaluated by light and electron microscopic, immunohistochemical, and morphometric analysis. *Cancer* 56:230, 1985.

53. Barrow DL, Tindall GT, Kovacs K, et al: Clinical and pathological effects of bromocriptine on prolactin-secreting and other pituitary tumors. *J Neurosurg* 60:1, 1984.

54. Bassetti M, Spado A, Pezzo G, Gianmattasio G: Bromocriptine treatment reduces the cell size in human macroprolactinomas: A morphometric study. *J Clin Endocrinol Metab* 58:268, 1984.

55. Tindall GT, Kovacs K, Horvath E, Thorner MO: Human prolactin-producing adenomas and bromocriptine: A histological, immunocytochemical, ultrastructural, and morphometric study. *J Clin Endocrinol Metab* 55:1178, 1982.

56. Landolt AM, Minder H, Osterwalter V, Landolt TA: Bromocriptine reduces the size of cells in prolactin-secreting pituitary adenomas. *Experientia* 39:625, 1983.

57. Hardy S: Transsphenoidal microsurgery of the normal and pathological pituitary. *Clin Neurosurg* 16:185, 1969.

58. Wilson CB: A decade of pituitary microsurgery. The Herbert Olivecrome lecture. *J Neurosurg* 61:814, 1984.

59. Randall RV, Laws ER Jr, Abboud CF, et al: Transsphenoidal microsurgical treatment of prolactin-producing pituitary adenomas. Results on 100 patients. *Mayo Clin Proc* 58:108, 1983.

60. Thompson JA, Treasdale GM, Gordon D, McGruden DC, Davies DL: Treatment of presumed prolactinoma by transsphenoidal operation; Early and late results. *Br Med J (Clin Res)* 292:1002, 1985.

61. Saitoh Y, Mori I, Arita N, et al: Treatment of prolactinoma based on the results of transsphenoidal operation. *Surg Neurol* 26:338, 1986.

62. Serri O, Rasio E, Beauregard H, Hardy J, Somma M: Recurrence of hyperprolactinemia after selective transsphenoidal adenomectomy in women with prolactinoma. *N Engl J Med* 309:280, 1983.

63. Parl FF, Cruz VE, Cobb CA, Bradley CA, Aleshire SL: Late recurrence of surgically removed prolactinomas. *Cancer* 57:2422, 1986.

64. Thorner MO, Martin WH, Rogol AD, et al: Rapid regression of pituitary prolactinomas during bromocriptine treatment. *J Clin Endocrinol Metab* 51:438, 1980.

65. Thorner MO, Perryman RL, Rogol AD, et al: Rapid changes of prolactinoma volume after withdrawal and reinstitution of bromocriptine. *J Clin Endocrinol Metab* 53:480, 1981.

66. Corenblum B, Hanley DA: Bromocriptine reduction of prolactinoma size. *Fertil Steril* 36:716, 1981.

67. Spark R, Baker R, Bienfang DC, Bergland R: Bromocriptine reduces

pituitary tumor size and hypersecretion. Requiem for pituitary surgery? *JAMA* 247:311, 1982.
68. Wass JAH, Williams J, Charlesworth M, et al: Bromocriptine in management of large pituitary tumors. *Br Med J* 284:1908, 1982.
69. Wollesen F, Andersen T, Karkle A: Size reduction of extrasellar pituitary tumors during bromocriptine treatment. Quantitation on effect of different types of tumors. *Ann Intern Med* 96:281, 1982.
70. Weiss MH, Wycoff RR, Yadley R, Gott P, Feldon S: Bromocriptine treatment of prolactin-secreting tumors: surgical implications. *Neurosurgery* 12:640, 1983.
71. Zarate A, Canales ES, Cano C, Pilonieta CJ: Follow-up of patients with prolactinomas after discontinuation of long-term therapy with bromocriptine. *Acta Endocrinol* 104:139, 1983.
72. Johnston DG, Kendall-Taylor P, Watson M, et al: Effect of dopamine agonist withdrawal after long-term therapy in prolactinomas. Studies with high-definition computerized tomography. *Lancet* 2:187, 1984.
73. Warfield A, Finkel DM, Schatz NJ, Savino PJ, Snyder PJ: Bromocriptine treatment of prolactin-secreting pituitary adenomas may restore pituitary function. *Ann Intern Med* 101:783, 1984.
74. Molitch ME, Elton RL, Blackwell RE, et al: The bromocriptine study group. *J Clin Endocrinol Metab* 60:698, 1985.
75. Liuzzi A, Dallabonzana D, Oppizzi G, et al: Low doses of dopamine agonists in the long-term treatment of macroprolactinomas. *N Engl J Med* 313:656, 1985.
76. Van't Verlaat JW, Croughs RJM, Hendriks MJ, et al: Bromocriptine treatment of prolactin-secreting macrodenomas: A radiological, ophthamological and endocrinological study. *Acta Endocrinol* 112:487, 1986.
77. Sieck JO, Niles NL, Jinkins JR, et al: Extrasellar prolactinomas: Successful management of 24 patients using bromocriptine. *Horm Res* 23:167, 1986.
78. Quigley ME, Judd SJ, Gilliand GB, Yen SSC: Functional studies of dopamine control of prolactin secretion in normal women and women with hyperprolactinemic pituitary microadenoma. *J Clin Endocrinol Metab* 50:994, 1980.
79. Ayers JWT: Reversible "hypopituitarism" and disappearance of microadenoma in a prolactinoma patient treated with bromocriptine. *Fertil Steril* 40:846, 1983.
80. Landolt AM: Cerebrospinal fluid rhinorrhea: A complication of therapy for invasive prolactinoma. *Neurosurgery* 11:395, 1982.
81. Clayton RN, Webb J, Health DA, et al: Dramatic and rapid shrinkage of a massive invasive prolactinoma with bromocriptine: A case report. *Clin Endocrinol* 22:573, 1985.
82. Breidahl HD, Topliss DJ, Pike JW: Failure of bromocriptine to maintain reduction size of a macroprolactinoma. *Br Med J* 287:451, 1983.
83. Dallabonzana D, Spelta B, Opizzi G, et al: Reenlargement of macroprolactinoma during bromocriptine treatment: Report of two cases. *J Endocrinol Invest* 6:47, 1983.
84. Van Roon E, van der Vijver JCM, Gerretsen G, Hekster REM, Wattendorff RA: Rapid regression of a suprasellar extending prolactinoma after bromocriptine treatment during pregnancy. *Fertil Steril* 36:173, 1981.
85. Maeda T, Ushiroyama T, Okuda K, et al: Effective bromocriptine treatment of a pituitary macroadenoma during pregnancy. *Obstet Gynecol* 61:117, 1983.
86. Bergh T, Nillius SJ, Enoksson P, Wide L: Bromocriptine-induced regression of a suprasellar extending prolactinoma during pregnancy. *J Endocrinol Invest* 7:133, 1984.
87. De Wit W, Bennink HJTC: Prophylactic bromocriptine treatment during pregnancy in women with macroprolactinoma: Report of 13 pregnancies. *Br J Obstet Gynaecol* 91:1059, 1984.
88. Ylikorkala D, Kivinen S, Ronnberg L: Bromocriptine treatment during early human pregnancy: Effect on the levels of prolactin, sex steroids and placental lactogen. *Acta Endocrinol* 95:412, 1980.
89. Goodman LA, Chang RJ: Pregnancy after bromocriptine-induced reduction of an extrasellar prolactin-secreting pituitary adenoma. *Obstet Gynecol* 64:2S, 1984.
90. Kletzky OA, Marrs RP, Davajan V: Management of patients with hyperprolactinemia and normal or abnormal tomograms. *Am J Obstet Gynecol* 147:528, 1983.
91. Falsetti L, Roggia A, Loda G, et al: Metergoline and bromocriptine in the management of tumoral and idiopathic hyperprolactinemia. *Horm Metab Res* 15:380, 1983.
92. Moriondo P, Travaglini P, Nissim M, Conti A, Faglia G: Bromocriptine treatment of microprolactinomas: Evidence of stable prolactin decrease after drug withdrawal. *J Clin Endocrinol Metab* 60:764, 1985.
93. Archer DF, Lattanzi DR, Moore EE, Harger JH, Herbert DL: Bromocriptine treatment of women with suspected pituitary prolactin-secreting microadenomas. *Am J Obstet Gynecol* 143:620, 1982.
94. Larrea F, Villanueva C, Cravioto MC, Escorza A, del Real O: Further evidence that big, big prolactin is preferentially secreted in women with hyperprolactinemia. *Fertil Steril* 44:25, 1985.
95. Rasmussen C, Bergh T, Nillius SJ, Wide L: Return of menstruation and normalization of prolactin in hyperprolactinemic women with bromocriptine-induced pregnancy. *Fertil Steril* 44:31, 1985.
96. Bergh T, Nillius SJ, Wide L: Menstrual functions and serum prolactin levels after long-term bromocriptine treatment of hyperprolactinemic amenorrhea. *Clin Endocrinol* 16:587, 1982.
97. Burrow GN, Worthman NB, Rewcastle NB, Holgate RC, Kovacs K: Microadenomas of the pituitary and abnormal sellar tomograms in an unselected autopsy series. *N Engl J Med* 304(3):156, 1981.
98. March CM, Kletzky DA, Davajan V, et al: Longitudinal evaluation of patients with untreated prolactin-secreting pituitary adenomas. *Am J Obstet Gynecol* 139:835, 1981.
99. Koppleman MCS, Jaffe MJ, Reith KG, Caruso RC, Loriaux DL: Hyperprolactinemia, amenorrhea and galactorrhea. A retrospective assessment of twenty-five cases. *Ann Intern Med* 100:115, 1984.
100. Pituitary Adenoma Study Group: Variation in assessing sella turcica tomograms for pituitary microadenomas. *Obstet Gynecol* 60:700, 1982.
101. Vance ML, Ridgway EC, Thorner MO: Follicle-stimulating pituitary tumor treated with bromocriptine. *J Clin Endocrinol Metab* 61:580, 1985.
102. Lamberts SWJ, Verleun T, Oosterom R, et al: The effects of bromocriptine, thyrotropin-releasing hormone, and gonadotropin- secreting pituitary adenomas in vivo and in vitro. *J Clin Endocrinol Metab* 64:524, 1987.
103. Johnston DG, Hall K, McGregor A, et al: Bromocriptine therapy for "nonfunctioning" pituitary tumors. *Am J Med* 71:1059, 1981.
104. Verde G, Oppizzi G, Chiodini PG, et al: Effect of chronic bromocriptine administration on tumor size in patients with "non-secreting" pituitary adenomas. *J Endocrinol Invest* 8:113, 1985.
105. Klibanski A, Neer RM, Beilins JZ, et al: Decreased bone density in hyperprolactinemic women. *N Engl J Med* 303:1511, 1980.
106. Schlechte J, Sherman B, Martin R: Bone density in amenorrheic women with and without hyperprolactinemia. *J Clin Endocrinol Metab* 56:1120, 1983.
107. Bikle DD, Spencer EM, Burke WH, Rost CR: Prolactin but not growth hormone stimulates 1,25-dihydroxyvitamin D_3 production by chick renal preparation in vitro. *Endocrinology* 107:81, 1980.
108. Matsumoto T, Horivchi N, Suda T, et al: Failure to demonstrate stimulatory effect of prolactin on vitamin D metabolism in vitamin D-deficient rats. *Metabolism* 28:925, 1979.
109. Pahuja DN, Deluca HF: Stimulation of calcium transport and bone calcium mobilization by prolactin in vitamin D-deficient rats. *Science* 214:1038, 1981.
110. Ziliotto D, Luisetto G, Heynen G, et al: Decrease in serum prolactin levels after acute intravenous injection of salmon calcitonin in normal subjects. *Horm Metab Res* 13:64, 1981.
111. Clementi G, Nicoletti F, Patacchioli F, et al: Hyproprolactinemic action of calcitonin and the tuberoinfundibular dopaminergic system. *J Neurochem* 40:885, 1983.
112. Rubinscci A, Scotti A, Tessari L: The effect of long-term treatment with L-dopa on bone mass of post-menopausal women. *Calcif Tissue Int* 35(5):A4, 1983.
113. Klibanski A, Greenspan SL: Increase in bone mass after treatment of hyperprolactinemic amenorrhea. *N Engl J Med* 315:542, 1986.
114. Caraceni MP, Corghi E, Ortolani S, et al: Increased forearm bone mineral content after bromocriptine treatment in hyperprolactinemia. *Calcif Tissue Int* 37:687, 1985.
115. Furtterweit W: *Polycystic Ovarian Disease.* New York, Springer-Verlag, 1984, pp 104–105.
116. Falaschi P, del Pozo E: Effects of bromocriptine on LH secretion in the polycystic ovary syndrome, in Calve DB, McDonald RJ, Horowski R. Wuttke TV (eds): *Lisuride and other Dopamine Agonists. Basic Mechanism and Endocrine and Neurological Effects.* New York, Raven, 1983, pp 325–330.
117. Rocco A, Falashi P, Pompei P, del Pozo E, Frajese G: Chronic anovulation in polycystic ovary syndrome: Role of hyperprolactinemia and its suppression with bromocriptine, in Zichella L, Pancheri P, (eds): *Psychoneuroendocrinology in Reproduction.* New York, Elsevier-North Holland, 1979.
118. Quigley ME, Rakoff JS, Yen SSC: Increased luteinizing hormone

sensitivity to dopamine inhibition in polycystic ovary syndrome. *J Clin Endocrinol Metab* 52:231, 1981.

119. Kazer RR, Kessel B, Yen SSC: Circulating luteinizing hormone pulse frequency in women with polycystic ovary syndrome. *J Clin Endocrinol Metab* 65:233, 1987.

120. Gambacciani M, Mellis GB, Paoletti AM, et al: Pulsatile luteinizing hormone release in postmenopausal women: Effect of chronic bromocriptine administration. *J Clin Endocrinol Metab* 65:465, 1987.

121. Moult PJA, Rees LH, Besser GM: Pulsatile gonadotropin secretion in hyperprolactinemic amenorrhea and the response to bromocriptine therapy. *Clin Endocrinol* 16:153, 1982.

122. Sander SE, Frager M, Case GD, Kelch RP, Marshall JC: Abnormal pattern of pulsatile luteinizing hormone secretion in women with hyperprolactinemia and amenorrhea: Response to bromocriptine. *J Clin Endocrinol Metab* 59:941, 1984.

123. Spruce BA, Kendall-Taylor P, Dunlop W, et al: The effect of bromocriptine in the polycystic ovary syndrome. *Clin Endocrinol* 20:481, 1984.

124. Corenblum B, Taylor PJ: The hyperprolactinemic polycystic ovary syndrome may not be a distinct entity. *Fertil Steril* 38:549, 1982.

125. Peillon F, Vincens M, Cesselin F, Doumith R, Mowszowicz I: Exaggerated prolactin response of thyrotropin-releasing hormone in women with ovulatory cycles: Possible role of endogenous estrogens and effect of bromocriptine. *Fertil Steril* 37:530, 1982.

126. Mudge TJ, Blight L, White GH, Judd SJ: Influence of prolactin on serum androgen in normoprolactinemic women. *Clin Reprod Fertil* 2:19, 1983.

127. El Tabbakh GH, Loufti IA, Azab I, et al: A controlled clinical trial for the effect of bromocriptine on the adrenal contribution in polycystic ovarian disease. *Acta endocrinol* 114:161, 1987.

128. Lobo RA, Kletzky OA: Normalization of androgen and sex hormone-binding globulin levels after treatment of hyperprolactinemia. *J Clin Endocrinol Metab* 56:562, 1982.

129. Evans WS, Schiebinger RJ, Kaiser DL, et al: Serum adrenal androgens in hyperprolactinemic women prior to, during, and after chronic treatment with bromocriptine. *Acta Endocrinol* 101:235, 1982.

130. Parker LN, Suckjoo C, Odell WD: Adrenal androgens in patients with chronic marked elevation of prolactin. *Clin Endocrinol* 8:1, 1978.

131. Seibel MM, Oskowitz S, Kamrava M, Taymor ML: Bromocriptine response in normoprolactinemic patients with polycystic ovary disease: A preliminary report. *Obstet Gynecol* 64:123, 1984.

132. Pehrson JJ, Langcope CL, Orczyk G, Vaitukaits JL: Effect of bromocriptine on polycystic ovary syndrome. Presented at the 7th International Congress of Endocrinology, Quebec City, Canada, July 1–7, 1984.

133. Buvat J, Buvat-Herbavt M, Marcolin G, et al: A double-blind controlled study of the hormonal and clinical effects of bromocriptine in the polycystic ovary syndrome. *J Clin Endocrinol Metab* 63:119, 1986.

134. Polson DW, Mason HD, Franks S: Bromocriptine treatment of women with clomiphene-resistant polycystic ovary syndrome. *Clin Endocrinol* 26:197, 1987.

135. Espersen T, Thomsen AC: Controlled study of bromocriptine and

136. Giampietro MG, Brunori CR, Teti GC: High rate of conception by cyclophenil-bromocriptine regimen in infertile women with normal prolactin levels. *Int J Clin Pharmacol Res* 2:301, 1982.

137. Pepperell RJ, Evans JH, Brown JB, et al: Serum prolactin levels and the value of bromocriptine in the treatment of anovulatory infertility. *Br J Obstet Gynaecol* 84:58, 1977.

138. Amos WL: Successful treatment of infertility with bromocriptine mesylate after failure of clomiphene in anovulatory patients. *Adv Ther* 1:343, 1984.

139. Suginami H, Hamadd K, Yano K, Kuroda G, Matsuura S: Ovulation induction with bromocriptine in normoprolactinemic anovulatory women. *J Clin Endocrinol Metab* 62:899, 1986.

140. Lenton EA, Sobowale OS, Cooke ID: Prolactin concentration in ovulatory but infertile women: Treatment with bromocriptine. *Br Med J* 2:1179, 1977.

141. McBain JC, Pepperell RJ: Use of bromocriptine in unexplained infertility. *Clin Reprod Fertil* 1:145, 1982.

142. Wright CS, Steale SJ, Jacobs HS: Value of bromocriptine in unexplained primary infertility: A double-blind controlled study. *Br Med J* 1:1037, 1979.

143. Ben-David M, Schenker JG: Transient hyperprolactinemia: A correctable cause of idiopathic female infertility. *J Clin Endocrinol Metab* 57:642, 1983.

144. del Pozo E: Management of borderline hyperprolactinemia. *Horm Res* 22:204, 1985.

145. McNeilly AS: Prolactin and the corpus luteum, in Jeffcoate SL (ed): *The Luteal Phase*. Chichester, Wiley, 1985.

146. Espinoza-Campos J, Butler WR, Knobil E: Inhibition of prolactin secretion in the rhesus monkey. Presented at the 57th annual meeting of the American Endocrine Society, New York, June 18–20, 1975.

147. Asch RH, Abou-Samra M, Braunstein GD, Pauerstein CJ: Luteal function in hypophysectomized rhesus monkeys. *J Clin Endocrinol Metab* 55:154, 1982.

148. McNatty KP, Sawers RS, McNeilly AS: A possible role for prolactin in control of a steroid secretion by the human graafian follicle. *Nature* 250:653, 1974.

149. Garcea N, Campo S, Siccardi P, et al: Effect of drug-induced hyper and hypoprolactinemia on human corpus luteum. *Acta Eur Fertil* 14:35, 1983.

150. Bohnet HG, Muhlenstedt D, Hanker JPF, Schneider HPG: Prolactin oversuppression. *Arch Gynecol* 223:173, 1977.

151. Godo G, Sas M, Falkey GY: Bromocriptine therapy of luteal insufficiency. *Acta Med Acad Sci Hung* 37:283, 1980.

152. Fredricsson B, Carlstrom, Bjork G, Messinis I: Effects of prolactin and bromocriptine on the luteal phase in infertile women. *Eur J Obstet Gynecol Reprod Biol* 11:319, 1981.

153. Sarris S, Swyer GIM, McGarrigle HHG, et al: Prolactin and luteal insufficiency. *Clin Endocrinol* 9:543, 1978.

PART VIII

Surgical Treatment of Female Infertility

CHAPTER 27

Diagnostic and Operative Hysteroscopy

Patrick J. Taylor

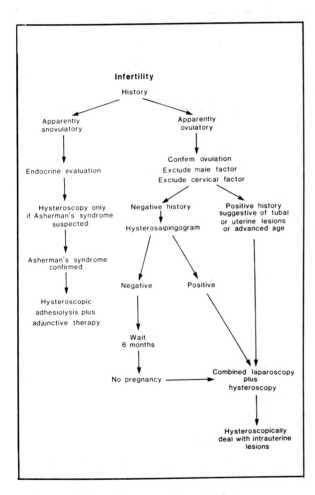

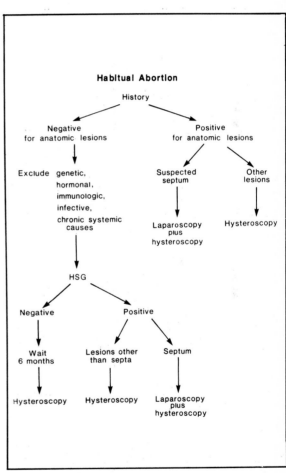

A vaginal speculum recovered from the ashes of Pompeii and now exhibited in the Archeological Museum in Naples in the first example of an instrument used to visualize the interior of the female genital tract. In 1805 Nelson won his great victory off Cape Trafalgar. In the same year Bozzini (cited by Lindemann)[1] was reprimanded by the medical faculty of Vienna for "undue curiosity" in attempting to visualize the interior of the urethra of a living human being. He also observed the cervix using a tubular speculum, light from a candle being reflected with a mirror.

Aubinais (cited by Lyon)[2] is credited incorrectly with the first hysteroscopy in 1864. In fact he observed the emergence of the fetal head from the cervix.

A 12-mm device with which the urethra could be investigated was introduced by Desormeaux.[3] The first true hysteroscopy was performed using Desormeaux's device in 1869 by Panteleoni,[4] who inspected and cauterized with silver nitrate polyps within the uterine cavity of a 60-year-old woman complaining of intractable uterine bleeding. The first modern endoscope was demonstrated by Nitze[5] in

1879. It possessed a proximal and distal lens and an integral source of illumination, principles fundamental to all modern endoscopes. This advance was ignored for 29 years, until 1908 when David[6] adapted the Nitze endoscope by adding a built-in magnifying lens and began to perform hysteroscopy.

The size of the instruments (David's model was 10.5 mm in diameter), poor illumination, inability to distend the uterus, and constant obscuring of the distal lens with blood and mucus did not encourage the practitioners of the time to embrace the procedure with enthusiasm. Indeed, Munde[7] felt that as much useful information could be obtained with the tip of the finger. The ingenious attempts to overcome these difficulties are described in detail elsewhere.[1,8,9]

Distention of the uterine cavity with carbon dioxide and improvement in the manufacture of lenses permitted better visualization with finer instruments, but the major impetus for all medical endoscopy came with the invention of the cold light source, which was based on the ability of stretched silica fibers, even if arranged in an incoherent fashion, to transmit light. Such fibers could be connected to an external light source, thus making it possible to transmit the light but not the heat generated from an incandescent bulb. This development led to an explosion in medical endoscopy.[10] Although laparoscopy[11,12] gained rapid acceptance, the development of modern hysteroscopy has been slower.

INSTRUMENTS

Since the early 1960s, hysteroscopic technology has advanced in three parallel directions, and several techniques have evolved. The three types of hysteroscopes in current use are contact, panoramic, and Hamou microcolpohysteroscope (MCH). Accessory equipment includes a viewing system, a gaseous or liquid distention medium where indicated, and ancillary instruments.

Contact Hysteroscope

Contact hysteroscopy is performed without uterine distention, with the distal lens of the telescope placed in contact with the surface to be observed. The Hysteroser (Fig. 27–1) (developed by the Institut d'Optiques de Paris, United States distributor Advanced Biomedical Instruments, Woburn, MA) has done away with the need for an external light source. The proximal end is a cylindric chamber that acts as a light trap and concentrates ambient room illumination. The proximal eyepiece magnifies the image 1.6 times. The telescope is a glass rod that possesses the optical properties of a thick lens, the magnifying property of which is inversely proportional to its length.[13,14] Models of 6 and 8 mm external diameter are used. An external sheath, which is equipped with biopsy forceps, is available. Although this instrument offers some advantages, such as use in an outpatient setting, it has not been employed widely in the area of infertility. We have not had the opportunity to use it extensively, and it is not discussed further.

Panoramic Hysteroscope

The term *panoramic hysteroscopy* describes the modern application of the older instruments used in conjunction with uterine distention and visualization of the uterine cavity without magnification.

Viewing Systems. The 150-watt cold light source connected by either a fiberoptic or alcohol-filled cable is adequate for all purposes with the exception of photography, which requires a xenon light source for

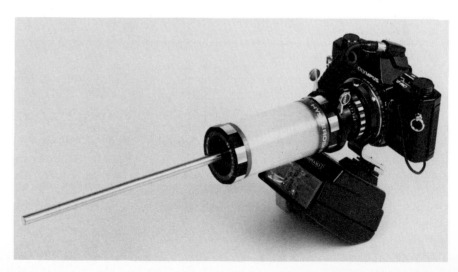

Figure 27–1. The contact hysteroscope (Hysteroser) with camera and flash attachments.

optimum results. The telescopes are adapted cysto-scopes and have external diameters that range from 4 to 6 mm. Both 180-degree and foroblique viewing systems are available. The range of models that is produced by the various instruments makers has been reviewed extensively.[15] All panoramic hysteroscopes are equipped with a stainless steel external sheath through which the telescope, distention medium, and ancillary instruments may be introduced. Introduction is performed through tap or rubber nipple systems.

Distention Media. The distention media have been reviewed extensively.[16] Because the uterine cavity is a potential space, for effective panoramic viewing the walls must be separated by a distention medium. The most widely used media are carbon dioxide (CO_2),[17] dextrose 5% in water (D_5W),[18] and high-viscosity substances.[19] The perfect distention medium would be easy to handle and immiscible with blood, and would pose no risk of local or systemic effects. Each of these media meets the specifications to a greater or lesser degree.

Carbon Dioxide. We have largely abandoned the use of carbon dioxide for conventional panoramic hysteroscopy. A gas-tight seal is required at the cervix, and the specially designed suction cups tend to be somewhat cumbersome. If this approach is to be used, only insufflation equipment specifically designed for hysteroscopy is safe. Insufflators designed for laparoscopy must *never* be used to perform hysteroscopy. Whereas the hysteroscopic insufflators deliver 100 mL of carbon dioxide/minute, the minimum flow rate of the laparoscopic insufflator is 1 L/minute. Such volumes of carbon dioxide carry a substantial risk of causing a lethal gas embolism.

Intrauterine pressure should not exceed 100 mm Hg. At these pressures, flow rates of 40 to 60 mL/minute are safe.[20] The view is clear, sharp, and excellent for photography if CO_2 is used. Trouble-

some gas bubbles can form and obscure the view if there is fluid or mucus within the uterine cavity. Bleeding also becomes a hindrance, making surgical manipulations difficult.

Dextrose 5% in Water. Dextrose 5% in water is particularly useful for outpatient hysteroscopy. The large volumes required as it flows freely from the cervix are offset by the fact that D_5W is inexpensive. Dissection is difficult, however, because of the ease with which D_5W mixes with blood. Therefore, mucus and blood must be flushed from the uterine cavity. This can be achieved by introducing a fine polyethylene catheter through the operating channel; injection of D_5W through this catheter results in pressures than can be achieved with the flow from the hysteroscopic sheath itself (Fig. 27–2). It is instilled by connecting one in-flow channel of the sheath to a 500-mL plastic bag wrapped in a blood pressure cuff that is inflated to a pressure of 80 to 120 mm Hg. Approximately 150 mL will be used in 10 minutes. With this system the usual intrauterine pressure is 40 mm Hg, but pressures of 100 to 110 mm Hg are required to visualize the tubal ostia.[21] These higher intrauterine pressures may be achieved by further inflating the blood pressure cuff.

High-Vicosity Fluids. Polyvinyl prolidene (4% Luviskol K-90), a mixture of different polymers, was originally proposed as a uterine distention medium.[21] It proved to be unsuitable.

Hyskon (Pharmacia, Piscataway, NJ) is a dextran with an average molecular weight of 70,000, made to 32% in 10% dextrose. It is electrolyte free, nonconductive, and biodegradable. No special instruments are required and it can be instilled through a 20-cc syringe connected either directly or by means of a short piece of polyethylene tubing to one of the in-flow taps of the sheath. It is particularly valuable for performing operative procedures because it does not mix with blood. Its major disadvantage is its

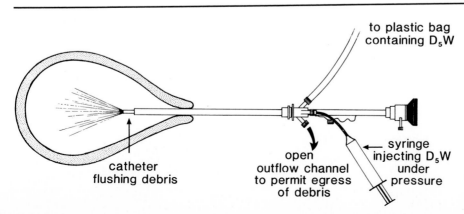

to plastic bag
containing D_5W

catheter
flushing debris

open
outflow channel
to permit egress
of debris

syringe
injecting D_5W
under
pressure

Figure 27–2. Catheter used to flush debris from the uterus; D5W is flowing in through one channel. The catheter is introduced through the operative stopcock, and the outflow channel is left open to permit egress of the debris.

stickiness as it dries. It must be rinsed thoroughly from all the moving parts of the instruments to prevent them from jamming. If such jamming occurs, the stopcock should not be forced but rather soaked for a few minutes in hot water.

Ancillary Instruments. Minimum equipment for routine diagnostic work includes a calibrated probe, fine suction irrigation catheters, soft tubal probes, scissors, and biopsy forceps. These instruments may be flexible, semiflexible, or rigid. For diagnostic work, flexible instruments are adequate and can be introduced through a somewhat smaller external sheath. If operative work is to be undertaken, rigid instruments are required and must be introduced directly along the axis of the operating sheath, necessitating the use of a hysteroscope with an offset eyepiece. The external sheath, by necessity, must be larger.

Both the shaft and handle of electrosurgical instruments should be insulated. Neuwirth and Amin[22] described a modification of the urologic resectoscope that accommodates a standard hysteroscope. A cutting loop is powered by a transistorized unit set to 60 to 80 W of cutting current. The depth of burn with this instrument is not greater than 2 mm.

Fine laser probes have become available. Although we find the modification of the MCH (described below) to be the instrument of choice for diagnostic work, if operative procedures are to be undertaken, the resectoscope or the operating panoramic hysteroscope equipped with rigid instruments is preferable.

Hamou Microcolpohysteroscope

The Hamou MCH[23] (Karl Storz Endoscopy America, Culver City, CA) is a compound instrument that can be used as a panoramic hysteroscope, a contact hysteroscope, or a microscope. The microscopic properties are made possible by a lens system that permits magnification of 1, 20, 60, and 150 times. Although the higher magnifications are of value in investigating premalignant disease of the cervix and endometrium, they have little role procedures for infertility. A second model, the Hamou II, was introduced that dispenses with the turret lens and the higher magnifications (Fig. 27–3). Both models can be focused by use of a knurled wheel. Both the Hamou I and II hysteroscopes come equipped with a diagnostic sheath and a larger operative sheath. This latter has been adapted to accept miniature flexible biopsy forceps, electroprobes, and scissors. An external sheath into which dissecting scissors are incorporated is also available. Our experience has been that the flexible instruments are too fragile for performing many operative procedures.

Illumination for the Hamou I and II instruments is once again provided by the standard 150-W cold light source connected by a light conducting cable.

When the Hamou MCH is used for panoramic viewing of the uterine cavity, carbon dioxide should be the distention medium. No special cervical occlusive cups are required. Although the standard constant pressure/variable flow or constant flow/variable pressure insufflators are quite adequate, Hamou has perfected an elegant electronic variable pressure/variable flow insufflator (see Fig. 27–2). This device uses an electronic molecular counter that allows for programmable control of both the flow and the pressure of carbon dioxide. Because pressure and flow are always in equilibrium, uterine distention is gentle and gradual.

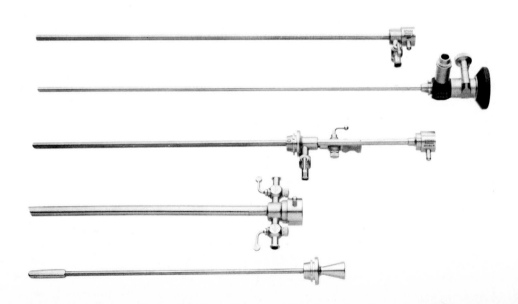

Figure 27–3. The Hamou II microhysteroscope.

HYSTEROSCOPY TECHNIQUE

Techniques differ for panoramic and Hamou MCH hysteroscopy. This section describes the step-by-step techniques of diagnostic hysteroscopy, many aspects of which are particular to each instrument; others are shared.

Procedures Common to Both Instruments

Preoperative Investigation.   Prior to performing hysteroscopy a complete history and physical examination should be carried out. In the patient complaining of infertility or habitual abortion, endoscopy should be one of the last procedures after other causes of these complaints have been excluded by less invasive means.

Preliminary investigations should include the blood group and hemoglobin of both partners. The woman's degree of immunity to rubella should be ascertained. We have abandoned veneral disease research laboratory (VDRL) testing as we have not discovered a single positive result in the last 1,700 examinations.[24] Cervical, vaginal, and seminal cultures should be performed for both the common infective organisms and for *Chlamydia* and *Mycoplasma*. If an infective agent is detected, appropriate antibiotic therapy should be instituted.

If general anesthesia is planned, the patient's fitness for this must be evaluated. Informed consent for the procedure must be obtained.

Timing.   Optimum evaluation of the uterine cavity in the patient complaining of infertility or habitual abortion can be achieved during the follicular phase of the menstrual cycle. If, however, hysteroscopy is to be combined with laparoscopy, there are advantages to performing the latter procedure in the immediately postovulatory phase, when, for example, evidence of ovulation can be sought. There is no contraindication to performing hysteroscopy at this time.

Positioning the Patient.   Hysteroscopy is performed in the dorsal lithotomy position with the patient's feet in stirrups. Although every attempt should be made to achieve asepsis, no antiseptic solution should be introduced into the vagina if carbon dioxide is to be used as the distention medium. All of the antiseptic solutions are soapy and will dirty the distal lens of the instrument, and usually are carried into the uterine cavity. Although the bubbles that are produced are quite spectacular, they absolutely hinder adequate visualization. Because the patient is instructed to void before the procedure, catheterization is rarely necessary.

A bimanual examination is performed to determine the position and mobility of the uterus. This elementary precaution protects against perforation of an unsuspectedly retroverted uterus. The cervix is exposed with a speculum and the anterior part of the cervic grasped with a single-toothed tenaculum. This tenaculum is placed in the vertical plane when the Hamou MCH is used.

Anesthesia.   The great majority of Hamou MCH hysteroscopies can be performed without anesthesia,[25] as opposed to conventional panoramic hysteroscopy, which requires some form of anesthesia. If the procedure is to be performed in the outpatient department, paracervical blockade with 1% bupivacaine, 10 mL injected on each side of the cervix, provides adequate analgesia, provided that 10 minutes are allowed to elapse from the time of injection.[26] Indications for general anesthesia include patients who are unduly apprehensive, those few in whom attempted procedures have proved to be too uncomfortable in the outpatient setting, and instances when hysteroscopy is to be combined with laparoscopy, either as a diagnostic procedure or when laparoscopic monitoring of intrauterine surgical procedures is indicated.

Techniques Particular to the Individual Instruments

Panoramic Hysteroscopy.   Insertion of the standard panoramic hysteroscope requires prior cervical dilatation. The uterus should be sounded and the cervix dilated to a size of dilator just smaller than the external diameter of the hysteroscope sheath. With the majority of instruments this requires dilatation to a Hegar #7 or #8. Once dilatation has been completed the hysteroscope is connected to the light source, and the distention medium and the sheath are filled with either carbon dioxide or fluid, depending on the medium used. With the distention medium flowing, the hysteroscope is inserted to the level of the internal os and the speculum is removed.

Viewing commences as the uterine cavity is entered, and should not proceed if the lens is obscured by mucus or blood. A red appearance over the end of the lens suggests that the telescope is in contact with the uterine wall and should immediately be withdrawn a few centimeters. If the examination is difficult and the pressure very low despite a high flow rate, a leak in the system or uterine perforation should be suspected.

An excellent view will be obtained as the uterine cavity distends. A systematic inspection should be made beginning with the fundus, identifying in turn each tubal ostium and the anterior, posterior, and

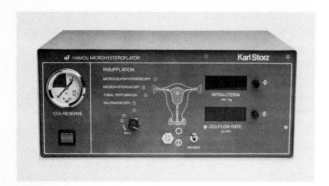

Figure 27–4. The Microhysteroflator.

lateral uterine walls. Inspection of the cervical canal is completed and the instrument is withdrawn.

Hamou Microcolpohysteroscopy. The hysteroscope is inserted through the sheath and connected to the light source (Fig. 27–3). Carbon dioxide is used as the distention medium and the in-flow valve is connected to the insufflator (Fig. 27–4). The carbon dioxide is present at a flow rate of 30 mL/minute and at a pressure of 90 mm Hg. Once the gas is flowing, the tip of the telescope is inserted to the external os. The flow of carbon dioxide produces a microcavity in the cervical canal immediately distal to the tip of the hysteroscope. As the cervical canal is distended, the instrument is gradually advanced into the microcavity. But this method of introduction under direct vision, atraumatic advance is possible, which is usually pain free and bloodless. The length, morphology, and any pathologic features of the cervical canal can be evaluated. As the instrument enters the

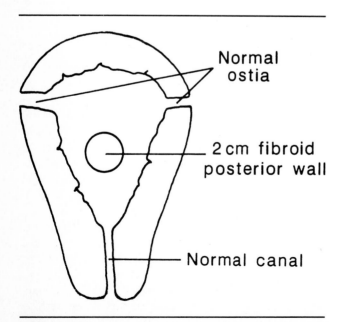

Normal ostia

2 cm fibroid posterior wall

Normal canal

Figure 27–5. Sketch documents hysteroscopic findings.

uterine cavity, an excellent, clear, panoramic view will be obtained. The cavity is surveyed in exactly the fashion described for conventional panoramic hysteroscopy.

It is important to document all findings.[27] Both still and videophotography provide elegant records. Nevertheless, the dictated operative report and a free-hand sketch of the uterine cavity and any associated lesions are simple and inexpensive, and may be of inestimable value (Fig. 27–5).

CONTRAINDICATIONS

Hysteroscopy should not be performed during menstruation. Not only does the blood make visualization more difficult, but at least a theoretical risk exists that the passage of endometrial fragments through the fallopian tubes may predispose the patient to subsequent endometriosis. A history of recent or present acute pelvic infection[25] and any suggestion of early pregnancy constitute absolute contraindications. Great care must be taken in patients suffering from Asherman's syndrome.[28] These uteri are unusually friable and easily perforated.

COMPLICATIONS

It is clear that diagnostic hysteroscopy in infertile patients or women complaining of habitual abortion is a low-risk procedure. Complications may arise, however, due to the anesthetic or the distention medium, during cervical dilatation, and during the performance of both diagnostic and operative hysterscopy. Failure to complete the procedure must also be considered as a complication.

Anesthesia
The risks of anesthesia, either general or local, are no different for hysteroscopy than for any other surgical procedure. Clearly, any risk of general anesthesia can be avoided if the procedure is performed without this approach. Hypersensitivity may occasionally occur even with local anesthetic agents, however.

If a local anesthetic has been augmented by administration of parenteral hypnotics, hallucinations may occur. This is particularly likely with the use of ketamine, diazepam, and droperidol.

Distention Medium
The use of D5W is essentially risk free. Rare cases of anphylaxis to dextran have been reported.[29] This usually occurs if the uterine cavity has been traumatized, allowing high volumes of dextran to enter the systemic circulation. Although carbon dioxide use may be associated with postoperative shoulder tip pain, hypercarbia and cardiac arrhythmias do not

occur unless the method of insufflation is inappropriate.[30]

Risks of Cervical Dilatation

During cervical dilatation it is possible to form a false passage or perforate the uterus. Fortunately, these events are rare.

More frequently the tenaculum tears free. Such an event occurred in 4 of 836 women who underwent panoramic hysteroscopy as part of an infertility investigation.[31] Although in this series we recorded only those cases that required suturing to control bleeding, dislodgement of the tenaculum is frequent although trivial. As cervical dilatation plays no part in MCH hysteroscopy, cervical lacerations are a rarity.

Uterine perforation may be caused by the sound, the dilator, or the hysteroscope. It should be suspected when the instrument has passed to a great depth, and be considered probable if large volumes of distention medium instilled at low pressures result in no uterine distention. Perforation occurred in 2 of 1,014 patients undergoing hysteroscopy. In both cases the instrument was employed by a learner under instruction.[32] Lindemann[33] reported 6 perforations in a total of 5,200 carbon dioxide hysteroscopies. Perforation is extremely unlikely to occur when the Hamou MCH is used because the instrument is advanced under constant visual control. Uterine perforation does not appear to be a major complication. Previously[25] we recommended assessment laparoscopy should it occur; however, we now recommend watchful expectancy unless there is a genuine reason to fear hemorrhage or bowel damage.

Those rare instances in which obvious hemorrhage is noted require immediate attention. Otherwise, the patient is observed for 2 to 3 hours, a baseline hematocrit is obtained, and her vital signs are monitored. If her condition is stable, she is discharged and asked to return for a follow-up visit in the office on the next day. At that time she is reexamined, her temperature and pulse are recorded, and hematocrit is repeated. Signs of peritonitis or intraperitoneal hematoma formation require readmission and treatment. It is wise to explain to the patient the nature of such complications and instruct her to call immediately should she experience pain, bleeding, or fever.

Acute infection after diagnostic hysteroscopy appears to be a rare complication. In a series of 1,000 Hamou MCH hysteroscopies, only 1 severe and 7 mild pelvic infections were identified.[34] The severe infection occurred during removal of a tubal stent after a tuboplasty. These same authors did not record a single instance of infection in 3,000 subsequent evaluations.

We previously cautioned against the risk of blind diagnostic curettage in infertile patients, having apparently demonstrated a correlation between curettage and the subsequent formation of intrauterine adhesions.[35] The question arose, does diagnostic hysteroscopy pose a similar risk? We have now had the opportunity to conduct 112 second-look hysteroscopies. These patients underwent laparoscopy and hysteroscopy prior to tubal reconstructive surgery, and second-look laparoscopy and hysteroscopy 6 weeks after the original procedure. No patients were determined to have intrauterine adhesions preoperatively and none showed fresh adhesion formation at the time of the second-look procedure. It was concluded that diagnostic hysteroscopy does not pose a risk of intrauterine adhesion formation.

Minor complications have been reported, including perforation of a thin-walled hydrosalpinx[36] at the time of carbon dioxide hysteroscopy. We noted a similar occurrence when dextran was used.[23] We reported a total complication rate in 1,014 combined laparoscopies and hysteroscopies to be less than 1%.[32]

The complications related to intrauterine surgery include bleeding, infection, and uterine perforation, and are discussed in more detail later in the chapter.

Failure to complete hyteroscopy has been reported in between 0 and 8% of patients.[26] Such failure occurred in 21 (2.2%) of 1,010 patients[32] due to inability to dilate the cervix in 11, blood obscuring the view in 4, and air bubbles hindering visualization in 6. The disastrous inadvertent visualization of an early pregnancy in one patient was described elsewhere.[37] The most common cause of failure is inability to dilate the cervix. This almost never occurs when using the Hamou MCH.

THE ROLE OF DIAGNOSTIC HYSTEROSCOPY IN INFERTILE PATIENTS AND THOSE WITH HABITUAL ABORTION

The role of diagnostic hysteroscopy in the management of patients complaining of infertility or habitual abortion is to detect the presence and confirm the exact nature of any intrauterine lesions that may be contributing to the condition.

Timing

Infertility. The investigation of the infertile couple should be concluded as rapidly, accurately, inexpensively, and noninvasively as possible. Based on these criteria, in most instances endoscopic evaluation should be one of the later investigations. At the first visit, a simple examination of the woman's menstrual pattern permits triage into two large groups, those in which the woman is (1) apparently ovulatory and (2) apparently anovulatory.

The Ovulatory Woman. When the woman apparently is ovulatory, ovulation should be confirmed by basal body temperature graph and measurements of serum progesterone levels. Two properly collected semen samples should be analyzed, and the sperm–cervical interaction determined by performing a postcoital test. If a male factor or cervical factor is detected and there is no history of tubal or uterine disease, these should be treated appropriately for 6 months before further investigation of the uterine cavity and fallopian tubes; only if such treatment is unsuccessful should evaluation of the female lower genital tract be undertaken. If in such couples the woman's history is suggestive of tubal or uterine disease, or if she is of advanced reproductive age (older than 35 years), the lower genital tract should be evaluated before any additional therapy is undertaken.

If the preliminary evaluation demonstrates normal ovulation, male factor, and sperm–cervical mucus interaction, the lower genital tract should be evaluated. The initial procedure should be hysterosalpingography.[38]

The Anovulatory Woman. The detailed workup of the anovulatory woman complaining of amenorrhea was described in Chapter 4. The role of hysteroscopy in such patients is largely restricted to those in whom a diagnosis of Asherman's syndrome is suspected. These patients may have amenorrhea, normal levels of gonadotropin and prolactin, and negative withdrawal bleeding when challenged with an estrogen–progestin combination. In such patients, diagnosis and treatment can be carried out during one procedure. We have now abandoned hysterosalpingography in favor of primary hysteroscopy.

Habitual Abortion. Strictly speaking, the diagnosis of habitual abortion should only be employed when 3 consecutive pregnancy losses of less than 20 weeks' gestation have occurred with a fetus weighing less than 500 g. A theoretical study by Malpas in 1938[39] predicted a 75% chance of subsequent spontaneous abortion in such patients. More likely, however, these women probably have a 70% chance of carrying any subsequent pregnancy to term.[40] Nevertheless, they have an increased likelihood of a specific cause for abortion, such as genetic, hormonal, anatomic, immunologic, infective, or chronic systemic disease.

Hysteroscopy's role is to detect anatomic uterine lesions. The uterine cavity should be investigated by both hysterosalpingography (HSG) and hysteroscopy. If the history is suggestive of an anatomic lesion, as may be the case when the surgeon performing curettage during a previous abortion has noted the probable presence of an intrauterine septum, HSG and hysteroscopy should be performed early. If no such history exists, investigation of the uterine cavity should be delayed until the karyotype of both partners has been determined and the female has undergone appropriate evaluation, including assessment of her thyroid status, and luteal phase adequacy, cervical and endometrial cultures for *Chlamydia* and *Mycoplasma,* and assessment of her toxoplasmosis titer.[41] The possible role of shared HLA antigens between partners[42] is beyond the scope of this chapter.

Complementary Role Hysterosalpingography and Hysteroscopy

In most instances the preliminary investigation of the lower genital tract should be by HSG. Advantages of initial HSG include (1) identification of uterine anomalies and intrauterine lesions; (2) identification of cornual occlusion or lesions, even in the presence of cornual patency; (3) immediate identification of distal tubal occlusion and assessment of intratubal architecture; and (4) planning of laparoscopic reparative surgery if distal tubal occlusion is noted.[38]

Just as wide discrepancy has been reported between hysterosalpingographic and laparoscopic findings,[43] similar incongruence between HSG and hysteroscopy has been noted. Siegler[44] compared the results of 104 patients complaining of infertility in whom both HSG and hysteroscopy were performed. Hysteroscopy failed in 8 patients. Uterine abnormalities were suggested by HSG in 19 patients; 2 of these were entirely normal at the time of hysteroscopy. Septa were confirmed by HSG in 6, adhesions in 5, and submucous fibroids in 2. An unsuspected uterine lesion was noted in 30 (38.9%) of 77 hysteroscopic examinations. One hundred forty-two patients were evaluated hysteroscopically, in 63 of whom results of previous HSG had been reported as abnormal. Hysteroscopic evaluation was normal in 20 (31.7%).[45]

Comparison of HSG and hysteroscopy in 91 infertile patients resulted in a divergence of opinion in 40%.[46] In a study by Snowden and associates,[47] in 16 (21%) of 77 women HSG indicated an abnormality. On hysteroscopy, findings were confirmed in 11 and refuted in 5. Of 61 patients who had a normal HSG, hysteroscopy detected an unsuspected lesion in only 1 (1%). The discrepancy between Snowden's study and that of other authors may be accounted for by the fact that the majority of lesions apparently missed by HSG are small, and the ability to detect such lesions depends on the care with which the HSG is performed. In Snowden's[47] series, 21% of patients had radiologic evidence of intrauterine abnormalities, a frequency that is considerably higher than that reported elsewhere.[48]

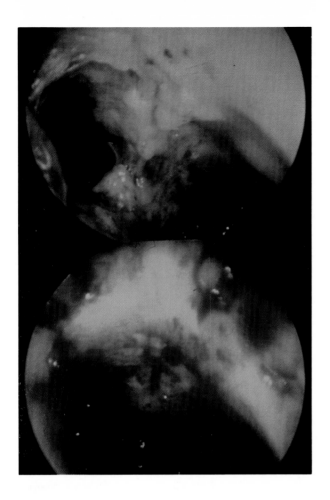

Figure 27–8. Dense intrauterine adhesions (top) before and (bottom) after removal. (Courtesy of Dr. J. Hamou.)

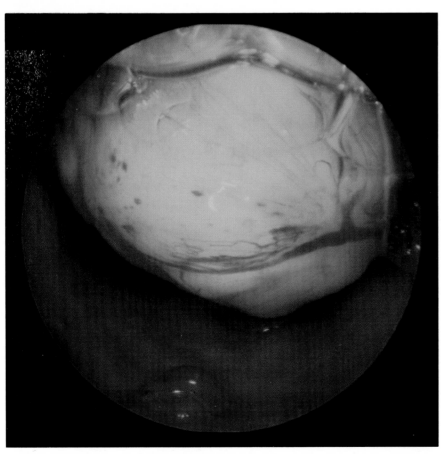

Figure 27–9. A large submucous fibroid. (Courtesy of Dr. J. Hamou.)

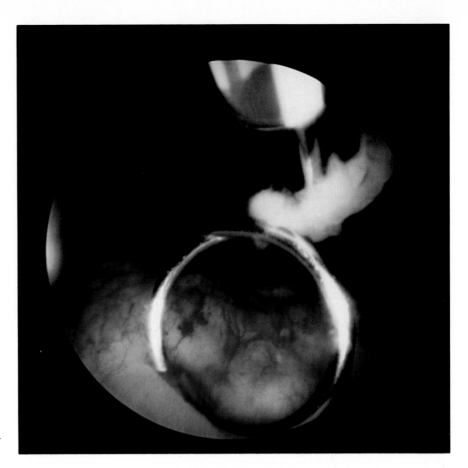

Figure 27–10. Electrosurgical snare is used to remove submucous fibroids. (Courtesy of Dr. J. Hamou.)

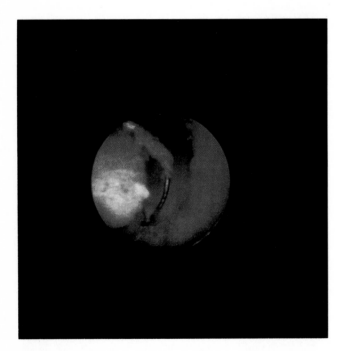

Figure 27–11. The resectoscope loop in use to divide a septum. (Courtesy of Dr. A.H. DeCherney.)

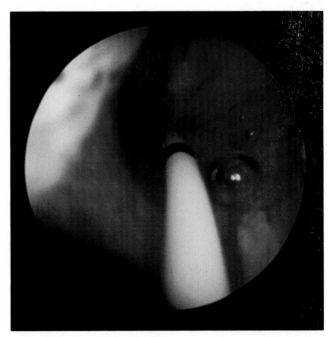

Figure 27–12. Cannulation of the tubal ostium.

TABLE 27–1. COMPARISON OF HYSTEROSALPINGOGRAPHIC AND HYSTEROSCOPIC FINDINGS

| Hysteroscopic Findings | Normal (*n* = 232) | Hysterosalpingographic findings Abnormal (*n* = 22) | | | |
		Filling Defect (*n* = 16)	Adhesions (*n* = 2)	Polyps (*n* = 1)	Septa (*n* = 3)
Normal	166	3	—	—	—
Adhesions	45	4	2	—	—
Polyps	18	9	—	1	—
Myomata	3	—	—	—	—
Septa	0	—	—	—	3

We compared HSG and hysteroscopic findings in 254 women[32] (Table 27–1). Correlation between the findings was good when results of the HSG were positive. Hysteroscopy is of particular value in identifying the exact nature of a lesion when the radiologic report notes a "filling defect." Although hysteroscopy may be more accurate in identifying small polyps and filmy adhesions, congruence between the HSG and endoscopic findings is excellent with respect to uterine malformations.[49]

Combined Laparoscopy and Hysteroscopy

In the infertile patient it has been our practice to combine hysteroscopy with laparoscopy. Both procedures can be carried out safely under the same general anesthesia. In 677 infertile women in whom both procedures were performed successfully, the results of both were considered to be normal in 156 (23.1%) and the findings of one or both were abnormal in 521 (76.9%). We believe the combination of laparoscopy and hysteroscopy offers the most complete evaluation of the lower reproductive tract.[31]

We were unable to correlate the hysteroscopic with the laparoscopic findings in 497 patients.[50]

The most frequently detected intrauterine lesion in the patient complaining of habitual abortion is a uterine septum. Hysteroscopy is unable to differentiate between the septate and bicornuate uterus. When evaluating the malformed uterus, combined laparoscopy and hysteroscopy is of inestimable value.

Findings

Table 27–2 demonstrates the hysteroscopic findings in five series of infertile patients. Untile recently, we performed all of our diagnostic hysterscopies using dextran 70 as the distention medium. We had the opportunity to compare the specific findings in 992 women evaluated using this method with those in 335 women in whom hysteroscopy was performed using the Hamou 1 instrument and carbon dioxide as the distention medium[54] (Table 27–3). In all instances the apparent detection rate was considerably higher when dextran was used. We were forced to conclude from these data that many of the findings in our

TABLE 27–2. HYSTEROSCOPIC FINDINGS IN FIVE SERIES OF INFERTILE WOMEN

Findings	1977*[52]	1977*[53]	1980[45]	Taylor et al[†]	1984[‡]
Number of cases	34	167	142	701	128
Failed	2	0	0	24	0
Normal cavities	20	68	54	419	45
Polyps or polyposis	2	60	34	89	6
Adhesions	4	19	28	155	27
Uterine malformations	2	9	9	9	2
Fibroids	2	11		5	4
Scarred cavity	4	—	—	—	—
Cervical stenosis	—	—	3	—	6
Cesarean section			3		
Scar defect	—	—			—
Vascular abnormalities	—	—	—	—	6
Endometritis	—	—	—	—	10
Bone metaplasia	—	—	—	—	1
Abnormalities (%)	43.7	59.0	62.0	41.6	64.8

*Panoramic hysteroscopy.
†Unpublished data.
‡Contact microhysteroscopy.
(Adapted from Hamou and Taylor.[25] Reproduced with permission.)

TABLE 27–3. SPECIFIC HYSTEROSCOPIC FINDINGS IN TWO GROUPS OF WOMEN IN WHOM HYSTEROSCOPY WAS SUCCESSFULLY PERFORMED

Distention Medium Group and Findings	Primary Infertility ($n = 493$)	Secondary Infertility ($n = 344$)	Reversal ($n = 155$)
Dextran 70			
Normal	350 (71%)	188 (55%)	104 (67%)
Adhesions	74 (15%)	103 (30%)	28 (18%)
Polyps	59 (12%)	40 (12%)	19 (12%)
Fibroids	6 (1%)	7 (2%)	2 (1%)
Septa	4 (0.8%)	6 (2%)	2 (1%)
Total abnormalities	143 (29%)	156 (41%)	51 (33%)
CO_2	($n = 160$)	($n = 118$)	($n = 57$)
Normal	153 (95.6%)	105 (89%)	54 (94.7%)
Adhesions	4 (2.5%)	5 (4.2%)	1 (1.75%)
Polyps	2 (1.25%)	0—	0 (1.75%)
Fibroids	1 (0.62%)	0—	1 (1.75%)
Septa	0—	8 (6.8%)	1 (1.75%)
Total abnormalities	7 (4.4%)	13 (11%)	3 (5.3%)

From Taylor PJ, Lewinthal D, Leader A, Pattinson HA: A comparison of dextran 70 with carbon dioxide as a distention medium for hysteroscopy in patients with infertility or requesting reversal of a prior tubal sterilization. *Fertil Steril* 47:861, 1987. Reproduced with permission from the publisher, the American Fertility Society.

preliminary studies were artifactual and that although fibroids and septa were detected with roughly the same prevalence, adhesions and polyps were noted much less frequently when carbon dioxide was used. On the basis of these findings, we now use carbon dioxide exclusively when performing hysteroscopy for diagnostic purposes.

Nevertheless, despite these somewhat unsettling findings, the most frequently noted lesions in patients complaining of infertility are polyps, adhesions, fibroids, and septa.

Polyps. For the following discussion, refer to Figs. 27–6 through 27–12 (27–8–27–12 on color page). Mucous polyps (Fig. 27–6) are noted within the uterine cavity and must be differentiated from dislodged strips of endometrium and myomata. In contrast, to myomata, which are fixed, polyps undulate gently with the flow of the distention medium. The final histologic diagnosis may be difficult to substantiate, and may reflect the fact that after removal, the typical histologic characteristics of polyps may be lost. The Hamou MCH, if used at high magnification, permits in-situ histologic diagnosis. Polyps may also be noted at the tubocornual junction (Fig. 27–7).

Adhesions. Although the patient with the classic amenorrhea traumaticum of Asherman[28] complains of amenorrhea, adhesions (Fig. 27–8) may occur in the woman with no disturbance of menstrual function. In 69 patients in whom intrauterine adhesions were detected, 23 had normal cyclic menses.[55] The formation of these adhesions is usually preceded either by pregnancy or some intrauterine manipulation. Vascularization and fibrosis probably have a role

in placental fragments after either spontaneous abortion or delivery.[55] In 192 women the probable etiologic event was puerperal curettage in 39, spontaneous abortion in 72, therapeutic abortion in 59, molar abortion in 9, diagnostic curettage in 1, myomectomy in 5, and cesarean section in 7. The use of intrauterine contraceptive devices has been implicated.[45] We have also remarked upon the role of diagnostic curettage.[35]

Histologically, these adhesions may be composed of endometrial, myofibrous, or connective tissue,[56] and they may be noted as lying centrally within the uterine cavity or projecting laterally as shelves from the uterine walls.[57] They can be distinguished hysteroscopically by the surface appearance and the force required to divide them. At 60 times magnification, with the Hamou MCH the exact histologic nature can be determined in vivo. The great majority are either endometrial or myofibrous and be seen lying centrally within the uterine cavity. This subject has been reviewed extensively.[58]

Fibroids. Fibroids (Fig. 27–9) bulge into the uterine cavity. The endometrium over them is thin and they are frequently covered with obvious vessels. They are smooth, firm, pale, and rounded, and may be pedunculated or sessile. They may be removed using an electrosurgical snare (Fig. 27–10).

Septa. The appearance of a septum is characteristic (Fig. 27–11). The dark uterine cornua are obviously separated by a central fibrous band. The surface appearance of the septum is dependent on the effect of the reproductive steroids on the endometrium, and varies throughout the menstrual cycle.

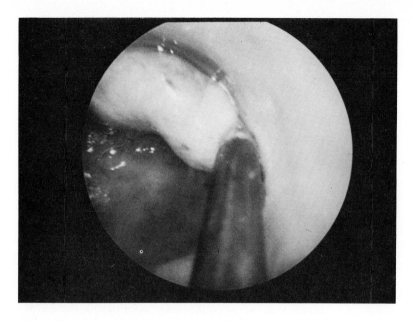

Figure 27–6. A large mucous polyp. The miniaturized electrode has been placed preparatory to electrocoagulation of the base. (Courtesy of Dr. J. Hamou.)

Significance of Hysteroscopically Detected Lesions

Polyps. It is probable that the finding of submucous polyps in patients with infertility and habitual abortion is simply incidental. We were unable to demonstrate any statistically significant difference in the prevalence of hysteroscopically detected polyps in women with primary or secondary infertility, or those requesting reversal of tubal sterilization. This last group, while not perfect, have served in all our studies as potentially fertile controls.[32,35,43,54]

Adhesions. Undoubtedly, the adhesions of Asherman's syndrome are a recognizable cause of infertility. The exact significance of less dense adhesions noted in regularly cyclic women has yet to be ascertained, and although in our earlier studies[35] we demonstrated a statistically significantly higher prevalence in patients complaining of secondary infertility, our most recent observations[54] have cast some doubts on the validity of these studies. This then clearly is an intriguing problem that remains to be resolved.

It may well be that adhesions play a role in habitual abortion. An improved live delivery rate was demonstrated in a group of women in whom such adhesions were diagnosed by hysterosalpingography.[59] Adhesions were noted in 51 women with a history of habitual abortion.[57] Subsequently, 18 remained infertile, 12 conceived and aborted, and 19 delivered at term. Although these studies do not permit the conclusion that intrauterine adhesions are a cause of habitual abortion, they certainly raise the suspicion.

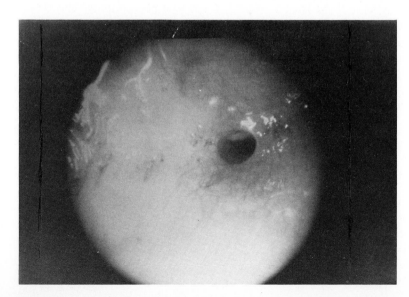

Figure 27–7. Intratubal polyp. (Courtesy of Dr. J. Hamou.)

Fibroids. It is probable that uterine leiomyomata are not a cause of infertility.[60] They do, however, predispose to habitual abortion. From a review of Hicks's series, it was demonstrated that in 441 women who suffered from uterine leiomyomata, 41% experienced spontaneous abortion.[60]

Uterine Malformations. It is unlikely that anomalies of the reproductive tract are a cause of infertility, but they have been implicated in the etiology of habitual abortion. In one study, the abortion rate was 33.8% in women with a bicornuate uterus, 22% in those with a septate uterus, and 34.6% in women with a single uterine horn.[61] Such malformations occur in 1 of every 700 women.[62]

OPERATIVE HYSTEROSCOPY

Not only does hysteroscopy permit accurate diagnosis of intrauterine lesions, in many instances it provides an avenue by which therapeutic maneuvers can be performed. Polyps, fibroids, adhesions, and septa all can be managed by hysteroscopic means, and the procedure also has other potential therapeutic uses.

Polyps

Although removing small intrauterine polyps may not influence the outcome in patients with infertility or habitual abortion, it seems appropriate that this be done when polyps are detected. Single polyps can be removed simply with a small hysteroscopic snare or by cauterizing the base (see Fig. 27–6). Multiple polyps are best dealt with by removing the hysteroscope, performing curettage, and immediately revisualizing the uterine cavity. If residual lesions are noted, they can be removed with the snare or by a second curettage. This approach ensures much more complete uterine emptying.

In 164 women previously undergoing curettage for abnormal uterine bleeding, hysteroscopy revealed residual lesions in 101.[63] Of these 101 patients, 51 had not obtained relief from bleeding. After hysteroscopic evaluation and repeat curettage controlled by hysteroscopy, only 2 of these patients returned with that complaint within 1 year.

Adhesions

Filmy adhesions frequently rupture under the pressure of the distention medium, or may be dislodged with the tip of the hysteroscope. If they are more dense they can be divided with the use of hysteroscopic scissors. Another technique is target abrasion.[55] The distal tip of the Hamou MCH is angled and somewhat sharp. In target abrasion, the tip is brought under direct visual control against one pole of the adhesion and is used to abrade progressively the attachment of the adhesion to the uterine wall. This procedure is repeated at the opposite pole (see Fig. 27–8). This technique was successful in 59 of 69 patients as an office procedure. The remaining 10 patients required general anesthesia because the procedure was too painful or the adhesions were remarkably dense.

Although target abrasion can indeed be carried out in the office, it has been our practice to do it under general anesthesia with laparoscopic monitoring. Undoubtedly, patients with adhesions have a very friable uterus that is prone to perforation.[21] Others[64] have recommended a similar approach.

Once the adhesions have been removed in all but the most minor cases, particularly if there has been any diminution in menstrual flow, an intrauterine device (IUD) should be placed within the uterine cavity and the patient should take premarin, 2.5 mg daily for 60 days, during the last 10 days of which she also takes medroxyprogesterone (Provera), 5 mg twice daily. Once these medications are discontinued and withdrawal bleeding occurs, the intrauterine device should be removed. An alternative approach to this regimen, made necessary by the fact that use of IUDs has been virtually discontinued in North America, is to administer premarin medroxyprogesterone only, and to perform a second-look hysteroscopy weeks after the initial procedure. This follow-up can be performed on an outpatient basis using the Hamou MCH. Any residual adhesions can be removed at that time.

It must be remembered that removal of intrauterine adhesions predisposes the patient to a number of potential difficulties in any ensuing pregnancy. In a series of 192 patients in whom adhesions were treated by hysteroscopic lysis, 79 (41.2%) became pregnant; of these, 29 (36.7%) aborted spontaneously, 2 had premature delivery, and 45 experienced at least 1 term delivery.[57] Eight patients who delivered required manual removal of the placenta or postpartum curettage. There is a distinct risk of placenta accreta after lysis of intrauterine adhesions. Of 3 such women, 2 required treatment by cesarean hysterectomy.[65]

Fibroids

Small submucous fibroids can be managed by hysteroscopic excision using the previously described resectoscope.[22] Pedunculated tumors are easily dealt with by dividing the pedicle. Small sessile lesions can be shaved until flush with the surrounding endometrium. Probably this procedure is best carried out under laparoscopic control. When hysteroscopic excision of fibroids is performed, dextran should be the distention medium. Postoperative bleeding can be controlled by the insertion of a Foley catheter. While the catheter is in place the patient should receive systemic antibiotics.

In the patient with more extensive tumors who must undergo formal abdominal myomectomy, preoperative hysteroscopy greatly aids in the identification of intracavity lesions and allows accurate planning of the uterine incisions. If no intrauterine lesions are noted, opening into the uterine cavity can be avoided.

Ultimately, such lesions may be effectively dealt with by the use of long-acting gonadotropin-releasing hormone analogs. Such an analog was used for 6 months in 6 patients.[66] In all 6, the uterus demonstrably shrank, as shown by ultrasonography, and did not increase in size for follow-up periods as long as 7 months after discontinuation of therapy.

Septa

When a uterine septum is detected by HSG, particularly in patients with habitual abortion, the next step should be to perform combined laparoscopy and hysteroscopy. It is only by these means that the exact configuration of the uterus can be determined. No septum with a base greater than 1 cm should be resected hysteroscopically; nor is hysteroscopy of any value in the surgical management of a patient with a bicornuate uterine deformity.

If the septum has a base less than 1 cm thick it can be dealt with very effectively by hysteroscopy. Once the lesion has been visualized, it is divided with hyteroscopic scissors. This is a remarkably bloodless procedure. While both the argon and YAG (yttrium, argon, garnet) laser have been used to divide uterine septa, performing the procedure with scissors or the resectoscope[67] is simpler, quicker, and requires less expensive equipment (Fig. 27–11). DeCherney and co- workers[67] treated 103 patients by this method. All were treated during the proliferative phase of the menstrual cycle. Dextran 70 was the distention medium and all patients were monitored laparoscopically. The septum was incised with a cutting current of 30 W/second. The operating time varied between 20 and 40 minutes. Resection was carried out successfully in 72 patients; 31 were considered inoperable. Only 1 uterine perforation occurred. After 72 successful hysteroscopic procedures, 58 resulted in successful delivery. The hysteroscopic procedure clearly is simpler than the Tomkins or Jones metroplasty and can be performed on an outpatient basis.

Potential Therapeutic Uses

Infertility, particularly unexplained infertility or that due to oligozoospermia or poor sperm–cervical mucus penetration, may now be managed by one form or another of gamete manipulation. Intrauterine insemination, in-vitro fertilization (IVF), and gamete intrafallopian transfer (GIFT), are finding ever-wider

roles. Of these, GIFT[68] may be of particular value in unexplained infertility and in women with hostile cervical mucus. It does require the performance of laparoscopy. The essential component underlying all forms of gamete manipulation has been the juxtaposition of sperm and oocyte, initially in the laboratory in cases of IVF, and in the ampulla of the fallopian tube with GIFT.

We demonstrated[69] that it is simple to visualize and cannulate the fallopian tube hysteroscopically as an office procedure requiring no anesthesia (Fig. 27–12). In 72 studied cycles it was possible in all cases to deposit previously capacitated spermatozoa at the tubocornual junction. Our protocol called for synchronization of ovulation on a predetermined regimen of Provera–clomiphene citrate. No pregnancies resulted from this approach, and subsequent follow-up studies demonstrated that our stimulation regimen more often than not produced luteinized unruptured follicle syndrome. This approach, which we called SHIFT (synchronized hysteroscopic insemination of the fallopian tube), is technically feasible and, given effective ovarian stimulation, may open an avenue to the future that could, if successful, provide an alternative to GIFT.

CONCLUSION

Hysteroscopy is no longer a "procedure looking for an indication." It has a small but definite role in evaluating the uterine cavity of patients suffering from infertility and habitual abortion. It offers an alternative approach to the management of intrauterine lesions (particularly septa and adhesions) and may find a place in alternative forms of gamete manipulation.

REFERENCES

1. Lindemann HJ: One hundred years of hysteroscopy, in Siegler AM, Lindemann HJ (eds): *Hysteroscopy: Principles and Practice*, Philadelphia, Lippincott, 1984.
2. Lyon SA: Intra-uterine visualization by means of hysteroscope. *Am J Obstet Gynecol* 90:443, 1964.
3. Desormeaux AJ: *De l'endoscopie et ces applications au dignostic et au traitement des affections de l'urethre et de la venrie.* Paris Balliere, 1855.
4. Silander T: Hysteroscopy through a transparent rubber balloon in patients with carcinoma of the uterine endometrium. *Acta Obstet Gynecol Scand* 42:284, 1963.
5. Nitze M: Ueber eine neue Beleuchtungsmethods der Hohlen des menschlichen Korpers. *Med Pres Wien* 20:851, 1879.
6. David C: L'endoscopie uterine (Hysteroscopie), applications au diagnostic et au traitement des affections inttra-uterine. Master's degree thesis, University of Paris, 1908.
7. Munde PF: *Minor Surgical Gynecology.* New York, W Wood, 1880.
8. Reuter HJ: *One Hundred Years of Cystoscopy.* Tuttlingen, Richard Wolff GmbH, 1979.
9. Van der Pas H: Historical aspects, in Van der Pas H, Van Herendal B, Van Lith D, Keith L (eds): *Hysteroscopy.* Boston, MPP Press, 1983.
10. Fourestier M, Gladu A, Vulmiere J: Perfectionnement à l'endoscopie medical. *Presse Med* 60:129, 1952.

11. Palmer R: La coelioscopie gynecologique. *Med Acad Chir* 72:36, 1946.

12. Steptoe PC: *Laparoscopy in Gynecology.* Edinburgh, Livingstone, 1967.

13. Baggish MS: Contact hysteroscopy: A new technique to explore the uterine cavity. *Obstet Gynecol* 54:350, 1979.

14. Barbot J, Parent B, Dubuisson JB: Contact hysteroscopy: Another method of endoscopic examination of the uterine cavity. *Am J Obstet Gynecol* 136:721, 1980.

15. Valle RF, Sciarra JJ: Current status of hysteroscopy in gynecologic practice. *Fertil Steril* 32:619, 1979.

16. Siegler AM, Kemmann E: Hysteroscopy. *Obstet Gynecol Surv* 30:567, 1975.

17. Lindemann HJ: Ein neue Unterschungsmethods fur die Hysteroskopie. *Endoscopy* 4:194, 1971.

18. Norment WB: Improved instruments for diagnosis of lesions by hysterogram and later hysteroscopy. *NC Med J* 10:646, 1949.

19. Edstrom K, Ferstrom I: The diagnostic possibilities of a modified hysteroscopic technique. *Acta Obstet Gynecol Scand* 49:327, 1970.

20. Quinones CR, Albarado BA, Azmar RR: Tubal catheterization: applications of a new technique. *Am J Obstet Gynecol* 114:674, 1972.

21. Menken FS: Eine neues Verfahren mit Vorrichtung zur Hysteroskopie. *Endoscopy* 3:200, 1971.

22. Neuwirth RS, Amin HK: Excision of submucus fibroids with hysteroscopic control. *Am J Obstet Gynecol* 126:95, 1976.

23. Hamou J: Hysteroscopy and microhysteroscopy with a new instrument, the microhysteroscope. *Acta Eur Fertil* 12:1, 1981.

24. Leader A, Taylor PJ, Daudi FA: The value of routine rubella and syphylitic serology in the infertile couple. *Fertil Steril* 42:140, 1984.

25. Hamou J, Taylor PJ: Panoramic, contact, and microcolpohysteroscopy in gynecologic practice. *Curr Probl Obstet Gynecol* 2:1, 1982.

26. Sciarra JJ, Valle RF: Hysteroscopy: Clinical experience with 320 patients. *Am J Obstet Gynecol* 127:340, 1977.

27. Yuzpe AA, Gomel V, Taylor PJ, Rioux JE: Endoscopic documentation, in Gomel V, Taylor PJ, Yuzpe AA, Rioux JE (eds): *Laparoscopy and Hysteroscopy in Gynecologic Practice.* Chicago, Year Book, 1986.

28. Asherman JG: Amenorrhea traumaticum (atretica). *J Obstet Gynaecol Br Emp* 55:23, 1948.

29. Knudtson ML, Taylor PJ: Uberempfindlichkeitsreaktion auf Dextran 70 (Hyskon) wahrend einer Hysteroskopie. *Geburtshilfe Frauenheilkd* 36:263, 1976.

30. Obstetrician convicted in sterilization death is placed on probation. *Ob/Gyn News* 9:4, 1974.

31. Taylor PJ, Leader A, Pattinson HA: Diagnostic hysteroscopy, in Hunt RB (ed): *Atlas of Female Infertility Surgery.* Chicago, Year Book, 1986, pp 182–197.

32. Taylor PJ: The significance of hysteroscopically detected intrauterine adhesions in the eumenorrheic infertile female. Doctor of medicine degree thesis submitted to the Queen's University of Belfast, 1985.

33. Lindemann HJ: CO_2 hysteroscopy today. *Endoscopy* 11:94, 1979.

34. Salat-Baroux J, Hamou JE, Maillard G, Chouraqui A, Verges P: Microhysteroscopy complications, in Siegler AM, Lindemann HJ (eds): *Hysteroscopy: Principles and Practice* Philadelphia, Lippincott, 1984, pp 112–118.

35. Taylor PJ, Cumming DC, Hill PJ: Significance of intra-uterine adhesions detected hysteroscopically in eumenorrheic infertile women and the role of antecedent curettage in their formation. *Am J Obstet Gynecol* 139:239, 1981.

36. Siegler AM, Kemmann E, Gentile GP: Hysteroscopic procedures in 257 patients. *Fertil Steril* 27:126, 1976.

37. Taylor PJ, Cumming DC: Hysteroscopy in 100 patients. *Fertil Steril* 31:301, 1979.

38. Taylor PJ, Gomel V: Endoscopy in the infertile patient, in Gomel V, Taylor PJ, Yuzpe AA, Rioux JE (eds): *Laparoscopy and Hysteroscopy in Gynecologic Practice.* Chicago, Year Book, 1986, p. 75.

39. Malpas P: A study of abortion sequences. *J Obstet Gynaecol Br Emp* 45:932, 1938.

40. Poland BJ, Miller JR, Jones DC, Trimble BK: Reproductive counselling in patients who have had a spontaneous abortion. *Am J Obstet Gynecol* 127:685, 1977.

41. DeCherney A, Polan ML: Evaluation and management of habitual abortion. *Br J Hosp Med* 261, 1984.

42. Scott JR: Immunologic aspects of recurrent spontaneous abortion. *Fertil Steril* 38:301, 1982.

43. Taylor PJ, Cumming DC: Laparoscopy in the infertile female. *Curr Probl Obstet Gynecol* 2:3, 1979.

44. Siegler AM: Hysterography and hysteroscopy in the infertile patient. *J Reprod Med* 18:143, 1977.

45. Valle RF: Hysteroscopy in the evaluation of female infertility. *Am J Obstet Gynecol* 137:425, 1980.

46. Labastida R, Dexeus S, Arias A: Infertility and hysteroscopy, in Siegler AM, Lindemann HJ (eds): *Hysteroscopy: Principles and Practice* Philadelphia, Lipincott, 1984, p. 175.

47. Snowden EU, Jarret JC, Dawood YM: Comparison of diagnostic accuracy of laparoscopy, hysteroscopy and hysterosalpingography in evaluation of female infertility. *Fertil Steril* 41:709, 1984.

48. Zondek BM, Rozin S: Filling defects in the hysterogram simulating intra-uterine synechiae which disappear after denudation. *Am J Obstet Gynecol* 88:123, 1964.

49. Rock JA: Diagnosing and repairing uterine anomalies. *Contemp Obstet Gynecol* 17:43, 1981.

50. Taylor PJ, Leader A, George RE, Fick G: Correlations between laparoscopic and hysteroscopic findings in 497 women with otherwise unexplained infertility. *J Reprod Med* 29:137, 1984.

51. Cohen M, Dmowski WP: Modern hysteroscopy: Diagnostic and therapeutic potential. *Fertil Steril* 24:905, 1977.

52. Mohr J, Lindemann HJ: Hysteroscopy in the infertile patient. *J Reprod Med* 19:161, 1977.

53. Hamou J, Salat-Baroux J: Advanced hysteroscopy and microhysteroscopy: Our experience with 1000 patients, in Siegler AM, Lindemann HF (eds): *Hysteroscopy: Principles and Practice* Philadelphia, Lippincott, 1984, p 63.

54. Taylor PJ, Lewinthal D, Leader A, Pattinson HA: A comparison of dextran 70 with carbon dioxide as the distention medium for hysteroscopy in patients with infertility or requesting reversal of a prior tubal sterilization. *Fertil Steril* 47:861, 1987.

55. Hamou J, Salat-Baroux J, Siegler AM: Diagnosis and treatment of intra-uterine adhesions by microhysteroscopy. *Fertil Steril* 39:321, 1983.

56. Foix A, Bruno RO, Davision T, Lem AB: The pathology of postcurettage intra-uterine adhesions. *Am J Obstet Gynecol* 96:1027, 1966.

57. Sugimoto O: Diagnostic and therapeutic hysteroscopy for traumatic intra-uterine adhesions. *Am J Obstet Gynecol* 96:1027, 1966.

58. Schenker J, Margalioth EJ: Intra-uterine adhesions: an updated appraisal. *Fertil Steril* 37:593, 1982.

59. Oelsner G, Amnon D, Insler V, Ferr DM: Outcome of pregnancy after treatment of intra-uterine adhesions. *Obstet Gynecol* 44:341, 1974.

60. Buttram VC Jr, Reiter RC: Uterine leiomyomata: Etiology, symptomatology and management. *Fertil Steril* 36:433, 1981.

61. Jones WS: Obstetric significance of female genital anomalies. *Obstet Gynecol* 10:1039, 1957.

62. Glass RH, Golbus MS: Habitual abortion. *Fertil Steril* 29:257, 1978.

63. Englund G, Ingleman-Sundberg A, Westin B: Hysteroscopy in diagnosis and treatment of uterine bleeding. *Gynaecologia* 143:217, 1957.

64. March CM, Israel R, March AD: Hysteroscopic management of intrauterine adhesions. *Am J Obstet Gynecol* 130:653, 1978.

65. Georgakopoulos P: Placenta accreta following lysis of uterine synechia (Asherman's syndrome). *J Obstet Gynaecol Br Commonw* 81:730, 1974.

66. Coddington CC, Collins RL, Shawker TH, et al: Long-acting gonadotropin hormone releasing hormone analogue used to treat uteri. *Fertil Steril* 45:624, 1986.

67. DeCherney AH, Russell JB, Giaebe RA, Polden ML: Resectoscopic management of mullerian fusion defects. *Fertil Steril* 45:726, 1986.

68. Asch RH: Ellsworth LR, Balmaceda JP, Wong PC: Pregnancy after translaparoscopic gamete intra-fallopian transfer. *Lancet* 2:1034, 1984.

69. Brooks JH, Mortimer D, Taylor PJ: Failure of hysteroscopic insemination of the fallopian tube in synchronized cycles. *J Fertil* in press.

CHAPTER 28

Operative Laparoscopy

Robert B. Hunt

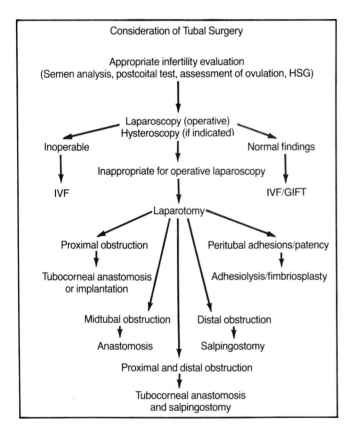

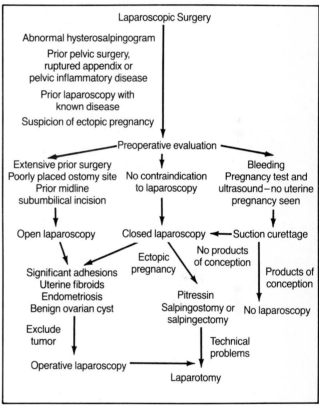

Mistakes occur when a person is over-worked or over-confident.

> *William Feather*

He who stops being better stops being good.

> *Oliver Cromwell*

"The obituary of laparotomy for pelvic reconstructive surgery has been written; it is only its publication that remains."[1] These prophetic words directed toward most infertility operations are, in my opinion, true. Laparotomy will remain the operation of choice for treating tubal anastomosis and a few other conditions for the foreseeable future. The remainder will be approached by operative laparoscopy (pelviscopy), in vitro-fertilization (IVF), and gamete intrafallopian transfer (GIFT).

This chapter will acquaint the reader with the operative laparoscopy techniques I currently use, based on 2 years' experience with some 400 patients. The techniques are a compilation of ideas worked out by my colleagues and me. They are highly effective and reproducible. Complication rates have been low.

PREPARATION OF THE OPERATING TEAM

To perform skillful operative laparoscopy, the surgeon must make a commitment to study and practice the techniques. To learn the procedures it is recommended that the surgeon attend workshops such as the ones sponsored by the American Association of

Gynecological Laparoscopists. Time spent performing laparoscopies with another surgeon is most helpful. It is also advisable to hone skills on a model such as the Pelvi-Trainer (Fig. 28–1). Such training not only perfects an individual's operative technique, but provides practice in identifying ureters, the rectosigmoid colon in its retroperitoneal location, and remaining pelvic structures, which is essential to successful outcomes.

The surgeon should select less difficult cases initially—for example, adhesiolysis for relatively minor adhesions. To distinguish these from diagnostic laparoscopy cases, the surgeon should schedule them as operative laparoscopies or pelviscopies and ask for 2 hours of operating time. The surgeon should arrange for coverage of his or her practice.

The operating team should preferably include an assistant in addition to the scrub nurse and circulator. Conducting an in-service course for operating room personnel is of enormous value; usually several sessions are required. This will ensure that the staff becomes as enthusiastic as the surgeon as they understand they are each valuable and totally necessary in performing these innovative techniques.

PATIENT PREPARATION

Operative laparoscopy is scheduled to be performed in the proliferative phase of the patient's cycle but after the menses have ceased. This permits a tubal lavage to be performed safely, avoids the potential of operating during pregnancy, and eliminates the problem of a bleeding corpus luteum. Each patient is mailed an informed consent (Fig. 28–2) and instructed to read it, initial each page, sign the last page to signify that she understands the consent, and return it to us. In addition, she is instructed to remain on a clear liquid diet and take a strong laxative (magnesium citrate) the day before the procedure, and take nothing by mouth after midnight before the procedure. Appropriate laboratory studies are performed, including chest radiograph and electrocardiogram when indicated.

INSTRUMENTATION

Light Source and Photography

The standard light source is a 150-W halogen lamp. Although this is adequate for operative laparoscopy, I prefer a xenon light source, as it provides brighter illumination and adequate light for video. I have found the xenon light inadequate for still photography, however. The exposure time is too long, resulting in blurred slides. I use a strobe flash built into the light source for still photographs, in conjunction with ASA 400 daylight film (Fig. 28–3). The resulting 35-mm slides are reproducibly excellent. Technology is rapidly evolving in the fields of video and still photography, and the surgeon should consult with the supplier before deciding on the equipment to be purchased.

I photograph every case, taking 3 exposures each of the uterus and the adnexae. I send 1 set to the patient and 1 to the referring doctor, and keep 1 in the patient's record. This policy makes good sense from legal, medical, and public relations standpoints.

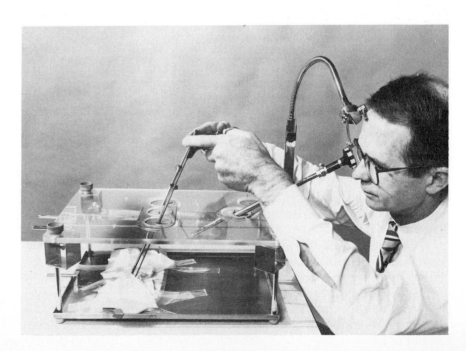

Figure 28–1. The Pelvi-Trainer is an excellent training model for suturing and other techniques requiring fine eye-to-hand coordination (WISAP/USA, Box 324, Tomball, TX 77375; 800–233–8448).

Purpose—Laparoscopy is an extremely valuable procedure in gynecology. It may be performed diagnostically or therapeutically, for example, to determine causes of pelvic pain or infertility, to divide adhesions, or to perform a tubal ligation. Pregnancy must be avoided during the menstrual cycle when the operation is to be performed.

Procedure—The operation is usually performed with the patient asleep (general anesthesia). Having attained satisfactory anesthesia, an instrument known as a cannula is inserted into the cervical canal and held in place with a tenaculum. These instruments enable the surgeon to position the uterus and thus aid in evaluation. An incision is made at the navel through which a telescope (laparoscope) is placed. One to three incisions are then made in the lower abdomen. These incisions aid the surgeon in moving structures in performing operative procedures. The incisions leave scars from one-quarter to one-half inch in length. To aid in visualization of pelvic and abdominal structures, the abdomen is inflated with gas to enlarge the space to be examined. Photographs are taken of the pelvic structures to augment the operative report. At the conclusion of the procedure, the gas is let out, all equipment is removed, and the abdominal wounds are closed with stitches. It is necessary sometimes to perform a dilatation and curettage (D&C) to assess the pelvic structures further. Laparoscopy may be performed as an outpatient procedure. In this case, the patient must arrange for someone to take her home.

Postoperative care—The patient will experience discomfort in her right shoulder due to referred pain from the right diaphragm created by the gas placed in the abdomen. The discomfort is usually gone within 2 days. There is invariably bruising and tenderness in the areas of the incisions. These usually disappear within 2 weeks.

Complications

1. Anesthesia: Anesthesiology has been refined so that it is a safe specialty. Anesthetic accidents do happen that may produce complications, however. The anesthesiologist will discuss these with you.
2. Phlebitis: The patient may experience tenderness at the site of the intravenous line. This responds to heat and is usually gone over several days. On occasion, a small lump will persist in that area.
3. Incisions: Occasionally, an incision will become infected or red-

dened. This should respond to warm showers or baths with gentle cleansing of the area with alcohol. If it does not respond within 2 days, the patient should notify Dr. Hunt.
4. Pelvic infections: The patient who has had previous pelvic infections or adhesions is predisposed to developing pelvic infections after any pelvic procedure. I usually administer an antibiotic to lessen the possibility of such an infection.
5. Allergic reactions: Several medications are used during hospitalization, including anesthetic agents, often antibiotics, and sometimes high-molecular-weight dextran, a solution made of sugar beets. Allergic reactions may develop to any of these agents.
6. Hemorrhage: When placing the various laparoscopic instruments through the abdominal wall or performing intraabdominal surgery, bleeding can occur. This is usually of a minor degree, but can be more serious and require major surgery to correct.
7. Gastrointestinal injuries: Injuries to the intestinal tract occur in approximately 1 per 500 procedures. They most often develop when placing the laparoscopic equipment through the navel because the surgeon cannot see what is within the abdominal cavity until the instrument has been placed. This is a major complication requiring immediate repair through a larger incision.
8. Failed procedure: Occasionally, I am unable to accomplish the procedure for any of a number of reasons.
9. Death: Each year, a few deaths are reported throughout the United States associated with laparoscopic procedures. They have been caused by such things as gas traveling to the lungs and infection. Fortunately, these are rare, but nevertheless, this procedure must be considered an operation with all its attendant complications.

Conclusion—I feel we have a very advanced operative team, including anesthesiologist, nurse anesthetists, and operating room nurses. Our equipment is modern. We are constantly aware of potential complications and are continually reviewing techniques to make all of our operative procedures safer.
(Modified from Hunt RB (ed): *Atlas of Female Infertility Surgery.* Chicago, Year Book, 1986, appendix A. Reprinted with permission.)

Figure 28–2. Consent form for laparoscopy.

Insufflator

Multiple puncture sites are necessary in operative laproscopy. One consequence of this is leakage of intraperitoneal gas through the wounds. To offset this, a rapid insufflator is desirable. It also ensures that the procedure does not become unnecessarily long and tedious. The standard insufflator for diagnostic work delivers 1 L of gas/minute. The insufflator shown in Figure 28–4 delivers up to 6 L/minute and is adjusted not to exceed a pressure of 8 mm Hg. The surgeon must be absolutely certain that intraabdominal pressure does not exceed a certain value; a maximum pressure of 15 mm Hg is recommended.

Laparoscope

We are fortunate in having a variety of excellent instruments from which to choose. I recommend a 1-cm laparoscope with a 30-degree lens. I have found this design to provide a superb undistorted field of view. It allows excellent documentation by video or still photograph (see Fig. 28–3). The angle lens makes it possible to work in otherwise inaccessible

places such as beneath the ovary. By placing the distal end of the laparoscope close to the structure being worked on, one can achieve 4 to 6 magnifications. Frequently I find visibility better and the surgery performed more precise than would have been the case of laparotomy.

Bipolar Coagulator

A bipolar coagulator and generator must be available at all times (Figs. 28–5 and 28–7). I have found this instrument to be extremely valuable in controlling arterial and venous bleeding. The vessel is identified by irrigation, lifted with the bipolar instrument, and coagulated. Energy is delivered to the immediate area with little lateral spread. I have used this technique with no complications in controlling open vessels adjacent to the ureter, bowel, and other major structures.

Endocoagulator

The endocoagulator is a simple, unique instrument, and is one of the most valuable. The generator heats

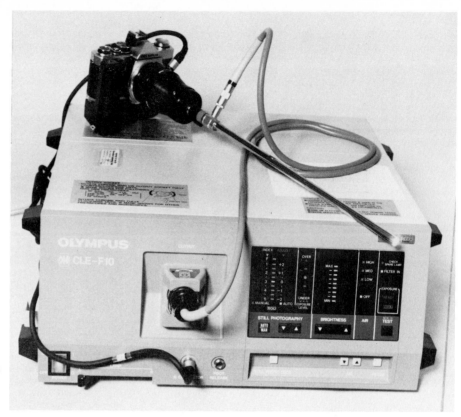

Figure 28–3. The Olympus halogen light source with built-in flash unit and associated laparoscope are excellent units. The xenon light source is model CLV-F10 (Olympus Corp., 4 Nevada Drive, Lake Success, NY 11042).

the tip of the coagulator or a predetermined temperature. After a preset time, this foot-operated instrument will shut itself off. In addition, it emits a tune so that the surgeon knows when the generator is activated. I set the generator at 100°C for everting the

mucosal flaps during a salpingostomy and 120°C for coagulating adhesions and endometrial implants.

Figures 28–6 and 28–7 show the crocodile forceps for broad adhesions and the point coagulator used for most other tasks where coagulation is required. The instruments are safe in that the depth of destruction is approximately 2 mm. This advantage makes the coagulator relatively ineffective against

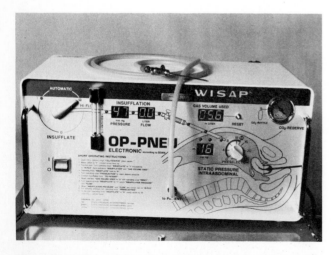

Figure 28–4. This rapid insufflator delivers between 1 and 6 L of gas/minute WISAP/USA). The intraperitoneal pressure is set not to exceed 8 mm Hg pressure. A less expensive and also superb unit is the Variflow (Laser, 1303 Keefer St, Tomball, TX 77375; 713–351–0424).

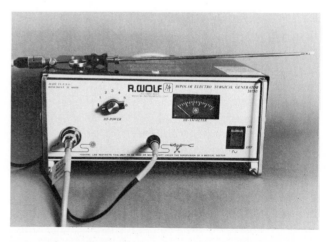

Figure 28–5. Kleppinger bipolar forceps are connected to a Wolf bipolar generator (model 2075U, Richard Wolf Medical Instruments, 7046 Lyndon Avenue, Rosemont, IL 60018; 312–298–3150, TELEX 72–6408).

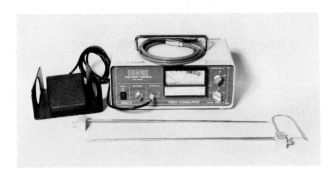

Figure 28-6. The endocoagulator generator is pictured together with a crocodile forceps and a point coagulator (WISAP/USA; and Karl Storz, 10111 W Jefferson Blvd, Culver City, CA 90230; 800-421-0837, 213-558-1500, or 800-252-2008 if in California).

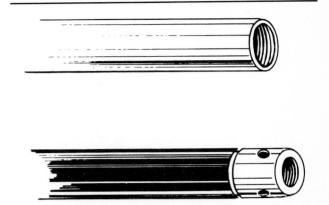

Figure 28-8. Top. The suction/irrigation cannula tip for the Aqua-Purator (WISAP/USA). **Bottom.** A standard suction/irrigation cannula tip (order no 8384.72, Richard Wolf; order no 26178U, Karl Storz).

large open vessels. I have found the crocodile forceps, however, to be efficient in sealing vessels in the mesosalpinx during salpingectomy.

Unipolar Coagulation

I have not found it necessary to use a unipolar generator in operative laparoscopy. Colleagues use the unipolar knife for such tasks as opening the fallopian tube in ectopic pregnancies and dissecting bowel off the posterior aspect of the uterus in endometriosis. Although they report satisfactory re-

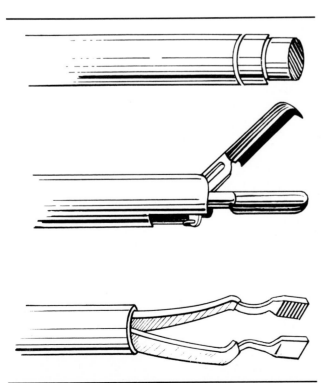

Figure 28-7. Top. Point coagulator (order no 7515, WISAP/USA). **Middle.** Crocodile forceps (order no 7510, WISAP/USA). **Bottom.** Kleppinger bipolar forceps (order no 8383.24, Richard Wolf).

sults, I am concerned about potential extension of destruction from the active electrode (knife) to adjacent tissues as electrical current makes it way to the passive electrode (ground pad). The disastrous bowel injuries associated with the unipolar generator in laparoscopic tubal ligations are well known.

Irrigation

For irrigation I use lactated Ringer's solution. The circulating nurse provides lactated ringer's warmed to body temperature. As 2 to 3 L are used in each case, an efficient irrigating system is essential.

The most readily available system is a 50-cc syringe attached to a standard irrigating cannula with plastic tubing (Fig. 28-8). Although it is seemingly inexpensive, the increased operating time required makes it prohibitively expensive. Also, it is difficult to use for suctioning the large blood clots frequently encountered in ectopic pregnancies.

An extremely cost-effective system is shown in Figures 28-8 and 28-9. This instrument is an absolute pleasure to use. By applying pressure on the two buttons on the handle of the cannula, the surgeon may alternately lavage and aspirate. Time saved in the operating room will quickly pay for the instrument.

Cervical Cannula

The standard cannula used in diagnostic laparoscopy is perfectly adequate in operative procedures (Fig. 28-10). Occasionally, a uterus is too bulky or too fixed in retroversion to be mobilized effectively by the cervical cannula. In this case the intraabdominal probe is placed against the back of the uterus to give sufficient pressure to allow the procedure to be safely carried out (Fig. 28-11).

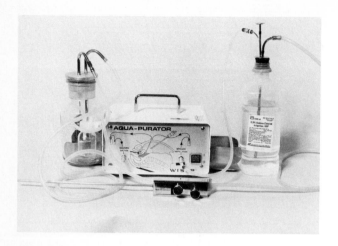

Figure 28–9. The Aqua-Purator is shown in its operational mode.

Scissors

Scissors of at least two different designs should be available. Figure 28–12 shows hooked and dissecting scissors. They must be kept sharp and in excellent working order, as they are the mainstay in performing dissections. A third type of scissors (Fig. 28–13) is useful for cutting sutures but is not used in dissections.

Grasping and Dilating Instruments

Pictured in Figure 28–14 are three important instruments used in performing procedures on the fallopian tubes.

Biopsy Forceps

The surgeon should have available biopsy forceps of two different designs (Fig. 28–15).

Needle Holders

Suturing through the laparoscope is a technique well worth mastering. I frequently do so when performing a salpingostomy or closing an ovary after removing an ovarian cyst. Figure 28–16 shows the two needle carriers I use.

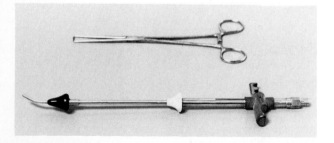

Figure 28–10. A Cohen cannula (order no 8378, Richard Wolf; order no 40-3510, Laser) and a tenaculum (order no 8370.14, Richard Wolf).

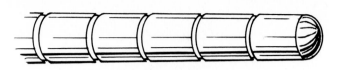

Figure 28–11. A palpation probe is calibrated in centimeters (order no 7656-3, WISAP/USA; order no 26175T, Karl Storz).

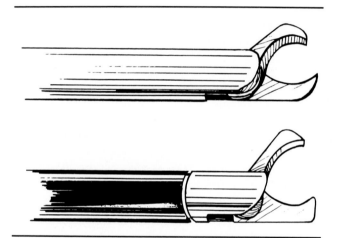

Figure 28–12. Top. Hooked scissors are excellent for opening a hydrosalpinx or opening the fallopian tube to remove an ampullary ectopic pregnancy (order no 7652, WISAP/USA; order no 26175 EH, Karl Storz; order no 8384.02, Richard Wolf; order no A5264, Olympus Corp; order no 6614, Reznik Instruments, 7308 N Monticello, Skokie, IL 60076). **Bottom.** Standard dissecting scissors (order no 8383.02, Richard Wolf).

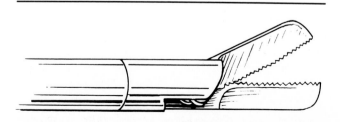

Figure 28–13. Serrated scissors are useful for cutting sutures (order no 26174-PS, Karl Storz; order no 7653, WISAP/USA).

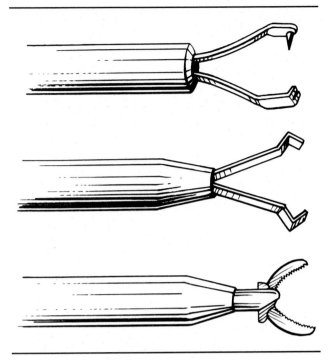

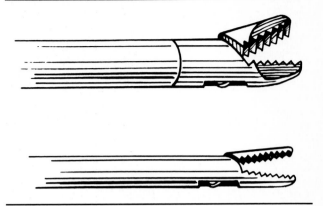

Figure 28-16. The 5-mm **(top)** and 3-mm **(bottom)** needle carriers are designed for placing intraabdominal sutures (order no 7668-1 [5-mm] and 7668 [3-mm], WISAP/USA).

Secondary Cannula

The 5.5-mm cannula is an open cannula and preferred over those with valves. This design allows free passage of instruments without causing damage to delicate tips. The 11-mm cannula is necessary when using large instruments through secondary incisional sites (Fig. 28-17).

Morcellator

Occasionally it is necessary to morcellate large tissue specimens to remove them from the abdomen. A tissue punch performs the task quite well (Fig. 28-18).

Claw and Spoon Forceps

These instruments are designed to remove large tissue specimens from the abdomen (Fig. 28-19 and 28-20).

Figure 28-14. **Top.** Toothed grasping forceps are useful in stabilizing the fallopian tube when performing a salpingostomy (order no 26177G, Karl Storz). **Middle.** Ampullary dilator is helpful in dilating a phimotic fimbrial ostium (order no 7651, WISAP/USA; order no 8384.14, Richard Wolf). **Bottom.** Atraumatic grasping forceps are effective for lifting the fallopian tube by its serosa while performing delicate dissection (order no 7655, WISAP/USA).

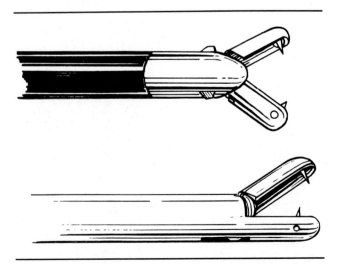

Figure 28-15. **Top.** The double-action biopsy forceps are excellent for removing adhesions as well as performing biopsies of ovaries and peritoneal surfaces (order no 8383.10, Richard Wolf; order no 6613, Reznik instruments; order no A5261, Olympus). **Bottom.** The single-action biopsy forceps has a spring-loaded handle that allows the surgeon to hold tissue without applying pressure to the handles. This feature is excellent for stabilizing the cut edge of the ovary while removing a cyst or fixing a cyst of Morgagni while the base is being coagulated and cut (order no 7654, WISAP/USA).

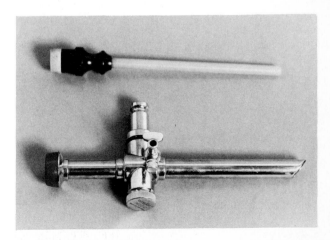

Figure 28-17. **Top.** The open cannula prevents damage to delicate instrument tips inserted through it (order no 8351.03, Richard Wolf). **Bottom.** The 11-mm cannula is used for large secondary instruments (order no 7620-1, WISAP/USA).

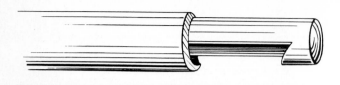

Figure 28–18. The tissue punch is used for morcellating large specimens such as a leiomyoma or an ovary (order no 7674, WISAP/USA).

OPERATIVE PROCEDURES

Initiation of the Procedure

Each procedure is performed with the patient under general endotracheal anesthesia. Local and regional anesthetics provide inadequate analgesia. The patient is placed in the standard position for diagnostic laparoscopy. After the preparation and draping, a Foley catheter is placed in the urinary bladder. Once the bladder is empty, the surgeon applies a catheter plug. This allows the scrub nurse to drain the bladder as necessary throughout the procedure. After the anesthesia examination is done, the cervical cannula is placed and secured with a tenaculum applied to the anterior portion of the cervix. The various generators are connected to their respective sterile cords and checked to ensure proper function.

It may add to the surgeon's comfort to wear a back brace and use a shoulder support placed over the patient's chest and lean on this while performing these delicate procedures (not shown, available through WISAP/USA). Another aid to comfort is to operate with a video monitor. In spite of this advantage, I currently perform most laparoscopic procedures under direct visualization.

Visualization of pelvic structures is accomplished through a periumbilical incision. At least 2 additional incisions for placing of secondary cannulas are made in either lower quadrant just lateral to the deep

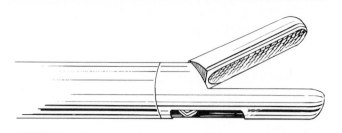

Figure 28–20. The spoon forceps is used to remove such tissue samples as an ectopic pregnancy and tissue fragments (order no 7675, WISAP/USA).

epigastric vessels. The periumbilical incision is large enough to allow passage of a 1-cm laparoscope and the 2 secondary incisions large enough to accept 5.5-mm cannulas.

Salpingo-Ovariolysis

The anatomic derangement most commonly encountered in infertility surgery is adhesion formation. This condition disturbs the tubo-ovarian relationship and thus impairs ovum pickup. Operative laparoscopy techniques have the special advantage of lessening adhesion reformation once adhesiolysis has been accomplished. My colleagues and I have often observed sometimes massive adhesions reforming after adhesiolysis by laparotomy.

Typical pelvic findings are shown in Figure 28–21. Note obliteration of the posterior cul-de-sac in addition to extensive adhesions anterior to the uterus and involving each adnexa. A key point is the separation between structures. Some separation is

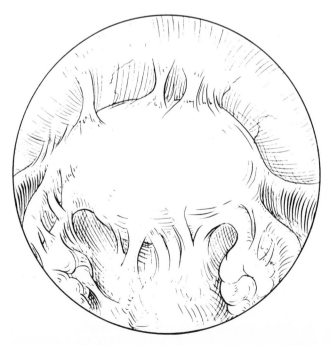

Figure 28–21. Characteristic appearance of major pelvic adhesions.

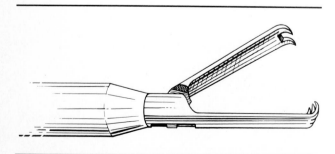

Figure 28–19. The claw forceps is a superb instrument for removing large tissue specimens such as leiomyoma, fallopian tube, or ovary (order no 7672, WISAP/USA).

required for successful and safe adhesiolysis. Dissection begins in the posterior cul-de-sac. It is best to leave the adhesions anterior to the uterus until last, as they support the uterus and facilitate the dissection. I sometimes leave the anterior adhesions altogether to keep the uterus suspended, provided the patient is asymptomatic.

The uterus is anteflexed by the nurse, and the adhesions are placed on stretch by the probe (Fig. 28–22). A crocodile forceps is used to coagulate the adhesions at 120°C. A point coagulator or bipolar forceps may be used instead. With the adhesions still under tension they are divided with scissors approximately 2 mm from the uterus (Fig. 28–23). They will retract toward the bowel and posterior pelvis when divided and do not have to be excised. Adhesions generally are arranged in layers. The surgeon works step by step, layer by layer, until the posterior pelvis has been totally freed of adhesions, thus providing access to the adnexa.

The nurse deflects the uterine fundus to the patient's left, exposing the right adnexa. With the left hand the nurse holds the right ovary laterally with the probe. The surgeon supports the laparoscope in the right hand (the reverse is the case for a left-handed surgeon) and operates with the left, standing at the patient's left side (Fig. 28–24). The adhesions have been coagulated with the point coagulator and are being divided. Sometimes it is advantageous to divide adhesions peripherally, as shown here. At other times they can be divided close to the ovary. The dissection continues until the ovary is completely free of medial, posterior, and lateral attachments. The surgeon seldom needs to enter the retroperitoneal

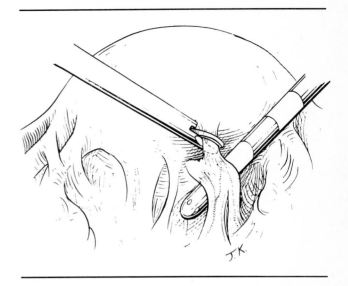

Figure 28–23. Adhesions are cut near the uterine serosa.

space and must keep the ureter in view at all times.

At this point the adhesions between the fallopian tube and the ovary are coagulated as necessary with the point coagulator, and divided close to the fallopian tube. The adhesions will retract to the surface of the ovary. They are kept under constant tension as the dissection proceeds (Fig. 28–25). To free the distal tube, the nurse lifts the tube with an atraumatic grasping forceps. Adhesions are incised close to the fimbriae, being careful not to cut the fimbriae as brisk bleeding will ensue (Fig. 28–26).

To remove ovarian adhesions, they are coagulated at 100 to 120°C. The coagulator is placed just on

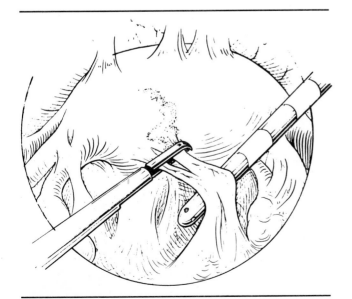

Figure 28–22. Broad adhesions are coagulated with crocodile forceps at 120°C.

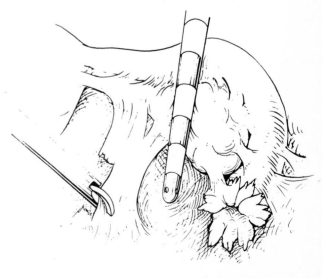

Figure 28–24. Coagulated adhesions are cut, releasing adnexal structures from the lateral pelvic sidewall.

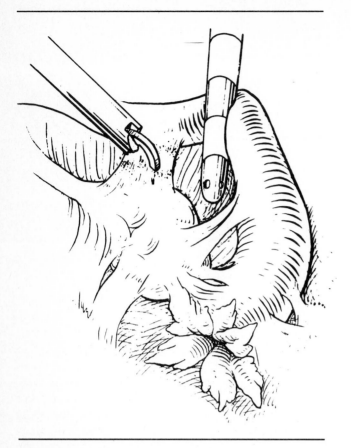

Figure 28–25. Adhesions are incised near the tubal serosa, thus releasing the fallopian tube from the ovary.

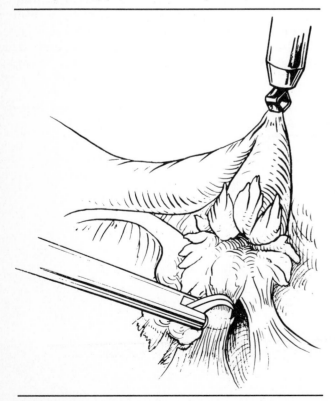

Figure 28–26. Tubal fimbriae are carefully released by sharp dissection.

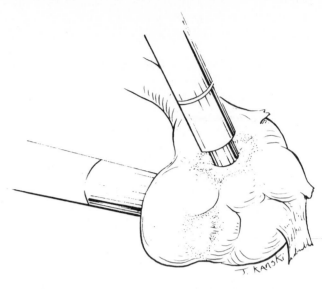

Figure 28–27. Adhesions attached to the ovary are coagulated with the point coagulator, being careful not to damage the ovarian cortex.

the adhesions and not on the ovarian surface itself (Fig. 28–27). This causes adhesions to shrivel and aids greatly in their removal. Using a biopsy forceps the surgeon strips away the adhesions by grasping and pulling them along the surface of the ovary (Fig. 28–28). To complete the adhesiolysis and fimbrioplasty, the surgeon irrigates the pelvis copiously, checks and halts any bleeding, takes necessary photographs, instills adjunctive agents (see below), and closes the three incisions with 4-0 sutures placed in an interrupted manner.

Salpingostomy

Figure 28–29 shows a hydrosalpinx after adhesiolysis has been completed. The nurse lifts the fallopian tube

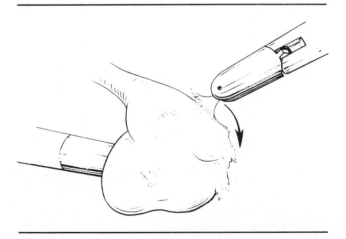

Figure 28–28. Using biopsy forceps, adhesions are stripped from the ovarian surface.

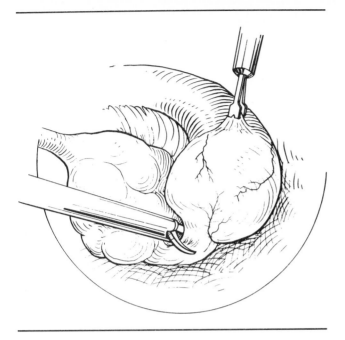

Figure 28–29. The fallopian tube is lifted superiorly and dissected from its firm attachment to the ovary.

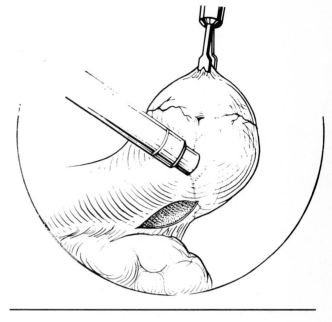

Figure 28–30. To be incised may be coagulated with the point coagulator at 100°C.

anteriorly as the surgeon begins dissecting the distal tube from the right ovary. It is better to dissect closer to the ovary than to the tube, as only a potential space exists between them. Some surgeons inject dilute vasopressin about the distal tube to decrease blood loss. Dissection stops when the site of the original tubo-ovarian ligament is reached. Although this point is recognized by the appearance of a relatively normal vascular pattern in the mesosalpinx, the surgeon often must choose the site arbitrarily, as anatomic landmarks may be distorted.

The surgeon may elect to coagulate along lines where the salpingostomy incisions are to be made (Fig. 28–30). I no longer do this, but rather distend the fallopian tube by transcervical lavage of indigo carmine and incise the tube with hooked scissors. My initial incision is vertical, directed toward the antimesenteric side of the tube (Fig. 28–31). This prevents my becoming disoriented when planning additional distal tubal incisions. Although I follow mucosal patterns, I fashion the incisions so that they resemble an inverted Y.

The mucosal flaps can be everted in several ways. A defocused carbon dioxide (CO_2) laser beam may be directed toward the serosal side of the flaps. This contracts the serosa and cleanly everts a thin flap. Using the same principle, the point coagulator at 100°C is placed adjacent to the serosa and the flap everts (Fig. 28–32). A third technique is to suture the flaps (Fig. 28–32). I prefer the second and third techniques.

When the salpingostomy is completed, an ampullary dilator is placed inside the tubal ostium, the dilator is opened, and the open instrument is withdrawn to evert the mucosa a little more (Fig. 28–33). After work on the opposite adnexa has been completed, the surgeon irrigates, checks for bleeding, instills adjunctive agents, and closes the abdomen.

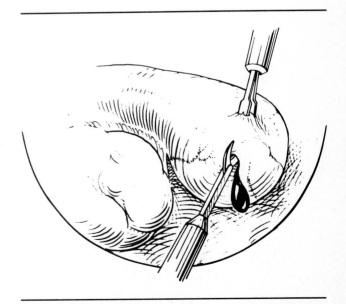

Figure 28–31. The distal fallopian tube is initially opened by incising toward the antimesenteric surface with hooked scissors.

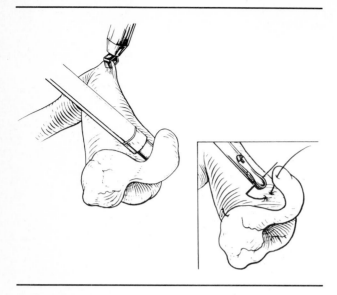

Figure 28–32. The salpingostomy is completed by everting the mucosa with the point coagulator at 100°C or suturing with 4-0 polydioxanone (order no Z-420, Ethicon, Rt 22 West, Somerville, NJ 08876; 201–524–0400).

Endometriosis

One of the most challenging diseases confronting the infertility surgeon is endometriosis. Its uncanny ability to invade pelvic tissues made reconstructive surgery difficult, stretching the operator's judgment and technical skills to the limit.

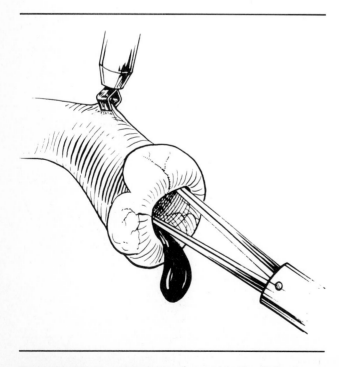

Figure 28–33. The salpingostomy is completed by dilating the tubal ostium with an ampullary dilator.

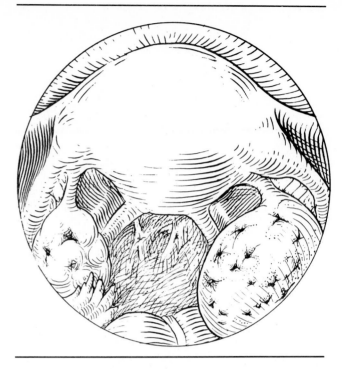

Figure 28–34. Typical appearance of severe endometriosis.

Pictured in Figure 28–34 are the pelvic structures of a patient with severe endometriosis. Disease involves the posterior cul-de-sac, the left ovary superficially, and the right ovary deeply (endometrioma). Adhesiolysis is first performed to open all compartments in the pelvis. The rectosigmoid colon and both ureters must be identified accurately. Particular note is made of the rectosigmoid in its extraperitoneal location. The ureters are best identified as they traverse the pelvic brim. They can be traced along the pelvic sidewalls from the brim in most instances.

After the adhesioloysis is completed, surgery is begun in the posterior cul-de-sac. The surgeon may choose several modalities of treatment, including laser ablation, bipolar coagulation, unipolar coagulation, coagulation with the endocoagulator, or excision. I use all except unipolar coagulation. Placing the tip of the laparoscope within 2 cm of the peritoneum, the surgeon can inspect the tissue at 4 to 6 magnifications for endometrial implants. The smaller implants and those near the rectosigmoid colon and ureters are coagulated with the point coagulator at 120°C. The 2-mm depth of penetration allows a comfortable margin of safety (Fig. 28–35). Larger implants are excised by grasping them with a biopsy forceps. The peritoneum is opened and undermined with scissors, and the implant excised. Laser ablation may be used for both smaller and larger implants.

Attention is directed to the left adnexa. Any implants on the fallopian tube or ovary are excised, coagulated with the point coagulator, or removed with the CO_2 laser. An alternative method of removal

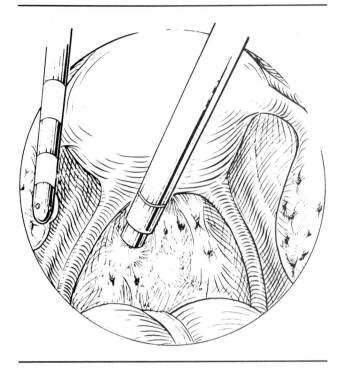

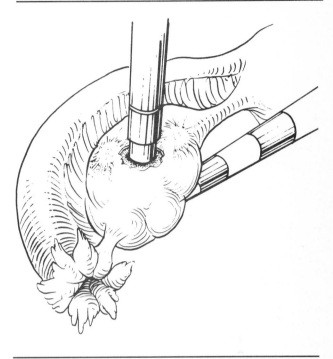

Figure 28–35. Cul-de-sac endometriosis is coagulated with a point coagulator at 120°C. The surgeon must be aware of the location of the extraperitoneal rectum and ureters.

Figure 28–37. The biopsy site is coagulated with the point coagulator at 120°C.

from the ovary is to grasp the lesion with the biopsy forceps (Fig. 28–36) and close its jaws around the implant, slowly lifting the jaws away and simultaneously sliding the cannula over the jaws. The cannula cuts the lesion away from the ovary. The base of the site is coagulated for hemostasis and to remove any remaining endometriotic tissue (Fig. 28–37).

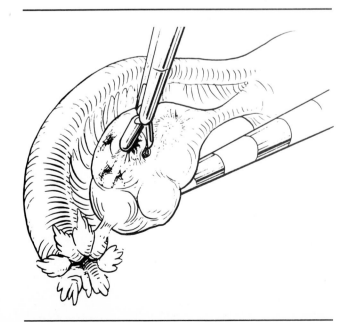

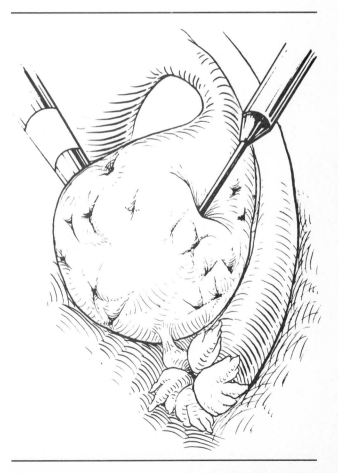

Figure 28–36. An endometrial implant is removed by biopsy forceps.

Figure 28–38. An endometrioma is partially collapsed by aspiration.

The right ovarian endometrioma is then examined. Frequently the endometrioma drains as the ovary is lifted away from the pelvic sidewall. If not, the cyst may have to be drained partially to decompress it (Fig. 28–38). The ovary is grasped laterally with a biopsy forceps and the cortex is incised well posterior (Fig. 28–39). This keeps the incisions remote from the fallopian tube and allows the cut edges of the ovary to coapt more easily. The surgeon places the tip of the laparoscope near the ovary, irrigates the cyst cavity, and carefully inspects it for any evidence of malignancy. If the cyst appears benign, the surgeon proceeds to remove it laparoscopically. If malignancy is suspected, the surgeon must consider converting to an immediate laparotomy. If there is any doubt as to the diagnosis, a frozen section examination is performed on the tissue in question.

To remove a benign cyst, the cyst wall is grasped with a second biopsy forceps and is removed by rotating the forceps (Fig. 28–40). This particular maneuver is sometimes difficult to perform. If it is impossible to establish a plane of dissection between the cyst wall and normal ovarian tissue, the surgeon may incise normal ovarian tissue, dissect down to the cyst wall, and then remove the cyst wall. A third, lower abdominal incision may be required to accomplish the dissection. The cyst wall is removed from

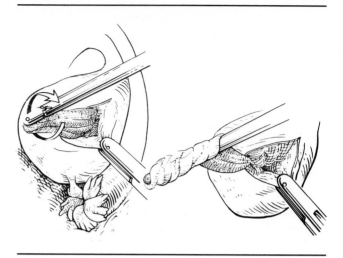

Figure 28–40. After visual inspection, the endometrial cyst wall is removed.

the abdomen with an 11-mm claw forceps. If it is difficult to resect the cyst wall, the surgeon may elect to remove as much as possible with biopsy forceps and coagulate the cyst cavity thoroughly with the point coagulator at 120°C.

To remove a smaller endometrioma (<2 cm), the cyst wall at the site where it approaches the ovarian capsule is biopsied away together with its overlying ovarian cortex, thus exposing the entire remaining cyst wall. After obtaining tissue for histology, the surgeon thoroughly coagulates the cyst wall at 120°C with the point coagulator.

Once the endometrioma has been removed, the ovary should be released and inspected. If the cut surfaces of the ovary fall together, nothing further needs to be done. If the cut surfaces gape, the surgeon should consider suturing them (Fig. 28–41).

The completed procedure is shown in Figure 28–42. The surgeon next instills adjunctive agents and closes the abdominal incisions.

Myomectomy

The surgeon sometimes encounters leiomyomata, which must be removed. Those less than 5 cm and subserosal (or intramural) but not involving the fallopian tube, urinary bladder, rectum, or uterine vessels, can be removed safely and efficiently by operative laparoscopy.

Figure 28–43 shows a subserosal leiomyoma. The surgeon may insert a spinal needle through the abdominal wall into the uterine wall and inject 3 U of vasopressin. I have found this step necessary in removing intramural leiomyomata, and it is an excellent way to control uterine hemorrhage from such conditions as a uterine perforation.

The leiomyoma is grasped with an 11-mm claw forceps. If desired, the base may be coagulated with

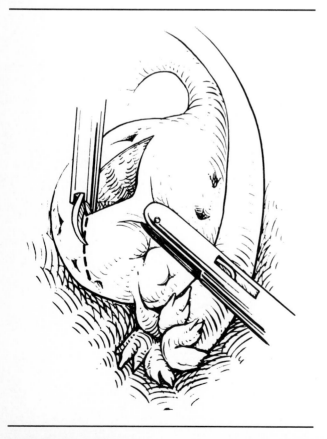

Figure 28–39. The endometrioma is opened by scissors.

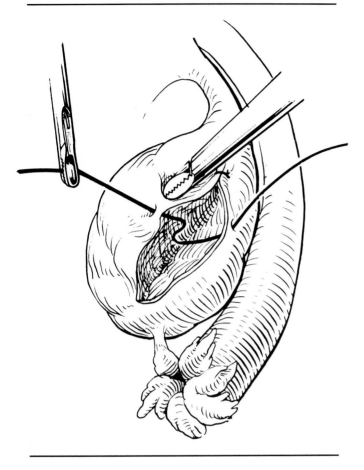

Figure 28–41. The gaping ovarian defect is closed with 4-0 poly-dioxanone.

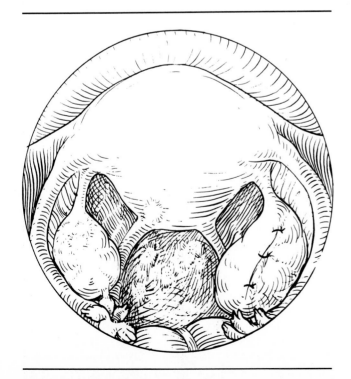

Figure 28–42. View of pelvis after the operation is completed.

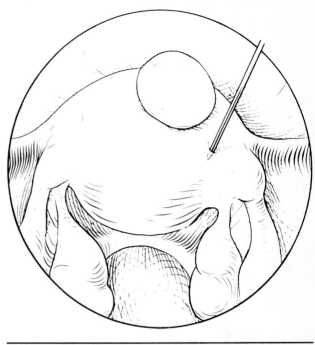

Figure 28–43. Vasopressin, 3 U, is injected into the myometrium with a 4½-inch 22-gauge spinal needle. It is best to dilute the vasopressin. I use 20 U/50 cc of lactated Ringer's.

the point coagulator at 120°C (Fig. 28–44) If the base is broad, the surgeon may incise the serosa with a scissor (Fig. 28–45). This is usually not necessary. The surgeon next rotates the claw forceps either clockwise or counterclockwise. The leiomyoma will be dissected from the uterine muscle and come away cleanly (Fig. 28–46). The surgeon then transfer the tumor to a 5-mm biopsy forceps. The claw forceps is replaced with a tissue morcellator and the leiomyoma removed piece by piece (Fig. 28–47). I have found that trapping the leiomyoma against the posterior aspect of the uterus or by withdrawing it against a 5 mm cannula aids in the morcellation process. Once the tumor has been removed from the abdomen, the defect is coagulated at 120°C with the point coagulator (Fig. 28–48). If bleeding is not controlled, a Kleppinger bipolar forceps can be substituted to achieve hemostasis. Suturing may be required with an intramural leiomyoma. The myomectomy is now complete.

Ectopic Pregnancy

One of the major complications for infertile patients in ectopic pregnancy. Although management may eventually be nonsurgical, current treatment is surgical excision. Operative laparoscopy has established a proved record in the surgical management of ectopic pregnancy.[2]

This section illustrates the step I take in dealing with the most common variation in ectopic pregnancy that I see—the unruptured ampullary gesta-

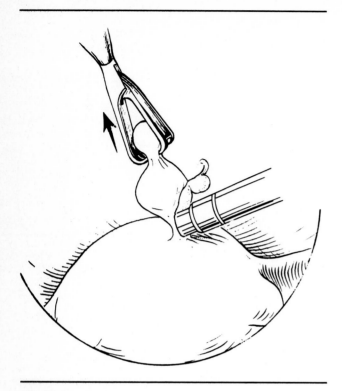

Figure 28–44. The leiomyoma is grasped with an 11-mm claw forceps and the base of the lesion coagulated with the point coagulator at 110°C.

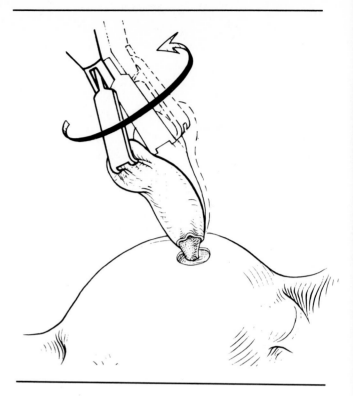

Figure 28–46. The leiomyoma is removed by rotating the claw forceps.

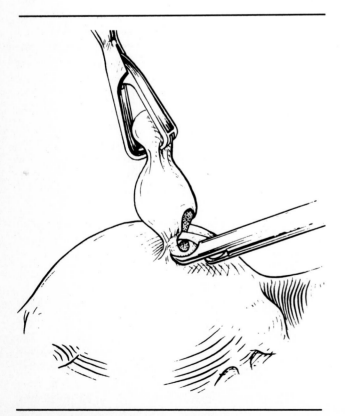

Figure 28–45. The uterine serosa is incised.

tion. One major problem is diagnosing ectopic pregnancy before it can be visualized at surgery. My present policy after tubal surgery is to follow every patient who has conceived by measuring serial quantitative levels of human chorionic gonadotropin (HCG), performing vaginal probe ultrasound studies, and following the patient's signs and symptoms. As soon as an ectopic gestation is supected based on results of these observations, laparoscopy is done.

Occasionally, a cornual pregnancy occurs or a very large ectopic gestation with a fetal heartbeat is detected on ultrasound. I often perform laparotomy on these patients, usually conserving the fallopian tube. In the case of an isthmic pregnancy, I perform a partial salpingectomy laparoscopically. If during a conservative operation for tubal ectopic pregnancy I cannot control bleeding from the implantation site, I do a partial salpingectomy or coagulate that segment of the fallopian tube, leaving enough tube for subsequent repair. The patient must be alerted to the possibility of a subsequent ectopic pregnancy in this unrepaired distal segment. If she does not wish to have the tube saved or if the tube is irreparable, I frequently perform a salpingectomy by laparoscopy.

In planning and carrying out the correct procedure, informed consent is extremely important. Postoperatively the patient must be followed with serial

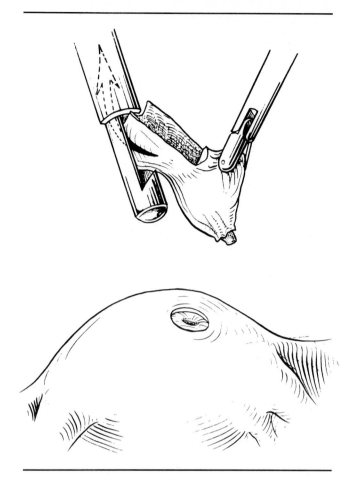

Figure 28–47. The leiomyoma is morcellated with the 11-mm tissue punch.

quantitative HCG studies if a partial or complete salpingectomy is not done. This will alert the surgeon to any persistent trophoblastic tissue.[2] In addition, the surgeon should administer hyperimmune globulin when appropriate and check the pathology to confirm removal of the pregnancy.

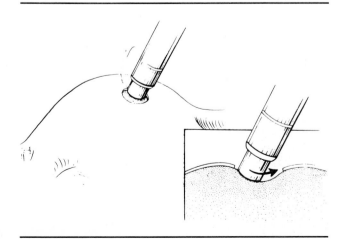

Figure 28–48. The uterine defect is coagulated with the point coagulator at 120°C.

Technique

Figure 28–49 shows an ectopic pregnancy in the midampulla of the right fallopian tube. A spinal needle is passed through the abdominal wall into the mesosalpinx and approximately 3 U of vasopressin is injected, raising a bleb. Next, the site of the ectopic is determined. A 1.5-cm track is coagulated over the site with the point coagulator at 100°C (Fig. 28–50). The tube is opened with hook scissors along the coagulated track (Fig. 28–51). An 11-mm spoon forceps is inserted, and the pregnancy extracted (Fig. 28–52). Using the Aqua-Purator, the placental site is irrigated copiously with lactated Ringer's solution (Fig. 28–53). During irrigation the distal end of the laparoscope is placed just over the salpingostomy site to search for retained products of conception; these fragments are removed.

The surgeon may extend the tubal incision if necessary. If the placental site continues to bleed, additional vasopressin may be injected and pressure applied to the site with a Kleppinger forceps. Whereas I coagulate the seromuscular layer of the tube for bleeding, I refrain from coagulating the interior of the fallopian tube, as extensive mucosal damage will result. Although the salpingostomy site may be sutured to close it, I prefer to leave it open or sutured loosely.

At the end of the operation, clots are suctioned out with the Aqua-Purator and the pelvis irrigated until suctioned fluid is clear. Adhesiolysis or other needed corrections may be performed at this time as appropriate. The procedure is completed by placing approximately 2 L of lactated Ringer's solution with

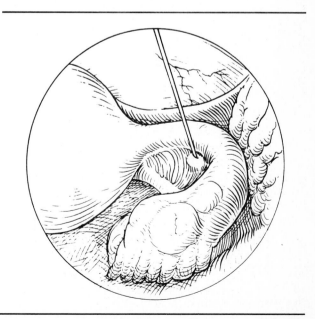

Figure 28–49. Vasopressin, 3 U, is injected into the mesosalpinx of a fallopian tube containing an ampullary ectopic pregnancy.

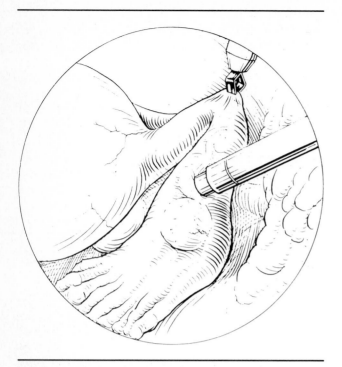

Figure 28–50. The seromuscular layer of the fallopian tube is coagulated with the point coagulator at 100°C immediately superior to the ectopic gestation.

adjunctive agents into the abdomen, releasing the pneumoperitoneum, and effecting a secure closure.

ADJUNCTIVE AGENTS

One of the greatest obstacles to obtaining an ideal anatomic result after an infertility operation is the formation of adhesions. My colleagues and I have noted a relative paucity of adhesions after operative laparoscopy relative to those found after laparotomy. In spite of this, we must be concerned with keeping adhesions to a minimum. I use the following regimen.

Antibiotics

Each patient receives prophylactic antibiotics, generally doxycycline given intravenously, immediately preoperatively and one additional dose approximately 3 hours later. Approximately 10 cc of 4.2% sodium bicarbonate is added to the bag of intravenous fluid containing the doxycycline. The sodium bicarbonate must never be added directly to the vial containing doxycycline, as this results in a small explosion. A large antecubital vein is used for the infusion to prevent superficial phlebitis. In the absence of active pelvic infection, antibiotics have not been shown to be of benefit.[3]

Steroids

I administer 20 mg of dexamethasone intraabdominally at the conclusion of an operative laparoscopy.

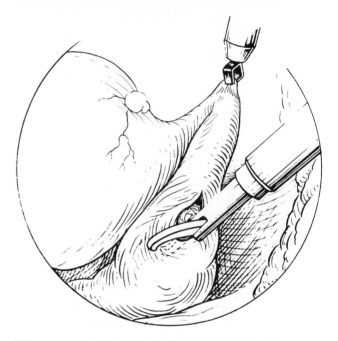

Figure 28–51. The fallopian tube is incised with hooked scissors along the coagulated track.

In patients undergoing laparotomy for ectopic pregnancy, Swolin[4] found adhesions to be less in those who received 2,000 mg hydrocortisone intraabdominally at the time the abdomen was closed as compared with patients not receiving the steroid. He graded the adhesions at the time of follow-up laparoscopy. I use the steroid regimen based on Swolin's work.

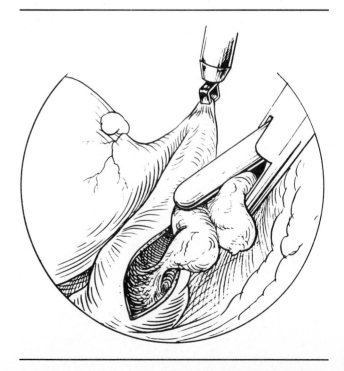

Figure 28–52. The ectopic gestation is removed with 11-mm spoon forceps.

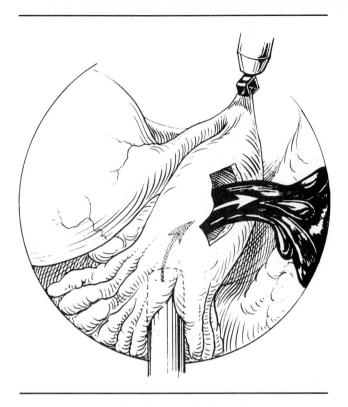

Figure 28–53. The fallopian tube is copiously irrigated with lactated Ringer's and carefully searched for retained products of conception.

Antihistamines
Promethazine 25 mg is added intraabdominally when the abdomen is closed after operative laparoscopy. Antihistamines used alone to prevent adhesions have not been studied in humans.[5] They have been studied in conjunction with steroids in primates, with no definite benefit being demonstrated.[6]

High-Molecular-Weight Dextran
The use of high-molecular-weight dextran has generated a great deal of interest. The rationale for its use are its siliconizing and hydroflotation properties. The Adhesion Study Group did find it of benefit in preventing adhesions.[7] I rarely use it in patients undergoing operative laparoscopy, however, as I am concerned over its anticoagulant properties when it comes in contact with pelvic structures having just undergone extensive dissection.

Lactated Ringer's Solution
I enthusiastically endorse the use of lactated Ringer's solution for preventing adhesions. In fact, all irrigation I use consists of warm lactated Ringer's. I generally use approximately 2 L during the operation and leave 1 to 2 L in the abdomen at the conclusion of the procedure. The purpose is to obtain a physiologic solution for irrigation and for hydroflotation. Although heparin prevents clot formation, in my experience, it has been associated with delayed bleeding

after operative laparoscopy.[8] Blandau[9] showed that a balanced salt solution is clearly superior to normal saline in pelvic surgery. The latter produced edema in rabbit fallopian tubes, whereas the former caused this edema to disappear.

Those of us involved in reconstructive surgery are and should continue to be concerned with the problem of postoperative adhesion formation. We applaud those conducting research in preventing their occurrence.

SURGICAL RESULTS

Salpingo-Ovariolysis
Gomel[10] reported on results in 92 patients undergoing salpingo-ovariolysis by operative laparoscopy. Each patient had been infertile for at least 20 months and each was judged to have moderate to severe adhesions. Ovum pickup was either greatly hampered or impossible in every case. After operative laparoscopy each patient was followed at least 9 months. Of this group 54 (58.7%) experienced at least 1 term pregnancy and 5 (5.4%) suffered an ectopic pregnancy. Of 123 patients undergoing salpingo-ovariolysis at laparotomy using the operating microscope, 28.4% were delivered of a term infant and 3.3% experienced an ectopic pregnancy.[11]

Salpingostomy
The numbers of patients reported having had salpingostomy by operative laparoscopy are small. Of 9 patients so treated, 4 had intrauterine pregnancies.[12] Eight of these 9 had experienced tubal closure after salpingostomy by laparotomy.

Laparoscopic salpingostomy was performed on 38 patients.[13] Of these, 10 (26%) developed pregnancy. The number of ectopic gestations and outcome of the pregnancies were not reported. Of 18 patients who underwent this procedure, 6 (33%) had term pregnancy, 2 (11%) experienced ectopic pregnancy, and 1 (6%) had a spontaneous abortion.[14]

Terminal salpingostomy by laparotomy using the operating microscope was performed on 143 patients.[11] Of these, 19.6% enjoyed term delivery and 2.1% experienced ectopic pregnancy. Seventy-eight patients underwent the same procedure.[15] Of these, 14 were lost to follow-up and presumed not pregnant. Seventeen (22%) had viable pregnancy and 4 (5%) ectopic gestation.

Endometriosis
The largest series we have for management of endometriosis by laparoscopy used the CO_2 laser. A combined series of 851 patients managed with this modality yielded the following pregnancy rates: 278 (58%) of 483 with mild endometriosis, 156 (51%) of

304 with moderate endometriosis, and 33 (52%) of 64 with severe disease.[16] Large series for destruction or resection of endometriosis using operative laparoscopic techniques other than the CO_2 laser are yet to be published. In 214 patients undergoing laparotomy for endometriosis, the conception rates were 70% for mild, 66% for moderate, and 61% for severe disease.[17] Of 107 patients treated similarly, conception rates were 75% for mild, 50% for moderate, and 33% for severe disease.[18] It should be noted, however, that in the former study, these percentages were calculated based on life-table comparisons of cumulative pregnancy rates, and in the latter they included only women who had not undergone previous surgical therapy for endometriosis. Therefore the reported results cannot be compared absolutely to the operative laparoscopy group.

Ectopic Pregnancy

That tubal pregnancies can be removed by operative laparoscopy has been clearly shown. Of 295 patients undergoing this procedure, only 15 (4.8%) required a second procedure to remove retained trophoblastic tissue. Seven of these underwent operative laparoscopy as the second procedure. Included in this series were 24 patients in whom the ectopic gestation occurred in a solitary tube. The fallopian tube was conserved, and each patient attempted a subsequent pregnancy. Of these 24, 11 (45.8%) had an intrauterine and 7 (29.1%) an ectopic pregnancy.[2]

CONCLUSIONS

Many laparoscopic techniques are currently available to correct pelvic diseases that contribute to infertility. These procedures can be performed reproducibly with low complication rates by the skilled laparoscopist using properly designed and maintained equipment. The real question is whether these techniques applied to the properly selected patient offer this patient a significant advantage. The answer is an enthusiastic yes. Economically, the cost is less than half that of laparotomy.[19] Other important savings are the patient's ability to return home on the day of surgery in most instances, experience decidedly less discomfort, and resume full-time activities within 1 week. Pregnancy rates with laparoscopy appear to equal or better those obtained by laparotomy for

salpingo-ovariolysis, salpingostomy, and endometriosis. A critic may argue correctly that our numbers are small and follow-up has been short. With this I agree, and I encourage those who perform operative laparoscopy to monitor carefully and report honestly the results in terms of ectopic, abortion, and viable pregnancies, using all patients operated on as the denominator.

Acknowledgments. My special thanks go to Jean Kanski-Bittl for the drawings, James F. Green for the photographs, and Sarah Jeffries for her editorial assistance.

REFERENCES

1. DeCherney AH: The leader of the band is tired. *Fertil Steril* 44(3):299, 1985.
2. Pouly JL, Mahnes H, Mage G, Canis M, Bruhat MA: Conservative laparoscopic treatment of 321 ectopic pregnancies. *Fertil Steril* 46(6):1093, 1986.
3. Holtz G: Prevention and management of peritoneal adhesions. *Fertil Steril* 41(4):497, 1984.
4. Swolin K: Die Einwirkung von grossen, intraperitonealen Dosen Glukokortikoid auf die Bildung von postoperativen Adhäsionen. *Acta Obstet Gynecol Scand* 46:204, 1967.
5. Pfeffer WH: Adjuvants in tubal surgery. *Fertil Steril* 33(3):245, 1980.
6. DiZerega GS, Hodgen GD: Prevention of postsurgical tubal adhesions: Comparative study of commonly used agents. *Am J Obstet Gynecol* 136:173, 1980.
7. Adhesion Study Group: Reduction of postoperative pelvic adhesions with intraperitoneal 32% dextran 70: A prospective, randomized clinical trial. *Fertil Steril* 40(5):612, 1983.
8. Holtz G, Hunt RB: Adjunctive agents in infertility surgery, in Hunt RB (ed): *Atlas of Female Infertility Surgery*. Chicago, Year Book, 1986, p 372.
9. Blandau RJ: Comparative aspects of tubal anatomy and physiology as they relate to reconstructive procedures. *J Reprod Med* 21(1):7, 1978.
10. Gomel V: Salpingo-ovariolysis by laparoscopy in infertility. *Fertil Steril* 40(5):607, 1983.
11. Verhoeven HC, Hunt RB, Schlosser HW: Salpingostomy, fimbrioplasty, and adhesiolysis, in Hunt RB: *Atlas of Female Infertility Surgery*. Chicago, Year Book, 1986, p 302.
12. Gomel V: *Recent Advances in Surgical Correction of Tubal Diseases Producing Infertility*. Chicago, Year Book, 1978.
13. Mettler L, Giesel H, Semm K: Treatment of female infertility due to tubal obstruction by operative laparoscopy. *Fertil Steril* 32(4):384, 1979.
14. Leventhal JM: Laparoscopy in female infertility, in Hunt RB (ed): *Atlas of Female Infertility Surgery*. Chicago, Year Book, 1986, p 213.
15. Hunt RB, Cohen SM: *Discussions of Salpingostomy*. Current Problems in Obstetrics, Gynecology, and Fertility. Chicago, Year Book, 1986, vol 9.
16. Martin DC (ed): *Intra-abdominal Laser Surgery*. Memphis, Resurge Press, 1986.
17. Rock JA: The conservative surgical treatment of endometriosis: Evaluation of pregnancy success with respect to the extent of the disease as categorized using contemporary classification systems. *Fertil Steril* 35(2):131, 1981.
18. Buttram VC Jr: Conservative surgery for endometriosis in the infertile female: A study of 206 patients with implications for both medical and surgical therapy. *Fertil Steril* 31(2):117, 1979.
19. Levine RL: Economic impact of pelviscopic surgery. *J Reprod Med* 30(9):655, 1985.

CHAPTER 29

Technical Aspects of Tubal Surgery

Robert B. Hunt

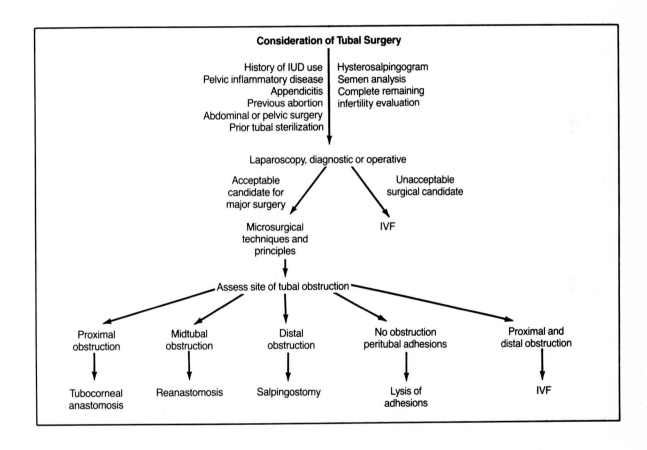

Nothing in life is to be feared. It is only to be understood.

Marie Curie

The most important factor in the successful pregnancy outcome in a given series of patients undergoing a particular tubal operation by a skilled surgeon is patient selection. For example, it has been shown that the chance of a successful pregnancy in a patient undergoing salpingostomy is poor if the better ovary is greater than 50% covered with dense adhesions.[1] Other poor prognostic findings in salpingostomy are a thick-walled tube, a large hydrosalpinx, extensive loss of tubal mucosa, lack of mucosal patterns on hysterosalpingogram, and a previous failed salpingostomy.[2-5]

The success of tubal implantation depends largely on the amount of damage to the fallopian tube. Successful outcomes after an implantation performed for reversal of a ligation are nearly twice those obtained when pathologic cornual occlusion exists.[6] In contrast, the pregnancy rates were similar when cornual anastomosis was performed in patients with cornual obstructions secondary to ligation and those with pathologic occlusion.[7] Other considerations are physiologic, such as the length of the ampulla after anastomosis for tubal reversal. An ampulla that is less than 2 cm long probably carries a reduced chance of success. Another important consideration is the presence of other unfavorable infertility factors, such as oligoovulation and reduced sperm motility.

The surgeon and the couple must have completed and carefully reviewed these many factors before mutually deciding on the best course of action in dealing with the tubal factor, whether it be reconstructive surgery or an alternative such as in-vitro fertilization (IVF). Surgery offers the best change of a successful pregnancy for most patients affected by tubal disease.

INSTRUMENTS

Retractor
The low-profile Kirschner retractor is a superb choice (Fig. 29–1). The curved blades minimize the chance of femoral nerve injury, and the square frame serves as a support for other surgeon's forearms. In addition, there are no screws and other small parts to break or get lost.

Silicone Mat
A silicone mat is placed beneath the fallopian tubes and ovaries when preparing the fallopian tubes for surgery (Fig. 29–2). The mat provides a smooth surface on which to work and a clean background when photographs are taken.

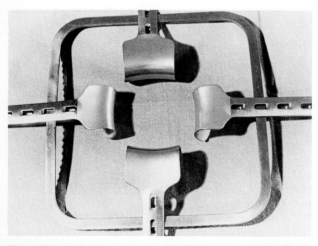

Figure 29–1. Kirschner retractor. (Available through Downs Surgical, 2500 Park Center Boulevard, Decatur, GA 30035, 404–987–0440; ELMED, 60 West Fay Avenue, Addison, IL 60101, 312–543–2792; Martin USA, 35 Melrose Place, Stamford, CT, 203–323–7087 or 800–243–5135; Zinnanti Surgical Instruments, 6311 Desoto Avenue, #M, Woodland Hills, CA 91367, 818–700–0090.) (From Hunt.[8] Reproduced with permission.)

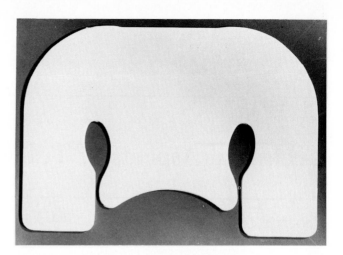

Figure 29–2. Silicone mat. (Available through Accurate Surgical and Scientific Instruments, 300 Shames Drive, Westbury, NY 11590, 516–433–4900 or 800–645–3539; Downs Surgical.) (From Hunt.[8] Reproduced with permission.)

Unipolar Coagular and Microelectrode
The unipolar coagulator should be a high-frequency, low-power unit and must be capable of delivering both the standard power needed for general surgery and the very low power required for the microelectrode. Figure 29–3 shows a typical microelectrode and the larger-needle electrode.

Bipolar Coagulator and Forceps
A separate unit for bipolar coagulation is desirable (Fig. 29–4). Many electrosurgical units that combine unipolar and bipolar generators require the unit to be manually switched to change from one to the other. This is impractical because both instruments are frequently used at the same time. I use three bipolar forceps: a long bayonet forceps and two standard forceps, one with fine and one with broad tip (Fig. 29–5).

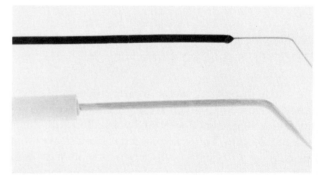

Figure 29–3. Top. Fine microelectrodes (available through Cameron Miller, 3939 South Racine, Chicago IL 60609, 312–523–6360; Martin USA) and **(bottom)** needle electrodes (usually standard operating room equipment). (From Hunt.[8] Reproduced with permission.)

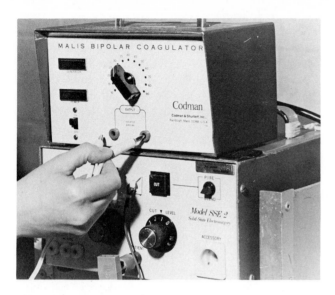

Figure 29–4. Top Bipolar and **(bottom)** unipolar generators. (From Hunt.[8] Reproduced with permission.)

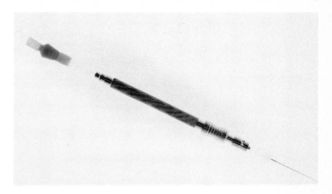

Figure 29–6. Gomel irrigator. (Available through ELMED; Martin, USA.) (From Hunt.[8] Reproduced with permission.)

Irrigator

The Gomel irrigator is well designed and useful (Fig. 29–6). It is connected to 500 cc warm lacted Ringer's containing 2,500 U heparin. If the Gomel irrigator is not available, a 30-cc syringe containing the irrigation solution and equipped with a 20-gauge blunt needle may be used.

Stangel Retrograde Lavage Cannula

When preparing the distal fallopian tube for anastomosis, the Stangel retrograde lavage cannula is most helpful (Fig. 29–7).

Dissecting Rods

Several dissecting rods are available (Fig. 29–8). They are extremely useful when performing adhesiolysis and preparing the fallopian tube for anastomosis. If the CO_2 laser is used, the laser beam must not strike these Teflon-coated rods, as it will destroy them.

Iris Scissors

This readily available instrument should be kept sharp; it is useful in transecting the fallopian tube.

Microsurgical Needle Carriers

The surgeon should try several designs of needle carriers before selecting the most desirable one. I prefer the Vickers-Owens (Fig. 29–9). A suture larger than an 8-0 should never be used with these delicate instruments, to avoid deforming their jaws.

Microsurgical Forceps

As with the needle carrier, the surgeon should exercise care when selecting forceps. I prefer the

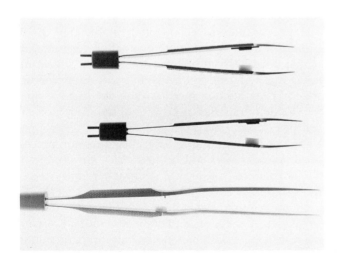

Figure 29–5. Top Bipolar forceps with fine and coarse tips and **(bottom)** long bayonet forceps forceps. (Available through Codman and Shutleff, Randolph, MA 02368, 617–961–2300 or 800–225–0460.) (From Hunt.[8] Reproduced with permission.)

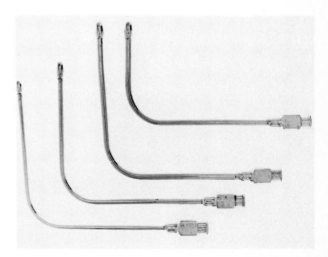

Figure 29–7. Stangel retrograde lavage cannulas. (Available through J Sklar Manufacturing Co, Long Island City, NY 11101, 212–429–1900.) (From Hunt.[8] Reproduced with permission.)

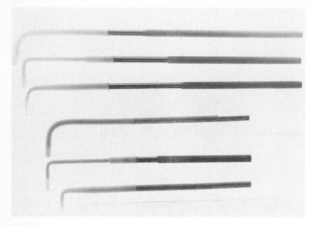

Figure 29-8. Teflon-coated dissecting rods. (Available through ELMED; Martin USA.) (From Hunt.[8] reproduced with permission.)

Vickers-Owens ring forceps (Fig. 29-10). An additional sturdy, toothed forceps should be available for lifting adhesions or a portion of the fallopian tube to be excised.

Microscissors

I have found the best designed scissors for tubal microsurgery is one with gently curved blades and blunted tips (Fig. 29-11). The length should be approximatley 12 cm. This design allows the surgeon to dissect atraumatically and effectively.

Scalpel

When preparing the cornu for anastomosis, I use an ophthalmic scalpel (Fig. 29-12). It is extremely sharp, has an ideal configuration, and is disposable.

Reamer

When the occasional tubal implantation procedure is required, I use the 1-cm Cohen reamer (Fig. 29-13). It must be kept sharp, preferably with the distal end covered when not in use.

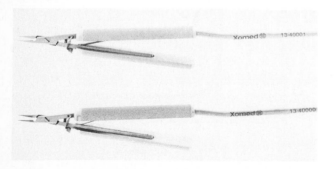

Figure 29-9. Vickers-Ownes needle carriers. (Available through ELMED; Keeler Instruments, 456 Parkway, Lawrence Park Industrial District, Broomall, PA 19008, 215-353-4350 or 800-523-5620; Martin USA.) (From Hunt.[8] Reproduced with permission.)

Camera

I obtain before and after photographs of every microsurgical operation. The Nikon camera with an 85 or 105-mm macrolens is an excellent choice. I send 1 set of the 35-mm slides to the patient and 1 to the referring physician, and keep 1 in the patient's record. This makes good sense from both medicolegal and public relations standpoints.

Instrument Box

The surgeon should purchase a sturdy box in which to store microsurgical instruments (Fig. 29-14).

Microscope

This expensive item is probably already available in the operating room. If possible, the surgeon should recommend purchase of a microscope with, or modify the existing microscope to contain, the following features: an extension on the microscope arm, an X-Y axis, foot pedal for remote control, automatic focus and zoom controls, separate opposing binocular lens, and inclinable binocular lens for the surgeon and assistant. When not in use, the microscope head should be kept covered with a large sail bag to prevent dust collecting on the instrument.

Loupes

Loupes save a great deal of time in performing adhesiolysis and other steps in the initial phases of the tubal operation, before higher magnification is required. I prefer those with 2.5 magnification, enhanced by additional light provided by a headlamp. Loupes are relatively inexpensive.

OPERATIVE PROCEDURES

Initiation of the Procedure

The patient enters the hospital on the day of the procedure. The appropriate evaluation for infertility would have been completed. In addition, she would have received and returned her informed consent sheet.[9] The previous afternoon she would have taken one bottle of magnesium citrate to induce a mechanical bowel prep and refrained from taking anything by mouth after midnight. After the admission process is complete, blood and urine studies are done, and she is taken to the surgical suite, where intravenous fluid is started and final preparations are made.

Once either general endotracheal or regional anesthesia is induced, a pelvic examination is accomplished, a Foley catheter and intrauterine catheter are inserted, and a vaginal pack is positioned.

The abdomen is prepared. I prefer the Hunt-Acuna incision.[10] It gives excellent pelvic exposure, protects the ilioinguinal nerve from injury, and

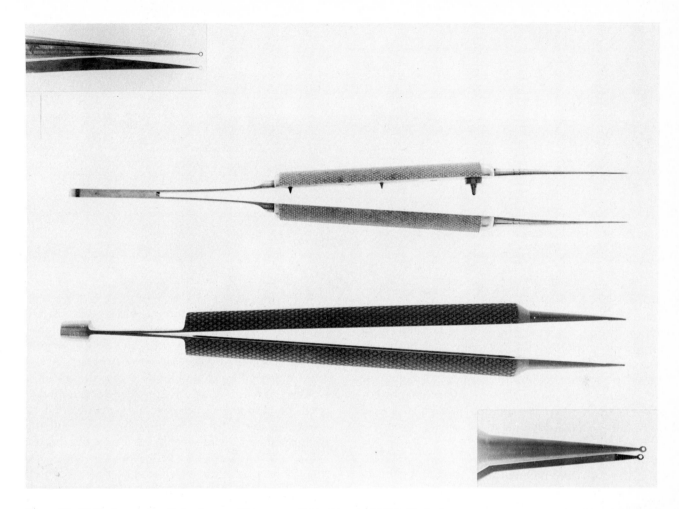

Figure 29–10. Two examples of ring forceps. They are available through ELMED, Keeler Insruments, and Martin USA **(top)** and Codman and Shurtleff **(bottom).** (From Hunt.[8] Reproduced with permission.)

results in a less painful postoperative course than the Pfannensteil incision. If the patient has had a previouis Pfannensteil, the Hunt–Acuna incision allows the surgeon to dissect in unscarred tissue. If the patient has a low midline scar, I use the old incision.

Adhesiolysis

Once the peritoneal cavity is open, the surgeon assesses for adhesions. Loupes are used for this part of the operation. The peritoneum in the lower

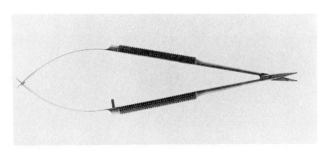

Figure 29–11. Microscissors. (Available through ELMED; Martin USA) (From Hunt.[8] Reproduced with permission.)

abdomen and the anterior and posterior cul-de-sac are cleared of bowel and omental adhesions (Fig. 29–15). If the omentum appears unhealthy, it is resected, with each significant omental vessel ligated individually. If the omentum is healthy but adhesed, an omentopexy is performed (Fig. 29–16).

Using dissecting rods and a needle electrode, the ovaries and fallopian tubes are dissected from the pelvic sidewall (Fig. 29–17). I feel it is unwise to use electrosurgery adjacent to the intestines. Sharp or occasionally blunt dissection is safer. Bleeding is controlled with bipolar coagulation.

Once the adhesiolysis is completed, a Jackson–Pratt sump drain, connected to its own suction, is positioned in the post cul-de-sac and Kerlex gauze placed. The silicone mat is laid over this (Fig. 29–18).

Pathologic Cornual Occlusion

In my experience, histologic studies of tissues removed for cornual occlusion have revealed the most common etiologies to be salpingitis isthmica nodosa, endometriosis, and fibrosis. The concept of repair is to excise all abnormal tissue and restore patency by

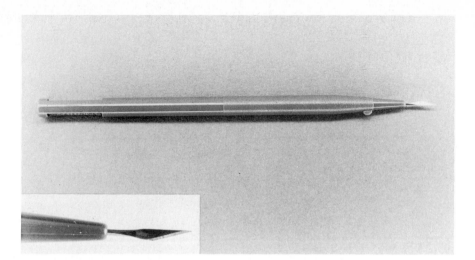

Figure 29–12. Ophthalmic scalpel. (Available through Sharpoint, PO Box 187, Mohnton, PA 19540, 215–670–2060.)

effecting a tension-free anastomosis or tubal implantation. I choose the latter procedure only if the entire intramural portion of the fallopian tube has been destroyed, an uncommon finding. The surgeon should personally review the hysterosalpingogram films, taking particular note of the intramural portion of the fallopian tube. Of great help is the appearance of the tubal ostia at the time of prior hysteroscopy.

Tubal Implantation

I use the cork bore method developed by Levinson for posterior uterine implantation.[6] The circulating nurse removes the intrauterine catheter after the surgeon has made final check to document tubal obstruction. The fallopian tube is transected in the midisthmus and the proximal tube excised. The lateral segment is dissected until healthy tissue is obtained, usually near the ampullary–isthmic junction. After patency is documented by retrograde lavage, the cut tube is incised with microscissors to produce a fish mouth (Fig. 29–19). A suture of 2-0 or 3-0 absorbable material is placed in either tubal flap, and each suture held with a fine hemostat, removing

the needle from each suture. A similar procedure is carried out on the opposite tube. The operating microscope is used for preparing the tubal segments.

Approximately 3 cc of dilute vasopressin (20 U in 50 cc lactated Ringer's) is injected into the posterior wall of the uterus (Fig. 29–20). Using the 1-cm cork bore, the surgeon selects the sites of implantation, usually at the level of the utero-ovarian ligaments. Each opening is made in the uterus by rotating the sharp cork bore, with a slight angle to the midline (Fig. 29–21). A sudden decrease in resistance indicates entry into the uterine cavity. The cork bore is withdrawn and the plug of myometrial tissue removed from it. A similar procedure is performed on the opposite side.

Focusing attention on one fallopian tube, the surgeon threads a #4 Mayo needle on the loose end of each suture. Each needle is passed through the

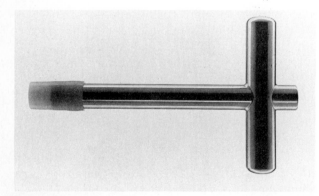

Figure 29–13. A 1-cm Cohen reamer. (Available through Zinnanti Surgical Instruments.) (From Hunt.[8] Reproduced with permission.)

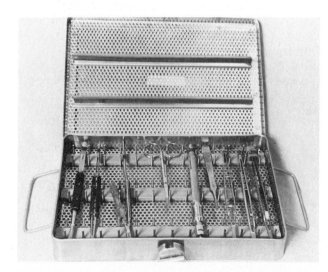

Figure 29–14. Microsurgical instrument box. (Available through Zinnanti Surgical Instruments.) (From Hunt.[8] Reproduced with permission.)

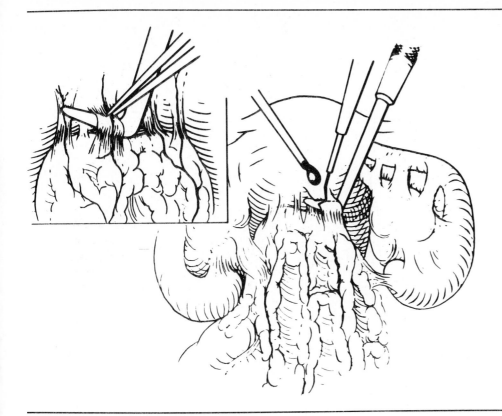

Figure 29–15. Posterior cul-de-sac dissection. Note bipolar coagulation **(inset).** (From Hunt.[8] Reproduced with permission.)

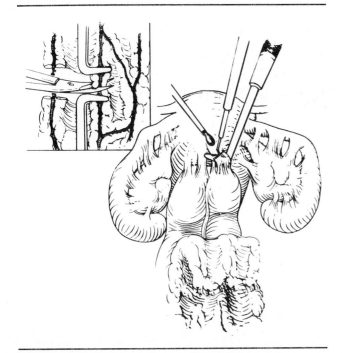

Figure 29–16. Omentopexy and partial omentectomy **(inset)**. Note bowel protected from the unipolar electrode by Teflon-coated dissecting rod. (From Hunt.[8] Reproduced with permission.)

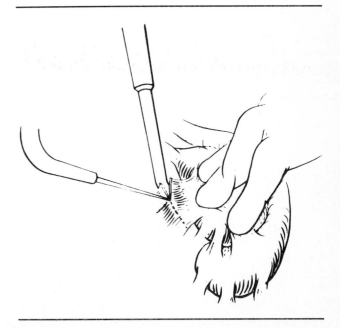

Figure 29–17. Mobilizing the right adnexa from the pelvic sidewall. (From Hunt.[8] Reproduced with permission.)

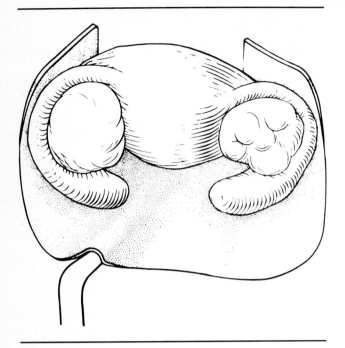

Figure 29–18. The pelvic structures are mobilized and exposed. (From Hunt.[8] Reproduced with permission.)

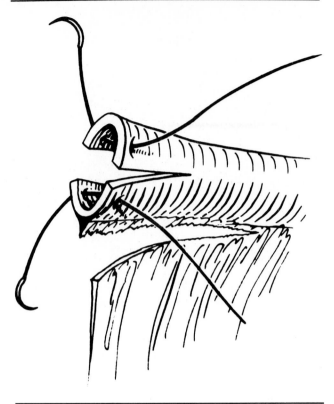

Figure 29–19. Fallopian tube prepared for implantation. (From Hunt.[8] Reproduced with permission.)

uterine openings, the eye of the needle first. The eye penetrates the endometrium and exits the serosa of the uterus. The sutures are gently tightened and the fallopian tube flaps guided into the uterine operning with ring forceps (Fig. 29–22). The sutures are gently tied, and additional sutures are placed, approximating tubal uterine serosa (Fig. 29–23). This relieves tension. A similar procedure is carried out on the opposite side.

If the uterus is retroverted, a uterine suspension is performed to prevent adhesions between the sites of implantation and the posterior cul-de-sac. The pelvis is copiously irrigated, adjunctive agents are added, and the abdomen closed. When pregnancy occurs, delivery by caesarian is recommended.[7]

Cornual Anastomosis

Approximately 3 cc of dilute vasopressin (20 U in 50 cc lactated Ringer's) is injected into the cornu for hemostasis (Fig. 29–24). With the aid of the operating microscope, the fallopian tube is transected in the midisthmus and the proximal segment dissected from the mesosalpinx until the uterotubal junction is reached. Care is taken to preserve the longitudinal vessels just beneath the tube. Bipolar coagulation is used for hemostasis. A peritoneal track is made over the fallopian tube and the tube divided with iris scissors (Fig. 29–25). Even though the tube may be patent at this level, it is seldom normal.

A 6-0 polypropylene suture is passed through the tube in a figure of 8 pattern. The suture ends are

held with a fine hemostat and an incision is made around the circular muscle fibers surrounding the intramural tubal segment (Fig. 29–26). When a 2-mm segment has been dissected, it is excised (Fig. 29–27) and the intramural segment of fallopian tube again is checked to make certain it is free of fibrosis, has a healthy mucosa, and is patent (Fig. 29–28). This dissection can be carried to the uterine cavity if necessary, although this makes for a difficult anastomosis. Also, the surgeon may have to excise crescents of myometrium superiorly to improve visibility.

Working laterally, the surgeon similarly separates the tube from its mesosalpinx until healthy

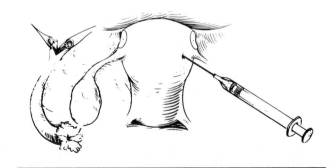

Figure 29–20. Dilute vasopressin is injected into them myometrium. (From Hunt.[8] Reproduced with permission.)

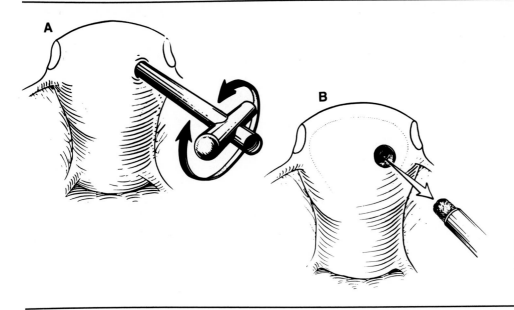

Figure 29–21. A. Cohen reamer applied to the uterus. **B.** A core of tissue is removed. (From Hunt.[8] Reproduced with permission.)

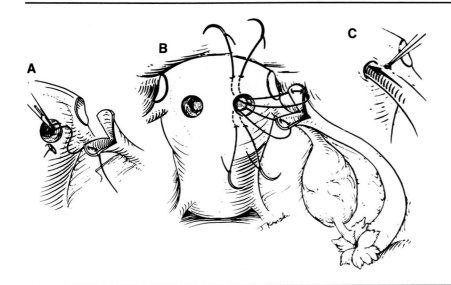

Figure 29–22. (A) Suturing is begun, **(B)** completed, and **(C)** the tube is implanted. (From Hunt.[8] Reproduced with permission.)

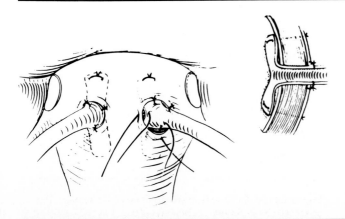

Figure 29–23. Serosal sutures are placed. Sagittal view of the implanted tube **(inset).** (From Hunt.[8] Reproduced with permission.)

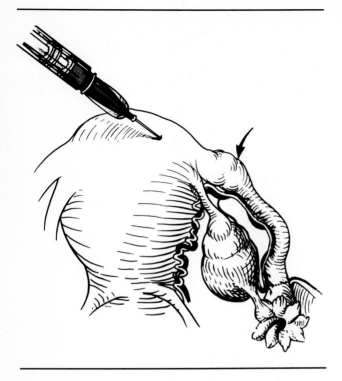

Figure 29–24. Dilute vasopressin is placed at the cornu. (From Hunt.[8] Reproduced with permission.)

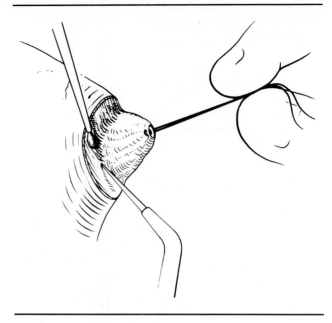

Figure 29–26. Intramural segment of the tube is dissected. (From Hunt.[8] Reproduced with permission.)

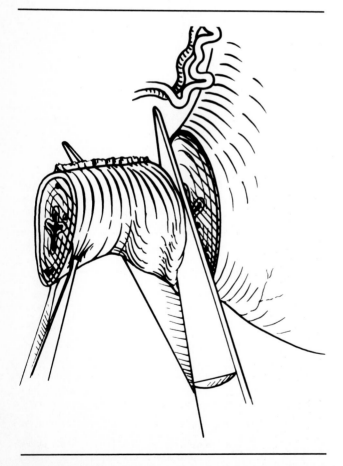

Figure 29–25. Proximal tube transected at its junction with the uterus. (From Hunt.[8] Reproduced with permission.)

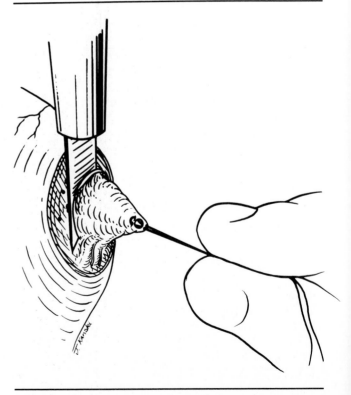

Figure 29–27. Intramural segment of the tube is excised. (From Hunt.[8] Reproduced with permission.)

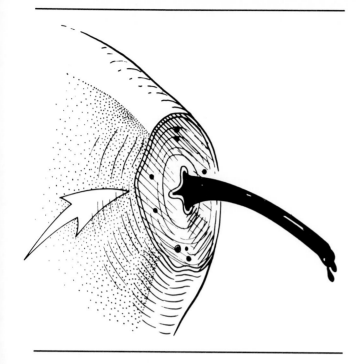

Figure 29–28. Tubal patency is established. (From Hunt.[8] Reproduced with permission.)

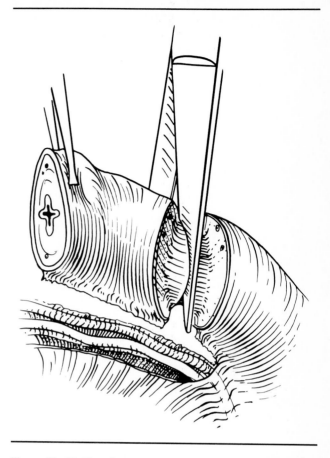

Figure 29–29. The tube is transected laterally. (From Hunt.[8] Reproduced with permission.)

tissue is encountered (Fig. 29–29). Patency is documented by retrograde lavage, using dilute indigo carmine (Fig. 29–30).

Having prepared the tube for anastomosis, the surgeon places stay sutures of 6-0 polypropylene to align the lumina. Great care must be taken to compensate for an asymetrically located tubal ostium in the cornu as well as to keep the tubal lumina at the same level. When the stay sutures are tightened, the lumina should align perfectly (Fig. 29–31).

The anastomosis is then performed using 8-0 sutures of synthetic absorbable or nonabsorbable material. I prefer nylon on a 130-μm taper-cut needle. Usually the tube is sutured in 4 places, avoiding the mucosa medially (Fig. 29–32). A small amount of mucosa is incorporated if the ampullary segment is being sutured, but avoided if the anastomosis involves the isthmus.

After the inner layer and stay sutures are tied, the fallopian tube is tested for patency. A watertight anastomosis is not necessary, but patency must be confirmed. If the anastomosis is satisfactory, the uterine and tubal serosa are approximated with 8-0 material, and additional stay sutures are placed if desirable (Fig. 29–33). A similar procedure is performed on the opposite side. After careful pelvic lavage, packing is removed, adjunctive agents are added, and the abdomen is closed.

Midtubal Anastomosis

The most frequent indication for isthmic–isthmic,

isthmic–ampullary, or ampullary–ampullary anastomosis, in my experience, is reversal of a tubal ligation. The second most frequent indication is tubal closure secondary to a previous ectopic pregnancy. The aim of the procedures is the same: to excise diseased tissue and perform a tension-free, precise anastomosis. Obviously, judgment is important. For example, the surgeon will occasionally encounter an extensively diseased ampulla, requiring a compromise. Then it is necessary to adhere to the above concept, yet leave enough ampulla for a successful pregnancy to occur. I believe the surgeon should leave at least 2 cm of ampulla with its fimbriae.

Studies have shown that the proximal fallopian tube adjacent to the ligation site is diseased in the majority of patients.[11] I recommend removing 0.5 to 1 cm of tube when preparing the proximal segment for anastomosis. To prevent excessive luminal disparity, the surgeon should open the most medial portion of the lateral segment when the ligation involves the ampulla (Fig. 29–34). It is seldom necessary to excise ampulla lateral to the site of ligation.

When the tubal segments have been prepared for anastomosis, stay sutures of 6-0 polypropylene are

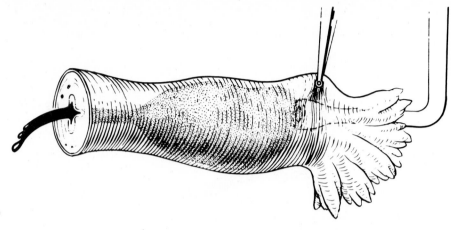

Figure 29–30. Patency is established. (From Hunt.[8] Reproduced with permission.)

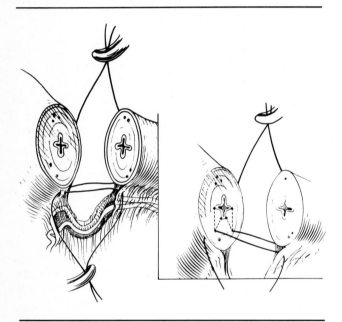

Figure 29–31. Stay sutures are placed. (From Hunt.[8] Reproduced with permission.)

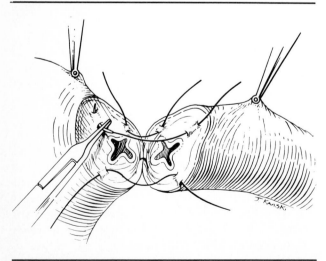

Figure 29–32. Inner layer of sutures is placed. (From Hunt.[8] Reproduced with permission.)

placed, and the inner layer of 9-0 synthetic absorbable or nonabsorbable sutures are placed and tied (Fig. 29–35). The surgeon should avoid the mucosa in the isthmic segment but may incorporate a small amount of mucosa in the ampullary segment. After stay sutures are tied, the tube is tested for patency and the serosa is approximated with 8-0 material. Additional stay sutures are placed if necessary. A similar procedure is carried out on the opposite tube.

If a great deal of luminal disparity exists, several steps may be taken to reduce this. The smaller segment may be transected at an angle and the larger segment may be narrowed with 9-0 sutures (Fig. 29–36). A standard anastomosis is then carried out (Fig. 29–37).

The pelvic cavity is cleansed, adjunctive agents are placed, and the abdomen is closed. A follow-up hysterosalpingogram is obtained 4 months after the procedure if pregnancy has not occurred.

Fimbrioplasty

Although the CO_2 laser may be used for the fimbrioplasty, I prefer the microelectrode and microscissors. Aided by magnification, the surgeon carefully

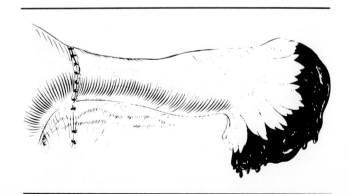

Figure 29–33. Anastomosis is complete. (From Hunt.[8] Reproduced with permission.)

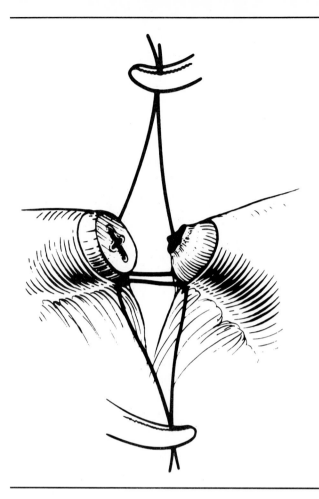

Figure 29–34. Tubal segments are prepared for anastomosis. (From Hunt.[8] Reproduced with permission.)

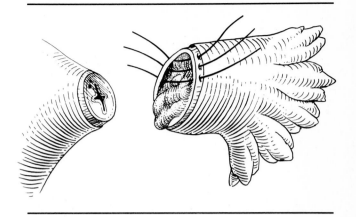

Figure 29–36. Correcting great luminal disparity. (From Hunt.[8] Reproduced with permission.)

excises adhesions from the fallopian tube and ovary. Accessory fimbrial stalks, cysts of Morgagni, and paratubal cyst are also removed where appropriate. If an accessory tubal ostium is present in the distal ampulla, the bridge of tissue separating it from the main ostium may be divided, converting the ostia into a single tubal ostium.

If fimbriae are covered by adhesions, the adhesions are gently excised, taking care not to damage the fimbriae (Fig. 29–38). A phimosis is corrected by incising along the antimesenteric side of the tube (Fig. 29–39), and the incised tissue is everted (Fig. 29–40).

When dissecting in the vicinity of the fimbriae, care must be taken not to grasp them but rather the serosa just proximal to them. The dissecting rod is a superb instrument for delineating and incising mucosal bridges (Fig. 29–41).

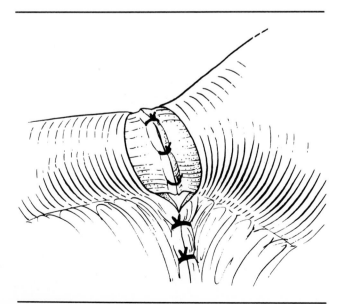

Figure 29–35. Inner layer of anastomosis is completed. (From Hunt.[8] Reproduced with permission.)

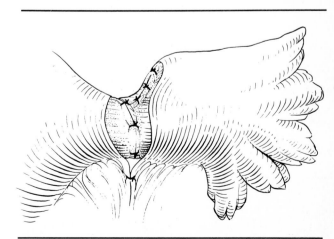

Figure 29–37. Inner layer of anastomosis is completed. (From Hunt.[8] Reproduced with permission.)

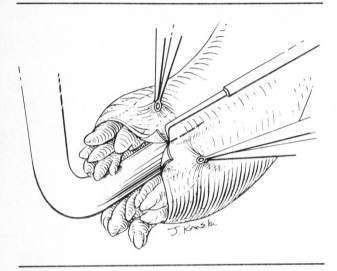

Figure 29–38. Excising scar tissue. (From Hunt.[8] Reproduced with permission.)

SALPINGOSTOMY

Once adhesiolysis has been accomplished (Figs. 29–42 and 29–43), the fallopian tube is dissected from its respective ovary to restore proper tuboovarian relationships (Fig. 29–44). With the tube distended with dilute indigo carmine, approximately three to five incisions are made in the most distal portion, following the most avascular lines (Figs. 29–45 and 29–46). The mucosal flaps are everted, and with use of the dissecting rods, the incisions are continued between arterioles (Figs. 29–47 and 29–

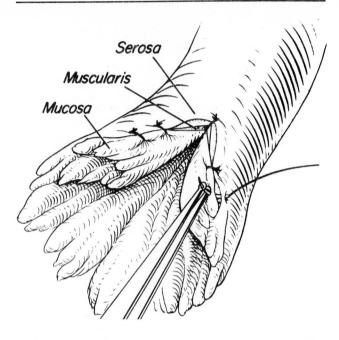

Figure 29–40. Fimbrioplasty nears completion. (From Hunt.[8] Reproduced with permission.)

48). After hemostasis has been obtained with bipolar coagulation, the serosa of the mucosal flaps is sutured to the serosa of the fallopian tube, just enough to keep the mucosal flaps everted (Fig. 29–49). I prefer 6-0 or 8-0 synthetic absorbable or nonabsorbable material. The surgeon then reconstructs the undersurface of the fallopian tube and the denuded ovarian surface (Fig. 29-50).

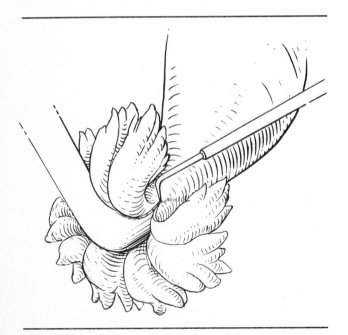

Figure 29–39. Correcting tubal phimosis. (From Hunt.[8] Reproduced with permission.)

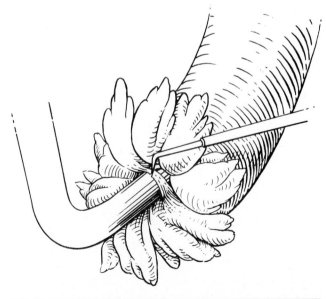

Figure 29–41. Mucosal bridge is divided. (From Hunt.[8] Reproduced with permission.)

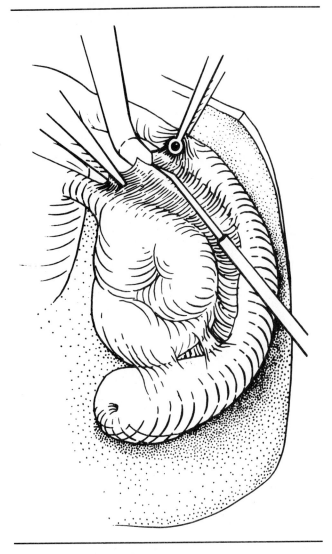

Figure 29–42. Dividing adhesions between tube and ovary. (From Hunt.[8] Reproduced with permission.)

Bipolar Block

Many believe concomitant cornual and distal fallopian tubal blockage is a contraindication for surgical correction. I disagree. My present policy is as follows. At the time of assessment laparoscopy, I perform an adhesiolysis of all pelvic structures. I then open the distal ends of the fallopian tube and perform a tuboscopy. If the tubal mucosa appears in relatively satisfactory condition, I conclude the procedure with a hysteroscopy to inspect the tubal ostia and attempt to open the proximal segment with a small wire-guided catheter. If unsuccessful, I then schedule the patient for salpingostomy and cornual anatomosis 2 months later. In a small series of 6 patients, 2 have delivered successfully. In a series of 8 patients undergoing correction of bilateral bipolar blocks, there were 2 pregnancies.[2]

RESULTS

Tubal Implantation

The success of tubal implantation depends on the disease process. An implantation performed to reverse tubal sterilization has an excellent prognosis. Of 38 patients in whom sterilization was reversed using the Levinson technique, 26 (68.4%) had a viable pregnancy. Of 30 patients with pathologic cornual occlusion, 11 (36.7%) achieved a viable pregnancy. In the total series of 68 patients, 4 (5.9%) suffered an ectopic pregnancy.[6]

Using a slightly different technique, one author reported a 50% pregnancy in 16 patients.[12] In a brief report 8 years later, subsequent results were much poorer, and the author concluded that posterior wall tubal implantation has a limited role in the management of cornual occlusion.[13]

A series of 60 patients underwent posterior wall implantation either to reverse of sterilization or correct pathologic cornual occlusion. In this group, 45% achieved a pregnancy.[7]

Tubal Anastomosis

Cornual anastomosis has yielded excellent results. Of 43 patients undergoing the procedure for reversal of sterilization, 26 (61%) achieved a pregnancy. There was one ectopic gestation.[14] Eighteen (64.3%) of 28 patients had term pregnancy after cornual anastomosis for mixed indications.[15] Of 48 patients undergoing the procedure for pathologic cornual occlusion, 27 (56.2%) had a term pregnancy. There were 3 (6.2%) ectopic pregnancies.[16] A recent series of 27 patients with pathologic cornual occlusion underwent microsurgical anastomosis. Of these 53.2% had viable pregnancy and 11% (3) ectopic pregnancy[17]. I believe each patient with pathologic cornual occlusion should have an initial effort, unless contraindicated, to establish patency by passing a small wire-guided catheter into the tube by radiologic or hysteroscopic techniques.

Tubal anastomosis for reversal of a previous sterilization has superb overall results. Of 118 such patients 93 (78.8%) patients achieved term pregnancy. Two (1.7%) sustained ectopic gestations.[16] Of 31 patients undergoing anastomosis to reverse previous sterilizations, 22 (71%) had intrauterine pregnancy; 19 (61%) delivered term infants.[18] Although none of these patients had ectopic pregnancies, the rate is generally thought to be approximately 5%.

Fimbrioplasty

Definitions of *fimbrioplasty* vary considerably. The word is sometimes used loosely to include correction of all distal tubal problems, including hydrosalpinges. Other series might include patients with removal of adhesions from the fallopian tube not

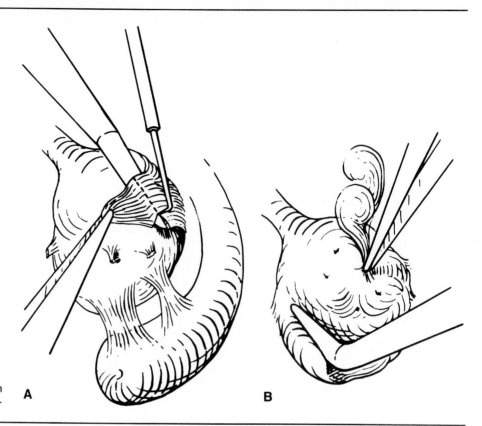

Figure 29–43. (A) Excising scar tissue and **(B)** shrinking small tufts of scar with the bipolar coagulator. (From Hunt.[8] Re-

involving the fimbriae or those with unilateral disease. The word should include only patients with diseased fimbriae bilaterally, or with an absent or inoperable opposite tube.

Of 130 patients undergoing fimbrioplasty and meeting the criteria of "pure" cases, 30% achieved a term pregnancy. The rate of ectopic gestation was 3.2%.[19] Of 35 patients undergoing a pure procedure, 21 (60%) achieved an intrauterine and 1 (3%) an ectopic pregnancy.[20]

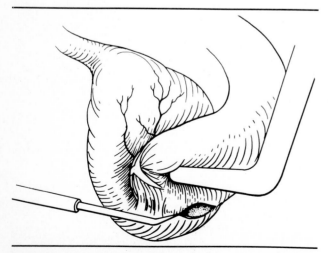

Figure 29–44. Mobilizing the distal end of a hydrosalpinx from the adjacent ovary. (From Hunt.[8] Reproduced with permission.)

Salpingostomy

Like fimbrioplasty, definition of *salpingostomy* may vary. It should refer only to patients who have surgical correction of bilateral hydrosalpinges, or who have correction of one tube when the other tube is absent or inoperable.

One such pure series included 143 patients undergoing terminal salpingostomy. Of these, 28 (19.6%) had term pregnancy and 3 (2.1%) ectopic gestation.[2] Of 78 patients undergoing salpingostomy, 14 were lost to follow-up and considered not pregnant. Seventeen (22%) of the 78 patients had viable and 4 (5%) ectopic pregnancies.[21]

ADHESION PREVENTION

Ischemia is a potent stimulus to intraabdominal adhesion formation.[22] All pelvic reconstructive procedures should be performed with this in mind. Another important fact is that peritoneal defects heal from the base and not from the edges.[23] Based on this valuable information, I discourage closing peritoneal defects under tension, using peritoneal grafts, and tying sutures tightly. In addition, several surgical procedures and therapeutic regimens have been devised to prevent postoperative adhesion formation.

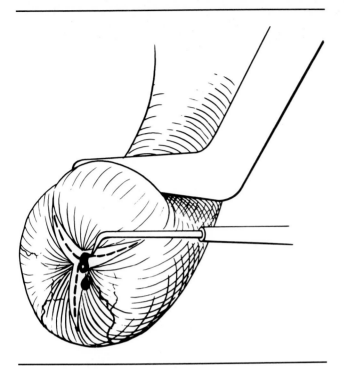

Figure 29–45. Salpingostomy is begun. (From Hunt.[8] Reproduced with permission.)

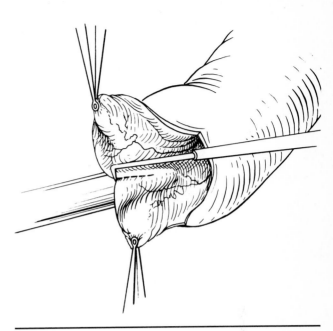

Figure 29–47. Dissection proceeds on the mucosal side. (From Hunt.[8] Reproduced with permission.)

Uterine Suspension

If the posterior cul-de-sac has been cleared of significant adhesions and the uterus is retroverted, the surgeon should consider performing a uterine suspension. Another indication is a posterior wall implantation in a patient with a retroverted uterus. I prefer triplication of the round ligaments, using 0 polypropylene (Fig. 29–51).

Peritoneal Platforms

Sometimes it is advisable to develop peritoneal platforms beneath each ovary after an extensive

adhesiolysis. I use 2-0 or 3-0 polydioxanone (Fig. 29–52). This procedure minimizes the chance of the ovary adhering to the pelvic sidewall.

Omentopexy or Omentectomy

If the omentum is involved in extensive adhesions, the surgeon may wish to remove the distal omentum

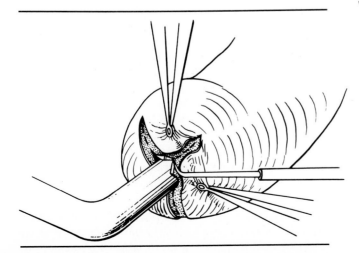

Figure 29–46. Dissection proceeds. (From Hunt.[8] Reproduced with permission.)

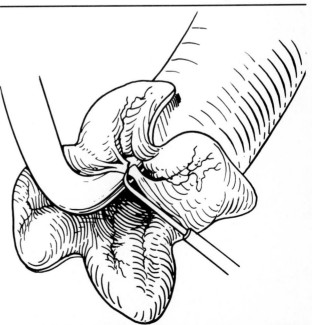

Figure 29–48. A mucosal bridge is divided. (From Hunt.[8] Reproduced with permission.)

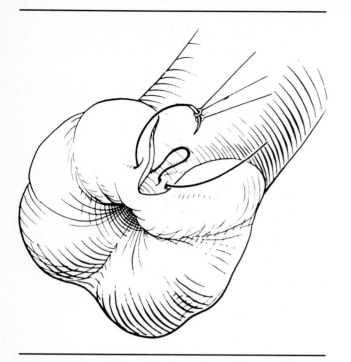

Figure 29–49. Mucosal flaps are sutured. (From Hunt.[8] Reproduced with permission.)

or perform an omentopexy. The latter is reserved for patients with a relatively normal-appearing omentum, and the former for those with a badly diseased one. If an omentectomy is performed, the surgeon must take care to ligate each omental artery individually to prevent a postoperative hemorrhage (see Fig. 29–16).

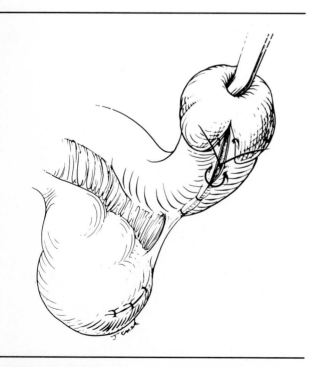

Figure 29–50. Denuded areas are repaired. (From Hunt.[8] Reproduced with permission.)

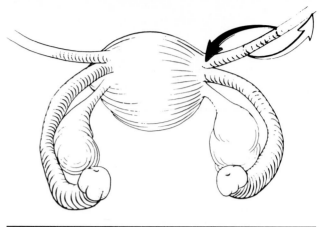

Figure 29–51. Triplication of round ligaments. (From Hunt.[8] Reproduced with permission.)

Irrigation

Saline produces edema of the fimbriae in animal fallopian tubes, and balanced salt solutions do not.[24] For this reason I use warm lactated Ringer's for irrigation; 5,000 U heparin is added to each L of irrigant to prevent blood clots in the operative sites. Whereas blood clots alone do not produce adhesions, their formation in the presence of tissue drying does.[25]

Steroids

A controlled study placed 2 g hydrocortisone intraperitoneally after removal of ectopic pregnancies in one group of patients. The second group received no steroids. A second-look laparoscopy 3 months later revealed fewer adhesions in the patients receiving hydrocortisone.[26]

Although widely used, steroids have not been shown by all animal studies to reduce adhesions.[27–29] The impetus for their use in North America came from a study using dexamethasone and promethazine.[30] The study involved many different surgeons, institutions, and infertility operations, and did not have a control group. The Horne regimen consisted of 20 mg dexamethasone and 25 mg promethazine given intramuscularly preoperatively, intraperitoneally at the completion of the operation, and every 4 hours intramuscularly for an additional 12 doses.

I use a modified Horne regimen consisting of 10 mg dexamethasone and 12.5 mg promethazine given intramuscularly preoperatively, intraperitoneally at the conclusion of the operation, and intramuscularly 4 hours postoperatively. Patients then receive 7 additional doses orally every 4 hours.

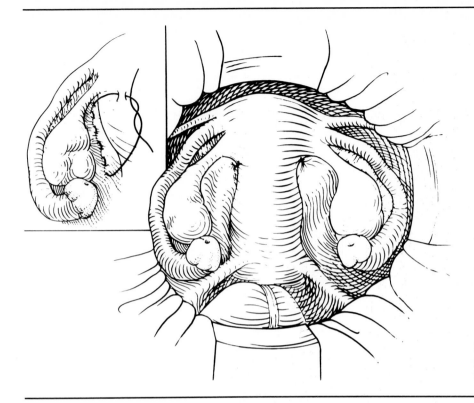

Figure 29–52. Peritoneal platforms are placed **(inset)** and view after completion. (From Hunt.[8] Reproduced with permission.)

High–Molecular—Weight Dextran

Intraperitoneal high-molecular-weight dextran is used by some surgeons. It has the ability to expand the volumes of intraperitoneal fluid by a factor of 5 to 1. If 100 cc dextran is added to the intraperitoneal cavity at the completion of the operation, 500 cc volume will result. This in turn produces hydroflotation, a desirable effect in preventing adhesions. The regimen lessened adhesion formation in a multicenter study using a control group.[31] Some believe it siliconizes peritoneal surfaces, thus reducing adhesions. High-molecular-weight dextran has not been approved for this use, however, and adverse reactions can occur.

At the time of wound closure, I instill 1L of lactated Ringer's solution intraperitoneally by means of a large rubber catheter. I do not use dextran for adhesion prevention.

Antibiotics

Many surgeons use antibiotics in the perioperative period in reconstructive tubal operations.[32] There has not ben any proof that results are improved by this practice.

I administer 100 mg doxycycline intravenously preoperatively and 1 dose postoperatively. The medication should be given in the antecubital vein if possible, to prevent phlebitis. I usually continue doxycycline, 100 mg orally twice daily, until the patient is discharged.

Antiprostaglandins

Antiprostaglandins have been studied as possible adhesion preventives. The one that has received the most attention is ibuprofen. Results of animal studies have been inconsistent.[33] I do not use these agents.

Hydrotubation

One study showed a markedly improved pregnancy rate in patients undergoing multiple hydrotubations after salpingostomy.[34] This finding has not been reproduced by others, and most colleagues no longer do this.[32]

Early Laparoscopy

Some have advocated laparoscopy to be performed as early as 8 days after adhesiolysis in the hope of separating postoperative adhesions before they have matured. One study showed a reduction in subsequent ectopic pregnancies but no increase in cumulative pregnancy rates when this practice was carried out.[35]

I previously preformed laparoscopies 3 weeks after adhesiolysis in most patients. I no longer do this, but rather recommend operative laparoscopy 12 to 18 months postoperatively, if indicated.

CONCLUSION

There have been enormous advances in the field of infertility. The most striking examples are in-vitro fertilization (IVF), gamete intrafallopian transfer (GIFT), ovulation-induction methods, and medical therapy for endometriosis. Although not as sensational, evolutionary progress is being made in the surgical management of infertility. Examples are our better understanding of normal and abnormal peritoneal healing, judicious use of the operating microscope, and refinement of operative laparoscopy. We are proud of our contributions to reconstructive surgery for infertile females, but we are challenged by our failures. With continued assessment of these failures, our efforts, in concert with those of our colleagues in related fields, will result in a greater chance for infertile couples' ultimate goal—a healthy baby.

REFERENCES

1. Hulka JF: Adnexal adhesions: A prognostic staging and classification system based on a five-year survey of fertility surgery results at Chapel Hill, North Carolina. *Am J Obstet Gynecol* 144:141, 1982.
2. Verhoeven HC, Berry H, Frantzen C, Schlosser HW: Surgical treatment for distal tubal occlusion. *J Reprod Med* 28(5):293, 1983.
3. Henry-Suchet J, Tesquiter L, Pez JP, Loffredo V: Prognostic value of tuboscopy vs hysterosalpingography before tuboplasty. *J Reprod Med* 29(8):609, 1984.
4. Young PE, Egan JE, Barlow JJ, et al: Reconstructive surgery for infertility at the Boston Hospital for Women. *Am J Obstet Gynecol* 108(7):1092, 1970.
5. Ozaras H: The value of plastic operations on the fallopian tubes in the treatment of female infertility. *Acta Obstet Gynecol Scand* 47:489, 1968.
6. Levinson CJ: Tubal implantation, in Hunt RB (ed): *Atlas of Female Infertility Surgery*. Chicago, Year Book, 1986, pp. 261–262.
7. Musich JR, Behrman SJ: Surgical management of tubal obstruction at the uterotubal junction. *Fertil Steril* 40(4):423, 1983.
8. Hunt RB (ed): *Atlas of Female Infertility Surgery*. Chicago, Year Book, 1986.
9. Hunt RB: Informed consent for pelvic reconstructive surgery using the operating microscope and/or carbon dioxide laser, in Hunt RB (ed): *Atlas of Female Infertility Surgery*. Chicago, Year Book, 1986, pp 406–408.
10. Hunt RB, Acuna HA: Pelvic preparation and choice of incision, in Hunt RB (ed): *Atlas of Female Infertility Surgery*. Chicago, Year Book, 1986, pp 125–142.
11. Vasquez G, Winston RML, Boeckx W, Brosens I: Tubal lesions subsequent to sterilization and their relation to fertility after attempts at reversal. *Am J Obstet Gynecol* 138:86, 1980.
12. Peterson EP, Musich JR, Behrman SJ: Uterotubal implantation and obstetric outcome after previous sterilization. *Am J Obstet Gynecol* 128(6):662, 1977.
13. Peterson EP: Uterotubal implantation—A reappraisal. *Fertil Steril* 39(3):401, 1983.
14. Winston RML: Reversal of tubal sterilization. *Clinical Obstet Gynecol* 23(4):1261, 1980.
15. Diamond E: A comparison of gross and microsurgical techniques for repair of cornual occlusion in infertility: A retrospective study, 1968–1978. *Fertil Steril* 32(4):370, 1979.
16. Gomel V: An odyssey through the oviduct. *Fertil Steril* 39(2):144, 1983.
17. Patton PE, Williams TJ, Coulam CB: Microsurgical reconstruction of the proximal oviduct. *Fertil Steril* 47(1):35, 1987.
18. Hunt RB: Tubal anastomosis, in Hunt RB (ed): *Atlas of Female Infertility Surgery*. Chicago, Year Book, 1986, p 265.
19. Verhoeven HC, Hunt RB, Schlosser HW: Salpingostomy, fimbrioplasty, and adhesiolysis, in Hunt RB: *Atlas of Female Infertility Surgery*. Chicago, Year Book, 1986, p 302.
20. Patton GW Jr: Pregnancy outcome following microsurgical fimbrioplasty. *Fertil Steril* 37(2):150, 1982.
21. Hunt RB, Cohen SM: Discussion of salpingostomy. In *Current Problems in Obstetrics, Gynecology and Fertility*, in Leventhal JM (ed). Chicago, Year Book, 1986, vol 9, p 3.
22. Ellis H: The cause and prevention of postoperative intraperitoneal adhesions. *Surg Gynecol Obstet* 133:497, 1971.
23. Raftery AT: Regeneration of parietal and visceral peritoneum: An electron microscopical study. *J Anat* 115:375, 1973.
24. Blandau RJ: Comparative aspects of tubal anatomy and physiology as they relate to reconstructive procedures. *J Reprod Med* 21(1):7, 1978.
25. Ryan GB, Grobety J, Majno G: Postoperative peritoneal adhesions. *Am J Pathol* 65:117, 1971.
26. Swolin K: Die Einwirkung von grossen, intraperitonealen Dosen Glukokortikoid auf die Bildung von postoperativen Adhäsionen. *Acta Obstet Gynecol Scand* 46:204, 1967.
27. Liao S, Surhiro GT, McNamara JJ: Prevention of postoperative intestinal adhesions in primates. *Surg Gynecol Obstet* 137:816, 1973.
28. Seitz HM Jr, Schenker JG, Epstein S, et al: Postoperative intraperitoneal adhesions: A double-blind assessment of their prevention in the monkey. *Fertil Steril* 24(12):935, 1973.
29. diZerega GS, Hodgen GD: Prevention of postoperative tubal adhesions: Comparative study of commonly used agents. *Am J Obstet Gynecol* 136:173, 1980.
30. Horne HW Jr, Clyman M, Debrovner C, et al: The prevention of postoperative pelvic adhesions following conservative operative treatment for human infertility. *Int J Fertil* 18:109, 1973.
31. Adhesion Study Group: Reduction of postoperative pelvic adhesions with intraperitoneal 32% dextran 70: A prospective, randomized clinical rial. *Fertil Steril* 40(5):612, 1983.
32. Hunt RB: Survey results, in Hunt RB (ed): *Atlas of Female Infertility Surgery*. Chicago, Year Book, 1986, pp 318–320.
33. Holtz G: Prevention and management of peritoneal adhesions. *Fertil Steril* 41(4):497, 1984.
34. Grant A: Infertility surgery of the oviduct. *Fertil Steril* 22(8):496, 1971.
35. Trimbos-Kemper TCM, Trimbos JB, van Hall EV: Adhesion formation after tubal surgery: Results of the eight-day laparoscopy in 188 patients. *Fertil Steril* 43(3):395, 1985.

CHAPTER 30

Additional Aspects of Tubal Surgery: A British Perspective

Robert M.L. Winston

Additional Aspects of Tubal Surgery

The Development of Tubal Microsurgery
Indications for Tubal Microsurgery
Types of Operations
Instruments
    Methods of Magnification
    The Operating Microscope
    Features of Loupes
    Diathermy
    Microsurgical Instruments
Surgical Principles
Abdominal Incision
Principles of Adhesiolysis
Salpingostomy

Cornual Anastomosis
Tubal Implantation
Reversal of Sterilization
    Excessive Scarring of the Tubal Stumps
    Joining Segments of Tubes of Widely Disparate Diameter
Preparation of the Ovaries Before In-Vitro Fertilization
Surgical Management of Ectopic Pregnancy
Appendix: Manufacturers of Microsurgical Equipment

Tubal disease is thought to be responsible for between 18 and 32% of fertility problems.[1,2] Indeed, in some parts of the world it is by far the most common cause of infertility; for example, it accounted for 87% of cases in parts of New Guinea.[3] It is remarkable that, until comparatively recently, it was often felt that once a woman had tubal damage, there would be little hope of pregnancy. A survey of the global results of tubal surgery done without microsurgical technique up to 1974[4] showed that only 9.5% of patients had a live baby after salpingostomy. Two advances that were developed in the last decade have changed this perspective somewhat. One, of course, is in-vitro fertilization (IVF). The other is tubal microsurgery, which is now the standard procedure used for reconstructive operations in infertile women. Microsurgery also has a place during incidental laparotomy in young women, who may only too easily be made infertile by adhesion formation after clumsy surgery.

Many physicians are of the opinion that IVF has almost entirely replaced tubal microsurgery. Although I am a strong advocate for IVF, I sometimes feel that the zeal for this complex and demanding treatment is not justified. The truth is that there is an important place for both, and very often, microsurgery is a much more successful and satisfactory treatment for tubal damage. The key of course, is careful selection of appropriate patients. Moreover, in so many countries where high technology is limited, microsurgery is of vital importance.

Microsurgery implies surgery performed with

the help of magnification, although from time to time it may be that only the principles of a refined atraumatic technique are really needed. The primary reason for magnification was initially the small size of the tubal lumen. At the narrowest part of the fallopian tube, the interstitial portion (which commonly becomes blocked) is usually less than 0.5 mm in diameter. It is not possible to anastomose this area accurately with the unaided eye. Microsurgery is not employed just because the tubes are small, however. Few surgeons have such myopia that they cannot clearly see the ovary or the periotoneal attachments of the genital tract, yet microsurgery is just as important when operating on the ovary or dividing peritoneal adhesions. An essential feature of microsurgery is that it avoids microscopic damage of delicate serosal and coelomic surfaces. Magnification when handling tissue gives immediate awareness of any trauma that may result.

THE DEVELOPMENT OF TUBAL MICROSURGERY

Wolfgang Walz was the first surgeon to use a microscope for tuboplasty.[5] He described a relatively crude technique to improve tubal implantation, and gave the opinion that the microscope might be used for salpingostomy. He made the important observation that the microscope would reduce iatrogenic damage. He correctly pointed out that improvements in technique alone would not greatly improve the results of tubal surgery; this, he stated, would be achieved with more careful selection of patients. Magnification with loupes was used by Swolin,[6] who introduced the important concept of electrosurgery for tubal operations. Gomel[7] also used loupes, but remained rather unconvinced of the value of the microscope until after 1977.[8] Refined microsurgical methods were introduced in 1974 in animal work.[9,10] These workers also used microsurgery for clinical work, and by the late 1970s it was apparent that magnification, whether by loupes or by microscope, gave improved surgical results. Tubal microsurgery became increasingly widespread for all infertility surgery and many reviews were published.[11-13] Various attempts to refine the techniques have been made (such as use of the laser), but improvement in results has been rather static.

INDICATIONS FOR TUBAL MICROSURGERY

The main indications for tubal microsurgery are tubal block, tubal constriction with scarring, and peritubal adhesions. The most common cause of blockage and

scar tissue is inflammatory disease. Even if the tubes are not actually blocked, surgery may sometimes be justified. For many years we have tended to think of tubal disease in terms of occlusion; however, before occlusion occurs there must be scarring and narrowing. Complete blockage is really only an end point in the disease process, and it may be justified on occasions to remove damaged but patent areas of the tubes in order to improve fertility.

The fimbrial end and the intramural portion are the common sites of blockage. Midtubal block is comparatively rare and is usually associated with very severe scarring or tuberculosis. Endometriosis may occasionally cause tubal blockage, most frequently at the cornual end. Congenital anomalies are an important cause of block, but are frequently misdiagnosed. They may result in hydrosalpinx formation, although cornual block can also be congenital. Blockage may also follow iatrogenic damage, such as previous sterilization.

TYPES OF OPERATIONS

Blockage at the fimbrial end leads to hydrosalpinx formation. Hydrosalpinges have the best surgical prognosis if they are thin walled. Thick-walled, fibrous, and hypertrophic hydrosalpinges do not lend themselves to a microsurgical approach and may reocclude even after careful surgery. When a hydrosalpinx is of long standing, the mucosa tends to become flattened and the ciliated epithelium lost. This is associated with a poor prognosis,[14] and some surgeons therefore feel that patients with hydrosalpinges should not be left indefinitely on waiting lists. Several standard operations are performed to repair fimbrial damage.

By international agreement, *salpingostomy* (salpingoneostomy) is the word used for surgical procedures to open a totally blocked fimbrial end. The block may be either terminal, if no part of the tube is resected and the opening is made at the most terminal part of the tube, or ampullary, if some tubal tissue is removed, or if the end is so damaged that the ostium has to be fashioned in the ampullary sidewall. Isthmic salpingostomy refers to similar operations on the isthmus when the whole ampulla has been removed.

Fimbrioplasty refers to similar procedures but should be used only if the tube is already partly open. Typically, it is employed for fimbrial phimosis or when a fibrous ring partly obstructs the fimbrial end. It is important that fimbrioplasty is not confused with salpingostomy. Fimbrioplasty carries a generally better prognosis. Unless proper terminology is used when publishing results, there is a risk of giving misleading information.

Salpingolysis is division of adhesions around the tube. Occasionally, it may be used in conjunction with fimbriolysis if the adhesions involve the fimbrial end. The word *tuboplasty* is a loose description of tubal surgery and is best avoided. It simply refers to plastic operations on the tube, and its use in publications makes it impossible to evaluate reported results. Blockage at the uterine end is usually in the interstitial portion itself, in the wall of the uterus, or in the first part of the isthmus. Most blocks are due to old infection, usually after miscarriage or pregnancy. The great majority of cases of cornual block can be treated by joining the healthy isthmic or ampullary segment onto the cornu, having first resected the blocked segment. The following terminology is widely accepted.

Cornual anastomosis may be deep if the whole of the intramural tube requires excision, or superficial if little of the interstitial tube is damaged. The procedure may be either isthmic–cornual or ampullary–cornual, depending on the amount of distal tube that requires resection.

In about 10% of patients there is no tissue on the uterine side for anastomosis, in which case tubal implantation may be indicated. *Tubal anastomosis* is the term for operations such as reverals of sterilization, when the tube may be blocked somewhere between cornu and fimbriae. The word *reanastomosis* is generally wrongly employed and should be reserved for repeat attempts at joining the tubes, after failed surgical reconstruction.

An exploratory operation on the tube may also be indicated, the most common being conservative surgery for ectopic pregnancy. The most important of these procedures (apart from salpingectomy) is *salpingotomy*. This refers to incision in the tube wall and inspection of the lumen, usually with evacuation of its contents. This is a better procedure for eccyesis than expressing the tubal contents through the fimbrial ostium, as it causes less mucosal damage and the implantation site can be resected if necessary.

Microsurgery is also valuable for operations on the ovary, uterus, and supporting structures when the tubes are intrinsically healthy. In these cases there may be adhesions around the ovaries, ovarian cysts, ovarian or peritoneal endometriosis, or uterine disease such as fibromyomata or adenomyosis. Many of these procedures do not require the use of a microscope, and application of microsurgical principles is usually sufficient.

INSTRUMENTS

Methods of Magnification

A decision has to be made whether to use a microscope or loupes (magnifying spectacles). The advantages of a proper operating microscope are really overwhelming. For certain procedures, particularly cornual surgery, a microscope is essential; loupes do not give sufficient magnification. Loupes may be an advantage for simple ovarian surgery when low magnification is helpful.

The Operating Microscope

The operating microscope should give variable magnification and high optical resolution; good, preferably coaxial, illumination is also necessary. Most modern microscopes are reasonably adequate in these respects. A major decision is whether to buy a single or two-operator microscope (diploscope). Diploscopes give the surgical assistant a stereoscopic view of the same field as the first surgeon, but are more cumbersome. This disadvantage may outweigh the advantages; but if surgical training is to be an important part of the unit's work, a diploscope is invaluable. Several types of microscopes are available.

Manually Operated Single-Operator Microscope. These microscopes are by Carl Zeiss (West Germany), Wild (Switzerland), Applied Fibroptics (Randolph, MA) and Olympus (Japan) (Appendix 30–1). The best buys in this category are perhaps the Zeiss OPMI-1, or the rather overpriced Wild. The Applied Fibroptics machine is excellent but not mounted quite as rigidly as the two European ones. The advantages of manual microscopes (especially that of Zeiss) are that they are easily moved in and out of the operating field, are very robust and not given to tremor, are quick to use, and are relatively cheap. Little can go wrong, as they can be focused even if there is a total power failure. I prefer a simple hand-operated microscope for most routine surgery. Their main disadvantage is that the surgeon's hands must be removed from the operative field to make adjustments. This can lead to inadvertent contamination of the operative field unless care is taken. It is also difficult to attach cameras, assistant's viewing arms, and other accessories to most manual microscopes without causing loss of stability.

Electrically Controlled Single-Operator Microscope. Perhaps the best microscope of this sort is the Zeiss OPMI-6, although Wild produces one that is in many respects its equal. Most electrically driven microscopes are controlled remotely by either a foot pedal or by switches on the microscope body. They allow the surgeon to change magnification without removing the hands from the surgical field; most of them also have electrically controlled focusing as well. The great advantage of these microscopes is that there is less risk of wound contamination. I am not convinced that they make surgery much faster, although this is widely claimed. It is far easier to take good photographs through an electrically driven microscope, and if closed-circuit videophotography is envisaged, these machines are almost indispensable. However, they are bulkier and more cumbersome than manual microscopes. The microscope body tends also to be longer so that the working distance may be less (there is a risk that a long surgical instrument may momentarily touch the microscope). The biggest disadvantage is that most of these microscopes cannot usually be focused or adjusted in case of power failure or if the switching gear fails. Switch failure is not uncommon. Switches in foot pedals are particularly vulnerable and tend to collect dirt or get damp. These microscopes are also more expensive.

Diploscope. Diploscopes are all electrically controlled by foot pedal. The most successful are made by Zeiss, the OPMI-7 and the OPMI-6D. The surgeon and assistant can sit opposite each other and view the same field stereoscopically. This is helpful for teaching and if an active assistant is required to cut sutures or take some of the strain of operating. The disadvantage is that these machines are all large. Moreover, the height of one set of binoculars is often most comfortable for one surgeon when the height of the eyepiece opposite leads to the other surgeon being very uncomfortable. Because all these microscopes are vertically mounted, lateral tilt is limited and none of them is as mobile as a single-operator microscope. For two people to have the same field of view, a beam splitter must be employed. This means that the available light is halved. This may be a problem if closed-circuit television or photography is being used, as yet another beam splitter is needed, which can lead to quite dim images and rather poor visual acuity.

Whatever microscope is used, it is important that it has certain accessories:

1. An objective of a focal length between 200 and 300 mm. Lenses with a shorter focal length give greater magnification. If the focal length is too short there is a risk of instruments being contaminated. Lenses with longer focal length give weaker illumination.
2. Low-power eyepieces. Usually × 10 eyepieces are best.
3. An extension to the carriage arm. This allows the microscope stand to be well away from the microscope body, which gives better access to the pelvis. An alternative is to have a ceiling-mounted microscope, but this is costly to install. The Zeiss range are probably the best buys. They have interchangeable accessories but are rather expensive. The Wild microscopes give rather better

illumination and a very flat field of view but are bigger and clumsy to use.

Features of Loupes

Loupes are magnifying eyeglasses that are attached to a headband or a pair of spectacles. Many people regard loupes as an alternative to the microscope. They should be used rather as an adjunct, when the higher magnifications offered by a microscope are a disadvantage. Loupes are ideal for ovarian cysts, endometriosis, and adhesiolysis, especially in preparing the pelvis for IVF. They give inadequate magnification for most tubal surgery, such as anastomosis or salpingostomy. Loupes are portable and relatively cheap, costing perhaps $400 to about $1,850 depending on the degree of sophistication. They are easy to learn to use as they have a fixed focus and magnification. They also give a wider field of view than some low-power microscopes, and this is a considerable help when working in a badly distorted pelvis.

Loupes have disadvantages. Their optical resolution is not as good as that of the microscope. They do not provide direct coaxial illumination, so the image is rather dim. This can make identification of pathologic tissue impossible. Alternatively, the surgeon can wear a powerful headlamp, but this can be ungainly and uncomfortable for long periods of time. High-power loupes magnify up to × 8 but are very difficult to use. Because loupes have a fixed focal length, the surgeon has to keep his or her head static, which is tiring. Moreover, the telescopic lenses themselves tend to obscure normal vision, and this can be infuriating.

In spite of these various shortcomings, loupes are useful if they are employed for the most appropriate procedures. The cheapest good loupes are manufactured by Keeler of London. Better, lighter ones are made by Carl Zeiss and by Designs for Vision. Designs for Vision also manufactures a headband to which can be fixed a fiberoptic light. I personally find these restricting and uncomfortable. These companies can make a pair of loupes that is permanently fixed to spectacles with lenses according to prescription, if needed. It is wise to buy a pair with no more than about × 4.5 magnification. An ideal focal length for most people is about 28 to 34 cm.

Diathermy

It may seem strange to emphasize diathermy, but this is a crucial instrument. Fine electrosurgery has proved to be one of the most important innovations in infertility surgery. Diathermy dissection of pelvic tissues and adhesions gives very clean results and can be largely bloodless. There is no doubt that it is greatly superior to cutting with sharp instruments or blunt dissection. Various authors have tried other instruments, such as the CO_2 laser, but microsurgical diathermy is definitely better (and cheaper). In spite of some rather exaggerated claims, there really is not the slightest evidence that laser surgery gives superior anatomic or clinical results to diathermy. It is essential that the right diathermy instrument is used, however. Conventional units cause a great deal of tissue damage, and an instrument that gives a very weak output is mandatory.

A suitable unit must generate both cutting and coagulation currents, and it is sometimes useful if there is a facility for blended diathermy. Cutting diathermy should be unipolar, through a fine needle used for dissection. As little as 4 to 5 W power is often all that is necessary or desirable. A unit with added bipolar coagulation is also useful for dealing with larger blood vessels during cornual surgery.

Several good instruments are available. The Valleylab Surgistat is cheapest and is adequate, though unsophisticated. The blend facility is limited and there is no bipolar outlet. Nonetheless, it is possible to achieve high-quality surgery with this machine that costs only about $1,000. Valleylab also makes excellent and more sophisticated instruments having a full range of facilities at a price. Martins of West Germany also makes a satisfactory machine, although I have found a certain amount of charring with the cutting output. The best machine, which is also very expensive (currently about $4,000), is made by Bard. This is perhaps the best microsurgical diathermy instrument made so far and has the advantage (like the more expensive Valleylab machines) that its output can be increased for conventional surgical requirements so that over 300 W can be delivered.

Although laser surgery has the reputation of being very valuable, hemostasis is better with fine diathermy and dissipation of the burn is minimal. Diathermy is much quicker to use, and the clinical results that have been published are equal to or better than those achieved with lasers. The most expensive microsurgical diathermy costs less than one tenth of the cost of a laser, and the running costs are only those required to replace the hand switch and the electrode needles periodically.

Microsurgical Instruments

Instruments for microsurgery must be of high quality and simple. Stainless steel is preferable, although titanium is in vogue at present. Steel is easier to repair if an instrument is damaged, and is far less costly. The lightness of titanium may also be a disadvantage, as many surgeons prefer some feeling of weight in the hand. Even the smallest instruments should be at least 10 cm in length. The following are essential instruments.

1. A minimum of two pairs of straight forceps are needed. One pair at least should be 18 cm long for dissection in deeper places. One pair should have a platform at the tip to grasp fine suture material easily. In addition, one pair of fine-toothed forceps is required to get hold of fibrous tissue when performing cornual surgery or when operating on the ovarian capsule.

2. Two pairs of scissors are needed, one of which should have curved blades. The best length is about 18 cm. Microsurgical scissors must be able to cut along the length of their blades. It is very important that the blades close with using uniform pressure, or fine dissection will be impossible.

3. One fine pair of microsurgical needleholders is required and should be reserved only for microsurgical needles; that is, needles less than 150 μm in diameter (a fine 6-0 needle). If bigger needles are grasped the blades will deform, and they will not hold fine sutures during knotting. Needleholders with a round grip are easier to use for long periods without getting cramped fingers. A second microvascular needleholder is also needed for large 6-0 or 4-0 needles, and this can be used with the naked eye only.

4. Fine metal probes are useful during anastomosis. Beginners will find that splinting helps to approximate cut tubal ends, although splints should not be left in the tube after surgery. Much thicker probes, made of Teflon, plastic, or glass, are useful for handling tissues and supporting them during dissection. They reduce abrasion or trauma that would be caused by handling with gloved fingers.

   A set of fine lachrimal probes may be used to dilate the narrowed intramural tube. If the isthmic segment requires probing, for example, to introduce a splint, the probe should be no thicker than 0.5 mm in diameter, otherwise there is a risk of damaging the tube. An ideal probe is made by Spingler-Tritt (S & T; see below). They also manufacture one for the ampullary end of the tube that is introduced through the fimbrial end.

5. A silicone operating pad, available from S & T, can be slid into the pouch of Douglas over a damp swab to support the uterus and appendages. It keeps the appendages in a fixed plane under the microscope. The pad should be a neutral color and should not cause glare.

6. Small tubal clamps may occasionally be a slight help during anastomosis. They should compress the cut tubal end circumferentially without damaging it. They are hemostatic and aid identification of the tissues during suturing.

7. A standard cervical clamp is the Shirodkar pattern, which is applied over the uterine fundus. It is rather bulky and tends to get in the way; a

similar alternative is the Buxton clamp. A different pattern is the clamp designed by Winston, which is usually applied laterally across the supravaginal cervix, compressing the uterine blood vessels. It greatly aids hemostasis during cornual surgery, and helps elevate and steady the uterus from behind without getting in the surgeon's way.

8. The best retractor has four blades. The biggest exposure is gained with a modified Kirschner retractor, which compresses the wound edge very effectively, maintaining hemostasis. This is better than the O'Connor–O'Sullivan pattern more commonly used by gynecologists. It can be obtained from Down's Surgical.

   The Steridrape with a 5-inch plastic ring (3M's catalog no. 1074) can be inserted inside the wound at the start of laparotomy. It prevents leakage of blood into the abdominal cavity from the wound edge, and keeps the peritoneal edge moist and free from trauma. It reduces the risk of serious peritoneal abdominal wall adhesions after surgery.

9. To ensure a clean cut across the tube prior to anastomosis, we find two cheap additions to the surgical set-up particularly useful. The first is the Thatcher, a small, hand-held tubal clamp that compresses the tube during transection. It contains an integral groove into which a fine blade (or Denis) is inserted. In a quick guillotine action the blade is pushed down the groove, and a very clean cut results. This facilitates anastomosis. A full description of these instruments is in the S & T catalog.

10. Nonabsorbable suture is preferable for fine work, such as 8-0 nylon on a thin 3/8 needle. The needle should be about 140 μm diameter. The most suitable is made by S & T; Ethicon and Davis & Geck make satisfactory alternatives, although their needles may be somewhat thicker and less well fixed onto the thread. Thicker sutures of polypropylene amide (Prolene) are also needed. This material is ideal because of its lack of tissue reaction. The 6-0 or 4-0 Prolene made by Ethicon on different needle sizes is suitable.

SURGICAL PRINCIPLES

Adhesion formation and excessive scarring are risks of pelvic surgery. Both adhesions and scar tissue tend to be extremely fibrous after surgical intervention unless great care has been taken to avoid wanton damage. Not only will clumsy surgery tend to make matters worse, but iatrogenic surgical damage leads to thick adhesions around the ovaries; this may not only lead to failure of tuboplasty but also to poor

ovarian function. Molloy and associates[15] clearly demonstrated that once the ovaries are incarcerated, the response to superovulation is much less satisfactory and IVF is less likely to succeed. It is therefore mandatory that great care be taken to ensure restoration and preservation of pelvic anatomy. Good tubal surgery requires not only the use of magnification, but also sound judgment and meticulous dissection.

Microsurgery is designed to reconstruct tissues in the best possible anatomic relationship. This requires knowledge of tubal physiology and anatomy as well as an understanding of pathology, particularly the pathology of pelvic inflammatory disease. It simply is not enough to think of tubal disease in terms of blockage. Merely unblocking the tubes does not produce good surgical results. The important principles are as follows.

1. Inadequate surgical exposure leads to unnecessary trauma because of the need to grasp tissues to pull them into view.
2. Excessive bleeding prevents the surgeon obtaining a good view of what he is going. Persistent blood clot and fibrin lead to adhesion formation after abdominal closure.
3. Irrigation with isotonic fluids, such as Ringer's lactate, keeps tissues moist and free of clot. Dry tissue is easily traumatized.
4. Raw areas, bruising, and necrotic tissue all can lead to adhesion formation or fibrosis. Avoid causing unnecessary peritoneal damage.
5. Some authors claim that deperitonealized areas will heal spontaneously, but there is good evidence from laparoscopic examinations performed after microsurgery that the fewer raw areas, the better. It is true that the abdominal peritoneum can be left unsutured after major abdominal surgery; most patients do not suffer serious consequences such as bowel obstruction. Nevertheless, check laparoscopy clearly shows that healing is more predictable with thorough peritoneal closure.
6. Nonabsorbable suture should be used. Absorbable sutures are gradually broken down by a process of rotting, which can lead to excessive fibrosis.
7. It is important to take as much care over closing the abdominal peritoneum as any other part of the procedure. It is worth everting cut peritoneal edges using a mattress suture. Relatively thin suture material should be employed.
8. Infection is a real hazard because it encourages poor healing, adhesion formation, and fibrosis. Care should be taken not to lengthen procedures unduly. Antibiotic cover should be considered if surgery has taken longer than usual. Never operate if there is any suspicion of active inflammatory disease; this must be treated first.

ABDOMINAL INCISION

Although a midline incision used to be favored by many tubal surgeons, perfectly adequate exposure can be achieved with a transverse suprapubic incision. This heals better and looks more sightly, important considerations in young women. Although the Pfannenstiel is the most popular transverse incision, it may not give really adequate exposure in all women unless it is extended laterally or unless the rectus muscles are at least partly transected. This is particularly the case in patients who have previously had a laparotomy performed through a Pfannenstiel approach. In these circumstances, I now sometimes prefer a modified Czerny incision, particularly in women who have already had a Pfannenstiel incision that is very scarred. This involves dissecting between the rectus sheath and rectus muscle down to the pubis (there is no need to dissect above the line of incision). The rectus muscle is now resected from the back of the pubis and reflected upward. Once the fundus of the bladder has been exposed, the peritoneal cavity can be entered through a transverse incision. The advantage of this approach is that it is bloodless, particularly if diathermy is employed. If especially wide exposure is required, the recurrent epigastric vessels can be ligated.

Careful closure of the abdominal incision is very important. When closing the abdominal peritoneum, a good surgeon will ensure that the cut edge of the peritoneum is everted with a mattress stitch, so that no raw area is presented to the abdominal contents. This is an effective method for preventing omental and bowel adhesions. Once the peritoneal cavity is closed, it is wise to use interrupted sutures to repair the rectus sheath. Full relaxation of the patient is essential until this part of the operation is accomplished, and there must be a good understanding between surgeon and anesthetist.

PRINCIPLES OF ADHESIOLYSIS

There is an increasing vogue for avoiding laparotomy in women with peritubal adhesions. Indeed, many patients with relatively limited avascular adhesions are particularly suitable for adhesiolysis done under laparoscopic control.[16] Many surgeons use the laser for this but I have had excellent results using "cold" instruments only. Appropriate instruments, designed by Semm, are available through Storz of West Germany.

A full description of the approach is beyond the scope of this chapter. When adhesions are very extensive, an open approach is generally preferred. Although salpingolysis and oophorolysis are the simplest microsurgical procedures, considerable dam-

age can result if they are done badly. Like all tubal surgery, the first operation has the best chance of success. The main principles, which are equally relevant to virtually all tubal surgery, include the following.

1. Whenever possible avoid picking up tissues with the fingers. Never grasp any peritoneal surface with crushing instruments.
2. Use a glass or plastic probe to dissect adhesions. Adhesions are best elevated on the tip of the probe and then divided using fine diathermy.
3. It is usually best to leave adhesions slightly long on the tubal serosa, so as not to leave a raw area. They can always be trimmed once division is completed; cut adhesions tend to roll back on themselves, making further resection unnecessary.
4. Usually try to suture raw serosa on the tube with 8-0 nylon. The ovarian capsule usually requires a slightly thicker suture, such as 6-0 Prolene.
5. Secure a good relationship betwen the fimbriae and the ovary. This may necessitate vigorous dissection between the end of the tube and the ovary, particularly if there are fibrous adhesions in this region. The fimbrial blood supply must not be damaged; scissors may be safer for this part of the operation than diathermy. Raw areas on the ovarian capsule should be excised and sutured once the tube is free.
6. Periovarian adhesions frequently produce fibrous scar tissue between the ovary and the lateral pelvic wall (the ovarian fossa). Quite vigorous dissection is usually required, and it is often necessary to create a large raw area before the ovary can be freed. One should not be nervous about this, provided that the ureter has been carefully identified. Raw peritoneum can be sutured vertically using 4-0 Prolene to cover the lateral pelvic wall. The raw ovarian surface can be excised before carefully suturing the capsule.
7. Adhesions in the pouch of Douglas should be removed if possible. This seems to improve the chance of an egg being picked up from the pouch.
8. It is a mistake to divide adhesions that do not appear to be interfering with tubal mobility or egg pickup. Extra dissection carries extra risk of recurrent adhesion formation.
9. Ventrosuspension, or shortening of the round ligaments, is generally unnecessary and may cause problems. It is best reserved for those cases where there is a high risk of dyspareunia after operation.
10. Steroids seem to be the most effective adjunctive treatment. An insoluble suspension of hydrocortisone acetate (1.0 to 1.5 L) can be left in the pelvis before the peritoneum is closed. Our

impression is that steroids are much more effective than hydroflotation or dextran in preventing recurrent adhesion formation.

SALPINGOSTOMY

It has been suggested that salpingostomy has been made redundant by in-vitro fertilization. This is not the case; provided patients are selected carefully, good results—certainly better than those currently reported with IVF in nearly all units—can be achieved, and about half those conceiving will have a second spontaneous conception and live birth (Fig. 30–1). If the tubes are thin walled, with little muscle fibrosis and reasonable mucosa, over one third of patients will achieve a live birth afterward.[17] This compares extremely favorably with the results achieved by IVF. In Britain, the report of the IVF Voluntary Licensing Authority[18] showed that only 8.5% of IVF treatment cycles ended with a live birth. Moreover IVF is complex, expensive, and emotionally demanding, and when it fails it leaves no increased chance of a successful conception afterward. Consequently, in our unit a combination of both treatment by surgery and later IVF, only if necessary, has proved a very satisfactory strategy. We no longer generally offer salpingostomy to women with severely fibrotic tubes or who have are very severe adhesions; unfortunately, only a minor proportion of our patients with hydrosalpinges have tubes that are not severely damaged (Fig. 30–2).

Salpingostomy is technically more difficult than is sometimes supposed. Although it is quite easy to open a closed ampulla, experience is needed if a functional tube is to be obtained. Generally, the best instrument for actual incision in the tube is the fine needle-point diathermy, which should be used at just sufficient intensity to allow cutting without charring. Once the tube is opened, a very few sutures—preferably of 8-0 nylon—are all that is needed to keep the margin of the tube everted. If the walls are fibrotic or hypertrophied (but the patient does not wish to have IVF) a somewhat thicker suture (such as 6-0) may be required. Very often, if the salpingostomy has been made properly, the tubal end everts itself and suturing is unnecessary.

The principles of salpingostomy are as follows. First, the anatomic relationship between the ampulla and the ovary must be restored before opening the tube. This requires identification of the ovarian end of the mesosalpinx and careful dissection so as not to damage the tubal blood supply. Once this has been achieved, the tube should be opened at its most terminal part. Usually a fibrous line can be clearly seen at this point, very often where little blood vessels run radially away from a so-called pucker point. Any incision made elsewhere is an incision in the wall of the tube and not where the fimbrial end was originally; it may heal spontaneously so that the tube may become blocked again within a few weeks.

When opening the tube, one should try to avoid cutting across any residual mucosal folds. Transection of the epithelial folds may damage the blood

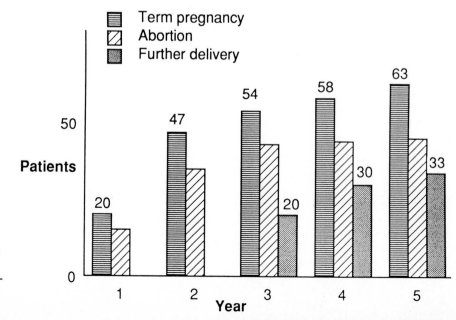

Figure 30–1. Follow-up results in 274 cases of primary microsurgical salpingostomy at Hammersmith Hospital 1971–1981: 63 women had at least 1 live infant (24%), and 33 of these women have had between 2 and 5 term deliveries of singleton pregnancies. Abortion rate is 16% in those followed.

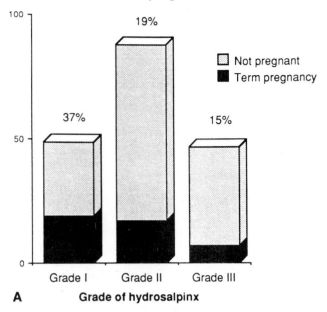

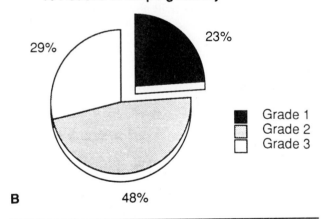

Figure 30–2. Grade of pathology in 184 patients with complete hydrosalpinges undergoing salpingostomy. Classification according to Boer-Meisl et al.[17] **A.** Just over one third of patients with grade I disease gave birth. **B.** Only 23% of Hammersmith patients have grade I disease.

supply. Moreover, as egg transport is likely to be mediated by interaction of two ciliated epithelial folds, the integrity of these folds may be an important factor in the success of surgery. Adhesions between mucosal folds should be deliberately divided. Eversion of the tubal mucosa should be continued just enough until there is a stable ostium. Too much eversion may devitalize the fimbrial lip by reducing venous drainage. The reconstructed ostium should be positioned so that it is capable of movement over the whole ovarian surface.

During salpingostomy (or fimbrioplasty) a few other points should be borne in mind:

1. Tubal tissue should not be resected unless it is obviously redundant. It is common to find that involution of even very large and "floppy" hydrosalpinges occurs after salpingostomy.
2. The fimbria ovarica should be reconstructed whenever possible. It may be an important channel of communication between the tube and ovary.
3. It is very easy to cause inadvertent damage to the ampullary blood supply in the region of the fimbria ovarica. Fimbrial vessels must be identified before dissecting or suturing in this region.
4. All raw areas near the newly constructed fimbria should be carefully repaired, usually with 8-0 nylon. It may even be necessary to place a free peritoneal graft in this region if dissection was extensive.
5. Maximize the amount of the surface area of the ovary available for ovulation. Good fimbrial surgery also usually means ovarian surgery.

CORNUAL ANASTOMOSIS

When simple cornual block is present, there is no doubt that the preferred treatment is by surgery, rather than by IVF. Cornual anastomosis[19] after inflammation is highly successful. When the ampulla is undamaged, between 50 and 60% of patients have a live birth (Fig. 30–3). The results are not nearly as good when the cornua are very expanded, fibrotic, and nodular, and are poor in most cases associated with fimbrial occlusion or severe ampullary adhesions. For these patients we offer IVF as the first line of treatment.

A microscope is essential for all cornual surgery because of the small diameter of the lumen in this region. The surgery can be very demanding indeed, particularly if there is much fibrosis in the uterine muscle or considerable nodularity and expansion of the cornu, or if the block is deep in the myometrium. If the whole isthmus is diseased and needs excision, the surgeon has the difficult job of joining two segments of tube with widely disparate luminal sizes. Very often the choice between surgery and IVF is predicated on the skills or interests of the team delivering treatment.

It is often more comfortable to perform cornual surgery sitting down. This is because quite high magnification is needed and the hands are steadier when operating in a seated position with the forearm supported. The surgeon should operate on the side of the table corresponding to the tube being repaired, changing sides when one anastomosis is finished. The first stage is to free the tubes from adhesions.

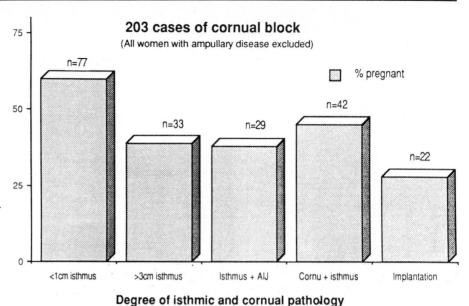

Figure 30–3. The results of microsurgical treatment of cornual block. In this personal series, all patients with ampullary lesions or major ovarian adhesions were excluded. The type of pathology (e.g., salpingitis isthmica nodosa, congenital block, adenomyosis) did not matter as much as the amount of tube that was involved in the pathologic process.

The cervix is now secured from above using a Shirodkar or Winston clamp. The Winston clamp is preferable because bleeding is controlled by the clamp's position across the uterine arteries. Dye should now be injected, preferably transfundally, using a 19-gauge needle attached to a plastic tube and a 20-mL syringe. This confirms that the cornua are blocked; they expand under the pressure of the dye in the uterine cavity, which helps dissection of the interstitial portion.

Once the microscope is in place, the isthmic portion of the tube is dissected from the cornu. Using magnification, the isthmic portion is inspected and all blocked or pathologic tissue carefully resected. The vascular arcades in the mesosalpinx should not be damaged unless this is unavoidable. The subtubal artery bleeds vigorously when cut across and can be controlled with diathermy or possibly a tubal clamp. If diathermy is used to make the initial cut, this should be "freshened up" with a fine scalpel blade so that no charred, compromised tissue is included in the anastomosis.

Diseased tissue is now sliced away from the cornu. It is important to remove it all and thus avoid risk of reocclusion. Mere patency is insufficient. The signs that all diseased tissue have been removed are 4 or 5 mucosal folds visible in the cornual lumen, no mucosal polyps visible, or any hypertrophied mucosa; fine blood vessels running in the epithelium close to its cut edge; the circular muscle coat showing regular striations around the tube; resection of all white, gritty, fibrous tissues; no extravasation of dye on transfundal dye injection; and no diverticulae present.

Care must be taken not to denude peritoneum by making the cornual incision too broad. Dithermy is extremely helpful to control bleeding, and an injection of oxytocin, 20 IU, will also reduce bleeding.

The block may be deep in the myometrium and access to the patent interstitial portion difficult. Under these circumstances it may be very helpful to open up the cornu. A vertical incision can be made for about 2 cm above the cornu toward the midline of the uterine fundus. This will be sutured at the end of the procedure in an inverted Y. If access is still a problem, two stay sutures of 6-0 Prolene can be placed behind and in front of the interstitial portion to hold the edges of the incision apart.

Once all pathologic tissue has been removed and interstitial patency to dye has been established, repair can commence. Beginners may find it easy to perform the anastomosis over a polyethylene splint. Certainly this helps to get rough approximation of the cut ends. A stay suture of 6-0 Prolene placed in the mesosalpinx just beneath the tube will relieve tension between the two cut ends. It is helpful to depress the uterus toward the side being operated while tying this suture, as this also relieves tension.

Once the cut ends are roughly approximated, the fine cardinal sutures can be placed. The first anastomotic suture layer should join the circular muscle coat, and these sutures should be placed as close to the mucosa as possible without actually entering the lumen of the tube. Usually 4 or 5 sutures are all that are required, the first to place being that at the base of the anastomosis at the six o'clock position. Wherever possible, 8-0 nylon should be used; sometimes there is too much tension for such fine needlework and 7-0 or 6-0 Prolene is required. It is a matter of preference whether these sutures should be tied as they are placed or all tied at the end. If the anastomosis is deep, it may be easier to tie them when they are all in position.

At this stage it is wise to test the join. The splint in the tube should be pulled out through the fimbriae and dye injected into the uterus with the cervix still clamped. The tube should be patent, and retrograde spill should occur without much leakage at the join. If there is excessive leakage or if the anastomosis is not patent, the sutures should be unpicked and a fresh start made. Once the surgeon is satisfied that the join is functional, a second anastomotic layer can be placed. This layer should take the longitudinal muscle coat together with a bite of serosa. If the anastomosis is very deep in the myometrium and stay sutures have been employed, these should be removed. It may also be necessary to remove a little of the peritoneum from the isthmic end of the tube, so that peritoneum is not buried in the join. The second layer of sutures can be continuous or interrupted; the aim is to give some strength to the join without kinking it—at the conclusion of the second layer, there should be no raw surfaces. If an inverted Y incision has been made, it can be closed at this stage and dye injected once again to confirm patency.

Healing is usually good after this surgical procedure. The cornu is quite strong enough to maintain a growing pregnancy, and rupture is unknown in my experience of over 200 cases. Consequently, cesarean section is usually not indicated. Adequate follow-up is important. Although it is considered unnecessary to perform hysterosalpingogram on patients after cornual surgery, a second-look laparoscopy should certainly be undertaken if conception has not occurred after a year. It seems that rather a high proportion of pregnancies miscarry after cornual anastomosis; the reason for this is unclear. Because reocclusion after pregnancy is not uncommon, it is important that these patients should have broad-spectrum antibiotic cover in the event of a threatened miscarriage.

There can be no doubt that cornual surgery is highly technical, and from time to time taxes the skill and patience of the most experienced surgeon. This is particularly so when the cornu has not been inflamed, but there is adenomyosis or cornual endometriosis. In such patients we occasionally defer tubal surgery, particularly in younger women. In a handful of patients whose laparoscopy showed bilateral cornual block but who had no macroscopic or historic evidence of infection or a congenital lesion, we have considered medical treatment worth trying. To be sure that a block is indeed present in both tubes, we invariably check this by hysterosalpingography. In 32 women we then administered danazol, usually 400 to 600 mg orally for 2 months. At the end of this period, hysterosalpingography was repeated. If this showed evidence that the block was improving, danazol was continued for an additional 3 months. If there was no change, medical treatment was regarded as unlikely to succeed, and the patient was offered tubal surgery. The pregnancy rate after 5 months of continuous danazol is recorded in Figure 30-4.

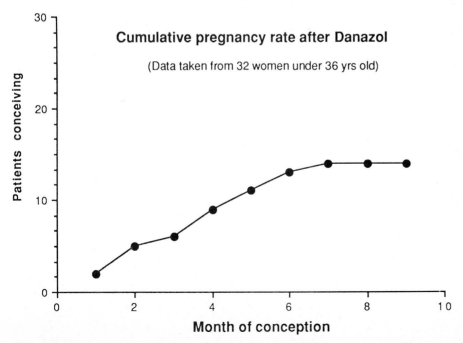

Figure 30–4. Cumulative pregnancy rate after danazol treatment in patients with (mostly deep) bilateral cornual block and presumed endometriosis. The mean length of infertility was 4.4 years.

TUBAL IMPLANTATION

On some occasions cornual anastomosis is impossible, most commonly when dense fibrosis in the cornual muscle extends throughout the full thickness of the myometrium. On rarer occasions, when there is a congenital abnormality, for example, there may simply be no intramural tube present. Very infrequently the uterus may be small and immobile and well down in a deep pelvis. In such cases cornual anastomosis may be impracticable. For these patients, tubal implantation may have to be considered.

Various methods of implanting the fallopian tube have been described. All have the disadvantage that the uterine wall is somewhat weakened and that tubal patency is difficult to guarantee. Two basic approaches are widely used. The first involves reaming or boring out the diseased intramural area and then introducing the cleaned transected stump of the tube through this hole. The second approach involves cutting a wedge of tissue from the uterine cornu with a knife or diathermy and then laying the cut tubal end in the defect; it is usual to suture the cut periphery of the tube onto the endometrial surface if possible. A microscope may be used for this in an attempt to achieve more accurate apposition of the mucosal surfaces. Another method of implantation involves transecting right through the uterine fundus from cornu to cornu, but this is done only rarely because of the substantial damage caused to the uterus. Now that IVF is widely available, it is important to consider that whichever method of implantation is done, the uterine cavity and muscle are disrupted as little as possible. Excessive distortion and scarring of the cavity may reduce the chances of subsequent embryo transfer being successful.

Of the implantation methods using a reamer, I find that described by Janacek (personal communication, 1982) best. We have used it with modest results in women with congenital uterine disease where the cornu is damaged. In a small personal series of 17 patients, 7 (41%) delivered a term or premature viable baby.

The Janacek method of implantation involves dividing the tube cleanly, close to the cornu. Bleeding vessels running under the tube and in the cornual mesentery may require treatment with diathermy. Once there is reasonable hemostasis, a suitably sized Janacek reamer is selected and attached to a 20-mL syringe. For most operations, the largest-diameter reamer is best (5 mm), although if the uterus is very small, it may be an advantage to try a smaller one. The reamer is pushed through the uterine wall in the region of the cornu until less resistance is encountered. Once the uterine cavity is entered, firm suction is applied to the syringe and redundant cornual tissue is aspirated well into the lumen of the reamer. The reamer is removed and the core of tissue ejected into a bottle of formalin for histologic examination. The cut end of tube is then prepared for implantation. Because better long-term patency is obtained when the lumen at the cut end is reasonably large, I tend to resect a good length of the isthmus (if not all of it), even if this segment is not obviously diseased. Subtubal vessels are again treated with bipolar diathermy, and a rim of the peritoneal coat is removed from the last 0.5 cm of the part of the tube to be implanted. The lateral margins of the cut end of tube are now secured with two 4-0 doubled-ended Prolene sutures, one at the 3 o'clock and one at the 9 o'clock position. A 5-mm glass rod is inserted into the cornual defect. This acts as a guide to ensure that the suture needles are placed right into the uterine cavity while anchoring the tube. The two 4-0 needles from each suture are passed into the uterine cavity and out through the uterine wall. One should be passed through the anterior, and one through the posterior wall. They are then tied over the uterine serosa. As the tension is taken up, the cut end of the tube will slide into the reamed hole and into the cavity. The final stage is to suture serosa of tube to uterine serosa; for this I prefer 6-0 Prolene.

I am uncertain whether or not cesarean section is really required after this procedure. At least 3 patients under our care have achieved a vaginal term delivery.

Implantation through a cornual wedge has the advantage that the join between the cut end of the tube and the edge of the endometrium can be seen during the procedure. Indeed, magnification can be used and, theoretically at least, approximation of the tissues should be more accurate. The cervix should be taken in a Winston clamp to control bleeding, and syntocinon, 20 U, or pitressin may be injected. Once the tube is resected from the cornu, a wedge is removed through an inverted Y incision. Stay sutures of 6-0 Prolene may be used to hold the cornual myometrium apart; alternatively, an ophthalmic lachrimal retractor of the self-retaining type may be helpful. Once the cut end of the tube has been carefully prepared it can be laid into the wedge and the cut edge sutured to the endometrium and basal layers. It may be helpful to fishtail its end slightly first so as to expose more mucosal surface. A satisfactory suture for all layers of this joint is 6-0 Prolene on an 8-mm needle.

Some authors advocate using a splint during this procedure, but this does not seem to make much difference to subsequent success. Approximately 75% of implanted tubes have remained patent after this procedure, but in my experience, only about one third of patients have achieved a pregnancy.

REVERSAL OF STERILIZATION

Reversal of female sterilization is usually the most straightforward of all tubal operations. Most of these patients, of course, are of proved fertility so it is hardly surprising that these operations are relatively very successful when done carefully. They are easiest when the ampulla is completely preserved, and isthmic–isthmic anastomosis is the most satisfactory procedure. Many of these patients are relatively old by the time they request reversal surgery, and age undoubtedly is major factor in failure. Figure 30–5 gives our global pregnancy rate in 480 reversal operations. Patients under age 35 years are very likely to conceive; with advancing years fertility declines sharply, and we have never seen any patient pregnant successfully when the operation has been conducted over age 43. The graph gives dramatic evidence of declining fertility and could serve as a model for many other procedures offered to the infertile woman, especially when one considers that this procedure is generally far more successful than nearly any other performed regularly for childlessness.

The principles and technique are very similar to those of cornual surgery, but more simple.[20] This is because access to both ends of the tube is easier and dissection into the muscular intramural portion of the cornu, which has many blood vessels, is seldom required. The preparation of the cut ends of the tube is a key factor in success, and it is mandatory to remove fibrotic and devitalized tube as far as possible if a good joint is to be obtained.

Even when the tubes are quite short, reversal can produce good results. Provided there is at least 4 to 5 cm of adhesion-free ampulla with healthy fimbrial mucosa, at least 50% of patients will conceive (Fig. 30–6). The length of residual isthmus seems relatively unimportant. The method of sterilization is not in itself important, although excessive diathermy can cause quite severe fibrosis, particularly in the region of the cornu.

Because the basic technique to reverse sterilization is very similar to that used for cornual anastomosis, a detailed description of the microsurgical procedure would be repetitive. Attention is confined in this chapter to methods for dealing with common problems.

Excessive Scarring of the Tubal Stumps

When the tubes have been ligated for more than about 5 years, the segment medial to the ligation often becomes dilated and the isthmic stumps become replaced by small, fibrous hydrosalpinges. Sometimes this dilation extends into the intramural

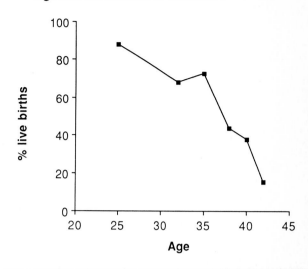

Age and the success of sterilization reversal

Figure 30–5. The relationship between the success of sterilization reversal by anastomosis and age of the patient. Only 15% of women between 41 and 42 years of age had a live birth.

portion of the tubes; quite often this may be associated with endometriotic changes in the medial tube,[21] possibly because endometrial fragments are regurgitated through an incompetent uterotubal junction repeatedly into the blind tube.

This can complicate tubal anastomosis because, unless all the fibrotic and scarred tubal tissue is removed, the joint may not allow ovum transport. Alternatively, an ectopic pregnancy may follow conception. Consequently, the microscope must be used to ensure that all fibrotic tubal tissue, especially that overlaid with flattened or avascular epithelium, is resected. Resection of the isthmus up to the dilated intramural segment may lead to the necessity of joining two segments of disparate luminal diameter, the narrower lumen being that on the lateral side of the anastomosis. This usually requires extra sutures in the inner layer to achieve a water-tight joint.

Joining Segments of Tubes of Widely Disparate Diameter

Some authors advocate artificially widening the mouth of the narrower segment of tube by fishtailing it. This is not very satisfactory. Others plicate the wide ampullary lumen, reducing its diameter with several circumferential sutures of 8-0 nylon. Prolapsed mucosal folds can be trimmed if they get between the cut edges of the tube.

For a better method,[21] a grooved, 1-mm probe (S & T catalog no. SG1) can be inserted through the fimbrial end of the tube toward the blind end of the ampulla. The tip of the probe, which is smooth and

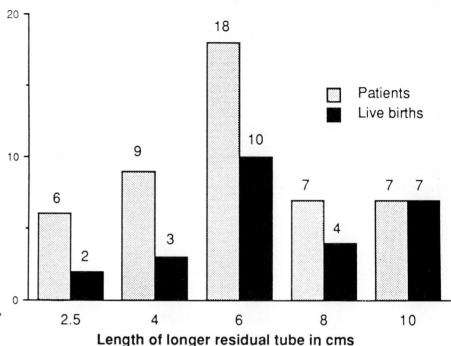

Figure 30–6. The length of the longer residual tube after anastomosis in 73 cases of reversal of sterilization. Over 50% of women will have a live birth if one tube is at least 5 cm in length.

bulbous, is gently pushed into the blind end stretching the tissue. The peritoneal coat of this segment is circumcised 4 to 5 mm from the tip of the tube and is then stripped from the muscle coat at this point. The very tip of the tube is then transected and the end of the probe advanced through this hole. This small incision leaves the diameter of the cut ampulla about that of the transected isthmic portion. The probe is advanced a little farther, a polyethylene splint is placed in the groove of the probe, and the probe is then withdrawn through the fimbriae. This movement cannulates the ampullary segment. The other end of the splint is then passed into the isthmus, and the anastomosis can be made over the splint without difficulty. Anastomosis is simple unless the ampullary side of the joint is very scarred.

PREPARATION OF THE OVARIES BEFORE IN-VITRO FERTILIZATION

One indication for surgery is the presence of many adhesions around the ovaries and so much damage of the tubes that reconstructive tuboplasty alone is unlikely to benefit the patient. Many of these women may be suitable for egg collection for IVF by ultrasonically guided follicular puncture. At the time of writing, however, this method seems less successful in some hands than laparoscopic egg collection.

Moreover, in spite of data suggesting that simple periovarian adhesions do not impair follicular development,[22] incarcerated ovaries[15] do not always respond well to superovulatory drugs, and surgical clearance may improve this. A comparatively high success rate has been achieved in some centers by preparing the pelvis for egg collection by preliminary oophorolysis.[23] This may be particularly indicated if the ovaries are cystic or damaged by old endometriosis, or if bowel is plastered firmly over the ovaries.

The principles of this surgery have been fully described[23] and include careful lysis of omental adhesions, often combined with partial omentectomy, elevation of the ovaries with wedge resection of raw areas of ovarian surface, repair of all raw peritoneal surfaces with Prolene sutures, free peritoneal grafting of the larger damaged peritoneal surfaces, and sometimes ventrosuspension of the uterus. Oophoropexy using 4-0 Prolene sutures to attach the ovaries to the cornu is also helpful in many cases, and in our experience seldom interferes with the view of the ovaries subsequently using ultrasound. Ultrasonic egg collection performed by the vaginal route may be difficult after oophoropexy, however. It is a moot point whether salpingectomy should also be undertaken. Even the most severely damaged tubes may work occasionally, and a surprising number of spontaneous pregnancies have been recorded after such "last-ditch" surgery when it was thought that IVF would be the only possible chance for pregnancy. Moreover, total salpingectomy may be bad psychologically for infertile patients and it does not guarantee freedom from ectopic pregnancy; eccyesis can still occur in the residual intramural portion of the tube after extracorporeal fertilization and embryo transfer.

SURGICAL MANAGEMENT OF ECTOPIC PREGNANCY

A full description of the management of tubal pregnancy is beyond the scope of this chapter. Interest in the use of laparoscopically guided aspiration of small ectopic pregnancies is increasing, and some authors claim excellent immediate results where there is tubal rupture, a pelvic hematoma, or both. Preservation of fertility is claimed to be surprisingly good after this approach, and most authors note no obvious increase in the frequency of recurrent ectopic pregnancy. More controlled data are needed, however, in particular information on the follow-up of patients after conservative surgery on the sole remaining fallopian tube (see below). Clearly, the presence of an apparently normal tube on the contralateral side gives follow-up data that are difficult to interpret. More recently still, some authors have attempted to treat tubal pregnancy in its early stages using vaginal or abdominal ultrasound to guide a needle to the pregnancy sac. Once the needle is in place, suitable material such as potassium chloride or methotrexate can be delivered to the sac in the hope of subsequent absorption of the pregnancy. These methods have obvious risks, and no long-term prognostic data are available.

Surgical management therefore remains the treatment of choice. Evidence suggests that milking an ectopic gestation through the fimbrial end increases tubal damage. This seems to give a high chance of a second ectopic pregnancy. We prefer to use a salpingotomy whenever possible. The antimesenteric border of the tube is excised over its expanded segment, and the pregnancy and blood clot are carefully removed. Bleeding can invariably be controlled with a few sutures of 4-0 or 5-0 Prolene in the region of the implantation site. A decision is then made whether to remove the implantation segment, ligate the tube, and leave the patient for subsequent tubal reconstruction, if she wishes. This approach has the advantage that the patient knows for certain that she will not risk another ectopic pregnancy in that tube. Alternatively, the salpingotomy incision can be repaired with a few interrupted sutures of 5-0 Prolene to restore immediate tubal continuity.

In general, we are not in favor of resecting the ectopic pregnancy with immediate anastomosis. This is difficult to do accurately with good tubal apposition

TABLE 30–1. LONG-TERM RESULTS OF OPEN CONSERVATIVE SURGERY FOR ECTOPIC PREGNANCY IN PATIENTS WITH ONLY ONE TUBE REMAINING

	Patients	Delivered	Recurrent Ectopic
Fimbrial expression	6	2	4 (66%)*,†
Salpingotomy	18	6 (33%)	7 (39%)*
Resection with later anastomosis	35	16 (46%)	6 (17%)†,‡,§

*One patient with repeated ectopic pregnancy.
†One patient with intrauterine and ectopic pregnancy.
‡Two patients with intrauterine and ectopic pregnancy.
§Three patients with more than one term pregnancy.

and cannot be discussed sensibly beforehand with the patient. Our results with conservative surgery for ectopic pregnancy are recorded in Table 30–1. A total of 69 patients with an eccyesis in their one remaining fallopian tube were operated since 1972. Microsurgical methods were used throughout but a microscope was only used for tubal anastomosis after the acute emergency, in most cases 6 to 24 months later. Tubal anastomosis was never done at the time of eccyesis. Although follow-up was somewhat incomplete, only 24 (35%) had documented term deliveries after open conservative surgery; 17 (25%) had at least one recurrent ectopic pregnancy. From these figures it appears that resection with subsequent anastomosis, although giving rather disappointing results, is superior to treating ectopic pregnancy conservatively with retention of the implantation site.

REFERENCES

1. Newton J, Craig S, Joyce D: The changing pattern of a comprehensive infertility clinic. *J Biosoc Sci* 6:477, 1974.
2. Raymont A, et al: Review of 500 cases of infertility. *Int J Fertil* 14:141, 1969.
3. Campbell GR, Roberts-Thomson K: Infertility in the Highlands. *Papua New Guinea Med J* 17(4):347, 1974.
4. Winston RML: Is microsurgery necessary for salpingostomy? *Aust NZ J Obstet Gynaecol* 21:143, 1981.
5. Walz W: Fertilitäts Operationen mit Hilfe eines Operationenmikroskopes. *Geburtshilf Gynakol* 153:49, 1959.
6. Swolin K: Electromicrosurgery and salpingostomy: Long-term results. *Am J Obstet Gynecol* 121:418, 1975.
7. Gomel V: Tubal anastomosis by microsurgery. *Fertil Steril* 28:59, 1977.
8. Gomel V: Salpingostomy by microsurgery. *Fertil Steril* 29:380, 1978.
9. Paterson P, Wood C: The use of microsurgery in the reanastomosis of the rabbit fallopian tube. *Fertil Steril* 25:757, 1974.
10. Winston RML, McClure Browne JC: Pregnancy following autograft transplantation of the fallopian tube and ovary in the rabbit. *Lancet* 2:494, 1974.
11. Siegler AM, Kontopoulos V: An analysis of macrosurgical and microsurgical techniques in the management of tubo-peritoneal factor in infertility. *Fertil Steril* 32:377, 1979.
12. Winston RML: Microsurgery of the fallopian tube: From fantasy to reality. *Fertil Steril* 34:521, 1980.
13. Bateman BG, Nunley WC, Kitchin JD: Surgical management of distal tubal obstruction—Are we making progress? *Fertil Steril* 48:523, 1987.
14. Vasquez G, Boeckx W, Winston RML, Brosens IA: Human tubal mucosa and reconstructive microsurgery, in Crosignani A, Rubin BL (eds): *Microsurgery in Female Infertility*. London, Academic Press, 1980, p 41.
15. Molloy D, Martin M, Speirs A, et al: Performance of patients with a frozen pelvis in an in vitro fertilization program. *Fertil Steril* 47:450, 1987.

16. Murphy AA: Operative laparoscopy. *Fertil Steril* 46:1, 1987.
17. Boer-Meisl ME, te Velde ER, Habbema JDF, Kardaun JWPF: Predicting the pregnancy outcome in patients treated for hydrosalpinx: A prospective study. *Fertil Steril* 45:23, 1986.
18. Voluntary Licensing Authority for Human In Vitro Fertilization and Embryology: *Third Annual Report.* London, VLA Secretariat, 1988.
19. Winston RML, Margara RA: Infertility surgery in the female, in Insler V, Lunenfeld B (eds): *Infertility: Male and Female.* London, Churchill Livingstone, 1986, pp 450–477.
20. Brosens I, Winston RML: *Reversibility of Female Sterilization.* London, Academic Press, 1978.

21. Vasquez G, Winston RML, Boeckx W, Brosens IA: Ultrastructural changes in the tube following sterilization. *Am J Obstet Gynecol* 138:86, 1980.
22. Diamond MP, Pellicer A, Boyers SP, DeCherney AH: The effect of periovarian adhesions on follicular development in patients undergoing ovarian stimulation for in vitro fertilization–embryo transfer. *Fertil Steril* 49:100, 1988.
23. Winston RML, Margara RA, Hillier SG: Technique and results of ovariolysis in preparation for in vitro fertilization. *Eur J Obstet Gynaecol* 18:381, 1984.

APPENDIX 30–1.
MANUFACTURERS OF
MICROSURGICAL EQUIPMENT

Applied Fiberoptics, Inc, c/o Codman and Shurtleff, Inc, Randolph, MA 02368, USA.

Bard Electro Medical Systems, Bard Ltd, Pennywell Industrial Estate, Sunderland, SR4 9EW, UK. Telex 537092.

Designs for Vision, Inc, 120 East 23rd Street, New York, NY 10010, USA.

Down's Surgical, Church Path, Mitcham, Surrey, CR4 3UE, UK. Telex 927045.

Keeler Instruments, 21–27 Marylebone Lane, London, W1M 6DS, UK. Telex 847565.

Olympus, Japan.

Spingler-Tritt (S & T), Surgical Needles and Instruments, Allmendweg 2, D-7893 Jestetten, Postfach 1104, West Germany.

Valleylab, Inc, PO Box 9015, Boulder, CO 80301, USA.

Wild Instruments, 48 Park Street, Lutton, LU1 3HPO, UK. Telex 825475.

Carl Zeiss (Oberkochen) Ltd, 31–36 Foley Street, London, W1P 8AP, UK. Telex 24300.

CHAPTER 31

The Role of the Laser

Augusto P. Chong

The Role of the Laser

Physical Principles	Ovarian Wedge
Practical Laser Physics	Resection
Laser Power Density	Myomectomy
Laser–Tissue	Metroplasty
Interaction	Adhesiolysis
Operative Principles	Tubal Surgery
Intrabdominal Use of the	Pelvic Endometriosis
Laser	**Laparoscopy**
Laparotomy	

The word *laser* is an acronym for light amplification by stimulated emission of radiation. Lasers may be considered one of the most important technicologic advances in this half-century due to their vast applications in industry, medicine, and other areas.

Prior to 1917 no one could conceive that light could be amplified as it is in the laser. In that year Albert Einstein laid the path for the creation of the laser by proposing the concept that "stimulated emission" must exist in nature. Credit for inventing the first laser is given to Maiman,[1] who generated the beam by exciting a ruby rod with intense pulses of light from a photographic flash lamp. In 1961 Javan and associates[2] developed the first gas laser using a mixture of helium and neon. In the same year Johnson[3] developed the neodymium:yttrium-aluminum-garnet (Nd:YAG) laser, which operated in the near infrared portion of the light spectrum. It was not until 1964 with the invention of the carbon dioxide (CO_2) laser, which emitted energy in the far infrared portion of the spectrum (10.6 mm), that the laser beam became invisible (Table 31–1).[4]

TABLE 31-1. CHARACTERISTICS OF MEDICALLY SUITABLE LASERS

Laser	Type	Wavelength	Mode	Delivery System
CO_2	Gas	10.600	CW, pulsed	Articulated arms, direct couple to microscope, fiberoptics (experimental)
Nd:YAG	Solid	1.060	CW, Q-switched	Fiberoptics
Ruby	Solid	694	Pulsed	Direct couple to microscope
Argon	Gas	515	CW, pulsed	Fiberoptics
KTP	Solid	532	CW, Q-switched	Fiberoptics
Helium-neon	Gas	632	CW	

PHYSICAL PRINCIPLES

To produce laser light, four components are required: an active medium composed of gas or gases, a source of energy (electrical current), an optical system, and ability to create a population inversion. The laser light has special properties. It is highly coherent, directional, highly collimated, and monochromatic. When a light exhibits complete coherence, there is a predictable connection, or correlation, between the amplitude and phase at any one point on the light wave with any other point. An immediate consequence of coherence is the appearance of "speckle," which is the reflection of laser light from rough surfaces, giving a sparkling or speckled pattern quite unlike any others. Perhaps the most unique property of laser light is its directionality. Because the light is contained between two highly reflective mirrors, the light wave is reflected many times, with only a small portion being transmitted by the mirrors. The many reflections increase the distance the light travels. The curvature of the waves is very small; therefore, the light waves emerging from the laser are nearly planar. Thus highly collimated light is created.

Another distinct property of the laser light is that it is monochromatic. A light from a light bulb passing through a prism gives out a mixture of several colors, in contrast to the laser light's projection of the closest to one single color.

PRACTICAL LASER PHYSICS

The interior of a laser tube represents an optically resonant tube with a totally reflective mirror in one end and a partially reflective mirror in the other (95%). Typically, this tube contains positively and negatively charged ions, whereas the CO_2 laser contains a mixture of three gases: CO_2, nitrogen (N_2), and helium (He). A high-voltage electric current energizes this plasma (active medium), which then promotes collision of gas molecules, raising them (at upper energy states, higher than the ground state) and creating a population inversion.

Figure 31–1 illustrates the laser action of the CO_2 molecule.[5] The molecule is raised in vibrational modes from the ground state (000) to an excited energy level (001). This same molecule can then be stimulated to fall from the higher energy level to a lower one (100 or 020), producing electromagnetic radiation (the laser beam) at 10.6 μm. This emission lies in the far infrared range of the light spectrum and is invisible. As the laser light wave reflects between the two mirrors, it grows in intensity until a steady state is reached. The beam then passes out through the partially reflective mirror. Nitrogen gas is added to facilitate movement of the CO_2 molecule from the

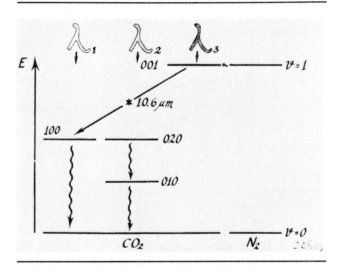

Figure 31-1. Lowest vibrational levels of the ground electronic state of an N_2 and CO_2 molecule. Energy diagram illustrates the dynamics of the nitrogen, helium, and CO_2 mixture in the laser tube. The CO_2 molecule is raised from the ground state, or rest (000), to an excited state, or energy level (001). The molecule is stimulated to drop to a lower energy level (100–020), and laser light is given off. The nitrogen gas facilitates excitation of the CO_2 molecule and the helium gas returns the molecule to the ground state.

ground to the excited state (that is, the energy of the N_2 molecule is imparted to the CO_2 molecule). After the transfer, the N_2 returns to the ground state so that the process can be repeated. Because the CO_2 laser produces an invisible beam (10.6 mm), most laser machines incorporate a coincident helium–neon (red beam) visible target onto which the CO_2 beam is aimed.

Laser Power Density

The power of the laser is relative to the focused beam, the spot diameter of the beam, the time exposure of the target area, and the actual wattage generated. A simple formula can easily explain how the spot diameter of the beam is so fundamental in modifying the laser power.

$$\frac{\text{Power density} = \text{watts power} \times 100}{\text{spot diameter}^2 \text{ (in mm)}} = \text{W/cm}^2.$$

Laser–Tissue Interaction

When the CO_2 laser beam hits tissue cells, the light energy is absorbed by the water in the cells and is converted to thermal energy. The intracellular temperature rapidly rises to 100°C or more, boiling the cell water and producing steam. The expansion of the steam makes the cell explode into a mist, a process called explosive evaporation (Fig. 31–2). The impact zone of the laser wound is a craterlike area composed of three major zones: vaporization, which is devoid of cellular material; thermal necrosis, consisting of irreversibly damaged tissue and sealed vascular chan-

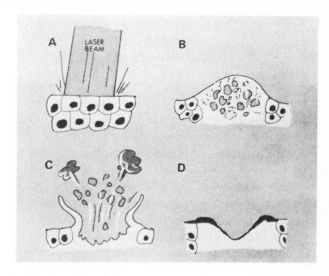

Figure 31–2. As the laser beam strikes the cells (A), the light energy is instantaneously converted to heat (B). The ultimate effect is vaporization of the cells into a mist of smoke by a process called explosive evaporation. (C) The end result is a crater or (D) spot.

nels; and injury, surrounding the zone of necrosis, within which cells may regenerate. Electron microscopy studies to assess and compare the effects of laser cutting versus conventional scalpel incisions using light, and scanning and transmission electron microscopy in the human fallopian tube show the impact zone (Fig. 31–3). The scanning electron microscopy photomicrograph shows a normal epithelial pattern at 1 mm (Fig. 31–4), while 500 μm distal to the laser-vaporized impact point a transitional zone shows evidence of some thermal damage epithelium,

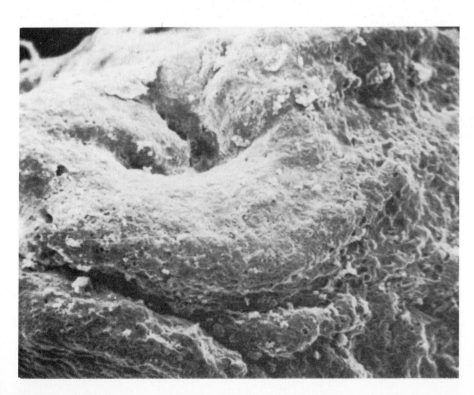

Figure 31–3. Scanning and transmission electron microscopy of the laser zone of impact in the human fallopian oviduct.

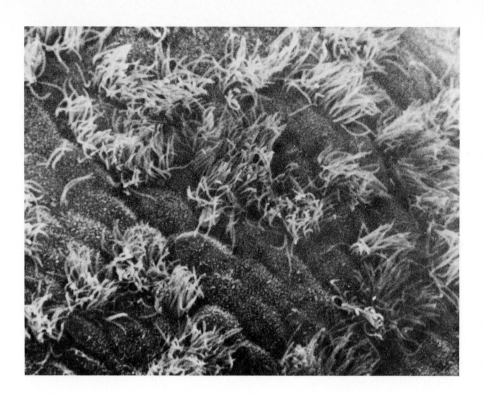

Figure 31–4. Scanning electron microscopy of a normal epithelial pattern 1 mm distal to the point of laser impact.

with few residual distorted cilia, secretory blebs, and no microvilli (Fig. 31–5). The power density used for excision in these studies was approximately 700 W/cm². The use of higher-power densities with smaller beam spot diameter (0.1 to 0.2 mm) produces less lateral thermal damage and less charring, enabling one to encounter normal tissue as close as 300 μm distal to the impact laser point. For incisions and excisions the superpulse laser has a maximum peak power that greatly exceeds continuous wave power. The power (watts) is intermittently produced in bursts at precise and rapidly repetitive rates and pulse duration.[6] Intermittent superpulse lasers cut more slowly; however, they are more precise and cause substantially less thermal damage to surrounding tissue,[7] probably because tissue is cooled between all pulses. More detailed discussions of laser physics appear elsewhere.[8,9]

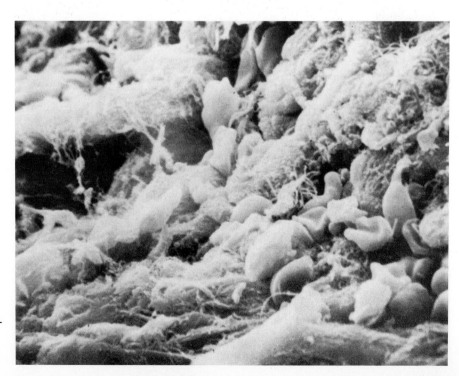

Figure 31–5. Scanning electron microscopy shows evidence of some thermal epithelial damage with some distorted cilia, secretory blebs, and no microvilli 500 μm distal to the impact.

OPERATIVE PRINCIPLES

Before using the laser intraabdominally or firing the beam on living tissue, the operator should calibrate the laser at different power settings, using a moistened, wooden tongue depressor to check the spot size and the accuracy of the helium–neon aiming beam used in conjunction with the CO_2 laser. Alignment should be as perfect as possible (Fig. 31–6). The instrument may be operated by means of an articulated arm and free handpiece, or it may be attached to a microscope and controlled by a micromanipulator. The laser output is controlled by a series of shutters; as the foot pedal is depressed, a shutter opens, allowing the laser beam to be transmitted to the tissue. Single-mode lasers produce a column of light with a roughly gaussian distribution. The center of the beam is more intense than the periphery, so that the wound produced on the tissue is V-shaped: the crater is deep in the center and shallow on the periphery.

Traction and countertraction are extremely important when incising tissue with the laser. The CO_2 laser is not the best instrument for coagulation purposes; however, small bleeding points (vessels <1 mm in diameter) may be sealed by defocusing the beam to produce a coagulation effect.

Intraabdominal laser surgery requires a basic set of accessory instruments. Backstop instruments, manipulating rods, mirrors, and anodized microsurgical instruments are the minimal equipment (Fig. 31–7). Backstop rods should absorb laser light, have minimal reflection, and be nonflammable, nonbreakable, and easy to manipulate. Manipulating rods should be relatively smoothe, nonreflective (round, irregular

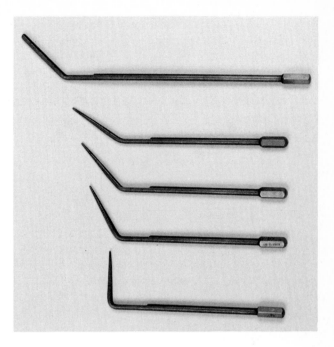

Figure 31–7. Backstop instruments of titanium.

surface), absorb heat and light, and be nonbreakable. Microsurgical instruments (anodized or titanium) should absorb light.

Laser machines for use in the abdominal cavity must be equipped with an articulated arm and must have a single-mode output. The focused laser beam should be able to attain a spot of less than 0.5 mm in diameter, unless it is used for laparoscopy, in which case a spot diameter of 1 to 2 mm is acceptable. The articulated arm has an autoclavable handpiece that can be attached. Every laser must be able to be attached to a double-headed operating microscope by means of a micromanipulator, enabling the laser beam to be controlled.

Manipulating and backstop instruments are required when the laser is used intraabdominally. Although glass or quartz rods are easy to manipulate and are quite frequently used as backstop instruments, it is important to remember that the laser light beam fatigues glass and can lead to unpredictable fracture. We prefer light-absorbing titanium rods. The laser's articulated arm is draped with 6-inch, sterile, double-thickness stockinette. A small opening is made in the stockinette to allow the sterile handpiece to be attached.

Early work showing the effectiveness of the CO_2 laser in human fallopian tubes stimulated wide interest, which was followed by numerous early publications on laser microsurgery of the fallopian tubes[11-16] and other pelvic structures.[17-21] Most procedures leading to improvement in reproductive performance have been accomplished with the CO_2 laser; however, argon,[22,23] Nd:YAG,[24] and potas-

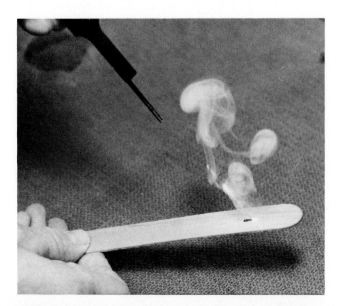

Figure 31–6. Calibrating and aligning the CO_2 laser at different power settings.

sium-titanyl-phosphate (KTP/532) lasers have been used for the photocoagulation or ablation of pelvic endometriosis.[25]

Selecting the machine for beginning a hospital program requires thorough research and full hospital commitment. This includes expending significant amounts of money, forming a committee to recommend the purchase of a specific machine with accessory instruments, and initiating a credentialing process and laser safety rules.[26,27]

INTRAABDOMINAL USE OF THE LASER

The CO_2 laser is the most suitable and versatile laser for the use in the abdomen, especially by laparotomy, because of its predictability for coagulation, vaporization, incision, and reflection.

Laparotomy

Ovarian Wedge Resection. Current theories have helped to expand our understanding of the pathophysiology of polycystic ovary disease, so that ovarian wedge resection is being performed with less frequency. Nevertheless, occasionally bilateral ovarian wedge resection is indicated when clomiphene citrate, gonadotropin-releasing hormone, and pure follicle-stimulating hormone have failed to induce ovulation and achieve subsequent pregnancy. When the decision to operate is made, the gynecologic surgeon must have in mind the important principles needed to avoid adhesion formation: careful handling of tissues, constant irrigation with an isotonic solution (preferably mixed with heparin to minimize fibrin deposition), proper and careful hemostatis, and minimal trauma to the immediate surrounding tissues. All of these principles can be maintained by using the CO_2 laser.

Technique. The enlarged ovaries must be appropriately exposed by isolating them between moist laparotomy pads. Low-power settings (3 to 5 W with a focused beam of 0.2 to 0.4 mm spot diameter) are used to trace the area of the ovary that is to be removed. After the tracing has been completed, the power density must be increased to 20 to 30 W with a focused beam to excise the desired area. Hooks (neurology or skin hooks) are used both for traction and good exposure. It is important to remember that there is an inverse relationship between power density and lateral heat damage; therefore, for excision purposes, high-power densities are required. With the CO_2 laser, excision of the wedged ovarian tissue is almost bloodless, especially if dilute vasopressin mixed with normal saline 1:30 is used to infiltrate the area. When minor bleeding occurs, small vessels (1.0 to 1.5 mm) can be coagulated by defocusing the laser beam. Vessels less than 1.0 mm in diameter are usually sealed while cutting with the CO_2 laser.

After the wedge resection, the edge is approximated with 5-0 polyglactin (deep) and 6-0 polyglactin (cortical) sutures in two layers, using a baseball stitch in the cortical layer. Sutures of 6-0 or 7-0 white braided nylon (Surgilon) can also be used in the cortical layer. Second-look laparoscopy performed on a few patients in our practice showed little or no evidence of adhesions using this technique.

Myomectomy. No absolute data support the contention that leiomyomata are the cause of infertility. This lack of correlation is particularly evident in subserosal myomata, among which the only rare exceptions are those that are so large that they disrupt the ovumpickup mechanism bilaterally. Large intramural myomata capable of deforming the uterine cavity or producing obstruction of the interstitial segment of the fallopian tubes can be a more credible cause of infertility. When they are present, it is difficult not to be inclined to excise them if they are the only apparent reason for the couple's infertility.

Submucosal myomata that deform the uterine cavity or cause menometrorrhagia could cause infertility by interfering with implantation.

Technique. Small myomata of less than 1.5 cm can be totally vaporized with the CO_2 laser very simply. The power density is 500 to 800 W achieved by defocusing the 0.2-mm laser beam on continuous mode to about 2 mm with 16 to 24 W of power:

$$\text{Power density} = \frac{20 \times 100}{(2)^2} = 500 \text{ W/cm}^2.$$

Applying this formula for power density, the charred tissue at the base of the vaporized myoma is cleaned off by gently rolling a cotton-tipped applicator moistened with heparinized Ringer's lactate solution (5,000 μ heparin in 1000 ml Ringer's lactate) over it. Suturing the base is not required.

Larger uterine myomata can be removed by first injecting dilute vasopressin mixed with normal saline (1:30) using a 27-gauge, 1-inch needle and a tuberculin syringe in the area where the incision will be made and in the base. This maneuver allows further hemostasis. After 1 minute, the vasopressin will throw small vessels into spasm. A lozenge incision is made (Fig. 31–8a). Using power densities of approximately 1,200 to 2,000 W/cm,[2] an incision is made about 1.5 to 2.0 mm in depth using continuous mode, dissecting the capsule off the myoma (Fig. 31–8b). Lower-power densities are achieved by defocusing the laser to 200 to 300 W/cm[2]. Skin hooks provide better

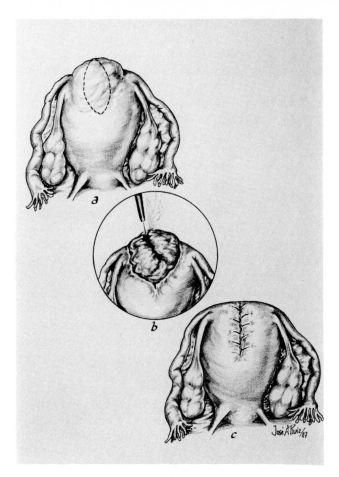

Figure 31–8. A. Tracing a lozenge incision with the CO_2 laser. **B.** Incision and dissection of the myoma. **C.** Approximation of the serosal surface with a baseball stitch.

exposure, and towel clips help to grasp the myoma and get traction. As previously stated, traction and countertraction are essential when the laser is used to excise, dissect, or transect tissues. A similar technique is described for myomectomies elsewhere.[28]

When the myoma has been removed, the defect is repaired by interrupted sutures of 4–0 polyglactin. The serosa is repaired by using 5-0 polyglactin employing a tapered gastrointestinal needle in a baseball stitch (Fig. 31–8c). It is important not to make the lozenge incision too large, as this creates excessive tension in the suture line.

Metroplasty. When the etiology of repetitive pregnancy loss is a septate (or subseptate) uterus, the septum can be excised with minimal blood loss using the CO_2 laser.

Technique. The technique is similar to the Jones metroplasty,[29] with the only difference being in the excision of the septum after infiltrating the traced areas with vasopressin in normal saline (1:30), as described for myomectomy. Tracing is done with 3 to

5 W of power and slightly defocused beam (about 3 feet away from the target area). The septum is excised with superpulse using high-power density (15,000 to 30,000 W/cm²). The edges are approximated to create a symmetric uterine cavity by suturing them in three planes, anteroposteriorly, not lateral to lateral. Edging the myometrium with the laser at the lower-power densities (2,000 to 4,000 W/cm²) divides the myometrium into two areas, making it easier to approximate by using 4-0 polyglactin for the deeper plane (close to the endometrium), 3-0 polyglactin for the middle part, and 5-0 polyglactin for the serosa in a baseball stitch. Tapered gastrointestinal needles must be used.

Adhesiolysis. Infections, endometriosis, and previous pelvic surgery are the three major causes of pelvic adhesions in the female. Adhesions can produce infertility only if they disrupt the normal pickup mechanism, whether they lie between the tube and the ovary like a veil or curtain, encase the whole ovary (or most of it), or fix the fimbriae in such a way that the fallopian tube cannot pick up the ovulating oocyte. This condition is also referred to as peritoneal factor.

When the reason for infertility is adhesions, the prognosis with adhesioloysis is good provided the reproductive surgeon meticulously follows well-known practices to prevent or minimize reformation and de novo adhesions.

Gentle handling of tissues, maintaining pelvic organs moist with isotonic solution containing heparin to decrease fibrine adhesiveness, precision hemostasis, and minimal (or no) bleeding when dividing adhesions, are always helpful.

Technique. Laser adhesiolysis can be accomplished using either the hand-held piece of the articulated arm or the microscope. The former had the advantages of great range of motion, the ability to change power densities from high to low quickly by simply defocusing the laser beam, and no need for extra training or time for the surgeon to become familiar with the different perspectives one has to obtain while operating with the microscope. One of the disadvantages is the available range of power densities, especially when using high densities, because it is impossible to keep the laser beam in focus at all times when incision or excision is performed. Small changes in focal length (such as 1 cm out of focus) results in a 93% loss of power density compared to tight, constant focus.[7] As the power density decreases, the time of incision increases, increasing tissue necrosis, ischemia, and fibrosis.[30]

Microscope laser adhesiolysis has the advantages of requiring minimal retraction and tissue handling, as well as enabling the operator to perceive the cutting depth most clearly.

When lysing adhesions with the CO_2 laser, a backstop instrument or barrier must be placed behind the adhesions to stop the beam from penetrating deeper and to prevent inadvertent damage to surrounding organs or structures. Backstop instruments must fulfill the requirements listed above; rods can be made of pyrex, quartz, or durable, extremely hard metals such as titanium (see Fig. 31–7). Although quartz and pyrex rods are quite versatile and offer the advantage of smooth surfaces, they should not be less than 5 mm in diameter.

The power densities used for adhesiolysis depend on the adhesion. If the adhesions are a veil and not vascular, densities for vaporization (400 to 1200 W/cm^2) are optimal and superpulse may be used. If the veil of adhesions is vascular, low-power densities (200 to 300 W/cm^2) using continuous mode coagulate the vessels by defocusing the beam; the veil is divided with vaporization powers. The backstop instrument is placed away from the adhesions to prevent it from becoming sticky.

When the adhesions are thick and not so vascular, high-power densities (1,200 to 4,000 W/cm^2) are used to divide them. Traction is not advisable unless the adhesions are extremely thick, in which case the laser is used to create a plane of dissection between organs.

One of the clear advantages of the CO_2 laser is its ability to reach poorly accessible areas with its reflecting power, by bouncing the beam off mirrors or highly smooth, reflective metal surfaces. When using mirrors, the laser beam is aimed directly at the desired target areas viewed in the mirrors, which makes the laser easier to manipulate without having to worry about mirror images. Many varieties of mirrors for laser use are available. We find a dental mirror with a 35-degree angle the most versatile. Others made of stainless steel and gold are available that offer the added advantage of longevity.

Tubal Surgery. The use of microsurgical techniques for the treatment of tubal occlusion has significantly improved pregnancy success rates and outcome over earlier techniques. The CO_2 laser is reported to be a valuable addition to these techniques.[10,11,14,19]

Technique. Initial animal studies showed that the laser could be used for tubal anastamosis.[10] Tubal "welding" is possible with low-power densities. Later studies[14,15] using numerous intermittent bursts at 0.1 to 0.2-second intervals, however, showed dehiscence of the tubal edges. Those observations indicated that laser welding of the fallopian tubes has little or no value. Midsegment occlusion: isthmic–isthmic, isthmic–ampullary, and ampullary–ampul-

lary anastomoses. After general anesthesia has been induced, a HUI uterine injector (Unimar, Canoga Park, CA) or a pediatric Foley catheter is placed in the uterine cavity for transcervical chromopertubation. At laparotomy, the pelvic organs are exposed. The laser instrument is attached to a double-headed operating microscope, with the beam controlled by a micromanipulator. The operative area should be exposed under good light, with 300 mm focal length. It is advised that microsurgical instruments be nonreflective titanium.

Once the fallopian tubes are exposed adequately, it is advisable to excise the obliterated areas while using high-power densities (maximum or close-to-maximum effective power density) with continuous mode. This decreases lateral heat damage and minimizes charred tissue deposition. The use of superpulse lasers[32] is very helpful in performing incisions and excisions of the fallopian tubes because they cause less lateral heat damage and less accumulation of charred tissue. It is important to remember to make the incision with the laser beam in focus, with the smallest spot diameter.

Alignment of the CO_2 laser beam with the coincident helium–neon laser should be near perfect, with adequate protection with the use of a backstop instrument for excisions or incisions. After the obliterated areas are excised, including a reasonable extended area of fibrosis (2 to 3 mm), 3 or 4 anastomotic stitches in two planes are placed (muscularis-to-muscularis and serosa-to-serosa), using 8-0 or 9-0 nylon or polyglactin. Chromopertubation is then performed to evaluate the anastomotic site.

Proximal obstruction. Interstitial, or cornual, obstruction is best handled by interstitial–isthmic anastomosis. The proximal portion of the tube is prepared by serially shaving the occluded portion until patency is identified. Shaving cannot be accomplished adequately with the CO_2 laser, however, and is not recommended. The best method is to use a new #11 blade for each cornual shaving. More precise and fine-cutting lasers may become available to excise precise areas, greatly improving the anastomotic site. Where indicated, tubal implantation can be performed with the CO_2 laser (for drilling purposes).

Distal occlusion of the fallopian tubes. When hydrosalpinx is present, as well as distal occlusion of the fallopian tubes with total or partial absence of fimbriae, the CO_2 laser is a versatile and useful instrument. It is capable of performing precision surgery with minimal bleeding and maximum speed.

In the cuff technique for salpingoneostomy, laser adhesiolysis is performed to free the fallopian tube (Fig. 31–9a). The end of the tube is held up with a stay suture of 6-0 polyglactin in a small, tapered

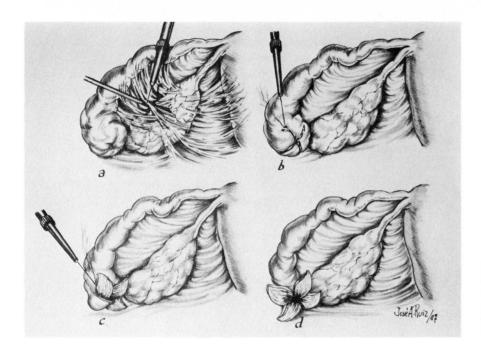

Figure 31–9. A. Laser adhesiolysis using a backstop instrument. **B.** The incision is made with high-power density. **C.** Low-power density is applied to the serosa of the free folds for eversion purposes. **D.** Finished distal salpingoneostomy.

needle. If a dimple can be identified, the face of the hydrosalpinx is infiltrated within the serosa using a 27-gauge needle with 2 to 3 mL of vasopressin and normal saline (1:30 solution).

Methylene blue is instilled to distend the fallopian tube further, and a symmetric Y incision is made with the laser using high-power density (10,000 to 30,000 W/cm^2). If available, we prefer to use an electronically superpulsed CO_2 laser because it produces minimal thermal injury, inflammation, and adhesion formation.[31] To protect the rest of the tube while making the incision, backstop instruments must be used. Once the incision has been made (Fig. 31–9b), the new stoma is maintained by suturing the edges of tubal (ampullary) wall to the serosa using 8-0 or 9-0 nylon.

When the distal portion of the hydrosalpinx is thin and there is complete (or almost complete) absence of fimbriae, the tubal wall can be everted to the serosa of the free folds by defocusing the CO_2 laser beam after incision and creating flaps using low-power density (50 to 200 W/cm^2) (Fig. 31–9c). Applying low-power density to these areas causes retraction of the peritoneal serosa with spontaneous eversion[9–11] and neatly finished terminal salpingoneostomy without the need for sutures (Fig. 31–9d). This is known as the Mage–Bruhat technique.

In the past, prosthetic devices such as Rock–Mulligan silastic hoods were used, but they required a two-stage surgical technique (two laparotomies). These devices showed a conception rate of 22%.[32,33] Microsurgical techniques have improved the pregnancy rates to over 30%[34,35] without the need for a second laparotomy. The use of the CO_2 laser with the Mage–Bruhat technique showed similar pregnancy

rates to the microsurgical techniques described by others.[36,67] It seems that pregnancy success rates for reconstructive surgery in bilateral terminal tubal occlusion are similar whether microsurgical techniques are used with electrosurgery or CO_2 laser; however, the interval between surgery and conception is shorter when the laser is used.[37,38]

The CO_2 laser for tubal surgery seems to be best suited in terminal salpingoneostomy using microsurgical techniques. Whether cuff salpingostomy or eversion technique is used depends on the morphohistologic characteristics of the tubal wall.

Pelvic Endometriosis. Endometriosis is an interesting and relatively common disease of unknown etiology. Its association with infertility is well documented, although it may not always be the absolute cause. Among women undergoing exploratory laparotomy, the frequency of pelvic endometriosis is approximately 15 to 25%.[39] When laparoscopy is performed for infertility reasons, the frequency is about 25% and in some studies approaches 50%.[39] Together with medical therapy with progestins, danazol, antiestrogens, and gonadotropin-releasing hormone agonists, conservative surgical management has been a well-accepted treatment of this condition. The precision, predictable destruction, hemostatic properties, and ability to reach poorly accessible areas have made the CO_2 laser an exceedingly appealing tool to treat this disease.

Technique. At laparotomy, endometrial implants can be vaporized easily by directly lasing the desired areas, using the free handpiece of the articulated arm with power densities of 500 to 1,200 W/cm^2 and

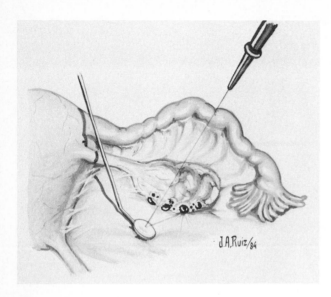

Figure 31–10. The CO₂ beam is deflected to reach poorly accessible areas.

continuous wave at rapid bursts. After complete vaporization, a moist cotton tip is used to remove the charred tissue by gently and firmly rolling it over the vaporized areas.

Dental mirrors, or beam deflectors made of shiny metals, are used to visualize poorly accessible areas (Fig. 31–10). The CO₂ laser beam is directed with precision and minimal manipulation, thus causing little trauma to tissues.

Small endometriomas, less than 1.5 cm, can be vaporized completely with the CO₂ laser by first using intermediate power densities (100 to 1,500

W/cm²) followed by lower densities (400 to 800 W/cm²) after the small amount of "chocolate" material has been washed out. This simple technique is bloodless and does not require suturing of the small surgical defect. At second-look laparoscopies, these areas have shown no adhesions (personal observation).

Larger endometrial cysts within the ovary can be treated without removing the ovary by first infiltrating the ovarian capsule (in the area to be excised) with vasopresin to minimize bleeding (Fig. 31–11A) and then tracing a lozenge area with lower-power densities to allow more precision (Fig. 31–11B). High power densities of 4,500 to 8,000 W/cm² are used to excise this after suction evacuation of the cystic contents and thorough lavage with Ringer's solution. The walls of the endometrioma are at that time systematically vaporized using 400 to 800 W/cm² (Fig. 31–11C). The defect is closed in two layers with 4-0 or 5-0 polyglactin, employing a superficial baseball stitch, as described earlier (Fig. 31–11D).

This method conserves the affected ovary(s) and produces pregnancy success rates of 40% for stage 4 pelvic endometriosis.[40,41] Table 31–2 shows the frequency of pregnancy in different stages of pelvic endometriosis after the use of the CO₂ laser in laparotomy.[41,42]

The pregnancy success rates for patients with endometriosis who were treated with CO₂ laser laparotomy compare favorably in the preliminary reports with a relatively short follow-up[20,40] with those for conventional surgical techniques.[42–45] Only time and well-controlled studies will allow us to

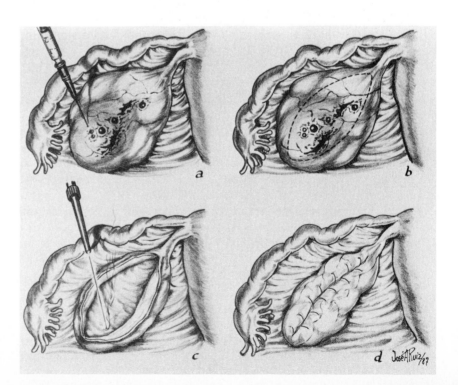

Figure 31–11. A. Infiltration of vasopressin. **B.** The lozenge area is traced with low-power density. **C.** The walls of the endometrioma are vaporized. **D.** The ovarian defect is closed with a baseball stitch.

TABLE 31-2. SEVERITY OF ENDOMETRIOSIS AND OCCURRENCE OF PREGNANCY IN INFERTILE PATIENTS TREATED BY CO_2 LASER

Stage of Endometriosis	No. of Patients	No. (%) Pregnant	
1	—	—	—
2	49	31	(63.3)
3	17	9	(52.9)
4	5	2	(40.0)
Totals	71	42	(59.2)

Source: From reference 40. Reprinted with permission.

compare the results of laser versus nonlaser techniques.

Laparoscopy

Endoscopy is one of the most significant advances in reproductive medicine. The original application of the laparoscope for diagnostic purposes has now been expanded to include a wide range of therapeutic options. The laser has further enhanced these therapeutic purposes by adding different dimensions to laparoscopic surgery. The hemostatic capability of the argon and Nd:YAG lasers is one example. The clinical uses of the CO_2 laser laparoscope include vaporizing endometriosis, ablating the uterosacral nerve, vaporizing hydatid cysts of Morgagni, and performing pelvic adhesiolysis, terminal salpingoneostomy, and salpingostomy for ectopic pregnancy.

Bruhat,[46] Tadir,[47] Daniel,[17] and their associates were the pioneers who developed instruments for the laparoscopic CO_2 laser. The basic instruments include a laparoscope with an operating channel of 4 or 5 mm diameter and a second puncture trochar for the use of a nonreflective probe or operating forceps. In the absence of an operating channel, a second puncture for the probe or forceps and a third

puncture for the laser instrument can be used (Fig. 31-12). The laser beam can either be directed with a micromanipulator or fixed, going straight through the operating channel.

The use of backstop instruments for adhesiolysis and beam deflectors (Fig. 31-12) to reach poorly accessible areas has greatly expanded the therapeutic potential of laser laparoscopy. Laparoscopy with the CO_2 laser is an effective and easy way to treat minimal, mild, moderate, and (occasionally) severe pelvic endometriosis.

Adhesiolysis is performed successfully in patients who do not require dissection between the bowel or vessels, as well as in those whose adhesions are not extremely thick or difficult to reach. Among the most exciting applications of the CO_2 laser is terminal salpingostomy, which can be accomplished with or without adhesiolysis using the Mage–Bruhat technique. With the laparoscope, laser systems can be adapted satisfactorily to perform several operations in the pelvis with the aim of improving or solving the impairment in the reproductive organs.

The CO_2 laser can be used through an operative channel or through an accessory trocar. The operator must not feel intimidated about using 3 or 4 punctures, if necessary, to adequately expose and manipulate the pelvic organs. Recovery and length of hospital stay are the same as with 2 or 3 punctures, and the results of adequate exposure and gentle manipulation warrant additional puncture(s).

I find CO_2 laser laparoscopy extremely helpful in treating adhesions, occasionally distal tubal disease, and especially endometriosis. When either large endometiomas or thick, severe adhesions are encountered, the surgeon must use judgment in deciding whether this problem can be approached with the laparoscope without compromising the patient's chances for pregnancy. This judgment should be based on both the extent of the disease and the

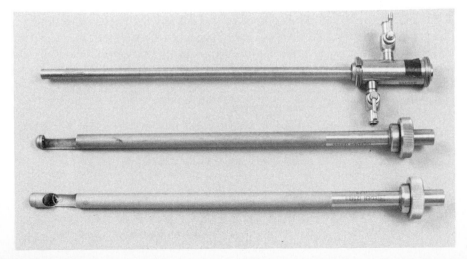

Figure 31-12. Accessories for CO_2 laser laparoscopy.

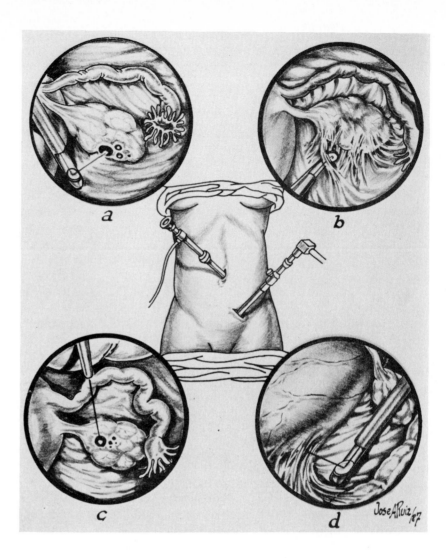

Figure 31–13. A. Laparoscopic use of beam deflectors. **B.** Laparoscopic use of the built-in backstop instrument. **C.** Direct vaporization of endometriosis. **D.** The beam deflector is used to vaporize filmy adhesions.

capabilities and skills of each individual surgeon. Excessive enthusiasm that could bias and blindly promote the use of an instrument or technique not proved to be far superior to others, and that could prove to be potentially harmful, is to be condemned.[48] The CO_2 laser is capable of vaporizing or ablating areas of endometriosis with precision and minimal bleeding (Fig. 31–13c) almost anywhere by using beam deflectors (Fig. 31–13a,d), and it can gently vaporize adhesions using the backstop instruments designed for that purpose (Fig. 31–13b). Meticulous fimbrolysis with the laparoscope can certainly avoid a laparotomy if complete (or close to complete) restoration of the ovum pickup mechanism is able to be accomplished with the laparoscope.

In addition to the CO_2 laser, the argon,[24] YAG,[49] and the KTP/532[26] lasers can be used for the photocoagulation or ablation of pelvic endometriosis by means of flexible fibers that pass easily through the operating channel of the laparoscope. A flexible CO_2 fiber is being developed.

All of this new technology is extremely exciting. Because of the versatility of the CO_2 laser as an operating tool, the initial enthusiasm to use this surgical method was so overwhelming that some investigators vehemently claimed it to be superior to existing techniques. This fervor promoted antagonism toward and created detractors of laser therapy among many leading infertility surgeons who achieved excellent results with conventional procedures. Now that the dust is settling, it is hoped that we can determine objectively the best applications of the CO_2 and other types of lasers in infertility surgery to teach and disseminate sound scientific knowledge as the only seed for academic and clinical excellence.

REFERENCES

1. Maiman TH: Stimulated optical radiation in ruby. *Nature* 187:493, 1960.
2. Javan A, Bennet WR Jr, Herriott OR: Population inversion and continuous optical laser oscillation in a gas discharge containing a HeNe mixture [letter]. *Physiol Rev* 6:106, 1961.
3. Johnson LF: Optical laser characteristics of rare-earth ions in crystals. *J Appl Physiol* 34(8):94, 1961.
4. Patel CKN, McFarlane RA, Faust WL: Selective excitation through vibrational energy transfer and optical laser action in N_2–CO_2. *Physiol Rev* 13:617, 1964.
5. Baggish MS, Chong AP: Intraabdominal surgery with the CO_2 laser. *J Reprod Med* 28:269, 1983.

6. Laakman KD: Laser physics II, in Baggish MS (ed): *Basic and Advanced Laser Surgery in Gynecology*. E Norwalk, CT, Appleton-Century-Crofts, 1984, p 38.
7. Fuller TA: Laser–tissue interaction: The influence of power density, in Baggish MS (ed): *Basic and Advanced Laser Surgery in Gynecology*. E Norwalk, CT, Appleton-Century-Crofts, 1984, p 58.
8. Dixon JA: *Surgical Application of Lasers*. Chicago, Year Book, 1983.
9. O'Shea DC, Callen WR, Rhodes W: *Introduction to Lasers and Their Applications*. Reading, MA, Addison-Wesley, 1978.
10. Klink F, Grosspietzsch R, Klitzing L, et al: Animal in vivo studies and in vivo experiments on human tubes for end-to-end anastomotic operation by CO_2 laser technique. *Fertil Steril* 30:100, 1978.
11. Bruhat MA, Mage G: Use of CO_2 laser in salpingoneostomy, in Kaplan I (ed): *Laser Surgery III*. Tel Aviv, Academic Press, 1979, pp 271–278.
12. Grosspietzsch R, Schultz BO, Endell W, et al: Reconsruktive Mikrochirurgie mit dem CO_2 Laser. *Res Exp Med* 174:239, 1979.
13. Bruhat MA, Mage G: Utilization du laser CO_2 en chirurgie tubaire. *Presse Med* 6:1, 1980.
14. Baggish MS, Chong AP: Carbon dioxide laser microsurgery of the uterine tube. *Obstet Gynecol*, 55:371, 1981.
15. Fayez JA, Jobson VW, Lentz SS, et al: Tubal microsurgery with the carbon dioxide laser. *Am J Obstet Gynecol* 146:371, 1983.
16. Bellina JH: Reconstructive microsurgery on the fallopian tube with the carbon dioxide laser: Procedures and preliminary results. *Reproduction* 5:1, 1981.
17. Daniel JF, Brown OH: Carbon dioxide laser laparoscopy: Initial experience in experimental animals and humans. *Obstet Gynecol* 59:761, 1982.
18. McLaughlin DS: Micro-laser myomectomy technique to enhance reproductive potential: A preliminary report. *Lasers Surg Med* 2:107, 1982.
19. Kelly RW, Roberts DK: Experience with the carbon dioxide laser in gynecologic microsurgery. *Am J Obstet Gynecol* 146:585, 1983.
20. Chong AP, Baggish MS: Management of pelvic endometriosis by means of intraabdominal carbon dioxide laser. *Fertil Steril* 41:14, 1984.
21. Diamond MP, Daniel JF, Martin DC, et al: Tubal patency and pelvic adhesions of early second-look laparoscopy following intraabdominal use of the carbon dioxide laser: Initial report of the intraabdominal laser study group. *Fertil Steril* 42:717, 1984.
22. Keye WR, Matson GA, Dixon J: The use of the argon laser in the treatment of experimental endometriosis. *Fertil Steril* 39:26, 1983.
23. Keye WR, Dixon J: Photocoagulation of endometriosis by the argon laser through the laparoscope. *Obstet Gynecol* 62:383, 1983.
24. Lomano JH: Photocoagulation of early endometriosis by the Nd:YAG laser through the laparoscope. *J Reprod Med* 30:77, 1985.
25. Daniell JF, Miller W, Tosh R: Initial evaluation of the use of the potassium-titanyl-phosphate (KTP/532) laser in gynecologic laparoscopy. *Fertil Steril* 46:3783, 1986.
26. Dorsey JH: Initiating a hospital CO_2 laser program. Part I. *Colposc Gynecol Laser Surg* 1:103, 1984.
27. Dorsey JH, Baggish MS: Initiating a CO_2 laser program, in Baggish MS (ed): *Basic and Advanced Laser Surgery in Gynecology*. E Norwalk, CT, Appleton-Century-Crofts, 1985, p 373.
28. Lashgari M, Tummillo M, Keene M: Myomectomy with the carbon dioxide laser. *Colposc Gynecol Laser Surg* 3:107, 1987.
29. Jones HW, Wheeless CR: Salvage of the reproductive potential of women with anomalous development of the mullerian ducts. *Am J Obstet Gynecol* 104:348, 1969.
30. McCoy TD, Martin DC, Poston W: Reanastomosis of rat uterine horn following laser and sharp incisions. *Fertil Steril* 41:805, 1984.
31. Baggish MS, Elbakry MM: Comparison of electronically superpulsed and continuous-wave CO_2 laser on the rat uterine horn. *Fertil Steril* 45:120, 1986.
32. Garcia CR, Aller J: Surgical approach to tubal disease. *Clin Obstet Gynecol* 17:102, 1974.
33. Roland M, Leisten D: Tuboplasty in 130 patients. Improved results due to stents and preoperative endoscopy. *Obstet Gynecol* 39:57, 1972.
34. DeCherney AH, Kase N: A comparison of treatment for bilateral fibrial occlusion. *Fertil Steril* 35:162, 1981.
35. Gomel V: Salpingostomy by microsurgery. *Fertil Steril* 29:380, 1978.
36. Mage G, Bruhat MA: Pregnancy following salpingostomy: Comparison between CO_2 laer and electrosurgery procedures. *Fertil Steril* 40:472, 1983.
37. Tulandi T, Farag R, McInnes RA, Golfand MM, Wright CV, Vilos GA: Reconstructive surgery of hydrosalpinx with and without the carbon dioxide laser. *Fertil Steril* 42:839, 1984.
38. Tulandi T, Vilos GA: A comparison between laser surgery and electrocautery for bilateral hydrosalpinx: A 2-year followup. *Fertil Steril* 44:846, 1985.
39. Bayer SR, Seibel MM: Endometriosis: Clinical symptoms and infertility, in Rolland R, Chada DR, Willemsen WNP (eds): *Gonadotropin Down-Regulation in Gynecological Practice*. New York, Liss, 1986, pp 103–133.
40. Chong AP, Keene M: Management of infertility patients with moderate to extensive pelvic endometriosis by intra-abdominal carbon dioxide laser. *Colposc Gynecol Laser Surg* 2:99, 1986.
41. American Fertility Society: Classification of endometriosis. *Fertil Steril* 32:633, 1979.
42. Acosta AA, Butram VC Jr, Malinak CR, Franklin RR, Vanderheyden JD: A proposed classification of pelvic endometriosis. *Obstet Gynecol* 41:1, 1973.
43. Garcia CR, David SS: Pelvic endometriosis: Infertility and pelvic pain. *Am J Obstet Gynecol* 129:740, 1977.
44. Schenkin R, Malinak LR: Reoperation after initial treatment of endometriosis with conservative surgery. *Am J Obstet Gynecol* 131:416, 1978.
45. Buttram VC Jr: Surgical treatment of endometriosis in the infertile female: A modified approach. *Fertil Steril* 32:635, 1979.
46. Bruhat M, Mage G, Mankes M: in Kaplan I (ed): *Laser Surgery III*. Tel Aviv, Academic Press, 1979, p 235.
47. Tadir Y, Ovadia J, Zuckerman Z, Kaplan I: in Atsumi K, Nimsakul N (eds): The 4th congress of international society for laser surgery, Tokyo, 1981, p 25.
48. Blackwell RE, Carr BR, Chang RJ, et al: Are we epxloiting the infertile couple? *Fertil Steril* 48:735, 1987.
49. Lomano JM: Laparoscopic ablation of endometriosis with the YAG laser. *Lasers Surg Med* 3:179, 1983.

CHAPTER 32

Diagnosis and Management of Ectopic Pregnancy

Michael P. Diamond, Gad Lavy, and Alan H. DeCherney

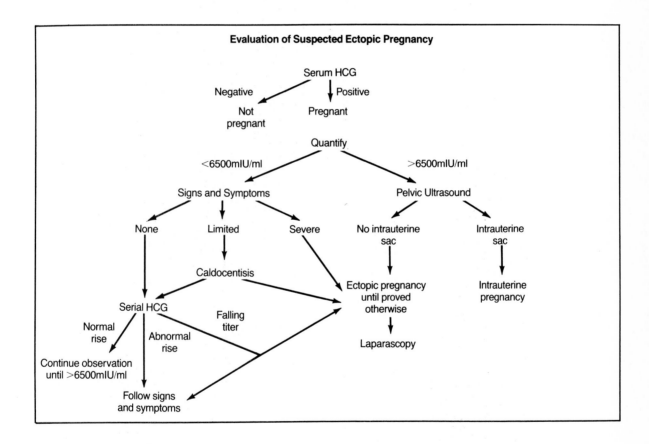

Ectopic pregnancies represent a leading cause of morbidity and mortality for women of reproductive age. In addition to the disruption they cause at the time of their occurrence, they leave permanent sequelae: an association with subsequent infertility, increased likelihood of recurrence, and psychologic trauma induced by these possibilities.

The potential dire consequences of an ectopic pregnancy cannot be overlooked. From 1979 to 1980, 86 deaths occurred in 102,100 ectopic pregnancies in the United States, a rate of 0.8 per 1,000.[1] The causes of death in these women were blood loss (85%), infection (5%), anesthesia complications (2%), and a variety of other factors in the remaining cases.[2] Misdiagnosis, which may have contributed to failure in identifying ectopic pregnancies earlier, occurred in at least 42 of these women (Table 32–1). Thus suspicion of an ectopic pregnancy must be followed by a concerted effort either to rule in or rule out the diagnosis.

From 1970 to 1980 the rate of ectopic pregnancies increased more than twofold, from 4.5 to 10.5 per

TABLE 32–1. MISDIAGNOSES OF FATAL ECTOPIC PREGNANCY

Misdiagnosis	Occurrence* No.	Occurrence* (%)[†]
Gastrointestinal disorder	14	(25)
Intrauterine pregnancy	10	(18)
Pelvic inflammatory disease	8	(14)
Psychiatric disorder	5	(9)
Spontaneous abortion	5	(9)
Sequelae of recent induced abortion	4	(7)
Urinary tract infection	4	(7)
Adnexal cyst	2	(4)
Dysfunctional uterine bleeding	2	(4)
Fetal death in utero	1	(2)
Placental abnormality (placenta previa, (abruptio placentae)	1	(2)
Totals	56	(100)

*Based on all recorded diagnostic errors. Misdiagnoses did not occur in some cases and occurred more than once in others.

[†]These percentages do not add up to 100 because of rounding.

Source: From Misdiagnosis for fatal ectopic pregnancies,United States, 1979 to 1980. Dorfman SF, et al.: Ectopic pregnancy Mortality, United States, 1979 to 1980: Clinical aspects. *Obstet Gynecol* 64:386 1984. Reprinted with permission from the American College of Obstetricians and Gynecologists and the author, Sally Faith Dorfman, MD.

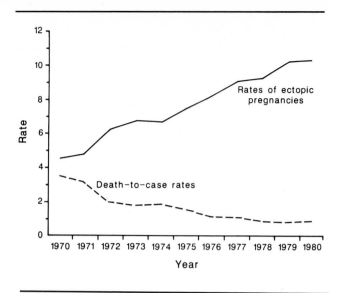

Figure 32–1. Rates of ectopic pregnancies* and death-to-case rates[+] by years. (From Ectopic pregnancies—United States, 1970–1980. *JAMA* 251:2327, 1984. Reproduced with permission of the American Medical Association, © 1984, American Medical Association.)

1,000 reported pregnancies (Fig. 32–1).[3] Over this same time period, advances in the early diagnosis and appropriate treatment of such gestations has resulted in a major reduction in the death:case ratio to nearly one fourth of its initial rate of 3.5 per 1,000. Nevertheless, the risk of maternal death in association with an ectopic pregnancy is approximately 10 times greater than that associated with childbirth, and more than 50 times greater than that associated with legally induced abortion.

Nontubal ectopic pregnancies represent only a small fraction of ectopic eccyeses, less than 5% (Fig. 32–2). Most occur in the ampullary portion of the fallopian tube, followed by the infundibular, isthmic, and interstitial segments. Although nontubal and interstitial gestations are rare, they represent nearly 20% of the deaths associated with ectopic pregnancies.[2] This disparity most likely results from difficulty in diagnosing gestations in these locations, and from their clinical features. Signs and symptoms of interstitial ectopic pregnancies often occur with more

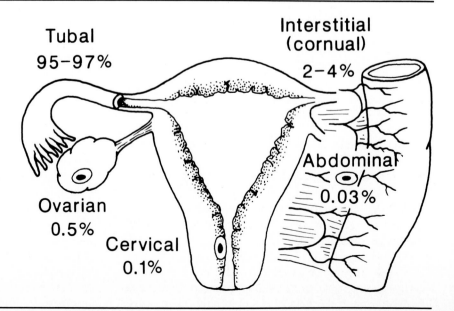

Figure 32–2. Sites and incidence of ectopic pregnancies. (From Mattingly.[4] Reproduced with permission.)

TABLE 32–2. SUMMARY: ECTOPIC PREGNANCY AFTER TUBAL SURGERY

Procedure	Technique	% Total Pregnancy	Pregnancy Range	% Ectopic	Ectopic Range
Salpingostomy	Macr*	42	35–65	3.4	1–20
	Micr†	52	31–69	1.8	0–16
Fimbrioplasty	Macr	42	36–50	14	10–18
	Micr	59	26–68	6	4–11
Neosalpingostomy	Macr	27	20–38	4.2	2–20
	Micr	26	17–44	7.7	0–18
Tubal anastomosis	Macr	44	25–83	9.2	0–15
	Micr	62	35–78	2.3	1–6.2
Removal of ectopic pregnancy	Salpingectomy	42	38–49	12	8–17
	Salpingostomy	57	39–73	11	0–20

*Macr, macrosurgery.
†Micr, microsurgery.
Source: From Lavy G, Diamond MP, DeCherney AH: Ectopic pregnancy: its relationship to tubal reconstructive surgery. *Fertil Steril* 47:543, 1987. Reproduced with permission of the American Fertility Society.

advanced gestations in association with cornual rupture and extensive hemorrhage.

A direct relationship between a history of prior pelvic inflammatory disease and subsequent ectopic pregnancies has been described.[5,6] Although it was considered that such prior infections represented the sequelae of gonorrheal infections, several studies implicated *Chlamydia trachomatis*.[7,8] The presence of these organisms is suggested by demonstration of serum IgG *Chlamydia* antibodies, cervical cultures, and polymorphonuclear infiltration of fallopian tube tissue. Although correlations have been noted between gross morphologic evidence of previous tubal infections and demonstration of chlamydial infections, many women with such gross manifestations do not recall previous clinical episodes of pelvic infection. Thus, infectious destruction of tubal anatomy and predisposition to an ectopic pregnancy can occur without being recognized by the individual.

The possible contribution of intrauterine devices (IUDs) to ectopic pregnancy has been a source of controversy. Although it was suggested that IUDs per se are associated with increased ectopic rates, one group demonstrated that the risk remains the same as that in women without IUDs.[9] The ratio of intrauterine to ectopic gestations is decreased, but this is due to a reduction of intrauterine pregnancies with IUDs.

Microsurgical techniques are used increasingly in reproductive pelvic surgical procedures to restore tubal patency and to treat tuboperitoneal disease. Ectopic pregnancy raes after neosalpingostomy have actually increased using microsurgical techniques as compared to prior macrosurgial procedures (Table 32–2).[10] This increased rate may be due to the "improvement" in maintaining tubal patency with such procedures. This improvement, although sufficient to allow union of the male and female gametes, may be insufficient to allow normal transit of the zygote to the uterine cavity.

Other factors that have been suggested to increase the risk for ectopic pregnancies include vaginal douching,[11,12] diethylstilbestrol (DES) exposure,[13] salpingitis isthmica nodosa,[14] and induced abortions.[15]

ETIOLOGY

The etiologies of ectopic pregnancies are diverse. Anatomic and hormonal factors have been implicated repeatedly; less clearly established are the possible contributions of semen abnormalities and chromosomal aberrations (Table 32–3).[16]

The most widely accepted etiology of tubal ectopic pregnancies is tubal scarring. This scarring may represent prior infection, prior tubal surgery, or

TABLE 32–3. ETIOLOGIES OF ECTOPIC PREGNANCIES

Anatomic	Hormonal	Controversial
Altered tubal transport	Ovulation induction	Endometriosis
Inflammatory changes	In vitro fertilization	Congenital abnormalities
Tubal ligation	Delayed ovulation	Blind pouches
Previous surgery for an ectopic pregnancy	Ovum transmigration	Semen quality
Induced abortion		Abnormal prostaglandin levels in semen
Diethylstilbestrol exposure		Chromosomal abnormalities

Source: From Russell JB: The etiology of ectopic pregnancy. *Clin Obstet Gynecol* 30:181, 1987. Reproduced with permission of the publisher, Lippincott/Harper & Row, Philadelphia.

the presence of pathologic processes in the pelvis, such as endometriosis or appendicitis. Such damage may be present both on the tubal serosa as well as inside the lumen. Although the former is readily identifiable at laparotomy or laparoscopy, the latter has traditionally been implicated by findings on hysterosalpingogram. The introduction of tuboscopy has allowed for direct examination of the luminal surfaces of the tube up to the isthmic–ampullary junction.

CLINICAL FEATURES

Signs and symptoms of ectopic pregnancy include abdominal pain, abnormal or absent menses, vaginal bleeding, adnexal mass, adnexal pain, pregnancy-related symptoms, nausea, vomiting, breast tenderness, dizziness, shoulder pain, and passage of tissue. In addition, individuals with ruptured ectopic pregnancies can experience syncope and hemorrhagic shock. Fortunately, as examination for and recognition of ectopic pregnancy have advanced over the last several decades, the ratio of ruptured to unruptured ectopic gestations at the time of diagnosis has decreased.

Tests used to diagnose ectopic pregnancies suggested by history and physical examination are shown in Table 32–4. The diagnoses that must be differentiated by these tests include a persistent corpus luteum (ruptured or unruptured), intrauterine pregnancy (viable gestation versus complete, incomplete, and threatened abortion), endometriosis, pelvic inflammatory disease, degenerating fibroid, appendicitis, adnexal torsion, and kidney stones.

Both urine and serum pregnancy tests are available. In the emergency room, urine tests are most frequently performed because the results can be available in minutes. Some are sensitive to levels as low as 50 mIU/mL, making the likelihood very rare that a clinically significant ectopic pregnancy would not be identified. False negative results can occur, however, due to dilution or to the presence of an older ectopic pregnancy that is outgrowing its blood supply and thus making only small amounts of human chorionic gonadotropin (HCG). Both positive and negative results in clinically suspicious situations should be followed by obtaining a serum sample to determine the level of the β-subunit of human chorionic gonadotropin (β-HCG).

Probably the most common test employed to identify the presence of an early pregnancy, its location, and its well-being is measurement of serum β-HCG levels. Titers of β-HCG are identifiable in serum beginning approximately 1 week after ovulation and continue to rise until approximately 10 menstrual weeks, at which time the mean level is

TABLE 32–4. DIAGNOSING ECTOPIC PREGNANCIES BY HISTORY AND PHYSICAL EXAMINATION

Sampling Period	No. of Patients	Doubling Time (days)
10–22 days after BBT nadir	57	1.4
11–21 days after administration of hCG	7*	1.7
11–32 days after insemination	27	1.9
0–20 days after detection of hCG	4	2.0
29–64 days after LMP	26	2.0
12–30 days after BBT shift	189	2.2
28–60 days after LMP	20	3.3
28–60 days after LMP	57	3.5†
13–20 days after BBT shift	18	1.5
13–25 days after BBT shift	26	1.9
13–30 days after BBT shift	30	2.2
13–39 days after BBT shift	35	2.7
28–35 days after LMP	17	1.4
28–42 days after LMP	35	2.2
28–49 days after LMP	40	2.5
28–56 days after LMP	42	2.9

BBT = Basal body temperature; LMP = Last menstrual period.
*One spontaneous abortion.
†Calculated from the authors' data.
Modified from reference 22.

100,000 mIU/mL (Fig. 32–3). The false negative rate (failure to identify an ectopic pregnancy) with this test has been reported to be 0% among 234 women with suspected ectopic gestations.[18] Among these women, 188 had negative pregnancy tests, and subsequent laparoscopy or laparotomy was able to be avoided in 149. Individuals with positive pregnancy tests can be placed in a high-suspicion group and subjected to further assessment in order to determine the location of the pregnancy.

When the serum β-HCG level in our laboratory exceeds 6,500 mIU/mL, abdominal pelvic ultrasound examination can identify the presence of an intrauterine pregnancy. In a series of 383 women with suspected ectopic pregnancies, an absent intrauterine gestational sac with a titer of over 6,500 mIU/mL was indicative of an ectopic pregnancy.[19] This test had 100% sensitivity, and 86% positive predictive value. Although the precise level of β-HCG might vary from laboratory to laboratory, in our hands a patient with a possible ectopic pregnancy with a level over 6,500 mIU/mL and no intrauterine gestational sac is considered to have an ectopic pregnancy until proved otherwise. Such women should undergo laparoscopy for diagnosis.

Among women with a suspected ectopic pregnancy but a β-HCG titer less than 6,500 mIU/mL who are clinically stable, observation is appropriate. This includes serial determination of β-HCG.[20–23] If with serial levels the titer comes to exceed 6,500 mIU/mL, ultrasonography should be performed to identify

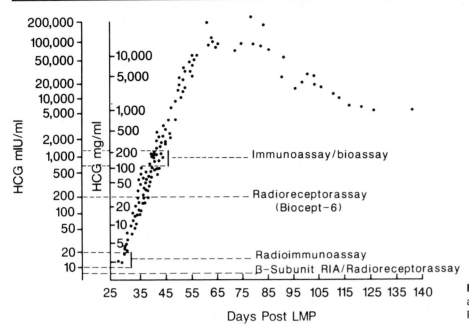

Figure 32–3. Limits of detection of blood and urine pregnancy tests. (From Batzer.[17] Reproduced with permission.)

whether the pregnancy is intrauterine. Generally, the doubling time has been said to take 2 days, although ranges of 1.4 to 3.5 days have been identified (Table 32–5).[22] This variability may reflect the gestational age at which the observations are made or the

TABLE 32–5. DOUBLING TIMES OF HCG IN EARLY PREGNANCY

Sampling Period	No. of Patients	Doubling Time (days)
10–22 days after BBT nadir	57	1.4
11–21 days after administration of hCG	7*	1.7
11–32 days after insemination	27	1.9
0–20 days after detection of hCG	4	2.0
29–64 days after LMP	26	2.0
12–30 days after BBT shift	189	2.2
28–60 days after LMP	20	3.3
28–60 days after LMP	57	3.5+
13–20 days after BBT shift	18	1.5
13–25 days after BBT shift	26	1.9
13–30 days after BBT shift	30	2.2
13–39 days after BBT shift	35	2.7
28–35 days after LMP	17	1.4
28–42 days after LMP	35	2.2
28–49 days after LMP	40	2.5
28–56 days after LMP	42	2.9

BBT = basal body temperature; LMP = last menstrual period.
*One spontaneous abortion.
†Calculated from the authors' data.

Source: From Pittaway DE, Reish RL, Wentz AC: Doubling times of human chorionic gonadotropin increase in early viable intrauterine pregnancies. *Am J Obstet Gynecol* 152:299, 1985. Reproduced with permission of the publisher, C.V. Mosby Company, St. Louis, MO.

viability of the developing embryo. In addition, it may reflect sampling bias, as peaks in serum β-HCG levels can be identified at 2 to 4-hour intervals.[24]

A minimum rise of serial titers in 48 hours of 66%, in 72 hours of 114%, and in 96 hours of 175% allowed identification of 90% of ectopic pregnancies.[23] Individuals whose titers rise at this rate and do not have intervening changes in their clinical features should have continued serial β-HCG monitoring until the level exceeds 6,500 mIU/mL, or the rate of rise falls below these rates. Titers that continue to rise but do not achieve these rises are thus highly suspicious of representing an ectopic pregnancy or a nonviable intrauterine pregnancy; they are, however, associated with a 10% false positive rate.

Management of women with slowly rising titers must be individualized based on clinical features, patient concern and anxiety, and the distance the persons would have to travel should the clinical situation worsen. Frequently, we hospitalize obese women for close monitoring. When serial β-HCG titers fall, it is thought to represent a nonviable pregnancy, either a missed or incomplete abortion, or an ectopic pregnancy. In women in whom the former is thought to be present, close observation and continued monitoring can frequently avoid the necessity of operative intervention. When an ectopic pregnancy is considered to be most likely, operative intervention is indicated. Our most frequent management plan is to perform a uterine curettage. If frozen sections fail to identify trophoblastic villi, laparoscopy is performed to evaluate the possibility of an ectopic gestation.

Culdocentesis is frequently performed, particularly in emergency room settings, to identify a hemoperitoneum. The presence of a positive urine pregnancy test with a positive culdocentesis (the presence of nonclotting blood) in a patient thought to be clinically suspicious for an ectopic pregnancy must be considered to suggest an ectopic pregnancy until proved otherwise.

From a series of 77 women with ectopic pregnancies, it was concluded that results of culdocentesis frequently are positive without coexistent hypotension, tachycardia, low hematocrit, or signs of peritoneal irritation.[25] In that series, positive culdocenteses were associated not only with ruptured but with unruptured ectopic pregnancies. In the latter patients, blood entered the peritoneal cavity from the tubal ostia. Other etiologies of positive results that can occur in the absence of an ectopic pregnancy include ruptured ovarian cysts, retrograde menstruation, and endometriosis.[26] Pseudo-false-positive results can be reported if recovered blood is not reexamined after allowing sufficient time for clotting to occur. If clotting does occur, it indicates that the blood is from a site punctured during culdocentesis.

A negative result of culdocentesis (obtaining clear or straw-colored fluid) is not diagnostic of the absence of an ectopic pregnancy, as an unruptured tubal eccyesis may be present. Women with positive urine pregnancy tests and negative culdocentesis can usually be observed while awaiting the serum β-HCG level. A nondiagnostic culdocentesis (failure to obtain either bloody or nonbloody fluid) does little to help identify the location of a pregnancy and should not be considered to be reassuring. Nondiagnostic taps were described in 16% of women with ectopic pregnancies.[26] Finally, results of culdocentesis were positive in 45% of women without classic peritoneal signs associated with an ectopic pregnancy.[26] Thus it appears reasonable, even with the ability to obtain serum β-HCG titers and ultrasonography, to have a low threshold for performing this test.

Laparoscopy confirms the diagnosis of ectopic pregnancy in most clinical situations. Because laparotomy is associated with greater morbidity than laparoscopy, it should be avoided to establish this diagnosis. An exception is the hemodynamically unstable patient in whom laparotomy is indicated.

At the time of laparoscopy the gestation is identified visually. In tubal ectopic gestations, the tube looks distended and has a bluish to purplish hue. When an ectopic tubal pregnancy is identified early by β-HCG titers and ultrasound scans, however, it is possible to perform a laparoscopy and not identify the site of the pregnancy. This is particularly true in women with tuboperitoneal disease who may have tubal scarring. Thus the decision of when to intervene surgically can be difficult. If done too early, the ectopic pregnancy may not be identifiable; if done too late, there may be extensive tubal damage, increased morbidity, and possible mortality.

Other serum markers have been proposed as possible indicators of ectopic pregnancies. Serum progesterone levels were measured in women with early intrauterine pregnancies and women with ectopic pregnancies.[27] In 20 normal pregnancies, with a mean gestational age of 4.4 ± 1.4 weeks and a β-HCG of 1,444 ± 2,343 mIU/mL, the mean progesterone level was 30.9 ± 6.9 ng/mL, with all values over 20 ng/mL. In contrast, in 29 ectopic pregnancies with a mean gestational age of 7.3 ± 2.7 weeks and a β-HCG titer of 866 ± 1,536 mIU/mL, the progesterone level averaged 5.7 ± 3.6 ng/mL, with the highest value being 12.9 ng/mL. Thus if progesterone levels can be determined rapidly, concomitant measurement of progesterone with β-HCG may be of benefit.

Two proteins produced by trophoblastic tissue have been evaluated as possible markers for ectopic pregnancies: pregnancy-specific β-1 glycoprotein (SP1) and pregnancy-associated plasma protein-A (PAPP-A).[28] The SP1 levels become detectable approximately 1 week after ovulation and have been used to identify ectopic pregnancies; however, they are less sensitive than serum β-HCG titers.[28] The PAPP-A can be detected approximately 1 month after conception, and has been variably reported to be either more discriminatory than HCG and SP1, or less discriminatory than HCG.[28] Thus clinical utility of these proteins as markers of ectopic pregnancies remains unestablished.

Free β-HCG is identifiable 3 to 4 weeks after conception.[29] Its clinical utility in the diagnosis of ectopic pregnancies as compared to nonviable intrauterine pregnancies has not been established.

At our center, three technologies are undergoing examination to identify their possible utility in the diagnosis of ectopic pregnancies. Vaginal ultrasound examinations performed using a 5-MHz vaginal transducer have identified an intrauterine sac in intrauterine pregnancies with a titer of 3,000 mIU/mL.[30] The location of the ectopic gestation has also been identified in some of these patients. Magnetic resonance imaging has identified extrauterine gestations, and Doppler flow studies examine blood flow to adnexal structures. It is hoped that these techniques will allow greater accuracy in identifying both intrauterine and extrauterine gestations.

TREATMENT

Appropriate treatment of ectopic pregnancies depends on the desires of the patient for future childbearing, clinical features, location of the gestation, anatomic status of the pelvis, available operating room equipment, and the skill and expertise of the surgeon. The options of the therapy include hysterectomy, salpingectomy, linear salpingostomy, milking technique, methotrexate (or other chemotherapeutic agent), and expectant management.

Hysterectomy should probably be limited to those individuals with a cornual ectopic pregnancy who have extensive destruction of the myometrium. For ectopic pregnancies in other locations within the tube, an operative technique with less morbidity can be performed. Because in-vitro fertilization centers are increasingly available, any woman who still desires to have a child should have the uterus conserved, even if both tubes are surgically absent. In a patient with a cornual ectopic pregnancy, however, a major concern with leaving the uterus in place is the risk of uterine rupture associated with future pregnancies. Prognostic factors to determine the risk of subsequent rupture are not well delineated.

The choice of surgical procedure for ectopic pregnancy in other parts of the fallopian tube depends on the location. In the ampullary segment, the ectopic trophoblastic tissue is thought, at least in part, to be between the lumen and the serosa.[31] Thus the gestation is not within the lumen, as it is in ectopic pregnancies located in the isthmic segment.[32] Larger ectopic pregnancies at any site within the tube that have caused extensive disruption of the tube are best treated by excision. If this represents only a small segment of the tube, partial excision is satisfactory. Alternatively, if the ectopic gestation represents an extensive portion of the tube, or if it has occurred in a woman who desires no future childbearing, salpingectomy can be performed.

More controversial is the appropriate surgical management of ectopic pregnancies that occupy only a small portion of the fallopian tube. For those in the infundibular segment, milking the tube has been suggested. Although it was suggested that this technique results in extensive scarring,[33] others have not identified poorer pregnancy outcome after the procedure.[34] The alternative conservative technique at this segment is to perform an antimesenteric incision over the distal aspect of the tube over the area of the ectopic pregnancy.

Ampullary ectopic pregnancies may be treated by linear salpingostomy. Tubal patency after such procedures is high, as usually the products of conception are not within the tubal lumen itself. Isthmic ectopic pregnancies also may be treated by this method; however, this is more controversial because of their intraluminal location. After such a conservative technique, the likelihood of fistula formation or tubal occlusion is greater than when linear salpingostomy is performed at the ampullary segment. Thus it has been suggested that segmental resection of the fallopian tube is the preferred conservative management of isthmic ectopic pregnancies.[32] A case may be

made, however, for performing linear salpingostomy with a subsequent hysterosalpingogram to establish the patency of the involved tube. If occlusion or fistula is identified, reanastomosis can subsequently be performed under controlled circumstances just as if segmental resection has been performed previously. This remains an area of contention.

For those wishing to preserve fertility, a major concern in the management of ectopic pregnancy is subsequent pregnancy outcome after either conservative or radical surgical management. Pregnancy outcome was compared in 50 women who underwent salpingectomy or salpingo-oophorectomy with that in 48 women who underwent salpingostomy for treatment of tubal ectopic pregnancy.[35] Among those who underwent the radical technique, the subsequent viable pregnancy rate was 42%, with 12% repeat ectopic pregnancies. These results were nearly indistinguishable from women who underwent salpingostomy, in whom the pregnancy rate was 39.6% and the repeat ectopic pregnancy rate 11.6%. Thus, in view of the possibility of future ectopic pregnancies in these women, necessitating subsequent tubal surgery including possible salpingectomy, it appears that conservative management is desirable when possible.

Among women with a sole remaining patent fallopian tube, treatment of ectopic pregnancy by linear salpingostomy has been followed by a viable pregnancy rate of 53% and a recurrent ectopic pregnancy rate of 20%.[36] A subsequent report noted an intrauterine pregnancy rate in this group of 47.6%, with a repeat ectopic pregnancy rate of 42.8%.[37] Because these pregnancy rates are greater than those currently available with alternative methods of conception, it appears to be reasonable to perform conservative procedures on women with a sole remaining fallopian tube.

Several groups reported treatment of ectopic pregnancies by linear salpingostomy at the time of laparoscopy.[38-40] The ability to perform such procedures at the same time as establishing the diagnosis has the obvious advantages of requiring a reduced amont of surgical intervention and of reduced patient morbidity. Patients are frequently able to be discharged either the day of surgery or the next day, thus also reducing patient costs. In our series of 79 women, 43 (62%) of 69 who were trying to conceive were able to do so.[38] Seven had repeat ectopic pregnancies, 3 in the ipsilateral tube and 4 in the contralateral tube. The term pregnancy rate of women trying to conceive was 38%. One group treated 321 tubal pregnancies conservatively with laparoscopic techniques. Fifteen women (48%) required a subsequent laparotomy or second laparoscopy because of retained trophoblastic tissue. Of 118 patients desiring subsequent pregnancy, 76 (64.4%)

had an intrauterine pregnancy and 26 (22%) had a second ectopic pregnancy. Eleven (48.8%) of 24 women attempting conception after conservative laparoscopic removal of an ectopic gestation from the sole remaining tube achieved an intrauterine pregnancy and 7 (29.2%) had a second ectopic.[39] Thus conservative management of tubal ectopic pregnancies at laparoscopy appears to be a viable clinical alternative.

Another topic of discussion is the management of a second ectopic pregnancy. Although the number of patients in such groups are small, one report identified a 31% term intrauterine pregnancy rate and a 20% third ectopic gestation rate.[41]

Ectopic pregnancy may persist after conservative surgery.[42] This is a possible sequela of both laparotomy and laparoscopic operative treatment, and indicates retention of residual trophoblastic tissue. Because linear salpingostomy techniques involve careful removal of the products of conception but do not disturb the bed from which these tissues arose, continuation of the pregnancy is not expected. One possible solution to decrease its likelihood would be more aggressive removal of necrotic-appearing tissue from this bed; however, this could induce bleeding, with subsequent requirements for cautery or salpingectomy. Such procedures could result in greater tubal damage and subsequent reduction in fertility potential. It is because of the possibility of such an occurrence that monitoring β-HCG levels after conservative treatment of tubal ectopic pregnancies is mandatory. These levels should be measured approximately once weekly, until the titers fall below the level of the sensitivity of the assay.

After linear salpingostomy, the β-HCG half-life is approximately 24 hours.[43] The HCG titers can persist after removal of ectopic pregnancies for 30[44,45] or more days. In a comparison of ectopic pregnancies treated by either salpingectomy or partial resection of the fallopian tube with those treated by linear salpingostomy or fimbrial expression, patients tended to have similar HCG disappearance curves.[44] The length of time it took for the titers to fall below the level of sensitivity in part depended on the initial HCG titer.

Among women in whom HCG titers do not fall to negative values, treatment for persistent trophoblastic tissue must be contemplated. These patients can often be followed for up to 1 to 2 months. Subsequently, the traditional method of management has been a repeat operative procedure, usually salpingectomy.[42] Others have treated ectopic pregnancies with chemotherapeutic agents. The most commonly suggested agent is methotrexate with leukovorum rescue.[46] Methotrexate has also been suggested for treatment of cornual ectopic pregnancies,[47] and as an alternative to conservative surgical

therapy after a laparoscopic diagnosis.[48] It is our belief that, in centers where operative management is a viable alternative, initial therapy with chemotherapeutic agents is not indicated; however, such treatment of persistent ectopic pregnancy in an attempt to avoid reoperation may be an alternative.

The surgical techniques involved in the management of an ectopic pregnancy have been reviewed[49] and are not discussed in detail here. Several areas of contention with regard to surgical management are briefly summarized.

In performing a linear salpingostomy, some individuals prefer to inject dilute vasopressin solution, 1 ampule in 20 to 30 cc saline, into the antimescenteric border of the fallopian tube, the tubal mesentery, or both. This has the advantage of reducing blood flow to the area of the ectopic gestation and thus makes the procedure less hemorrhagic. Others suggest that administration of vasopressin might allow a vessel to begin bleeding at a later time after the completion of the procedure and thus lead to postoperative hemorrhage. Although this remains a theoretical concern, it does not appear to be a major clinical issue.

A second issue is the choice of instruments for performing a linear salpingostomy. Instruments include a scalpel, electrocautery, and one of a wide variety of lasers. All but the scalpel allow some degree of hemostasis in the process of making the salpingostomy incision. To date, no studies have assessed the clinical utility of electrocautery versus any of the lasers in making this incision.

A third issue is whether or not to include a cornual resection as a part of the procedure. The advantage is that it reduces the likelihood that a subsequent ectopic pregnancy will form in the residual portion of the tube. The disadvantage is that incisions into the myometrium perhaps predispose to subsequent cornual rupture. The likelihood of this occurrence in part depends on the amount of cornual tissue resected. It is our clinical practice to make only a very small cornual resection, 2 to 3 mm, if at all.

SUMMARY

Since the 1960s major advances in the diagnosis of ectopic pregnancies have been achieved through the serial measurement of β-HCG levels and ultrasonography. Other techniques, including vaginal ultrasonography, are promising for continuing advances in the ability to identify ectopic pregnancies at an early gestational age prior to extensive tubal damage. Great advances have also been made in the management of ectopic pregnancies; in contrast to radical procedures involving salpingectomy or salpingo-oophorectomy, many individuals now perform conservative surgical procedures such as linear salpingostomies and segmental resections. Many of these procedures are performed at the time of laparoscopy rather than requiring a laparotomy. The role of chemotherapeutic agents such as methotrexate is being examined. Use of agents that impair ovarian steroidogenesis may be useful for nonsurgical management of ectopic pregnancies.

REFERENCES

1. Dorfman SF: Deaths from ectopic pregnancy, United States, 1979 to 1980. *Obstet Gynecol* 62:334, 1983.
2. Dorfman SF, Grimes DA, Cates W, et al: Ectopic pregnancy mortality, United States, 1979 to 1980: Clinical aspects. *Obstet Gynecol* 64:386, 1984.
3. Centers for Disease Control: Ectopic pregnancies, United States, 1970–1980. *MMWR* 33:2327, 1984.
4. Mattingly RF: Ectopic pregnancy, in TeLinde (ed): *Operative Gynecology,* ed 5. Philadelphia, Lippincott, 1977, p 369.
5. Westrom L: Effect of acute pelvic inflammatory disease on fertility. *Am J Obstet Gynecol* 121:707, 1975.
6. Westrom L, Benatsson LH, Mardl PA: Incidence, trends, and risks of ectopic pregnancy in a population of women. *Br Med J* 282:15, 1981.
7. Svensson L, Mardh P-A, Ahlgren M, Nordenskjold F: Ectopic pregnancy and antibodies to *Chlamydia trachomatis. Fertil Steril* 44:313, 1985.
8. Brunham RC, Binns B, McDowell J, Paraskevas M: *Chlamydia trachomatis* infection in women with ectopic pregnancy. *Obstet Gynecol* 67:722, 1986.
9. Ory HW, Women's Health Study: Ectopic pregnancy and intrauterine contraceptive devices: New perspective. *Obstet Gynecol* 57:137, 1981.
10. Lavy G, Diamond MP, DeCherney AH: Ectopic pregnancy: Its relationship to tubal reconstructive surgery. *Fertil Steril* 47:543, 1987.
11. Neumann HH, DeCherney A: Douching and pelvic inflammatory disease [letter]. *N Engl J Med* 295:789, 1976.
12. Chow W-H, Daling JR, Weiss NS, Moore DE, Soderstrom R: Vaginal douching as a potential risk factor for tubal ectopic pregnancy. *Am J Obstet Gynecol* 153:727, 1985.
13. DeCherney AH, Cholst I, Naftolin F: Structure and function of the fallopian tubes following exposure to diethylstilbestrol (DES) during gestation. *Fertil Steril* 36:741, 1981.
14. Majmudar B, Henderson PH, Semple E: Salpingitis isthmica nodosa: A high-risk factor for tubal pregnancy. *Obstet Gynecol* 62:73, 1983.
15. Daling JR, Chow HW, Weiss NS, Metch BJ, Sodersom S: Ectopic pregnancy in relation to previous induced abortion. *JAMA* 253:1005, 1985.
16. Russell JB: The etiology of ectopic pregnancy. *Clin Obstet Gynecol* 30:181, 1987.
17. Batzer FR: Hormonal evaluation of early pregnancy. *Fertil Steril* 34:1, 1980.
18. Schwartz RO, DiPietro DL: β-HCG as a diagnostic aid for suspected ectopic pregnancy. *Obstet Gynecol* 56:2, 1980.
19. Romero R, Kadar N, Jeanty P, et al: Diagnosis of ectopic pregnancy: Value of the discriminatory human chorionic gonadotropin zone. *Obstet Gynecol* 66:357, 1985.
20. Cartwright PS, DiPietro DL: Ectopic pregnancy: Changes in serum human chorionic gonadotropin concentration. *Obstet Gynecol* 63:76, 1984.
21. Holman JF, Tyrey EL, Hammond CB: A contemporary approach to suspected ectopic pregnancy with use of quantitative and qualitative assays for the β-subunit of human chorionic gonadotropin and sonography. *Am J Obstet Gynecol* 150:151, 1984.
22. Pittaway DE, Reish RL, Wentz AC: Doubling times of human chorionic gonadotropin increase in early viable intrauterine pregnancies. *Am J Obstet Gynecol* 152:299, 1985.
23. Romero R, Kadar N, Copel JA, et al: The value of serial human chorionic
24. Owens OM, Ryan K, Tulchinsky D: Episodic secretion of human chorionic gonadotropin in early pregnancy. *J Clin Endocrinol Metab* 53:1307, 1971.
25. Cartwright PS, Vaughn B, Tuttle D: Culdocentesis and ectopic pregnancy. *J Reprod Med* 29:89, 1984.
26. Romero R, Copel JA, Kadar N, et al: Value of culdocentesis in the diagnosis of ectopic pregnancy. *Obstet Gynecol* 65:519, 1985.
27. Matthews CP, Coulson PB, Wild RA: Serum progesterone levels as an aid in the diagnosis of ectopic pregnancy. *Obstet Gynecol* 68:390, 1986.
28. Seppala M, Purhonen M: The use of HCG and other pregnancy proteins in the diagnosis of ectopic pregnancy. *Clin Obstet Gynecol* 30:148, 1987.
29. Cole LA, Restrepo-Candelo H, Lavy G, DeCherney AH: HCG free β-subunit as marker of outcome of in vitro fertilization clinical pregnancies. *J Clin Endocrinol Metab* 64:1328, 1987.
30. Shapiro BS: The nonsurgical management of ectopic pregnancy. *Clin Obstet Gynecol* 30:230, 1987.
31. Budowick M, Johnson TRB Jr, Gendry R, Parmley TH, Woodruff JD: The histopathology of the developing tubal ectopic pregnancy. *Fertil Steril* 34:169, 1980.
32. Boyers SP, DeCherney AH: Isthmic ectopic pregnancy: Segmental resection as treatment of choice. *Fertil Steril* 44:307, 1985.
33. Timonen S, Nieminen U: Tubal pregnancy, choice of operative method of treatment. *Acta Obstet Gynecol Scand* 46:327, 1967.
34. Sherman D, Langer R, Herman A, Bukovsky I, Caspi E: Reproductive outcome after fimbrial evacuation of tubal pregnancy. *Fertil Steril* 47:420, 1987.
35. DeCherney AH, Kase N: The conservative surgical management of unruptured ectopic pregnancy. *Obstet Gynecol* 54:451, 1979.
36. DeCherney AH, Maheaux R, Naftolin F: Salpingostomy for ectopic pregnancy in the sole patent oviduct: Reproductive outcome. *Fertil Steril* 37:619, 1982.
37. Oelsner G, Rabinovitch O, Morad J, Mashiach S, Serr DM: Reproductive outcome after microsurgical treatment of tubal pregnancy in women with a single fallopian tube. *J Reprod Med* 31:485, 1986.
38. DeCherney AH, Diamond MP: Pregnancy following laparoscopic linear salpingostomy. *Obstet Gynecol* 70:948, 1987.
39. Pouly JL, Mahnes H, Mage G, Canis M, Bruhat MA: Conservative laparoscopic treatment of 321 ectopic pregnancies. *Fertil Steril* 46:1093, 1986.
40. Cartwright PS, Herbert CM III, Maxson WS: Operative laparoscopy for the management of tubal pregnancy. *J Reprod Med* 31:589, 1986.
41. DeCherney AH, Silidker JS, Mezer HC, Tarlatzis BC: Reproductive outcome following two ectopic pregnancies. *Fertil Steril* 43:82, 1985.
42. Rivlin ME: Persistent ectopic pregnancy: Complication of conservative surgery? *Int J Fertil* 30:10, 1985.
43. Holtz G: Human chorionic gonadotropin regression following conservative surgical management of tubal pregnancy. *Am J Obstet Gynecol* 147:347, 1983.
44. Kamrava MM, Taymor ML, Berger MJ, Thompson IE, Seibel MM: Disappearance of human chorionic gonadotropin following removal of ectopic pregnancy. *Obstet Gynecol* 62:486, 1983.
45. Steier JA, Bergsjo P, Myking OL: Human chorionic gonadotropin in maternal plasma after induced abortion, spontaneous abortion, and removed ectopic pregnancy. *Obstet Gynecol* 64:391, 1984.
46. Cowan BD, McGehee RP, Bates GW: Treatment of persistent ectopic pregnancy with methotrexate and leukovorum rescue: A case report. *Obstet Gynecol* 67:50S, 1986.
47. Tanaka T, Hayashi H, Kutsuzawa T, Fujimoto S, Ichinoe K: Treatment of interstitial ectopic pregnancy with methotrexate: Report of a successful case. *Fertil Steril* 37:851, 1982.
48. Ory SJ, Villaneuva AL, Sand PK, Tamura R: Conservative treatment of ectopic pregnancy with methotrexate. *Am J Obstet Gynecol* 154:1299, 1986.
49. Diamond MP, DeCherney AH: Surgical techniques in the management of ectopic pregnancy. *Clin Obstet Gynecol* 30:200, 1987.

gonadotropin testing as a diagnostic tool in ectopic pregnancy. *Am J Obstet Gynecol* 155:392, 1986.

inner cells have homogeneous surfaces and lack intracellular polarity.[22,23] The outer cells then begin to differentiate into trophectoderm cells (Fig. 33–1E,F) that eventually give rise to the placenta and other extraembryonic tissues; cells at internal positions contribute to the inner cell mass (Fig. 33–1E,F) of the blastocyst.[24,25] The inner cell mass cells give rise primarily to the tissues of the fetus. The blastocyst expands (Fig. 33–1F) during the fourth day of gestation due to fluid accumulation within the blastocoel that is stimulated by an increased active transport of solutes across the trophectoderm layer and into the intercellular space.[26]

The trophectoderm cells of the expanded mouse blastocyst become further differentiated into polar and mural trophectoderm cells (Fig. 33–2). The polar trophectoderm are those cells lying over the inner cell mass at the embryonic pole, while the remainder of the trophectoderm cells are referred to as mural. As implantation proceeds, the inner cell mass undergoes differentiation into endoderm and ectoderm.[14] In the

mouse, the polar trophectoderm along with some of the adjacent inner cell mass cells begin proliferating rapidly, giving rise to the ectoplacental cone. Meanwhile, the mural trophectoderm cells terminally differentiate into primary giant cells. Giant cell formation begins in the region farthest away from the embryonic pole.[14,27] As cells of the ectoplacental cone are displaced away from the inner cell mass, they form secondary giant cells.[14] It is the giant trophoblast cells that invade the uterine endometrium during implantation.[11] In the human, these early events are less well known. In the classic study by Hertig and Rock,[10] it appeared that a peripheral layer of primitive syncytiotrophoblast, formed by the fusion of polar trophectoderm cells, surrounded an inner layer of proliferating cytotrophoblast. Together these cells give rise to the structure of the primitive villi of the invading conceptus. Although the organization of rodent and human trophoblast differs and endoreduplication of DNA rather than cell fusion leads to giant cell formation in the rodent, both systems are characterized by a group of mononucleated, proliferating trophoblasts surrounded by terminally differentiated, giant trophoblast cells.

STAGES OF IMPLANTATION

Human fertilization and early preimplantation development occur in the oviduct or fallopian tube. The embryo enters the uterus approximately 72 hours after ovulation in the mouse and probably at that same time in the human.[19,28] At the time implantation begins, embryo development has proceeded through approximately 6 or 7 divisions, compaction has occurred and apical junctional complexes have formed, and the blastocyst has undergone expansion. The mouse embryo hatches and begins the process of attachment by the end of the fourth gestational day, while the human blastocyst remains in the uterus for an additional 2 or 3 days before implanting.[10,28] The precise time of hatching in the human is unclear.

Implantation begins as the blastocyst lodges in a crypt of the uterine folds and hatches from the zona pellucida.[6] The ensuing multistep process may be divided into several stages: (1) hatching from the zona pellucida, (2) apposition of the blastocyst and the uterine wall, (3) adhesion of the trophoblast and the uterine luminal epithelium, and (4) penetration of the luminal epithelium by the trophoblast, leading to invasion of the underlying stroma.[6] During this process the blastocyst undergoes a developmental program whereby its nonadherent trophectoderm cells become adhesive trophoblast a few hours after the embryo hatches from the zona pellucida.[6,29,30]

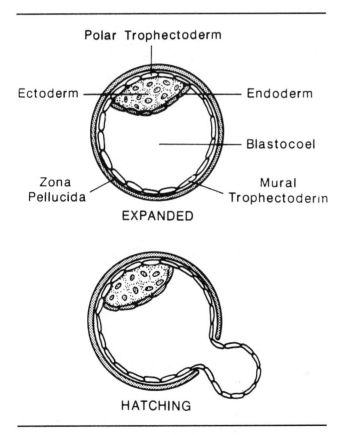

Figure 33–2. Hatching of the expanded blastocyst. Shortly before implantation the zona pellucida is shed, allowing contact between the trophectoderm cells, now the trophoblast, and the uterine epithelia. Further cell differentiation of the trophectoderm into polar and mural trophectoderm and of the inner cell mass into endoderm and ectoderm begins. When cultured in vitro, the mural trophectoderm forms a slitlike opening in the zona pellucida and progressively squeezes through it.

Hatching

Observations of hatching in vitro have demonstrated that the blastocyst repeatedly expands (over 2 to 3 hours) and rapidly contracts (4 to 5 minutes) within the zona pellucida,[31] eventually forming a small slitlike opening at the surface of the zona pellucida. The trophectoderm cells squeeze through the zona opening and reexpand outside, producing a figure 8 shape during the intermediate stages of hatching (see Fig. 33–2). At the completion of hatching in vitro, the empty zona with a slit through half of its circumference remains. Hatching in vivo appears to be accompanied by degradative enzymes secreted by the uterus that facilitate the breakdown of the zona. The nature of the agents responsible for hatching is discussed further below.

Apposition

Apposition, as described by Schlafke and Enders,[6] refers to the period when the embryo comes into contact with the receptive portion of the endometrium and the progressive onset of adhesion begins. The mouse and human embryo both lodge antimesometrially[32] in a crypt created by the uterine folds, forming an implantation chamber.[6] During this period fluid is absorbed by the uterus, facilitating the collapse of the uterine wall around the blastocyst, and promoting intimate contact between trophoblast and uterine epithelial cells.[6] Also during the apposition phase the trophoblast cells transform into giant cells and attain adhesive properties required for subsequent implantation. The trophectoderm cells of the human embryo presumably begin to fuse into a syncytium during the latter part of the apposition period.

Attachment

Previous reviews[3,6,33] described the next phase of implantation as one characterized by the adhesion of the trophoblast cells with the uterine luminal epithelium; however, the exact nature of the adhesion between these two cell types is unclear. Microvilli present on the surfaces of both trophoblast and epithelial cells interdigitate extensively, and the intercellular distances at these sites appear reduced upon electron microscopic examination,[6] suggesting the presence of junctional complexes. In mammals that exhibit superficial implantation,[6–8] this interaction is probably highly adhesive, because it forms the only connection between the placenta and maternal support. During interstitial implantation, however, the epithelial cells are penetrated by the trophoblasts either by sloughing and engulfment, as in the rodent, or by the breakdown of epithelial junctional complexes, as in the human, allowing the trophoblast cells to move into the underlying stroma.[6,9,13,34] Therefore it would appear that during interstitial

implantation adhesion between the trophoblast and uterine epithelial cells is transient and culminates in aggression toward the epithelium on the part of the trophoblast.

Invasion

As mentioned earlier, the trophoblast penetrates the endometrium shortly after attachment to the epithelium is observed. The invasion of the endometrium by the human embryo is illustrated in Figure 33–3. Schlafke and Enders[6] categorized the mechanisms of trophoblast invasion used by various animals into three groups: (1) intrusive, which includes humans, wherein the trophoblast moves between luminal epithelial cells that remain viable; (2) displacement, which includes the rodents, wherein the epithelial cells slough from the underlying basement membrane and die; and (3) fusion, exemplified by the rabbit, wherein the epithelial cells fuse with the trophoblast to form an invasive heterosyncytial mass. The loosening or soughing of the epithelial cells observed in humans and rodents occurs throughout the area near the implantation site,[6,13,34] suggesting that, in addition to the trophoblast, actions of the underlying decidual cells may play a role in compromising the integrity of the epithelium.[35] In human implantation, the parted epithelium reforms above the invading embryo, forming a plug.[10] The mouse embryo remains partially exposed above the epithelium, freeing the ectoplacental cone to extend across the lumen and adhere to the mesometrial wall at the opposite side of the lumen.[6] In each type of invasion, once past the epithelium, the trophoblast adheres to the basal lamina and penetrates into the underlying connective tissue of the decidualized endometrium.[36,37]

STRUCTURE OF THE UTERUS AND DECIDUALIZATION

The wall of the human uterus consists of three layers: an inner endometrium, a middle myometrium, and an external serosal covering. The endometrium consists of simple tubular glands set in a vascular, cellular stroma.[38] During the early proliferative phase of the menstrual cycle, the glands are small, straight, tubular, and round in cross-section. Their epithelium is cubocolumnar, while stromal cells are elongated and compact with indistinct cytoplasm. Gradually, under the influence of estrogen, the glands multiply and their epithelium becomes taller and pseudostratified.[38] By the midsecretory phase, progesterone is abundant and intraglandular glycogen secretion reaches a peak. Stromal edema and spiral artery development reach a peak on day 22 or 23 in response to progesterone (Fig. 33–4). The blood vessels prolif-

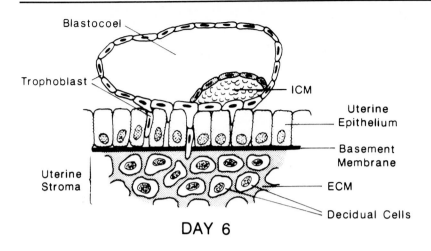

DAY 6

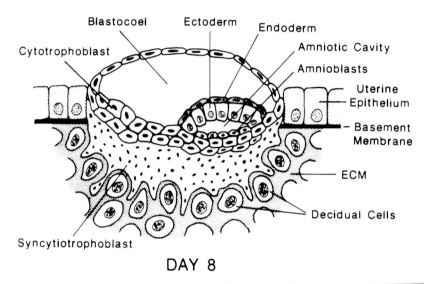

DAY 8

Figure 33–3. Implantation of the human blastocyst. Illustrated, on day 6 of pregnancy, is the intrusive movement of trophoblast cells past the uterine epithelial layer, through the basement membrane, and into the extracellular matrix material that surrounds the decidual cells. By day 8 of pregnancy, some of the trophoblasts have fused to form a syncytium, which invades further through the basement membrane and into the stroma, and other trophoblasts near the inner cell mass have become proliferative cytotrophoblast cells. Meanwhile, the inner cell mass has undergone further development into an embryonic disk composed of endoderm, ectoderm, and amnioblasts with the beginnings of an amniotic cavity.

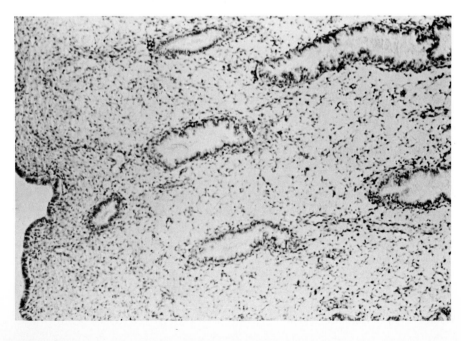

Figure 33–4. Histologic specimen of midsecretory endometrium, approximately day 22.

erate and the myofibrils differentiate. The perivascular stromal cells show increased eosinophilia and density; these are predecidual cells.[39]

Implantation of the blastocyst normally occurs during the midsecretory phase of the cycle. After implantation, glandular secretion continues and stromal edema persists. After the 14th day of gestation, or 15 days after ovulation, a fully formed decidua emerges with almost the entire endometrial stroma being converted into pavement-like sheets of epithelial cells.[40]

The human endometrium or decidua in the late luteal phase consists of three layers.[40] Beginning with the luminal surface they are the zona compacta in the region of the mouths of the glands, a middle zona spongiosa containing the tortuous and dilated glands, and a zona basalis adjacent to the myometrium. The zona compacta and the zona spongiosa combine to form the zona functionalis, and are shed at menses. The zona basalis remains intact after menstruation, and the endometrial lining is regenerated from this layer by the outgrowth of epithelium from the glands. The decidua is thus the endometrium of the uterus during pregnancy and receives its name because most of it is cast off after birth.[41]

Decidualization is the hormone-induced response occurring in the endometrial stroma prior to nidation. It occurs sequentially after estrogenic priming, followed by progesterone stimulation of stromal elements. It is characterized by transformation of fibroblastic stromal cells into large polygonal cells containing glycogen and lipid, and demonstrating basophilic cytoplasm with euchromatic, vesicular nuclei.[42] This so-called decidual reaction is noted to occur first around stromal blood vessels, gradually spreading throughout the endometrium.[43] Thus a distinct functioning unit termed *decidua* is formed between fetal and maternal components.

Additional stromal components arising during pregnant and nonpregnant cycles have been described.[44] The function of these cellular components ranges from synthesis of protein macromolecules to enzymatic degradation to phagocytosis. At least 11 or more stromal cell types have been classified according to their permanent or transient existence within uterine stroma. Fibroblasts, mast cells, lymphocytes, and stem cells are resident cells, while decidual cells, monocyte macrophages, lymphocytes, and others occur transiently within the endometrium.[45]

The portion of the decidua directly beneath the site of implantation is called the decidua basalis, while the decidual portion overlying the developing ovum and separating it from the rest of the uterine cavity is the decidua capsularis. The remainder of the uterus is lined by the decidua vera. The decidua basalis contributes to the formation of the basal plate of the placenta.[46] The basalis is invaded extensively by trophoblastic giant cells that appear at the time of implantation. The degree of penetration of these giant cells is variable and at times may penetrate the myometrium.[6,35] Where the invading trophoblasts encounter the decidua, there occurs a zone of fibrinoid degeneration called the Nitabuch layer.[46] When the integrity of the decidua is breached, as in placenta accreta, the Nitabuch layer is usually absent.[47]

The myometrium is the smooth muscle of the uterine wall and is arranged in bundles separated by cellular connective tissue containing vessels. The innermost layers are distributed in a sphincterlike fashion around the intramural portions of the fallopian tubes. The intermediate myometrial layer has a spongy texture and is interspersed with many large venous channels.[39] The outer layer of the myometrium consists of intermingled longitudinal and circular fibers. The uterine serosa, a thin, glistening capsule, lies external to the myometrium except laterally at the attachment of the broad ligament.

EMBRYONIC SIGNALS AND UTERINE RECEPTIVITY

The development of both embryo and endometrium must be synchronous so that successful implantation can occur.[48] The blastocyst stage must be attained by the developing embryo, and the endometrium must be in the receptive or sensitized state. Uterine readiness can be characterized by several biochemical and histologic features such as decidualization, vascular permeability, and luminal surface changes.[48,49]

Invasion by the trophoblast is limited by the formation of the decidual cell layer in the uterus, with fibroblastlike cells in the stroma being transformed into glycogen- and lipid-rich cells. In humans, decidual cells surround uterine blood vessels late in the menstrual cycle, but extensive decidualization does not occur until pregnancy is established.[43,48] Ovarian steroids direct decidualization, and in humans a combination of estrogen and progesterone is critical.[50,51] In animals, implantation is preceded by an increase in uterine stromal capillary permeability at the site where the blastocyst will attach.[52] This localization and subsequent decidualization as observed in rodents raise the possibility that a signal from the embryo might be an important triggering mechanism.[52] An important unanswered question associated with implantation concerns the mechanism by which the mother rejects a genetically abnormal embryo or fetus. One possibility is that the abnormal embryo is incapable of producing a signal in early pregnancy that is recognizable by the mother.[53,54]

It has been suggested that the release of carbon dioxide by the embryo in the form of bicarbonate raises the pH of the embryo surface, which in turn increases its adhesiveness. Carbon dioxide also may act as a signal for decidual response in the mother.[55] The physical presence of the embryo may be adequate for triggering a decidual response in the uterus, since the presence of an oil drop in a hormonally primed rodent uterus induces localized decidualization.[54]

The human conceptus produces human chorionic gonadotropin (HCG) that is detectable in serum at about the time of implantation on day 6 of pregnancy.[56,57] It is presently not known whether the release occurs before or after the embryo invades the endometrium; however, HCG has been detected in human preimplantation embryos cultured in vitro.[56] Human chorionic gonadotropin is luteotrophic and stimulates the corpus luteum to produce progesterone. Functioning of the corpus luteum is critical during the first 7 to 9 weeks of pregnancy, and luteectomy early in human pregnancy can precipitate abortion.[58] Similarly, early pregnancy loss in animals can be induced by injections of anti-HCG antiserum.[59]

Another early-acting signal produced by embryos has been found in studies of pregnancy in sheep. The luteotropic effects of the prostaglandin (PG), $PGF_{2\alpha}$, and luteotropin, that act upon the ovary during the luteal phase must be blocked if pregnancy is to continue. Cultured extracts of 14 to 16-day-old sheep embryos produced ovine trophoblastic protein-1 (OTP-1) that acts on the maternal endometrium and may elicit maternal responses that contribute to the maintenance of pregnancy in the sheep.[60] This protein has a molecular weight of 18,000 daltons and is thought to be a translation product of sheep conceptus mRNA. The OTP-1 cDNA has been cloned and its amino acid sequence determined. There is evidence that this protein exhibits a 40% homology to the interferon-α family and a 75% homology with the bovine interferon-α-II subfamily.[61] It is believed that this substance (or group of substances) may directly or indirectly prolong the life span of the corpus luteum and prevent a return to ovarian cyclicity during pregnancy.

Shelesnyak suggested that histamine may initiate the decidual response of the endometrium.[62] Antihistamines administered directly into the uterus prevent the decidual response in rats. It has subsequently been shown that there are two different receptors for histamines, H_1 and H_2. It is likely that early experiments demonstrating a lack of effect of systemic antihistamines may have achieved a block to only one of the receptors. When both receptors are blocked in rats, the number of implantation sites decreases.[63] Mast cells in the uterus are a major source of histamine, but it is possible that the embryo can also synthesize histamine, causing the localized increase in capillary permeability and decidualization of the endometrium.[62]

The embryonic signals that trigger decidualization are effective only in a proper hormonal milieu.[53] Much of the knowledge concerning the steroid hormone requirements for implantation in animals has been gained from studies of delayed implantation.[64] In a number of species, preimplantation embryos normally lie dormant in the uterus for periods as long as 15 months before implantation is initiated. In other species, delayed implantation can be induced by postpartum suckling or by performing ovariectomy on day 3 of pregnancy.[65] Delayed implantation is characterized by a marked decrease in synthesis of DNA and protein by the blastocyst. The embryo can be maintained at the blastocyst stage by injecting the mother with progesterone.[64] In mice the endometrium is first primed by basal-level estrogen, and then maintained during a progesterone-dependent sensitization stage that is finally attenuated by an estrogen surge shortly prior to the blastocyst's entry into the uterus.[63] In other species the nidatory surge of estrogen is not required. On the basis of these findings, the steroid hormonal requirements for implantation have been determined.

Prostaglandins play an important role in mediating vascular changes and decidualization of the endometrium. Their importance is related to their stimulatory effect on the uterus. Prostaglandin production in the pregnant or pseudopregnant rat uterus peaks on day 5, when uterine tissue is most sensitive to stimuli. Maximal uterine response to PGE_2, an isomer of PGE, may be due to endometrial receptors for these substances.[66] High-affinity PGE_2-binding sites may represent PGE_2 receptors, although equivalent binding sites for $PGF_{2\alpha}$ have not been detected. Alternatively, the changes in endometrial vascular permeability may require other mediators in addition to prostaglandins, and it may be the production, release, or action of these compounds that determines maximum uterine sensitization.[67] As a result of the heightened responsiveness to PGE_2 and other stimuli, the sensitized uterus can undergo the decidualization process. During decidualization, the stromal cells of the endometrium undergo growth and differentiation into decidual cells that ultimately give rise to the maternal component of the placenta in pregnancy. It is always preceded by increased endometrial vascular permeability, which in the rodent occurs during a limited time, after pregnancy or pseudopregnancy.[43] Its occurrence can be detected by intravenously injecting rats with Evans blue on day 6 of pregnancy. After removing the uterus, implantation sites are clearly seen as well-defined blue stripes indicating the regions of increased capillary permeability.[68]

In rodents, implantation can be interrupted by injection of prostaglandin inhibitors, such as indomethacin, which prevent the increase in endometrial vascular permeability.[49] Additional evidence for a role for prostaglandins in the earliest stages of implantation is the finding of increased concentrations of these substances at prospective implantation sites.[43,67] The source of these prostaglandins is not known, but it is likely that their synthesis may be stimulated by the tissue damage that accompanies implantation.

The sequential maturation of uterine epithelium in the mouse model is closely linked to the hormonal conditioning effects of estrogen and progesterone.[50] During the prereceptive or neutral period, progesterone stimulation for 48 hours exerts a priming effect on the uterus. This produces an increase in estrogen receptors in the stromal layer of the endometrium and redirects the effect of estrogen from the epithelial to the stromal layer. During this period of progesterone priming, the uterus shows suboptimal sensitivity for the decidual reaction, allowing the blastocyst to survive in dormancy. The subsequent action of estrogen then serves to produce a state of uterine receptivity, followed in 36 hours by a state of uterine refractoriness.[50,51] During the latter period an environment hostile to the embryo develops, accompanied by inhibition of the decidual reaction.

Maintenance of the uterus in the neutral state requires the continuity of progesterone administration. The antiprogesterone RU-486 given on day 1 of pregnancy in the rat extends the receptive phase beyond the normal timing and postpones establishment of uterine refractoriness.[69] Increasing the dose of RU-486 adversely affects fertility by reducing egg survival.[52]

HATCHING ENZYMES

The emergence of the blastocyst from the zona pellucida prior to attachment to the uterus is probably the result of at least three forces. These include a degradative enzyme at the surface of the blastocyst, a degradative enzyme secreted by the uterus, and the physical expansion and contraction of the blastocoele. It appears that an absolute requirement for the uterine protease does not exist, owing to the ability of blastocysts to hatch in culture.[28,70] However, hatching in vitro does not occur for about 24 hours after the collection of mouse blastocysts on day 4 of gestation, while blastocysts free of their zona pellucida may be found in the uterus late on day 4.[71] Therefore,

intrauterine enzymes may affect the time sequence of hatching.

The zona pellucida is composed of three glycoproteins secreted by the oocyte, and possibly the granulosa cells, as well, during early egg maturation.[72,73] These glycoproteins are assembled into an extracellular matrix that surrounds the ovum and remains throughout preimplantation embryogenesis. In addition to providing the ovum with physical protection, the zona pellucida glycoproteins serve as species-specific sperm-recognition molecules and induce the acrosome reaction after sperm binding.[74] The zona pellucida is subject to dissolution by several agents, including proteases, low pH, and reducing agents.[75] The mouse has been shown to produce a 74,000 daltons trypsinlike enzyme called strypsin, which is localized at the surface of particular blastomeres.[76] The localization of strypsin in the mural trophectoderm correlates with the location of the corresponding linear slit that forms in the zona pellucida during hatching in vitro. In addition to strypsin and the physical movements of the embryo, factors secreted by the uterus may facilitate the breakdown of the zona pellucida in vivo. There is evidence that in some mammals proteases capable of lysing the zona pellucida are secreted by the uterus.[77] The lowering of the local pH by released carbon dioxide from the embryo or the secretion of a reducing agent such as glutathione in the vicinity of the blastocyst would also accelerate zona lysis; however, evidence for these mechanisms is lacking. Acting in concert, proteases of both embryonic and uterine origin, together with other factors, may assure rapid hatching in utero.

TROPHOBLAST–EPITHELIAL INTERACTIONS

As the embryo comes into close contact with the endometrium, the microvilli on its surface flatten and interdigitate with those on the luminal surface of the epithelial cells.[6] The epithelial surface of the endometrium is thrown into folds, providing ample surface area for contact with the blastocyst. Eventually the cell membranes are in intimate contact, and junctional complexes are formed. At this point, the embryo can no longer be dislodged from the surface of the epithelial cells by flushing the uterus with physiologic solution. Schlafke and Enders[6] described three types of subsequent interactions between the implanting trophoblast and the uterine epithelium. In the first type, trophoblast cells intrude between uterine epithelial cells and make their way to the basement membrane. In the second type, the epithelial cells lift off from the basement membrane, thus allowing the trophoblast to insinuate itself underneath the epithelium. In the third type, fusion of trophoblast cells with individual uterine epithelial cells occurs, as described in the rabbit.[78] This last process of gaining entry into the epithelial layer poses interesting theories regarding the immunologic consequences of mixing cells of two different genotypes.

Trophoblast cells co-cultured with uterine epithelial monolayers fail to display the cell–cell interactions seen in vivo, and instead displace the epithelia and adhere to the substratum.[16,17,79] An alternative model system for studying the initial interaction of mouse trophoblast cells with the uterine epithelium has been described[80] wherein vesicles are formed from sheets of isolated epithelium and incubated with mouse blastocysts in hanging-drop culture. Observations of these cells by electron microscopy revealed features found in vivo,[6] such as interdigitation of surface microvilli, junctional formation, phagocytosis of dead epithelia, and invasion.[80] In future studies of cell–cell interactions during this phase of implantation, such models should prove superior to the co-culture of embryos with monolayers of epithelia.

INVASION OF
THE ENDOMETRIUM

During invasion of the stromal layer of the endometrium by the trophoblast giant cells (mouse) or syncytial trophoblast (human), the extracellular matrix surrounding decidual cells is penetrated. A similar, albeit uncontrolled, process occurs during metastasis by cancer cells in many tissues. Although the two processes are not completely analogous, metastasis is more easily studied experimentally than implantation, and it is useful to consider the abundant information that has been gathered on the subject of tumor cell invasion.

Composition of the
Extracellular Matrix

The extracellular matrix is composed primarily of three classes of macromolecules: proteoglycans, collagens, and adhesion glycoproteins (Table 33–1). Proteoglycans are composed of a small protein core and a large sulfated carbohydrate called a glycosaminoglycan, whereas collagens and glycoproteins are synthesized as proteins that are subsequently glycosylated with various amounts of carbohydrate (approximately 5 to 40% of total weight). Extracellular matrix both surrounds cells and is arranged as basement membrane.[81,82] A basement membrane is present between the epithelial layer and underlying stroma in most tissues, including the uterus. The composition and arrangement of the extracellular

TABLE 33–1. COMPONENTS OF THE EXTRACELLULAR MATRIX

Components and Examples	Associated Cell Type
Glycosaminoglycans of proteoglycans	
Hyaluronic acid	Loose connective tissue
Chondroitin sulfate	Cartilage, aorta
Dermatan sulfate	Skin
Heparin sulfate	Basement membrane, organs
Keratan sulfate	Cornea, cartilage, bone
Collagen	
I and III	Connective tissue, organs
II	Cartilage, vitreous humor
IV	Epithelial (basement membrane)
V	Tendon
VI	Blood vessels, placenta
VII	Amnion
Adhesion glycoproteins	
Fibronectin	Fibroblast cells
Laminin	Epithelial (basement membrane)
Vitronectin	Fibroblasts
Chondronectin	Chondrocytes

Source: From references 81, 110, and 111.

matrix varies among tissue types and within tissue layers. Therefore, as a cell invades a tissue it encounters extracellular matrix of varying composition and supramolecular structure. The basement membrane or basal lamina characteristically contains collagen type IV, heparin sulfate proteoglycan, and the glycoprotein laminin, while stroma is characterized as having an extracellular matrix with predominantly collagen types I and III, chondroitin sulfate proteoglycans, and the glycoprotein fibronectin. This description is very generalized, and content varies from tissue to tissue, and may include other components. During differentiation of the uterine stroma fibroblasts into decidua, increased synthesis and secretion of type IV collagen, laminin, and heparin sulfate proteoglycan has been observed,[83,84] making it more similar to the overlying basement membrane. Fibronectin and hyaluronic acid are also present in the decidualized endometrium.[83–85]

The macromolecules that make up the extracellular matrix interact with each other as well as with receptors located at the surface of cells that come in contact with the matrix.[81,82] The adhesion glycoproteins have several structural domains capable of binding to other matrix components and cell surface receptors. One of the best studied is fibronectin, which has binding domains for heparinsulfate, hyaluronic acid, collagen types I and III (gelatin), and a cell surface receptor glycoprotein, integrin, present in a variety of fibroblasts and transformed cells.[81,82] Integrin has been identified and shown to be composed of two glycoproteins with molecular weights of about 140,000 daltons.[86,87] In addition, the cell-binding site of fibronectin has been isolated and sequenced.[88] Through the binding interactions of these many components the extracellular matrix assumes various arrangements that influence the cells that come in contact with it. It has been shown that the interaction of cells with certain extracellular matrix components can be chemotactic and can influence the differentiation of those cells.[82,89,90]

Models of Invasion Based on Metastasis

A useful paradigm for developing an understanding of implantation is the metastasis of tumor cells. Trophoblast cells invading the endometrium must carry out some of the same processes as tumor cells invading host tissues. Whereas cancer is an uncontrolled cellular proliferation, trophoblast proliferation is self-limited and does not normally metastasize through the circulatory system.[11] Regardless, both trophoblasts and tumor cells invade by passing through an epithelial layer, penetrating the basement membrane, and migrating within the extracellular matrix of the underlying stroma.

During metastasis, secondary tumor deposits are formed by tumor cells that have left the primary tumor, traveled in the circulation, and initiated a secondary tumor in a distant organ. To carry out this process, the tumor cells must traverse the basement membrane surrounding the primary tumor as well as that of the invaded organ, and then move into the extracellular matrix surrounding the interstitial stromal cells at the secondary site. Liotta and co-workers[91] described this process and studied it in vitro using cultured carcinoma cells. The tumor cells move through the peripheral blood to a new site where they attach to the endothelial cells lining a venule or capillary wall. The tumor cells are able to extend cell processes between the endothelial cells and gain access to the underlying basement membrane.

Liotta and associates[91] outlined a three-step hypothesis to explain the biochemical basis of the subsequent invasion of the basement membrane and underlying extracellular matrix. Tumor cells initially attach to the basement membrane or stromal extracellular matrix, degrade it locally to gain access through it, and finally migrate through it to a new location where the process is repeated. In this manner they invade and proliferate at the new location. These three activities can be studied separately in vitro.[91] Trophoblast cells must accomplish an analogous task when establishing a site for placentation during pregnancy.

The elements of the three-step hypothesis of tumor invasion have been supported by experiments

with tumor cells cultured in vitro. Specific glycoproteins isolated from the extracellular matrix, such as fibronectin and laminin, have been used in cell attachment assays to demonstrate the ability of tumor cells to recognize these glycoproteins and adhere to them.[81,91] Analysis of the culture medium from tumor cells grown in vitro demonstrated their ability to secrete high concentrations of hydrolytic enzymes capable of degrading the matrix components.[91] In vivo these enzymes may work locally, becoming diluted by diffusion and inactivated by natural protease inhibitors present in the serum and interstitial fluid. Therefore the capacity for very localized degradation of the matrix by tumor cells has been shown to be feasible. Locomotion of tumor cells into the new site may be directed by chemotactic factors, facilitating continued invasion inward. Laminin has been shown to elicit a chemotactic response from tumor cells in vitro.[89,90] The preference of certain cells for metastasizing to particular organs may be a function of chemotactic factors arising from cells in those organs.[91] Trophoblast cells cultured in vitro and blastocysts in outgrowth culture have been used to study similar biochemical processes that may occur during implantation.[13,15,18,29,33,85,92-95]

In-Vitro Biochemical Studies of Trophoblast Invasion

Because of the number of cell types involved, inaccessibility, and the limited amount of material comprising the embryo itself, cell biologic and biochemical studies of implantation have been limited. Implantation and placenta formation is a unique feature of mammals, and so, unlike many other aspects of embryogenesis, there is no model of this process in lower organisms where large numbers of embryos can be produced for biochemical analysis. Attempts have been made to isolate and focus on specific facets of implantation by artificially inducing the decidual response in the absence of an embryo,[54] by inducing pseudopregnancy through ovariectomy and steroid hormone stimulation,[96,97] and through delayed implantation.[65] A successful model for studying the ability of the blastocyst to grow and differentiate in the absence of maternal influences has been in-vitro outgrowth culture.[13] It is important, however, that caution be used when extrapolating information gained through in-vitro experimentation to the whole animal unless confirming experiments have been performed in vivo.

Until recently, little was known about the adhesive properties of the blastocyst at implantation, although it was hypothesized early that the prominent glycocalyx observed at the surface of trophoblast and endometrial cells was involved.[6] Studies of early embryo development leading up to implantation have indicated that glycoprotein synthesis by the blastocyst is critical for attachment competence in vitro. An inhibitor of N-glycosylation of proteins, tunicamycin, will prevent embryos at the blastocyst stage from attaching in vitro.[98,99] The drug appears to block the synthesis of a major class of large-molecular-weight oligosaccharides that are added to glycoproteins by morulae and blastocysts.[100] Enzymes essential to the initial assembly of N-linked oligosaccharides increase in their specific activity as development proceeds toward implantation,[99] further indicating the important role for this class of macromolecules at implantation. It is still unclear what constitutes the molecular mechanism of trophoblast adhesion; however, studies of implantation using in vitro models have begun to shed some light on this topic.

When blastocysts are cultured in complex, serum-containing medium they attach to the plastic or glass substratum by the mural trophoblast cells and, as in utero, the giant cells become polyploid through endoreduplication.[12,15] They then spread on the substratum, forming a monolayer, much like tissue culture cells (Fig. 33–5). Although several notable differences between implantation and in vitro outgrowth of blastocysts have been identified,[13,15] it is nevertheless possible to produce somewhat normal fetuses of very advanced developmental stages in vitro.[101] The outgrowing trophoblast cells demonstrate numerous ectoplasmic developments, including filopodia, lobopodia, and lamellipodia.[13] These activities are reminiscent of the early implantation period in vivo when trophoblasts extend flanges of

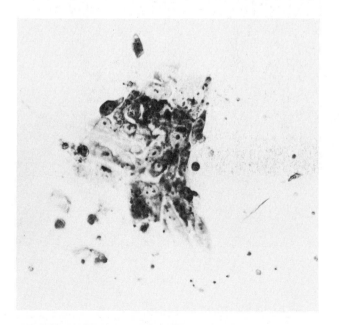

Figure 33–5. A mouse blastocyst cultured in vitro on a substratum precoated with fibronectin by the method of Armant el al.[93] The trophoblast cells have undergone differentiation into giant cells that contain large nuclei with many nucleoli. These cells migrate extensively on the substratum and are morphologically similar to trophoblasts cultured in serum-containing medium.[13]

cytoplasm between the luminal epithelium and into the underlying basement membrane.[13] In the in-vitro outgrowth model, however, there is clearly no contact with the uterine epithelium, as occurs in utero.[6] Indeed, co-culture of blastocysts and uterine epithelial cells results in a clearing of the epithelial cells in the vicinity of the embryo, perhaps due to the release of cytolytic agents.[16,17,79] In view of this aggressive trophoblast behavior in vitro, it is most likely that trophoblast outgrowth is a model for the invasive phase of implantation.

The ability of blastocysts to attach and outgrow in medium supplemented with serum has been shown to be developmentally regulated and not merely a consequence of the loss of the zona pellucida.[29,30] The media requirements for this activity have been found to include certain amino acids,[102–104] glucose,[105] and a macromolecular component of serum.[106] It was recognized early that the macromolecular component of serum may serve to provide a coat of one or more proteins on the surface of culture dishes.[29] In early studies, outgrowth-promoting activity was provided by collagen[29] and fetuin[92] preparations that were probably impure mixtures of several proteins. Studies undertaken in recent years have demonstrated that mouse embryos will outgrow in serum-free media on substrata containing highly purified preparations of extracellular matrix components present in the stroma during trophoblast invasion,[84,107–109] including fibronectin, laminin, vitronectin,[93,94] or hyaluronate.[84]

The components of the extracellular matrix have been extensively studied biochemically.[81,82,86,90,91,110,111] Studies of cells in tissue culture reveal that in addition to cell adhesion and spreading, these molecules have been associated with cell migration and tumor cell invasion during metastasis.[90,112,113] Fibronectin, laminin, and vitronectin can bind to a number of other extracellular matrix and cell surface macromolecules (collagens, proteoglycans, and membrane glycoprotein receptors) through specific structural domains within the glycoproteins.[81,82,90,91] The receptor-binding sites of fibronectin and vitronectin are identical and have been identified as the amino acid sequence Arg-Gly-Asp-Ser.[88] Synthetic peptides containing this sequence will competitively inhibit fibronectin and vitronectin-mediated cell adhesion through specific interaction with the cell surface receptors (integrins).[114,115] A synthetic peptide of this structure will block blastocyst adhesion on either fibronectin or vitronectin-coated substrata.[94] Furthermore, blastocyst outgrowth is prevented by an antiserum raised against a group of membrane glycoproteins,[95] including one of 140,000 daltons, which is the molecular weight of integrins.[86] These results suggest that receptors for extracellular matrix components may play an important role in the developmental regulation of trophoblast adhesion during blastocyst outgrowth in vitro.

It can only be speculated that the molecular events uncovered in the in vitro outgrowth model play a role during the process of implantation in utero. The glycoconjugates found to promote blastocyst outgrowth are secreted by the decidual cells into the extracellular matrix,[107,108] and increases in the production of hyaluronate in the mouse[85] and laminin in the human[83,84] occur in the uterus at the time it becomes receptive to an implanting embryo. It is not clear, however, as to what molecules are produced by the trophoblast cells that allow their adhesion to these extracellular matrix molecules, because the active matrix components have binding sites for a number of ligands, including unique cell surface receptors for each of the outgrowth-promoting substances. Perhaps the trophoblast must produce several receptors that are used at different times as it comes in contact with various components of a heterogeneous matrix during its invasion of the endometrium (see Fig. 33–3). It also must be shown that a molecule putatively involved in the adhesion of trophoblasts during the peri-implantation stage is developmentally regulated in a way that corresponds with the changing adhesive properties of the trophoblast cells. Furthermore, proof is still needed that the adhesiveness of trophoblasts in vitro corresponds with attachment during implantation in vivo through the use of specific molecular probes to perturb implantation in animals. Once the molecular basis of implantation is better understood, it will be possible to exploit the clinical relevance of the process to infertility.

REFERENCES

1. Rock JA, Zacur HA: The clinical management of repeated early pregnancy wastage. *Fertil Steril* 39:123, 1983.
2. Glass RH, Golbus MS: Habitual abortion. *Fertil Steril* 29:257, 1978.
3. Webb PD, Glasser SR: Implantation, in Wolfe DP, Quigley MM (eds): *Human In Vitro Fertilization and Embryo Transfer.* New York, Plenum, 1984, pp 341–364.
4. Lala PK, Kearns M, Parkar RS, Scodras J, Johnson S: Immunological role of the cellular constituents of the decidua in maintenance of semiallogenic pregnancy. *Ann NY Acad Sci* 476:183, 1986.
5. Weiser RS: Pregnancy as an experimental system for the study of immunologic phenomena, in Blaudau RJ (ed): *Biology of the Blastocyst.* Chicago: University of Chicago Press, 1971, pp 523–535.
6. Schlafke S, Enders AC: Cellular basis of interaction between trophoblast and uterus at implantation. *Biol Reprod* 12:41, 1975.
7. Finn CA: Species variation in implantation. *Prog Reprod Biol* 7:253, 1980.
8. Wimsatt WA: Some comparative aspects of implantation. *Biol Reprod* 12:1, 1975.
9. Pijnenborg R, Robertson WB, Brosens I, Dixon G: Review article: Trophoblast invasion and the establishment of haemochorial placentation in man and laboratory animals. *Placenta* 2:71, 1981.
10. Hertig AT, Rock J: Two human ova of the pre-villous stage having a developmental age of about seven and nine days respectively. *Contri Embryol* 31:65,1945.
11. Ilgren EB: Review article: Control of trophoblastic growth. *Placenta* 4:307, 1983.
12. Barlow PW, Owen DJ, Graham CF: DNA synthesis in the pre-implantation mouse embryo. *J Embryol Exp Morphol* 27:431, 1972.
13. Enders A, Chavez DJ, Schlafke S: Comparison of implantation in utero and in vitro, in Glasser SR, Bullock DW (eds): *Cellular and Molecular Aspects of Implantation.* New York, Plenum, 1981, pp 365–382.
14. Gardner RL: Origin and differentiation of extraembryonic tissues in the mouse. *Int Rev Exp Pathol* 24:63, 1983.
15. Jenkinson EJ: The in vitro blastocyst outgrowth system as a model for the analysis of peri-implantation development, in Johnson M (ed): *Development in Mammals.* Amsterdam, Elsevier-North Holland, 1978, vol 2, pp 151–172.
16. Sherman MI, Solomon DS: The relationships between the early mouse embryo and its environment, in Market CL, Papaconstantinou J (eds): *Developmental Biology of Reproduction.* New York, Academic Press, 1975, pp 277–309.
17. Salomon DS, Sherman MI: Implantation and invasiveness of mouse blastocysts on uterine monolayers. *Exp Cell Res* 90:261, 1975.
18. Glass RH, Aggeler J, Spindle A, Pedersen R, Werb Z: Degradation of extracellular matrix by mouse trophoblast outgrowths: A model for implantation. *J Cell Biol* 96:1108, 1983.
19. Johnson MH: Membrane events associated with the generation of a blastocyst. *Int Rev Cytol Suppl* 12:1, 1981.
20. Pratt HPM, Ziomek CA, Reeve WJD, Johnson MH: Compaction of the mouse embryo: An analysis of its components. *J Embryol Exp Morphol* 70:113, 1982.
21. Ducibella T: Surface changes of the developing trophoblast cell, in Johnson MH (ed): *Development in Mammals.* Amsterdam, Elsevier-North Holland, 1977, vol 1, pp 5–30.
22. Reeve WJD, Ziomek CA: Distribution of microvilli on dissociated blastomeres from mouse embryos: Evidence for surface polarization at compaction. *J Embryol Exp Morphol* 62:339, 1981.
23. Ziomek CA, Johnson MH: Cell surface interaction induces polarization of mouse 8-cell blastomeres at compaction. *Cell* 21:935, 1980.
24. Tarkowski AK, Wroblewska J: Development of blastomeres of mouse eggs isolated at the 4- to 8-cell stage. *J Embryol Exp Morphol* 18:155, 1967.
25. Hillman N, Sherman MI, Graham C: The effect of spatial arrangement on cell determination during mouse development. *J Embryol Exp Morphol* 28:263, 1972.
26. Benos DJ, Biggers JD, Balaban RS, Mills JW, Overstrom EW: Developmental aspects of sodium-dependent transport processes of preimplantation rabbit embryos, in Graves JS (ed): *Regulation and Development of Membrane Transport Processes.* New York, Wiley, 1985, pp 211–235.
27. Dickson AD: The form of the mouse blastocyst. *J Anat* 100:335, 1966.
28. Diaz S, Ortiz ME, Croxatto HB: Studies on the duration of ovum transport by the human oviduct. III. Time interval between the luteinizing hormone peak and recovery of ova by transcervical flushing of the uterus in normal women. *Am J Obstet Gynecol* 137:116, 1980.
29. Jenkinson EJ, Wilson IB: In vitro studies on the control of trophoblast outgrowth in the mouse. *J Embryol Exp Morphol* 30:21, 1973.
30. Sherman MI, Atienza-Samols S: In vitro studies on the surface adhesiveness of mouse blastocysts, in Ludwig H, Tauber PF (eds): *Human Fertilization.* Littleton, MA, PSG, 1978, pp 179–183.
31. Borghese E, Cassini A: Cleavage of mouse egg, in Rose GG (ed): *Cinemicrography in Cell Biology.* New York, Academic Press, 1963, p 274.
32. Mossman HW: Orientation and site of attachment of the blastocyst: A comparative study, in Blandau RJ (ed): *The Biology of the Blastocyst.* Chicago, University of Chicago Press, 1971, pp 49–57.
33. Chavez DJ: Cellular aspects of implantation, in Van Blerkom J, Motta PJ (eds): *Ultrastructure of Reproduction.* The Hague, Martinus Nijhoff, 1984, pp 247–259.
34. Nilson BD: Electron microscopic aspects of epithelial changes related to implantation. *Prog Reprod Biol* 7:70, 1980.
35. Schlafke S, Welsh AD, Enders AC: Penetration of the basal lamina of the uterine luminal epithelium during implantation in the rat. *Anat Rec* 212:47, 1985.
36. Boyd JD, Hamilton WI: The giant cells of the pregnant human uterus. *J Obstet Gynaecol Br Emp* 67:208, 1960.
37. Billington WD: Biology of the trophoblast, in Bishop MW (ed): *Reproductive Physiology.* London, Logos, 1971, vol 5, pp 27–47.
38. Sundstrom P, Nilsson O, Liedholm P: Scanning electron microscopy of human preimplantation endometrium in normal and clomiphene/hCG-stimulated cycles. *Fertil Steril* 40:642, 1983.

39. Bloom W, Fawcett DW: *A Textbook of Histology*. Philadelphia, Saunders, 1986, pp 877–888.

40. Wynn RM: Ultrastructural development of the human decidua. *Am J Obstet Gynecol* 118:652, 1974.

41. Kelly DE, Wood RI, Enders AC: *Bailey's Textbook of Microscopic Anatomy*, ed 18. Baltimore, Williams & Wilkins, 1984, pp 743–747.

42. Glasser SR: The uterine environment in decidualization and implantation, in Balin H, Glasser SR (eds): *Reproductive Biology*. Amsterdam, Excerpta Medica, 1972, pp 776–833.

43. Kennedy TG: Prostaglandins and uterine sensitization for the decidual cell reaction. *Ann NY Acad Sci* 476:43, 1986.

44. Padykula HA: Cellular mechanisms involved in cyclic stromal renewal of the uterus. III. Cells of the immune response. *Anat Rec* 184:49, 1976.

45. Padykula HA, Tansey TR: The occurrence of uterine stromal and intraepithelial monocytes and heterophils during normal late pregnancy in the rat. *Anat Rec* 193:329, 1979.

46. Parr MB, Parr EL: Permeability of the primary decidual zone in the rat uterus: Studies using fluorescein-labeled proteins and dextrans. *Biol Reprod* 34:393, 1986.

47. Pritchard JA, MacDonald PC, Gant NF: *Williams Obstetrics*, ed 7. E Norwalk, CT, Appleton-Century-Crofts, 1985, pp 98–106.

48. Cove H: *Surgical Pathology of the Endometrium*. Philadelphia, Lippincott, 1981, pp 26–36.

49. Kasamo M, Ishikawa M, Yamashita K, Sengoku K, Shimizu T: Possible role of prostaglandin F in blastocyst implantation. *Prostaglandins* 31:321, 1986.

50. De Hertogh R, Ekka E, Vanderheyden I, Glorieux B: Estrogen and progestogen receptors in the implantation sites and interembryonic segments of rat uterus endometrium and myometrium. *Endocrinology* 119:680, 1986.

51. Gidley-Baird A, O'Neill C, Sinosich MJ, Porter RN, Pike IL: Failure of implantation in human in vitro fertilization and embryo transfer patients: The effect of altered progesterone/estrogen ratios in humans and mice. *Fertil Steril* 45:69, 1986.

52. Phychoyos A: Uterine receptivity for nidation. *Ann NY Acad Sci* 476:36, 1986.

53. Heap RB, Flint AP, Gadsby JE: Role of embryonic signals in the establishment of pregnancy. *Br Med Bull* 35:129, 1979.

54. Dey SK, Johnson DC: Embryonic signals in pregnancy. *Ann NY Acad Sci* 476:49, 1986.

55. Boving BG: Implantation. *Ann NY Acad Sci* 75:700, 1959.

56. Fishel SB, Edwards RG, Evans CJ: Human chorionic gonadatropin secreted by preimplantation embryos cultured in vitro. *Science* 223:816, 1984.

57. Shutt DA, Lopata A: The secretion of hormones during the culture of human preimplantation embryos with corona cells. *Fertil Steril* 35:413, 1981.

58. Csapo AI, Pulkkinen MD, Wiest WG: Effects of luteectomy and progesterone replacement therapy in early pregnant patients. *Am J Obstet Gynecol* 115:759, 1973.

59. Joshi NJ, Nandedkar TD: Effects of intrauterine instillation of antiserum to hCG during early pregnancy in mice. *Acta Endocrinol* 107:268, 1984.

60. Godkin JD, Bazer FW, Roberts RM: Ovine trophoblast protein 1, an early secreted blastocyst protein, binds specifically to uterine endometrium and affects protein synthesis. *Endocrinology* 114:120, 1984.

61. Imakawa K, Anthony RV, Kazemi M, et al: Interferon-like sequence of ovine trophoblast protein secreted by embryonic trophectoderm. *Nature* 330:377, 1987.

62. Shelesnyak MC: Inhibition of decidual cell formation in the pseudopregnant rat by histamine antagonists. *Am J Physiol* 170:522, 1952.

63. Shelesnyak MC: A history of research on nidation. *Ann NY Acad Sci* 476:5, 1986.

64. Evans CA, Kennedy TB: Blastocyst implantation in ovariectomized, adrenalectomized hamsters treated with inhibitors of steroidogenesis during the preimplantation period. *Steroids* 36:41, 1980.

65. Van Blerkom J, Chavez DJ, Bell H: Molecular and cellular aspects of facultative delayed implantation in the mouse, in Ciba Foundation Symposium: *Maternal Recognition of Pregnancy*. Amsterdam, Excerpta Medica, 1979, p 141.

66. Kabawat SE, Mahpareh MZ, Driscoll SG, Bhan AK: Implantation site in normal pregnancy. A study with monoclonal antibodies. *Am J Pathol* 118:76, 1985.

67. Malathy PV, Cheng HC, Dey SK: Production of leukotrienes and prostaglandins in the rat uterus during preiimplantation period. *Prostaglandins* 32:605, 1986.

68. Martel D, Psychos A: Estrogen receptors in the nidatory sites of the rat endometrium. *Science* 211:1454, 1981.

69. Rider V, Heap RB, Wang MY, Feinstein A: Anti-progesterone monoclonal antibody affects early cleavage and implantation in the mouse by mechanisms that are influenced by genotype. *J Reprod Fertil* 79:33, 1987.

70. Cole RJ: Cinemicrographic observations on the trophoblast and zona pellucida of the mouse blastocyst. *J Embryol Exp Morphol* 17:481, 1967.

71. Rumery RE, Blandau RJ: Loss of zona pellucida and prolonged gestation in delayed implantation in mice, in Blandau RJ (ed): *The Biology of the Blastocyst*. Chicago, University of Chicago Press, 1971, pp 115–129.

72. Bleil JD, Wasserman PM: Structure and function of the zona pellucida: Identification and characterization of the proteins of the mouse oocyte's zona pellucida. *Dev Biol* 76:185, 1980.

73. Bleil JD, Wasserman PM: Synthesis of zona pellucida proteins by denuded and follicle-enclosed mouse oocytes during culture in vitro. *Proc Natl Acad Sci USA* 77:1029, 1980.

74. Bleil JD, Wasserman PM: Mammalian sperm-egg interaction: Identification of a glycoprotein in mouse egg zonae pellucidae possessing receptor activity for sperm. *Cell* 20:837, 1980.

75. Wolf DP: The mammalian egg's block to polysperm, in Mastroianni L, Biggers JD (eds): *Fertilization and Embryonic Development in Vitro*. New York, Plenum, 1981, pp 183–197.

76. Perona RM, Wasserman PM: Mouse blastocysts hatch in vitro by using a trypsin-like proteinase associated with cells of mural trophectoderm. *Dev Biol* 114:42, 1986.

77. Denker HW: Role of proteinases in implantation. *Prog Reprod Biol* 7:28, 1980.

78. Larsen JF: Electron microscopy of the implantation site in the rabbit. *Am J Anat* 109:319, 1961.

79. Glass RH, Spindle AI, Pedersen RA: Mouse embryo attachment to substratum and interaction of trophoblast with cultured cells. *J Exp Zool* 208:327, 1979.

80. Morris JE, Potter SW, Rynd LS, Buckley PM: Adhesion of mouse blastocysts to uterine epithelium in culture: A requirement for mutual surface interactions. *J Exp Zool* 225:467, 1983.

81. Yamada K: Cell surface interactions with extracellular materials. *Annu Rev Biochem* 52:761, 1983.

82. Hynes RO, Yamada KM: Fibronectins: Multifunctional modular glycoproteins. *J Cell Biol* 95:369, 1982.

83. Kisalus LL, Herr JC, Little CD: Immunolocalization of extracellular matrix proteins and collagen synthesis in first-trimester human decidua. *Anat Rec* 218:402, 1987.

84. Wewer UM, Faber M, Liotta LA, Albrechtsen R: Immunochemical and ultrastructural assessment of the nature of the pericellular basement membrane of human dedidual cells. *Lab Invest* 53:624, 1985.

85. Carson DD, Dutt A, Tang JP: Glycoconjugate synthesis during early pregnancy: Hyaluronate synthesis and function. *Dev Biol* 120:228, 1987.

86. Pytela R, Pierschbacher MD, Ruoslahti E: Identification and isolation of a 140 kd cell surface glycoprotein with properties expected of a fibronectin receptor. *Cell* 40:191, 1985.

87. Brown PJ, Juliano RL: Selective inhibition of fibronectin-mediated cell adhesion by monoclonal antibodies to a cell-surface glycoprotein. *Science* 228:1448, 1985.

88. Pierschbacher MD, Ruoslahti E: Cell attachment activity of fibronectin can be duplicated by small synthetic fragments of the molecule. *Nature* 309:30, 1984.

89. McCarthy JB, Furcht LT: Laminin and fibronectin promote the haptotactic migration of B16 mouse melanoma cells in vitro. *J Cell Biol* 98:1474, 1984.

90. Martin GR, Timpl R: Laminin and other basement membrane components. *Annu Rev Cell Biol* 3:57, 1987.

91. Liotta LA, Rao CN, Wewer UM: Biochemical interactions of tumor cells with the basement membrane. *Annu Rev Biochem* 55:1037, 1986.

92. Rizzino A, Sherman MI: Development and differentiation of mouse blastocysts in serum-free medium. *Exp Cell Res* 121:222, 1979.

93. Armant DR, Kaplan HA, Lennarz WJ: Fibronectin and laminin promote in vitro attachment and outgrowth of mouse blastocysts. *Dev Biol* 116:519, 1986.

94. Armant DR, Kaplan HA, Mover H, Lennarz WJ: The effect of hexapeptides on attachment and outgrowth of mouse blastocysts

cultured in vitro: Evidence for the involvement of the cell recognition tripeptide Arg-Gly-Asp. *Proc Natl Acad Sci USA* 83:675, 1986.

95. Richa J, Damsky CH, Buck C, Knowles BB, Solter D: Cell surface glycoproteins mediate compaction, trophoblast attachment, and endoderm formation during early mouse development. *Dev Biol* 108:513, 1985.

96. Psychoyos A: Hormonal control of ovoimplantation. *Vitam Horm* 31:20, 1973.

97. Finn CA, Martin L: The control of implantation. *J Reprod Fertil* 39:195, 1974.

98. Surani MAH: Glycoprotein synthesis and inhibition of glycosylation by tunicamycin in preimplantation mouse embryos: Compaction and trophoblast adhesion. *Cell* 18:217, 1979.

99. Armant DR, Kaplan HA, Lennarz WJ: N-linked glycoprotein biosynthesis in the developing mouse embryo. *Dev Biol* 113:228, 1986.

100. Iwakura Y, Nozaki M: Effects of tunicamycin on preimplantation mouse embryos: prevention of molecular differentiation during blastocyst formation. *Dev Biol* 112:135, 1985.

101. Hsu YC: In vitro development of individually cultured whole mouse embryos from blastocyst to early somite stage. *Dev Biol* 68:453, 1979.

102. Gwatkins R: Amino acid requirements for attachment and outgrowth of the mouse blastocyst in vitro. *J Cell Physiol* 66:335, 1966.

103. Spindle A, Pedersen RA: Hatching, attachment, and outgrowth of mouse blastocysts in vitro: Fixed nitrogen requirements. *J Exp Zool* 186:305, 1973.

104. Sherman MI, Barlow PW: Deoxyribonucleic acid content in delayed mouse blastocysts. *J Reprod Fertil* 29:123, 1972.

105. Wordinger RJ, Brinster RL: Influence of reduced glucose levels on the in vitro hatching, attachment and trophoblast outgrowth of the mouse blastocyst. *Dev Biol* 53:294, 1976.

106. Gwatkins R: Defined media and development of mammalian eggs in vitro. *Ann NY Acad Sci* 139:79, 1966.

107. Wartiovaara J, Leivo I, Vaheri A: Expression of the cell surface-associated glycoprotein, fibronectin, in the early mouse embryo. *Dev Biol* 69:247, 1979.

108. Leivo I, Vaheri A, Timpl R, Wartiovaara J: Appearance and distribution of collagens and laminin in the early mouse embryo. *Dev Biol* 76:100, 1980.

109. Grinnell F, Head JR, Hoffpauir K: Fibronectin and cell shape in vivo: Studies on the endometrium during pregnancy. *J Cell Biol* 94:597, 1982.

110. Roden L: Structure and metabolism of connective tissue proteoglycans, in Lennarz WJ (ed): *The Biochemistry of Glycoproteins and Proteoglycans.* New York, Plenum, 1980, pp 267–371.

111. Maye R: The different types of collagen and collagenous peptides, in Trelstad RL (ed): *The Role of Extracellular Matrix in Development.* New York, Liss, 1984, pp 33–42.

112. Thiery JP, Duband J, Tucker GC: Cell migration in the vertebrate embryo: Role of cell adhesion and tissue environment in pattern formation. *Annu Rev Cell Biol* 1:91, 1985.

113. McCarthy JB, Hagen S, Furcht LT: Human fibronectin contains distinct adhesion- and motility-promoting domains for metastatic melanoma cells. *J Cell Biol* 102:179, 1986.

114. Akiyama SK, Yamada KM: Synthetic peptides competitively inhibit both direct binding to fibroblasts and functional biological assays for the purified cell-binding domain of fibronectin. *J Biol Chem* 260:10402, 1985.

115. Pytela R, Pierschbacher MD, Ruoslahti E: A 125/115-kDa cell surface receptor specific for vitronectin interacts with the arginine-glycine-aspartatic acid adhesion sequence derived from fibronectin. *Proc Natl Acad Sci* 82:5766, 1985.

CHAPTER 34

Gamete Intrafallopian Transfer

Alexander M. Dlugi

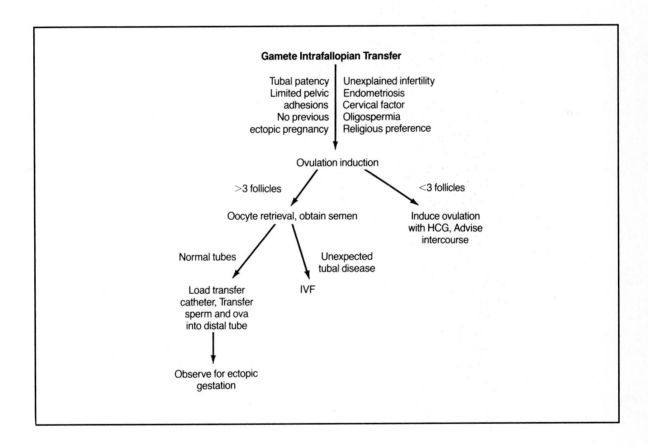

Gamete intrafallopian transfer (GIFT) is a procedure in which preovulatory oocytes and washed sperm are transferred directly into the fallopian tubes. By placing both gametes at the normal site of human fertilization, this technique attempts to mimic the natural physiologic process leading to implantation of an embryo(s) within the uterine cavity. Since its original description by Asch and associates[1] in 1984, over 1,000 GIFT patient cycles have been reported in the literature.

PATIENT SELECTION

Prior to being considered for the GIFT procedure, every couple should undergo a thorough and complete infertility evaluation, including semen analysis, hysterosalpingogram, postcoital test, and timed endometrial biopsy. Although a diagnostic laparoscopy completes the workup, some patients prefer to combine this procedure with a potentially therapeutic maneuver such as GIFT or in-vitro fertilization (IVF).

The pharmacologically stimulated and enlarged ovaries, however, may interfere with visualization of the pelvis in its entirety and thus compromise the diagnostic aspect of the procedure. In addition, endoscopic surgery, if indicated, might have to be postponed to another time so as not to compromise the fragile ovaries or interfere with GIFT.

Of the 609 reported patients to whom an etiology for infertility has been ascribed, the majority (33.7%) fall into the category of unexplained infertility (Table 34–1). Mild endometriosis (16.3%) and male factors (29.7%) (usually oligospermia) account for the two other largest diagnostic groups. These, as well as patients with infertility of an immunologic origin in either partner that has not responded to less invasive measures, and women with cervical factor or ovulatory dysfunction refractory to treatment, might benefit from GIFT. Patients with unilateral tubal damage or with a sole ovary and tube on the contralateral side similarly might be candidates for this procedure.

Normalcy of at least one fallopian tube, if not both, has been stressed by numerous authors as a prerequisite for GIFT.[2–5] One group specifically excluded any patient with a history of tubal disease or surgery, or with an apparent tubal abnormality seen on laparoscopy.[3] Other authors, however, have performed the GIFT procedure in patients with adnexal (including peritubal) adhesions.[6–8] Of primary concern is the possibility of establishing an ectopic pregnancy in these compromised tubes. Although the exact risk is unknown, the two ectopic pregnancies in a series of 276 cycles occurred in patients with tubal disease.[8] One patient had previously undergone bilateral neosalpingostomies, with the remaining endosalpinx described as being grossly normal. The second patient had pelvic adhesions, a hydrosalpinx, and one "normal" tube. Clearly, caution

should be exercised before transferring gametes to a potentially damaged fallopian tube.

While GIFT is an attractive alternative to IVF, it does not address the question of whether the female's oocytes are fertilizable by the male's spermatozoa unless pregnancy occurs. The answer may be of particular importance in cases of unexplained, immunologic, or male-factor infertility. The sperm-penetration assay was recommended as a predictive test for successful IVF[9]; by extension, this could also apply to GIFT. Others, however, found this test of little use.[10]

The results of simultaneous IVF and GIFT were reported in 16 couples.[4] Only 1 patient achieved a pregnancy with GIFT. In addition, only 50% had any oocytes fertilized in vitro. The authors concluded that an important percentage of patients with infertility probably have spermatozoa or oocyte dysfunction, and suggested that GIFT be performed only in couples in whom there is conclusive proof that the woman's oocytes can be fertilized by the man's spermatozoa. Similarly, 1 pregnancy was reported among 6 couples with male-factor infertility and documented IVF.[11] Two of 5 women whose husbands' sperm failed to fertilize the oocyte in vitro subsequently conceived when donor sperm were used. Three pregnancies occurred in 9 cycles when IVF was documented, but none occurred in 9 cycles when IVF did not occur.[12] On the other hand, when supernumerary oocytes in a GIFT program were treated with IVF, there was no correlation between IVF and the likelihood of GIFT pregnancies; 5 women became pregnant even though the supernumerary oocytes did not fertilize in vitro.[13] Thus the usefulness of an IVF cycle as a screening method prior to patient selection for GIFT is not clear. Nevertheless, until more information is available, an initial IVF cycle in cases of male-factor infertility or one after several GIFT cycles in which pregnancy does not ensue may be warranted to examine sperm–egg interaction.

OVULATION INDUCTION

The goal of any regimen of ovulation induction is to achieve the growth of numerous follicles that yield numerous preovulatory oocytes suitable for transfer into the fallopian tube. Many protocols have been described, all virtually identical to those used for IVF cycles. Although human menopausal gonadotropin (HMG) alone is preferred by some, clomiphene citrate alone or in some combination with HMG, and follicle-stimulating hormone (FSH) with HMG, have also been used (Table 34–2).

As with IVF cycles, no one protocol has proved to be more beneficial than another. One group reported the retrieval of more oocytes when HMG

TABLE 34–1. DISTRIBUTION OF DIAGNOSES OF PATIENTS UNDERGOING THE GIFT PROCEDURE

Diagnosis	No. (%) of Patients Reported	
Unexplained	205	(33.7)
Male factor	181	(29.7)
Polycystic ovaries	1	(0.16)
Immune	7	(1.1)
Cervical factor	28	(4.6)
Anovulation	8	(1.3)
Endometriosis	104	(17.1)
Luteal phase defect	2	(0.33)
Failed TID	10	(1.6)
Adnexel adhesions	49	(8.0)
Tubal damage to one tube	8	(1.3)
Several factors	6	(0.99)

TABLE 34-2. EXAMPLES OF FOLLICLE-STIMULATION PROTOCOLS USED IN GIFT CYCLES

Stimulation	HCG	Criteria for HCG	Reference
HMG 150 IU beginning day 3	10,000	2 or more follicles $\geq$ 16 mm and $E_2 \geq$ 300-500 pg/ml for each main follicle	2
Clomiphene 100 mg beginning day 3 or 4 × 5 days and HMG 150 IU starting day 6-8	5000 IU	?	3
or Clomiphene 100 mg beginning day 3 or 4 × 5 days	—	Used spontaneous LH surge	3
or HMG 150 IU beginning day 3 or 4	5000 IU	?	3
FSH 150 IU in AM, 150 IU in PM on days 3 and 4 with HMG 150 IU daily from day 5	10,000 IU	2 or more follicles $\geq$ 16 mm and $E_2 \geq$ 400 pg/ml	5
or HMG 150 IU from day 3 or 5	10,000 IU	"	5
or Clomiphene 100 mg daily from day 3-7 or day 5-9 and HMG 150 IU from fourth day of CC administration	5000 IU	"	5
Clomiphene 100 mg daily from day 2-6 and FSH 75 IU daily	5000 IU	2 or more follicles $\geq$ 19 mm	21
Clomiphene 150 mg/day × 5 days starting day 3 or HMG 150-300 IU day 3	5000 IU	2 or more follicles $\geq$ 18-20 mm	6
or Clomiphene 150 mg/day days 3-7 and HMG from day 8 or 9	"		
Clomiphene 100 mg/day × 5 days starting 10 days before average cycle midpoint and HMG 150 IU starting on day 2 of clomiphene	5000 IU	Given at optimal time or withheld if LH surge	13
Clomiphene 100 mg/day × 5 days starting day 4 and HMG 75 IU on days 4-8 HMG 75-225 IU then continued	?	Sixth day of E_2 rise	4

was used alone or in conjunction with clomiphene as compared to clomiphene alone. In a later paper, these same authors[8] noted that 80% of cycles stimulated with clomiphene alone failed to reach laparoscopy. They also noted that the majority of their GIFT pregnancies occurred at serum estradiol (E_2) levels of 300 to 500 pg/preovulatory follicle, or with a mean serum E_2 level of 1,190 ± 18 pg/mL (7 of 10 transfers). At higher (2,683 ± 20 pg/mL) levels of serum E_2, more than half of the early pregnancies were biochemical, without clinical evidence. The two ectopic pregnancies in their series also fell into the group with high E_2 levels.

THE PROCEDURE

Sperm Collection and Preparation

Sperm are typically collected by masturbation 2 to 2.5 hours prior to oocyte retrieval, although some au-

thors [7,8] prefer a longer interval of time before the actual transfer.

To comply with the doctrines of the Roman Catholic church, sperm can be collected during intercourse while using a perforated condom. In this fashion, neither contraception nor masturbation is employed, and any ensuing pregnancy results as an extension of the conjugal act.

The semen specimen is allowed to liquefy over the next 30 minutes, after which the sperm are washed, centrifuged, and allowed to swim up to the final collectable pool. The media used for sperm washing vary according to the individual investigator. The following are examples:

1. Ham's F-10 with 10% fetal cord serum (1:3 vol/vol) containing streptomycin, 6,000 $U/10^4$ mL and penicillin, 12,000 $U/10^2$ mL[2]
2. Ham's F-10 with 7.5% fetal cord serum[3]
3. Ham's F-10 with 7.5% patient's serum containing

penicillin G, 75 mg/L, streptomycin sulfate, 75 mg/L, calcium lactate, 252 mg/L, and sodium bicarbonate, 2.1 g/L at a pH of 7.35 and osmolarity of 280 to 285 mOsm[7]

4. Earle's medium[14]

No one method has thus far been shown to be superior to another, although it was suggested that Percoll gradient centrifugation might yield sperm of better morphologic quality as determined by transmission electron microscopy.[15] The final specimen is incubated at 37°C in an atmosphere of 5% carbon dioxide and 95% air until ready for transfer catheter loading.

Oocyte Retrieval

Thirty-four to 36 hours after the administration of human chorionic gonadotropin (HCG), oocytes are retrieved. This is generally accomplished by laparoscopy under general anesthesia. Standard laparoscopic equipment and techniques are used (Fig. 34–1). Several puncture sites may be necessary to attain access to all the ovarian follicles. These sites are usually placed lateral to the lower midline incision, either at the same level or higher. Both fallopian tubes may later be cannulated from a single right lower quadrant insertion of the aspirating cannula.[4] In our experience, however, it is easier to use two separate insertions to facilitate easy cannulation of the tubes. Each pelvis should be assessed individually for appropriate placement of the aspirating cannula in order to minimize the number of puncture sites.

An alternative to laparoscopic retrieval is direct ovarian follicle aspiration through minilaparotomy.

In this instance, a 2 to 3-cm transverse incision may be made at the level at which the uterine fundus reaches the anterior abdominal wall, as determined by bimanual pelvic examination. Once the peritoneal cavity is entered, the enlarged, fragile ovaries are often directly in view, and the individual follicles can be aspirated serially using the same needle used during a laparoscopic procedure. As the follicles shrink in size, the ovary often falls back into the pelvis. When this occurs, further aspirations may be technically difficult. Gentle digital elevation of the suspensory ligament of the ovary or the ovary itself often restores the ovary to a more favorable position. Extreme care must be exercised to avoid bursting the follicle walls during this maneuver. Alternatively, oocyte retrieval may be performed by laparoscopy or ultrasound to avoid inadvertently rupturing follicles, and the gamete transfer performed by minilaparotomy (see below).

Once the oocytes have been retrieved, they are placed in culture medium and graded for maturity. Several culture media are used, as follows:

1. Ham's F-10 with 50% fetal cord serum under silicon oil[2]
2. Ham's F-10 with 7.5% fetal cord serum[2]
3. Menezo B$_2$ medium with 50% inactivated maternal serum[6]
4. Follicular fluid[7]
5. Ham's F-10[16]
6. Ham's F-10 with 50% maternal serum[5]
7. Earle's medium[14]

Although most authors use prepared media, some place oocytes in a Petri dish containing clear follicular

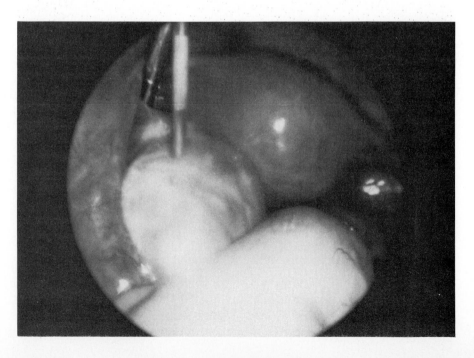

Figure 34–1. Laparoscopic oocyte retrieval. (Courtesy of Machelle M. Seibel.)

TABLE 34–3. TRANSFER CATHETER LOADING

Reference	Space	Space	Sperm (μl)	Space	Oocytes	Space	End	Total Transferred Volume (μl)
2	Air	None	5	5 μl air	25 μl medium	5 μl air	10 μl medium	45
3	Medium	25 μl air	25	10 μl air	50 μl medium	10 μl air	25 μl medium	145
6	10 μl medium	20 μl air	25	20 μl air	30 μl medium	20 μl air	10 μl medium	135
7	Follicular fluid	5 μl air	5–30	None	5–15μl follicular fluid	5 μl air	5 μl follicular fluid	45
16				4–5 μl of media containing both oocytes and spermatozoa				4–5
5	Medium	5 μl air	50	None	25 μl medium	None	5 μl medium	85
4	Air	10 μl medium	?	Air	?	Air	5–10 μl medium	40–75
8	Follicular fluid	5 μl air	4–15	None	1–2 μl follicular	4–5 μl	5μl follicular	50
1	10 μl medium	5 μl air	25	5 μl air	40 μl medium	5 μl air	10 μl medium	95

fluid usually obtained from the first aspirated follicle.[7] No advantage of this method or any other has been demonstrated thus far.

Transfer

Some of the different types of transfer catheters available are as follows:

1. Deseret Intracath (no 3132, Deseret Co, Sandy, UT)[2]
2. 16-gauge 24-inch Deseret Intracath[3]
3. Semar Catheter (Wisap, Munich, West Germany)[6]
4. Teflon embryo transfer catheter (#5 French) with side-open tip cut off[7]
5. Stirrable GIFT catheter (#7 French) and oocyte catheter (#3 French)[16]
6. 16-gauge end-hole Teflon catheter (HT Barnaby, Baltimore, MD)[5]
7. Cook Catheter (no NRT 5.0-VT-50-P-NS-GIFT, William A. Cook Australia Pty, Ltd, Melbourne, Australia)[4,13]

Methods of loading are described in Table 34–3 and Figure 34–2. Most authors use separate transfer catheters for each fallopian tube. The number of sperm transferred is generally 10,000 per tube, although one group[4] used 150,000 to 200,000. In cases of oligospermia, this may be increased up to any amount from 200,000 to 800,000.[7,17] The number of oocytes transferred per tube is usually 2 or 3, although up to a total of 6 have been used.[3] The ideal number has not been determined, although it was suggested that the transfer of 4 oocytes results in a higher pregnancy rate compared to the transfer of fewer oocytes.[7] The pregnancy rate per cycle was 52.6% when 3 oocytes were transferred, compared to 30.7% when only 2 were transferred. It is also unclear whether only mature oocytes should be used or whether the transfer of immature oocytes has any detrimental effect.

In every case of GIFT, sperm and oocytes are separated in the transfer catheter by a space of air or medium (see Fig. 34–2). This ensures that fertilization does not take place until the gametes are deposited within the fallopian tube. The fact that the embryo is never extracorporeal renders the GIFT procedure acceptable to most orthodox religions. Juxtaposing the fluid columns containing sperm and oocytes has been proposed, however, to allow the onset of sperm penetration of the cumulus oophorus within the confines of the catheter.[8] Furthermore, those authors stripped a portion of the cumulus oophorus with 18-gauge needles prior to catheter loading in order to decrease the thickness of the barrier to penetration. The possibility that fertilization may occur in the transfer catheter may raise serious ethical dilemmas for some religious groups, although human fertilization has been shown not to occur in vitro before two hours.

The gametes are readily transferred into the fallopian tubes under laparoscopic visualization (Fig. 34–3). The transfer catheter may be threaded down the aspirating cannula or through an appropriate-size

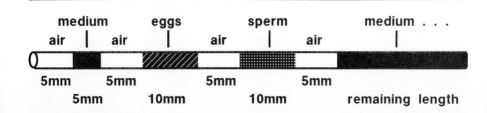

Figure 34–2. Schematic drawing of a GIFT transfer catheter. Notice that gametes are separated by air or medium. (Courtesy of Machelle M. Seibel.)

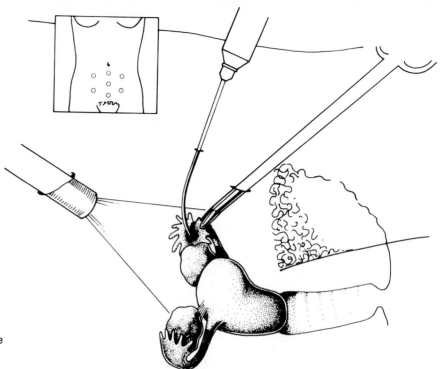

Figure 34–3. Schematic description of the GIFT procedure. Inset illustrates potential locations for additional puncture sites.

trocar cannula. Using an atraumatic grasping forceps, the serosa is picked up and the fimbriated portion of the tube aligned with the advancing cannula. Straightening the tube often helps to identify its lumen. It is important to approach the tube from the correct angle to ensure proper placement of the cannula and the catheter within the tube. A flexible, maneuverable catheter has been described that may allow for easier entry into the tubal ostium. The metal cannula is placed in the tubal lumen to a distance of 1 to 2 cm. The catheter is then advanced another 1 to 2 cm beyond the end of the cannula, and the gametes are gently injected into the ampulla. The same process is then repeated for the other tube.

Gamete transfer is also easily accomplished by minilaparotomy (Fig. 34–4). A finger or an atraumatic tube holder can be used to elevate the tube and its fimbriated end into the opening of the incision.

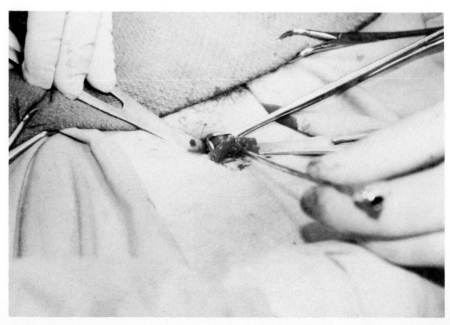

Figure 34–4. Gamete transfer by minilaparotomy. (Courtesy of Machelle M. Seibel.)

TABLE 34-4. OUTCOMES OF GIFT PROCEDURE

Reference	No. of Retrievals	Current or Delivered Pregnancy	No. of Abortions	No. of Chemical Pregnancies	Ectopic Pregnancies (%)	Continuing Pregnancy/Retrieval (%)
2	10	2	2			20
3	19	3		1		15.8
6	44	14	2		1	31.8
7	59	9	3	18		15.3
16	8	1	2			7.7
5	70	16	3	4		22.9
4	16	1				6.3
8	59	18	1	19	2	30.5
13	42	7				16.7
15	18	4				22.2
19	1	1				100.0
11	1	—	—	—	9.1	
12	18	3	—	—	—	16.7
21	6	2	—	—	—	33.0
Totals	1156	246	59	49	11	21.3

Under direct visualization, the tubal lumen can then be cannulated and the catheter threaded down to an appropriate position. This approach can always be used when laparoscopic cannulation is difficult. Unfortunately, scarring may make repeat procedures more difficult.

More recently, ultrasound guided transuterine gamete transfer has been described. Although more technically difficult, the ability to perform both the oocyte retrieval and gamete transfer under local anesthesia will undoubtedly make this the method of choice in the future.

RESULTS

The outcomes of GIFT procedures are shown in Table 34-4. There have been 354 (30.6%) reported pregnan-

cies out of 1,156 retrievals. Two hundred forty-six are in progress or have delivered, representing a 21.3% pregnancies per retrieval. Fourteen percent of all the pregnancies were chemical, and 16.7% ended in clinical abortion. Eleven ectopic pregnancies (3.1% of all pregnancies) have been reported. Twenty-nine multiple gestations, representing 8.2% of all pregnancies, have been reported. Of these, 12 resulted in twins, 3 triplets, and 1 quadruplets. One of the triplet pregnancies reverted to a twin gestation at 8 weeks.[7]

The etiology of infertility has some bearing on the success of GIFT (Table 34-5). Patients with mild endometriosis or unexplained infertility appear to fare well. Pregnancy rates per cycle of 26% (27 cycles) for unexplained infertility, 66.6% for mild endometriosis (3 cycles), and 66.6% (9 cycles) for adhesions were reported in patients who failed to conceive after standard donor insemination.[6] No pregnancies were

TABLE 34-5. PREGNANCY RATES BASED ON ETIOLOGY OF INFERTILITY

Reference	Unexplained (%)	Endometriosis (%)	Cervical Factor (%)	Male Factor (%)	Adhesions (%)
6	66.6	26.0	0	0	66.6
7	27.0	0.0	0	15.0	40.0
8	37.5	28.5	14.2	16.6	50.0
17	—	—	—	0	—
23	40.0	26.0	—	21.0	—
26	47.0	30.0	—	36.0	—

achieved in patients with hostile cervical mucus or when a male factor was present. Of 2 pregnancies in 3 patients with adnexal adhesions, one ended in a miscarriage and the second was ectopic.

Favorable clinical pregnancy rates per retrieval also were reported for patients with unexplained infertility (27%).[7] Poorer rates were noted in the presence of oligospermia (15%), endometriosis (0%), and cervical factor problems (0%). One of 2 patients with immune factor infertility conceived, as did 2 of 3 with ovulatory dysfunction. Eight of 20 patients with adnexal adhesions or tubal disease also were successful in achieving intrauterine pregnancy. In a follow-up series, those authors reported continued success among patients with unexplained infertility (37.5% pregnancy/transfer), pelvic adhesions (50%), and tubal disease (33.3%).[8] Lower rates were found among patients with endometriosis (28.5%), oligospermia (16.6%), and cervical factor infertility (14.2%). No pregnancies occurred among patients who were anovulatory or had an immune factor.

No pregnancy was achieved with GIFT among 9 patients whose partners were oligospermic ($< 12 \times 10^6$/mL), while 4 of 9 normospermic couples conceived.[18] These data must necessarily be interpreted with caution, as the total number of patients in each diagnostic category is low.

MODIFICATIONS OF GIFT

As discussed previously, the GIFT procedure does not indicate whether fertilization has occurred unless a pregnancy ensues. In couples with oligospermia, for whom the answer to this question is particularly relevant, it was proposed that fertilization be allowed to take place in vitro.[17] If fertilization were under way, as judged by the presence of 2 pronuclei 18 hours after insemination of an oocyte, the pronuclear oocytes would be transferred into the fallopian tubes by GIFT. Of 5 patients undergoing this modified procedure, only 1 demonstrated in-vitro fertilization of 1 out of 4 oocytes, while 3 of another woman's oocytes were fertilized by donor sperm. No pregnancies were reported. On the other hand, a twin pregnancy was achieved in a patient whose serum contained sperm antibodies when 3 oocytes were fertilized in vitro and the zygotes were later transferred into one fallopian tube.[19] While fertilization is confirmed and the early embryo is allowed to be nurtured in its natural physiologic environment with this technique, it remains to be determined whether the method improves pregnancy rates compared to standard GIFT of IVF protocols. Again, because of extracorporeal fertilization, serious religious objections may arise.

Intratubal insemination has been proposed as an extension to intracervical and intrauterine insemination.[20] In this procedure, only sperm are placed within the fallopian tube under laparoscopic guidance. Five pregnancies were achieved among 20 women undergoing 28 such treatment cycles. In a similar vein, hysteroscopic insemination of the fallopian tube has been described.[21] No pregnancies were achieved in 52 cycles. More extensive experience with these methods is required before judgment can be passed concerning their efficacy.

SUMMARY

The rationale for performing GIFT is that it allows gametes to be placed directly into the natural physiologic environment appropriate for fertilization. The placement of several ova retrieved from pharmacologically stimulated ovaries may increase the chances that one will indeed be fertilized. Potentially defective ovum pickup mechanisms of the fallopian tube are bypassed. Similarly, introduction of motile spermatozoa within the ampulla of the tube may overcome compromised sperm transport and hostile cervical mucus. Although an overall 22% pregnancy rate is respectable, it remains to be defined whether it is significantly better than that achieved with standard IVF cycles. Some combination of sequential GIFT–IVF cycles may ultimately prove to be the best approach to investigate the intricacies of sperm–egg interaction while maintaining a high therapeutic value.

REFERENCES

1. Asch RH, Ellsworth LR, Balmaceda JP, Wong PC: Pregnancy after translaparoscopic gamete intrafallopian transfer. Lancet 2:0134, 1984.
2. Asch H, Balmaceda JP, Ellsworth L, Wong PC: Preliminary experiences with gamete intrafallopian transfer (GIFT). Fertil Steril 45:366, 1986.
3. Corson SL, Batzer F, Eisenberg E, et al: Early experience with the GIFT procedure. J Reprod Med 31:219, 1986.
4. Quigley MM, Sokoloski JE, Withers DM, Richards SI, Reis JM: Simultaneous in vitro fertilization and gamete intrafallopian transfer. Fertil Steril 47:797, 1987.
5. Molloy D, Speirs A, du Plessis Y, McBain J, Johnston I: A laparoscopic approach to a program of gamete intrafallopian transfer. Fertil Steril 47:289, 1987.
6. Guastella G, Comparetto G, Palermo R, et al: Gamete intrafallopian transfer in the treatment of infertility: The first series at the University of Palermo. Fertil Steril 46:417, 1986.
7. Nemiro JS, McGaughey RW: An alternative to in vitro fertilization-embryo transfer: The successful transfer of human oocytes and spermatozoa to the distal oviduct. Fertil Steril 46:644, 1986.
8. McGaughey RW, Nemiro JS: Correlation of estrogen levels with oocytes aspirated and with pregnancy in a program of clinical tubal transfer. Fertil Steril 48:98, 1987.
9. Rogers BJ: The sperm penetration assay: its usefulness reevaluated. Fertil Steril 43:821, 1985.
10. Wolf DP, Sokoloski JE, Quigley MM: Correlation of human in vitro fertilization with the hamster egg bioassay. Fertil Steril 40:53, 1983.

11. Grunert GM, Gibbons W, Rodriquez-Rigau LJ, Steinberger E: Combined gamete intrafallopian transfer (GIFT) and in vitro fertilization in male factor infertility. Presented at the 5th world congress on in vitro fertilization and embryo transfer, Norfolk, VA, April 1987.

12. Chang SP, Ng HT, Chao HT, Chen SC, Tzeng CR: Early experience with a combined procedure of GIFT and IVF. Presented at the 5th world congress on in vitro fertilization and embryo transfer, Norfolk, VA, April 1987.

13. Matson PL, Yovich JM, Bootsma BD, Spittle JW, Yovich JL: The in vitro and fertilization ability of human sperm capacitated by swim up and Percoll gradient centrifugation. Presented at the 43rd annual meeting of the American Fertility Society, Reno, NV, 1987.

14. Imoedemhe DAG, Wafik AA, Chan RCW: Gamete intrafallopian transfer (GIFT): The Solimon Fakeeh Hospital preliminary experience. Presented at the 5th world congress on in vitro fertilization, Norfolk, VA, April 1987.

15. Tanphaichitr N, Agulnick A, Seibel MM, Taymor ML: Comparison of the in vitro fertilization rate by human sperm capacitation by multiple-tube swim-up and Percoll gradient centrifugation. *J IVF/ET* 5:119, 1988.

16. Confino E, Friberg J, Gleicher N: A new stirrable catheter for gamete intrafallopian tube transfer (GIFT). *Fertil Steril* 46:1147, 1986.

17. Blackledge DG, Matson PC, Willcox DC, et al: Pro-nuclear stage transfer and modified gamete intrafallopian transfer techniques for oligospermic cases. *Med J Aust* 145:173, 1986.

18. Yovich JC, Matson PL, Turner SR, Richardson P, Yovich JM: Limitation of gamete intrafallopian transfer in the treatment of male infertility. *Med J Aust* 144:444, 1986.

19. Devroey P, Braeckmans P, Smitz J, et al: Pregnancy after translaparoscopic zygote intrafallopian transfer in a patient with sperm antibodies. *Lancet* 1:1329, 1986.

20. Berger GS: Intratubal insemination. *Fertil Steril* 48:328, 1987.

21. Brooks JH, Taylor PJ, Mortimer D: Synchronized hysteroscopic insemination of the fallopian tube (SHIFT). Presented at the 5th world congress on in vitro fertilization and embryo transfer, Norfolk, VA, April 1987.

CHAPTER 35

In-Vitro Fertilization

Neri Laufer, Lawrence Grunfeld, and G. John Garrisi

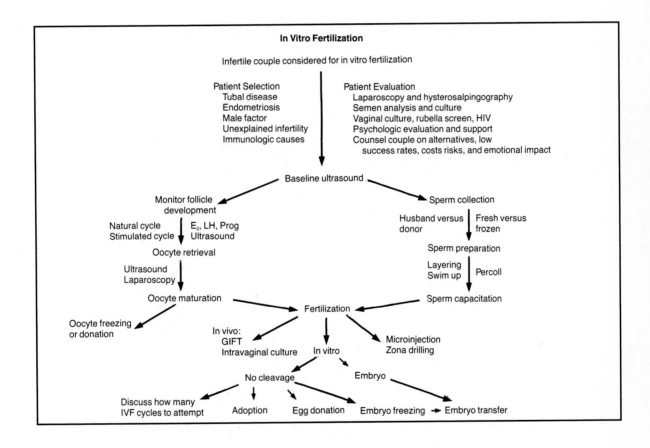

The first successful human pregnancies and births after in vitro fertilization (IVF) were reported by Steptoe and Edwards in 1978[1] and by Lopata and co-workers in 1980.[2] This achievement was a culmination of scientific efforts that stretched over almost a century. Walter Heape in 1891 was the first to demonstrate the possibility of recovering a preimplantation-stage embryo from flushings of a rabbit oviduct and transferring the embryo to a foster mother, in which normal development continued.[3] As a result of Heape's pioneering work and successful embryo transfers in other species, scientific inter-est focused on culturing embryos in the laboratory. Hammond[4] in 1949 developed a complex medium that supported the growth of 8-cell mouse embryos to blastocysts, and Whitten[5] in 1956 demonstrated that a simple, chemically defined medium could be equally effective. The discovery of sperm capacitation by Austin[6] and Chang[7] in 1951, coupled with simple culture techniques, resulted in the first successful fertilization of rabbit eggs in vitro reported by Chang in 1959.[8]

The birth of Louise Brown, the first IVF-embryo transfer (ET) baby, in 1978, triggered a succession of medical, biologic, and technical developments that have simplified the procedure, increased its efficiency, and expanded its indications. In the 1970s IVF-ET was transformed from an experimental procedure to one that is integral to the reproductive endocrinologist's practice. It has become a medical discipline in which clinicians and reproductive biologists team closely to treat patients and gain better insights into problems associated with human reproduction, and has dramatically affected almost all the traditional treatment modalities of infertility.

PATIENT SELECTION

Originally, IVF was developed for patients with absent or irrepairably damaged fallopian tubes.[2] As IVF evolved and became more commonly available its indications widened. Currently, it is performed in women with infertility due to such disorders as unexplained infertility, immunologic infertility, male-factor infertility, and endometriosis. The minimal requirements are that the patient have a normal uterine cavity, a source of oocytes, and enough sperm to achieve fertilization. Although IVF may be an alternative in the therapy of most infertility disorders, it may not always be the best treatment. Therefore it is imperative that the infertility evaluation be complete, that alternative therapies be considered, and that success rates for all forms of treatment be discussed honestly with the couple.

Tubal Disease

Advances in microsurgical techniques have resulted in excellent outcomes for many types of tubal dysfunction. As a result, obstructed fallopian tubes are usually repaired surgically. The success of surgical repair depends on the extent of tubal destruction, however.[9] When the fimbriae are preserved and the tube is not dilated, lysis of adhesions may be followed by pregnancy in over 50% of individuals.[10] In contrast, when the fimbriae are closed, a neosalpingostomy must be performed, resulting in a favorable outcome in only 15 to 20% of patients.[9] For comparison, a single cycle of IVF results in pregnancy in approximately 20% of women. Fewer than 10% of patients with dense adnexal adhesions, fixation of the ovary and tube, absence of fimbriae, bipolar disease, and presence of a hydrosalpinx greater than 30 mm diameter[11] become pregnant after surgical repair.

Sterilization procedures that retain more than 6 cm of fallopian tube and preserve the fimbriae are best treated with microsurgical anastomosis. A midsegment tubal anastomosis offers a pregnancy rate of over 60%, while a tubocornual anastomosis results in pregnancy in 45 to 50% of patients.[9,10] Even several cycles of IVF cannot match these success rates.

Patients initially treated by a microsurgical procedure and who do not conceive, however, are best treated by IVF, because the success rate for repeat tuboplasty after a microsurgical procedure is under 10%.[12]

After a surgical procedure it is important to wait an appropriate length of time for pregnancy to occur. Eighty-five percent of intrauterine pregnancies occur within 2 years of distal tubal obstruction repair; there are as many successes during the second year as certainly plays a role in the choice of therapy for women in whom surgery fails, it is prudent not to initiate IVF before an adequate trial at conception has passed.

Endometriosis

Endometriosis is present in 20 to 40% of women with infertility.[13] The mechanism of infertility in severe disease is mechanical obstruction of the fallopian tube and encasement of the ovary. In mild disease the etiology of the infertility is less clear,[14] however, pregnancy rates of 50% occur with no treatment in the 6 months after diagnostic laparoscopy.[15-18]

Infertility due to moderate and severe endometriosis treated by surgical correction combined with either danazol or a gonadotropin-releasing hormone (GnRH) agonist results in pregnancy rates above 50% in women with moderate endometriosis and 30 to 40% for those with severe disease.[13] When conception does not occur within an adequate follow-up interval, IVF should be considered.

Male Factors

Although a lower fertilization rate can be anticipated when the male partner is oligospermic, once the oocyte fertilizes, implantation rates may be normal.[19] Seventy-five percent of couples with oligospermia had at least one embryo transferred and achieved an overall pregnancy rate of 45%.[20] The implantation rate in oligospermic couples is higher than that in normospermic couples (57 versus 22%),[21] which is not surprising, because procedures performed with oligospermic men are biased toward normal reproductive function in the female partner. One should be cautious in interpreting this finding, however, because fertilization rates are lower in oligospermic couples and the pregnancy rate per cycle is markedly diminished.

The hamster-egg-penetration test described by Yanagimachi in 1976 is considered useful in screening sperm prior to IVF.[22,23] Although in most cases a positive result is well correlated with human oocyte fertilization, in cases of oligospermia the test is less predictive. A poor test result was associated with human oocyte fertilization in only 63% of oligospermic couples.[24] In normospermic couples, 90% of those with normal hamster-egg-penetration results fertilize in vitro. Sperm-penetration assays are useful prior to IVF as a screen for unexplained infertility in normospermic couples. Oligospermic couples should not be rejected from attempts at IVF solely on the basis of poor results of this test.

Fifteen percent of infertile couples do not have an identifiable cause of their infertility. Before the condition is classified as unexplained, a thorough evaluation is mandatory. Of the couples for whom no explanation is found, 20% will become pregnant each year for 3 years, with a cumulative pregnancy rate of 58% after 4 years.[16] When expectant management is no longer appropriate, IVF can be useful both as a treatment and as a diagnostic tool. Some couples who undergo IVF demonstrate abnormal fertilization, which can be due to defective sperm penetration, abnormal oocyte development, or abnormalities in sperm–oocyte interaction. Those in whom poor or no fertilization has occurred usually achieve normal fertilization when donor sperm is substituted for the partner's sperm.

Immunologic Causes

The presence of antibodies to sperm in the female reproductive tract or on the sperm surface adversely affects fertility.[25] Antibodies directed against the sperm tail and midpiece can alter sperm motion, while antibodies directed against the sperm head can affect sperm–oocyte interaction.[26]

Women with antisperm antibodies fertilize fewer oocytes than do those whose sera do not contain antibodies to sperm.[27,28] Some of these patients have abnormal binding to the zona pellucida.[29] As a result, their fertilization rate is decreased. If IVF is performed in a woman with antisperm antibodies, it is important that her serum not be used in preparing the medium. If the oocytes do fertilize, the expected implantation rate of these embryos is identical to that of patients with tubal disease.[25]

GIFT VERSUS IVF

The patient with patent fallopian tubes poses a special problem with respect to IVF. It was demonstrated in women with at least one normal tube that transferring gametes into the ampullary portion (gamete intrafallopian transfer, or GIFT) achieved higher pregnancy rates than IVF.[30] It is not entirely surprising that pregnancy rates are improved with in-vivo fertilizing procedures, since in-vitro culture conditions attempt to simulate the fallopian tube, although they cannot totally reproduce it. It is important to remember that this procedure is only appropriate when at least one tube is normal. If patients are appropriately selected, pregnancies can be achieved in 19% of those with idiopathic disease and 33% of those with male-factor infertility.[31]

One problem with GIFT is that one cannot observe oocyte fertilization. When there is concern that poor fertilization may occur, such as in male-factor, immunologic, or idiopathic infertility, it would be appropriate to save some oocytes to test for evidence of fertilization. A convenient way to achieve an enhanced fertilization rate with GIFT and still obtain information about sperm–oocyte interaction is to combine the two procedures. If more than 4 oocytes are recovered, 4 of them can be placed into the fallopian tube and the rest can be fertilized in vitro. If normal fertilization occurs, these embryos are cryopreserved.

STIMULATION OF FOLLICULAR GROWTH

The first pregnancies obtained by IVF in humans were achieved with oocytes from unstimulated natural cycles.[1,2] The disadvantages of this approach were numerous: the necessity for frequent measuring of blood or urine luteinizing hormone (LH) level, the need for 24-hour commitment of staff and facilities, a low (0 to 60%) chance of aspirating at least 1 oocyte, and a low mean number of oocytes aspirated per woman.[32,33] This approach was abandoned in 1981, when it was shown that ovulation induction with clomiphene citrate (CC) coupled with either a naturally occurring LH surge or the administration of human chorionic gonadotropin (HCG) resulted in an 8% rate of viable pregnancies and the first twin gestation.[32,34]

Since the early 1980s the number of ovulation-inducing agents in IVF has grown and includes clomiphene, human menopausal gonadotropins (HMG) and HCG, "pure" follicle-stimulating hormone (FSH), GnRH, and GnRH analogs or contraceptive pills in conjunction with gonadotropins. Although no single agent or combination is optimal, a trend is emerging suggesting an advantage of some combination therapies over others.

Clomiphene Citrate–HMG

Clomiphene citrate alone, 50 to 150 mg/day on cycle days 5 to 9, has been largely abandoned and replaced by clomiphene–HMG regimens that capitalize on the synergistic effect of the two agents. Clomiphene, 50 to 100 mg/day, is given from days 2 to 6, or 5 to 9; and HMG, 2 to 4 ampules, is added from day 2, 5, or 7 for 3 to 4 days. When at least 1 follicle reaches a diameter greater than 18 to 20 mm, HMG is discontinued and HCG administered.[35-37]

In a summary of almost 1,000 IVF pregnancies from Australia and New Zealand, obtained between 1979 and 1984 and published by the Australian

National Perinatal Statistics Unit in 1985, the combination of clomiphene–HMG was used in over 75% of cycles.[38] The overall pregnancy rate reported for these agents is in the range of 15 to 17% per aspiration, or 20% per transfer,[36,39] with a 25% multiple pregnancy rate.[35] The pregnancy rate almost doubled to over 30% if oocytes aspiration followed an endogenous LH surge rather than the administration of HCG.[35] In another report, no difference was found between spontaneous LH and exogenous HCG administration, but the best results were obtained when the addition of HMG to clomiphene was tailored to individual responses.[36]

Clomiphene citrate in this combination has been hypothesized to enhance follicular recruitment and to act as an antiestrogen, preventing a short luteal phase caused by HMG.[37] Its protective effect against high midluteal luteolytic estradiol (E_2) levels was also suggested.[40] Comparing clomiphene to the HMG cycles, the luteal phase was significantly shorter in HMG cycles (14.9 versus 17.3 days, respectively), and late luteal progesterone levels were significantly lower in the HMG group. When HMG cycles were compared to CC-HMG regimens, the latter demonstrated the following: (1) a faster growth rate, so that at the time of aspiration, follicles are larger and easier to aspirate, especially when ultrasound-guided technique is used; (2) a higher E_2 response; (3) a large preovulatory progesterone rise; (4) a high percentage of LH initiation; and (5) a higher frequency of poor or abnormal endocrine response.[41] Manipulating the initiation of CC-HMG to either day 2 or 4 of the cycle did not change any of these drawbacks: a spontaneous LH surge occurred in nearly 50% of patients on day 2 and 36.5% on day 4. Similarly, conception rates did not differ between the groups.[42]

One must bear in mind, however, that a considerable body of data exists to suggest that clomiphene citrate may have undesirable effects in the reproductive tract. This estrogen antagonist seems to have a dose-dependent antiestrogenic effect on the endometrium[43] and is associated with a decrease in endometrial cytosol estrogen receptors.[44] It was demonstrated histologically that clomiphene administered in the follicular phase induces premature secretory changes in the rabbit oviduct and uterine mucosa,[45] and human endometrium.[46] Asynchronous endometrial development may interfere with uterine receptivity in the early stages of implantation. Moreover, in rats the drug was shown to induce premature meiotic-like changes in oocytes and inhibit in-vitro follicular steroidogenesis.[47] It has also been found to decrease fertilization and development of mouse oocytes in vivo and in vitro.[48] Similarly, studies in humans have demonstrated that clomiphene inhibits progesterone production by granulosa–lutein cells in culture (Fig. 35–1).[49,50]

Clinically, clomiphene is effective in inducing ovulation in over 70% of anovulatory women, but there is an estimated 50% discrepancy between apparent ovulation and actual conception rates. In addition, 25% of clomiphene-related conceptions terminate in abortion, apparently because of corpus luteum deficiency.[51] In view of these laboratory and clinical data suggesting an undesired effect of clomiphene on the endometrium, follicle, and oocyte, in our opinion the use of menotropins alone appears advantageous for IVF.

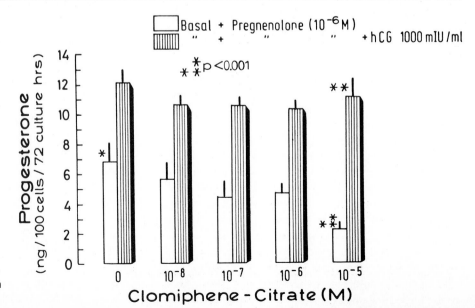

Figure 35–1. The effect of clomiphene citrate on in vitro progesterone secretion by human granulosa–lutein cells.

HMG–FSH

Mild ovarian stimulation with HMG for oocyte retrieval in IVF was pioneered by Steptoe and Edwards[37] but later abandoned. The first viable pregnancies resulting from the use of ovulation induction with HMG were achieved by Jones and co-workers.[52] This group employed a relatively small dosage of HMG (approximately 10 ampules per cycle) with the objective of maturing about 3 large follicles. Monitoring of this regimen takes into consideration not only follicular size and serum E_2 level, but also two additional clinical variables: cervical score and vaginal cytology. The rationale behind clinical monitoring is to determine the occurrence of the biologic shift, assuming that it represents similar changes throughout the reproduction tract, including the endometrium.

The HCG is administered either 28 to 36 or 52 to 60 hours after discontinuation of HMG, depending on the individual response. Use of this regimen in over 400 cycles resulted in an average of 2.3 mature cleaving oocytes, a pregnancy rate of about 25%, an abortion rate of 26.5%, and a cancellation rate of 15% due to either low response or premature LH surge.[53] We have chosen to intervene more aggressively in the normal cycle with a high dose of HMG at the time of follicular recruitment and selection in order to recruit 4 to 5 large follicles. The protocol is summarized in Figure 35–2. Three ampules of HMG are administered beginning on day 3 of a 28 to 32-day cycle. On the 6th day of medication, ovarian sonography and E_2 levels are monitored; 3 to 4 ampules a day are then administered until HCG injection.[54,55] The minimal criteria for HCG administration 24 hours after the last HMG injection are at least 2 follicles with a diameter greater than 1.5 cm and E_2 levels exceeding 500 pg/mL. With this regimen, it was possible to obtain an average of 6 mature oocytes, with 18% clinical pregnancies per transfer and 15% abortions. Other groups using a similar protocol reported an 11 to 31%

clinical pregnancy rate per transfer with an abortion rate of about 18%.[56-58]

Pure FSH was introduced in the late 1980s[59] and is used either in combination regimens with HMG[60] or alone,[61] followed by HCG. In a preliminary report comparing various combinations of HMG-FSH, a higher pregnancy rate was reported in patients undergoing their first IVF attempt with a combination of HMG-HCG than for those receiving FSH alone (30 versus 21%, respectively).[56] In an extended study of over 1,300 cycles, the highest pregnancy rate (25%) was achieved in combination 1 (2 HMG + 2 FSH on day 3–4 and 2 HMG thereafter), in which FSH was used to augment the recruitment phase.[62] The success rate was lower for the fixed protocol of 2 HMG/day (21.5%) and lowest (17%) for 2 FSH. Similarly, the viable pregnancy rate was low (12.2%) for 2 FSH and high (18%) for combination 1, although not statistically significant. The Yale program has reported a small series of 27 patients undergoing FSH stimulation for IVF. Of significance, more rapidly cleaving embryos were obtained and a higher, but not significantly higher, conception rate was achieved with FSH than with HMG (36 versus 22%).[63] It was suggested that a healthier intrafollicular environment for oocyte development was achieved by FSH stimulation due to a decrease in androgen:estrogen ratio and a lower follicular fluid testosterone level.[64]

It is concluded that HMG and FSH regimens seem to offer the same clinical conception rates per transfer (20%) as CC-HMG cycles but are associated with a lower clinical abortion rate (18 versus 25%) and consequently a slightly higher number of live births. The occurrence of a spontaneous LH surge is twice as high in CC-HMG cycles (30%) as in HMG cycles (15%), necessitates close LH monitoring, and is probably associated with a higher rate of cancelled cycles.

Because no prospective, randomized, clinical

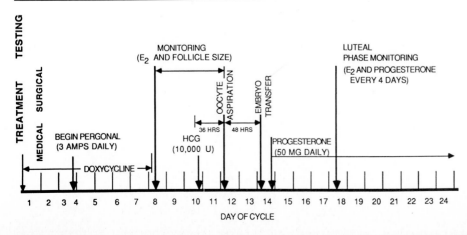

Figure 35–2. High-HMG stimulation protocol.

trial of these two main treatment schedules has been performed, it is impossible to conclude whether one is superior to the other. It is recommended that new centers that must choose between the two main modalities adhere to one regimen and acquaint themselves with its specific response pattern. Centers that use HMG may choose to use the "sweetened" FSH-HMG protocol as a first or second-line ovulation-induction protocol. In this case too, the theoretical advantages of FSH have not translated into clear, practical, clinical benefits.

Programmed Oocyte Retrieval: Contraceptive Pills– Clomiphene-HMG-HCG

An interesting and innovative approach to planned ovulation induction includes trying to preprogram the date of follicular aspiration 2 to 3 months in advance.[65] In the cycle prior to oocyte recovery, women were treated by triphasic contraceptive pills. This treatment was discontinued arbitrarily and ovulation induction with CC-HMG started; HCG was administered on day 11 so that retrieval was always carried out on day 13. This protocol achieved 23% conceptions per transfer.

A similar approach taken by another group used 2 months of combined contraceptive pills prior to the treatment cycle. They achieved similar results to nontreated cycles, and demonstrated that patient scheduling could be predetermined well in advance and that the contraceptive pills had no untoward effects on the endometrium.[66] These authors also concluded that stimulated ovaries that have been in a resting state due to previous pretreatment may achieve better follicular growth. In this respect, it seems that GnRH analogs are more effective than contraceptive pills.

GnRH and GnRH Analogs

One of the difficulties encountered when menotropins are used to stimulate the growth of several follicles is asynchronous development. Follicles mature at different rates because not all are at the same stage of development when menotropin treatment is

started. Follicular development is a random event that begins at least 60 days prior to the onset of the rise of FSH that indicates the onset of a given menstrual cycle.[67] This development is not gonadotropin dependent and occurs even in women who are gonadotropin deficient. When menotropins are administered, some follicles are more advanced than others, and therefore of different sizes and producing variable quantities of estrogen.[68] Thus, since oocytes must be aspirated simultaneously, not all are ready for fertilization.

Another problem with endogenous pituitary secretion is the premature LH surge. Under ordinary circumstances the pituitary responds to sustained elevations of estrogen levels with a positive feedback response in LH secretion. Although this physiologic response is necessary for single ovulation to occur, LH surges prior to the administration of HCG in stimulated cycles can result in ovulation prior to egg retrieval. Even if ovulation does not occur, exposure to high levels of LH prior to ovulation can have detrimental effects on the developing oocyte.[69] Premature LH surges are troublesome in stimulated cycles and are evident by a decline in estrogen levels.

These observations led to a search for a method to eliminate gonadotropin secretion in normally ovulating women. One method to achieve this goal and avoid a premature LH surge is to administer a GnRH agonist (GnRHa). Several GnRH analogs have been synthesized; however, only leuprolide (Lupron, TAP Inc) is approved by the Food and Drug Administration in the United States, and only for prostate cancer. Some of the GnRH agonists that are currently undergoing clinical trials are shown in Table 35–1.[70]

A GnRHa was initially used in IVF to pretreat normally menstruating women who experienced premature LH surges in superovulation cycles. Delivering HOE-766 (Hoechst, North Somerville, NJ) by nasal spray, 1,000 μg 5 times daily, together with progressively increasing doses of HMG, resulted in complete elimination of premature luteinization as measured by serum progesterone concentration.[71] Similar results were reported with fewer cancelled cycles, more mature oocytes, and higher pregnancy

TABLE 35–1. CURRENTLY AVAILABLE GnRH ANALOGS

Compound	Name	Administration	Company
[D-Leu^6,Pro^{9}NEt]GnRH	Leuprorelin*	Daily injection	TAP
[D-Trp^6]GnRH	Tryptorelin	Injection	Lederle
[D-Trp^6,Pro^{9}NEt]GnRH	Lutrelin	Injection	Wyeth
[D-Ser(tBu)^6,Pro^{9}NEt]GnRH	Buserelin	Nasal	Hoechst
[D-Ser(tBu)^6,Aza-Gly^{10}]GnRH	Zoladex	Implant	ICI
[D-His(Bzl)^6,Pro^{9}NEt]GnRH	Histrelin	Injection	Ortho
[D-Nal(2)^6]GnRH	Nafarelin	Nasal	Synthex

*Available in the United States.

rates (29 versus 13%) when women undergoing IVF were premedicated with [D-TRP⁶]- GnRH.[72] At Mount Sinai Hospital 10 women whose cycles were cancelled because of premature LH surges were treated with leuprolide beginning in the luteal phase of the cycle prior to HMG stimulation. After withdrawal bleeding, leuprolide was continued, and progressively increasing doses of HMG were administered until an ovarian response was achieved. None of these patients experienced a decline in estradiol prior to HCG administration; 3 pregnancies occurred in this group (Fig. 35–3).

Administration of a GnRH analog for IVF is also indicated in poorly responsive women. A group of women in whom fewer than 3 oocytes were aspirated experienced a twofold increase in the number of oocytes recovered.[73] Buserelin (Hoechst) resulted in fewer abandoned cycles because of inadequate folliculogenesis (14 versus 53%).[74] A high response was obtained in 3 of 5 women who had suboptimal responses to menotropins with [D-His⁶, Pro⁹-NEt]-GnRH pretreatment.[75]

Although low responders have improved cycles with GnRHa pretreatment, perimenopausal women pose a special problem. Women with elevated gonadotropin levels respond poorly to menotropins because of diminished FSH receptors on their granulosa cells. Their cycles are marked by a shortened follicular phase due to elevated FSH secretion. Theoretically, decreasing FSH secretion should result in stimulation. Although some patients who were classified as low responders may have had elevated gonadotropin levels, as yet no large series of perimenopausal women exists. Six of 8 women with elevated gonadotropins were stimulated with high-dose pulsatile GnRH.[76]

When the analog is first administered, a brief agonist effect is seen initially prior to down-regulation. Hyperstimulation with GnRHa alone was reported secondary to this agonist effect, but is not common.[75] It seems that most of the LH that is

secreted immediately is immunoactive, but not bioactive, and does not stimulate the ovaries.[77]

The best time to begin the GnRHa pretreatment seems to be in the midluteal phase. Beginning in the follicular phase after the FSH level has already risen prolongs the duration of therapy required to achieve suppression. In preliminary studies performed with GnRHa administered in the midluteal phase, suppression usually occurred by the time the next menstrual period was due.[78,79]

One of the disadvantages of using GnRHa for down-regulation is the length of time required for this effect to occur. By altering the amino acid substitutions in the native GnRH molecule, antagonists can be synthesized that have high-affinity binding to the GnRH receptor without any agonistic properties. Antagonists of GnRH have not yet been studied in large clinical trials in humans because of their tendency to cause histamine release. Primates pretreated with GnRH antagonists had a more homogeneous response to HMG therapy.[80] In the future, more of these compounds may become available.

The luteal phase of patients pretreated with GnRHa is characterized by deficient progesterone secretion. Cycles in which GnRHa was used had 70% of the progesterone secretion in the luteal phase compared to cycles in which menotropins and clomiphene were administered.[81]

In summary, premedication with a GnRHa as a pretreatment to HMG therapy for superovulation may potentially improve IVF results by inducing better interfollicular synchronization. The elimination of premature LH surges is sufficient justification to use these agents in appropriately selected patients.

CLINICAL MONITORING OF OVULATION INDUCTION

An optimal system of ovulation induction is probably the most important factor affecting the success of IVF,

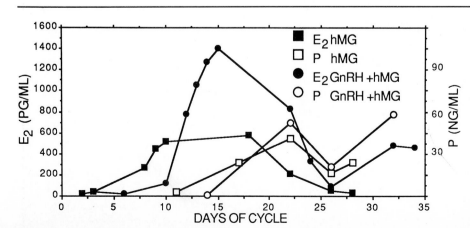

Figure 35–3. Combined GnRH analog + HMG conception cycle compared to a previous aborted HMG cycle in the same patient.

because it determines the quality of oocytes, the completeness of endometrial responsiveness, and corpus luteum function. The two most widely used peripheral markers for monitoring ovarian activity in IVF and ovulation induction are estradiol-17β (E_2) to assess follicle development (mostly in combination with ovarian ultrasonography), and progesterone as a marker of luteinization and corpus luteum function. Some centers also measure LH in urine or serum as a means of intercepting a premature LH surge.

The programmed succession of steps involved in follicular growth and maturation, as well as in endometrial development, are maintained through a delicate balance of steroid and nonsteroidal signals. Because of this apparent complexity it is necessary to weigh the relative importance of these steroid markers and to determine whether E_2 and progesterone are sufficient by themselves to act on their main target organ, the endometrium, to induce morphologic and functional changes compatible with successful embryo implantation. Women with primary ovarian failure who conceived after the transfer of donated embryos to the uterus serve as a unique model to address this question. We[82,83] and others[84,85] performing oocyte donation have demonstrated conclusively that artificially induced endometrial maturation is coupled with functional receptivity. Pregnancies resulting from the transfer of donated embryos to fallopian tubes demonstrate that it is also possible artificially to mimic functional changes within the tubes that support normal growth and propagation of an embryo to the implantation site solely by administering E_2 and progesterone.[86]

These clinical trials clearly suggest that serum levels of the two markers might be sufficient to assess follicular growth and endometrial responsiveness if they are properly interpreted. The monitoring and consequent titration of medication in the original embryo-donation protocols were geared to mimic an unstimulated cycle. During the normal ovulatory cycle follicular growth is linear and is paralleled by an increase in circulating E_2. In these cycles, ultrasound measurements of follicles correlated well with serum E_2 levels, and both these variables were shown to be equally effective predictors of follicle growth.[87,88] In natural cycles, 95% of circulating E_2 levels were shown to emanate from the growing follicle[89] and ovulation to occur at a fairly narrow range of 22 to 27 mm.[90]

In induced cycles, the normal monofollicular quota is disturbed, creating radical changes in the intraovarian milieu.[91] When serum E_2 levels and follicle size, determined by ultrasound, were correlated in normally ovulating women treated with clomiphene for IVF, both increased linearly, but the correlation between separate pooled values was significantly lower than that reported for the normal cycle.[92] Similarly, in HMG cycles for IVF, no correlation was found between serum E_2 and the size of the largest follicle.[93] We found that E_2 alone on the day of HCG administration could not differentiate between women developing 1 large (> 15 mm) follicle (635 ± 47 pg/mL) and those developing 3 large follicles (687 ± 86 pg/mL).[90] The mean follicular volume did not differ in these cycles. We therefore concluded that the individual follicle contributes more to peripheral E_2 levels in monofollicular cycles than in multifollicular cycles. This observation, coupled with our demonstration that mature oocytes are not necessarily aspirated from large follicles, strongly suggests an asynchrony between follicular growth and functional maturation.[68]

The crucial decision in every IVF cycle is the timing of HCG administration, which triggers the cascade of luteal phase events. Premature administration disrupts preovulatory follicular development and results in failure to ovulate.[94] Delay in HCG administration was associated with a reduced fertilization rate and an increased percentage of degenerated oocytes caused by prolonged oocyte retention in follicles undergoing atresia.[95] Due to close monitoring to IVF cycles, further insight was gained into ovulation induction, and better criteria were established for the timing of HCG administration and cancellation of cycles.

The absolute level of E_2 at the time of HCG administration seems to play an important part in IVF success. Low responders have been shown to do poorly, and arbitrary high cutoff levels have been retrospectively correlated with better success rates. In the Norfolk program, high responders (> 600 pg/mL) had a higher conception rate than low responders (< 300 pg/mL) (23 and 15%, respectively).[96] Using the same protocol or ovulation induction, cycles that did not reach an E_2 level of over 700 pg/mL were aborted.[97] A significantly higher conception rate was shown in CC-HMG cycles when E_2 levels were above 1,000 pg/mL on the day of HCG (20 versus 4%, respectively) and 17 and 13% in high-HMG IVF cycles.[58] Similar findings were reported for E_2 levels exceeding 1,000 pg/mL in "programmed" cycles (50 and 5.6%, respectively).[98] In a retrospective analysis of 242 IVF cycles employing high-HMG and ultrasound-guided aspiration, a higher cutoff point (1,500 pg/mL) was associated with a doubling of conception rates (20.5 and 10.4%, respectively; $p < 0.5$).[99] It is concluded that absolute E_2 levels greater than 1,000 pg/mL for CC-HMG cycles, over 800 pg/mL for high HMG, and above 500 to 700 pg/mL in low-HMG cycles, are associated with a better clinical conception rate. Because the success of IVF is multivariant, it may be that a higher cutoff point with a subsequent higher number of oocytes and embryos may compensate for deficiencies in growth conditions in a given

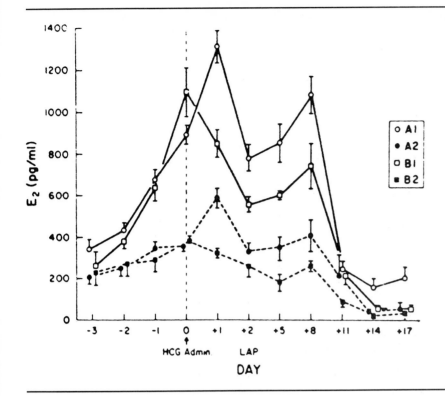

Figure 35–4. The pattern of E_2 response in IVF patients treated by a high-HMG protocol.

laboratory environment. It is therefore mandatory for each program to establish its own criteria for minimal serum E_2 levels on the day of HCG, below which it would be justified to abort a cycle.

It appears that in addition to the absolute E_2 level, the pattern of the E_2 response may serve as a relatively good predictor of oocyte quality and the success of IVF. We identified two basic patterns of E_2 response in a retrospective analysis of 144 patients receiving high-dose HMG-HCG treatment: group A showed an increase in E_2 levels ($\geq$ 10% over the previous day's determinations) on day +1 (the day after HCG administration); group B had a decrease in E_2 levels on day +1. Each of these groups was further subdivided into high responders ($E_2 > 500$ pg/mL on day 0) designated A_1 and B_1, and low responders ($E_2 < 500$ pg/mL on day 0) designated A_2 and B_2 (Fig. 35–4). Group A_1 patients had a higher E_2 level from days 0 through +8, developed a larger number of follicles on the day of laparoscopy, and attained a higher number of fertilized oocytes. Group A patients had the highest rate of pregnancies per aspiration rate and the highest continuing pregnancy rate (Table 35–2). Over 90% of continuing pregnancies occurred

TABLE 35–2. THE ASSOCIATION BETWEEN CONCEPTION RATE AFTER IVF AND THE PATTERN OF E_2 RESPONSE

Results of IVF E_2 Pattern	Classified by A_1	Follicular A_2	Serum E_2 Pattern B_1	B_2	Total
Follicles/woman	6.3	4.8	5.7	3.4	5.6
Oocytes/woman	5.±2.3	3.5±1.8	4.4±2.4	2.4±1.4	4.3±2.1
Oocytes recovered/follicle (%)	80	73	76	70	77.1
Transfer/laparoscopy	95	90	82	64	88.0
Pregnancy/transfer (%)	20	15	16	0	17
Pregnancy/laparoscopy (%)	19	14	13	0	15
Continuing pregnancy/laparoscopy (%)	13	7	3	0	8
Continuing pregnancy/transfer (%)	13	8	3	0	9

Source: From Laufer et al.[100] Reproduced with permission.
Dunan's test analysis of oocytes per woman:
A_1 vs B_1 (p<0.05); A_1 vs B_1 (p<0.05); A_2 vs B_2 (p<0.05); A_1 vs B_1 (NS); B_1 vs A_2 (NS); B_1 vs B_2 (NS).

in women with a type A pattern, and of these, 80% had an A_1 response.[100] Similar findings were reported in CC- HMG[36] and low-HMG cycles.[96]

The association between E_2 pattern and oocyte maturity and development was further evaluated. Decreasing E_2 levels on the day of HCG administration or the day after its injection correlated with decreased fertilization and cleavage when compared with cycles with increasing E_2.[101] Similarly, the number of atretic oocytes and the percentage of polyspermic fertilization were higher, suggesting postmaturity of oocytes derived from cycles with a decreasing E_2 pattern. Furthermore, an A pattern was associated with a better developmental potential— that is, a higher percentage of regular embryos and a higher conception rate.[102] Other observations[103–105] corroborated the fact that a continuous daily estradiol rate is associated with a better IVF outcome. The pattern of E_2 seems to be important also in patients classified as group II (World Health Organization) undergoing HMG ovulation induction. In these patients we found that women with type A_1 response had a significantly greater chance of conceiving than those with a B_1 response (55 and 14%, respectively). Moreover, of all conceptions, 78% occurred in type A_1 responders and the rest in type B.[106] In the natural ovulatory cycle the spontaneous LH surge is followed by a fall in E_2 levels. In contradistinction, during HMG induction of ovulation, an increase in E_2 after HCG is associated with a significantly higher conception rate.

These retrospective studies strongly suggest that oocyte maturation, normalcy of fertilization, and morphology of embryos and their subsequent developmental potential are already determined before oocyte recovery. Furthermore, high E_2 levels that continue to increase after HCG administration positively affect oocyte quality and endometrial receptiveness.

The value of monitoring IVF cycles with progesterone levels in addition to E_2 is not clear. The two markers were investigated as the sole monitoring variables in CC-HMG cycles, omitting follicular ultrasound. When HCG was administered 2 days after E_2, levels were higher than 800 pg/mL, and progesterone levels did not exceed 1.5 ng/mL.[107] With this simplified monitoring system, 30% clinical pregnancy and 9% cancellation rates were achieved. These authors did not find any difference in E_2 or progesterone levels between conception and nonconception cycles. A comparison of the progesterone:E_2 ratio in 5 pregnant and 8 nonpregnant patients after clomiphene-HMG stimulation for IVF revealed no difference on the day of HCG administration (day 0) and 4 days prior to day 0.[108] In a larger group of 79 patients treated by high-dose HMG-HCG, we compared the progesterone:E_2 ratio in 13 patients who conceived, 8

who had an early pregnancy loss, and 58 who did not conceive. Neither E_2 nor progesterone individually differed between the pregnant and nonpregnant groups, but ratio on day 0 was significantly lower for conception cycles (0.69 versus 1.24; $p < 0.08$). It may be hypothesized that an optimal ratio is necessary for the development of a receptive endometrium or is an indirect marker of optimal follicular development.

Alternatively, a higher ratio may be associated with a premature LH surge or high tonic levels of LH. Measurement of urinary LH in CC-HMG cycles revealed that high urinary LH levels before oocyte recovery were associated with a high cancellation and lower fertilization rates, and a poor quality of embryos.[109] In a group of 63 similarly treated women, those whose basal LH values were more than 1 SD above the mean had decreased fertilization and cleavage rates, and did not achieve pregnancy.[69] This phenomenon was attributed to premature oocyte maturation or aging. Both the progesterone:E_2 ratio and the tonic levels of LH need further corroboration before a more conclusive decision can be made as to their value in routine monitoring IVF cycles.

Serial ultrasound scanning of the ovaries is a standard procedure in monitoring follicular growth in every IVF program. The transition from abdominal to vaginal sectors has increased the resolution and obviated the need for a full bladder. Several transducers have been devised to facilitate both imaging and vaginal oocyte aspiration.[110] With the increase in ultrasound resolution, it became possible to document not only size but also intrafollicular elements, such as loosening of the mural granulosa cells and the expanded cumulus mass. Evaluation of the detection of cumulus oophorus in IVF cycles revealed that when a cumulus mass was seen, it could be taken as a sign of oocyte maturity.[111] Mature oocytes were also found where no cumulus was seen, however. At present, the value of assessing intrafollicular structures seems to be limited.

Ultrasound may be used also to assess endometrial development indirectly. In spontaneous cycles, endometrial thickness was found to correlate well with E_2 and progesterone levels; however, this was not always the case in induced cycles.[112–114] In 47 IVF cycles (37 nonconception and 10 conception) we found three consecutive growth patterns: an accelerated growth rate of about 0.5 mm/day from 9 mm on day 3 to 12 mm on day +2; a second decreased rate of 0.1 mm/day until day +11; and an accelerated rate with the establishment of conception. No conception occurred with an endometrial thickness less than 13 mm on day +11, but 64% of nonconception cycles have also attained this value.[115] Endometrial thickness does not seem to be of any predictive value.

A modality that currently has a limited clinical application for routine monitoring is magnetic resonance imaging (MRI). In normal cycles we demonstrated that on ultrasound and MRI, endometrial development showed similar patterns (Fig. 35–5). A distinct feature of MRI was the demonstration of a junction zone located immediately beneath the endometrium (Fig. 35–6). From its anatomic location, it best correlates with the arcuate vessels. Because its maximum growth rate is between days 8 and 16 of a cycle—the time of maximal E_2 production—it may be that high E_2 levels have an angiogenic effect on junction zone vasculature, which in turn affects endometrial development.[116]

With the evolution of sonographic and Doppler techniques to measure blood flow, it may be that monitoring ovarian and uterine vasculature will increase the sensitivity of monitoring modalities and increase the success of ovulation induction and IVF.

OOCYTE ASPIRATION

Oocyte retrieval in humans was first performed in 1966 through a laparotomy.[117] A nonsurgical approach was described in 1972 in which oocytes were flushed from the endometrial cavity.[118] With further refinement of techniques, Edwards and Steptoe successfully fertilized human oocytes recovered laparoscopically in 1977.[1] Laparoscopy allows for direct visualization of the follicles as they are aspirated, and is the gold standard by which other methods are judged. In general, recovery rates with this technique range from 60 to 90% (Table 35–3).

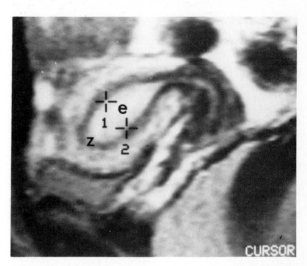

Figure 35–6. MRI of the uterus demonstrating the junctional zone (Z). Endometrial thickness is marked by crosshairs.

Improvements in ultrasound imaging have resulted in ultrasound-guided oocyte retrieval replacing laparoscopic retrieval. Oocytes can be aspirated through the anterior abdominal wall or through the urethra with an abdominal transducer, or through the vagina with either an abdominal or a vaginal transducer. One of the difficulties encountered with ultrasound-guided retrievals is proper spatial orientation. When the needle is not in the path of the ultrasound beam it is not visible, and its movement is difficult to control. Therefore both abdominal and vaginal transducers are equipped with guides that directly couple the path of the needle to the plane of the ultrasound beam.

The first ultrasound-guided aspiration of oocytes was performed transabdominally by Lenz and Lauritsen in Denmark.[119] Their approach was transabdominal with a transvesicle puncture. Oocyte recovery rate in this series was 53%, which compares favorably with laparoscopically performed procedures. Transurethral[120] and transvaginal[121] approaches to the ovary using an abdominal transducer have also been used.

A major improvement in ultrasound retrieval occurred with the development of transvaginal transducers. Ovaries that are surrounded by dense adhesions tend to be fixed to the cul-de-sac, a location that is most easily reached transvaginally (Fig. 35–7). The absence of bowel gas in this location allows the ovaries to be visualized directly without the need of a sonic window to enhance transmission.[122,123] Transabdominal and transvaginal ultrasound-guided follicular aspirations have resulted in oocyte retrieval rates of 60 to 75%, which are comparable to those obtained by laparoscopy (see Table 35–3).[122,124–130] In addition to easier access to the ovaries with vaginal aspiration, the risks of bladder injury, hematuria, and

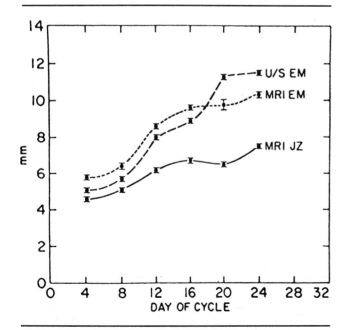

Figure 35–5. Comparison of ultrasound (U/S) and MRI pattern of endometrial (EM) and junctional zone (JZ) development in 5 natural cycles.

TABLE 35-3. COMPARISON OF LAPAROSCOPIC AND ULTRASOUND ASPIRATION TECHNIQUES

| | Recovery Rate (% of follicles aspirated no. of eggs) | | | Fertilization Rate % | | |
Reference	Laparoscopy	Transvesicle	Transvaginal	Laparoscopy	Transvesicle	Transvaginal
124	91/3.0	70 1.7		72	88	
Levy et al, unpublished data, 1987	83/5.7		73/6.0 Vag scan	60		63
125			43/2.2 Abd scan			37
126	92/3.7		75/4.7 Abd scan	69		68
127	86/2.3		74/2.6 Vag scan	75		54
128	60/4.0	74/5.3		71	63	
129	62/2.1	69/1.57		68	86	
130		68/5.5			75	

infection that are associated with transvesical puncture[130] are reduced.

The needle used for oocyte recovery has also received a great deal of attention. It is the goal to recover the maximum number of oocytes with minimal trauma. If the inner diameter of the needle is too small, shearing off of the cumulus cells and possible damage to the oocytes may occur. A better yield during laparoscopy was achieved using a 2.16-mm (14-gauge) needle as compared with a 1.2-mm (19-gauge) needle.[131] Smaller diameters were also used successfully, however, and a fine needle with an inner diameter of 1.4 mm was reported to be more efficient than a coarse needle with an inner diameter of 2.2 mm.[132]

In our IVF program laparoscopic retrievals are performed with a 14-gauge needle. It is modified

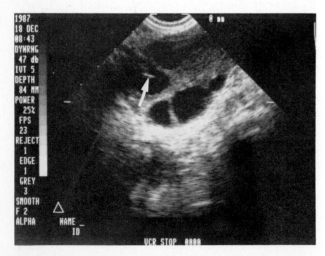

Figure 35-7. Transvaginal ultrasonically guided oocyte aspiration. The echogenic tip of the needle is visualized within a follicle (arrow).

from a Tru-cut biopsy needle and allows easy attachment of a DeLee suction trap for the collection of follicular fluid. The large diameter does not disrupt the cumulus cells from the oocyte and results in recovery rates of 83%.[55] Transvaginal retrievals are performed with a smaller needle with an outer diameter of 17 gauge, while transvesicle procedures are performed with 14-gauge needles.

Suction pressures are usually controlled at 100 to 170 mm Hg. Although the recovery rate increases when vacuum is raised from 120 to 200 mm Hg, this is compromised by a higher rate of damaged oocytes.[133] At suction pressures of over 200 mm Hg there was damage to the ocrona radiata and the vitelline membrane resulting in "fractured oocytes." Aspiration with a syringe provides uncontrolled suction pressure that also is likely to result in damage to the oocyte.[134] Better recovery rates were noted for all needle sizes tested when suction pressures under 150 to 200 mm Hg were compared to those over 200 mm Hg.[103] Flushing the follicle enhances oocyte recovery rates by approximately 10 to 20%.[135] Whether flushing should be performed is a decision each program must make based on its oocyte recovery rates.

Laparoscopy is performed under general anesthesia, while ultrasound aspirations have less anesthetic requirements. Transvesicle aspirations have been performed with local anesthesia and sedation, but the posterior bladder wall cannot be anesthetized and the transvesicle puncture is often quite painful.[119] Regional anesthesia is recommended by some authors for transvesicle recoveries.[136] Transvaginal approaches to the ovary are less painful, and some perform this procedure on an ambulatory basis with only a paracervical block and intravenous sedation.[137,138]

Patients who have transvaginal ultrasound aspirations under local anesthesia tolerate the procedure well. In fact, unanimous preference was voiced by patients for this method of retrieval.[139] Although 90% of patients experienced some pain or no pain, none described the procedure as very painful.[140] Premedication with a sedative and paracervical block was sufficient anesthesia for 70% and additional sedation was necessary for 20%; 10% found the procedure to be painful enough to require heavier anesthesia.[140]

No major complications were reported in over 800 transvaginal recoveries.[141] Reports of pelvic infection after vaginal retrieval are unpublished, but there appears to be less than 1 infection for every 100 procedures performed. Because of the proximity of the hypogastric vessels to the ovary, care should be taken to avoid lacerations. The major vessels are easily visualized and avoided with transvaginal ultrasound scanning (Fig. 35–8).

Most centers perform oocyte aspirations under the guidance of transvaginal ultrasound. Transvesicle retrievals are still appropriate for the occasional patient who may have had an ovarian suspension or whose ovaries are situated near the fundus of the uterus. The laparoscopic technique should not be entirely abandoned, as some patients may have oocyte retrieval at the same time as a diagnostic laparoscopy. This is currently also the procedure of choice for those who are having oocyte retrieval for IVF combined with GIFT. Physicians who perform oocyte retrieval should be familiar with all the techniques so that even patients with ovaries in unusual locations can have optimal oocyte recovery.

IN-VITRO FERTILIZATION AND EMBRYO CULTURE

Culture Medium

The procedures used for human IVF are derived largely from the extensive literature developed for mouse, rabbit, and hamster gamete and embryo culture. Several culture media have been used with

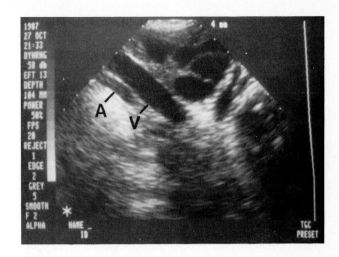

Figure 35–8. Vaginal ultrasonography demonstrates the proximity of the hypogastric vessels (A = artery, V = vein) to the follicles.

success for human IVF, ranging from Ham's F10[2], a complex solution of salts, vitamins, cofactors, and amino acids, to simple balanced salt solutions (Whittingham's T6,[142] Quinn's HTF,[143] and Earle's solutions).[144] None of these culture media has been demonstrated to have a clear advantage over the others. We examined the performance of Ham's F10 and human tubal fluid (HTF) in a prospectively randomized clinical study. Although we found no significant difference in the clinical pregnancy rate, we did observe a difference in the morphologic appearance and in the rate of cleavage of embryos grown in the two media. Embryos grown in HTF contained blastomeres that were more consistently regular in size and shape than their counterparts grown in Ham's F10 (Fig. 35–9). Furthermore, the rate of cleavage, judged by the proportion of embryos that developed past the 4-cell stage in a 40-hour culture period, was significantly increased by culture in HTF.

In addition to the formulation of the medium, the purity of the water used for its preparation is critical. In most laboratories, deionized water is glass-distilled two to five times prior to use.[145]

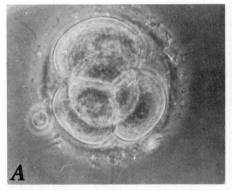
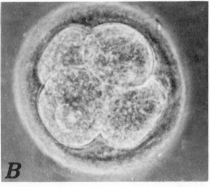

Figure 35–9. Morphologic comparison of human embryos cultures in Ham's F10 and HTF medium. **A.** A 4-cell embryo after 40 hours of culture in HTF medium. **B.** A 4-cell embryo after 40 hours of culture in Ham's F10; note the slight increase in cytoplasmic granularity and the slightly irregular cellular outlines in the blastomeres of this embryo.

Commercially available high-pressure liquid chromatography (HPLC)-grade water is also widely used,[146] especially in heavily industrialized areas where organic impurities may persist even in rigorously redistilled water.

High-molecular-weight serum macromolecules have been shown to enhance fertilization and cleavage rates,[147] although the value of adding protein supplementation to the medium has been questioned.[148] A source of protein is routinely used as a medium supplement in most IVF laboratories. Homologous maternal serum,[149] fetal cord serum,[52] human serum albumin (HSA),[150] bovine serum albumin (BSA),[145] and human amniotic fluid[151] have been used successfully as protein supplements. Maternal and fetal cord sera are used most commonly as medium supplements; no well-controlled clinical studies have shown either of these serum sources to provide a significant advantage. Although individual samples of maternal serum have been shown to be deleterious to mouse embryos cultured in vitro,[152] their use for human IVF has not resulted in a significant decrease in the pregnancy rate.[153] Supplementation with heat-inactivated, sterile-filtered serum is usually 7.5 to 10% for insemination medium, and, after pronuclei are identified, 15 to 20% for the 24-hour period after fertilization. When HSA or BSA is used, it is added at a level of 3 to 5 mg/mL. Studies of serum substitutes (defined preparations of growth factors, hormones, and nutrients) on the development of mouse embryos have failed to demonstrate an advantage over current procedures.[154,155]

Culture Conditions

Environmental conditions are important to the culture of gametes and embryos. The pH of the medium is maintained in the range of 7.35 to 7.4 by culture is an environment of 5% carbon dioxide. Phenol red is used in most media formulations as a sensitive pH indicator in the range of 6.5 to 8. The establishment and strict maintenance of physiologic pH in the culture medium is an absolute requirement for human IVF. The amount of time that the oocytes or embryos are exposed to other than optimum pH should be carefully monitored and minimized.

The optimum oxygen concentration in the culture environment is a matter of some debate. In early mouse work, in-vitro culture of 1-cell embryos to the blastocyst stage in certain strains could only be achieved in the presence of a reduced oxygen tension (5% CO_2, 5% O_2, 90% N_2).[156] Also, some evidence indicates that the oxygen tension in the oviduct is lower than atmospheric oxygen pressure. Nevertheless, human embryos, as well as embryos from a variety of experimental and domestic animals, develop well in an atmosphere of 5% carbon dioxide in air (20% O_2). No comparative studies have shown

that culture in either this or the triple mix offers a significant advantage in human IVF.

Embryos are normally grown at a temperature of 37°C. A slight increase in this temperature (to about 37.3°C) results in a modest increase in the developmental rate of the embryos. There is no evidence that this increase is beneficial to the establishment of human pregnancies, however. Maintaining the appropriate temperature and minimizing deviations from that temperature during observation and handling are essential. The choice of incubator design is important in this regard. Water-jacketed incubators are designed to minimize the decrease in internal temperature when the door is opened; however, recovery of the designated temperature also occurs more slowly in these incubators. Although incubators that do not employ water jackets may have a greater loss of temperature when the door is opened, the recovery time is relatively quick. In a busy laboratory, when the incubator door is unavoidably opened with some frequency, rapid temperature recovery may have a significant benefit over the slow loss and slow recovery design. It has been shown that slow recovery of temperature in an incubator can have an adverse effect on the rate of embryo cleavage in a human IVF program.[157]

Plastic organ culture dishes, plastic or glass test tubes, and drops of medium under paraffin oil have all been used with success for human IVF and embryo culture. Each of these vessels has relative advantages and disadvantages. Culture in organ culture dishes is widely practical, because a relatively large volume (1 to 3 mL) of medium can be used to minimize osmotic changes and local depletion of metabolites. Care must be exercised to minimize handling time of dishes, because it has been shown that the pH rises above physiologic levels in less than 2 minutes in room air.[158] Temperature and pH recover to appropriate levels relatively rapidly after the dishes are replaced in the incubator. The advantage of culture in tubes is that the surface area is minimized, so that the loss of pH and temperature equilibration is minimized. A layer of paraffin oil over drops of medium prevents osmotic changes due to evaporation, and slows the loss of pH and temperature equilibration. Return to the appropriate temperature and pH is also slowed by the layer of oil, which must be tested carefully for toxicity.

Maintaining quality control standards, both for medium preparation and for any other component of the IVF process, is of primary importance. Routine medium testing by mouse embryo culture reveals irregularities in a preparation prior to its exposure to human material. The most common test of medium suitability employs mouse embryos fertilized in vivo, collected at the 2-cell stage, and cultured to the hatched blastocyst stage.[159] Mouse embryos are quite easily cultured in this manner, and it is not uncommon to observe a developmental rate of 2-cell embryos exceeding 90%. The culture of 1-cell mouse embryos has been employed by many groups to increase the sensitivity of the assay[160]; this test provides a more reliable indicator of the suitability of the medium.

A more crude quality control check is the sperm-survival assay, wherein sperm are maintained in vitro for 72 hours, after which their survival and motility are assessed. The advantages of this test are that it is readily available as a by-product of each IVF cycle, and that each batch of serum can be tested with little difficulty. These quality control assays are readily adaptable to determine embryo toxicity of individual components of the IVF process, or to assess procedural differences in embryo handling or culture.

Taking these factors into account, we currently use either Ham's F10 or HTF, prepared fresh weekly with HPLC water, and supplemented with human maternal serum at a level of 10% for insemination medium and 20% for growth medium. In the event of sperm-directed antibodies in the maternal serum, we use BSA (3 mg/mL) as a medium supplement. We use a dry-jacketed incubator, with the capability to produce a reduced oxygen environment (5% CO_2, 5% O_2, 90% N_2). Organ culture dishes contain 2 cc of medium, without an oil overlay. In choosing these conditions, we have opted for a system in which equilibration is rapidly lost and rapidly recovered, as opposed to one in which it is slowly lost and slowly recovered.

Oocyte Maturation

The mammalian oocyte undergoes a complex series of structural and metabolic changes prior to ovulation. The most obvious of these is the resumption of meiosis. The germinal vesicle, characteristic of the prophase I stage of meiosis, is broken down, and the oocyte progresses to metaphase II, resulting in the extrusion of the first polar body. These chromosomal changes are accompanied by a variety of other events, including transcription, protein synthesis, changes in energy metabolism, and differential membrane transport.

It is important to assess the maturity of the preovulatory oocyte obtained by follicular aspiration so as to optimize the rate of fertilization. Immature (germinal vesicle stage) oocytes should be allowed to mature in vitro prior to insemination.[161] Similarly, metaphase II oocytes should be inseminated soon after retrieval. Insemination of either immature or postmature oocytes results in a decreased rate of fertilization and in an increased rate of polyspermy.[162]

Because it is difficult to visualize cytoplasmic markers of maturity through the cumulus cell mass and the dense corona cell layer surrounding the oocyte, several schemes have been devised to assist the determination. The least invasive of these procedures is an assessment of the degree of disassociation of the oocyte-corona-cumulus complex (OCCC). In a natural cycle, when an oocyte is aspirated from a mature follicle a few hours before ovulation, the corona-cumulus cell mass around it has undergone a process of mucification and dispersal, which is paralleled by the resumption of meiosis and oocyte maturation. In stimulated cycles, asynchrony exists between the appearance of the cumulus cell mass and the actual maturity of the oocyte. Only 38% of oocytes judged as mature according to their OCCC morphology at the time of aspiration were found to contain a polar body. It was possible by removing the OCCC enzymatically (hyaluronidase, 300 IU/mL) to observe that after 8 hours of preincubation an additional 30% attained a polar body.[163] In the absence of a precise determination of the meiotic state of the oocyte, it has been empirically determined that an in-vitro culture period of 5 to 8 hours between aspiration and insemination optimizes the rate of fertilization and subsequent embryo cleavage.[161]

Sperm Preparation and Insemination

At the time of ejaculation, human sperm are incapable of fertilization. As they make their way through the cervical mucus, the "decapacitation factor" is stripped away from them and capacitation is allowed to occur. Therefore when sperm are collected for IVF, it is important to separate them from the seminal proteins in order to facilitate capacitation. Several methods have been devised to do this. Most IVF centers use a two-step washing procedure combined with a swim-up separation.

After liquefaction, a sperm count and estimation of motility are made. The semen is diluted with insemination medium and then centrifuged at 300 g to pellet the spermatozoa. The supernatant is removed and the pellet is resuspended in insemination medium. After a second centrifugation, the sperm pellet is gently overlaid with insemination medium. During a subsequent incubation period of 1 hour, the motile sperm from the pellet swim into the medium. In this manner, the most highly motile sperm can be isolated from the ejaculate. The swim-up procedure may be a crude mimicry of the type of selection of motile sperm that probably occurs in the cervical mucus in natural cycles.

One variation of this procedure is to perform the swim-up prior to washing by carefully layering the insemination medium over the more dense semen. This technique has the advantage of providing a greater yield, because the sperm are not swimming from a densely packed pellet, and results in a cleaner preparation. A disadvantage is that the removal of the seminal proteins is delayed by up to 1 hour. Another variation is to resuspend the sperm after washing, and to underlay a column of insemination medium with the suspension.[164]

When motility is low, a swim-up may not provide sufficient numbers of sperm for insemination. Selection of motile sperm in a discontinuous Percoll gradient is frequently used in these cases. The Percoll technique, first developed by Gorus and Dipelecos[165] and refined by Forster and associates,[166] separates the cells that are present in the ejaculate according to density. The seminal fluid and most other seminal cells are excluded from layers containing more than 60% Percoll. In layers containing more than 80% Percoll, there is a significant enrichment of motile spermatozoa (up to 90%).[167] Discontinuous gradients are created by pipetting 1-mL aliquots of decreasing concentrations of isotonic Percoll (made by diluting the aqueous Percoll with concentrated culture medium) in a centrifuge tube. Many different specific schemes are in use; a typical pattern is, from the top to the bottom of the tube, 55, 80, and 95% Percoll in insemination medium. Semen is gently placed on the top of the gradient, followed by centrifugation at 300 g for 45 minutes. The upper two layers are discarded, and the lower two layers (80 and 95% Percoll) are washed twice to remove residual Percoll.

Occasionally, the initial percentage of motile sperm in a given sample is so low that the typical losses due to processing either by swim-up or Percoll gradients yield insufficient numbers. In such cases, a simple two-step washing technique is used to minimize the loss of motile spermatozoa. It also may be feasible to collect sperm specimens over a number of days and pool the washed spermatozoa for insemination. It was shown that motility is maintained in at least half of the sperm for a mean of 153 hours when held at room temperature in equilibrated, serum-containing medium.[168] This value varied among patients from 24 to 290 hours.

Insemination for human IVF is usually carried out in a final concentration of 50,000 to 100,000 sperm/mL. As few as 10,000 and as many as 1 million sperm/mL have been used with success. In cases of severe oligospermia, we increase the number of sperm from 100,000 to 500,000.

Embryo Development In Vitro

The ova are transferred from insemination medium to growth medium 16 to 18 hours after insemination. If cumulus or corona cells obscure visualization of pronuclei, they are removed by repeated gentle pipetting with hand-drawn pipettes. Pronuclei may be located either centrally or ecentrically, and contain up to 8 nucleoli.[169] The male and female pronuclei are generally indistinguishable. It is important to verify the presence of only 2 pronuclei in order to prevent the transfer of triploid embryos. Triploid embryos are observed in 4 to 12% of oocytes fertilized in vitro,[170] and after syngamy they are indistinguishable from their diploid counterparts. Triploid embryos are capable of development for a variable period in utero.[171] Care should be taken in assessing triploidy, however. Because cellular vacuoles may be confused with pronuclei, presumed triploid oocytes were examined with the electron microscope, and vacuoles that resembled pronuclei but that did not contain chromosomes frequently appeared in the cytoplasm of fertilized oocytes.[172] These investigators suggest that the presence of nucleoli be used as a definitive diagnostic criterion of a pronucleus.

Methods to assess the viability of embryonic cleavage stages are largely noninvasive. Cleavage rate, and the size, number, and general appearance of the blastomeres, have been used as the principal indicators of viability. Neither the rate of development nor the morphology of the embryos is a precise indicator of developmental potential. There is a correlation between the transfer of the more rapidly dividing embryos and in increased frequency of implantation; however, slowly dividing embryos may also produce viable fetuses.[173]

Embryonic morphology is also not a completely reliable indicator of developmental viability, as several irregularities have been observed in human embryos. When anucleate cytoplasmic fragments are observed and comprise only a small proportion of the embryo, they appear to have no effect on the subsequent viability of the embryo. More extensive fragmentation usually indicates reduced viability. Similarly, the degree of cytoplasmic granulation in human embryos is variable, with no clear indication that this factor is related to embryonic quality. Intermediate cleavage stages (3 and 5 cells) may indicate that cleavage was arrested prior to the completion of the next cell division, but usually these embryos continue to divide normally.

Other noninvasive techniques may provide information on the developmental potential of human embryos. Evidence exists that the presence of a relatively thick zona pellucida around the oocyte at the time of recovery indicates increased potential for cell division in vitro.[174] Zona thickness may be a function of oocyte maturity, because it has been shown to increase in thickness as the follicle develops.[175]

It may also be possible to differentiate among embryos with varying developmental potentials by measuring the uptake or release of critical metabolites from the culture medium.[176,177] It is possible to accurately determine oxygen[178] and pyruvate[176] uptake and lactic acid production by human embryos[179] without affecting further development in vitro. Platelet-activating factor has also been detected in media conditioned by fertilized, but not unfertilized, oocytes.[180] A significantly higher level of this factor was observed in media from embryos that resulted in pregnancy. It remains to be determined whether these specific uptake or release assays are of any value in determining embryo potential in terms of establishment of pregnancy. These types of studies hold great promise for diagnosis of embryo development.

Genetic Aspects of Fertilizationin Vitro

It has been estimated that fewer than 10% of the embryos that are transferred to the uterus after human IVF implant successfully.[180] A significant proportion fail to develop due to chromosomal abnormalities. As many as 40% of oocytes that are recovered in stimulated cycles have abnormal chromosome complements.[181] This proportion increases to 65% when only oocytes that fail to fertilize normally are analyzed,[182] indicating that oocyte chromosomal deficiencies are responsible for some failures to fertilize. Because spermatozoal chromosomal abnormalities are estimated to be in the 10% range,[183] a significant proportion of fertilized oocytes can also be expected to be aneuploid. A study analyzing 3 human embryos found that 2 of them were chromosomally abnormal.[182] Subsequent studies on larger numbers of cleaving embryos showed that approximately 20% displayed some chromosomal abnormality,[171,184] although one report noted no abnormalities among 30 analyzable spreads.[185] Multinucleated blastomeres in cleaving human embryos have been reported[186,187]; it is proposed that extra nuclei, or pseudonuclei, arise either by defective migration of chromosomes at mitotic anaphase,[187] or by karyokinesis without cytokinesis.[186] Because the pseudonuclei contain chromatin, determined both by electron microscopic appearance and [^{3}H]thymidine incorporation, the presence of these structures probably also indicates aneuploidy.

Several factors may contribute to the presence of chromosomal abnormalities in oocytes and embryos observed during IVF cycles. Overmaturation of oocytes, high average maternal age, and the hormonal induction of superovulation have all been suggested as possible causative factors. However, a high percentage of embryos that are flushed from the uterus at 4.5 days of gestation during natural cycles are developmentally retarded or arrested.[188] It is entirely possible, therefore, that the chromosome abnormalities that have been described are unrelated to IVF manipulations.

Embryo and Oocyte Cryopreservation

Since the first report of a pregnancy from a cryopreserved human 8-cell embryo,[189] pregnancies have been established in several IVF centers from embryos frozen at the zygote,[190] early cleavage,[189,191] or blastocyst[192] stages. Embryo cryopreservation is now considered to be a routine component of the IVF-ET process.

Several factors have contributed to the need to develop cryobiologic techniques for human embryos. Because the transfer of numerous embryos provides a significant advantage in establishing pregnancy, ovarian-stimulation protocols have been designed in many programs to recruit large numbers of mature oocytes. The transfer of many embryos also results in an increased risk of multiple pregnancy, however, with the attendant potential for obstetric complications. Therefore, most programs have chosen to limit the number of embryos transferred to 3 or 4, with the remaining embryos frozen for transfer in future cycles. Because pregnancy rates do not increase substantially when more than 4 embryos are transferred,[193] embryo cryopreservation has the additional advantage of increasing the pregnancy rate per oocyte retrieval. By eliminating the need for repeated stimulation and oocyte retrieval in subsequent transfer cycles, the expense and risk to the patient are reduced.

Another advantage of embryo cryopreservation is that frozen and thawed embryos can be transferred to the uterus in a natural cycle at the appropriate time after ovulation. This will eliminate any deleterious effect that the hormones used for ovulation induction may have on the uterus, and allow for synchronous embryonic and uterine development. Because of these advantages, it was recommended that only those embryos that are judged unlikely to survive the freeze–thaw procedure be transferred fresh, and all of the remaining ones be frozen for future transfer in natural cycles.[194]

Embryo cryopreservation is also beneficial in other procedures related to IVF. Frequently, oocyte retrieval at the time of GIFT results in more oocytes than are necessary for transfer. The availability of cryofacilities makes it reasonable to fertilize the remaining oocytes in vitro, culture them to the appropriate stage, and freeze them for future transfer. On occasions of oocyte or embryo donation, cryopreservation may help to facilitate cycle synchronization between donor and recipient. Finally, the advent of preimplantation diagnosis techniques may increase the need for reliable embryo freezing methods.

Methods of Cryopreservation

Several different embryo-freezing procedures, using different cryoprotectants, have been employed successfully. The use of a cryoprotectant solution is essential to minimize the lethal formation of intracellular ice. Early work on mouse embryos established the technique of slow freezing in an aqueous dimethyl sulfoxide (DMSO) solution to −80°C, followed by slow thawing. With modifications, this procedure has been used successfully in several human IVF programs to freeze embryos of 4 to 16 cells (Fig. 35–10).[189,191,195] The requirements for slow thawing can be obviated by cooling to the relatively high subzero temperatures of −30 to −40°C prior to plunging into liquid nitrogen.[196] An ultrarapid freezing method, in which embryos are exposed briefly to high concentrations of DMSO (3 to 4 M) in 0.25 M sucrose and then plunged into liquid nitrogen, has been shown to be as efficient as more conventional methods for freezing mouse embryos.[197]

The use of 1,2 propanediol (PROH) and sucrose as a cryoprotectant agent for human embryos has also been described.[190,194,198] This protocol involves rapid freeze and rapid thaw, and unlike DMSO protocols, in which optimum survival is seen after freezing 4 to 16-cell embryos, best results are obtained when embryos of 1 to 4 cells are frozen. These authors reported pregnancy rates after transfer of 1 or 2 frozen embryos equal to that after transfer of 3 fresh embryos during the same period (21%).[194]

Glycerol has also been used as a cryoprotective agent for human embryos.[192,199] It is primarily used for freezing blastocysts in a relatively rapid freeze–thaw program. Although the reported pregnancy rates per thaw cycle are high (35%), there is a significant loss of viable embryos during the extended culture period to the blastocyst stage.[199]

Vitrification has been proposed as a rapid method of cryopreserving embryos.[200] Concentrated cryoprotectant solutions (up to 40% w/v) are used to allow extensive supercooling of the solution. This method results in solidification of the solution without concomitant formation of ice crystals. Its utility for human IVF has yet to be established.

In summary, the choice of cryoprotectant and method of cryopreservation depend largely on the developmental stage of the embryos. The stage-dependent variations in effectiveness of each cryoprotectant probably is a result of a difference in the size of the cells at each stage and the relative permeabilities of the cryoprotectants. Although high pregnancy rates have been obtained from the transfer of embryos frozen at an early developmental stage in PROH, modifications of the DMSO protocol are still widely used. We employ a variation of the PROH procedure, using a programmed, open freezing system. An example of a frozen and thawed embryo is shown in Figure 35–2.

Oocyte Cryopreservation

Cryopreservation of human oocytes has proved to be significantly more difficult than freezing embryos. The rates of survival after thawing, fertilization, and cleavage are very low.[201,202] Only a few pregnancies resulting from the transfer of embryos developed from frozen oocytes have been reported.[202] Apart from the difficulties of maintaining oocyte viability and function, there is a possibility that increased rates of aneuploidy may result from freezing eggs. At ovulation, the mature oocyte is arrested in metaphase of the second meiotic division, with the meiotic spindle in place. It has been shown that spindle microtubules depolymerize at temperature below 4°C.[203] It is possible, therefore, that chromosomes may be selectively lost on completion of meiosis after sperm penetration. Maintenance of euploidy after oocyte cryopreservation remains to be rigorously demonstrated.

EMBRYO TRANSFER

Although 70 to 80% of oocytes aspirated fertilize and cleave, only 20% of transferred embryos implant. The process of embryo replacement is vital to the success of IVF, but, unfortunately, it is a blind procedure.

The optimal stage of development of the embryo at the time of uterine transfer is not clear. Under normal circumstances the embryo reaches the uterus at least 96 hours from the peak LH surge at the 8-cell to 16-cell stage.[204,205] Development of embryos in in-vitro culture conditions is slightly delayed; most embryos at 48 hours from retrieval (84 hours from LH peak) are at the 2 to 6-cell stage. Although holding the embryo in culture longer than 48 hours and transferring at an advanced stage may more closely reproduce the natural condition, any increase in

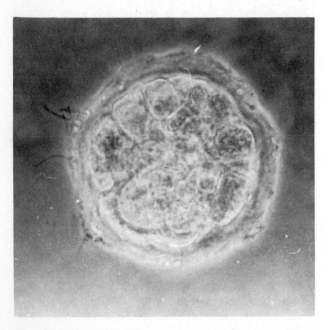

Figure 35–10. A 16-cell embryo after cryopreservation and thawing; while several blastomeres have lost cellular integrity, the majority are intact.

implantation rate would be offset by the loss of embryos due to inadequate culture conditions. Early transfer does not seem to affect the rate of implantation. No difference was noted in pregnancy rates in transfers performed 24 or 48 hours after retrieval.[127] However, another group reported an overall pregnancy rate of 37% with transfers performed 2 days after retrieval compared to a 25% rate when transfer occurred on the day after retrieval (25%).[206] Our center performs embryo replacement 48 hours after oocyte retrieval.

The state of the endometrium is also important in selecting an appropriate day for embryo replacement. Data derived from the replacement of donor embryos demonstrated that there is a window of uterine receptivity. When 2 to 8-cell embryos are replaced on day 20 (132 hours after peak LH) or later, pregnancy rarely develops. The optimal time of replacement is day 18 to 19 (84 to 108 hours from peak LH). This suggests that 84 hours is an appropriate time to replace embryos at this stage of development.[82]

In the early years of IVF-ET the optimum number of embryos to transfer into the uterus was not known. The chance of implantation is dependent on both the quality of the embryo and the receptivity of the endometrium. In a laboratory where embryo quality is poor, many embryos must be transferred for a single one to implant. In a laboratory of established quality, there seems to be no advantage in transferring more than 4. Exceeding this number increases the risk of multiple pregnancy. When four embryos are transferred the probability of a pregnancy resulting in twins is 15%, and in triplets, 2% (Table 35–4).[192,207–212]

Routinely, transfer is performed by passing a Teflon catheter loaded with embryos through the cervical os. The embryos are suspended in 50%–90% serum-supplemented media to enhance stickiness. The column with the embryos (20 to 30 μL) is placed between two smaller columns of media (5 to 10 μL) and air (5 to 10 μL). The catheter is passed through

TABLE 35–4. PREGNANCY RELATED TO NUMBER OF EMBRYOS TRANSFERRED

Reference	Number of Embryos						
	1	2	3	4	5	6	7
209	20	30	39				
206	20	23	29	39	19	50	
127	11	30	36				
210	10	11	15				
55	7	23	13	25	25	—	33
211	6	24		33	50		
212	9.5	14.6	19.3	24.1 (>4)			

the cervical os, usually with the aid of a rigid guide. It is advanced to the fundus of the uterus and withdrawn approximately 1 cm, where its contents are slowly expelled. Once the catheter is withdrawn, its contents are checked for the presence of residual embryos.

Many modifications of embryo transfer catheters have been developed, but all have either a side or an end opening. Two that are popular for embryo placement are the Jones and the Tomcat catheters. The former is relatively thick, with a side port and a closed end.[213] The internal diameter is 0.86 mm and the external diameter is 1.47 mm. This rather large and rigid catheter passes easily through the endocervical canal with minimal uterine manipulation. Its larger diameter, however, requires more fluid to suspend the embryos, and a total of 50 to 90 μL of media is loaded with each transfer. The Tomcat (Sherwood, Inc) catheter, introduced by Kerin and co-workers,[214] has an external diameter of 1 mm at its tip and 3 mm at the 8 cm mark. Its smaller diameter and its end port allows the embryos to be suspended in only 20 μL of media. Pregnancy rates improved when the loading technique reduced the volume of transfer media from 20 μL with 10 μL air, to 15 μL with only 4 μL air.

The importance of the transfer procedure to the retention of embryos has been documented by a few centers. When the cervix was examined 15 minutes after transfer, fluid was noted in the os in 22% of cases.[215] Examination of the cervical mucus of women who had embryos transferred into the uterus revealed that when only the catheter was inspected, 13% of the transfers had residual embryos in the catheter.[216] When the cervix was also inspected, 17% of transfers resulted in residual embryos, half being stuck in the cervical mucus. Embryos could be found in the cervical mucus even if no transfer fluid was present, implying a loss of embryos on withdrawal of the catheter. Examination of posthysterectomy specimens from women who preoperatively had 50-μL spheres placed transcervically revealed the spheres to be located within 1 cm of the area in which they were placed.[217] Thus it would seem that the fluid transferred with the embryos stays close to the site of introduction. Loss of embryos is probably caused by failure of proper entry into the endometrium or sticking to mucus on withdrawal of the catheter.

The technique of transfer may be important in avoiding ectopic pregnancies. A comparison of deep uterine insertion versus low insertion (5.5 mm from the external os) yielded similar pregnancy rates, with a decreased ectopic pregnancy rate in the lower transfer technique.[218] Pregnancy rates do not appear to differ when transfer depth ranges between 6 and 9 cm.[58] It is recommended that embryos be transferred at least 1 cm proximal to the uterine fundus.

The routine for replacing embryos in humans is through the cervix, although the procedure may be performed transfundally. (The latter is most common for cattle and horses.) The transcervical route has obvious advantages in patient comfort and ease of placement. Furthermore, manipulation of the uterus through a transfundal puncture may increase prostaglandin production and increase uterine tone, with adverse effects on the embryo. Two pregnancies have been reported in humans with ultrasound-guided, transfundal transfer.[219] Although this is not the standard practice, it may be useful in patients in whom abnormalities of the cervix make transcervical transfer impossible.

The position in which most patients are placed for transfer is one that results in dependency of the fundus of the uterus. Those with an anteverted uterus assume the knee–chest position, and those with a retroverted uterus are supine. No controlled studies demonstrate the superiority of either position, but patients are more comfortable supine. At Bourn Hall, pregnancies did not vary with the position of the uterus in a series of replacements all done in the lithotomy position.[220] Similarly, the duration of time that patients rest after transfer does not affect the conception site.[221] The position of the patient and the duration of bedrest after transfer appear to be the least important factors determining the success of embryo replacement.

THE LUTEAL PHASE AND EARLY GESTATION

Implantation failure after ET is a major problem in IVF cycles. The achievement of a pregnancy in an unstimulated cycle after transfer of thawed embryos, and the failure of pregnancy to occur in stimulated cycles after transfer of fresh embryos, emphasize the presence of three important factors in the recipient[221]: the adequacy of hormone production in the luteal phase, normal uterine milieu, and synchronization between endometrial and embryonal development at the time of transfer.

The corpus luteum may be vulnerable to damage, because thousands of granulosa cells are unavoidably aspirated during oocyte collection. In HMG-induced cycles we found that granulosa–lutein cells are composed of two subpopulations: small, nonluteinized cells with a few LH receptor-binding sites; and large, luteinized cells that contain an abundance of lipid droplets and LH receptor-binding sites.[222] Because these cells may contribute to the normal hormone output of the corpus luteum, assessing the effect of follicular aspiration on the luteal phase is important. The effect of aspiration has been controversial. Small but significant decreases in serum progesterone and estradiol levels have been noted in normal cycles in which embryo transfer was not accomplished.[223] Conversely, others demonstrated that follicular aspiration has no effect on either the length or hormone levels of the luteal phase.[224-226] Because only about 5 to 10% (3×10^6) of the total (50×10^6) granulosa cell complement is aspirated, it is highly unlikely that aspiration is a primary cause for corpus luteum insufficiency.

Corpus luteum deficiency around day 11 to 13 after HCG administration was documented in HMG-induced cycles for IVF. A short luteal phase was noted in all HMG-treated patients, and these authors consequently abandoned this treatment.[227] Some workers [223,228] reported that the luteal phase of their first pregnancies was characterized by a decline in progesterone level in the late luteal phase, and advocated the use of progesterone supplementation.[52]

We compared the pattern of luteal phase, progesterone, and estradiol in our patients who underwent HMG stimulation without follicular aspiration to that in those who underwent IVF with a similar ovulation-induction regimen and progesterone supplementation. The length of the luteal phase did not differ in these two groups and it was 14.4 and 15.8 days in length, respectively. Similarly, the pattern of progesterone and estradiol secretion did not differ between nonconceptual cycles of aspirated and nonaspirated cycles. In cycles resulting in a continuing IVF pregnancy, however a sharp decline in both estradiol and progesterone levels occurred from day 8 to day 12 of the luteal phase, with a subsequent increase in these hormones with the establishment of pregnancy. This was highlighted when the successful IVF cycles were compared with a failed IVF group in which the women were implanted with the same number of morphologically normal, cleaved embryos (Fig. 35–11). The pattern of declining estradiol and progesterone levels in the latter half of IVF conception cycles is in sharp contrast to the hormonal pattern of conception cycles in similarly treated women not undergoing IVF. In these women, a continuous rise in both estradiol and progesterone was shown to take place from the midluteal phase onward.[229] Similar observations on a nadir of progesterone production in the late luteal phase were demonstrated also in CC-HMG cycles.[230,231]

The relationship between early corpus luteum E_2 and progesterone production and the success of IVF is unclear. A comparison of 185 failed CC-HMG IVF cycles to 13 chemical and 37 continuing pregnancies revealed that the latter had a higher progesterone level and a lower E_2:progesterone ratio on day 5 after HCG administration.[230] Similar finding on higher progesterone level in the early luteal phase of conception cycles was reported[232] but not corroborated.[233,234] A possible luteolytic effect of

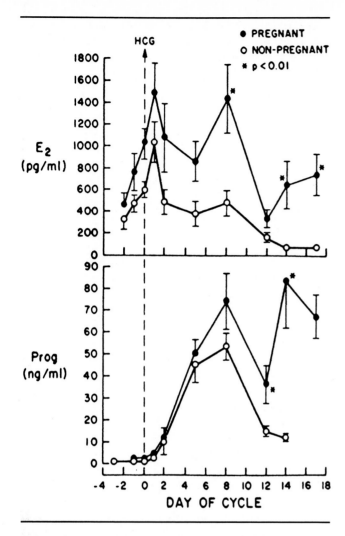

Figure 35–11. Comparison of serum E_2 and progesterone in 8 conception and 8 failed IVF cycles matched for the number of embryos transferred. (Adapted from Dlugi et al.[229] Reproduced with permission.)

high periovulatory estrogen levels was suggested by an inverse relationship between the levels of estrogen in the follicular phase and the length of the luteal phase.[227] Such a relationship in similar ovulation-induction protocols was not confirmed by others.[229,230]

Many IVF centers supplement the luteal phase in spite of the fact that no controlled study has shown any benefit from this as a routine practice. Proluton (Schering, Kenilworth, NJ) was used from day 7 to 16 after oocyte recovery and produced no effect on pregnancy rate.[233] The use of 1,000 to 2,000 IU of HCG on alternate days induced an increase in E_2 and progesterone levels and resulted in a prolongation of luteal phase.[231] This treatment did not affect IVF outcome. Dydrogesterone (Duphaston, Duphar, France) was evaluated and was not found to affect IVF outcome.[235] No increase in pregnancy rates occurred after supplementation with either medroxyprogesterone acetate or HCG.[236]

In an effort to counterbalance the possible negative effects of high E_2 levels around the time of ovulation, progesterone was administered immediately before[234] or after HCG administration.[83] Both studies documented an increase in progesterone in the early luteal phase with no adverse effect on embryos, but did not demonstrate increased likelihood of conception after IVF. The fact that manipulations of the luteal phase do not affect the outcome of IVF strengthens the assumption that the destiny of a given cycle is predetermined in the follicular phase. It seems that after HCG administration the developmental changes in the follicle and endometrium follow a preprogrammed, rigid course that does not lend itself to corrective measures.

Very few observations have evaluated the luteal phase by endometrial biopsy. The frequency of luteal phase defect (LPD) noted by investigators who employed an early luteal phase endometrial biopsy ranged from 28 to 76%.[226,237–241] Three groups[226,238,240] performed the biopsy at or near the time of ET (approximately day 16 to 18 of the menstrual cycle) and one[233] performed it at the time of supposed implantation (approximately day 21 of the cycle). When biopsy was done on day 17, normal luteal phase length and progesterone levels were noted in 25 patients.[226] Seven (28%) had abnormal endometrial histology. When biopsy was performed prior to ET (day 17 or 18), the pregnancy rate was not affected by the trauma; no pregnancy occurred if ET was performed into follicular phase endometrium.[237] Defining the day of follicle aspiration as day 14 of the cycle, biopsy was carried out in women who did not undergo ET on days 14 (2 patients), 15 (3 patients), and 16 (17 patients).[238] Proliferative endometrium was found in biopsies done days 14 and 15. The endometrium of 11 patients biopsied on day 16 was more "advanced" by 1 to 3 days later, and in 5 of these patients it was in phase. Because these biopsies were not dated from the onset of menses after laparoscopy, it is difficult to assess the extent of endometrial maturation.

Endometrial biopsy performed 2 to 4 days after laparoscopy in stimulated IVF cycles without ET revealed abnormal histology in 12 (63%) of 19 patients.[240] When performed on day 21, the biopsy was out of phase in 35% of women, with no change in endometrial estrogen or progesterone receptors or peripheral progesterone levels.[239] We evaluated the luteal phase by endometrial biopsy 11 to 13 days after HCG administration or initiation of an LH surge in 25 stimulated patients who did not undergo ET. Nineteen (76%) had LPD ranging from 3 to 7 days (Table 35–5). Analysis of the relationship of E_2 levels to endometrial histology demonstrated that 66% of patients with E_2 greater than 1,000 pg/mL had an in-phase biopsy, whereas only 26% with out-of-phase

TABLE 35–5. LUTEAL PHASE ENDOMETRIAL HISTOLOGY IN STIMULATED IVF CYCLES

Reference	Day of Endometrial Biopsy	Number of Patients	Abnormal Dating (%)
226	17	25	28
228	14–16	22	73
240	16–18	19	63
239	21	32	35
241	23–25	25	76

biopsy had an E_2 above that level on day 0. This study provides further evidence for the strong association between optimal follicular development and adequate endometrial maturation. It is also evident that ovulation induction is associated with a high rate of LPD, emphasizing the urgent necessity for better stimulation protocols.

Alternatively, LPD could be due to inadequate HCG production by the embryo. Serum E_2, progesterone, and β-HCG levels were measured in viable pregnancies, clinical abortions, biochemical pregnancies, and nonconception cycles.[242] The level of β-HCG started to increase significantly earlier in viable pregnancies than in clinical abortion, and suggested that delayed HCG production in women who are destined to abort may be a sign of early embryopathy. A similar study found that β-HCG secretion is delayed in conception after IVF by 2 to 3 days when compared to spontaneous conception of stimulated non-IVF cycles.[243] These observations were confirmed by the demonstration that aborting pregnancies had significantly lower β-HCG values until the 13th day after the last menstrual period, and that this disparity of value widened with time.[244] We found that at the 11th to 12th day after HCG administration, when the β-HCG levels are at their nadir, serum E_2 levels are valuable in predicting successful pregnancies. Estradiol levels on these days were significantly ($p < 0.01$) higher in conception (294 ± 20 pg/mL) than in failed cycles (72 ± 11 pg/mL). A level of E_2 over 100 pg on day 10 to 11 that increases on day 14 is an early sign of corpus luteum rescue by

conception.[245] A similar pattern of E_2 increase as an early signal of conception was reported by others.[246]

Successful initiation of pregnancy was shown to occur only in association with embryos that are capable of producing significant amounts of platelet-activating factor (PAF).[247] This compound causes a decrease in the maternal platelet count in early pregnancy, and it was suggested that the products derived from platelet breakdown play a role in initiating pregnancy. This group demonstrated that only 50% of IVF-derived embryos have the capacity to produce PAF. Only 50% of women who received embryos that produced PAF subsequently showed thrombocytopenia, and conception was initiated in half of them.

Taken together, these observations on late luteal function and early initiation of pregnancy strongly suggest that inappropriate follicular stimulation may result in an increased rate of embryos defective in biosynthesis ability, impaired corpus luteum function, and abnormal endometrial development.

RESULTS

Confusion exists concerning success rates of IVF because of a lack of standard definitions. Some centers report pregnancies as any positive pregnancy test, while others report only those that have an ultrasound diagnosis of a viable fetus. Approximately 20% of pregnancies are chemical pregnancies, and these would artificially inflate success rates.[38] With this caveat in mind, several reports are presented (Table 35–6).

The live infant rate for in IVF is significantly less than the overall pregnancy rate. Live births occur in approximately 55% of pregnancies, chemical pregnancies in 15 to 20%, and spontaneous abortions in 20 to 30%.[38,248–250] The spontaneous abortion rate is high in embryo transfer cycles, but this must be compared with the 20 to 30% seen in all infertile women.[251] The greatest risk of spontaneous abortion occurs in women over 40 years of age, which is reported as 60[252] and 45%.[38]

Ectopic gestation after ET occurs in approxi-

TABLE 35–6. ASSOCIATION BETWEEN DIAGNOSIS AND IVF OUTCOME

Reference	Tubal	Endometriosis	Male Factor	Unexplained	All Except Male
256	13.5	12.1	8.9	22.9	13.6
97	35	—	25	20	37
248	20	14	18	20	
212	10.7	8.2	6.9	8.7	7.8*
					11.5†

*Primary infertility.
†Secondary infertility.

mately 1 to 5% of pregnancies.[38,248–250] It probably occurs secondary to transfer of embryos into the fallopian tubes at the time of embryo replacement. Another possibility is that oocytes left behind at the time of follicular puncture may fertilize and implant in the tube. To prevent this complication, it is recommended that the cornual ends of the tubes be cauterized when laparoscopic evaluation discovers damage too severe to attempt further repair.

Pregnancies that progress to viability are complicated only by the risk of multiple gestation. If the number of embryos transferred is limited to 4 or fewer, the maximum risk of twins can be calculated as 15%, triplets 2%, and quadruplets less than 1%.[253] The risk of multiple birth increases as more embryos are replaced. When multiple births are excluded, the risk of prematurity is not increased over the general population. At Yale–New Haven Hospital the birth weights of the first 44 infants conceived in vitro were all appropriate or large for gestational age.[254] The risk of prematurity in multiple pregnancies conceived in vitro is 49% for twins and 94% for triplets.[38] Cesarean section in IVF pregnancies was 45 to 55%, but bias on the part of the obstetricians in performing early cesarean delivery probably accounts for this.[38,212,250]

The first babies delivered after in-vitro conception were closely scrutinized for abnormalities. At Norfolk, 3 of 115 infants had major congenital anomalies.[249] The rate of congenital anomalies in the Australian collaborative series was 2.6%, which is only slightly higher than that in the general population.[38] Although several cases of chromosomal anomalies have been reported, patients undergoing IVF do not seem to be at increased risk.[255]

The most important factor influencing IVF success is the patient's primary diagnosis. When the cumulative pregnancy rate as related to the indication for the procedure was calculated, tubal disease resulted in pregnancy in more than 70% of individuals, unexplained infertility in 65%, endometriosis in 59%, and male factor in 14%.[256] Each IVF cycle is independent, and the probability of implanting does not change from cycle to cycle. The pregnancy rate for a single cycle of IVF was approximately 14%, and more than 6 cycles were needed to achieve the maximum cumulative pregnancy rate. The World Collaborative Report found an overall pregnancy rate of approximately 11% per cycle if patients with male factors were excluded.[212] Both Guzick and the World Collaborative Report demonstrated decreased fertility in couples seeking IVF for male factors, with pregnancy rates of 8 and 7%, respectively. Patients with primary infertility have significantly lower pregnancy rates than those with secondary infertility.[212]

Age plays an important role in the outcome of IVF. Pregnancy rates fell from 20% in those age 25 to 29 years to 13% in those over 40 years.[209] The World

Collaborative Report of 1985 demonstrated a decrease in pregnancy rates from 13 to 7% as patients younger than 30 were compared with those over 40 (Table 35–7).[212] Women over 40 who do conceive have a spontaneous abortion rate of over 60%.[252]

In summary, IVF is most successful in young women who have had previous pregnancies, who have a diagnosis of tubal disease, and who have optimal stimulation cycles. In these women, if a good estradiol pattern results in the retrieval of several oocytes and the transfer of at least 4 embryos into the endometrial cavity, a clinical pregnancy rate of approximately 20% can be anticipated.

FUTURE ASPECTS OF IVF—MICROMANIPULATION

The technique of micromanipulation has been used with nonhuman mammalian cell gametes and embryos since the late 1970s. Embryo-manipulation techniques were developed as tools for the study of early embryonic development, cell differentiation, and regulation of development. In animals, several techniques, including nuclear injection, nuclear transplantation, embryo splitting, chimera production, and sperm injection, have been used.[257] The procedure is done using two glass micropipettes, one for holding the embryos and the other for microsurgery. Micromanipulation is performed under 100 to 400 X magnification. The pipettes are connected by plastic tubing to syringes, which in turn control the fluid movement in the micropipettes (Fig. 35–12).

Fertilization Enhancement

The most important barrier to sperm penetration into the ooplasm is the zona pellucida. Severe oligoasthenospermia and defective acrosome function are two examples of conditions that may benefit from procedures that enhance fertilization. Three methods of micromanipulation are under active investigation: injection of sperm directly into the ooplasm, insertion of sperm under the zona pellucida, and "zona drilling," a method whereby a gap is created through

TABLE 35–7. ASSOCIATION BETWEEN AGE AND IVF OUTCOME

Reference	Age (yrs)				
	25	25–29	30–34	35–39	40
209	21.0	19.0	19.0	13.0	
206		25.0	20.0	35.0	
252				35.0 (40)	27.0
272	—	8.5	13.0	14.0	9.0
212		13.6	12.5	11.8	7.2

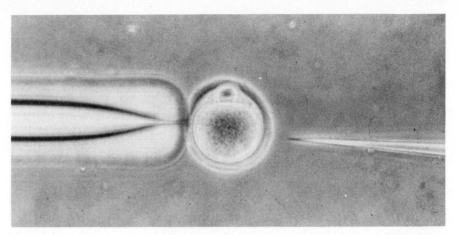

Figure 35–12. Micromanipulation demonstrates a holding pipette (left) and an injecting sharp pipette (right). (Courtesy of Dr. J. Gordon.)

the zona either mechanically or with solvents (Fig. 35–13).

Sperm microinjection is the most aggressive method. Individual sperm or sperm heads are chosen at random and thrust directly into the ooplasm. Extreme oligospermia is potentially treatable with this technique, and sperm need not be motile or capable of interacting normally with oocyte membrane. This procedure has a few major drawbacks. Because sperm must undergo acrosome reaction prior to entry, it may well be that those chosen randomly may have failed to undergo the process. Pretreatment of the sperm population prior to microinjection in order to achieve acrosome reaction may alter also other sperm structures. Cytoplasmic microinjection bypasses all natural barriers to sperm penetration and removes all biologic selectivity from the process. In addition, activation of the oocyte may fail to occur because all normal interaction between the gametes is bypassed. Finally, the micropipette may damage the ooplasm. Although it was possible to achieve fertilization and some cleavage, no live animals were born after the procedure, and it therefore should not be attempted presently in humans.[258,259]

Subzonal insertion of sperm involves microinjection of one or a few sperm under the zona and then allowing normal fusion to take place. Unlike microinjection, it allows for gamete surface interactions that lead to oocyte activation. A disadvantage of subzonal insertion is that when single sperm are chosen for manipulation, they must be treated to assure completion of the acrosome reaction. In addition, the technique cannot be used when sperm are unable to interact properly with the oocyte. Efforts to obtain fertilization by this method have been considerably more successful than with cytoplasmic microinjection. Hamster and human oocytes showed an appreciable fertilization rate when several sperm were inserted subzonally.[260] In these experiments sperm were not treated to induce acrosome reaction, and therefore the fertilization rate was low when fewer than 5 sperm were inserted. In addition, insertion of numerous sperm carried a risk of polyspermic fertilization. Five human oocytes fertilized by this method cleaved. In similar experiments, sperm were treated to induce the acrosome reaction, and then single cells were inserted under the zona.[261] Five of 7 oocytes formed 2 pronuclei, and 1 of 3

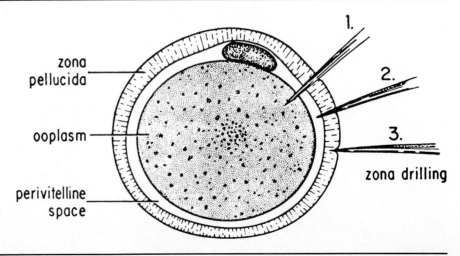

zona pellucida

ooplasm

perivitelline space

1.

2.

3.

zona drilling

Figure 35–13. Schematic representation of the three main methods used in micromanipulative enhancement of fertilization.

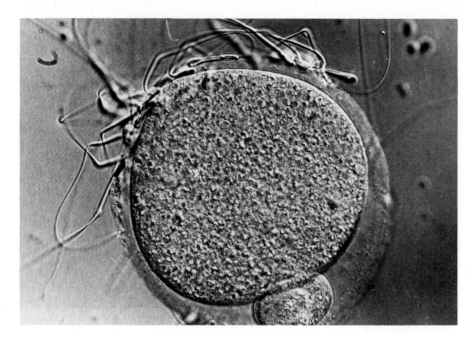

Figure 35–14. A drilled mouse oocyte demonstrates a window created in the zona. Sperm are attached to the exposed ooplasm. (Initial magnification X 400, Nomarski optics. (Courtesy of Dr. B. Talansky.)

cultured for a longer period reached the 4-cell stage. Two main problems are associated with this technique. First, the sperm used in the reported experiments were normal, and thus success with oligoasthenospermic samples is not clear. Second, no animal model is available to demonstrate that normal young animals can develop, and therefore the procedure's safety is not clear.[261,262]

In zona drilling[263] a gap, or window, in the zona is created through which sperm gain direct access to the ooplasm (Fig. 35–14). The main advantage of the procedure is that it is the least aggressive and leaves intact most of the natural barriers. With this procedure sperm must capacitate, undergo the acrosome reaction, swim to the oocyte, and participate normally in fusion. The disadvantages are that the most severe forms of infertility, particularly sperm immotility, cannot be treated, and that more than one sperm may find its way into the ooplasm. Animal studies with zona drilling demonstrated its potential, as live animals have been born after the procedure.[263] Moreover, oocyte survival rates were high, the frequency of polyspermy was low, and fertilization could be observed with a sperm:egg ratio as low as 10. A follow-up report provided preliminary evidence that infertile mice with morphologically abnormal sperm could be restored to fertility by zona drilling.[264]

As a consequence of these findings, we are conducting clinical trials with zona drilling in patients who did not achieve at least one fertilization in previous IVF attempts (Table 35–8). We have not yet obtained a pregnancy with this procedure. These micromanipulations offer a new approach to the treatment of male infertility, but must be thoroughly tested in an animal model before being applied to clinical trials. As with the first IVF pregnancies, the extent of risk to which fetuses will be exposed is unknown.

Embryo Biopsy

In animals it is possible by micromanipulation to remove a single blastomere from a 4 to 8-cell embryo. The zona-enclosed embryo will continue to develop normally, and the zona-free blastomere will continue to develop into a blastocyst and produce identical and normal offspring.[265–267] Similarly, it is possible to remove some of the mural trophectoderm at the blastocyst stage without hindering the normal development of the biopsied blastocyst.[268] Early or late preimplantation embryo biopsy material can then be subjected to genetic analysis. The embryo can be frozen until the genetic analysis is complete.

Karyotyping was performed successfully in human embryos,[269] and sexing is possible by the use of Y chromosome repeated-sequence probes.[270] Gene point mutation analysis such as in sickle cell disease necessitates the use of a DNA sequence probe. The

TABLE 35–8. PRELIMINARY RESULTS WITH HUMAN ZONA DRILLING

	Drilled No. (%)	Not Drilled No. (%)
Surviving oocytes	28(65)	—
Normal fertilization	7(25)	2(18)
Polyspermic fertilization	4(14)	2(18)
Unfertilized	17(61)	7(64)

All patients failed to fertilize oocytes in previous IVF cycles.

specific DNA sequence is used to label the gene and is detected by either fluorescent antibody or radioactivity. These techniques employ a relative large sample of DNA and consequently a large number of cells. To provide a sufficient quantity of DNA for analysis and amplify the amount from a few cells, several methods are under development. One strategy is to culture the biopsied blastomeres in conditioned medium that will allow them to develop beyond the stage of a blastocyst and provide enough cells and DNA for analysis. Another approach amplites a small amount of DNA by a factor of hundred thousands through in-vitro hybridization.[272] This should dramatically accelerate the development of this field of preimplantation genetic diagnosis. In turn, such development would permit women at significant risk for specific inherited disorders to undertake a pregnancy with unaffected embryos, and would obviate the need for further antenatal testing. It is beyond the scope of this chapter to address the ethical, legal, and religious aspects involved with these advanced modalities. Nevertheless, it is clear that an urgent need exists for developing new and clear guidelines to meet the serious concerns associated with these potential scientific breakthroughs.

REFERENCES

1. Steptoe PC, Edwards RG: Birth after re-implantation of a human embryo. Lancet 2:366, 1978.
2. Lopata A, Johnston IWH, Hoult IJ, Speirs AI: Pregnancy following intrauterine implantation of an embryo obtained by in vitro fertilization of a preovulatory egg. Fertil Steril 33:117, 1980.
3. Heape W: Preliminary note on the transplantation and growth of mammalian ova within a uterine foster-mother. Proc R Soc 48:457, 1891.
4. Hammond J: Culture of mouse embryos using an egg-saline medium. Nature 163:28, 1949.
5. Whitten WK: Culture of tubal mouse ova. Nature 177:96, 1956.
6. Austin CR: Observations of the penetration of the sperm into the mammalian egg. Aust J Sci Res 134:581, 1951.
7. Chang MC: Fertilizing capacity of spermatozoa deposited in the fallopian tubes. Nature 168:697, 1951.
8. Chang MC: Fertilization of rabbit ova in vitro. Nature 184:406, 1959.
9. Soules MR: Infertility surgery, in DeCherney AH (ed): Reproductive Failure. New York, Churchill Livingstone, 1986, p 117.
10. Bateman BG, Nunley WC, Kitchen JK: Surgical management of distal tubal obstruction—Are we making progress? Fertil Steril 48:523, 1987.
11. Trimbos-Kemper TCM, Trimbos JB, Van Hall EV: Conscientious evaluation of tubal surgery results, in DeCherney AH, Polan ML (eds): Reproductive Surgery. Chicago, Year Book, 1987, p 74.
12. Thie JL, Williams TJ, Coulam CB: Repeat tuboplasty compared with primary microsurgery for postinflammatory tubal disease. Fertil Steril 45:784, 1986.
13. Webster BW, Wentz AC, Maxson WS: Endometriosis, in DeCherney AH, Polan MI (eds): Reproductive Surgery. Chicago, Year Book, 1987, p 221.
14. Seibel MM, Berger MJ, Weinstein FG, et al: The effectiveness of danazol on subsequent fertility in minimal endometriosis. Fertil Steril 38:534, 1982.
15. Olive DL, Haney AF: Endometriosis, in DeCherney AH (ed): Reproductive Failure. New York, Churchill Livingstone, 1986, p 153.
16. Rousseau S, Lord J, Lepage Y, Campenhout JV: The expectancy of pregnancy for "normal" infertile couples. Fertil Steril 40:768, 1983.
17. Haney AF, Hughes CL, Whitesides DB, Dodson WC: Treatment independent, treatment associated pregnancies after additional therapy in a program of in vitro fertilization and embryo transfer. Fertil Steril 47:634, 1987.
18. Dodson WC, Whitesides DB, Hughes CL, Easley HA, Haney AF: Superovulation with intrauterine insemination in the treatment of infertility: A possible alternative to gamete intrafallopian transfer and in vitro fertilization. Fertil Steril 48:441, 1987.
19. Mahadevan MM, Trounson AO: The influence of seminal characteristics on the success rate of human in vitro fertilization. Fertil Steril 42:400, 1984.
20. Cohen J, Edwards R, Fehilly C, et al: In vitro fertilization: A treatment for male infertility. Fertil Steril 43:422, 1985.
21. Engler Y, Puissant F, Vekemans M, et al: Higher pregnancy rates after in vitro fertilization and embryo transfer in cases with sperm defects. Fertil Steril 48:254, 1987.
22. Yanagimachi R, Yanagimachi H, Rogers BJ: The use of zona-free animal ova as a test system for the assessment of the fertilizing capacity of human spermatozoa. Biol Reprod 15:471, 1976.
23. Rogers BJ: The usefulness of the sperm penetration assay in predicting IVF success. J IVF/ET 3:209, 1986.
24. Margalioth EJ, Navot D, Laufer N, et al: Correlation between the zona-free hamster egg-sperm penetration assay and human in vitro fertilization. Fertil Steril 45:665, 1986.
25. Aybaliotis B, Bronson R, Rosenfeld D, Cooper G: Conception rates in couples where autoimmunity to sperm is detected. Fertil Steril 43:739, 1985.
26. Bronson R, Cooper G, Rosenfeld D: Sperm antibodies: Their role in infertility. Fertil Steril 42:171, 1984.
27. Clarke GN, Lopata A, Johnston WIH: Effect of sperm antibodies in females on human in vitro fertilization. Fertil Steril 46:435, 1986.
28. Mandelbaum SL, Diamond MP, DeCherney AH: Relationship of antisperm antibodies to oocyte fertilization in in vitro fertilization–embryo transfer. Fertil Steril 47:644, 1987.
29. Bronson RA, Cooper GW, Rosenfeld DL: Sperm-specific isoantibodies and autoantibodies inhibit the binding of human sperm to the human zona pellucida. Fertil Steril 38:724, 1982.
30. Asch RH, Balmaceda JP, Ellsworth LR, Wong PC: Preliminary experiences with gamete intrafallopian transfer (GIFT). Fertil Steril 45:366, 1986.
31. Leeton J, Healy D, Rogers P, Yates C, Caro C: A controlled study between the use of gamete intrafallopian transfer (GIFT) and in vitro fertilization and embryo transfer in the management of idiopathic and male infertility. Fertil Steril 48:605, 1987.
32. Trounson AO, Leeton JF, Wood C, Webb J, Wood J: Pregnancies in human by fertilization in vitro and embryo transfer in the controlled ovulatory cycle. Science 212:681, 1981.
33. Testart J, Frydman R, DeMounzon J, Lassale B, Belaisch JC: A study of factors affecting the success of human fertilization in vitro. I. Influence of ovarian stimulation upon the number and condition of oocytes collected. Biol Reprod 28:415, 1983.
34. Wood C, Trounson AO, Leeton JF, et al: Clinical features of eight pregnancies resulting from in vitro fertilization and embryo transfer. Fertil Steril 38:22, 1982.
35. Kerin JF, Warner GM, Quinn PJ, et al: Incidence of multiple pregnancy after in vitro fertilisation and embryo transfer. Lancet 2:537, 1983.
36. Lopata A: Concepts in human in vitro fertilization and embryo transfer. Fertil Steril 40:289, 1983.
37. Edwards RG: In vitro fertilization and embryo replacement: Opening lecture. Ann NY Acad Sci 442:1, 1985.
38. In vitro fertilization pregnancies, Australia and New Zealand 1979–1984. Sydney, National Perinatal Statistics Unit, 1985.
39. Marrs RP, Vargyas JM, Saito H, et al: Clinical applications of techniques used in human in vitro fertilization research. Am J Obstet Gynecol 146:477, 1983.
40. Dlugi AM, Laufer N, Botero-Ruiz W, et al: Altered follicular development in clomiphene citrate versus human menopausal gonadotropin-stimulated cycles for in vitro fertilization. Fertil Steril 43:40, 1984.
41. Kerin J, Quinn P, Herriot D, Wilson L, Stone B: Effects of follicle induction on ovary and endometrium in DeCherney AH, Naftolin F (eds): The Control of Follicle Development, Ovulation and Luteal Function. Lessons from In Vitro Fertilization. New York, Raven, 1987, p 301.
42. Mahadevan MM, Fleetman J, Taylor PJ, Leader A, Pattinson AH: The effect of the day of initiation of ovarian stimulation on the day of luteinizing hormone surge and outcome of in vitro fertilization. Fertil Steril 47:976, 1987.
43. Lamb EJ, Colliflower WW, Williams JW: Endometrial histology and conception rate after clomiphene citrate. Obstet Gynecol 39:389, 1972.
44. Kokko E, Janne O, Kauppila A, Vihko R: Cyclic clomiphene citrate treatment lowers cytosol estrogen and progestin receptor concentra-

tions in the endometrium of postmenopausal women on estrogen replacement therapy. *J Clin Endocrinol Metab* 52:345, 1981.

45. Birkenfeld A, Weber-Benndorf M, Mootz V, Beier HM: Effect of clomiphene on the functional morphology of oviductal and uterine mucosa. *Ann NY Acad Sci* 442:153, 1985.

46. Birkenfeld A, Navot D, Levij IS, et al: Advanced secretory changes in the proliferative human endometrial epithelium following clomiphene citrate treatment. *Fertil Steril* 45:462, 1986.

47. Laufer N, Reich R, Braw R, Schenker JG, Tasafriri A: Effect of clomiphene citrate in preovulatory rat follicles in culture. *Biol Reprod* 27:463, 1982.

48. Laufer N, Pratt B, DeCherney AH, Naftolin F, Markert CL: The in vivo and in vitro effect of clomiphene citrate on the development. *Am J Obstet Gynecol* 147:633, 1983.

49. Laufer N, Barr I, Lewin A, et al: Clomiphene inhibits progesterone secretion of human granulosa luteal cells in long term culture. Proceedings of the fourth world congress on IVF, Melbourne, Australia, 1985.

50. Olsson JH, Nilsson L, Hillensjo T: Effect of clomiphene isomers on progestin synthesis in cultured human granulosa cells. *Hum Reprod* 2:463, 1987.

51. Garcia J, Seegar-Jones G, Wentz AC: The use of clomiphene citrate. *Fertil Steril* 28:707, 1977.

52. Jones HW, Jones GS, Andrews MC, et al: The program for in vitro fertilization at Norfolk. *Fertil Steril* 38:14, 1982.

53. Jones HW: Oocyte recruitment with human menopausal gonadotropin (HMG) and follicle stimulating hormone (FSH), in DeCherney AH, Naftolin F (eds): *The Control of Follicle Development, Ovulation and Luteal Function. Lessons from In Vitro Fertilization.* New York, Raven, 1987, p 211.

54. Laufer N, DeCherney AH, Haseltine FP, et al: The use of high-dose human menopausal gonadotropin (HMG) in an in vitro fertilization program. *Fertil Steril* 40:734, 1983.

55. Laufer N, DeCherney AH, Haseltine FP, et al: Human in vitro fertilization employing individualized ovulation induced by human menopausal gonadotropins. *J IVF/ET* 1:56, 1984.

56. Yven BH, Pride SM, Rowe TC, et al: Comparison of the outcome of ovulation induction therapy in an IVF program employing a low-dose and an individually adjusted high-dose schedule of HMG. *Am J Obstet Gynecol* 151:172, 1985.

57. David M, Barak Y, Amit A, et al: Interdepartmental unit of IVF/ET, Serlin-Hakirya Maternity Hospital, Tel Aviv, Israel. *J IVF/ET* 4:65, 1987.

58. Meldrum DR, Chetkowski R, Steingold KA, et al: Evolution of a highly successful in vitro fertilization embryo transfer program. *Fertil Steril* 48:86, 1987.

59. Jones GS, Garcia JE, Rosenwaks Z: The role of pituitary gonadotropins in follicular stimulation and oocyte maturation in the human. *J Clin Endocrinol Metab* 59:178, 1984.

60. Moasher SJ, Garcia JE, Rosenwaks Z: The combination of FSH and HMG for the induction of multiple follicular maturation for IVF. *Fertil Steril* 44:62, 1985.

61. Jones GS, Acosta AA, Garcia JE, Bernardus RE, Rosenwaks Z: The effects of FSH without additional LH on follicular stimulation and oocyte development in normal ovulatory women. *Fertil Steril* 43:696, 1985.

62. Navot D, Rosenwaks Z: The use of FSH for controlled ovarian hyperstimulation in IVF. *J IVF/ET* In press.

63. Russel JB, Jones EE, Polan ML, Boyers SP, DeCherney AH: The use of purified FSH in an IVF-ET program. Presented at the 42nd annual meeting of the American Fertility Society, Toronto, 1986.

64. Polan ML, Danielle A, Russel JB: Ovulation induction with HMG compared to pure FSH results in differences in FF androgen levels. Presented at the 42nd annual meeting of the American Fertility Society, Toronto, 1986.

65. Frydman R, Forman R, Rainhorn JD, et al: A new approach to follicular stimulation for IVF: Programmed oocyte retrieval. *Fertil Steril* 48:657, 1986.

66. Cohen J, Debache C, Solal P, et al: Results of planned in vitro fertilization programming through the pre-administration of estrogen–progesterone combined pill. *Hum Reprod* 2:7, 1987.

67. Hillier SG, Afnan AMM, Margara RA, Winston RML: Superovulation strategy before in vitro fertilization. *Clin Obstet Gynecol* 12:687, 1985.

68. DeCherney AH, Tarlatzis BC, Laufer N: Follicular development: Lessons learned from human in vitro fertilization. *Am J Obstet Gynecol* 153:911, 1985.

69. Stranger JD, Yovich JL: Reduced in vitro fertilisation of human oocytes from patients with raised basal luteinizing hormone levels during the follicular phase. *Br J Obstet Gynaecol* 92:385, 1985.

70. Vickery BH: Comparison of the potential for therapeutic utilities with gonadotropin-releasing hormone agonists and antagonists. *Endocr Rev* 7:115, 1986.

71. Fleming R, Coutts JRT: Induction of multiple follicular growth in normally menstruating women with endogenous gonadotropin suppression. *Fertil Steril* 45:226, 1986.

72. Barriere P, Lopes P, Dubourdier S, Lerat F, Charbonnel B: Short administration regimen of GnRH analogs in ovarian induction for IVF. Presented at fifth world congress on in vitro fertilization and embryo transfer, Norfolk, VA, April 5, 1987.

73. Porter RN, Smith W, Craft IL, Abdulwahid NA, Jacobs HS: Induction of ovulation for in vitro fertilisation using buserelin and gonadotropins. *Lancet* 2:1284, 1984.

74. Healy DL: Lessons from using LHRH analogs in IVF. Presented at fifth world congress on in vitro fertilization and embryo transfer, Norfolk, VA, April 5, 1987.

75. DeZiegler D, Cedars MI, Randle D, et al: Suppression of the ovary using a gonadotropin-releasing hormone agonist prior to stimulation for oocyte retrieval. *Fertil Steril* 48;807, 1987.

76. Jones GS, Muasher SJ, Rosenwaks Z, Acosta AA, Liu HC: The perimenopausal patient in in vitro fertilization: The use of gonadotropin-releasing hormone. *Fertil Steril* 46:885, 1986.

77. Meldrum DR, Tsao Z, Monroe SE, et al: Stimulation LH fragments with reduced bioactivity following GnRH administration in women. *J Clin Endocrinol Metab* 58:755, 1984.

78. Meldrum D: GnRH analogs in reproduction. Presented at 43rd annual meeting of the American Fertility Society, Reno, NV, Sept 28, 1987.

79. Palermo R, Amodeo G, Navot D, Rosenwaks Z, Cittadini E: Concomitant follicle-stimulating hormone and luteinizing hormone- releasing hormone agonists and menotropin treatment for the synchronized induction of multiple follicles. *Fertil Steril* In press.

80. Kenigsberg D, Littman BA, Hodgen GD: Induction of ovulation in primate models. *Endocrinology* 7:34, 1986.

81. Smitz J, Devroey P, Braeckmans P, et al: Management of failed cycles in an IVF/GIFT program with the combination of a GnRH analogue and HMG. *Hum Reprod* 2:309, 1987.

82. Navot D, Laufer N, Kapolovic J, et al: Artificially induced endometrial cycles and establishment of pregnancies in the absence of ovaries. *N Engl J Med* 314:806, 1986.

83. Laufer N, Navot D: Peripheral markers in IVF, in DeCherney AH, Naftolin F (eds): *The control of Follicular Development, Ovulation and Luteal Function. Lessons from In Vitro Fertilization.* New York, Raven, 1987, p 79.

84. Lutjen P, Trounson A, Leeton J, et al: The establishment and maintenance of pregnancy using in vitro fertilization and embryo donation in a patient with primary ovarian failure. *Nature* 307:175, 1984.

85. Rosenwaks Z: Donor eggs: Their application in modern reproductive technologies. *Fertil Steril* 47: 895, 1987.

86. Asch RH, Balmaceda JP, Ord T, et al: Oocyte donation and GIFT in premature ovarian failure. Presented at the 43rd annual meeting of the American Fertility Society, Reno, NV, Sept 28, 1987.

87. Hackeloer B, Fleming R, Robinson H, Adam A, Coults S: Correlation of ultrasonic and endocrinologic assessment of human follicular development. *Am J Obstet Gynecol* 135:122, 1979.

88. Kerin JF, Edmonds DK, Warms GM, Cox LW, Seamark RF: Morphological and functional relations of graafian follicle growth to ovulation in women using ultrasonic, laparoscopic and biochemical measurements. *Br J Obstet Gynaecol* 88:81, 1981.

89. Baird DT, Fraser IS: Blood production and ovarian secretion rates of estradiol and estrone in women throughout the menstrual cycle. *J Clin Endocrinol* 38:1009, 1974.

90. DeCherney AH, Laufer N: The monitoring of ovulation induction using ultrasound and estrogen. *Clin Obstet Gynecol* 27:993, 1984.

91. Lefevre B, Demoulin A, Testart J, et al: Absence of predictive value of follicular inhibin on the results of human IVF. *Fertil Steril* 46:325, 1986.

92. Vargyas JM, Marrs RP, Kletzky O, Mishell D: Correlation of ultrasonic measurement of ovarian follicle size and serum estradiol levels in ovulatory patients following clomiphene citrate for in vitro fertilization. *Am J Obstet Gynecol* 144:569, 1982.

93. Mantzavinos T, Garcia J, Jones HW: Ultrasound measurement of ovarian follicle stimulated by human gonadotropins for oocyte recovery and in vitro fertilization. *Fertil Steril* 40:461, 1983.

94. Williams RF, Hodgen GD: Disparate effects of human chorionic

gonadotropin during the later follicular phase in monkeys: Normal ovulation, follicular atresia, ovarian acyclicity and hypersecretion of FSH. *Fertil Steril* 33:64, 1980.

95. Laufer N, DeCherney AH, Tarlatzis BC, et al: Delaying human chorionic gonadotropin (HCG) administration in human menopausal gonadotropin (HMG) induced cycles decreases successful in vitro fertilization (IVF) of human oocytes. *Fertil Steril* 42:198, 1984.

96. Jones HW, Acosta A, Andrews MC, Garcia JF: The importance of the follicular phase to success and failure in in vitro fertilization. *Fertil Steril* 40:317, 1983.

97. Sher G. Knutzen V, Strattan C: In vitro fertilization and embryo transfer: Two-year experience. *Am J Obstet Gynecol* 67:309, 1986.

98. Frydman R, Forman R, Rainhorn JO, et al: High pregnancy rate following fixed schedule ovulation induction in an IVF program, in DeCherney AH, Naftolin F (eds): *The Control of Follicle Development, Ovulation and Luteal Function. Lessons from In Vitro Fertilization.* New York, Raven, 1987, p 239.

99. Laufer N, Less A, Lewin A, et al: A multivariate analysis for the prediction of conceptions following IVF-ET. Presented at the fifth world congress on in vitro fertilization and embryo transfer, Norfolk, VA, 1986.

100. Laufer N, DeCherney AH, Tarlatzis BC, Naftolin F: The association between periovulatory serum 17β-estradiol pattern and conception in human menopausal gonadotropin–human chorionic gonadotropin stimulation. *Fertil Steril* 46:73, 1986.

101. Ben Rafael Z, Kopf GS, Blasco L, Flickinger GL: Follicular maturation parameters associated with the failure of oocyte retrieval fertilization and cleavage in vitro. *Fertil Steril* 45:51, 1986.

102. Dor J, Rudak E, Mashiach S, et al: Periovulatory 17β-estradiol changes and embryo morphologic features in conception and non-conceptional cycles after human IVF. *Fertil Steril* 45:63, 1986.

103. Dirnfeld M, Lejeune B, Camus M, Vekemans M, Leroy F: Growth rate of follicular estrogen secretion in relation to the outcome of in vitro fertilization and embryo replacement. *Fertil Steril* 43:379, 1985.

104. Leerentveld RA, Zeilmaker GH, Van der Stoep M: Monitoring of clomiphene citrate stimulation by means of plasma 17β-estradiol determination and ultrasonographic follicle measurement in in vitro fertilization treatment cycles. *Hum Reprod* 2:187, 1987.

105. Yovich J, Stranger JD, Yovich JM, Tuvik AI, Turner SR: Hormonal profiles in the follicular phase, luteal phase and first trimester of pregnancies arising from IVF. *Br J Obstet Gynaecol* 92:374, 1985.

106. Navot D, Margalioth EJ, Laufer N, et al: Periovulatory 17β-estradiol pattern in conception and nonconceptional cycles during menotropin treatment of anovulatory infertility. *Fertil Steril* 48:57, 1987.

107. Wramsby H, Sundstrom P, Liedholm P: Pregnancy rate in relation to number of cleaved eggs replaced after in-vitro fertilization in stimulated cycles monitored by serum levels of estradiol and progesterone as sole index. *Hum Reprod* 2:325, 1987.

108. Gidley-Baird AA, O'Neil C, Sinosich MJ, et al: Failure of implantation in human IVF and ET: The effects of altered progesterone/estrogen ratios in humans and mice. *Fertil Steril* 45:69, 1986.

109. Howles CM, Macnamee MC, Edwards RG, Goswang R, Steptoe PC: Effects of high tonic levels of LH, on outcome of in-vitro fertilisation, *Lancet* 2:521, 1986.

110. Platt LD: New look in ultrasound: The vaginal probe. *Contemp Ob/Gyn* 30:99, 1987.

111. Cacciatore B, Liukkonen S, Koskimies A, Ylostalo P: Ultrasonic detection of a cumulus oophorus in patients undergoing IVF. *J IVF/ET* 2:224, 1985.

112. Hackeloer BJ: Ultrasound scanning of the ovarian cycle. *J IVF/ET* 1:217, 1984.

113. Smith B, Porter R, Ahuja K, Craft I: Ultrasonic assessment of endometrial changes in stimulated cycles in an in-vitro fertilization and embryo transfer program. *J IVF/ET* 1:233, 1984.

114. Fleischer AC, Pittaway DE, Beard LA, et al: Sonographic depiction of endometrial changes occurring with ovulation induction. *J Ultrasound Med* 3:341, 1984.

115. Rabinowitz R, Laufer N, Lewin A, et al: The value of ultrasonographic endometrial measurement in the prediction of pregnancy following IVF. *Fertil Steril* 45:824, 1986.

116. Wiczyk HP, Janus C, Richards CJ, et al: Comparison of magnetic resonance imaging and ultrasound in evaluating follicular and endometrial development through the normal cycle. *Fertil Steril* 49:969, 1988.

117. Edwards RG, Donahue RP, Baramaki TA, Jones HW: Preliminary attempts to fertilize human oocyte matured in vitro. *Am J Obstet Gynecol* 96:192, 1966.

118. Croxatto HB, Fuentealba B, Diaz S, Pastene L, Tatum HJ: A simple nonsurgical technique to obtain unimplanted eggs from human uteri. *Am J Obstet Gynecol* 112:662, 1972.

119. Lenz S. Lauritsen JG: Ultrasonically guided percutaneous aspiration of human follicles under anesthesia. A new method of collecting oocytes for in vitro fertilization. *Fertil Steril* 38:673, 1982.

120. Parsons J, Riddle A, Booker M, et al: Oocyte retrieval for in vitro fertilisation by ultrasonically guided needle aspiration via the urethra. *Lancet* 1:1076, 1985.

121. Gleicher N, Friberg J, Fullan N, et al: Egg retrieval for in vitro fertilisation by sonographically controlled vaginal culdocentesis. *Lancet* 1:508, 1983.

122. Feichtinger W, Szalay S, Beck A, Kemeter P, Janisch H: Results of laporoscopic recovery of preovulatory human oocytes from nonstimulated ovaries in an ongoing in vitro fertilization program. *Fertil Steril* 36:707, 1981.

123. Russel J, DeCherney AH, Hobbins J: A new transvaginal probe and biopsy guide for oocyte retrieval. *Fertil Steril* 47:350, 1987.

124. Robertson R, Picker R, O'Neill C, Ferrier A, Saunders D: An experience of laparoscopic and transvesicle oocyte retrieval in an in vitro fertilization program. *Fertil Steril* 45:88, 1986.

125. Dellenbach P, Nisand I, Moreau L, et al: Transvaginal sonographically controlled follicle puncture for oocyte retrieval. *Fertil Steril* 44:656, 1985.

126. Cohen J, Debache C, Pez JP, Junca AM, Cohen-Bacrie P: Transvaginal sonographically controlled ovarian puncture for oocyte retrieval for in vitro fertilization. *J IVF/ET* 3:309, 1986.

127. Feichtinger W, Kemeter P: Organization and computerized analysis of in vitro fertilization and embryo transfer programs. *J IVF/ET* 1:34, 1984.

128. Lewin A, Laufer N, Rabinowitz R, et al: Ultrasonically guided oocyte collection under local anesthesia: The first choice for in vitro fertilization—A comparative study with laparoscopy. *Fertil Steril* 46:257, 1986.

129. Janson PO, Wikland M: A comparison between patients randomly selected for either laparoscopic or ultrasound guided puncture of follicles. *Arch Androl* 11:212, 1983.

130. Riddle AF, Pampiglone JS, Sharma V, et al: Two years' experience of ultrasound-directed oocyte retrieval. *Fertil Steril* 48:454, 1987.

131. Jones HW, Acosta AA, Garcia J: A technique for the aspiration of oocytes from human ovarian follicles. *Fertil Steril* 37:26, 1982.

132. Renou P, Trounson AO, Wood C, Leeton JF: The collection of human oocytes for in vitro fertilization. I. An instrument for maximizing oocyte recovery rate. *Fertil Steril* 37:26, 1982.

133. Lopata A, Johnston IWH, Leeton JF, et al: Collection of human oocytes at laparoscopy and laparotomy. *Fertil Steril* 25:1030, 1974.

134. Cohen J, Avery S, Campbell S, et al: Follicular aspiration using a syringe suction system may damage the zona pellucida. *J IVF/ET* 3:224, 1986.

135. Honea KL, Stangel JJ, Parker A, et al: Improvement of retrieval rates in transvaginal ultrasound directed ovum retrieval using a follicle flushing system. Presented at fifth world congress on in vitro fertilization and embryo transfer, Norfolk, VA, April 5, 1987.

136. Kogowski A, Lessing J, Amit A, et al: Ultrasound guided oocyte retrieval. *Obstet Gynecol* 69:1, 1987.

137. Schulman J, Dorfmann A, Jones S, et al: Outpatient in vitro fertilization using transvaginal ultrasound guided oocyte retrieval. *Obstet Gynecol* 69:1, 1987.

138. Schulman J, Dorfmann A, Jones S, Joyce B, Hanser J: Outpatient in vitro fertilization using transvaginal oocyte retrieval and local anesthesia. *N Engl J Med* 312:1639, 1985.

139. Nero F, Diamond MP, Lavy G, et al: Patient survey of preferred method of oocyte recovery. Presented at the fifth world congress on in vitro fertilization and embryo transfer, Norfolk, VA, April 5, 1987.

140. Hammarberg K, Enk L, Nilsson L, Wikland M: Oocyte retrieval under the guidance of a vaginal transducer: Evaluation of patient acceptance. *Hum Reprod* 2:487, 1987.

141. Dellenbach P, Nisand I, Moreau L, et al: Update on experience with transvaginal method of oocyte retrieval. Presented at the fifth world congress on in vitro fertilization and embryo transfer, Norfolk, VA, April 5, 1987.

142. Trounson AO, Leeton JF, Wood L: In vitro fertilization and embryo transfer in the human, in Rolland R, Van Hall EV, Hillier SC, et al (eds): *Follicular Maturation and Ovulation.* Amsterdam, Excerpta Medica, 1982, p 312.

143. Quinn P, Kerin JF, Womes GM: Improved pregnancy rate in human in

vitro fertilization with the use of a medium based on the composition of human tubal fluid. *Fertil Steril* 44:493, 1985.

144. Steptoe PC, Edwards RG, Purdy JM: Clinical aspects of pregnancies established with cleaving embryos grown in vitro. *Br J Obstet Gynaecol* 87:757, 1980.

145. Marrs RP: Laboratory conditions for human in vitro fertilization procedures. *Clin Obstet Gynecol* 29:180, 1986.

146. Laufer N, Tarlatzis BC, Naftolin F: In vitro fertilization: State of the art. *Semin Reprod Endocrinol* 2:197, 1984.

147. Saito H, Berger T, Mishell DR, Marrs RP: The effect of serum fractions on embryos growth. *Fertil Steril* 41:761, 1984.

148. Caro CM, Trounson A: The effect of protein on preimplantation mouse embryo development in vitro. *J IVF/ET* 1:183, 1984.

149. Leuny PCS, Gronow MJ, Kellow GN, et al: Serum supplement in human in vitro fertilization and embryo development. *Fertil Steril* 41:36, 1984.

150. Menezo Y, Testart J, Perrone D: Serum is not necessary in human in vitro fertilization, early embryo culture, and transfer. *Fertil Steril* 45:750, 1984.

151. Gianalvoli L, Seracchioli R, Ferraretti A, et al: The successful use of human amniotic fluid for mouse embryo culture and human in vitro fertilization, embryo culture, and transfer. *Fertil Steril* 46:907, 1986.

152. Shirley B, Wortham JWE, Witmeyer J, Condon-Mahoney M, Fot G: Effects of human serum and plasma on development of mouse embryo in culture media. *Fertil Steril* 43:129, 1985.

153. Shirley B, Wortham JWE, People D, White S, Condon-Mahoney M: Inhibition of embryo development by some maternal sera. *J IVF/ET* 4:93, 1987.

154. Pope AK, Harrison KL, Wilson LM, Breen TM, Cummins JM: Ultra ser G as a serum substitute in embryo culture medium. *J IVF/ET* 4:286, 1987.

155. Caro CM, Trounson A, Kirby C: Effect of growth factors in culture medium on the rate of mouse embryo development and viability in vitro. *J IVF/ET* 4:265, 1987.

156. Whitten WK: Nutrient requirement for the culture of preimplantation embryos in vitro, in Raspe G (ed): *Advances in Biosciences.* London, Pergamon, 1971.

157. Abramczuk J, Lopata A: Incubator performance in the clinical in vitro fertilization program: Importance of temperature conditions for the fertilization and cleavage of human oocytes. *Fertil Steril* 46:132, 1986.

158. Chetkowski RJ, Nass TE, Matt DW, et al: Optimization of hydrogen ion concentration during aspiration of oocytes and culture and transfer of embryos. *J IVF/ET* 2:207, 1985.

159. Trounson A, Conti A: Research in human in vitro fertilization and embryo transfer. *Br Med J* 285:244, 1982.

160. Quinn P, Warnes GM, Kerin JF, Kirby C: Culture factors in relation to the success of human in vitro fertilization and embryo transfer. *Fertil Steril* 41:202, 1984.

161. Trounson AO, Mohr LR, Wood C, Leeton JF: Effect of delayed insemination on in vitro fertilization, culture, and transfer of human embryos. *J Reprod Fertil* 64:285, 1982.

162. Veeck LL, Wortham JWE, Witmyer T, et al: Maturation and fertilization of morphologically immature human oocytes in a program of in vitro fertilization. *Fertil Steril* 39:594, 1983.

163. Laufer N, Tarlatzis B, DeCherney AH, et al: Asynchrony between human cumulus-corona cell complex (CCC) and oocyte maturation after human menopausal gonadotropin (HMG) treatment for in vitro fertilization (IVF). *Fertil Steril* 42:366, 1984.

164. Tanphaichitr N, Randall M, Fitzgerald L, et al: An increase in the in vitro fertilization capability of low density human sperm capacitated by multiple tube swim-up. *Fertil Steril* 48:821, 1987.

165. Gorus FK, Dipelecos DG: A rapid method for the fractionization of human spermatozoa according to their progressive motility. *Fertil Steril* 35:662, 1981.

166. Forster MS, Smith WD, Lee WI, et al: Selection of human spermatozoa according to their relative motility and their interaction with zona free hamster eggs. *Fertil Steril* 50:655, 1983.

167. Berger T, Maris RA, Moyer DL: Comparison of techniques for selection of motile spermatozoa. *Fertil Steril* 43:268, 1985.

168. Fishel SB, Walters DE, Yodyinggaud V, Edwards RG: Time-dependent motility changes of human spermatozoa after preparation for in vitro fertilization. *J IVF/ET* 2:233, 1985.

169. Soupart P, Strong PA: Ultrastructural observations on human oocytes fertilized in vitro. *Fertil Steril* 25:11, 1974.

170. Wentz AC, Repp JE, Maxson WS, Pittaway DE, Torbit CA: The problem of polyspermy in in vitro fertilization. *Fertil Steril* 40:748, 1983.

171. Michelmann HW, Bonhoff A, Mettler L: Chromosome analysis in polyploid human embryos. *Hum Reprod* 1:243, 1986.

172. VanBlerkom J, Bell H, Henry G: The occurrence, recognition, and developmental fate of pseudo-multipronuclear eggs after in vitro fertilization of human oocytes. *Hum Reprod* 2:217, 1987.

173. Mohr LR, Trounson AO, Leeton JF, Wood C: Evaluation of normal and abnormal human embryo development during procedures in vitro, in Beier HM, Lindner HR (eds): *Fertilization of the Human Egg In Vitro.* Berlin, Springer Verlag, 1983.

174. Chan PJ: Developmental potential of human oocytes according to zona pellucida thickness. *J IVF/ET* 4:237, 1987.

175. Wolgemuth DJ, Celenza J, Bundman DS, Dunbar BJ: Formation of the rabbit zona pellucida and its relationship to ovarian follicular development. *Dev Biol* 106:1, 1984.

176. Leese HJ, Barton AM: Pyruvate and glucose up-take by mouse ova and preimplantation embryos. *J Reprod Fertil* 71:9, 1984.

177. Leese HJ: Analysis of embryos by non-invasive methods. *Hum Reprod* 2:37, 1987.

178. Magnusson C, Hillensjo T, Hamberger L, Nilsson L: Oxygen consumption by human oocytes and blastocysts grown in vitro. *Hum Reprod* 1:183, 1986.

179. O'Neill C, Saunders DM: Assessment of embryo quality. *Lancet* 2:1035, 1984.

180. Roger PWA, Milne BJ, Trounson AO: A model to show human uterine receptivity and embryo viability following ovarian stimulation for in vitro fertilization. *J IVF/ET* 3:93, 1986.

181. Wramsby H, Freda K, Liedholm P: Chromosome analysis of human oocytes removed from preovulatory follicles in stimulated cycles. *N Engl J Med* 316:121, 1987.

182. Martin RH, Balkan W, Burn K, et al: The chromosome constitution of 1000 human spermatozoa. *Hum Genet* 63:305, 1983.

183. Angell RR, Aitken RJ, Vanlook PFA, Lunsden MA, Templeton AA: Chromosome abnormalities in human embryos after in vitro fertilization. *Nature* 303:336, 1983.

184. Plachot M, Junca A, Mandelbaum J, et al: Chromosome investigations in early life. II. Human preimplantation embryos. *Hum Reprod* 2:29, 1987.

185. Wramsby H, Fredga K, Liedholm P: Ploidy in human cleavage stage embryos after fertilization in vitro. *Hum Reprod* 2:233, 1987.

186. Lopata A, Kohlman D, Johnston I: The fine structure of normal and abnormal human embryos developed in culture, in Beico HM, Lindner HR (eds): *Fertilization of the Human Egg in Vitro.* Heidelberg, Springer Verlag, 1983.

187. Tesarik J, Kopecny V, Plachot M, Mandelbaum J: Ultrastructural and autoradiographic observations on multinucleated blastomeres of human cleaving embryos obtained by in vitro fertilization. *Hum Reprod* 2:127, 1987.

188. Buster JE, Bastillo M, Rod I, et al: Biologic and morphologic development of donated human ova recovered by non-surgical uterine lavage. *Am J Obstet Gynecol* 153:211, 1985.

189. Trounson A, Mohr L: Human pregnancy following cryopreservation, thawing and transfer of an eight-cell embryo. *Nature* 305:707, 1983.

190. Lasalle B, Testart J, Renard JP: Human embryo features that influence the success of cryopreservation with the use of 1,2 propanediol. *Fertil Steril* 44:645, 1985.

191. Zeilmaker GH, Alberda AT, Van Gent I, Rijkmans CMPM, Drogendijk AC: Two pregnancies following transfer of intact frozen-thawed embryos. *Fertil Steril* 42:293, 1984.

192. Fehilly CB, Cohen J, Simons RF, Fishel SB, Edwards RG: Cryopreservation of cleaving embryos and expanded blastocysts in the human: A comparative study. *Fertil Steril* 44:638, 1985.

193. Croft I, Porter R, Green S, et al: Success of fertility, embryo number and in vitro fertilization. *Lancet* 1:732, 1984.

194. Testart J, Lassalle B, Forman R, et al: Factors influencing the success rate of human embryo freezing in an in vitro fertilization and embryo transfer program. *Fertil Steril* 48:107, 1987.

195. Marrs RP, Brown J, Sata F, et al: Successful pregnancies from cryopreserved human embryos produced by in vitro fertilization. *Am J Obstet Gynecol* 156:1503, 1987.

196. Willadsen SM: Factors affecting the survival of sheep embryos during deep-freezing and thawing, in *The Freezing of Mammal Embryos.* Amsterdam, Excerpta Medica, 1977.

197. Trounson AO, Peura A, Kirby C: Ultrarapid freezing: A new low-cost and effective method of embryo cryopreservation. *Fertil Steril* 48:843, 1987.

198. Testart J, Lassalle B, Belaisch-Allart J, et al: High pregnancy rate after early human embryo freezing. *Fertil Steril* 46:268, 1986.

199. Cohen J, Simons RS, Fehilly CB, Edwards RG: Factors affecting survival and implantation of cryopreserved human embryos. *J IVF/ET* 3:46, 1986.

200. Rall WF, Fahy GM: Ice-free cryopreservation of mouse embryos at −196°C by vitrification. *Nature* 313:573, 1985.

201. Feichtinger W, Benko I, Kemeter P: Freezing human oocytes using rapid techniques, in Feichtiger W, Kemeter P (eds): *Future Aspects in In Vitro Fertilization*. Berlin, Springer Verlag, 1987.

202. Deidrich K, Al-Hasami S, Van der Ven H, Krebs D: Successful in vitro fertilization in frozen-thawed rabbit and human oocytes, in Feichtinger W, Kemeter D (eds): *Future Aspects in In Vitro Fertilization*, Berlin, Springer Verlag, 1987.

203. Pichering SJ, Johnson MH: The influence of cooling on the organization of the meiotic spindle of the mouse oocyte. *Hum Reprod* 2:207, 1987.

204. Croxatto HB, Ortiz ME, Diaz S, et al: Studies on the duration of egg transport by the human oviduct. *Am J Obstet Gynecol* 132:629, 1978.

205. Bustillo M, Buster JE, Cohen SW, et al: Nonsurgical ovum transfer as a treatment in Fertile women. *JAMA* 251:1171, 1984.

206. Jones HW, Acosta AA, Andrews MC, et al: Three years of in vitro fertilization at Norfolk. *Fertil Steril* 42:826, 1984.

207. Gronow MJ, Martin MJ, McBain JC, et al: Aspects of multiple embryo transfer. *Ann NY Acad Sci* 442:381, 1985.

208. Jones HW: Embryo transfer. *Ann NY Acad Sci* 442:375, 1985.

209. Edwards RG, Fishel SB, Cohen J, et al: Factors influencing the success of in vitro fertilization for alleviating human infertility. *J IVF/ET* 1:3, 1984.

210. Bellaisch-Allart JC, Frydman R, Testart J, et al: In vitro fertilization and embryo transfer program in Clamart, France. *J IVF/ET* 1:51, 1984.

211. Kerin JF, Warnes GM, Quinn P, et al: In vitro fertilization and embryo transfer program, department of obstetrics and gynecology. University of Adelaide at the Queen Elizabeth Hospital, Woodville, South Australia. *J IVF/ET* 1:63, 1984.

212. Sepalla M: The world collaborative report on in vitro fertilization and embryo replacement: Current state of the art in January 1984. *Ann NY Acad Sci* 442:558, 1985.

213. Jones HW, Acosta AA, Garcia JE, Sandow BA, Veeck L: On the transfer of conceptuses from oocytes fertilized in vitro. *Fertil Steril* 39:241, 1983.

214. Kerin JF, Jeffrey R, Warnes GM, Cox LW, Broom TJ: A simple technique for human embryo transfer into the uterus. *Lancet* 2:726, 1981.

215. Schulman JD: Delayed expulsion of transfer fluid after IVF/ET. *Lancet* 1:44, 1986.

216. Poindexter AN, Thompson DJ, Gibbons WE, et al: Residual embryos in failed embryo transfer. *Fertil Steril* 46:262, 1986.

217. Liedholm P, Sundstrom P, Wramsby H: A model for experimental studies on human egg transfer. *Fertil Steril* 41:519, 1984.

218. Yovich JL, McColm SC, Turner SR, Murphy AJ: Embryo transfer technique as a cause of ectopic pregnancies in in vitro fertilization. *Fertil Steril* 44:318, 1985.

219. Parsons JH, Bolton VN, Wilson L, Campbell S: Pregnancies following in vitro fertilization and ultrasonographically directed surgical embryo transfer by prerurethral and transvaginal techniques. *Fertil Steril* 48:691, 1987.

220. Goswamy RK, Addo S, Steptoe PC: Does patient position for embryo replacement affect outcome of in vitro fertilization treatment? Presented at the fifth world congress on in vitro fertilization and embryo transfer, Norfolk, VA, April 5, 1987.

221. Feichtinger W, Kemeter P, Szalay S: The Vienna program of in vitro fertilization and embryo transfer—A successful clinical treatment. *Eur J Obstet Gynaecol Reprod Biol* 125:63, 1983.

222. Laufer N, Luborsky J, Tarlatzis B, et al: Asynchrony between oocyte-corona-cumulus complex maturation and mural granulosa cell luteinization in HMG-HCG cycles for IVF. Proceedings of the Society for Gynecologic Investigation, Phoenix, March 1985.

223. Jones GS, Garcia J, Acosta A: Luteal phase evaluation in in vitro fertilization, in Edwards RG, Purdy JM (eds): *Human Conception In Vitro*. London, Academic Press, 1982, p 297.

224. Kerin JF, Broom TJ, Ralph MM, et al: Human luteal phase function following oocyte aspiration from the immediately preovular graafian follicle of spontaneous ovular cycles. *Br J Obstet Gynaecol* 88:1021, 1981.

225. Kemeter P, Feichtinger W, Neumark J, et al: Influence of laparoscopic follicular aspiration under general anesthesia on corpus luteum progesterone secretion in normal and clomiphene-stimulated cycle. *Br J Obstet Gynaecol* 89:948, 1982.

226. Frydman R, Testart J, Giacomini P, et al: Hormonal and histological study of the luteal phase in women following aspiration of the preovulatory follicle. *Fertil Steril* 38:312, 1982.

227. Steptoe PC, Edwards RG, Purdy JM: Clinical aspects of pregnancies established with cleaving embryos grown in vitro. *Br J Obstet Gynaecol* 87:757, 1980.

228. Garcia J, Jones GS, Acosta A, Wright G: Corpus luteum function after follicle aspiration for oocyte retrieval. *Fertil Steril* 36:565, 1981.

229. Dlugi AM, Laufer N, DeCherney AH, et al: The preiovulatory and luteal phase of conception cycles following in vitro fertilization. *Fertil Steril* 41:530, 1984.

230. Lejeune B, Camus M, Deschacht J, Leroy F: Differences in the luteal phase after failed or successful in vitro fertilization and embryo replacement. *J IVF/ET* 3:358, 1986.

231. Mhadevan MM, Leader A, Taylor PJ: Effects of low-dose HCG on corpus luteum function after embryo transfer. *J IVF/ET* 2:190, 1985.

232. Yovich JL, McColm SC, Yovich JM, Matson PL: Early luteal serum progesterone concentrations are higher in pregnancy cycles. *Fertil Steril* 44:185, 1985.

233. Leeton J, Trounson A, Jessup D: Support of the luteal phase in IVF programs: Results of a controlled trial with intramuscular proluton. *J IVF/ET* 2:166, 1985.

234. Howles CM, Macnamel MC, Edwards RG: Follicular development and early luteal function of conception and non-conceptional cycles after human in vitro fertilization: Endocrine correlates. *Hum Reprod* 2:17, 1987.

235. Belaisch-Allart J, Testart J, Fries N, Forman RG, Frydman R: The effect of dydrogesterone supplementation in an IVF program. *Hum Reprod* 2:183, 1987.

236. Yovich JL, Stanger JD, Yovich JN, Tuvik AI: Assessment and hormonal treatment of the luteal phase of IVF cycles. *Aust NZ J Obstet Gynaecol* 24:125, 1984.

237. Abate V, Call A, Sanchi A: Endometrial biopsy at the time of embryo transfer: Correlation of histologic diagnosis with therapy and pregnancy rates [abstr]. *Fertil Steril* 41:43S, 1984.

238. Garcia JE, Acosta AA, Hsiu JG, Jones HW: Advanced endometrial maturation after ovulation induction with human menopausal gonadotropin/human chorionic gonadotropin for in vitro fertilization. *Fertil Steril* 41:31, 1984.

239. Salat-Baroux J, Giacomini P, Cornet D: Study of the luteal phase after ovulation and in vitro fertilization [abstr]. *Fertil Steril* 41:16S, 1984.

240. Cohen JJ, Debache C, Pigeau F, et al: Sequential use of clomiphene citrate, human menopausal gonadotropin, and human chorionic gonadotropin in human IVF. II. Study of luteal phase adequacy following aspiration of the preovulatory follicles. *Fertil Steril* 42:360, 1984.

241. Graf M, Reyniak V, Battle-Mutter P, Laufer N: Histologic evaluation of the luteal phase in women following follicle aspiration for oocyte retrieval. *Fertil Steril* In press.

242. Tarlatzis BC, Laufer N, DeCherney AH, et al: The value of β- HCG, estradiol, and progesterone levels in predicting the pregnancy outcome in IVF cycles. *J IVF/ET* 1:143, 1984.

243. Englert Y, Roger M, Belaisch-Allart J, et al: Delayed appearance of plasmatic chorionic gonadotropin in pregnancies after IVF-ET. *Fertil Steril* 42:835, 1984.

244. Yovich J, Stanger JD, Yovich JM, Tuvik AI, Turner SR: Hormonal profiles in the follicular phase, luteal phase, and first trimester of pregnancies arising from IVF. *Br J Obstet Gynaecol* 99:374, 1985.

245. DeCherney AH, Tarlatzis BG, Laufer N, Naftolin F: A simple technique of ovarian suspension in preparation for in vitro fertilization. *Fertil Steril* 43:659, 1985.

246. Emperaire JC, Ruffie A, Audebert AJ, Verdauger: Early prognosis for IVF pregnancies through plasma estrogen. *Lancet* 2:1151, 1984.

247. O'Neil C, Gidley-Baird AA, Pike CC, et al: Maternal blood platelet physiology and luteal phase endocrinology as a means of monitoring pre and post-implantation embryo viability following IVF. *J IVF/ET* 2:59, 1985.

248. Trounson A, Wood C: In vitro fertilization results, 1979–82, at Monash University, Queen Victoria, and Epworth Medical Center. *J IVF/ET* 1:42, 1984.

249. Andrews MC, Muasher SJ, Levy DL, et al: An analysis of the obstetric outcome of 125 consecutive pregnancies conceived in vitro and resulting in 100 deliveries. *Am J Obstet Gynecol* 154:848, 1986.

250. Frydman R, Belaisch-Allart J, Fries N, et al: An obstetric assessment of the first 100 births from the in vitro fertilization program at Clamart, France. *Am J Obstet Gynecol* 154:550, 1986.

251. Weir NC, Henricks CH: The reproductive capacity of an infertile population. *Fertil Steril* 20:289, 1969.

252. Romeu A, Muasher SJ, Acosta AA, et al: Results of in vitro fertilization attempts in women 40 years of age and older: The Norfolk experience. *Fertil Steril* 47:130, 1987.

253. Speirs AC, Lopata A, Gronow MJ, Kellow GN, Johnston W: Analysis of the benefits and risks of multiple embryo transfer. *Fertil Steril* 34:468, 1983.

254. Nero F, Diamond MP, DeCherney AH: Estimated gestational age (EGA) and birth weights in infants conceived in an in vitro fertilization (IVF) program. Presented at the fifth world congress on in vitro fertilization and embryo transfer, Norfolk, VA, April 5, 1987.

255. Biggers JD: Risks of in vitro fertilization and embryo transfer in humans, in Crosignani PG, Rubin BL (eds): *In Vitro Fertilization and Embryo Transfer*. London, Academic Press, 1983.

256. Guzick DS, Wilkes C, Jones HW: Cumulative pregnancy rates for in vitro fertilization. *Fertil Steril* 46:663, 1986.

257. Robl JM, First NL: Manipulation of gametes and embryos in the pig. *J Reprod Fertil* 33:101, 1985.

258. Uehara T, Yanagimachi R: Microsurgical injection of spermatozoa into hamster eggs with subsequent transformation of sperm nuclei into male pronuclei. *Biol Reprod* 15:467, 1977.

259. Markert CL: Fertilization of mammalian eggs by sperm injection. *J Exp Zool* 228:195, 1983.

260. Lassalle B, Courtot AM, Testart J: In vitro fertilization of hamster and human oocytes by microinjection of human sperm. *Gamete Res* 16:69, 1987.

261. Laws-King A, Trounson A, Sathanathan H, Kila I: Fertilization of human oocytes by microinjection of a single spermatozoon under the zona pellucida. *Fertil Steril* 48:637, 1987.

262. Barg PE, Wahrman MZ, Talansky BE, Gordon JW: Capacitated, acrosome reacted but immotile sperm, when microinjected under the mouse zona pellucida, will not fertilize the oocyte. *J Exp Zool* 237:365, 1986.

263. Gordon JW, Talansky BE: Assisted fertilization by zona drilling: A mouse mode for correction of oligospermia. *J Exp Zool* 239:347, 1987.

264. Gordon JW: Use of micromanipulation for increasing the efficiency of mammalian fertilization in vitro. Proceedings of the fifth world congress on IVF and embryo transfer. *Ann NY Acad Sci*, 541:601, 1988.

265. Tsunoda Y, McLaren A: Effects of various procedures on the viability of mouse embryos containing half the normal number of blastomeres. *J Reprod Fertil* 69:315, 1983.

266. Tarkowski AK, Wrablewska J: Development of blastomeres of mouse eggs isolated at the 4 and 8 cell stage. *J Embryol Exp Morphol* 18:155, 1967.

267. Barton SC, Adams CA, Norris ML, Surarni MAH: Development of gynogenetic and parthenogenetic inner cell mass and trophectoderm tissue in reconstituted blastocysts in the mouse. *J Embryol Exp Morphol* 90:267, 1985.

268. Edwards RG: Diagnostic methods for human gametes and embryos. *Hum Reprod* 2:415, 1987.

269. Verlinsky Y, Pergament E, Binor Z, Rawlins R: Genetic analysis prior to implantation: Future application of in vitro fertilization in the treatment and prevention of human genetic diseases, in Feichtinger W, Kenneth P (eds): *Future Aspects in Human IVF*. Berlin, Springer Verlag, 1987, p 262.

270. Jones KW, Singh L, Edwards RG: The use of probes for the Y chromosome in preimplantation embryo cells. *Hum Reprod* 2:439, 1987.

271. Embory SH, Scharf SJ, Saiki RK, et al: Rapid prenatal diagnosis of sickle cell anemia by a new method of DNA analysis. *N Engl J Med* 316:656, 1987.

CHAPTER 36

Ovum Donation

Daniel Navot, Zev Rosenwaks

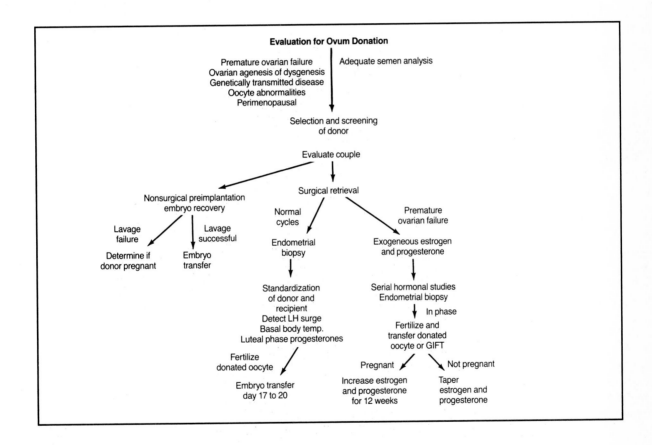

The successful reimplantation of a human embryo in 1978 marked the beginning of a new era in reproductive physiology and infertility therapy.[1] In-vitro fertilization (IVF) and related technologies have access to the microenvironment of the human oocyte, the subtleties of gamete interaction, and the intricacies of syngamy and early embryonic development. Egg and embryo donation is an obvious outgrowth of IVF. Essentially, the technique involves the transfer of embryo(s) or oocyte(s) from a fertile donor into the uterus of a phenotypically matched infertile recipient.[2-4] Successful transfer of donor embryos[4-6] and in-vitro-fertilized donor oocytes[2,3] has extended our ability to treat female infertility due to ovarian agenesis, oocyte depletion, inaccessibility of oocytes, and genetic abnormalities that preclude the use of disease-carrying gametes.[2,3,7]

Although oocyte donation is medically analogous to sperm donation, the relative inaccessibility of female gametes and the relative difficulty of synchronizing the ovulatory process in the donor with endometrial maturation in the recipient make the procedures quite different technically. Because the temporal window of endometrial receptivity and the window of transfer in the human are unknown, there is a tremendous clinical and scientific challenge—and reward—inherent in the practice of oocyte donation.

HISTORICAL PERSPECTIVES

Although the use of embryo transfer (ET) to alleviate infertility is relatively recent, this technology has been under investigation for a century since the first successful ET was performed in rabbits.[8] This was followed by experimentation in many species, with the greatest number of studies performed in the mouse, rabbit, sheep, and cow. The first successful bovine ET was reported in 1951,[9] and since then, many advances and refinements have led to a high success rate and the routine use of this technique in the cattle industry.[10] Briefly, the procedure involves the following steps: superovulation of the donor with gonadotropins, insemination (allowing fertilization to occur in vivo), embryo recovery, isolation of the embryo(s), and transfer of the embryo(s) to a recipient uterus. Thus, the donor is the genetic mother, while the host or recipient is the surrogate who carries and gives birth to the young.

It is evident that to optimize success in the bovine model, the recipient must be at the same stage of the estrus cycle as the donor. Asynchrony of 2 days or more in the luteal phase results in poor pregnancy rates.[11] In mice, synchrony must be within 6 hours for implantation to take place.[12] In sheep, when synchronization of donor and recipient is exact, 75% of all recipients become pregnant; a relatively high pregnancy rate is also obtained with asynchrony of up to 2 days. When there is a difference of 3 or more days, however, only 8% of ewes become pregnant.[13] In cattle, transfer efficiency approaches 70%.[14] A 36% pregnancy rate (4 of 11) was reported in oophorectomized recipient monkeys replaced with subcutaneous estradiol (E_2) and progesterone capsules,[15] with a tolerance of 3 days of asynchrony between embryo and endometrium.

Patient Selection and Indications

Women of reproductive age who lack ovaries, or whose ovaries are not functional, make up an important group of sterile patients who may benefit from ovum donation. These include women with the following diagnoses or indications:

1. Ovarian agenesis or dysgenesis
   Pure gonadal dysgenesis (46,XX)
   Turner's syndrome (45,X)
   Turner-like mosaics (variable karyotype)
   Swyer's syndrome (46,XY)
2. Premature ovarian failure
   Idiopathic (premature menopause)
   Autoimmune
   Iatrogenic (surgical ablation, radiation chemotherapy) or environmental (infections, drugs)
   Resistant ovary syndrome
   Genetic predisposition
3. Genetically transmitted diseases
   Maternal autosomal dominant
   Autosomal recessive, both partners
   X-linked recessive
4. Surgically inaccessible ovaries
5. Oocyte abnormalities
6. Perimenopausal

By far the most common complaint for which infertile women request ovum donation is the idiopathic form of premature ovarian failure (POF), or premature menopause. This is defined as permanent ovarian failure, and is characterized by elevated gonadotropin levels that occur after menarche but before the age of 35 or 40 years.[16,17] The condition is relatively common; approximately 4% of women reach menopause before age 30 years.[17] Undoubtedly, a sizable portion of these individuals may not have completed their families. A very important subgroup of patients, who need meticulous pretreatment evaluation, are those with Turner's syndrome and various other major chromosomal aberrations.

There is a strong correlation between autoimmune phenomena and POF, for example, Addison's disease,[18,19] Hashimoto's thyroiditis, myasthenia gravis, and systemic lupus erythematosus.[17] Further support that POF is due to an autoimmune phenomenon is provided by numerous reports of the presence of antibodies to specific ovarian components among these patients.[20,21] The other possible indications for ovum donation are self-explanatory.

The list of etiologic diagnoses discriminates two subgroups with regard to treatment strategy. Patients with genetically transmitted disease, inaccessible ovaries, or oocyte abnormalities are normally cycling women in whom an attempt at ovum donation takes place during a natural cycle. In contrast, those with ovarian dysgenesis or agenesis, or POF, require exogenous hormone replacement, because they are acyclic and lack any endogenous ovarian activity. Perimenopausal women make up a variable subgroup. They may still have cyclicity but it may be inadequate, and hormone replacement or augmentation may be required.

EVALUATION OF THE INFERTILE COUPLE PRIOR TO OVUM DONATION

Prerequisites for ovum donation include a normal uterus in the female, an adequate spermogram in her

TABLE 36–1. WORK-UP OF COUPLES WHO ARE CANDIDATES FOR OVUM DONATION

Female with Ovarian Failure	Male Partner
Baseline hormonal study	Spermatogram
Karyotype	
Hysterosalpingography	
Antiovarian antibodies*	
Cardiopulmonary work-up*	
Blood chemistry and hemotologic profile	
Rubella AB	
VDRL, hepatitus screen, HIV	Tay–Sachs*
HLA–AB typing	HLA–AB typing
Preparatory cycles(s)	
	Psychiatric and social evaluation
	informed consent

*If indicated

partner, and the absence of any contraindication for pregnancy.

Table 36–1 outlines the general guidelines for pretreatment evaluation. As a rule, programs that practice ovum donation are referral centers, and patients have already been through at least a preliminary diagnostic workup. Still, the need may arise to complete these tests and examinations. In patients with POF the karyotype should be scrutinized for the existence of a Y chromosome or fragment, which, if found, requires gonadectomy. In those with Turner's syndrome or a Turner-like mosaic, a thorough cardiopulmonary workup is warranted. The detection of associated congenital abnormalities should raise doubts about the advisability of pregnancy. The possible adverse effects on the already compromised cardiovascular system should be carefully assessed. In women with secondary ovarian failure of any etiology, the irreversibility of the phenomenon should be reassessed.

Finally, for optimal patient care and better clinical outcome, preparatory cycles should be evaluated for adequacy of the natural or exogenously stimulated endometrial cycle. During these preparatory cycles,[3,7] serial hormone studies and dated endometrial biopsies should be carried out. In the natural cycle a biopsy on day 26 is needed to rule out an inadequate luteal phase. During an exogenously supplemented cycle, a periimplantation (day 20 to 22) and a late luteal (day 26) biopsy should ascertain normalcy of the artificially induced cycle.

RECIPIENTS WITH NORMAL MENSTRUAL CYCLES

Patients who are carriers of genetically transmitted diseases, have surgically inaccessible ovaries, have oocyte abnormalities, or are perimenopausal and therefore unable to conceive despite cyclic ovarian function[11] are included in the category of recipients

with normal menstrual cycles. Embryo transfer, whether of in-vivo or in-vitro-fertilized oocytes, must be timed within a temporal window that is as yet incompletely defined.[23] Thus, the natural cycle must be closely monitored to detect the midcycle luteinizing hormone (LH) surge. Serum estradiol (E_2) and LH assays are performed during the early follicular phase and daily in the periovulatory phase of the cycle. A single daily LH measurement seems to be adequate for detecting the surge. It is recommended that a basal body temperature chart and daily progesterone determinations in the early luteal phase be used to confirm the timing of the LH surge and ovulation. The day of LH surge is arbitrarily defined as day 14, with day 15 designated as the day of ovulation.

Figure 36–1 represents an example of oocyte donation in the natural cycle. The recipient was a 40-year-old woman who had several IVF failures. The donor was a 32-year-old patient receiving IVF who agreed to donate all mature oocytes in excess of 5. Four donated oocytes were inseminated; 3 fertilized and were transferred on day 20 of the recipient's cycle, defined herein as day 19 relative to the LH peak, which occurred on day 15. Results of a test for human chorionic gonadotropin (HCG) were positive 8 days after transfer, and the patient delivered an infant at term.[24]

Another successful example was a 39-year-old woman with a 15-year history of infertility who had repeatedly failed IVF attempts because of an oocyte abnormality. A suitably matched donor was found who agreed to donated excess oocytes. Two 16-cell embryos were transferred on the 3rd day after the LH peak, designated herein as day 17 of the natural cycle. The recipient's LH surge occurred on the day of the donor oocyte harvest. To allow 1 more day of endometrial maturation, the embryos were placed in the uterus 3 days after in-vitro insemination rather than the customary 2 days. The 16-cell embryos implanted when placed into a histologic day-17 endometrium, and the patient delivered a healthy infant at term.

ARTIFICIALLY INDUCED ENDOMETRIAL CYCLES IN RECIPIENTS WITH OVARIAN FAILURE

Although various replacement protocols have been reported, they all endeavor to mimic the steroidal milieu of the normal menstrual cycle.[2,3,7] Essentially, estrogen, and estrogen plus progesterone, are administered sequentially.

The authors who reported the first pregnancy in a patient with POF used oral estradiol valerate (E_2V) (Progynova, Schering Corp, Kenilworth, NJ) and vaginal progesterone suppositories for steriod replace-

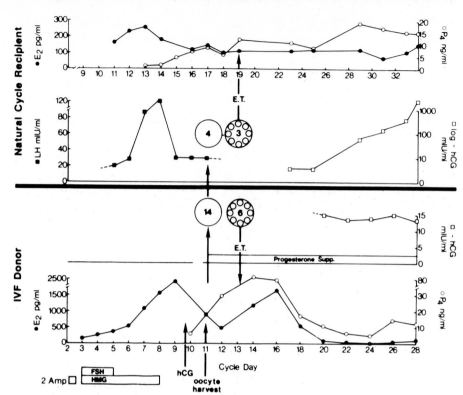

Figure 36–1. Oocyte donation of excess oocytes (from a patient undergoing IVF) to a natural-cycle recipient. The day of LH surge is defined as day 14. Four oocytes were inseminated with the spermatozoa of the recipient's husband. Three embryos were transferred on day 19. An 8-cell conceptus was the most advanced embryo transferred.

ment.[2] After ET, they used intramuscular progesterone injections and oral E_2V to maintain the pregnancy. A slight modification of this protocol resulted in satisfactory serum levels of both steroids and adequate endometrial development, as judged by luteal biopsy. Figure 36–2 details the protocol that we used initially.[3] Briefly, E_2V, 1 mg/day, was administered orally on days 1 through 5. The dosage was increased by 1 mg/day on days 6 through 9, and to 6 mg/day on days 10 through 13. The dosage was reduced to 2 mg/day on days 14 through 17, increased to 4 mg/day on days 18 through 26, and then reduced to 1 mg/day on days 27 and 28. It should be noted that the reduction on days 14 through 17 was used to mimic the drop in E_2, which is observed in the natural cycle after the LH surge. Progesterone was administered in a single intramuscular dose of 25 mg/day on days 15 and 16, increased to 50 mg/day on days 17 through 26, and reduced to 25 mg/day on days 27 and 28.

Intramuscular progesterone appears to be consistently absorbed, offering a predictable serum level and an unvarying action at the level of the target organ, the endometrium. Indeed, serum E_2 and progesterone levels closely simulated those of a normal 28-day cycle. The E_2 level rose gradually from a mean of 120 pg/mL in the early follicular phase to 900 pg/mL during the preovulatory phase. After a decrease in E_2 in the early luteal phase, a secondary rise corresponding to the midluteal phase was ob-

served (see Fig. 36–2). Serum progesterone also reached a peak at a mean level of 27 pg/mL. Endometrial thickness gradually increased from about 6 mm on day 6 to 12 mm on day 18 and remained constant thereafter.

A similar protocol using micronized E_2 (Estrace, Mead Johnson, Evansville, IN) was carried out in the donor egg program in Norfolk (Fig. 36–3).[7] An adequate luteal phase was induced by progesterone vaginal suppositories, 75 to 150 mg/day, or an intramuscular regimen. Additional acceptable routes of E_2 administration include vaginal rings[7] and transdermal patches (Estraderm, CIBA Pharmaceutical, Summit, NJ).

PATTERNS OF OTHER HORMONES IN THE REPRODUCTIVE SYSTEM

It is useful to view the clinical situation of ovum donation as a human in-vivo model in which ovarian function is substituted by exogenous estrogen and progesterone administration. In this model the positive feedback of very low endogenous estrogen levels is replaced by an incremental regimen of estrogen and progesterone isolated from any other ovarian regulatory substance that may affect the reproductive axis. In our model, a gradual decline in serum LH levels was observed. Pretreatment values of greater

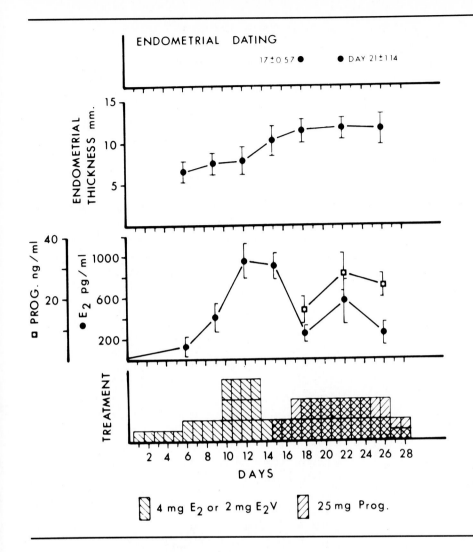

Figure 36–2. Exogenous hormonal treatment and serum estrogen and progesterone levels throughout the preparatory cycle in 8 patients. The endometrial response was evaluated by ultrasonography and morphology. Values are means ± SD. E_2 = estradiol; E_2V = estradiol valerate.

than 100 mIU/mL dropped to 44.3 ± 29.7 by midcycle and to 13.0 ± 8.4 when exogenous progesterone was added (Fig. 36–4). Follicle-stimulating hormone (FSH) behaved similarly; mean pretreatment values of 89.3 ± 7.3 mIU/mL declined by midcycle to 43.0 ±

27.7 and gradually fell further when exogenous progesterone was added. By day 18 the FSH level was 19.7 ± 24.5 mIU/mL, leveling off to 8.7 and 7.0 mIU/mL by days 25 and 31, respectively.

In contrast to our findings, others reported

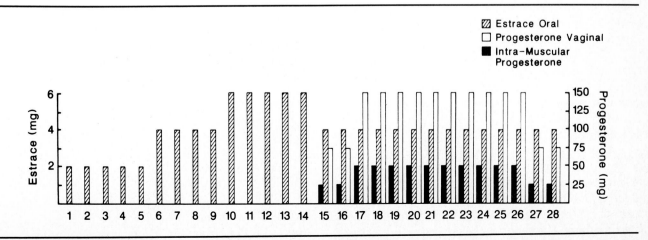

Figure 36–3. Estrogen and progesterone replacement protocols currently used in Norfolk.

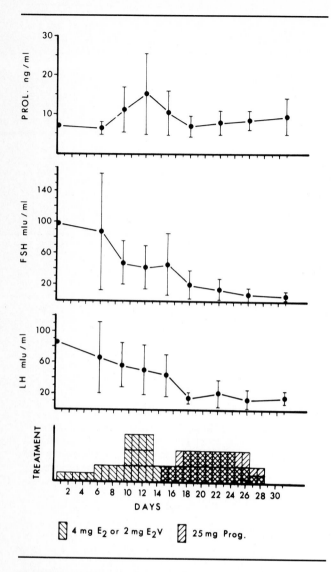

Figure 36–4. Serum gonadotropin and prolactin levels in response to exogenous estradiol and progesterone therapy in 8 patients with ovarian failure.

incomplete suppression of FSH levels, which was ascribed to lack of ovarian inhibin.[25] Our supraphysiologic E_2 and progesterone levels most likely compensated for the lack of inhibin. The same group reported on the occurrence of LH surges in 7 of 8 patients between days 12 and 14.[25] Only 3 of 8 had a detectable FSH surge concomitantly with the LH surge. These authors speculated that although an estrogen rise above a certain threshold is obligatory for triggering LH and FSH surges, progesterone is also required to trigger the FSH surge.[25]

Although physiologic or near physiologic levels of serum estrogen and progesterone are of considerable importance, final judgment of the suitability of a given replacement protocol depends on the histologic assessment of the endometrium. Secretory changes that compare favorably with the expected natural cycle day histology would be the desired end point.

ENDOMETRIAL MORPHOLOGY

Endometrial biopsies are performed during two replacement cycles. A preimplantation phase biopsy (day 20 to 22) is followed by a late (day 26 or 27) biopsy in a second estrogen and progesterone replacement cycle.

We have observed that biopsies performed on days 20 to 22 display the glandular architecture of day 17 to 18, together with a characteristic stroma of day 21 to 23. Histology of a typical early biopsy performed on day 21 is shown in Figure 36–5. The subnuclear vaculization and linear arrangement of nuclei characteristic of day 18 architecture are juxtaposed with edematous stroma suggestive of day 21 to 22 endometrium. This asychrony occurs despite seemingly adequate progesterone absorption. In contrast, biopsies performed on day 26 reveal the characteristic pseudodecidual changes in the stroma of day 25 to 26 endometrium. Thus, early development of the endometrial glands seems to lag behind that of the stroma, although the endometrium appears to catch up in the late luteal phase. It should be emphasized that the biopsy findings in the early luteal phase were confirmed on repeated biopsies, suggesting that the lag in glandular maturation was not due to first-cycle exposure to steroids. Rather, the glands may require a longer, albeit lower, threshold exposure to progesterone in order to achieve prompt and timely secretory changes. Except for the phenomenon of asychrony, endometrial morphology or ultrastructure conforms to that of a natural cycle. Electron microscopy of a day-18, artificially matured endometrium reveals the nucleolar channel system, a prominent feature of the early secretory endometrium.

Experience with a patch that delivers estrogen transdermally (Estraderm) reveals an equally adequate or even superior delivery system. Because the dermal route bypasses the portal system, the most potent estrogen, E_2, is not converted by gastrointestinal passage to the less potent estrone (E_1). Similarly, the potential adverse effects of estrogen on lipid metabolism and blood coagulation are minimized.

OOCYTE DONORS

Patients who undergo IVF and have excess oocytes are potential candidates for ovum donation. In the early days of the procedure, patients were advised not to attempt fertilization of more than 5 oocytes so as to minimize the occurrence of multiple gestations. The term "excess oocytes," however, became obsolete with successful cryopreservation of human embryos. Patients may now choose to inseminate all of their oocytes, transfer a prechosen number, and freeze the remaining concepti. Consequently, the

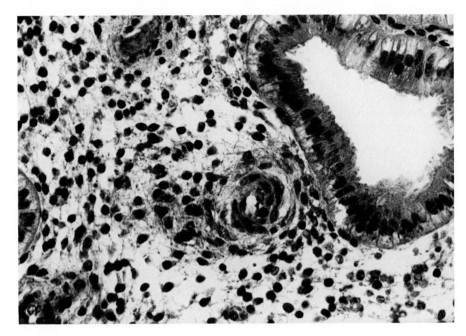

Figure 36–5. Histology of endometrial biopsy taken on day 21 after estrogen and progesterone replacement in a patient with ovarian failure. Note the subnuclear vacuolization and linear arrangement of nuclei characteristic of day-18 glands juxtaposed with edematous stroma and periarteriolar cuffing characteristic of day-22 to day-23 endometrium.

donor program depends on the availability of specific donors. In some instances a sister has provided oocytes. At other times a patient requesting tubal sterilization agrees to undergo gonadotropin stimulation before the surgical procedure.

Payment to donors should be discouraged, as recommended by the Ethics Committee of the American Fertility Society.[26]

A prospective donor and recipient are phenotypically matched. The donor should undergo complete psychologic and medical evaluations, and should be screened for hereditary and sexually transmitted diseases (Table 36–2).

To secure several fertilizable oocytes, ovarian stimulation must be carried out. Any stimulation of proved efficacy may be used.[2,3,7] Figure 36–1 illustrates a gonadotropin-stimulated cycle in the donor. Stimulation is typically begun on days 3 and 4 of the

cycle with the administration of 2 ampules of FSH in the morning, followed by 2 ampules of human menopausal gonadotropin (HMG) (Pergonal) in the afternoon. From day 5 onward, 2 ampules of HMG are administered daily until critical follicular development is achieved, as judged by daily measurement of serum E_2 levels are ultrasonograms.[27] Between days 8 and 11 of the cycle, HCG is administered, and oocyte harvest is scheduled for 34 to 36 hours later.[28] After harvest, the oocytes are inseminated with the sperm of the recipient's partner. The resulting embryos are kept in culture for 44 to 72 hours, when 2 to 16-cell embryos are transferred into the recipient's uterus.[29]

NONSURGICAL EMBRYO RECOVERY AND TRANSFER

As originally described by Seed and Seed[30] and mastered by others,[4–6] the technique of lavage is based on nonsurgical recovery of the in-vivo-fertilized preimplantation embryo. The fertile, naturally ovulating donor is inseminated by the semen of the infertile patient's partner. Transcervical uterine lavage is performed on the donor 5, 6, and 7 days after her LH peak with 60 mL of Dulbecco's medium supplemented with 5% human serum albumin. Recovery of an ovum terminates the lavage sequence. The embryo is then isolated and transferred into the recipient's uterus. One report includes 53 insemination cycles in which 25 ova (47%) were recovered.[31] Five (20%) of 25 attained the blastocyst stage, the only developmental stage associated with viable pregnancy. One ectopic and 3 intrauterine gestations were achieved in the recipients; 2 pregnancies carried

TABLE 36–2. GUIDELINES FOR SELECTION AND WORK-UP OF PROSPECTIVE OVUM DONORS

Clinical Appraisal	Laboratory Studies
Age (≤35 yrs)	Complete blood count and chemistry panel
Phenotype	HIV
Complete history and physical examination	Hepatitis screen
Family history of congenital or hereditary diseases	Tay–Sachs*
Detailed informed consent	Sickle cell screen*
Psychiatric interview	HLA–AB†

*As indicated.
†Optional.

to term. Two additional pregnancies were retained in the donors (lavage failures).

The overall efficiency of this technique is limited, and the hazard of a retained, undesired pregnancy is relatively high. Although the original indication for nonsurgical ET was tubal infertility, the procedure may be extended to acyclic women or those with POF. Augmentation of ovulation in the donor might improve the efficiency of ovum recovery.

TEMPORAL WINDOW OF ENDOMETRIAL RECEPTIVITY IN THE HUMAN

In the natural cycle, ovum transport is programmed in a way that allows fertilization, embryo transport, and embryo development to be synchronous with endometrial receptiveness. During IVF the embryo available for transfer is usually at the stage of 4 to 8 blastomeres. For this early developmental stage the optimal window of transfer or optimal endometrial receptivity has not been defined. At the inception of our donor egg programs,[3,7] clinical experiments were devised that would define this temporal window. In this experimental model, complete disassociation between the events leading to embryogenesis (donor) and endometrial development (recipient) allowed embryos of a definite blastomeric stage to be replaced into endometria at variable maturational stages. Endometrial receptivity was tested by replacing 2 to 16-cell embryos between days 16 and 24 of hormonally and histologically defined cycles.[7] In our preliminary experience (Table 36–3),[3] 2 of 8 recipients receiving transfer on days 16 to 21 conceived. Two conceptions occurred on days 18 and 19; others failed to occur on days 16, 17, 18 (2), 19, and 21. Experience has provided evidence of endometrial receptivity on days 18 to 19, and has extended the window of transfer to day 17.[7] Of 21 transfers performed with several concepti derived from mature oocytes, 7 patients became pregnant. All 7 (or 7 of 14) were

transferred on day 17 to 19 of an idealized cycle. None of the remaining 7 women transferred on day 20 or later became pregnant.

One group[2,25] typically performed ET on day 17 ± 1 of the replaced cycle. Most of their transfers were of embryos derived from patients undergoing IVF who were willing to donate excess oocytes. Thus single embryos were transferred in most donation cycles. Because it has been shown that the IVF success rate is increased by transfer of increasing numbers of embryos,[22] it is expected that transfer of several concepti to recipients would result in an improved success rate. Perhaps more important, excess oocytes obtained from patients undergoing IVF tend to be the least desirable morphologically, because the oocytes with the best morphology are saved for the IVF cycle. Therefore, clinics using excess oocytes may have a lower pregnancy rate than those using designated oocytes, although sisters and women undergoing sterilization have also been donors.

Based on our own experience and that of others,[23] transfer of frozen and thawed embryos has further extended the period of successful ET to day 16. A blastula was transferred successfully into a day-22 endometrium[33]; however, the report of this pregnancy did not precisely delineate the occurrence of the LH surge and ovulation, thus making the conclusions somewhat speculative.

If one considers that a 2 to 12-cell embryo requires approximately 3 or 4 days to reach the blastocyst stage, at which implantation takes place, then ET on day 19—the limit of the transfer window—would lead to implantation on day 22 or 23. It can therefore be speculated that after day 23 the endometrium is incompatible with implantation. It appears that ET as early as day 16 allows embryonic development to continue within the uterine cavity, enabling implantation to occur at a later stage when endometrial maturation catches up with embryonic development.

The temporal window for human ET extends

TABLE 36–3. PREGNANCIES ACHIEVED BY OVUM DONATION ACCORDING TO DIAGNOSIS AND TIMING OF TRANSFER

Primary Diagnosis	Day of Embryo Transfer	Number of Embryos Replaced	Stage of Embryonic Cleavage*
Surgically castrated[†]	19	4	(4)2 (6)2
Gonadal dysgenesis[†] (46,XX)	18	4	(4)3 (6)1
Premature menopause	18	2	(6)1 (8)1
Premature menopause	21	3	(4)2 (3)1
Premature menopause	19	2	(5)1 (6)1
Premature menopause	17	2	(5)1 (6)1
Balanced translocation	18	2	(2)1 (2PN)1
Turner's syndrome	16	3	(4)3

*Cell stage in parentheses, followed by number of embryos attaining that stage of embryonic cleavage.
†Conceived after embryo transfer.
PN = pronucleus.

between days 16 and 19 of a hormonally and morphologically defined 28-day cycle. Whether there is an optimum day of transfer within that time frame, or whether embryonic or endometrial tolerance for asynchrony is even greater, must await confirmation by additional data.

SYNCHRONIZATION BETWEEN DONOR AND RECIPIENT

The relatively restricted period available for implantation demands precise synchronization between donor and recipient. The strategy for synchronization is completely different for natural cycles and stimulated cycles. The first step is to standardize the cycles.

Natural Cycles

The day of LH peak is traditionally designated as day 14, or luteal day 0. An attempt was made to synchronize natural cycles in donor and recipient by synchronizing LH peaks at ± 2 days.[4–6] To facilitate proper timing, the recipients took oral contraceptives prior to the transfer cycle.

The concept of ± 2 days is probably correct. The embryo may survive in a uterine environment not yet suitable for implantation; however, an endometrium too advanced may preclude successful implantation. Moreover, proper timing is dependent on the predicted onset of menstrual flow in the donor, a prediction that is notoriously unreliable in times of stress. Of 12 transfer cycles, 4 (33%) were out of synchronization by ± 3 days, while 3 more (25%) were ± 2 days off; only 5 (42%) were aligned within ± 1 day.[5] An alternative technique uses progestational agents to prolong the luteal phase in donor or recipient. Theoretically, such intervention into the natural cycle may have less effect on the ensuing, actual donation cycle. This technique is as likely to fail as the other.[5]

Stimulated Cycles. Stimulation for multiple follicular recruitment and multiple ovulation is an obligatory step in the prospective ovum donor. When the donor is aligned with a recipient who has natural cycles, the problem of synchronization is complicated further by the fact that in the stimulated cycle the follicular phase is shortened by as much as 4 to 5 days. In a typical gonadotropin-stimulated cycle, HCG—as a surrogate LH surge—is given on day 9.[28] Figure 36–1 illustrates the point precisely. The recipient's menstrual cycle started 6 days prior to the donor's cycle. Because of a shortened follicular phase in the donor, however, at the time of the natural and surrogate LH surges there was a lag of only 1 day in the recipient. Embryo transfer on day 19 of the recipient's cycle resulted in a pregnancy that carried to term.

With a designated donor such as a patient undergoing tubal ligation, it is relatively easy to control the cycle with oral contraceptives or progestational agents. Although the actual stimulation cycle may have a relatively slow recruitment phase, this lag may be overridden by massive gonadotropin stimulation. The recipient with POF, in whom estrogen and progesterone supplementation mimics the natural 28-day cycle, presents a similar logistic dilemma; her supplementation must be initiated 2 to 5 days prior to the predicted onset of menses in the prospective donor. Figure 36–6 illustrates synchronization between a recipient with gonadal dysgenesis and a matched donor. The donor, who previously took oral contraceptives, received HCG on day 12, corresponding to day 14 in the recipient. On day 18, 4 embryos at the 4 to 6-blastomere stage were transferred. Ten days later conception was diagnosed, and subsequently the patient delivered a healthy female child at term.

A novel approach that provides complete control over the donor cycle uses gonadotropin-releasing hormone (GnRH) agonists. The drawbacks of this pretreatment include its cost, the prolonged treatment phase, and the still-unknown long-term side effects. All these points must be carefully considered before administration of a GnRH agonist to a healthy woman who volunteers to donate oocytes.

Another alternative, and an agreeable one, is to manipulate the recipient's artificial cycle. Initially, all replacement protocols were devised to mimic the natural cycle as closely as possible[2,3,7]; however, the need for better synchronization prompted us to create artificial cycles in which estrogen and progesterone stimulation was drastically changed. A short follicular phase protocol (6 days of estrogen stimulation) and a long follicular phase protocol (21 to 35 days of unopposed estrogen stimulation) were devised. Prolonged stimulation had no apparent adverse effect on endometrial morphology. The glandular and stromal elements seemed to be in phase with the chronologic age of the endometrium. It is of special interest that despite the prolonged exposure to high-dose estrogen, its known mitogenic and proliferative effects were not apparent on histologic examination. Similarly, a relatively short exposure to moderate E_2 levels appeared to be adequate for the induction of endometrial progesterone receptors and allowed for normal secretory transformation.

GAMETE INTRAFALLOPIAN TRANSFER IN PREMATURE OVARIAN FAILURE

Gamete intrafallopian transfer (GIFT) was performed with oocyte donations in 8 patients with POF.[34] Exogenous supplementation with estrogen and pro-

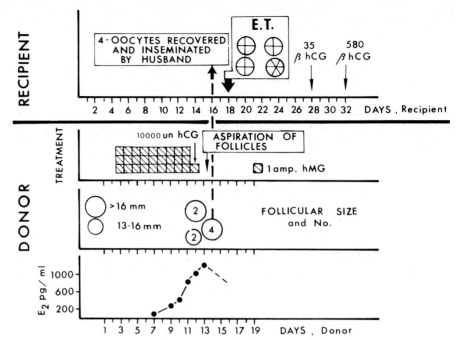

Figure 36–6. Synchronization between a recipient with ovarian failure and a matched donor. A singleton pregnancy was established after the transfer of 4 embryos in the 4 to 6-cell stage on cycle day 19. Cycle day 1 of the donor corresponds to cycle day 4 of the recipient. ET = embryo transfer; HCG = human chorionic gonadotropin; HMG = human menopausal gonadotropin; E_2 = estradiol.

gesterone was similar to our protocol.[7] One or 2 donated oocytes were transferred with 100,000 motile sperm per oviduct. All transfers were performed on cycle days 12 to 15 (not normalized for HCG). From the day of GIFT onward, supraphysiologic doses of estrogen (Estrace), 8 mg, and progesterone 50 mg in oil, were administered. The group reported 6 clinical pregnancies in the 8 patients, a remarkable 75%, which might justify the additional surgical procedure if the results prove to be reproducible in larger series.

PREGNANCY AND ITS MAINTENANCE IN OVARIAN FAILURE

As of May 1987, 18 centers around the world reported on 69 pregnancies resulting from ovum donation; 56 were achieved in patients with POF and 13 in natural cycles.[35]

Detailed experience describing requirements for pregnancy maintenance has been reported by several investigators.[2,3,7] A positive β-HCG titer can be expected on day 28, 10 days after ET. If results of the pregnancy test are negative, the dosage of estrogen and progesterone is tapered to allow endometrial shedding and menstruation to occur. If the results are positive, most investigators immediately and substantially increase the estrogen dosage. In one study, patients took 2 mg of E_2V in the luteal phase of the transfer cycle, increasing the dosage to 8 or 9 mg/day as soon as the β-HCG titer

became positive.[2] At the same time the patients received intramuscular progesterone, 50 to 100 mg/day. The authors suggested that this regimen maintained plasma steroid levels at concentrations that were within the normal ranges for pregnancy. The goal was to maintain E_2 concentrations at 100 to 500 pmol/L and within the progesterone range of 100 to 200 nM/L. Estrogen treatment was discontinued at 12 weeks of pregnancy, whereas progesterone injections were maintained through week 16.

Others rapidly increased exogenous estrogen and progesterone when pregnancy was diagnosed.[3] From weeks 7 and 8, when the hormones were kept at a fixed dosage, relatively stable blood levels were obtained. It was assumed that notable endogenous production of steroids would be reflected by a net increase in the artificially achieved steady state. During week 11 the anticipated surge in E_2 was observed, and stepwise withdrawal of exogenous estrogen was begun. The first 2 patients experienced a rise in progesterone level during week 12, and a stepwise withdrawal of exogenous progesterone was begun. By week 16, both pregnancies were maintained solely by placental E_2. By week 18, one patient no longer required exogenous progesterone.

These preliminary observations dated placental takeover to week 12 of gestation.[36] In contrast, more recent data (D. Navot, unpublished data) suggest that significant placental steroidogenesis may begin earlier. It appears that in humans, the dosage of estrogen and progesterone required for implantation and early pregnancy maintenance may be less than has been used. Nevertheless, gravid patients who lack ovarian function should be regarded as in-vivo models for the study of placental steroidogenesis isolated from ovarian hormonal function. These models should be used to determine specifically the time of luteoplacental shift, and the exact estrogen and progesterone requirements for initiating and maintaining pregnancy in patients with POF.

LEGAL AND ETHICAL ISSUES CONCERNING OVUM DONATION

Many legal and bioethical aspects of ovum donation may be inferred from the practice of sperm donation. Although practiced for over a century, sperm donation still lacks universal statutes to deal with its inherently complex legal issues. Thus it is understandable that ovum donation, which has been practiced for only 3 years, has scarcely more than guidelines in most countries. A few potentially controversial issues arising from ovum donation are as follows:

1. The legal status of children born as a consequence of ovum donation
2. The rights of the genetic mother
3. Anonymity of the donor and access of the child to information regarding his or her conception
4. Unwitting sibling marriage, and the problem of incest
5. The physician's responsibility with regard to the selection of donors, and liability to donor, recipient, and child

Oocyte donation has an advantage over sperm donation in that the nongenetic mother carries the child and gives birth, thereby allowing her to experience the desired pregnancy. A major disadvantage is the surgical procedure inherent in oocyte collection. The risks of the surgical procedure should be evaluated carefully when considering egg donation by a close relative[7] or when oocyte retrieval is coincidental to another surgical procedure. In the former instance the overall short and long-term risks must be assessed, while in the latter the added risk of oocyte retrieval during tubal ligation or diagnostic laparoscopy is minimal. The ability to use ultrasound-guided oocyte retrieval under local anesthesia will diminish the potential risks to elective donors.[37]

Ovum donation is permitted in the United States, the United Kingdom, Australia, Austria, Israel, and Italy.[38] Some countries hold the view that gamete donation in conjunction with IVF is beyond the limit of therapy permissible for infertile couples.[39] The Warnock Committee in the United Kingdom,[40] the Waller Committee in Australia,[41] and the Ethics Committee of the American Fertility Society (AFS)[26]

have elaborated on different aspects of the subject. The Waller Committee was the first in the world to proclaim that the recipient woman is the legal mother and that the donor has no legal rights or responsibilities to the child.[41] The AFS Ethics Committee recommended against compensation for oocyte donation and advocated meticulous confidentiality. The committee also stressed that when excess oocytes are donated during an IVF attempt, "every effort should be made not to diminish the donors' chances of becoming pregnant."[26] Until appropriate legislative measures are taken, it is strongly advised that artificial conception services should work in conjunction with well-established infertility clinics. These clinics should be equally able to provide medical care, counseling, and support. Their clinical and research activities should be open to peer and public scrutiny.

SUMMARY

Estrogen and progesterone replacement in patients with ovarian failure allows assessment of the relative roles of these steroids in endometrial proliferation and differentiation. The transfer of concepti of a defined stage into a specific endometrium has made possible the assessment of the human window of implantation. Precise manipulation of endometrial proliferation and differentiation, by varing the estrogen and progesterone regimen in patients with POF, will allow the separation of endometrial from ovarian factors. The ability to manipulate estrogen and progesterone dosage during pregnancy in these patients will precisely define the role of these steroids in establishing and maintaining pregnancy.

A donor oocyte program, although it is an exciting and gratifying treatment modality for infertility, has provided a unique human model for the study of the interaction among conceptus, endometrium, and steroids. It may also elucidate previously unapproachable questions of human reproduction and infertility.

REFERENCES

1. Steptoe PC, Edwards RG: Birth after the reimplantation of a human embryo. *Lancet* 2:336, 1978.
2. Lutjen P, Trounson A, Leeton J, et al: The establishment and maintenance of pregnancy using in vitro fertilization and embryo donation in a patient with primary ovarian failure. *Nature* 307:174, 1984.
3. Navot D, Laufer N, Kopolovic J, et al: Artificially induced endometrial cycles and establishment of pregnancies in the absence of ovaries. *N Engl J Med* 314:806, 1986.
4. Buster JE, Bustillo M, Thorneycroft IH, et al: Nonsurgical transfer of in vivo fertilized donated ova to five infertile women: Report of two pregnancies. *Lancet* 2:223, 1983.
5. Bustillo M, Buster JE, Cohen SW, et al: Nonsurgical ovum transfer as a treatment in infertile women: Preliminary experience. *JAMA* 25:1171, 1984.
6. Bustillo M, Buster JE, Cohen SW, et al: Delivery of a healthy infant following nonsurgical ovum transfer. *JAMA* 251:889, 1984.

7. Rosenwaks Z: Donor eggs: Their application in modern reproductive technologies. *Fertil Steril* 47:895, 1987.

8. Heape W: Preliminary note on the transplantation and growth of mammalian ova within a uterine foster mother. *Proc R Soc Lond* 48:457, 1890.

9. Wilett EL, Black WG, Casida LE, Stone WH, Buckner PJ: Successful transplantation of a fertilized bovine ovum. *Science* 113:247, 1951.

10. Seidel GEJ Jr: Superovulation and embryo transfer in cattle. *Science* 211:351, 1981.

11. Newcomb R, Rowson LE: Conception rate after uterine transfer of cow eggs in relation to synchronization of oestrus and age of eggs. *J Reprod Fertil* 43:539, 1975.

12. Beatty RA: Transplantation of mouse eggs. *Nature* 168:2995, 1951.

13. Rowson LEA, Moor RM: Embryo transfer in the sheep: The significance of synchronizing oestrus in the donor and recipient animal. *J Reprod Fertil* 11:201, 1966.

14. Rowson LEA, Lawson RAS, Moor RM, Baker AA: Egg transfer in the cow: Synchronization requirements. *J Reprod Fertil* 28:427, 1972.

15. Hodgen GD: Surrogate embryo transfer combined with estrogen-progesterone therapy in monkeys, implantation, gestation and delivery without ovaries. *JAMA* 250:2167, 1983.

16. Friedman C, Barrows H, Kim MH: Hypergonadotropic hypogonadism. *Am J Obstet Gynecol* 145:360, 1983.

17. Tulandi T, Kinch RAH: Premature ovarian failure. *Obstet Gynecol Surv* 36:521, 1981.

18. Turkington RW, Lebovitz HE: Extra-adrenal endocrine deficiencies in Addison's disease. *Am J Med* 43:499, 1967.

19. Irvine WJ, Chan MMW: Immunological aspects of premature ovarian failure associated with idiopathic Addison's disease. *Lancet* 1:883, 1968.

20. De Moraes-Ruehsen M, Blizzard RM, Garcia-Bunuel R, Jones GS: Autoimmunity and ovarian failure. *Am J Obstet Gynecol* 112:693, 1972.

21. Caldwell BV, Luborsky-Moore JL, Kase N: A functional LH agonist and LH receptor antagonist in serum from a patient with premature ovarian failure syndrome. Presented at the meeting of the Endocrine Society, Miami, June 15, 1978.

22. Navot D, Rosenwaks Z, Margalioth EJ: Prognostic assessment of female fecundity. *Lancet* 2:645, 1987.

23. Van Stierteghem AC, Van den Abbeel E, Braeckmans P, et al: Pregnancy with a frozen–thawed embryo in a woman with primary ovarian failure. *N Engl J Med* 317:113, 1987.

24. Trounson A, Leeton J, Besanka M, Wood C, Conti A: Pregnancy established in an infertile patient after transfer of a donated embryo fertilised in vitro. *Br Med J* 286:835, 1983.

25. Lutjen PJ, Findlay JR, Trounson AO, Leeton JF, Chan LK: Effects on plasma gonadotropins of cyclic steroid replacement in women with premature ovarian failure. *J Clin Endocrinol Metab* 62:419, 1986.

26. Jones HW Jr: Ethical considerations of the new reproductive technologies. *Fertil Steril* 46:suppl 1, 1986.

27. Muasher SJ, Garcia JE, Rosenwaks Z: The combination of follicle stimulating hormone and human menopausal gonadotropins for the induction of multiple follicular maturation for in vitro fertilization. *Fertil Steril* 44:62, 1985.

28. Rosenwaks Z, Muasher SJ: Recruitment of fertilizable eggs, in Jones HW Jr, Jones GS, Hodgen GD, Rosenwaks Z (eds): *In Vitro Fertilization–Norfolk*. Baltimore, Williams & Wilkins, 1986, p 30.

29. Veeck LL, Maloney M: Insemination and fertilization, in Jones HW Jr, Jones GS, Hodgen GD, Rosenwaks Z (eds): *In Vitro Fertilization—Norfolk*. Baltimore, Williams & Wilkins, 1986, p 168.

30. Seed RG, Seed RW: Artificial embryonation–human embryo transplant. *Arch Androl* 5:90, 1980.

31. Bustillo M, Buster JE: Nonsurgical ovum transfer: The Harbor, UCLA experience, in Feichtinger W, Kemeter P (eds): *Future Aspects in Human In Vitro Fertilization*. Berlin, Springer-Verlag, 1987, p 122.

32. Jones HW Jr, Acosta AA, Andrews MC, et al: Three years of in vitro fertilization at Norfolk. *Fertil Steril* 42:826, 1984.

33. Formigli L, Formigli G, Rocciio C: Donation of fertilized uterine ova to infertile women. *Fertil Steril* 47:162, 1987.

34. Asch RH, Balmaceda JP, Ord T, et al: Oocyte donation and gamete intrafallopian transfer in premature ovarian failure. *Fertil Steril* 49:263, 1988.

35. Schenker JG: Ovum donation: State of the art. *NY Acad Sci*, in press.

36. Ryan KJ: Placental synthesis of steroid hormones, in Tulchinsky D, Ryan KJ (eds): *Maternal–Fetal Endocrinology*. Philadelphia, Saunders, 1980, p 3.

37. Seibel MM: A new era in reproductive technology: In vitro fertilization, gamete intrafallopian transfer, and donated gametes and embryos. *N Engl J Med* 318:828, 1988.

38. Schenker JG, Frenkel DA: Medico-legal aspects of in vitro fertilization and embryo transfer practice. *Obstet Gynecol Surv* 42:405, 1987.

39. German Medical Association: Statement. *Dtsch Arzteibl* 22:91, 1985.

40. Committee of Enquiry into Human Fertilization and Embryology: *Report*. London, Her Majesty's Stationery Office, 1984.

41. Committee to Consider the Social, Ethical, and Legal Issues Arising from In Vitro Fertilisation: *Reports*. Melbourne, Australia, 1983, 1984.

CHAPTER 37

Cryopreservation and Infertility

Pierre Jouannet, Rene Frydman, A. Van Steirteghem, J. P. Wolf, F. Czyglik, and E. Van Den Abbeel

---

Cryopreservation and Infertility

HISTORICAL OVERVIEW OF CRYOPRESERVATION

Sperm Freezing

The first studies of the effect of very low temperatures on human spermatozoa were made by Spallanzani in 1776,[1] and the concept of sperm banking was discussed about a century later by Mantegazza.[2] It was known in the early 1940s that some spermatozoa could survive after freezing, and cryopreservation of spermatozoa became possible when Rostand[3] discovered the cryoprotective role of glycerol for biologic structures in 1946 and when Polge and co-workers[4] successfully used this procedure in 1949. The technique was rapidly and extensively used to breed farm animals, but application to humans was not undertaken for a long period of time. Bunge and Sherman[5] first obsrved in 1953 that human sperm, frozen in dry ice and later thawed, were able to fertilize and induce normal embryonic development. In the following years only a few births were reported after insemination with stored sperm. The first births after freezing of human spermatozoa with glycerol in liquid nitrogen were reported to 1964.[6] The same year it was shown that dimethylsulfoxide (DMSO) was toxic to spermatozoa.

Human sperm cryobanking really grew in the 1970s. In the United States, the hope of obtaining "fertility insurance" prior to vasectomy led to the development of commercial banks, with some banks also established in university hospitals. In France, the first Centre d'Etude et de Conservation du Sperme (CECOS) was set up in 1973. The American Association of Tissue Banks was created in 1976, and the first international meeting on human semen cryopreservation was held in Paris in 1978.

The concept of using frozen donor sperm for artificial insemination was not clearly understood in many countries until recently. It is only since the risk of disease transmission was demonstrated, especially acquired immunodeficiency syndrome, that it has been recommended to use only frozen semen for therapeutic insemination by donor (TID), as this procedure provides the necessary controls to contain this risk.

Embryo Freezing

Embryo cryopreservation was first performed successfully in the mouse.[7] The methods were later adapted to preserve embryos of other animal species at low temperature, and they became established means of commercially banking cattle and sheep embryos. In the mouse, this procedure allowed genetic conservation of different strains. In the mouse and other animal species it is reliable and safe with respect to genetic stability and occurrence of malformations at birth.

The techniques used to freeze human embryos were based on those used in animals, with the first human pregnancy reported after transfer of an 8-cell embryo frozen in DMSO. The pregnancy aborted at 24 weeks due to an obstetric complication.[8] The first pregnancies and live births using the DMSO protocol were reported in the mid-1980s.[9,10] Around the same time, the first birth after successful conservation at low temperature of a blastocyst frozen in glycerol was reported.[11] In addition to the DMSO and glycerol

protocols, pregnancies were reported with the use of propanediol as cryoprotective agent.[12]

Oocyte Freezing

In contrast with embryo freezing, fewer experimental data are available concerning oocyte freezing. Only three groups have reported pregnancies and the birth of 4 children after transfer of a previously frozen fertilized oocyte.[13-15] The survival rate after thawing was reduced in three protocols, and polyploidy is substantially increased.[14]

CONCEPTS

Long-term storage of biologic structures requires the arrest of cellular and molecular activity while maintaining the integrity of the structures necessary to restore normal cell function. This can be done by removing water from the cell either by lyophilization or by freezing; however, the former may be mutagenic. Lowering the temperature induces an important decrease or a complete stop of cell metabolism. Freezing and thawing can be toxic either directly through physical or chemical modifications of the cell, or indirectly due to damage of the cell structures by ice crystals.

The phenomena accompanying freezing and thawing are summarized in Figure 37–1. Basic as-

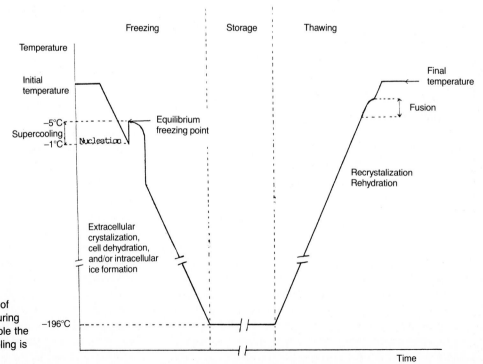

Figure 37–1. Schematic depiction of events occurring at the cell level during freezing and thawing. In this example the sample is not seeded, so supercooling is important before nucleation.

pects and consequences of low-temperature preservation have been extensively reviewed elsewhere.[16] The main consequence of freezing is the phase modification of water. The first event is the nucleation or formation of the first ice crystal at a temperature below the equilibrium freezing point. In biologic systems, nucleation begins in the extracellular environment usually between −5 and −15°C. The difference between equilibrium and nucleation temperature is supercooling. The degree of supercooling may be decreased by inducing physical seeding, which is the initiation of nucleation at a controlled temperature near the equilibrium point.

During freezing, the proliferation of ice crystals induces the development of a solid phase, whereas the solute concentration increases in the portion that remains liquid. Due to membrane permeability and the freezing rate, this leads to cell dehydration and shrinkage, and increased concentration of intracellular solute. Cell dehydration may be avoided by rapid freezing, but this does result in nucleation of large amounts of intracellular ice, which may damage the cell structure. Partial dehydration of the cells before freezing may reduce intracellular crystalization; for example, by incubating the cells in a sucrose solution. During thawing, an osmotic shock may also occur when water returns to the cell. Other damage may be the consequence of crystalization of the amorphous intracellular ice.

The addition of cryoprotective agents (CPAs) has been shown to diminish significantly the deleterious effect of freezing and thawing. These organic solvents modify the physical properties of a solution by lowering its freezing point. When they replace intracellular water, they reduce the adverse consequences of phase change during crystalization and fusion. Their action depends on their ability to penetrate the membranes, and also on their degree of toxicity to the cell. To prevent this toxicity, CPAs are often added to the solution at a very low temperature. Another way to avoid cell damage is to produce vitrification instead of water crystalization. Vitrification is the formation of amorphous ice, which can be achieved by very rapid freezing or by using a very high CPA concentration.

Finally, the success of the freezing–storage–thawing procedure is dependent on many factors. Some are linked to the cell, such as cell size, surface:volume ratio, membrane permeability, and resistance to osmotic or cold shock. Others are technical, such as the nature and concentration of the CPA, and the rate of freezing and thawing. Those various factors cannot be efficiently combined by mathematical formula, and the pragmatic approach of gamete and embryo cryopreservation has shown that optimum conditions have not yet been well defined and may be very different from one cell to another.

CRYOPRESERVATION IN ANIMAL REPRODUCTION

Cryopreservation of spermatozoa has been widely developed in domestic animal strains.[17] The protocol used is mainly derived from the method initially proposed by Polge and associates.[4] Because it permits almost indefinite conservation of semen, numerous sperm banks have been created, thus allowing dramatic improvements in reproduction techniques of domestic animals by genetic selection, preservation of various disappearing species, and creation of some new ones, such as cows that produce abundant milk and that resist bad climate conditions. Furthermore, progress in gene transfer has emphasized the interest in cryopreservation of breeds of genetic interest.

Semen of more than 50 different species has been frozen successfully. Artificial insemination with frozen semen in cattle is widely done, with more than 90% of dairy animals reproduced by this technique in developed countries. There is a great variability among species and among males with respect to freezability of semen, however.[18] In the pig, for instance, birth rates after artificial insemination with frozen sperm are about 10% less than those obtained with fresh semen,[19] while in the mare this level drops to 50% of the controls.[17,18]

Techniques for the cryopreservation of embryos have been used successfully to date in 9 species of domestic animals, including the cow, rabbit, and mouse. These are described in detail elsewhere.[20–23] Only minor changes have been introduced in the procedures. One modification is the use of sucrose prior to cooling the embryos and during the thawing process as an osmotic aid during dilution of the CPA.[12,23]

Hormonal stimulation of ovaries and the ability to increase by several times the mean number of viable embryos produced per cycle have led to advances in embryo cryopreservation. Under optimal conditions, the resulting pregnancy rate in cattle is only 10% lower than with fresh embryo transfer. The economic aspects are important because this technique allows the development of embryos of defined genetic origins in "surrogate cows." This may eventually help find a solution to the problem of disease transmission by embryos (such as bovine diarrhea virus), because evidences exists that several types of viruses are unable to cross the zona pellucida of frozen–thawed embryos.[24]

Cryopreservation of oocytes also has been proposed. In 1977, Whittingham reported the first study of fertilization of unfertilized mouse oocytes previously stored at $-196°C$.[25] Although survival of embryos is good because they can accommodate the loss of a few cells during the freezing–thawing procedure, that of oocytes is limited. The fact that mammalian oocytes are large cells arrested in meiosis increases the sensitivity of the cell skeleton to crystalization and the osmotic effects of cryopreservation. The use of cryoprotectant such as DMSO and 1,2-propanediol (PROH) with sucrose decreases the seeding temperature of the medium of 5 to 7°C and dehydrates the cells, reducing the deleterious effects of freezing. Techniques such as vitrification with very rapid freezing are under investigation. Nevertheless, it is doubtful that mouse, rabbit, hamster, and primate oocytes can be cryopreserved by DMSO freezing and thawing protocols.[25–29]

In most of these reports the viability and fertilizing potential after freezing were rather encouraging. In contrast to embryo freezing, however, no satisfactory answer has been given as to whether genetic consequences would occur after low-temperature conservation of oocytes. One group reported that the number of polyploid embryos derived after freezing oocytes was twice that of a control group.[29]

CRYOPRESERVATION OF HUMAN SPERMATOZOA

Technical Procedures
Since the first human pregnancy reported after insemination with cryopreserved sperm,[5] many different methods have been used to freeze human semen. Variations may concern the nature of the cryoprotective agent, the dilution medium, the temperature of CPA added to the semen, the semen container, the cooling, freezing, and thawing rates, and the storage temperature.

Technical procedures have been progressively improved in a pragmatic way. In most cases, they were not evaluated by studying the fertilization rate of cryopreserved sample, but by establishing the recovery or cryosurvival rate, which is the ratio of the percentage of motile sperm observed after thawing to the percentage of motile sperm in fresh semen × 100. The choice of technique may be a function of cryopreservation activity of a given center. A sperm bank that freezes many samples every day could use sophisticated methods, while a small center would employ more simple and inexpensive procedures.

Glycerol is the CPA most commonly used. It has a better cryoprotective effect than DMSO or ethylene glycol.[30,31] A final concentration of 6 to 8% glycerol gives the best postthaw motility and velocity of spermatozoa.[32] Although glycerol may be used alone, diluting it in a semen extender containing proteins and sugars seems to allow better recovery of postthaw motility[33,34] and should be recommended. Many different media have been described, most of them containing egg yolk, sucrose or glucose, citrate, glycine, and antibiotics.[30,35] A comparative study found that the best recovery rate of sperm motility was obtained with the following buffer: 48% Tetris, 30% citrate, 20% egg yolk, and 2% fructose.[33]

Usually, the semen is diluted 1:1 in the extender containing the CPA and incubated 15 minutes at room temperature. The temperature of this incubation step does not influence the recovery rate.[30] All kind of containers have been used to freeze human semen, such as ampules, syringes, pellets, and 0.5-mL or 0.25-mL plastic straws. The recovery rates of 0.5 and 0.25-mL straws are not significantly different.[36] We prefer the latter because they can store a much higher number of doses from a single ejaculate and therefore allow more inseminations.

The first pregnancies recorded were obtained with semen frozen in dry ice ($-80°C$).[5] The use of liquid nitrogen ($-196°C$) was proposed by Sherman,[37] and the first pregnancies after this deep-freezing procedure were recorded in 1964.[6] Liquid nitrogen is now widely available and used, at least in developed countries. At first, freezing was done by suspending the semen sample in the vapor of liquid nitrogen at approximately $-60°C$. Subsequently, investigators preferred to control the cooling and freezing temperatures more strictly.[31] Computerized automatic freezers are easily available. Generally, a slow cooling rate of 0.5 to 2°C/minute is used from room temperature to 4 or 5°C, and then a faster freezing rate of 3 to 5 or 10°C/minutes until reaching $-80°C$, when the semen is plunged into liquid nitrogen.[31,38,39] Incorporating a holding temperature at $-5°C$ for 10 minutes with seeding could improve postthaw sperm motility and the ability to penetrate zona-free hamster oocytes.[40] Thawing is done by bringing the semen to room temperature or to 37°C for 10 to 15 minutes before insemination.

Influence of Cryopreservation on Sperm Function
Whatever the CPA and the technique, the most important and spectacular effect of freezing on sperm is loss of motility.[30,32,33,40] It is mainly due to the cold shock, but dilution in cryoprotective medium before freezing is also partly responsible.[41] The mean motility recovery rate is between 60 and 70% according to most studies, but can be very different from one sample to another, depending on initial sperm concentration, motility, and morphology.[35] In a study of 15,364 insemination cycles with frozen semen, the most predictive variable of the conception rate was postthaw motility[42] (Fig. 37-2).

The main cellular alterations responsible for the

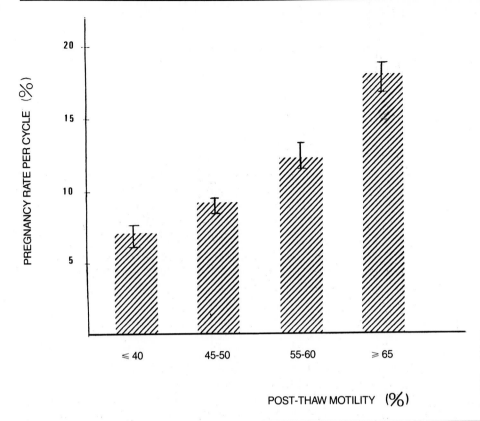

Figure 37–2. The influence of spermatozoa postthaw motility on pregnancy rate. These results were obtained from a program of artificial insemination with 1,438 donor ejaculates. (From Mayaux et al.[42] Reproduced with permission.)

loss of motility do not seem to be at the axonemal level; it is possible to restore normal movement of demembranated bull spermatozoa after freezing and thawing.[43] Loss of motility is more probably related to plasma membrane damage, which has been described in electron microscopic studies.[44-48] Important modifications of the acrosomal structure are also frequently observed, but frozen sperms' ability to penetrate zona-free hamster oocytes is not altered over that of fresh spermatozoa.[40,48] The mechanisms of sperm membrane cryoinjury are not well understood. It has been suggested that hyperproduction of superoxide radicals may be responsible.[49,50] The demonstration of a beneficial effect of adding dithiothreitol to the cryoprotective medium on sperm motility and viability recovery rate after freezing supports this hypothesis.[51]

There is no evidence of genetic alteration of spermatozoa by freezing, and the risks of abortion or malformation are not higher with frozen than fresh sperm.[52-54]

Clinical Use of Cryopreserved Semen

In cattle breeding, the use of frozen sperm allows genetic control of reproduction. Such possibilities were advocated by some of the pioneers who used frozen semen in humans. In 1964, one of them was

predicting a "genetic improvement through germinal choice to achieve human betterment of mind and body."[54] Fortunately, such strange, controversial, and unrealistic views were not adopted, and the clinical developments of human semen banking have been mainly limited to preserving fertility of men undergoing voluntary sterilization or treatment of malignancy, and TID in cases of infertility.

Semen Autopreservation. Semen autopreservation may be considered when a man is to be sterilized either intentionally, as in the case of vasectomy, or as a consequence of treatment, mainly chemotherapy and radiotherapy.

Accompanying the development of vasectomy in the United States, commercial banks were established in the 1960s. After that, controversy arose as to the efficiency of this procedure to restore fertility compared to vasovasostomy. Unfortunately, no clear data are available in the literature on these subjects. In France, about 500 men every year store their semen prior to vasectomy in the various CECOS banks. The sperm is stored only if the freezing test made on each ejaculate is positive; that is, if more than 2×10^6 spermatozoa/0.25-mL straw have progressive motility after thawing. The test is positive in only 70% of men, although most of them are fertile when they request a vasectomy.[55] As a rule, 50 straws are stored for each

TABLE 37–1. OVERVIEW OF THE USE OF SEMEN AUTOPRESERVED BY FREEZING (VASECTOMY EXCLUDED)

Reference	Period Under Study	Total Number of Men	Number of Men Using Their Semen	Number of Pregnancies
63	1969–1979	183	16	0
64	1973–1978	113	15	4
65	1975–1984	24	4	1
62	1976–1984	ND	22	8

man, and usually 2 or 3 ejaculates are sufficient to supply this stock.[55]

In the French experience, a little more than 1% of vasectomized men use their frozen semen. This low figure may be explained by the fact that most vasectomies were performed for stable couples with children. If the number of men who use their semen after vasectomy is so small, and "if the storage of first semen does not guarantee future fertility,"[56] one can wonder if it is necessary to store semen before a vasectomy. The CECOS experience shows that even if frozen semen should not be considered as fertility insurance, the delay together with various contacts with the medical team, caused by the need to collect several ejaculates before surgery, may be a significant help by giving men time to think about and discuss their options, and thus strengthen their decision on whether or not to undergo vasectomy. Having a "fertility potential" may also have some psychologic benefit even if men never use their stored semen.[57]

In the year after chemotherapy, the frequency of azoospermia varies from 14% for men with testicular tumors to 79% for those with Hodgkin's disease.[58] Semen freezing may offer the ability to preserve the fertility potential of young men with malignant disease. Unfortunately, semen quality is often altered in such men, and the minimum number of motile spermatozoa in a thawed straw estimated necessary to result in pregnancy is obtained in only a minority.[59,60] No pregnancy could be obtained with autopreserved semen when sperm concentration was under 40[59,61] or 55%[58] of the initial ejaculate. In the CECOS of Paris-Bicetre, the freezing test found more than 2×10^6 motile spermatozoa/thawed straw in 40% of men with Hodgkin's disease ($n = 580$) and 16% of men with testicular tumor ($n = 560$).[58] The

very low number of pregnancies obtained with frozen sperm of such patients (Table 37–1) may be explained by this poor quality. This was well demonstrated by Czyglik, who did not observe a pregnancy when less than 0.5×10^6 spermatozoa/straw were motile after thawing. On the other hand, pregnancy rates were identical to those observed in TID when the straw contained more than 2×10^6 motile spermatozoa after thawing (Table 37–2).

There is a clear need to improve semen autopreservation. At the CECOS Paris-Bicetre, 13% of the men whose semen was successfully frozen used it afterward, and 40% declared that they would have used it if necessary. New techniques must be developed to allow better cryopreservation of sperms' fertilizing ability. In addition, in-vitro fertilization (IVF) might facilitate fertilization and normal fetal development with thawed semen of poor quality.

A final question regarding autopreservation is the influence of long-term storage on sperms' fertilizing ability.[62–64] In 1973, a significant decline was reported in the motility of sperm thawed after 3 years in storage.[65] This result was not confirmed by others, who found that motility remained remarkably stable in sperm cryopreserved for more than 10 years.[66] Several men with cancer became fathers after their wives were inseminated with semen stored for more than 10 years.

Use of Frozen Donor Semen in TID. Therapeutic insemination with donor semen is widely used to help infertile couples have children. Since several studies have shown higher pregnancy rates with fresh semen, however, the use of cryopreserved semen has been increasing rather slowly. In a survey made in 1979, only 12.7% of physicians who were

TABLE 37–2. PREGNANCY RATES PER INSEMINATION CYCLE ACCORDING TO THE QUALITY OF THAWED SEMEN PRESERVED BEFORE CHEMOTHERAPY OR RADIOTHERAPY

	Number of Motile Spermatozoa/Thawed Straw(10^6)			
	<0.5	0.5–2	>2	Control*
Pregnancy rate (%)	0	3	11	10.4
Number of cycles	106	159	267	5022

*Control values are the result of a TID program.
Source: From reference 59. Reproduced with permission.

practicing TID in the United States used frozen semen.[67] A survey done in 1987 by the Office of Technology Assessment (OTA) of the U.S. Congress revealed that frozen semen was used by 78% of physicians.[68]

In France, since the early 1980s the nationwide CECOS network located in university hospitals receives about 3,000 requests for TID every year, representing about 90% of these procedures.[69] The French experience clearly demonstrates the advantages of using frozen semen: better organization of semen collection and screening of donors; disassociation of semen collection and TID to preserve donors' anonymity; the possibility of storing and transporting semen, thus allowing several inseminations to be performed per cycle, or permitting a couple to conceive several children from the same donor; greater choice of phenotype characteristics; and better medical control of donor screening in specialized centers, and better knowledge of the results.

From this last point of view, the results of the last OTA survey are informative. In 1986 the American Fertility Society recommended genetic screening of potential donors,[70] but in 1987 less than half of American physicians did this, and did it inefficiently in many cases.[68] Genetic screening is not always easy, however. Of 676 potential fertile donors interviewed by a geneticist and karyotyped between 1973 and 1983 in the CECOS Paris-Bicetre, 2.6% were excluded for cytogenetic reason and 3.4% for genetic reasons.[71] It appears that much of the difficulty lies in the subjectivity of the decision to reject donors.[71] These authors conclude that donors should be classified into three categories:

1. Those rejected because of a genetic risk regarded as being too high.
2. Those accepted without any particular conditions, whose semen can be used for every recipient.
3. Those accepted under certain condition because of a moderate genetic risk factor, whose semen can only be used for recipients without the same risk factor.

Of course such a policy could be set up in all cases, but it is easier to apply when the geneticist and a center using frozen semen collaborate closely.[71]

One main advantage of cryopreservation is that it offers the maximum guarantee of avoiding the transmission of sexual diseases. Of course, semen donors may be screened for medical history of sexually transmitted disease (STD) and bacteriologic tests may be performed on the sample used, but a complete evaluation cannot be done on the day of donation.[72] Furthermore, it is well known that seropositivity for the human immune virus (HIV) antibody may be delayed.[73] Therefore it is necessary to establish a quarantine between the collection and use of donated semen. According to the recommendations of the Food and Drug Administration and the Centers for Disease Control, this quarantine should be for 6 months.[74] The American Fertility Society modified its guidelines accordingly,[75] and the CECOS network is following the same practice. Donors must be screened for risk factors for HIV infection, with a blood sample taken at the time of semen collection and 6 months after. The semen can be used only if both samples are negative for HIV antibodies.[76]

If the primary purpose of a fertility clinic is to establish safe pregnancy,[74] only frozen semen should be used as long as simple and rapid tests are not available to detect STD on fresh samples. To establish pregnancy as quickly as possible, it is important to recruit large numbers of donors in order to use the semen having the best potential fertilizing ability, to improve cryotechnology to reduce alterations in spermatozoa induced by freezing, or both.

CRYOPRESERVATION OF HUMAN EMBRYOS

Embryo Survival After Thawing

The stage at which human embryos should be frozen to obtain optimal results is controversial; recommendations have included blastocyst,[77] 8-cell stage,[78] and pronucleate egg[12] using glycerol, DMSO, and PROH, respectively. In the experience of one group, no differences were found between DMSO and PROH (Table 37-3).

Embryo survival was correlated with morphologic features.[79] Optimum success was obtained by

TABLE 37-3. PREGNANCIES AFTER REPLACEMENT OF FROZEN-THAWED EMBRYOS

Freezing Procedure	Pregnancies					
	No./Transfer	%	No./Embryo			
			Replaced	%	Thawed	%
PROH	16/132	12.1	16/153	9.9	16/461	3.5
DMSO	25/204	12.3	25/281	8.9	25/759	3.3
Totals	41/336	12.2	41/443	9.3	41/1220	3.4

Outcome of 41 pregnancies: 19 healthy children born, including 7 children from the donation program; 15 continuing; 7 (early) abortions.
Source: From reference 85. Reproduced with permission.

TABLE 37–4. INFLUENCE OF LENGTH OF STORAGE OF CRYOPRESERVED EMBRYOS ON PREGNANCY RATE

Length of Cryostorage (months)	No. of Thawed Embryos	Transferred Embryos (% of thawed embryos)		Thawing Cycles	Pregnancies (% thawing cycles)	
<3	341	239	(70.1)	245	31	(12.6)
4–6	185	137	(74.1)	109	13	(11.9)
7–12	72	48	(66.7)	41	4	(9.8)
13–24	19	16	(84.2)	12	2	(16.7)
Totals	617	440	(71.3)	387	50	(12.9)

Source: From reference 84. Reproduced with permission.

selecting 1-cell embryos or 2 and 4-cell embryos with a favorable appearance.[80] Differences in ability to implant were not found between intact and nonintact embryos. Pregnancy was reported even if less than half of the cells were intact after thawing.[81]

The follicular response of the embryo recipient also influences success. Cleaving embryos had a higher chance of survival and implantation in women with 4 to 7 follicles.[82]

Stimulation treatment in the IVF cycle may result in embryos' resistance to cryopreservation or their ability to develop. Pregnancy rates tended to be higher for cryopreserved embryos in women who did not receive agonist therapy than in those who did.[82] The pregnancy rate per frozen embryo did not decrease with increased length of storage[83] (Table 37–4).

Survey of Cryopreservation of Human Embryos

A survey was conducted on human embryo and oocyte cryopreservation up to December 1986. The results, presented at the fifth world congress on IVF, summarized the experience of 24 centers.[84] As indicated in Table 37–5, about half of the 3,577 frozen and thawed embryos were judged suitable for transfer. They had a 4.6% chance to implant. A pregnancy rate of 13.4% per replacement was achieved. The abortion rate (26.4%) was similar to that in IVF and gamete intrafallopian transfer (GIFT).

TABLE 37–5. SURVEY OF RESULTS OF HUMAN EMBRYO CRYOPRESERVATION

Result	Number
Embryos frozen and thawed	3577
Embryos replaced	1794
Transfers	1219
Pregnancies	163
Abortions	43
Births or continuing pregnancies	123

Source: From reference 85. Reproduced with permission.

Clinical Importance of These Techniques

There is a positive correlation between the pregnancy rate per transfer and the number of embryos transferred. The pregnancy rate varies from 18% when only 1 embryo is transferred to approximately 30% for 3 embryos.[85] Multiple pregnancies occur with a frequency of 2% in natural cycles, but reach 20% after replacement of 2 or more embryos in IVF cycles.[86]

The perinatal mortality for multiple pregnancies is around 10 times greater than for singleton gestations. Therefore, it is recommended that the number of fresh embryos replaced in the course of the IVF cycles (3 to 4) be reduced to avoid the disadvantage of multiple pregnancies. The remaining (supernumerary) embryos are cryopreserved for later use. Even so, in GIFT, the number of oocytes replaced should be limited to 3 or 4. The remaining oocytes can be inseminated, and if they fertilize and cleave normally, they can be cryopreserved.

Freezing may be justified as a means to meet a couple's short-term procreative goal. It may be acceptable to the extent that it allows either the transplantation of embryos during the woman's subsequent cycle, or successive transplantations in the case of failure, without the necessity for further surgical interventions and without destroying the embryos not immediately transplanted. It has also been proposed that all the embryos obtained should be frozen and in this way possibly avoid their replacement in hyperstimulated cycles, which could adversely affect implantation. For a given number of embryos, however, there was no significant difference in pregnancy rates when they were all immediately transferred or when they were frozen and replaced successively.[87] Only the multiple pregnancy rate varies in these different circumstances.

Transfers can be carried out either in spontaneous cycles or in highly stimulated cycles in anovulatory patients (Fig. 37–3). Substitutive hormonal therapy after desensitization by a gonadotropin-releasing hormone (GnRH) agonist has been proposed.[88] Exact embryo–endometrium synchrony seems to give the best results in terms of pregnancy per transfer.

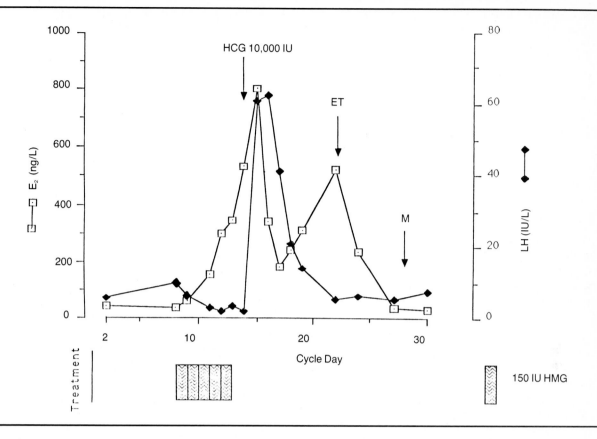

Figure 37–3. Concentrations of estradiol-17β and luteinizing hormone (LH) during the transfer cycle of a cryopre-served blastocyst. The patient received human menopausal gonadotropin (HMG), 150 IU daily, from day 8 to day 12 of the cycle. On day 14 ovulation was induced by the administration of 10,000 IU human chorionic gonadotropin (HCG). The frozen and thawed blastocyst was replaced on day 22. No pregnancy occurred.

Transfer takes place between 0 and 3 hours after thawing, except for pronucleate eggs, which are cultured for 1 day after thawing (Fig. 37–4).

The perinatal outcome of 50 pregnancies resulting from the transfer of human embryos that had been cryopreserved for up to 2 years was reported.[83] Early pregnancy losses after the use of these embryos did not appear different from those in IVF pregnancies transferring fresh embryos. One major fetal abnormality was recorded. Thirty-one healthy babies were born from 28 pregnancies, and a further 7 pregnancies are in progress. The caesarian section rate for these deliveries was only slightly higher than that in the general population.

The Fate of Supernumerary Cryopreserved Embryos

The de facto existence of extra embryos raises the ethical problems of their possible conservation by freezing, their donation to another patient, and their destruction without invasive examination.[89]

The donation of embryos from one couple to another is already possible, but although the technical aspects of these manipulations are relatively straightforward, the ethical dimensions are more complicated. The donation of frozen embryos, however, should not be regarded any differently from the donation of fresh embryos, such as is performed using uterine lavage procedures. Frozen embryos would most probably be donated when several embryos are obtained in an IVF cycle, and pregnancy, especially multiple gestations, results from the transfer of the fresh embryos. Such a couple might then donate their frozen embryos to a less fortunate couple.

OOCYTE FREEZING

Oocyte freezing is clearly useful from a practical standpoint, similar to that outlined above for embryo freezing. Furthermore, in some countries it might be more acceptable on ethical grounds than freezing and thawing embryos. It also would be beneficial to young women at risk to lose ovarian function due to chemotherapy, surgery, or certain pelvic diseases. This would be analogous to semen banks for men who are at risk to lose their reproductive function; when techniques of oocyte freezing become reliable, egg banks could offer similar alternatives.

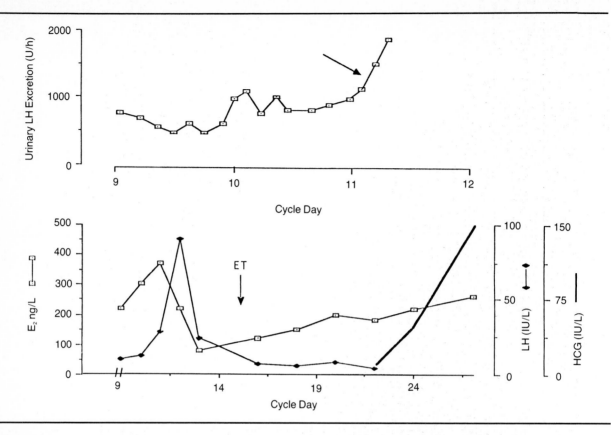

Figure 37–4. Urinary and serum endocrine profiles during the transfer cycle of a cryopreserved embryo. **Top.** The urinary concentration (U/hr) as determined by 3-hour urine correction. The level of LH starts to rise on day 11 of the cycle (arrow). **Bottom.** Serum levels of estradiol-17β, LH, and HCG in the periovulatory period and luteal phase. On day 15 of the cycle an 8-cell, frozen–thawed embryo was transferred; 9 days later the serum HCG level became positive.

Two centers reported detailed clinical results of human oocyte freezing. After freezing 228 oocytes, 70 were judged suitable for embryo replacement.[13,14] At the time of the survey, 33 transfers resulted in 4 pregnancies; 2 aborted and 3 resulted in healthy children, including one set of twins.

The success rate of IVF diminishes significantly with the use of thawed compared to fresh oocytes.[90] This may be due to cytoskeletal damage, especially at the spindle level, as demonstrated in several species.

Oocyte or embryo donation can alleviate the infertility of patients without ovarian function due to ovarian dysgenesis, premature menopause, or surgical castration. These women require steroid substitution therapy with estradiol valerate and progesterone to make their endometrium receptive.[91–94] Oocyte donation can also be indicated in patients with functional ovaries who have repeated ovarian stimulation failures, failed fertilizations in the course of several IVF cycles, the presence of genetic risk factor, or a medical contraindication to undergoing oocyte retrieval.

Oocytes and embryos can be donated by volunteers, patients undergoing laparoscopic sterilization, and women who are willing to donate their excess oocytes and embryos after IVF. A major difficulty in a donation program consists in the synchrony between the ovarian cycles of donor and recipient. If this synchrony is not present at the time donated material is available, the embryo can be cryopreserved to be replaced at an appropriate time in the course of a subsequent cycle[95,96] (Fig. 37–5). The availability of an adequate embryo cryopreservation program will increase the chance of establishing a donor program (Table 37–6).

ETHICAL CONSIDERATIONS

Cryopreservation, whatever its uses may be, results in a period of timelessness in the genesis of life. It may bring out the "reification" of the embryo in vitro and the risks of disassociation among gamete production, fertilization, and pregnancy. It may lead to the creation of stocks of gametes and embryos to be used by the person(s) from whom they issued or by others in order to help them have children. The introduction of a break in the normal timing or of a foreign procreator in the reproductive process, and the possibility for society (through medical and scientific

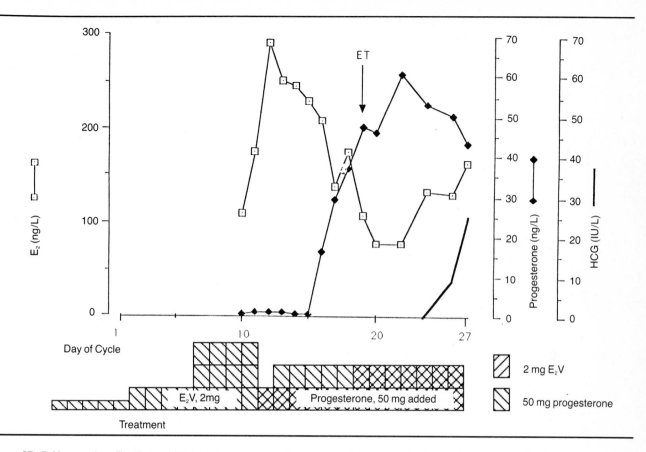

Figure 37–5. Hormonal profile of an artificial cycle substituted with oral estradiol valerate (E₂V) and intramuscular natural progesterone from a patient with primary ovarian failure. A 4-cell, frozen-thawed embryo was replaced on day 17 of the substituted cycle (arrow). The patient became pregnant 8 days after the transfer.

technology) to control it, are strongly disturbing the classic concepts of morality and social organization of the family.

Many countries and international organizations, and philosophical, political, religious, and professional authorities, have stated recommendations or enacted laws on cryopreservation.[97-99] The procedure should be carried out only in approved centers, giving all technical and scientific guarantees, and

TABLE 37–6. PREGNANCIES AFTER OOCYTE AND EMBRYO DONATION

Replacement	Number of Pregnancies/ Number of Transfers	
	Primary Ovarian Failure	Functional Ovaries
Fresh oocytes/embryos		
Intrauterine	7/30	6/25
GIFT*	1/20	—
ZIFT†	3/8	0/1
Cryopreserved embryos	4/23	5/17

*GIFT = Gamete intrafallopian transfer.
†ZIFT = zygote intrafallopian transfer.
Summarized at the Center for Reproductive Medicine at the Vrije Universiteit, Brussels.

considered to be fully capable to inform and assist couples who apply. These centers, which should operate without commercialization, must respect the principles that regulate procreation in-vitro in their country.

The ethical questions raised by cryopreservation of spermatozoa and oocytes are similar. When either is frozen to preserve a fertility potential of a given person, the only questions are who is allowed to use the gamete and when? The simplest and more logical answer is that the person who produced the cell is the only one able to decide its use, and that should be, of course, to procreate. This would deny the use of cryopreserved gametes after the death of the donor— for example, if the remaining partner wanted to have the child of the deceased individual. To permit this would change the purpose of cryopreservation, which was to preserve the fertility potential of the donor. As a rule, respect for the dignity of this person would allow him or her the right to decide on the use of the gametes, and of course, this can be done only if the person is alive. Thus the question arises as to whether gametes should be cryopreserved only for people facing possible sterility or for anybody who would like to procreate at any time.

When gametes are cryopreserved for donation,

fewer specific issues arise. It could be stressed that because freezing offers the best condition for detailed screening of donors and for matching donors and recipients most precisely, all programs of gamete donation should only use frozen specimens.

Embryo cryopreservation raises different questions because it concerns a unique entity able to develop into a human being. Human embryos should not be frozen independent of the desire for parenthood. The technique should be considered only as an extension of IVF for infertile couples. It is not freezing for convenience, but rather part of the infertility treatment.

According to the French National Ethical Committee, embryos may be cryopreserved only for a limited period of time and related to the immediate project of having a child, and not as part of an indeterminate parenthood program. This time limit should be no more than 1 year except for medical reasons. In the experience of the Clamart and Brussels groups, the great majority of patients ask for transfer of the remaining frozen embryos in the 6 months after unsuccessful transfer of a fresh one. This assures that freezing is only a prolongation of IVF.

During the limited period of preservation, frozen embryos belong to the genitor couple. The couple may request to have the embryos transferred in a later cycle, to destroy them with or without allowing them to be subjected to scientific research, or to donate them to another infertile couple. Problems arise when the time limit is exceeded and the embryos have not been reclaimed.

After the birth of a child and if the couple still has stored embryos, the question arises as to whether it is acceptable to transfer the embryos to attempt a second pregnancy. The idea of a stock of embryos subjected to the hazards of parental desire must be rejected. Our clinical experience indicates that after the first pregnancy, most patients desire a second baby. In Clamart, however, 9 problems arose among 150 couples. These occurred when the couple abandoned the project, or when a second pregnancy was unfeasable, for example, because of separation, illness, or death of one or both partners. In such cases should the embryos be destroyed when both genitors cannot agree on donation?

We think that gamete and embryo freezing are intended to help sterile people have children. Several principles should guide our thinking. One of the most important is that human gametes and embryos are the products of the human body and cannot be commercialized. Cryopreservation will lead to the birth of many children and, as is the case for atomic energy, this gametic energy must be regulated to avoid catastrophes. Society must define the rules; however, the medical community is not merely a technician, but is concerned with the conception and progress of humanity. As such, medical scientists and clinicians must offer society guidelines based on their experience and on their projections, however inchoate, of future capabilities.

REFERENCES

1. Spallanzani L: Opuscoli di fisca spermamtici, animale e vegatabile, opuscule II. Osservaziioni, a Sperienze intorno ai Vermicelli dell'Uomo et degli animali. Modena, Italy, 1776.
2. Mantegazza J: Fisiologia sullo sperma umano. Rendic Reale Instit Lomb 3:183, 1866.
3. Rostand J: Cole R Acad Sci Paris, 222:1534, 1946.
4. Polge G, Smith AU, Parkes AS: Revival of spermatozoa after vitrification and dehydration at low temperature. Nature 164:664, 1949.
5. Bunge RG, Sherman JK: Fertilizing capacity of frozen human spermatozoa. Nature 172:767, 1953.
6. Perloff WH, Steinberger E, Sherman JK: Conception with human spermatozoa frozen by nitrogen vapor technique. Fertil Steril 15:501, 1964.
7. Wittingham DG: Survival of mouse embryos frozen to −196°C and −269°C. Nature 178:411, 1972.
8. Trounson A, Mohr L: Human pregnancy following cryopreservation, thawing and transfer of an eight-cell embryo. Nature 305:707, 1983.
9. Zeilmaker GH, Alberda AT, Van Gent I, Rijkmans CMPM, Drogendijk AC: Two pregnancies following transfer of intact frozen–thawed embryos. Fertil Steril 2:293, 1984.
10. Downing BG, Mohr LR, Trounson AD, Freeman LE, Wood C: Birth after transfer of cryopreserved embryos. Med J Aust 142:409, 1985.
11. Cohen J, Simon RF, Fehily CB, et al: Birth after replacement of hatching blastocyst cryopreserved at expanded blastocyst stage. Lancet 1:647, 1985.
12. Lassalle B, Testart J, Renard JP: Human embryo features that influence the success of cryopreservation with the use of 1,2-propanediol. Fertil Steril 44:645, 1985.
13. Chen C: Pregnancy after human oocyte cryopreservation. Lancet 1:884, 1986.
14. Al-Hasani A, Diedrich K, Van Der Ven H, et al: Cryopreservation of human oocytes. Hum Reprod 2:695, 1987.
15. Van Uem JFHM, Siebzehnrubl ER, Schuh B, et al: Birth after cryopreservation of unfertilized oocytes. Lancet 1:752, 1987.
16. McGrath JJ: Preservation of biological material by freezing and thawing, in Shitzer H, Eberhart C (eds): Heat Transfer in Medicine and Biology. New York, Plenum, 1985, pp 185–238.
17. Renard JP, De Rochambeau H, Lauverq JJ: Utilization of gamete and embryo banking for the preservation and study of genetic resources in farm animals. Proc V WCAP 1:66, 1983.
18. Nishikawa Y: Studies on the preservation of raw and frozen horse semen. J Reprod Fertil 23:99, 1975.
19. Paquignon M, Bussiere J, Bariteau F, Courot M: Effectiveness of boar semen under practical conditions of artificial insemination. Theriogenology 14:217, 1980.
20. Ciba Foundation Symposium 52. Amsterdam, Excerpta Medica, 1979.
21. Wittingham DG: Principles of embryo preservation, in Ashwood-Smith MJ, Farrant J (eds): Low Temperature Preservation in Medicine and Biology. Baltimore, University Park Press, 1980, pp 65–83.
22. Wittingham DG, Leibo SP, Mazur P: Survival of mouse embryos frozen to −196°C and −269°C. Science 178:411, 1972.
23. Renard JP, n'Guyen B-X, Garnier V: Two-step freezing of two-cell rabbit embryos after partial dehydration at room temperature. J Reprod Fertil 71:573, 1984.
24. Eaglesome MD, Mitchell D, Betteridge KJ, et al: Transfer of embryos from bovine leukaemia virus-infected cattle to uninfected recipients: preliminary results. Vet Rec 3(6):122, 1982.
25. Whittingham DG: Fertilization in vitro and development to term of unfertilized mouse oocytes previously stored at −196°C. J Reprod Fertil 49:89, 1977.
26. De Mayo FJ, Rawlins RG, Dukelow WR: Xenogenous and in vitro fertilization of frozen/thawed primate oocytes and blastomere separation of embryos. Fertil Steril 43:295, 1985.
27. Critser JK, Arneson BW, Aaker DV, Ball GD: Cryopreservation of

hamster oocytes: Effects of vitrification or freezing on human sperm penetration of zona-free hamster oocytes. *Fertil Steril* 46:277, 1986.

28. Al-Hasani S, Tolksdorf A, Diedrich K, Van Der Ven H, Drebs D: Successful in vitro fertilization of frozen-thawed rabbit oocytes. *Hum Reprod* 1:309, 1986.

29. Glenister PH, Wood MJ, Kirby C, Whittingham DG: Incidence of chromosome anomalies in first-cleavage mouse embryos obtained from frozen-thawed oocytes fertilized in vitro. *Gamete Res* 16:205, 1987.

30. Mahadevan M, Trounson AD: Effect of cryoprotective media and dilution methods on the preservation of human spermatozoa. *Andrologia* 15:355, 1983.

31. Serafini P, Marrs RP: Computerized staged-freezing technique improves sperm survival and preserves penetration of zona-free hamster ova. *Fertil Steril* 45:854, 1986.

32. Pilikian S, Czyba JC, Guerin JF: Effect of various concentrations of glycerol on post-thaw motility and velocity of human spermatozoa. *Cryobiology* 19:147, 1982.

33. Weidel L, Prins GS: Cryosurvival of human spermatozoa frozen in eight different buffer systems. *J Androl* 8:42, 1987.

34. Harrison RF, Shepard BL: A comparative study in methods of cryoprotection for human semen. *Cryobiology* 17:25, 1980.

35. David G, Czyglik F: Tolérance à la congélation du sperme humain en fonction de la qualité initiale du sperme. *J Gynecol Obstet Biol Reprod* 6:601, 1977.

36. Emperaire JC, Czyglik F: Semen freezing in 0.15 and 0.25-mL straws, in David G, Price WS (eds): *Human Artificial Insemination and Semen Preservation*. New York, Plenum, 1980, pp 161–166.

37. Sherman JK: Improved methods of preservation of human spermatozoa by freezing and freezing-drying. *Fertil Steril* 14:49, 1963.

38. Mahadevan M, Trounson AO: Effect of cooling, freezing and thawing rates and storage condition on preservation of human spermatozoa. *Andrologia* 16:52, 1984.

39. Thachil JV, Jewett MAS: Preservation techniques for human semen. *Fertil Steril* 35:546, 1981.

40. Critser JK, Husebenda AR, Aaker DW, Arneson BW, Ball GD: Cryopreservation of human spermatozoa. 1. Effect of holding procedure and seeding motility, fertilizing ability and acrosome reaction. *Fertil Steril* 47:656, 1987.

41. Serres C, Jouannet P, Czyglik F, David G: Effects of freezing on spermatozoa motility, in David G, Price WS (eds): *Human Artificial Insemination and Semen Preparation*. New York, Plenum, 1980, pp 147–160.

42. Mayaux MJ, Schwartz D, Czyglik, F, David G: Conception rate according to semen characteristic in a series of 15,364 insemination cycles: Result of a multivariate analysis. *Andrologia* 17:9, 1985.

43. Lindemann CB, Fisher M, Lipton M: A comparative study of the effects of freezing and frozen storage on intact and demembranated bull spermatozoa. *Cryobiology* 19:20, 1982.

44. Pedersen H, Lebech PE: Ultrastructural changes in human spermatozoa after freezing for artificial insemination. *Fertil Steril* 22:125, 1971.

45. Escalier D, Bisson JP: Quantitative ultrastructural modification in human spermatozoa after freezing, in David G, Price WS (eds): *Human Artificial Insemination and Semen Preservation*. New York, Plenum, 1980, pp 107–122.

46. Mahadevan MM, Trounson AO: Relationship of fine structure of sperm head to fertility of frozen human semen. *Fertil Steril* 41:287, 1984.

47. Heath E, Jeyendran RS, Perez-Pelaez M, Sobrero AJ: Ultrastructural categorization of human sperm cryopreserved in glycerol and in TESTCY. *Int J Androl* 8:101, 1985.

48. Serafini PC, Hauser D, Moyer D, Marrs RP: Cryopreservation of human spermatozoa: Correlation of ultrastructural sperm head configuration with sperm motility and ability to penetrate zona-free hamster ova. *Fertil Steril* 46:691, 1986.

49. Jones R, Mann T: Damage to ram spermatozoa by peroxidation on endogenous phospholipids. *J Reprod Fertil* 50:261, 1977.

50. Aitken RJ, Clarkson JS: Cellular basis of defective sperm function and its association with the genesis of reactive oxygen species by human spermatozoa. *J Reprod Fertil* 81:459, 1987.

51. Rao B, David D: Improved recovery of post thaw motility and vitality of human spermatozoa cryopreserved in the presence of dithiothreitol. *Cryobiology* 21:536, 1984.

52. Schwartz D, Mayaux MJ, Guichard-Moscato ML, Czyglik F, David G: Abortion rate in AID and semen characteristics: A study of 1345 pregnancies. *Andrologia* 18:292, 1986.

53. Federation CECOS, Matte JF, Le Marec B: Genetic aspects of artificial insemination by donor (AID). Indication, surveillance and results. *Clin Genet* 23:132, 1983.

54. Sherman JK: Research on frozen human semen. Past, present and future. *Fertil Steril* 15:486, 1964.

55. Jouannet P, Jardin A, Czyglik F, David G, Fourcade R: Conservation du sperme et vasectomie. *Seminaire d'Uronephrologie no 5*. Paris, Masson, 1979, pp 113–120.

56. Behrman SJ: The preservation of semen. *Fertil Steril* 24:396, 1973.

57. Delaisi de Parseval G, Jouannet P: Semen storage, delayed fatherhood and vasectomy, in *Psychosomatic Obstetrics and Gynaecology*. Leiden, Boerhaave Committee for Postgraduate Medical Education, 1985, pp 45–50.

58. Czyglik F: Prévention des sterilites introgenes par la congélation du sperme, in *33rd Assises Francaises de Gynecologie*. Paris, Masson, 1987, pp 265–276.

59. Sanger WG, Armitage JO, Schmidt MA: Feasibility of semen cryopreservation in patients with malignant disease. *JAMA* 244:789, 1980.

60. Bergman S, Howards S, Sanger W: Practical aspects of banking patients' semen for future artificial insemination. *Urology* 13:408, 1979.

61. Scammel GE, Stedronska J, Edmonds DK, et al: Cryopreservation of semen in men with testicular tumors of Hodgkin's disease: Results of artificial insemination of their partners. *Lancet* 2:31, 1985.

62. Friedman S, Broder S: Homologous artificial insemination after long-term semen cryopreservation. *Fertil Steril* 35:321, 1981.

63. Czyglik F, Auger J, Albert M, David G: L'autoconservation du sperme avant thérapeutique sterilisante. *Nouv Presse Med* 11:2749, 1982.

64. Rhodes EA, Hoffman DJ, Kaempfer SH: Ten years' experience with semen cryopreservation by cancer patients: Follow-up and clinical considerations. *Fertil Steril* 44:512, 1985.

65. Smith K, Steinberger E: Survival of spermatozoa in a human sperm bank. *JAMA* 223:774, 1973.

66. David G, Czyglik F: Apparent improvement in human semen after long-term storage, in Andre J (ed): *The Sperm Cell*. The Hague, Martinus Nijhoff, 1983, pp 29–32.

67. Currie Cohen M, Luttrell L, Shapiro S: Current practice of artificial insemination by donor in the United States. *N Engl J Med* 300:585, 1979.

68. Anonymous: *Artificial Insemination Practice in the U.S. Summary of a 1987 Survey*. OTA Brief. Washington, DC, 1988.

69. David G: Artificial insemination by donor (AID), in Steinberger E, Frajese G, Steinberger A (eds): *Reproductive Medicine*. New York, Raven, 1984, pp 319–326.

70. American Fertility Society. New guidelines for the use of semen donor insemination: 1986. *Fertil Steril* 46(suppl 2):95S, 1986.

71. Selva J, Leonard C, Albert M, Auger J, David G: Genetic screening for artificial insemination by donor (AID). *Clin Genet* 29:389, 1986.

72. Maslola L, Guinan ME: Screening to reduce transmission of sexually transmitted diseases in semen used for artificial insemination. *N Engl J Med* 314:1354, 1986.

73. Ranki, Krohn K: Long latency precedes over seroconversion in sexually transmitted human immunodeficiency virus infection. *Lancet* 2:589, 1987.

74. Centers for Disease Control: Semen banking, organ and tissue transplantation, and HIV antibody testing. *MMWR* 37:57, 1988.

75. American Fertility Society: Revised new guidelines for the use of semen donor insemination. *Fertil Steril* 49:211, 1988.

76. Ball GD: Acquired immune deficiency syndrome and the fertility clinic. *Fertil Steril* 45:172, 1988.

77. Cohen J, Simons FR, Edwards RG, Fehilly CB, Fishel SB: Pregnancies following the frozen storage of expanding human blastocysts. *J IVF/ET* 2:59, 1985.

78. Freeman L, Trounson A, Kirby C: Cryopreservation of human embryos progress on the clinical use of the technique in human in vitro fertilization. *J IVF/ET* 3:53, 1986.

79. Mandelbaum J, Junca AM, Plachot P, et al: Human embryo cryopreservation, extrinsic and intrinsic parameters of success. *Hum Reprod* 2:709, 1987.

80. Testart J, Lassalle B, Forman RG, et al: Factors influencing the success rate of human embryo freezing in an in vitro fertilization and embryo transfer program. *Fertil Steril* 48:107, 1987.

81. Veiga A, Calderon G, Barri PN, Corleu B: Pregnancy after the replacement of a frozen thawed embryo with <50% intact blastomeres. *Hum Reprod* 2:321, 1987.

82. Testart J, Volante M, Gazangel A, et al: Development and clinical application of embryo cryopreservation. *Hum Reprod* in press.

83. Frydman R, Forman RG, Belaisch-Allart J, et al: An obstetric analysis of

50 consecutive pregnancies after transfer of human cryopreserved embryos. *Am J Obstet Gynecol*, 160:209, 1989.

84. Van Steirteghem A, Van Den Abbeel E: Survey on cryopreservation. *Ann NY Acad Sci*, in press.

85. Edwards RG, Steptoe PC: Current status of in vitro fertilization and implantation of human embryos. *Lancet* 2:1265, 1973.

86. Frydman R, Belaisch-Allart J, Fries N, et al: An obstetric assessment of the first 100 births from in vitro fertilization. *Am J Obstet Gynecol* 154:550, 1986.

87. Frydman R, Forman RG, Belaisch-Allart J, Hazout A, Testart J: An assessment of alternative policies for embryo transfer in an IVF-ET program. *Fertil Steril* 50:466, 1988.

88. Frydman R, Bouchard P, Parneix I: Les agonistes de la LHRH ont-ils un role dans le cycle de transfert des embryons congelés. *Contrib Fertil Sexualite* 16:29, 1988.

89. Jouannet P: Reflexion à propos des problèmes ethiques soulevés par la congélation d'embryons humains. *Med Sci* 2:345, 1986.

90. Mandelbaum J, Junca AM, Plachot M, et al: Cryopreservation of human embryos and oocytes. *Hum Reprod* 3:117, 1988.

91. Lutjen P, Trounson A, Leeton J, et al: The establishment and maintenance of pregnancy using in vitro fertilization and embryo donation in a patient with primary ovarian failure. *Nature* 307:174, 1984.

92. Navot D, Laufer N, Kopolovic J, et al: Artifically induced endometrial cycles and establishment of pregnancies in the absence of ovaries. *N Engl J Med* 314:806, 1986.

93. Rosenwaks Z: Donor eggs: Their application in modern reproductive technologies. *Fertil Steril* 47:895, 1987.

94. Devroey P, Braeckmans P, Camus M, et al: Pregnancies after replacement of fresh and frozen-thawed embryos in a donation program, in Feichtinger W, Kemeter P (eds): *Future Aspects of Human In Vitro Fertilization*. Berlin, Springer-Verlag, 1987, p 133.

95. Van Steirteghem AC, Van Den Abbeel E, Braeckmans P, et al: Pregnancy with a frozen-thawed embryo in women with primary ovarian failure. *N Engl J. Med* 317:113, 1987.

96. Van Steirteghem AC, Van Den Abbeel E, Camus M, et al: Cryopreservation of human embryos obtained after gamete intrafallopian transfer and/or in vitro fertilization. *Hum Reprod* 2:309, 1987.

97. Warnock M: *Report of the Committee of Inquiry into Human Fertilization and Embryology*. London, Her Majesty's Stationary Office, 1984.

98. Avis du Comite National d'Ethique. La Fabrique du corps humain: avis de recherche sur l'embryon. *Acte Sud-INSERM*, 1987.

99. American Fertility Society Ethics Committee: The cryopreservation of eggs: Ethical consideration of the new reproductive technologies. *Fertil Steril* 46(suppl 1):51, 1986.

CHAPTER 38

Legal Aspects of Infertility

Lori B. Andrews, Ami S. Jaeger

Legal Aspects of Infertility

**Constitutional Dimensions of
    Procreation**
**Embryo Research and
    Development of Infertility
    Therapies**
Informed Consent
    Considerations for IVF
    Considerations for
        Cryopreservation
    Considerations for Embryo
        Donation
Single Parenthood

Physician Involvement
Quality Assurance
    Personnel Qualifications
    Screening
**Record-Keeping and
Confidentiality**
    Record-Keeping
    Confidentiality
Legal and Biologic Parentage
Payment to Third Parties
**The Law, Responsibility, and New
    Reproductive Therapies**

Medical practice involving the diagnosis and treatment of infertility is influenced by a variety of factors, ranging from community attitudes to the personal moral judgments of the patients and the health care professionals involved. Not the least of the factors affecting medical efforts to overcome infertility is the law. Statutes, regulations, judicial decisions, and constitutional protection of the right to privacy to make procreative decisions can profoundly influence which infertility services are offered, and in what manner. The law in some cases shapes the standards by which health care professionals must practice; in other instances, it influences the rights and responsibilities of the infertile couple and of society with respect to the resulting child.

CONSTITUTIONAL DIMENSIONS
OF PROCREATION

There is a strong moral and legal basis in our society for protection of autonomy in reproductive decisions. Decisions about whether or when to have children are thought to be a matter of personal private concern, not a subject of governmental mandate. Such decisions are protected by the U.S. Constitution under the right to privacy.

The constitutional protection of reproductive decisions was addressed by the U.S. Supreme Court as early as 1942 in *Skinner v. Oklahoma*,[1] which struck down an Oklahoma statute authorizing the sterilization of habitual criminals convicted of crimes involving moral turpitude. The court stated, "[W]e are dealing with legislation which involves one of the basic civil rights of man. Marriage and procreation are fundamental to the very existence and survival of the race."[2]

In a later series of cases involving contraception and abortion, the Supreme Court delineated how an individual's decision about whether or not to bear or beget a child was constitutionally protected from governmental interferences.[3] The court has deemed childbearing and childrearing rights as "far more precious than property rights."[4] The court wrote, "[I]f the right of privacy means anything it is the right of the individual, married or single, to be free of unwarranted governmental intrusion into matters so fundamentally affecting a person as the decision whether to bear or beget a child."[5] For a governmental regulation that infringes on reproductive decisions to be upheld as constitutional, it must be necessary to further a compelling state interest, and it must regulate in the least restrictive manner possible.[6]

In reality, it is hard to imagine a state interest strong enough to justify a law prohibiting a person from choosing to become a parent. "The decision ranks in importance with any other a person may make in a lifetime; an attempt to imagine state interests that would justify governmental intrusions amounting to a practical prohibition on procreation and childbearing takes us out of our experience and into an imaginary world of Malthusian nightmare."[7] Various commentators and legislators have set forth particular state interests that they argue would justify regulating alternative reproduction. These include the fetus's interest in being free from pain; the potential child's interest in being physically and mentally healthy; the adult participant's interest in being free from undue physical and psychologic risk; the individual's interest in making decisions about his or her own body; the individual's and couple's interest in reproductive and parental autonomy; the donor's and surrogate's interest in being free from manipulation by other people; doctors' and researchers' interests in meeting their professional obligations to help patients and to further scientific knowledge; and society's interests in retaining values and maintaining institutions such as the family.[8]

The constitutional right to privacy protects the decision to reproduce coitally because of biologic and social importance of being a parent.[9] The rationales for reproductive autonomy similarly extend to decisions to reproduce noncoitally.[10] The New Jersey Supreme Court in the landmark Baby M case, dealing with a child conceived by artificial insemination of a surrogate mother, noted that alternative reproduction methods fall within the constitutional right of privacy.[11]

This right serves as the backdrop against which government actions (such as the adoption of state or federal laws) must be measured. It is a basis on which health care professionals and patients can challenge legislation that prohibits or otherwise restricts research or clinical practice in the area of medically assisted reproduction. It also provides the framework that guides the actions and decisions of individuals who use new technologies and of practitioners who provide them. For example, proposed state laws banning surrogate parenting are not the least restrictive means of regulating surrogate parenting and so may be declared unconstitutional. Similarly, total prohibition of embryo transfer under existing embryo research bans would probably be invalid as an unconstitutional interference with the fundamental right to procreate.[12]

EMBRYO RESEARCH AND DEVELOPMENT OF INFERTILITY THERAPIES

In-vitro fertilization (IVF) is the keystone of new reproductive technologies. It is a major therapy for infertility and it makes other reproductive innovations (such as surrogate gestational motherhood) possible. The development of IVF became a reality through research with embryos. Improved IVF pregnancy rates and the development of other infertility treatments will occur as such research continues. Yet the permissibility of undertaking such investigations is guided by state and federal laws (known as "fetal research laws") that govern research with conceptuses.

Used in the broadest sense, "fetal research" includes any untested or unproved procedure involving embryos or fetuses. According to the medical definition, "A human embryo becomes a fetus at about the end of the eighth week of fertilization."[13] In contrast, statutory language generally defines a fetus as any product of conception, which means the fertilized egg, zygote, morula, blastocyst, embryo, and fetus. Thus, many statutes that regulate fetal research would apply equally to what a physician would categorize as embryo research.

Just as the statutes cover a broad developmental range of fetuses, they cover a broad range of activities affecting not only basic research but the introduction of reproductive technologies into the clinical setting. With their advent, these technologies opened a vast range of therapies for infertility. They also opened up a window of opportunity for research on the embryo.[14] Extracorporeal embryos provide an opportunity for observation and discovery of disease or developmental processes that have no clinical application in the treatment of infertility. For example, embryo research could be important "for developing or testing contraceptives, studying early forms of malignant cancer, providing an in vitro screening system for teratogens, studying the mechanisms by which chromosomal abnormalities are produced, understanding normal and abnormal cell growth and differentiation."[15] Embryo research could also lead to better understanding of genetic disease, genetic screening, and gene therapy.[16] What should be the source of embryos to be used in research? Should only those spare ones created in the attempts to treat infertility be used, or should some be created specifically? Society must balance the potential scientific and social gains from such investigations with the ethical and moral value in protecting the embryo as the symbolic potential of human life. Statutory enactments have attempted to formulate a regulatory framework for these ethical issues.[17]

As of late 1988, states have laws specifically aimed at regulating fetal research.[18] Of these 25 laws, 24 impose some restriction on experimentation with live fetuses ex utero,[19] 6 prohibit or impose sanctions aimed at prohibiting any type of research on a live fetus,[20] and 12 prohibit nontherapeutic research on live fetuses.[21] The Louisiana statute prohibits an IVF embryo from being "farmed or cultured solely for research purposes or any other purposes."[22]

Some of these statutes were originally enacted as sections of an abortion statute. For example, of the 25 fetal research statutes, 12 apply to research performed on fetuses or embryos that are product of an abortion.[23] This distinction becomes important as reproductive technologies are introduced into the clinical setting. For example, if embryo lavage is considered to be an abortion, these statutes could regulate in-vivo fertilization followed by embryo transfer.

By performing new techniques, physicians begin to bridge the gap between research and accepted clinical procedures. Some commentators argue that IVF, despite a decade of clinical application, is experimental because its long-term medical, psychologic, and social effects have not been determined.[24] A more common viewpoint is that IVF is now an accepted clinical practice rather than an experimental technology. Some of the more recently applied adjuncts to IVF—such as embryo cryopreservation, donation of embryos, and in-vivo fertilization followed by embryo transfer—are sufficiently novel and untested to be considered research, however.

Clinicians' involvement with embryos is distinguishable from that of researchers who do not intend to transfer the embryo to a uterus, and whose inquiries go beyond the treatment of infertility. The former usually perform transfers to initiate pregnancy, and so safety to the potential offspring should be a major concern to them.[25]

Merely because physicians use a research procedure to treat infertility, however, does not exempt them from federal and state regulations on fetal research. Federal regulations cover the conceptus starting with implantation[26]; thus they would not address techniques such as IVF or in-vivo fertilization followed by embryo transfer. An additional set of regulations, however, bans funding of research involving IVF unless reviewed by the Ethics Advisory Board. The Ethics Advisory Board's term has expired and has not been reconstituted; thus there is a de facto moratorium on federally funded IVF research.

State laws extend beyond governmentally funded research, and could affect privately funded investigation and the private clinical practice of a number of infertility techniques involving embryos. Of the 25 states with such laws, 7 prohibit research involving preimplantation embryos.[27] These statutes probably do not apply to IVF, because it is now generally considered to be standard medical practice, and arguably is not experimental; however, they potentially could restrict extensions of IVF such as cryopreservation or embryo donation. A few states specifically address IVF in their fetal research statutes. For example, New Mexico defines clinical research to include research involving human in-vitro fertilization.[28] Illinois, on the other hand, specifically exempts IVF from the prohibition on fetal research.[29]

In-vivo fertilization followed by embryo transfer is not as well developed as is IVF, and thus statutory restrictions on embryo research will affect in-vivo fertilization differently. In this procedure, a second woman is artificially inseminated with the sperm of the husband of an infertile woman. Five days later the embryo is flushed out of the second woman by lavage and implanted into the wife.[30] Because embryo lavage may be considered an abortion (since it involves removing the embryo from the uterus), the procedure could run afoul of both the laws banning research on preimplantation embryos and those that ban research on a fetus in connection with an abortion.[31] These statutes could prohibit in-vivo fertilization followed by embryo transfer, or cryopreservation.

In the course of IVF or in-vivo fertilization a woman may produce more eggs and embryos than she can safely use for reproductive purposes. Questions arise whether these materials can be cryopreserved, discarded, donated to another woman, or used for research. The answer depends on statutory regulation and the wishes of the couple. The laws regulating fetal research prior or subsequent to a planned abortion would not affect cryopreservation after IVF because neither procedure involves an aborted fetus.[32] Because cryopreservation is still an experimental procedure, however, laws in 9 states that prohibit fetal research even in instances in which there is no abortion could prohibit its use.[33] Although regulation might be justified on the grounds that the goal of such legislation is to protect the resulting child, harm to the embryo itself would not justify a state ban on this technique.[34]

A second option the couple or individual may have is to discard any excess embryos. There are several reasons why the couple would make that choice; for example, the woman might not want to risk multiple pregnancies, or the embryo may show cellular damage. In the future, if genetic testing is done on embryos, pregnancy could be terminated to avoid the birth of a handicapped child. No law explicitly requires all fertilized eggs and preimplantation embryos to be transferred to a uterus[35]; however, several statutes imply that physicians could be prosecuted for discarding embryos. The Louisiana law that defines an embryo as "an in vitro fertilized human ovum"[36] states, "The use of a human ovum fertilized in vitro is solely for the support and contribution of the complete development of human in utero implantation."[37] A further provision states, "A viable in vitro fertilized human ovum . . . shall not be intentionally destroyed by any natural or other juridical person or through the actions of any other such person."[38] Thus under this statute, it seems that discarding embryos produced through IVF is prohibited.

A separate provision within the Louisiana statute creates responsibilities for the physician. It provides that "[a]ny physician or medical facility who causes in vitro fertilization of a human ovum in vitro will be directly responsible for the in vitro safekeeping of the fertilized ovum."[39] This statute forces physicians and health care institutions to be cautious in introducing new therapies because of the increased statutory responsibilities. The creation of extra liabilities and responsibilities impedes the availability of IVF and its adjuncts.

An earlier Illinois law created a similar responsibility for physicians performing IVF.[40] It raised so many questions about their duties and liabilities that a physician and couple he was treating brought a suit against the Illinois Attorney General and the prosecuting attorney to prevent its enforcement.[41]

In response, the defendants indicated they would not prosecute physicians for all potential risks to the embryo. A physician would be in violation of the law only if he or she willfully harmed the embryo through abuse, mutilation, extermination, or destructive laboratory experimentation. Even these limitations put a chill on IVF programs. Subsequently, the amended law was to provide an exception for IVF.[42] Unless cryopreservation is considered to be part of IVF, however, the law may make embryo freezing a criminal offense.

Physicians and clinics also face liability for discarding an embryo without the permission of the couple. That right belongs to the couple. In a 1973 case, physicians at Columbia Presbyterian Hospital in New York City attempted the in-vitro fertilization of a woman's egg with her husband's sperm. Without consulting with the physician or the couple, the department chairman removed the culture and destroyed it. The couple sued the department chairman and the hospital's trustees, charging conversion of personal property and intentional infliction of emotional distress.[43] The jury rejected the property claim but awarded plaintiffs damages for emotional distress.

A third option the couple has with respect to the excess embryos is to sell or donate them to another

woman. Sixteen states prohibit a woman from selling an embryo for experimentation[44]; 9 prohibit the donation of embryos or a fetus for research purposes.[45] As embryo transfer after IVF or in-vivo fertilization becomes standard clinical practice, these regulations would no longer restrict donation.

The restriction on the sale or donation of embryos for research must be distinguished from the bans in 3 states that restrict such sale or donation for any purpose.[46] The primary distinction between them is that, even if in-vivo fertilization followed by embryo transfer became a standard clinical procedure, the latter laws would still restrict the sale or donation of embryos.

A fifth circuit opinion questioned the continued validity of the statutory bans on embryo and fetal research.[47] The court declared unconstitutional an earlier Louisiana law that forbade experimentation on living or dead aborted fetuses unless the experimentation was therapeutic.[48] The court concluded that the word "experimentation" was impermissibly vague,[49] because physicians do not and cannot distinguish clearly between medical experiments and medical tests.[50] The court noted that "even medical *treatment* can be reasonably described as both a test and an experiment."[51] In light of the opinion, the Louisiana legislature drafted a new statute; whether or not it reconciles these distinctions remains to be seen through litigation.

Although the Louisiana statute prohibits the sale of eggs and embryos created through IVF,[52] it allows embryo donation.[53] It states, "If the in vitro fertilization patients renounce, by notarial act, their parental rights for in utero implantation, then the in vitro fertilized human ovum shall be available for adoptive implantation in accordance with written procedures of the facility where it is housed or stored."[54] No payment will be made to either party. A further provision prohibits the culture of an in-vitro-fertilized human ovum for research "or any other purposes."[55] The statute still seems to ban embryo research. Thus it seems that excess embryos may be donated, but only for implantation in another woman. Furthermore, the statute does not seem to resolve the ambiguity between research and treatment called into question by the fifth circuit case.

INFORMED CONSENT

The ultimate decision regarding the use of infertility therapies lies with the individual or couple. There is a legal basis for allowing the patient to decide which treatment plan to undergo. Founded both in statutory and case law, the doctrine of informed consent protects the patient's decision making and right to control his or her body.[56] It is the legal and ethical duty of the physician to communicate with the patient so that the patient fully understands the treatment options.

The informed consent doctrine requires health care professionals to provide sufficient information so that patients can make a knowledgeable decision about whether to proceed with a proposed procedure.[57] Studies show that patients benefit both physically and psychologically from having such information. These benefits include furthering self-determination, checking against unnecessary or inappropriate procedures, aiding physician decision making, improving the physician–patient relationship, and speeding recovery.[58] The goal of the communication is to ensure that patients receive relevant information so that they can evaluate the proposed procedure objectively and then apply personal values in order to reject or accept the recommendation.[59]

Early court decisions on informed consent held physicians liable for operating on patients without their consent. By the late 1950s and early 1960s the courts' notion of informed consent included the requirement that patients must be told about a proposed procedure's risk in order to make an informed decision.[60] The current doctrine requires the physician to discuss the patient's condition; the availability, risks, and alternatives of diagnostic procedures; and the availability, risks, and alternatives of treatment procedures.

The health care professionals providing infertility therapies should provide extensive information to the couple on the nature and risks as well as the potential success of the proposed procedure. Alternative means of treatment should also be discussed. The couple should be counseled together and individually to assure that one partner is not being pressured to undergo certain therapies. The institution should provide its success rates, because these differ widely for various programs, with many programs not yet reporting a pregnancy.[61] Information should be given to the patients concerning embryo discard, storage, donation, research, and cost to themselves.[62] The information should include which techniques are available; data on the risk of infection, spontaneous abortion, stillbirth, and so forth; an explanation of the psychologic risks of participating in the procedures; and the type and purpose of the research if it is being conducted. Finally, the discussion should be concluded with a solicitation of what the couple wants.

Considerations for IVF

In addition to the general types of information regarding risks, alternatives, and so forth that must be disclosed about all proposed procedures, each reproductive technology raises special informed consent considerations. For example, the IVF protocol involves stimulation of a woman's ovaries. This has resulted in some women providing as many as 17 or more eggs per laparoscopy.[63] If all eggs were fertilized and reimplanted into the woman's uterus, the risks of multiple pregnancies to her and to the potential offspring would be great. Usually only 3 or 4 embryos are implanted; hence the couple must decide what they want done with any excess embryos that are created. The couple may decide to implant all the embryos (at which point the risks of multiple gestation should be explained), freeze the embryos for subsequent implantation, terminate them, donate them to another woman,[64] or donate them for research. Most clinics currently limit the couple's choice to implantation or termination.[65]

Considerations for Cryopreservation

If the couple is considering cryopreservation, the physician should explain to them the institution's policies on how long preservation will be allowed, as well as the survival rate of embryos after thawing and any physical or psychologic risks to the resulting child that freezing might entail. The couple should also be asked for a written directive regarding the fate of the embryos if they divorce, decide against implantation, or if one or both die. If both die, or if they file for divorce without directives about what will be done with the embryos, it is unclear who should make the decision regarding the embryos' future. Louisiana, by appointing the physician as temporary guardian, might make him or her responsible for such decisions.[66]

If cryopreservation becomes more common, it might be considered negligent for a physician to discard embryos. For example, if 5 embryos are created, 3 are implanted, and the remaining 2 destroyed, but the 3 implanted embryos do not develop into a pregnancy, the woman might claim that her physician negligently interfered with her chances of creating a child by discarding the additional embryos rather than freezing them.[67] This could be especially critical if the eggs are obtained as the result of "last chance" surgery (for example, before a woman undergoes radiation therapy or a hysterectomy).

Considerations for Embryo Donation

The physician should discuss the risks involved with embryo donation with the donors. There are two types of donors: those who have completed their families and are donating embryos so another woman may have a family; and women undergoing infertility treatments who, through therapy procedures, have created excess embryos. Women who have fulfilled their own childbearing needs should be counseled about the physical risks associated with embryo donation, such as infection, permanent scarring, and other side effects. In addition to these physical risks, women who undergo infertility therapy must be counseled on the psychologic risks of donation. First the physician should make sure there is no coercion of the woman or the couple to donate an embryo; participation in an IVF program should not be limited to women or couples who agree to donate excess embryos. Second, the physician must counsel the woman to consider the emotional risk of donation in case she herself does not achieve a pregnancy. Donors also should consider the risk of the resulting child's potential emotional reaction on learning of the existence a biologic parent with whom he or she will have no contact.

These considerations for IVF, cryopreservation, and embryo donation arise in addition to the required informed consent disclosures. They point to the increased complexity of decision making in the area of medically assisted reproduction, as compared to that with other medical advances, because they involve caretaking decisions for potential or newly created life, in addition to the preservation of an existing life.

SINGLE PARENTHOOD

Originally intended to assist married couples, the new reproductive technologies can be used to facilitate single parenthood: single men may hire a surrogate; single women may be artificially inseminated. A majority of the artificial insemination statutes assume that a married couple will be using the procedure, but none make it illegal for an unmarried woman to do so.[68] The Ohio and Oregon statutes specifically acknowledge that a single woman might use donor sperm.[69]

No laws prohibit the insemination of unmarried women. Even if a state passed such a law it would be unlikely to be upheld as constitutional. The constitutional protection of reproductive decisions extends to individuals as well as married couples.[70] A single woman, denied artificial insemination at a clinic affiliated with a state or federal institution that will only inseminate a married couple, can claim that her privacy right to make procreative decisions and her equal protection right are violated by the clinic's policies. This has already happened in one case. The clinic associated with a state university settled the suit by agreeing to drop the marriage requirement and consider the woman as a candidate for insemination.[71]

The insemination of single women brings into question traditional notions of family.[72] It raises such issues as whether it is in the child's best interests to have two parents; and whether a single parent can meet the physical and emotional needs of the child, especially if the parent will have to work to support

the child. However, studies of children in single-parent, female-headed families have found that they have comparable cognitive abilities to those raised in two-parent homes.[73] In addition, children in single-parent homes have a level of self-esteem that is at least equal to that of children in two-parent families.[74] Children raised in lesbian-headed households do not differ from other children as to their gender-role behavior or their sexual preference.[75]

Societal interests, even those that concern the definition of family or suggest community intolerance, are not compelling enough to prohibit the insemination of single women. One court stated in a case involving an unmarried woman undergoing artificial insemination, "We wish to stress that our opinion in this case is not intended to express any judicial preference toward traditional notions of family structure or toward providing a father where a single woman has chosen to bear a child."[76]

The focal point of case law concerning the artificial insemination of single women has been paternity. An Ohio law tries to clarify this issue by providing that if an unmarried woman is artificially inseminated, "the donor shall not be treated in law or regarded as the natural father."[77] In contrast, a New Jersey case involving the home insemination of a single woman held that the man providing the semen was the legal father of the child.[78] This decision is based a unique set of facts, however (the donor, who was the woman's boyfriend, sued for visitation rights), and so it does not provide much guidance for other cases. The court held that the boyfriend who provided the sperm was the legal father and granted him visitation rights. In reaching its decision, the court distinguished this from previous artificial insemination cases because "there is no married couple [and because] there is no anonymous donor."[79] The court found that, "If an unmarried woman conceives a child through artificial insemination from semen from a known man, that man cannot be considered to be less a father because he is not married to the woman."[80] The court also stated that the decision was consistent with judicial policy "favoring the requirement that a child be provided with a father as well as a mother."[81] This decision has been read narrowly; there have been no cases in which an anonymous sperm donor has been held liable for child support against his wishes.

PHYSICIAN INVOLVEMENT

Physician involvement in artificial insemination by donor (AID)* is not medically necessary; nonetheless,

---

*Although the medical term has evolved to be *therapeutic insemination by donor* (TID), in legal language it is still AID, and that term is used in this chapter.

some statutory enactments require physician supervision. Arguably, this could clarify the parental status of the parties involved. At least 16 of the related statutes assume that AID will be performed by or under the supervision of a "licensed physician," "certified medical doctor," or person "duly authorized to practice medicine."[82] Because AID is a relatively simple procedure[83] and involves minimal risks, the statutes that require medical assistance raise questions about whether its performance by someone other than a physician (such as a husband, lover, donor, or friend) has different legal consequences that prevent the consenting husband from taking on, and the consenting donor from relinquishing, parental rights and responsibilities. For example, the California artificial insemination statute states "[I]f, under the supervision of a licensed physician and with the consent of her husband, a wife is inseminated artificially with the semen donated by a man who is not her husband, the husband is treated in law as if he were the natural father of a child thereby conceived."[84] This type of statutory language raises questions about whether the consenting husband is the legal father when a physician is not involved in the procedure.[85] In that case, however, more general statutory provisions regarding paternity would usually give paternity rights to the husband.

The statutory requirement for physician supervision, however, can create problems when AID performed by a nonphysician involves an unmarried woman. Some unmarried women have trouble finding physicians who will agree to perform the procedure for them.[86] Their alternative is to find a donor through a network of friends and acquaintances. In one case, an unmarried woman privately selected a sperm donor and performed the insemination in her home by herself.[87] The sperm donor was listed as the father on the child's birth certificate. He filed an action to establish paternity and visitation rights. The appellate court scrutinized the statute, which said, "The donor of semen provided to a licensed physician for use in artificial insemination of a woman other than the donor's wife is treated in law as if he were not the natural father of a child thereby conceived."[88] The court held that because the semen was not provided to a physician, the donor was the legal father, and granted him visitation rights.

The court noted that "nothing inherent in artificial insemination requires the involvement of a physician."[89] Physician involvement "might offend a woman's sense of privacy and reproductive autonomy, might result in burdensome costs to some women, and might interfere with a woman's desire to conduct the procedure in a comfortable environment such as her own home or to choose the donor herself."[90] A third reason for not using the services of a physician, not mentioned by the court, is that some

people feel that the medical screening of donors by infertility clinics is inadequate and thus they wish to choose their own donors.[91] The court also gave two reasons why physician involvement might be appropriate, however. The physician could obtain a medical history of the donor and screen him. Also, the physician "can serve to create a formal, documented structure for the donor–recipient relationship to avoid misunderstandings between the parties."[92] These reasons are particularly applicable to situations in which AID is used as part of a surrogate parenting arrangement.

QUALITY ASSURANCE

Personnel Qualifications
Traditionally, patients have relied on the tort system to ensure a minimal level of quality by bringing a medical malpractice claim. The guidelines of professional organizations such as the American Fertility Society and the American Association of Tissue Banks regarding the performance of reproductive technologies are evidence of the standard of care that must be met. A Louisiana law codifies such standards by specifically addressing the qualifications of professionals and standards for the facilities performing IVF[93]: The facilities must meet "the standards of the American Fertility Society and the American College of Obstetrics and Gynecologists"; the director of the facilities must be a "medical doctor licensed to practice medicine in this state and possessing specialized training and skill in in vitro fertilization"; and the physicians performing the technique are required to act "in conformity with the standards established by the American Fertility Society or the American College of Obstetricians and Gynecologists." In contrast, no state laws specifically set forth qualifications for personnel who are involved with artificial insemination or surrogate motherhood.

Screening
The statutes addressing reproductive technologies have generally paid no attention to medical, genetic, and psychologic screening of the participants. The development of surrogate motherhood has caused lawmakers to consider the issue and to rethink previous law about donor insemination to address screening in that context as well.[94] Medical and genetic screening of donors is necessary to protect the health of recipients and the resulting children. A psychologic assessment may be necessary to determine whether the participants are informed, and are voluntarily and competently entering into alternative reproduction.

At least 3 statutes address sperm donor screening. Laws in Idaho and Oregon provide that a person who knows he has a genetic defect or venereal disease may not be a sperm donor,[95] but they provide no requirement that the donors be screened. The Idaho law does require that sperm donors be screened for human immunodeficiency virus.[96] Under an Ohio law,[97] the donor of fresh semen must undergo a physical examination, give a medical and genetic history, and be tested for blood type and Rh factor. The donor of fresh sperm must undergo appropriate laboratory studies, which "may include, but are not limited to, venereal disease research laboratories, karyotyping, [gonococcus] culture, cytomegalo[virus], hepatitis, kem-zyme, Tay-Sachs, sickle-cell, ureaplasma, HTLV-III, and chlamydia."[98]

Although few statutory guidelines exist, physicians would face tort liability if they did not undertake proper screening of donors. Failure to do so could leave them liable for physical and emotional harm experienced by a recipient or her offspring as a result of the transmission of disease. In addition to the common law requirements, both the American Fertility Society (AFS)[99] and the American Association of Tissue Banks (AATB)[100] have developed extensive screening guidelines. These may be considered evidence of at least a minimal level of professional responsibility for screening. For example, the AFS suggests excluding sperm donors who are at risk of having a sexually transmitted disease. They also suggest rescreening every 6 months and are discontinuing the use of a donor if he has a new sexual partner or if there is a break in monogamy or abstinence.

The guidelines also recommended rejecting donors with a family history of certain enumerated genetic disorders as well as carriers of those disorders. The AATB Reproductive Council standards recommend selecting donors on the basis of a "personal, physical, and genetic examination and history" as well as in-depth semen analysis. The guidelines mandate rejection of a potential sperm donor if he is employed in a job involving chemical or radiation exposure, or if he is an alcohol or drug abuser.[101] Screening for infectious and genetic diseases should be done on egg or embryo donors as well.

RECORD-KEEPING AND CONFIDENTIALITY

Record-Keeping

Confidential medical records should be kept that identify all the parties, and include medical and genetic histories of donors and surrogates.[102] These histories should be available to the couples or individuals who use assisted reproduction and also to the children created through these techniques. An Ohio law requires substantial but nonidentifying disclo-

sures about sperm donors. The physician is required to provide to the recipient and her husband the medical and genetic history of the donor and persons related to him, blood type, Rh factor, race, eye and hair color, age, height, weight, educational attainment and talents, religious background, and any other information that the donor has indicated may be disclosed.[103]

Efforts at record-keeping on providers of gametes has been minimal. Failure to keep adequate records presents the chance of harm to all parties. If a child is conceived with donated egg or sperm and has a medical problem due to a genetic disorder passed on through the donated gamete, without adequate records there is no way of identifying the donor to prevent using him or her for subsequent pregnancies. If the resulting child develops a medical problem that requires donation of genetically compatible organic material (such as bone marrow), if records are incomplete the child may be prevented from contacting a potential donor.

Reluctance by clinicians to keep records may stem from the fear that if donors could be identified, they might be held financially liable for the child. Physicians may argue that record-keeping is a burdensome task that diverts resources away from treating the patient[104]; however, they may be best suited for accepting this responsibility and ensuring confidentiality. Their duty to keep records may be based on tort principles or professional ethics code.[105] A number of states require, by statute, that physicians keep records about donor insemination.[106] The Ohio law requires them to maintain a file for at least 5 years, separate from any regular medical chart, which includes the written consent form and information provided to the recipient.

Infertility programs should document whether they have in fact achieved a pregnancy and their pregnancy rates. An analysis of such records provides the data to meet the requirements for informed consent.[107]

In addition to physicians and clinics keeping records about the participants in medically assisted reproduction (including donors and surrogates) and about resulting children, the state might have an interest in keeping information about the extent of use of alternative reproduction, the number of attempts, and rates of pregnancy, miscarriage, stillbirths, live births, and birth defects. Finally, state record-keeping could include maintaining a voluntary registry so that if both sides agree, biologic children and their siblings or parents can be identified to each other.

Some states already have legislation that sets forth record-keeping requirements for specific procedures. For example, the artificial insemination statutes of 10 states require physicians to file with the appropriate state department the dates of all procedures they perform.[108] Three states require physicians to file information on the birth of children conceived through AID.[109]

Pennsylvania has such requirements for IVF, although not for AID. Anyone conducting IVF is required to file quarterly reports with the Department of Health, including the names of everyone assisting in the procedure, the location in which it is performed, names and addresses of sponsoring individuals or institutions (except the names of the donors or recipients of gametes), the number of ova fertilized, the number of embryos destroyed and discarded, and the number of women in whom the embryos are implanted.[110]

Confidentiality

State laws protect the physician–patient relationship by providing that the disclosure of confidential information is grounds for revocation of the physician's medical license or a basis for other disciplinary action. An ethical duty also exists, founded on the Hippocratic Oath or AMA's Judicial Ethics, that is paralleled by a legal duty set out in the disciplinary or testimonial privilege statutes in a majority of the states.

States that mandate filing a husband's consent to AID procedures also protect the confidentiality of such information and the privacy of the individuals. The information, generally confidential, may be opened by a court "for good cause shown." The extent and protection of confidentiality varies among jurisdictions. For example, the Ohio law provides that the physician maintaining a file on AID "shall not make this information available for inspection by any person" unless a court determines that inspection "is necessary for or helpful in the medical treatment of a child born as a result of artificial insemination."[111]

LEGAL AND BIOLOGIC PARENTAGE

Third-party involvement raises the potential for a distinction between legal and biologic parentage. In the context of AID, the courts recognized the consenting husband's legal parentage through a series of early cases that established the child's legal identity. Usually these cases arose out of a divorce proceeding. In one case the husband claimed he should not have to support the child because they were not genetically related.[112] In another, the wife tried to deny her husband visitation rights based on the same rationale.[113] Sometimes, in the earliest cases, the courts declared the child born as a result of artificial insemination to be illegitimate. It is well established,

however, that the courts will protect the child financially and emotionally by finding the consenting husband to be the legal father, with support responsibilities and visitation rights.

All of the 30 states regulating AID clarify the paternity of a child by providing that the sperm recipient and her consenting husband are the legal parents.[114] The consenting husband is the legal father for legitimacy, inheritance, and support purposes.[115] Some statutes, such as those of Minnesota, Montana, Nevada, New Mexico, Virginia, Wisconsin, and Wyoming, require the husband's written consent to the procedure for him to be recognized as the legal parent.[116]

It appears that in cases involving surrogate gestational mothers, courts are adopting the position that the couple who provides the gametes are the legal parents. In *Smith v. Jones*, a case involving a surrogate gestational mother who carried a couple's embryo, a district court recognized the genetic parents as the legal parents and granted them the right to have their names put on the birth certificate.[117] The gestational surrogate was not considered to be the mother, and the couple did not have to adopt the child.

A different result was reached by the New Jersey Supreme Court in the landmark Baby M decision. Here the court held that the man providing the sperm was the legal father, and the woman providing the egg and gestating the embryo was the legal mother.

Arkansas, Indiana, Kentucky, Louisiana, Nebraska, and Nevada specifically regulate surrogate motherhood arrangements.[118] Of these 6 states, only 1 specifically addresses paternity. The Arkansas statute presumes that the legal mother of a child, conceived by artificial insemination and born to an unmarried surrogate mother, is the intended mother. The Nevada law allows payment to a surrogate, while the Louisiana, Indiana, Kentucky, and Nebraska statutes void paid surrogacy contracts. If a dispute arose in the last 2 states or those that have no surrogacy statute, the existing AID, adoption, and parentage statues would provide a framework for determining paternity.

PAYMENT TO THIRD PARTIES

It is axiomatic in a market economy that providers of goods and services are compensated. Our society routinely compensates third parties for their time, effort, inconvenience, and availability in providing a service or product. The involvement of third parties in reproduction raises the question of compensating them for their efforts. Think, for example, of a surrogate who puts her own life at risk in order to give birth to a child for another couple. Should she be compensated, or does that commercialize the creation of life?

Sperm donors are routinely compensated for providing gametes. Payment to egg or embryo donors is often perceived to be different. One state explicitly forbids payment of egg donors in the context of in-vitro fertilization.[119] In addition, in 6 states the organ transplant laws are drafted so broadly that they could be used to ban payment to egg donors.[120] For example, a Virginia statute makes it "unlawful to sell, to offer to sell, to buy, to offer to buy or to procure through purchase" a human organ.[121] An organ is "any natural body part with the exception of hair, blood, or any other self-replacing body fluid."[122]

Some states regulate payment to an embryo donor rather than to an egg donor. Florida and Louisiana expressly prohibit payment to embryo donors.[123] In addition, 11 statutes that prohibit a woman from selling a fetus for experimentation employ language broad enough potentially to forbid payment to a woman who undergoes in-vivo fertilization followed by embryo transfer.[124]

Payment to surrogate mothers seems to have raised the most public discussion of reimbursing third parties for their assistance in medically assisted reproduction. Nevada exempts paid surrogacy contracts from the prohibition against payment in connection with an adoption.[125] Laws in at least 23 states prohibit payment in connection with an adoption, which could be interpreted as restricting commercial surrogate motherhood.[126] Because the adoption laws were drafted with a different purpose, they may be distinguished from surrogate parenting, and arguably may not restrict payment to a surrogate. Paying a surrogate a fee is distinguishable from paying an already pregnant woman for her child.

Courts have had to deal with payments to surrogates in the absence of legislative guidelines, and their reactions have been mixed. The New Jersey Supreme Court voided a surrogacy contract and held that statutes banning payment in connection with an adoption prohibited payment to a surrogate.[127] This is similar to an earlier decision in which a Michigan court held that the statutory ban that prohibited payment in connection with an adoption also prohibited payment to a surrogate under a surrogate contract.[128] Other courts, specifically those in New York and Kentucky, have allowed compensation to the surrogate.[129] The Kentucky court concluded that contracts to pay surrogate mothers did not violate the statutory prohibition against payment in connection with an adoption.[130] A subsequently-adopted Kentucky statute, however, voids paid surrogacy contracts.

Laws restricting payment to third parties must be assessed in light of the individual's or couple's rights of privacy to make procreative decisions. People with particular infertility problems may be forced to remain childless if payment is not allowed, because it may not be possible to recruit donors or surrogate mothers without paying them. As with other statutory regulations restricting alternative reproduction, laws denying payment to third parties would be upheld only if they further a compelling state interest. For example, because the decision to use a surrogate is protected by the right to privacy, moral disapproval of payment as the commercialization of motherhood would be an insufficient reason to ban payment.

THE LAW, RESPONSIBILITY, AND NEW REPRODUCTIVE THERAPIES

The new reproductive therapies offer the hope of children to infertile couples, but with the promise comes additional responsibilities for all parties. The researcher who uses the new opportunities for embryo and fetal research must comport with ethical standards. Clinicians' responsibilities include counseling and informing the participants in medically assisted reproduction, as well as screening the third parties involved. The individual or couple using the technologies will be faced with a host of new psychologic challenges. Society will be forced, in the course of questioning traditional notions of family, to decide how best to protect the fundamental rights of its citizenry. Finally, all those involved, from the researcher to society in general, must provide a safe, nurturing environment for the resulting children.

The law will play a part in shaping the impact of the new reproductive technologies by protecting constitutional rights, setting the standards for research and practice, defining the rights and responsibilities of the parties and society, and contributing to the ethical considerations.

REFERENCES

1. 316 U.S. 535 (1942).
2. *Skinner v. Oklahoma*, 316 U.S. 535, 541 (1942).
3. See, e.g., *Griswold v. Connecticut*, 381 U.S. 479 (1965); *Eisenstadt v. Baird*, 405 U.S. 438 (1972); *Roe v. Wade*, 410 U.S. 113 (1973).
4. *Stanley v. Illinois*, 405 U.S. 645, 651 (1972).
5. *Eisenstadt v. Baird*, 405 U.S. 438, 453 (1972).
6. *Roe v. Wade*, 410 U.S. 113, 155 (1973).
7. Karst: The freedom of intimate association. *Yale LJ* 89:624, 1980.
8. Andrews and Hendricks: Legal and moral status of IVF/ET, in C Fredericks, et al (eds): *Foundations of In Vitro Fertilization.* place, pub, 1987, p 312.
9. See Robertson: Embryos, families, and procreative liberty: The legal structure of the new reproduction. *So Cal L Rev* 59:939, 1986.
10. Andrews: The legal status of the embryo. *Loyola L Rev* 32:357, 1986.
11. *In re Baby M*, A-39-87, slip op. at 61 (N.J. Supreme Ct., February 3, 1988).
12. Robertson: Embryo research. *Univ W Ontario L Rev* 24:15, 1986.

13. *Second International Dictionary of Medicine and Biology*. New York: Wiley, 1986.
14. Clifford Grobstein introduced the notion of IVF opening a window to the embryo. C. Grobstein: *From Chance to Purpose: An Appraisal of External Human Fertilization*. 1981.
15. Robertson, Embryo research, *supra* n. 12 at 17.
16. Ibid at 17.
17. See, e.g. Louisiana statute which prohibits the creation of embryos solely for research. La. Rev. Stat. Ann. §9:122 (West Supp. 1987).
18. Ariz. Rev. Stat. Ann. §36–2302 (1986); Ark. Stat. Ann. §§82–436 to 442 (Supp. 1985); Cal. Health & Safety Code §25956 (West 1984); Fla. Stat Ann. §§390.001(6), (7) (West 1986); Ill. Ann. Stat. ch. 38, para. 81–26(7) (Smith-Hurd 1986); Ind. Code §35–1–58.5–6 (1986); Ky. Rev. Stat. Ann. §436.026 (Baldwin 1985); La. Rev. Stat. Ann. §9:122 (West Supp. 1987); Me. Rev. Stat. Ann. tit. 22, §1593 (1980); Mass. Ann. Laws ch. 112, §12J (Law. Co-op. 1985); Mich. Comp. Laws Ann. §§333.2685–.2692 (West 1980); Minn. Stat. Ann. §§145.421–.422 (West Supp. 1987); Mo. Ann. Stat. §188.037 (Vernon 1983); Mont. Code Ann. §50–20–108(3) (1985); Neb. Rev. Stat. §§28–342 to –346 (1985); N.M. Stat. Ann. 24–9A–1 (1981); N.D. Cent. Code §14–02.02–01 to –02 (1981); Ohio Rev. Code Ann. §2919.14 (Baldwin 1982); Okla. Stat. Ann. tit. 63, §1–735 (West 1984); Pa. Stat. Ann. tit. 18, §3216 (Purdon 1983); R.I. Gen. Laws §11–54–1 (Supp. 1986); S.D. Codified Laws Ann. §34–23A–17 (1986); Tenn. Code Ann. §39–4–208 (1982); Utah Code Ann. §§76–7–310 to –311 (1978); and Wyo. Stat. §35–6–115 (1977).
19. Only Utah does not have such a restriction.
20. Arizona, Indiana, Kentucky, Maine, Ohio, and Wyoming. All these laws, except for that in Maine, apply only to research on aborted fetuses.
21. Arkansas, California, Florida, Missouri, Nebraska, Oklahoma, and Pennsylvania, which apply only to live aborted fetuses; and Illinois, Massachusetts, Montana, North Dakota, and Rhode Island, which apply to live fetuses.
22. La Rev. Stat. Ann. §9:122 (West Supp. 1987).
23. Arizona, Arkansas, California, Florida, Indiana, Kentucky, Missouri, Nebraska, Ohio, Oklahoma, Pennsylvania, and Tennessee.
24. Robertson, Embryo research, *supra* n. 12 at 16.
25. Ibid at 16.
26. 45 C.F.R. §46.203(c) (1986).
27. Illinois, Maine, Massachusetts, Michigan, North Dakota, Rhode Island, and Utah.
28. N.M. Stat. Ann. §24–9A01(D) (1986).
29. Ill. Ann. Stat. ch. 38, para. 81–26(7) (Smith-Hurd Supp. 1987).
30. Bustillo, Buster, Cohen, et al: Delivery of a healthy infant following nonsurgical ovum transfer. *JAMA* 251:889, 1984.
31. Arizona, Arkansas, Indiana, Louisiana, Maine, Massachusetts, Michigan, Missouri, Montana, Nebraska, North Dakota, Ohio, Oklahoma, Pennsylvania, Rhode Island, Utah, and Wyoming. This includes both statutes that specifically apply to embryos and those that neglect to define "fetus" or the term used to refer to the subject of research, and might be interpreted to include preimplantation embryos.
32. Arizona, Arkansas, California, Florida, Indiana, Kentucky, Missouri, Nebraska, Ohio, Oklahoma, Tennessee, and Wyoming.
33. Illinois, Louisiana (applies to cryopreservation after IVF), Maine, Massachusetts, Michigan, North Dakota, Pennsylvania, Rhode Island, and Utah.
34. Robertson, Embryo, families, and procreative liberty, *supra* n. 9 at 994–995.
35. The American Fertility Society (AFS) considers it ethical to dispose of nontransferred embryos. Ethics Committee of the American Fertility Society: Ethical considerations of the new reproductive technologies. *Fertil Steril* 46 (suppl):1S, 1986.
36. La. Rev. Stat. Ann §9:121 (West Supp. 1987).
37. La. Rev. Stat. Ann §9:122 (West Supp. 1987).
38. La. Rev. Stat. Ann §9:129 (West Supp. 1987).
39. La. Rev. Stat. Ann §9:127 (West Supp. 1987).
40. The Illinois statute, now repealed, granted custody to the physician of an in vitro-fertilized egg. The physician was "deemed to have care and custody of a child" for purposes of an 1877 child abuse act. Ill. Ann. Stat. ch. 23, para. 2354 (Smith-Hurd 1968).
41. *Smith v. Hartigan*, 556 F. Supp. 157 (N.D. Ill. 1983).
42. Ill. Ann. Stat. ch. 38, para 81–26(7) (Smith-Hurd Supp. 1986).
43. *Del Zio v. Manhattan's Columbia Presbyterian Medical Center*, No. 74–3558 (S.D. N.Y. November 14, 1978).
44. Arkansas, Florida, Illinois (specifically exempts IVF), Kentucky, Loui-
siana (only involves embryos created through IVF), Maine, Massachusetts, Michigan, Minnesota, Nebraska, New Mexico, North Dakota, Ohio, Oklahoma, Rhode Island, and Utah.
45. Arkansas, Kentucky, Maine, Massachusetts, Michigan, Nebraska, North Dakota, Rhode Island, and Wyoming.
46. Fla. Stat. Ann. §873.05 (West Supp. 1987); Ill. Ann. Stat. ch. 81 para. 81–26(7) (Smith-Hurd Supp. 1987) (prohibits sale only); La. Rev. Stat. Ann §9:122 (West Supp. 1987) (prohibits sale of IVF embryos).
47. 794 F.2d 994 (5th Cir. 1986).
48. *Margaret S. v. Edwards*, 794 F.2d 994 (5th Cir. 1986).
49. Ibid at 999.
50. Ibid.
51. Ibid.
52. La. Rev. Stat. Ann. §9:122 (West Supp. 1987).
53. La. Rev. Stat. Ann. §9:130 (West Supp. 1987).
54. La. Rev. Stat. Ann. §9:130 (West Supp. 1987).
55. La. Rev. Stat. Ann. §9:122 (West Supp. 1987).
56. See Andrews: Informed consent statutes and the decisionmaking process. *J Leg Med* 5:163, 1984.
57. Andrews: The rationale behind the informed consent doctrine. *J Med Pract* 1:59, 1985.
58. See chapter entitled, Provision of genetic services—Informed consent and other duties to disclose, in L. Andrews: *Medical Genetics: A Legal Frontier*. Chicago, American Bar Foundation, 1987, pp 105–134.
59. Andrews, The rationale behind the informed consent doctrine, *supra* n. 57 at 60.
60. *Natason v. Kline*, 186 Kan. 393, 350 P.2d 1093 (1960), *reh'g denied* 187 Kan. 186, 354 P.2d 670 (1960). The case involved a woman who suffered extensive tissue and bone damage after a series of cobalt treatments for breast cancer. The court held that where there is a substantial risk of injury in administering a treatment and no emergency exists, the physician has a duty to make a reasonable disclosure to the patient of the known risks and would be subject to liability for a failure to do so.
61. AFS, *supra* n. 35 at Appendix D, 87S–88S.
62. Robertson, Embryos, families, and procreative liberty, *supra* n. 9 at 1036.
63. Andrews, The legal status of the embryo, *supra* n. 10 at 401.
64. An international review found that 60 live births have resulted from pregnancies involving donated eggs. Andrews, *Medical Genetics, surpra* n. 58.
65. Andrews and Hendricks, *supra* n. 8 at 315.
66. La. Rev. Stat. Ann. §9:126 (West Supp. 1987).
67. Andrews and Hendricks, *supra* n. 8 at 315.
68. Kritchevsky: The unmarried woman's right to artificial insemination: A call for an expanded definition of family. *Harvard Women's L J* 4:1, 1981.
69. Ohio Rev. Code Ann. §3111.31 (Baldwin 1987); Or. Rev. Stat. §677.365 (1977). The Ohio statute applies to artificial insemination for the purpose of impregnating a woman so that she can bear a child that she intends to raise as her child. The Oregon statute requires the consent of her husband "if she is married." Or Rev. Stat. §677.365 (1977).
70. As the U.S. Supreme Court noted, "It is the right of the *individual*, married or single, to be free of unwarranted governmental intrusion in matters so fundamentally affecting a person as the decision whether to bear or beget a child." *Eisenstadt v. Baird*, 405 U.S. 438, 453 (1972) (emphasis in the original).
71. *Smedes v. Wayne State University*, (E.D. Mich., filed July 16, 1980).
72. Similar issues are raised by an unmarried man's use of a surrogate mother.
73. McGuire and Alexander: Artificial insemination of single women. *Fertil Steril* 43:182, 1985.
74. Raschke and Raschke: Family conflict and children's self concept: A comparison of intact and single parent families. *J Marriage Fam* 41:367, 1979. Weiss: Growing up a little faster. *J Social Issues* 35:97, 1979.
75. McGuire and Alexander, *supra* n. 74 at 182.
76. *Jhordan C. v. Mary K.*, 179 Cal. Appl. 3d 386, 224 Cal Rptr. 530, 537–8 (1986).
77. Ohio Rev. Code Ann. §3111.37(B) (Baldwin 1987). The statue does not define "woman" as a married woman.
78. *C.M. v. C.C.*, 152 N.J. Super. 160, 377 A.2d 821 (1977).
79. *C.M. v. C.C.*, 152 N.J. Super. 160, 377 A.2d 821, 824 (1977).
80. *C.M. v. C.C.*, 152 N.J. Super. 160, 377 A.2d 821,824 (1977).
81. *C.M. v. C.C.*, 152 N.J. Super. 160, 377 A.2d 821,824 (1977).
82. Alabama, Alaska, California, Colorado, Idaho, Illinois, Minnesota, Montana, Nevada, New Jersey, New Mexico, Ohio, Virginia, Washington, Wisconsin, and Wyoming.

83. See e.g., Andrews: "Alternative modes of Reproduction," in Cohen S. and Taub N. eds. *Reproductive Laws for the 1990s*. Clifton, N.J. 1989, p. 377. Rutgers (forthcoming 1988), which demonstrates that artificial insemination may be accomplished in the privacy of one's own home with instruments no more sophisticated than a turkey baster. The Ohio law seems to anticipate this: "[s]upervision requires the availability of a physician for consultation and direction, but does not necessarily require the personal presence of the physician who is providing the supervision." Ohio Rev. Code Ann. §3111.32 (Baldwin 1987).

84. Cal. Civ. Code §7005(a) (West 1983).

85. Andrews, "Alternative reproduction," 30–1, 30–19, in *Disputed Paternity Proceedings* (MB) (1986).

86. A national survey of physicians providing artificial insemination found that 10% of the procedures were performed in unmarried women. Curie-Cohen, Luttrell, and Shapiroa: Current practice of artificial insemination by donor in the United States. *N Engl J Med* 300:585, 1979. One reason why most physicians, both those in private practice and in hospitals, refuse to inseminate unmarried women is that they erroneously fear the practice is illegal. A second reason is that some of the physicians believe that unmarried women and/or lebians should not be mothers. Kritchevsky, *supra* n. 68.

87. *Jhordan C. v. Mary K.*, 179 Cal. App. 3d 386, 224 Cal. Rptr. 530 (1986).

88. Cal. Civ. Code §7005(b) (West 1983).

89. *Jhordan C. v. Mary K.*, 179 Cal. App. 3d 386, 224 Cal Rptr. 530, 535 (1986).

90. *Jhordan C. v. Mary K.*, 179 Cal. App. 3d 386, 224 Cal Rptr. 530, 535 (1986).

91. Andrews: Yours, mine and theirs. *Psychol Today* 18: 20, 1984.

92. *Jhordan C. v. Mary K.*, 179 Cal. App. 3d 386, 224 Cal Rptr. 530, 535 (1986).

93. La. Rev. Stat. Ann. §9:128 (West Supp. 1987).

94. Andrews: The aftermath of Baby M: Proposed state laws on surrogate motherhood. *Hastings Center Report* 17:31, Oct/Nov 1987.

95. Idaho Code §39–5404 (Supp. 1986); Or. Rev. Stat. §677.370 (1981). See also a New York City ordinance that provides that carriers of genetic diseases or defects and men suffering from venereal disease or tuberculosis cannot be sperm donors. It also provides that the sperm donor and recipient must have compatible Rh factors. City of New York Health Code §§21.03, .05 (1973).

96. Idaho Code §39–5408 (Supp. 1986).

97. Ohio Rev. Code Ann. §3111.33 (Baldwin 1987).

98. Ibid.

99. AFS, *supra* n. 35 at Appendices B and C, 83S–86S.

100. American Association of Tissue Banks: Addendum 2: Specific standards—Reproductive council. *American Association of Tissue Banks Provisional Standards* 22, Sept 1984.

101. For a complete description of the screening guidelines developed by AFS and AATB, see Andrews, *Medical Genetics, supra* n. 68 at 168–171.

102. AFS, *supra* n. at Appendix B, para. IV 84S.

103. Ohio Rev. Code Ann. §3111.35(2) (Baldwin 1987).

104. In a 1979 survey, 83% of physicians offering artificial insemination by donor were opposed to the idea of a statutory requirement for keeping records on the child or the donors. Curie-Cohen, Luttrell, and Shapiro: Current practice of artificial insemination in the United States. *N Engl J Med* 300:585 1979.

105. Ontario Law Reform Commission: *Report on Human Artificial Reproduction and Related Matters*. 1985, p 184.

106. See, e.g., Cal. Civ. Code §7005 (West 1983); Ohio Rev. Code Ann. §3111.36 (Baldwin 1987).

107. Records should be available to the patients concerning embryo discard, storage, donation, research, and cost. Robertson, Embryos, families, and procreative liberty, *supra* n. 9 at 1039.

108. Alabama, Colorado, Minnesota, Montana, Nevada, New Jersey, New Mexico, Washington, Wisconsin, and Wyoming.

109. Connecticut, Idaho, and Oregon. Connecticut requires the information be filed with the Probate Court; Idaho and Oregon require the information be filed with the state registrar of vital statistics.

110. 18 Pa. Cons. Stat. Ann. §3213(e) (Purdon Supp. 1986).

111. Ohio Rev. Code Ann. §3111.36(C) (Baldwin 1987).

112. *Anonymous v. Anonymous*, 41 Misc. 2d 886, 246 N.Y.S.2d 1835 (1964).

113. *N.Y. v. Dennett*, 15 Misc. 2d 260, 184 N.Y.S.2d 178 (1958).

114. Similarly, laws of 16 of the 30 states explicitly provide that the man donating sperm to a woman who is not his wife is not the legal father of the child: Alabama, California, Colorado, Connecticut, Idaho, Illinois, Minnesota, Montana, Nevada, New Jersey (unless the woman and donor have entered into a contract to the contrary), New Mexico (unless the woman and donor have agreed in writing to the contrary), Oregon, Texas, Washington (unless the woman and donor have agreed in writing to the contrary), Wisconsin, and Wyoming.

115. Alabama, Alaska, Arkansas, California, Colorado, Connecticut, Florida, Georgia, Idaho, Illinois, Kansas, Louisiana, Maryland, Michigan, Minnesota, Montana, Nevada, New Jersey, New Mexico, New York, North Carolina, Ohio, Oklahoma, Oregon, Tennessee, Texas, Virginia, Washington, Wisconsin, and Wyoming.

116. Minn. Stat. Ann. §257.56(1) (West 1982); Mont. Code Ann. §10–6–106 (1985); Nev. Rev. Stat. §126.061 (1986); N.M. Stat. Ann. §40–11–6(A) (1986); Va. Code Ann. §64.1–7.1 (1980); Wis. Stat. Ann §767.48(9) (West 1981); §891.40 (West Supp. 1986); Wyo. Stat. §1402–103 (1985).

117. *Smith* v. *Jones*, No. 85 532014 02 (Michigan Cir. Ct., Wayne Co., March 14, 1986). There was a similiar case, with the same result in California, *Smith* v. *Jones*, No. CF 025653 (Los Angeles Superior Ct., Los Angeles Co., June 9, 1987).

118. Ark. Stat. Ann. §9–10–201 (1987); Ind. S.B. 98 (enacted 1988); Ky. S.B. 4 to be codified at Ky. Rev. Stat. Ann. §199.590 (1988); La. H.B. 327 to be codified at La. Rev. Stat. Ann. §9:2713 (1987); Neb. L.B. 674 (enacted 1988); Nev. S.B. 272 to be codified at Nev. Rev. Stat. ch. 773, §6(5) (1987).

119. La Rev. Stat. Ann. §9:122 (West Supp. 1987).

120. D.C., Michigan, Maryland, Minnesota, Texas, and Virginia.

121. Va. Code Ann. §32.1–289.1 (1985).

122. Va. Code Ann. §32.1–289 (1985).

123. Fla. Stat. Ann. §873.05 (West 1986); La. Rev. Stat. Ann. §9:122 (West Supp. 1987) (The Louisiana law applies to embryos created through in vitro fertilization).

124. Maine, Massachusetts, Michigan, Nebraska, North Dakota, Ohio, Oklahoma, Rhode Island, Tennessee, Utah, and Wyoming. Nebraksa, Ohio, Oklahoma, and Wyoming cover only aborted embryos.

125. Nev. S.B. 272 to be codified at Nev. Rev. Stat. ch. 773, §6(5) (1987).

126. Alabama, Arizona, California, Colorado, Delaware, Florida, Georgia, Idaho, Illinois, Indiana, Iowa, Kentucky, Maryland, Massachusetts, Michigan, New Jersey, New York, North Carolina, Ohio, South Dakota, Tennessee, Utah, and Wisconsin. One court interpreted the statutory prohibition against payment in connection with an adoption to include prohibiting payment to a surrogate. *Doe v. Kelley*, 106 Mich. App. 169, 307 N.W.2d 438 (Mich. App. Ct. 1981), *Cert. denied* 459 U.S. 1183 (1983).

127. In Re Baby M, A–39–87, slip op. (N.J. Supreme Ct., February 3, 1988).

128. *Doe v. Kelley*, 106 Mich. App. 169, 307 N.W.2d 438 (Mich. App. Ct. 1981) *Cert. denied* 459 U.S. 1138 (1983). In one court's analysis, "the net effect of the [Kelley] decision prohibits the use of surrogate mothers in the State of Michigan since few women other than perhaps a close family member would bear someone else's child without compensation." *In re Adoption of Baby Girl L.J.*, 132 Misc. 2d 972, 505 N.Y.S2d 813, 816 (1986).

129. *In re Baby M*, 217 N.J. Super. 313, 525 A.2d 1128 (1987); *In re Adoption of Baby Girl L.J.*, 132 Misc. 2d 972, 505 N.Y.S.2d 813 (1986); *Surrogate Parenting Associates, Inc. v. Kentucky*, 704 S.W.2d 209 (Ky. 1986).

130. *Surrogate Parenting Associates, Inc. v. Kentucky*, 704 S.W.2d 209 (Ky. 1986.).

CHAPTER 39

Ethical Considerations in Infertility: Human Generation—Fact, Foible, and Fable

John D. Biggers

Ethical Considerations in Infertility

Two Cultures
Critical Times of Development
History of Understanding Conception
Catholic Interpretation of Conception
The Life Cycle
Preembryos
Toward Ethical Solutions
Conclusion

It is inevitable that the thoughts of anyone who has worked on the subjects outlined in this article should turn to Aldous Huxley's fantasy Brave New World, *where he describes completely artificial fertilization and development of human embryos. Fortunately we are far removed from this frightening prospect.[1]*

We are still a long way from being able to cultivate embryos and fetuses completely in vitro. Nevertheless, since 1958, when these lines were written, new technologies have been produced for the manipulation of early mammalian embryos that can be applied for good or evil to human embryos. Perhaps the most spectacular of these has been human in-vitro fertili-

zation and embryo transfer (IVF-ET), first reported by Steptoe and Edwards in 1978.[2] From its inception this technique has raised debates about the ethical aspects of reproductive technologies,[3-5] and as recently as 1987 the Vatican formally denounced them all as amoral.[6] These debates are likely to intensify, for techniques being developed in the area of animal science are readily applied to human embryos. This has already occurred with respect to freezing and storing embryos for future use.[7,8] Other techniques are possible but have not as yet been employed, such as embryo splitting to produce identical twins, and sexing embryos to control the sex of offspring.

The range of ethical questions that has been raised about IVF-ET is shown by the following classification, which appeared in a 1983 editorial in the *Journal of Medical Ethics*[9]:

1. Ethical dilemmas originating in our taboos about sexuality
2. Ethical dilemmas associated with conflicts of interest among participants in the reproductive process, such as the donor of the gametes, the surrogate woman in whose uterus the fetus develops, and the fetus itself
3. Ethical dilemmas pertaining to the moral status of the embryo/fetus
4. Ethical dilemmas stemming from moral concern about the nature of mankind and whether we should interfere with natural reproductive processes
5. Ethical dilemmas relating to the resolution of moral conflicts that arise among individual members of a pluralistic society who hold different views on these issues

These areas have general applicability to all reproductive technology.

It is not surprising that the reactions to these issues have been very mixed. They range from strong approval of methods that can alleviate hitherto intractable forms of human infertility to outright condemnation. Unfortunately, the majority have been highly emotional, and as a result, ethical positions are often reached precipitously and uncritically. Such reactions make a very poor foundation for public policy.

TWO CULTURES

A basic question is, how can scientists help in the analysis of ethical issues? One of the difficulties in these analyses is that the issues transcend two different cultures—scientific and humanitarian—the members of which have great difficulty understanding each other.[10] Moore[11] pointed out that the power of the scientific way of knowing "is that whatever answers are obtained must be verifiable by all other scientists with equal wisdom, skill and open-mindedness. Thus the procedures of science are self-correcting." In this respect, the scientific method differs from other ways of knowing, such as in the humanities, for example, where interpretations and opinions often replace verifiable facts.

A primary role of science in ethical debates is in conceptual analysis,[12] that is, making clear the language used and the ideas developed by the scientific approach to a problem. Specifically, in the analysis of reproductive technologies the scientific way of knowing should clarify discussions about the biologic nature of life. It is particularly important to recognize and avoid what Professor Margaret Somerville called behavior-governing terms. These are terms that are deliberately based on apparently simple descriptions for the purpose of gaining popular support in an argument.[13] Terms of particular concern here are *life begins at conception*, used by the opponents of abor-

tion, and *pre-embryo* and *pro-embryo*, which have been introduced to regulate the use of early prenatal humans in scientific research. I believe that the proposal to use specific cutoff times in development as a basis for making ethical decisions is both uninformed and fraught with pitfalls.

CRITICAL TIMES OF DEVELOPMENT

A question that is frequently asked in discussions about abortion is, when does life begin? This is not a simple question, a fact recognized by the Committee of Inquiry into Human Fertilization and Embryology in a report prepared in 1984 for the British government, under the chairmanship of Dame Mary Warnock.[14] Their report stated, "Although the questions of when life or personhood begin appear to be questions of fact susceptible to straightforward answers, we hold that the answers to such questions in fact are complex amalgams of factual and moral judgements."

This complexity is often not recognized in scholarly works and in public and political discussions. For example, the theologian Maurice Reidy[15] enunciated the principle that *human life begins at fertilization.* Frequently the same idea is asserted by the news media and from the pulpit in the form, *life begins at conception.* Unfortunately, many individuals who make these statements believe that they have the unqualified support of science. I believe that this claim is false.

After the introduction of IVF-ET, several nations established committees to evaluate the ethical aspects of this technology. Their deliberations concluded that up to 14 days after fertilization the human embryo does not have to be protected absolutely and can therefore be disposed of under certain circumstances, including being used for research. In the United Kingdom, where this recommendation was made by the Warnock Committee, the Medical Research Council and the Royal College of Obstetricians and Gynaecologists established a Voluntary Licensing Authority for Human In Vitro Fertilization and Embryology.[16] Its main term of reference is "To approve a code of practice on research related to human fertilization and embryology."

At the first meeting of this body it was decided to introduce the word *pre-embryo* to denote the phase of life up to 14 days after fertilization. Most members of the committee "hoped that this term would be more easily understood by the lay public than the equally correct term 'conceptus' or 'zygote'." Since then, the Ethical Committee of the American Fertility Society has enthusiastically adopted the word and attempted to establish that it has sound biologic foundations.[17]

The word *pro-embryo* was suggested as an alternative to preembryo by Professor Roger Short to the Senate Select Committee of the Australian Government considering human embryo experimentation in Australia. The use of these words has not been without controversy. For this reason the Senate Select Committee preferred not to use them in favor of the word *embryo*.[13] In my view these efforts are unfruitful for an informed debate on ethical issues, and represent a misreading of scientific fact.

False claims or the misrepresentation of scientific facts should be of particular concern to scientists in the United States, because scientific respectability has been explicitly claimed for bills concerning human life that have been introduced before the United States Congress. In 1981 two so-called human life bills were introduced before the 97th Congress. The House of Representatives bill (H.R. 3225) contained the following clause: "Present day scientific evidence indicates that a human being exists from conception" (section 2(a)). The Senate bill (S. 158) stated, "The Congress finds that present day scientific evidence indicates a significant likelihood that actual human life exists from conception" (section 1). Note that the author of the Senate bill was not so sure that human life exists from conception and used the language of probability theory in this tentative assertion.

These two bills did not pass; however, similar bills continue to be introduced in which science is invoked in support of statements of this kind. A Senate bill (S. 1242) was before the recent 100th Congress that was called the "President's pro-life bill of 1987." Section 2 stated, "The Congress finds that—(1) *scientific* evidence demonstrates that abortion takes the life of an unborn child who is a living human being."

In the 1988 state of the union address, President Reagan substituted the word *scientific* with the word *medical*. The intended scope of this assertion is indicated by section 2 of a proposed amendment to the Constitution (H.J. Res. 104), which was also introduced before the 100th Congress, and which states, "With respect to the right to life guaranteed to persons by the fifth and fourteenth articles of amendment to the Constitution, the word 'person' applies to all human beings, including their unborn offspring at every stage of their biological development including fertilization."

When this amendment was first published in the *National Right to Life News,* a footnote explained that the amendment should apply from the beginning of fertilization. These proposals in Congress are attempts to legalize an axiom on which to base a moral code whose primary purpose is to outlaw abortion. The axiom is similar to that proposed by Reid.[15] It must be recognized by the public, however, that this action could have negative effects, for it would interfere with several aspects of reproductive medicine that many members of society find desirable even if they object to abortion.

HISTORY OF UNDERSTANDING CONCEPTION

Human beings have been interested in generation since ancient times, yet a verifiable scientific explanation of the mechanisms involved was only reached during the early part of the present century. If science is to be invoked in ethical debates and the formulation of public policy, the scientific history of how this understanding was reached must be clearly understood.

Conception is an old medieval word that first appeared in ecclesiastic writings. It is derived from the Latin root *capio*, which means to grasp, take hold, receive into the body. St. Thomas Aquinas, one of the great scholars of the 13th century, wrote, "the *conception* of a male is not completed *(non perficitur)* until about the fortieth day, . . . that of a female not until about the ninetieth day."[18] Three centuries later, in 1615, Cooke commented, "*Conception* is nothing els but the wombs receiuing and imbracing of the seede."[19]

Conception was used in these senses prior to the 1820s. Up to that time a wide variety of theories of generation were held with respect to how and when embryos were formed. The theories can be characterized under one of four headings: epigenesis, metamorphosis, pre-existence, and preformation.[20-22] Epigenesis, an idea with its origins in the writings of Aristotle, was defined in the 17th century by William Harvey as the sequential production of the parts of an embryo. He contrasted this mechanism with metamorphosis, in which all parts of the embryo appear simultaneously some time after conception. Pre-existence embraces all theories that held that organisms exist in the form of miniatures since the creation of the universe, stored up one generation within another. Preformation refers to theories that hold that a miniature that grows into a whole organism is formed within the body of the parent, which in its original version is through the agency of the soul.

There were also theories about the source of the embryo. The earliest was the twin-semen theory, originally due to Aristotle, which held that the embryo originates from the admixture of male and female secretions within the mother's body. This view was challenged in 1651 by Harvey[23] with his famous dictum, all individuals come from eggs. Then, after the invention of the microscope by Leeuwenhoek, and the first observation of human spermatozoa by his pupil Hamm in 1679,[24] a contrasting theory arose that all individuals come from spermatozoa.[25] Preformationists then fell into two groups, the ovists, who believed that miniatures were present in eggs, and the animaculists, who believed that miniatures were present in spermatozoa. The over-enthusiastic use of the microscope led to the publication of such illustrations as Hartsoeker's drawing of the homunculus (Fig. 39–1).

At this time, however, not all scientists accepted that spermatozoa were involved in reproduction even in the face of convincing evidence. In 1780 Spallanzani showed in frogs that if semen is filtered through paper it loses its ability to stimulate eggs to develop. If the material on the paper is washed into water containing eggs, the eggs are then activated. Despite this evidence Spallanzani was such a convinced ovist that he rejected the notion that spermatozoa are

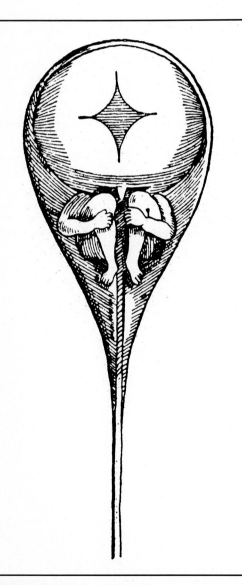

Figure 39–1. The homonculus—a 17th century representation of the human spermatozoon, drawn by Hartsoeker. (From Needham.[25] Reproduced with permission.)

concerned in generation.[26,27] It may not be surprising therefore that Linnaeus at about the same time classified spermatozoa in a group of "living molecules" under the name *Chaos infusorium.*[28] They included (1) the contagion of eruptive fevers, (2) the cause of paroxysmal fevers, (3) the moist virus of syphilis, (4) the airy mist floating in the month of blossoming, (5) Munchhausen's septic agent of fermentation and putrefaction, and (6) Leeuwenhoek's spermatic animalcules.

Thus, at the end of the 18th century the current understanding of generation was rudimentary. It was summarized by Haighton[29] in 1797 as follows: "Physiologists are by no means agreed concerning the immediate cause of conception. All admit the necessity of sexual intercourse. They acknowledge too the necessity of some part of the female being affected by the direct contact of a fecundating fluid, but what the precise part is which must receive the stimulus, has hitherto been involved in mystery and doubt."

It was over the next 80 years that two major questions were answered: what are the roles of spermatozoa and ova in the generation of sexually reproducing organisms? What is the anatomic site in mammals where the ova and spermatozoa interact?

Evidence that spermatozoa are specifically involved in generation was first produced by the French physiologists Prevost and Dumas.[20-32] Among several studies, they repeated the experiments of Spallanzini and obtained the same results. They were not ovists, however, and so they concluded correctly that spermatozoa are involved in generation, and produced quantitative evidence that only one spermatozoon is needed to initiate development. They also argued, with considerable perspicacity, that whatever leaves the mammalian ovary is considerably smaller than the graafian follicle. Three years later in 1827, Von Baer[33] confirmed this speculation when he observed a mammalian egg, that of a dog, for the first time.

None of these investigators understood the roles of the ovum and spermatozoon in fertilization, however. Another 12 years passed before further progress was made. In 1837 Martin Barry,[34-36] a graduate of Edinburgh Medical School, "spent some time in Germany for the purpose of becoming acquainted with the known facts on animal development and other objects of microscopic research." Among those who provided him with facilities was Theodor Schwann, one of the proponents of the cell theory, who in 1838 suggested that the ovum was a cell. Barry was clearly influenced by the "doctrine of the cells," for he used the ideas extensively in his papers on mammalian generation. In 1840 he published a diagram that he suggested showed that a spermatozoon actually penetrates an ovum at the time of fecundation (Fig. 39–2). It was at this time that the

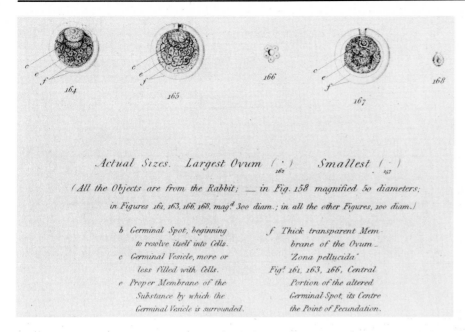

Figure 39–2. The first illustration, published in 1840, suggesting that a spermatozoon has entered an ovum. (From reference 36.)

word *fertilization* was introduced into the scientific literature. Fertilization originally meant to make land fruitful or productive. Its first use in a specific scientific sense, that I have been able to trace, is by the educator William Carpenter, another graduate of Edinburgh Medical School. He used the word in the first edition of his book *Principles of General and Comparative Physiology*, published in 1839, in a discussion of generation in plants.[37] It was Barry's illustration that caused Carpenter in the second (1841) edition of his textbook to suggest that the eggs of animals were stimulated to develop in a comparable manner.[38]

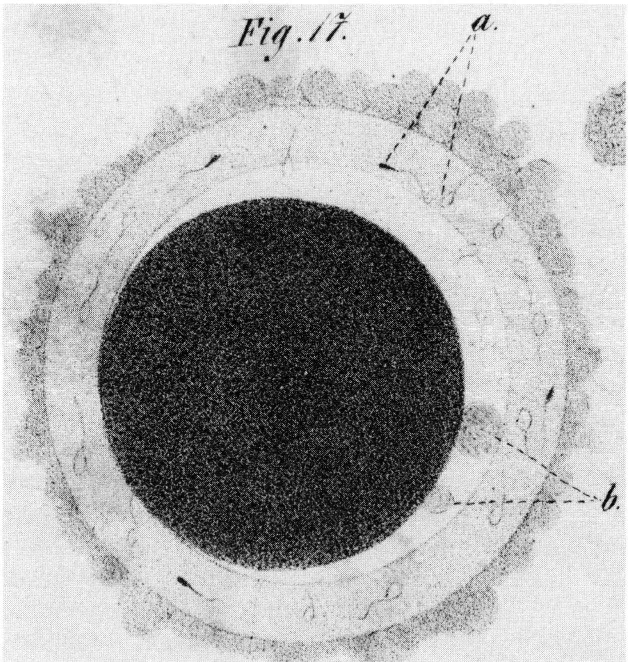

Despite Carpenter's enthusiasm, the suggestion that spermatozoa enter ova was met with skepticism. Certainly the diagram Barry published was not particularly convincing. A major critic was the German embryologist Theodore Bischoff. In a treatise on the early development of the rabbit,[39] he reported the association of spermatozoa with the egg, but his illustration shows them only in the zona pellucida (Fig. 39–3). He stated explicitly that he had been unable to convince himself that a spermatozoon comes to lie in the interior of the ovum. One year later Barry repeated his claim of sperm penetration and supported it with an illustration showing spermatozoa inside the ovum[41,42] (Fig. 39–4). It was not clear, however, whether the sperm were in the embryo proper or in the perivitelline space. In further studies on the early development of the dog, guinea pig, and deer, Bischoff maintained his skepticism, and his illustrations showing sperm in the zona pellucida seem to be merely decorative.[42–44] As a result, Barry and Bischoff entered into a bitter controversy.[45–48]

The ancient view of the seat of conception held that it was the uterus. In the 17th century, beginning with De Graaf, it was believed that conception occurred in the ovary.[49] This view persisted until the mid-19th century, but it did not go unchallenged. Prevost and Dumas[32] believed that the spermatozoa exert their influence in the fallopian tubes, and

Figure 39–3. Bischoff's drawing, published in 1842, of spermatozoa in the outer layers of the rabbit ovum. (From Bischoff.[39])

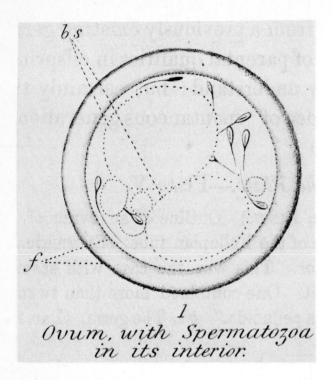

Figure 39–4. Barry's second illustration, published in 1843, shows spermatozoa within the ovum of a cleaving rabbit embryo. (From Barry.[41])

Ritchie[49] argued it was in the uterus, just as the ancients believed. The problem was considerably clarified in a pamphlet by Bischoff, written in German, which attracted sufficient attention in England and the United States that it was translated independently in both countries.[50,51] The regard with which the work was held is indicated by a statement of Louis Agassiz of Harvard, who wrote in recommending it for translation, "Never were experi-

ments upon this long vexed question conducted with more skill and success and never were the physiological views derived from them deduced with more accuracy and precision."[52]

In it, a so-called law of mammalian generation was developed:

> Both in mammals and in man, the self-forming ova undergo, in the ovaries of the female individuals, a periodical maturation, quite independently of the influence of the male seminal fluid. At this period these mature ova disengage themselves from the ovary, and are extruded. If copulation takes place, by the material influence of the semen upon the ovum, the fecundation of the latter results. If copulation does not take place, the ovum is nevertheless extruded from the ovary, and enters the fallopian tube, but there proves abortive. The influence of the semen must, however, always be exercised within the tube, in order to produce development of the ovum, which, indeed, first commences its evolution within that duct.

Ten years passed, however, before Bischoff accepted Barry's belief that spermatozoa penetrate the ovum.

Another 20 years elapsed before the true nature of fertilization was established in the rabbit by Van Beneden,[51] that is, that one spermatozoon fuses with one ovum and that the nuclear material from the two cells interacts. It was during these studies of rabbit generation that Van Beneden learned of the work of Oscar Hertwig[53] at the Stazione Zoologica, Naples, on the pronuclei of the sea urchin, and he immediately saw its relevance to his work. The understanding of the cytologic events in fertilization was finally completed by the work of Fol[54] on the starfish in 1877, during which he actually observed the entrance cone through which a spermatozoon enters an ovum (Fig. 39–5).

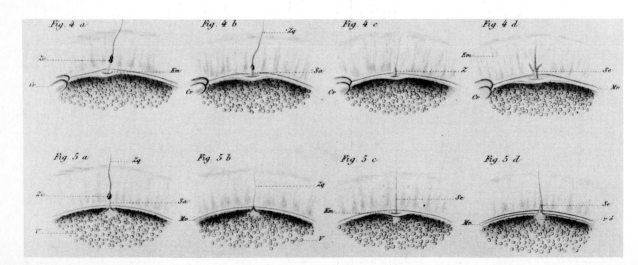

Figure 39–5. Fol's illustrations of spermatozoa entering an ovum in the starfish, published in 1879. (From Fol.[54])

The cell that results from the fusion of a spermatozoon and an ovum was called the *zygote* in 1891. Thus the basis was laid for a modern definition of conception found in 1966 in Webster's *Third New International Dictionary:* "Formation of a viable zygote (fertilization results in the conception of a new entity capable of developing into a being like its parent)." By this definition the meanings of conception and fertilization have converged, and for practical purposes the words are synonymous.

CATHOLIC INTERPRETATION OF CONCEPTION

The difference in the meanings of conception and fertilization is illustrated clearly in the history of the Catholic interpretation of conception.[19] The Aristotelian interpretation used by St. Thomas Aquinas regards it as a process. Although the beginning of conception is not identified, the end of conception is given by the elapsed time, which varies with the sex of the fetus (40 days for the male and 90 days for the female). Prior to completion of conception, the embryo was said to be *informis* and *inanimatus,* while after the completion of conception it was said to be *formatus* and *animatus.* The distinction was important. Until 1869, causing the death of an animate fetus was culpable, whereas causing the death of an inanimate embryo was not. For a brief period from 1588, as the result of a bill issued by Pope Sixtus V, the destruction of both inanimate and animate stages was condemned, the punishment being excommunication without the possibility of absolution. These structures were soon amended by Pope Urban VII, who in 1591 changed the bill to read, "The penalties for procuring the abortion of an inanimate fetus or for administering or taking potions to cause women to be sterile we revoke just as if that constitution so far as it concerns these things had never been issued."

By 1860 the Catholic teaching on this question was beginning to be reversed again to the more stringent position decreed by Pope Sixtus V. Thus in a letter to Horatio Storrer,[55] one of the leading opponents of abortion in the United States of the last century and chairman of a committee on abortion of the fledgling American Medical Association, Bishop Fitzpatrick of Boston wrote

> that the destruction of the human foetus in the womb of the mother, at any period from the first instance of conception, is a heinous crime, equal, at least, in guilt to that of murder. The very instant conception has taken place, there lies the vital germ of a man. It may already be a living man, for neither mothers nor physicians can tell when life is infused; they can only tell when its presence is manifested, and there is a wide difference between these two things.

In 1869 Pope Pius IX declared, "excommunicate all who procured abortion, without distinction either as to method, direct or indirect, intentional or involuntary, or as to gestational age of the fetus, whether it were formed or unformed, animate or inanimate." This ruling was introduced in response to the rapidly spreading practice of abortion in Europe and the United States. The prohibition stands today.

The declaration of Pope Pius IX was issued before the process of fertilization was finally understood in 1877. Once the meanings of conception and fertilization became synonymous, however, it was natural to assume that the prohibition applied from the time when fertilization occurs. Moreover, since a new adult human being will form from a fertilized egg, if all goes well, it is also natural, but naive, to conclude that life begins in the biologic sense at conception.

THE LIFE CYCLE

The problem with the proposal that life begins at conception is that it does not take into account the cycle of life.[56] A phenomenon known from the early part of the 19th century was the alternation of generations. First described by Chamisso in 1819,[57] it arose from the fact that some organisms occur in different alternate morphologic forms. Before this phenomenon could be explained, the existence of somatic cells and germ cells had to be discovered. Immediately after the discovery of fertilization, several investigators had the idea that two types of cells were in the early embryo. Weissman finally formulated a unified explanation in 1893 by applying the rapid advances in the newly emerging science of cytology.[58,59] His theory came to be known as the theory of the continuity of the germ plasm.

A key observation that led to the theory was made by Van Beneden[60] in studies on fertilization in *Ascaris,* showing that at fertilization each parent contributes an equal number of chromosomes, called the haploid number. Thus the total number of chromosomes in the zygote is twice the haploid number and is called the diploid number. Weissman,[61] among others, recognized that when gametes are formed again, the cells must undergo a unique type of division that reduces the number of chromosomes to the haploid number. The process that mediates this reduction was eventually shown to be a mechanism present in both sexually reproducing plants and animals, and was given the name meiosis.

The recognition of meiosis enabled Farmer and Moore[62] to partition the life cycle into the premeiotic phase, which begins at fertilization, and the postmeiotic phase, which ends at fertilization. Thus life never ends. In current language we speak of the premeiotic phase as the diploid phase and the postmeiotic phase as the haploid phase (Fig. 39–6).[63] In animals the haploid phase is very short and does not give rise to a haploid multicellular phase as in plants. Nevertheless, the unicellular haploid phase that exists in animal life cycles—the ovum and spermatozoon—is essential for the perpetuation of the species. The ovum and sperm are produced by the process of

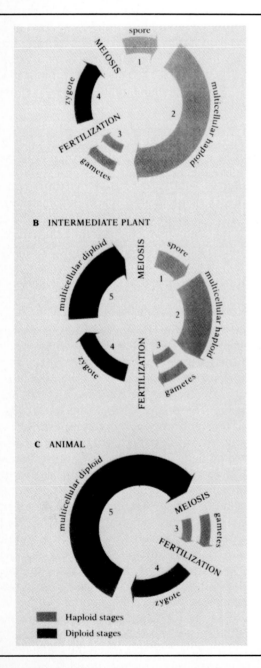

B INTERMEDIATE PLANT

C ANIMAL

▓ Haploid stages

█ Diploid stages

Figure 39–6. The phases of the life cycle of plants and animals, showing how fertilization and meiosis are transitions between the diploid and haploid stages. (From Keeton.[63] Reproduced with permission.)

meiosis, which marks the transition from the diploid to the haploid phase, and the zygote is produced by the process of fertilization, marking the return to the diploid phase from the haploid phase. All individuals of both phases are alive, and meiosis and fertilization are equally important transitions in the cycle of life. Also of importance is the fact that although human spermatozoa and ova are single cells, they are each genetically unique members of the haploid phase of human life. Similarly, human zygotes are single cells that are genetically unique members of the diploid phase of human life. Thus genetic uniqueness is not a property restricted to diploid life.

I reiterate that life, in the biologic sense, does not begin at conception or fertilization, for it never stops. It is a continuous process, a fact also emphasized by Mill.[64] To ask when life begins is the wrong question; the reply that life begins at conception is incorrect. Biologically correct statements would be, "diploid life begins as the result of fertilization," and, "haploid life begins as the result of meiosis." Then valid ethical questions would take the form, "are the moral values of haploid and diploid life equal?" and, "if not, are the moral values of all stages of diploid life equal?"

These are questions that science has helped to formulate. They are moral questions, however, whose answers fall outside the realm of science.

PRE-EMBRYOS

The word *pre-embryo* was introduced due to the perceived need for a term understandable by the public in the licensing of research on early prenatal human beings.[16] After considering several points of view as to how long an embryo should be kept alive in vitro, the Warnock Committee[14] recommended

> that no live human embryo derived from in vitro fertilization, whether frozen or unfrozen, may be kept alive, if not transferred to a women, beyond 14 days after fertilization, nor may it be used as a research subject beyond 14 days after fertilization. This 14-day period does not include any time during which the embryo may have been frozen. We further recommend that it shall be a criminal offense to handle or to use as a research subject any live human embryo derived from in vitro fertilization beyond that limit. We recommend that no embryo which has been used for research should be transferred to a woman.

The need for a specific time—14 days—in making this recommendation is a legal one. In making their choice of a cutoff time the committee was faced with options ranging from the beginning of implantation (about 7 days) to the first signs of development of a central nervous system (22 to 23 days). They selected 14 days after fertilization on the grounds that by then the primitive streak develops in the germinal disk, after which time the embryo begins its individual development. They also felt it met the suggestions of some individuals that the cutoff time should be when implantation is completed. That it should be associated with the completion of implantation was recommended in 1979 in the report of the Ethics Advisory Board of the former U.S. Department of Health, Education, and Welfare.[65] The definition of pre-embryo as applied to the human is a prenatal individual from fertilization to one that has developed a primitive streak, or from 1 to 14 days inclusive. Despite the recommendation of the Ethics Advisory Board that federally supported research on human embryos up to 14 days of age be allowed subject to certain restrictions, it has never been implemented because of the de facto moratorium on fetal research put in place in 1975 by the department of HEW.

The partitioning of prenatal development into developmental periods is not a new idea. In 1930 Arey[66] suggested three periods, those of the ovum, the embryo, and the fetus. He proposed that the period of the ovum in the human ends at the end of the second week after fertilization, when the embryonic disk forms by the apposition of the floor of the early amnion and the roof of the yolk sac. This critical time corresponds with the cutoff time recommended by the Warnock Committee. From a scientific point of view, however, it is important to recognize, as several embryologists have done, that the selection of this stage of development for the purpose of classification is arbitrary. For example, Patten[67] wrote, "Terms designating 'stages of development' are convenient in discussing the progress of events, and the relative uniformity which has gradually been established in their usage is a great aid in mutual understanding. It should be borne in mind, however, that the delimitation of 'stages' is purely arbitrary, for development is a continuous process and one phase merges into another without any real point of demarcation."

The word pre-embryo is rapidly being adopted in the medical and ethical literature, due in part to its strong endorsement by the Ethics Committee of the American Fertility Society.[17] In their report they attempted to attribute special features to a pre-embryo that set it apart from later stages, instead of recognizing the arbitrary nature of the word. The features described are first that the prenatal individual is largely extraembryonic in nature; that the descendents of most of its cells will give rise to the placenta and fetal membranes, which are only temporary organs discarded at birth. The second argument is that after the 14th day of development, identical twins cannot form by the process of polyembryony. In this process more than one primitive

streak is laid down in the germinal disk, which leads to the formation of two genetically identical individuals. Thus it is argued the human organism less than 14 days old is not committed to develop into a single individual.

These characteristics of the human organism less than 14 days old are unrelated and seem to provide little compelling scientific justification to set this period aside with the specific name of pre-embryo. The quantitative argument that the organism is largely extraembryonic overlooks the more important fact that by the time the blastocyst forms (about 4 days after fertilization), a few cells are irreversibly committed to the inner cell mass where organogenesis takes place.[68] Even if only one cell were committed in the blastocyst, the organism contains a cell whose descendents will participate in the development of an adult human being. Although it is scientifically correct to state that polyembryony cannot occur in the human organism that is more than 14 days old, it serves only to emphasize a fact that does not seem to be a profound occurrence in the life cycle, namely, that the organism can on rather rare occasions duplicate its genotype.

In my view there is little to recommend the use of pre-embryo as a scientific term. It has the disadvantage of being a potentially behavior-governing, prejudicial word in an ethical debate, because it suggests to many people that, because it is not an embryo, its moral value is lower than that of the embryo. This is an opinion that cannot be justified on scientific grounds.

TOWARD ETHICAL SOLUTIONS

Three arguments are sometimes invoked to justify the view that a zygote produced at fertilization acquires full moral status and must be protected absolutely: (1) the genetic argument, (2) the discontinuity–continuity argument, and (3) the individuality argument.[69] These were analyzed in detail by the Australian geneticist and bioethicist Dawson, who held that none of them is internally consistent, and that it is unconvincing to claim that fertilization is a determinant of moral status. I believe that all three arguments are deficient for failing to recognize that fertilization is a transition in the life cycle, and for failing to explain the assumption that the moral value of a diploid individual is greater than that of an haploid individual. I agree with Dawson that it is inappropriate to base public policy or legislation regulating reproduction technology on the claim that fertilization is a determinant of moral status.

A physiologic fact that seldom enters into debates on the moral status of the prenatal human embryo is its relationship with its mother. For the first few days after fertilization the maternal organism continues to function as though she is nonpregnant. Her reproductive processes are under the control of the hormones produced by her ovaries just as though she was in the second half of her menstrual cycle. Approximately 8 days after fertilization, a signal from the embryo passes to the mother that causes her ovaries to switch to a function characteristic of pregnancy. Thus the mother is not physiologically aware of the presence of an embryo until that time at the earliest. She cannot become conscious of the pregnancy until the first missed menstrual period. For this reason Bengt Boving[70] proposed that the word *conception* refer to the act of becoming pregnant, thus associating conception with the process of implantation. This is an alternative definition of conception, to be found in Webster's dictionary. Also it is the one adopted in 1972 by the nomenclature committee of the College of Obstetricians and Gynecologists.[71] At that time, the proposal came under fire from those who opposed the use of the intrauterine device as a contraceptive. They believed that it was a verbal maneuver to overcome their objections to the possibility that the devices kill very early embryos. In view of the difficulties of using fertilization to assess the moral status of an embryo, it seems worthwhile to reconsider the proposal of Boving in an impartial manner.

The way we think about life depends on the way we are educated, which in turn depends on our cultural heritage. Although I have reverence for all phases of the human life cycle and their individual members, and experience a sense of awe when I work with them, my own beliefs do not place equal moral value on haploid and diploid human life, nor do they give equal weight to the moral value of all phases of the diploid phase of the life cycle. From an adult perspective, as I contemplate the human life cycle I experience a type of what philosophers call moral distancing. For example, although I am concerned about death, I would be more affected by the loss of a close relative as the result of a car accident than by the death of people unknown to me dying from an earthquake on the other side of the globe. I have little concern about the disposal of human spermatozoa or unfertilized ova. I have more concern about human preimplantation embryos, but not sufficient to cause difficulties over their loss as, say, the result of having to dispose of spare embryos in the course of treating a woman for infertility by in-vitro fertilization, or by preventing their development by the use of an intrauterine device. Interrupting the development of an embryo that is undergoing organogenesis gives me more concern, while interfering with a fetus with the beginnings of an adult appearance gives me great concern. It is for these reasons that the selective reduction of multifetal pregnancies in the first

trimester[72] causes me uneasiness compared to the disposal of spare embryos.

The basis of these feelings is hard to justify, and they cannot stand alone as the basis for establishing the moral status of the different stages of embryonic life. If my moral judgements are based only on whether biologic life is present, I would assign equal moral value to all phases of the life cycle and not be prepared to allow destruction of any members, including spermatozoa and unfertilized ova. My judgments are perhaps made on another meaning of life, recognized by the use of different words in the ancient Greek language, which categorized "having a life" as distinct from "being alive."[73] An analysis of our moral attitudes to the early human embryo would be more rational if those attitudes were based on an examination of the role of moral distancing as applied to the life cycle, coupled with an examination of the times when, in the words of the Oxford philosopher Jonathon Glover,[74] it is permissible to cause death or save lives.

It is very likely that pure moral conservatives will not accept this approach and will insist that any discussion should accept the axiom that life begins at conception. Utilitarian moral conservatives will not be happy with this approach because of the flexibility it gives to defining the onset of "having a life." They fear that any relaxation will mark the beginning of a slippery slope in which more controversial reproductive technologies will be condoned. They argue, for example, that IVF-ET will pave the way for sex selection by transferring only embryos of one sex. Dealing with these different fundamental attitudes takes us back to the fifth category of ethical problem mentioned at the beginning of this chapter: How do we resolve moral conflicts that arise between members of a pluralistic society who hold different views on these issues?[75]

CONCLUSION

I would like to make a few general remarks concerning ways of approaching ethical issues involved in reproductive technology. Science is subject to a rigid discipline and is self-correcting. This discipline should be invoked when scientists see science being misused or misinterpreted in the establishment of ethical principles or public policy. The misinterpretation of science by special-interest groups in support of their cause cannot be tolerated. I have emphasized the central role of the life cycle and I have used it to argue that the selection of transitions in the cycle, such as fertilization, as cutoff points cannot be logically justified. I advocate therefore that the time has come for a different approach.

We should seek solutions to ethical problems in

reproductive technology that are acceptable in a pluralistic society. Instead of basing our solutions on some general theory about the nature of human life, such as life begins at conception or the doctrine that human life is begotten and not made.[76] we should adopt a multipartite approach.[77] We should consider separately, for example, the use of IVF-ET to treat infertility, the diagnosis of the sex of early embryos for sex control, the use of spare embryos for research, and the production of embryos for research. As an example, consider an infertile woman whose only chance of having a child is by means of IVF-ET. I think most of us would agree that giving her a chance to have her own child is good. It is a right recognized in the Charter of the United Nations. In the present state of the art, however, IVF-ET always has the potential of yielding more embryos than needed. Which do we prefer? Not treating the woman at all? Treating the woman but applying global principle that says all fertilized ova must be returned to the patient, with the attendant risks of multiple pregnancies and economic disruption of the family? Treating the woman but freezing and storing all spare embryos, thus putting off the ethical decision about their disposal to the indefinite future? Or treating the woman but applying a local principle that recognizes that very early embryos may not have the same moral value as older fetuses, and that the spare unused embryos were at least necessary to ensure the birth of a healthy baby?

We have come through several centuries of fables about generation into an era in which the facts of generation are understood scientifically in terms of the life cycle. All phases of the cycle are living and all members of the human life cycle are genetically unique. Do we now want to adhere to the nonscientific foible that life begins at conception in making ethical decisions?

REFERENCES

1. Biggers JD, McLaren A: "Test-tube" animals. The culture and transfer of early mammalian embryos. *Discovery* 19:423, 1958.
2. Steptoe PC, Edward RG: Birth after the reimplantation of a human embryo. *Lancet* 2:366, 1978.
3. McCormick RA: *How Brave a New World.* New York, Doubleday, 1981.
4. Walters L: The fetus in ethical and public policy: Discussion from 1973 to the present, in Bondeson WB et al (eds): *Abortion and the Status of the Fetus.* Dordrecht, Reidel, 1983, pp 15–30.
5. Edwards R, Steptoe P: *A Matter of Life.* London, Hutchinson, 1980.
6. Congregation for the Doctrine of the Faith: *Instruction on Respect for Human Life in its Origin and on the Dignity of Procreation.* Boston, Daughters of St Paul, 1987, pp 16–32.
7. Trounson A, Mohr L: Human pregnancy following cryopreservation, thawing and transfer of an eight-cell embryo. *Nature* 305:707, 1983.
8. Siebzehrubl E, Trotnow S, Weigel M, et al: Pregnancy after in vitro fertilization, cryopreservation and embryo transfer. *J IVF/ET* 3:261, 1986.
9. Editorial: In vitro fertilization. *J Med Ethics* 9:187, 1983.
10. Snow CP: *Public Affairs.* New York, Scribners, 1971, pp 13–79.
11. Moore JA: Science as a way of knowing—Genetics. *Am Zool* 26:583, 1986.
12. Regan T: Introduction, in Regan T (ed): *Matters of Life and Death.* New York, Random House, 1980, pp 3–27.
13. Senate Select Committee on the Human Embryo Experimentation Bill 1985: *Human Embryo Experimentation in Australia.* Australian Government Publishing Service, 1986, sect 2.14, p 11.
14. Department of Health and Social Security: *Report of the Committee of Inquiry into Human Fertilization and Embryology.* London, Her Majesty's Stationery Office, 1984.
15. Reidy M: Ethical issues in reproductive medicine: From the perspective of moral theology, in Reidy M (ed): *Ethical Issues in Reproductive Medicine.* Dublin, Gill & Macmillan, 1982, pp 118–145.
16. Voluntary Licensing Authority for Human In Vitro Fertilization and Embryology: *First Report.* London, Medical Research Council, 1986, p 8.
17. Ethics Committee of the American Fertility Society: Ethical considerations of the new reproductive technologies. *Fertil Steril* 46(suppl 1):1S, 1986.
18. Dunstan GR: The moral status of the human embryo: A tradition recalled. *J Med Ethics* 10:38, 1984.
19. Murray JAH, Bradley H, Craigie WA, Onions CT: Oxford English Dictionary. Oxford, Oxford University Press, 1933, pp 760–761.
20. Roger J: *Les sciences de la vie dans la pensée francaise du XVIII siècle.* Paris, Armand Colin, 1963, p 325.
21. Wilkie JS: Preformation and epigenesis: A new historical treatment. *Hist Sci* 6:138, 1967.
22. Bowler PJ: Preformation and pre-existence in the seventeenth century: A brief analysis. *J Hist Biol* 4:221, 1971.
23. Harvey W: *De Generatione.* London, 1651.
24. Leeuwenhoek A: Observationes D. Anthonii Lewenhoeck, de natis e semini genitali animalculis. *Philos Trans R Soc Lond (Biol)* 12:1040–1043, 1679.
25. Needham J: *A History of Embryology.* Cambridge, Cambridge University Press, 1959, pp 206–211.
26. Cole FJ: *Early Theories of Sexual Generation.* Oxford, Oxford University Press, 1930, pp 182–194.
27. Tyler A: Introduction: Problems and procedures of comparative gametology and syngamy, in Metz CB, Monroy A (eds): *Fertilization.* New York, Academic Press, 1967, vol 1, pp 9–19.
28. Dobell C: *Antony van Leeuwenhoek and His "Little Animals": Being Some Account of the Father of Protozoology and Bacteriology and his Multifarious Discoveries in these Disciplines.* New York, Dover, 1960.
29. Haighton J: An experimental inquiry concerning animal impregnation. *Philos Trans R Soc Lond (Biol)* 18:112, 1797.
30. Prevost JL, Dumas JBA: Nouvelle theorie de la génération. *Ann Sci Nat Paris* 1:1, 1824.
31. Prevost JL, Dumas JBA: Deuxieme memoire sur la génération. *Ann Sci Nat Paris* 2:100, 1824.
32. Prevost JL, Dumas JBA: De la génération dans les mammifères, et des premiers indices du developpement de l'embryos. *Ann Sci Nat Paris* 3:113, 1824.
33. Von Baer C: *De Ovi Mammalium et Hominis Genesi* (1827). Brussels, Impression Anastaltique, Culture et Civilation, Bruxelles, 1966, p 37.
34. Barry M: Researches in embryology. First series. *Philos Trans R Soc Lond (Biol)* 1:301, 1838.
35. Barry M: Researches in embryology. Second series. *Philos Trans R Soc Lond (Biol)* 2:307, 1839.
36. Barry M: Researches in embryology. Third series. *Philos Trans R Soc Lond (Biol)* 3:529, 1840.
37. Carpenter WB: *Principles of General and Comparative Physiology.* London, Churchill, 1839.
38. Carpenter WB: *Principles of General and Comparative Physiology,* ed 2. London, Churchill, 1841.
39. Bischoff TLW: *Entwicklungsgeschichte des Kaninchen-Eies,* Braunschweig, Friedrich Vieweg, 1842.
40. Barry M: Spermatozoa observed within the mammiferous ovum. *Philos Trans R Soc Lond (Biol)* 133, 1843.
41. Barry M: On fissiparous generation. *Edinb New Phil J* 35:205, 1843.
42. Bischoff TLW: *Entwicklungsgeschichte des Hunde-Eis.* Braunschweig, Friedrich Vieweg, 1845.
43. Bischoff TLW: *Entwicklungsgeschichte des Meerschweinchens.* Geissen, J. Ricker'sche Buchhandlung, 1845.
44. Bischoff TLW: *Entwicklungsgeschichte des Rehes.* Geissen, J. Ricker'sche Buchhandlung, 1854.
45. Keber F. *Eintritt der Samenzellen in das Ei.* Konigsberg, Kommission bei den Gebrudern Borntrager, 1854.
46. Barry M: Confirmation in two quarters of the discovery by Keber, of the

penetration of a remarkable body, believed by him to be a spermatozoon, into the ovum of the fresh water mussel. *Monthly J Med* 20:33, 1855.

47. Barry M: Meissner shown to have been the first who confirmed the fact that the spermatozoon penetrates into the interior of the ovum of the rabbit, the animal in which penetration was first observed. *Monthly J Med* 20:140, 1855.

48. Barry M: Postscript to a paper in the January number of this journal, confirming the discovery by Keber of a remarkable body penetrating the ovum of the fresh water mussel. *Monthly J Med* 20:313, 1855.

49. Ritchie C: Contributions to the physiology of the human ovary. *London Med Gaz* 36(1):509, 1845.

50. Bischoff TLW: The periodical maturation and extrusion of ova, independently of coitus, in mammalia and man, proved to be the primary condition to their propagation. *London Med Gaz* 35:443, 1844–1845.

51. Gilman CR, Tellkampf T: *Tracts on Generation*. New York, Wood, 1847.

52. Van Beneden E: Le maturation de l'oeuf, la fécondation et les primieres phases du developpement embryonnaire des mammiferes d'après des recherches faites chez le lapin. *Bull Acad Soc Lettres Beaux Arts Belg* 40:686, 1875.

53. Hertwig O: Beitrage zur Kenntniss der Bildung, Befruchtrung und Teilung des tierischen Eies. *Morphol Jahrb* 1:347, 1876.

54. Fol H: Recherches sur la fécondation et le commencement de l'henogenie chez divers animaux. *Men Soc Phys Hist Nat Geneve* 26:89, 1879.

55. Storrer HR: *On Criminal Abortion in America*. Philadelphia, Lippincott, 1860.

56. Biggers JD: When does life begin? *Sciences* Dec: 20, 1981.

57. Huxley TH: Observations upon the anatomy and physiology of *Salpa* and *Pyrosoma*. *Philos Trans R Soc Lond (Biol)* 2:567, 1851.

58. Weismann A: *The Germ-plasm: A Theory of Heredity*. New York, Scribner, 1893.

59. Wilson EB: *The Cell in Development and Heredity*. New York, Macmillan, 1925, pp 1–20.

60. Van Beneden E: Recherches sur la maturation de l'oeuf et la fécondation. *Arch Biol* 4:265, 1883.

61. Weismann A: *Essays upon Heredity and Kindred Biological Problems*. Oxford, Clarendon Press, 1887, vol 1, p 343.

62. Farmer JB, Moore JES: On the meiotic phase (reduction divisions) in animals and plants. *Q J Microbiol Sci* 48:489, 1905.

63. Keeton WT: *Biological Science*. New York, Norton, 1976, p 579.

64. Mill J: Some comments on Dr Iglesias's paper, In vitro fertilisation: The major issues. *J Med Ethics* 12:32, 1986.

65. Ethics Advisory Board, Department of Health, Education and Welfare: *HEW Support of Research Involving Human In Vitro Fertilization and Embryo Transfer*. Washington, DC, U.S. Government Printing Office, 1979.

66. Arey LB: *Developmental Anatomy*, ed 2. Philadelphia, Saunders, 1930.

67. Patten BM: *Human Embryology*. Philadelphia, Blakiston, 1946, p 62.

68. Pedersen RA: Potency, lineage, and allocation in preimplantation mouse embryos, in Rossant J, Pedersen RA (eds): *Experimental Approaches to Mammalian Embryonic Development*. Cambridge, Cambridge University Press, 1986, pp 3–33.

69. Dawson K: Fertilization and moral status: A scientific perspective. *J Med Ethics* 13:173, 1987.

70. Boving B: Implantation mechanisms, in Hartman CG (ed): *Mechanisms Concerned with Conception*. New York, Macmillan, 1963, pp 321–396.

71. Hughes EC: *Obstetric–Gynecologic Terminology*. Philadelphia, Davis, 1972. pp 299–304.

72. Berkowitz RL, Lynch L, Chitkar U, et al: Selective reduction of multifetal pregnancies in the first trimester. *N Engl J Med* 318:1043, 1988.

73. Kushner T: Having a life versus being alive. *J Med Ethics* 10:5, 1984.

74. Glover J: *Causing Death and Saving Lives*. Harmondsworth, Penguin, 1977.

75. Singer P, Wells D: *The Reproductive Revolution*. Oxford, Oxford University Press, 1984.

76. O'Donovan O: *Begotten or Made?* Oxford, Clarendon Press, 1984.

77. Held V: *Rights and Goods*. New York, Free Press, 1984.

PART X

Adoption

CHAPTER 40

The Adoption Alternative

Sharon Heim Jette

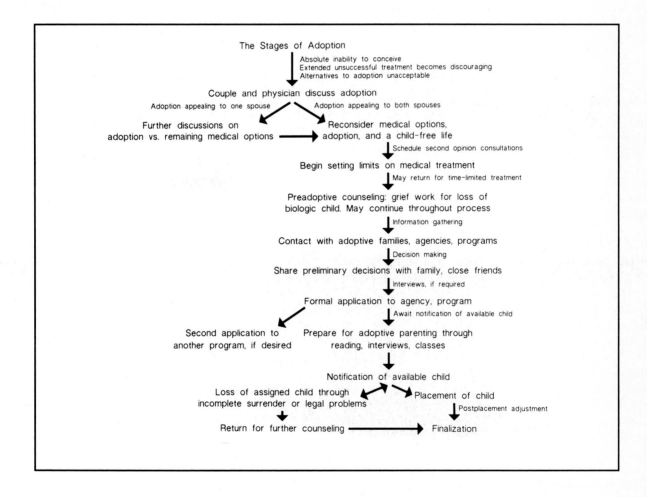

As a couple proceeds through extensive infertility tests and treatments without achieving a successful pregnancy, one or both partners may begin to consider adoption as an alternative way to build a family. The proliferation of adoption alternatives in the past decade has created an overlap of health and social services, called a "confluence of interest" in the field of adoption.[2] The practitioner must be prepared to give supportive information and referral without judgment. Assisting couples to gain current information and decide the merits of this alternative for themselves becomes an important role for the infertility practitioner.

ISSUES TO RESOLVE PRIOR TO ADOPTION

Rarely does the decision to adopt occur easily or spontaneously for infertile couples. Typically, one partner exhibits a readiness to adopt before the other, creating an unparallel course for decision making. While exploring adoption procedures, some couples express great relief that both members find this alternative acceptable; others learn that readiness to conceive does not guarantee readiness to adopt.

Second Choice or Second Best?

Although used interchangeably, the terms *second choice* and *second best* are not identical. If couples considering adoption can learn to differentiate between them, they can better acknowledge the facts and cope with feelings that will arise.[3]

Second choice indicates that a couple first elected to pursue biologic parenthood; adoption becomes, in fact, a second (or third or last) choice. Yet adoption need not be considered second best, as for many infertile couples it becomes the best possible and most realistic pathway to parenthood. In subsequent years successful parenting will depend upon the couple's ability to accept that, although acquired through an acknowledged second choice of method, their adopted children are not second best, but part of the best possible family.

While making the commitment to adopt, couples learn to break the cycle of failure produced by infertility or pregnancy loss. The challenge is to gain self-confidence as parents, regardless of their past history. Both partners must determine if, indeed, the child-free lifestyle would be a better alternative; both have to examine whether they can be satisfied with parenthood rather than pregnancy.

In addition, couples should determine if their decision to adopt is firm despite what others, even family and close friends, might think or say. Infertile couples are very much influenced by the reactions of families; adoption can intensify intergenerational conflict, with the infertile couple fearful of disappointing their parents.[3]

Shared Parenting

The traumas of loss and separation exist in adoption. The parents and child both experience loss; acknowledging these losses can help these families to bond. In a classic model of family development, adoptive parents are encouraged to identify the differences between their families and biologic families in order to cope with the losses.[5] A newer model acknowledges that adoption places unique stresses on the family's development, and again, encourages parents to face these differences rather than deny them.[6]

When considering an adoption, therefore, couples must decide whether they have the courage to be different. They must ask themselves if they can become parents without having exclusive parenting rights; the biologic parents have rights that may be exercised at the time of placement or much later in life. The adopted children also have rights. They have been separated through no fault of their own from their heritage and may wish to gain contact with their biologic family when they are older.

Couples often fear that they will inherit a set of problems beyond their ability to manage. Studies of the question of heredity versus environment indicate that substantial genetic transmission of cognitive ability does occur but is not predicatable for specific traits.[7] Environmental variables also significantly influence an adopted child's mental development and language ability, together with hereditary factors.[8] Although much more controlled research must be undertaken, other studies concluded that adopted children experience greater risk of psychologic and academic adjustment problems than comparable non-adopted children.[9,10] Adoptive parents can assist their children to develop their natural talents and gifts, however, and are advised to seek guidance to resolve any adjustment difficulties without assuming that they are caused by adoption.[11]

Concurrent Pursuit of Medical Treatment and Adoption

More and more often, couples initiate adoption proceedings while still undergoing infertility treatment. As one of the pair reaches age 40, they are pressured to push for aggressive treatment at the same time that many traditional adoption options are closing. Some couples become exhausted by the energy spent pursuing infertility treatment. Others express relief knowing they have a second plan on which to fall back. In either event, couples pursuing both options concurrently are at high risk for marital stress, with indications for supportive counseling during this fragile time of making decisions.

When the couple undergoes medical treatment, they share the mutual goal of a pregnancy. As they consider adoption, a new wave of feeling may follow the realization that this is another complex procedure with new limits to learn. Anger and resentment easily develop when they are required to prove themselves worthy to be parents. Many express the humiliation associated with asking perfect strangers at an agency for help. Financing the high cost of adoption also can exacerbate the feelings of inadequacy and jealousy of those whose obstetric costs are covered by insurance. The anxiety of an indefinite wait for an unknown child produces many opportunities for second-guessing the decision to adopt. All of these feelings added to the continual grief of infertility can over-whelm the couple considering adoption in the midst of treatment.

Expansion of Adoption Support Services

As adoption services have become more comprehensive and competitive, a large network of support services has evolved to assist infertile couples prior to and after adoption. Appendix 40–1 lists organizations that provide a wide range of services, including information and referral, preadoptive support groups, parent preparation programs, and postadoptive assistance.

TRADITIONAL VERSUS NONTRADITIONAL ADOPTIONS

Due to a growing demand for adoptive babies, adoption is rapidly expanding from being a traditional family service to a business.

Established, licensed agencies historically have accepted applications, approved the parents, processed the paperwork, and placed available children from local, out-of-state, and foreign sources. This process now takes from 2 to 6 years for domestic infants but less than 2 years, usually, for foreign-born children. Alternatively, a family could accept an available child for foster care and hope to adopt later. Since the early 1980s, private, independent arrangements have become more common than agency-facilitated adoptions of infants.[12] Several nontraditional but legal approaches are popular and offer their own advantages.

Private adoption is the process of locating, independently or through an intermediary, birth parent(s) willing to place a child with the couple. Public advertising is allowed in some states; private letters of solicitation are otherwise sent to physicians, clinics, lawyers, schools, and so on, in search of a source. In most cases this type of adoption can be arranged within a year.

In the few states where private adoption is outlawed to protect adoptive parents from unscrupulous baby-selling schemes, a licensed agency must act as intermediary to supervise the proceedings. This is called an *identified* or *cooperative adoption*, in which agencies actively recruit and support birth mothers.[13]

An adoption may be termed *open* if by mutual consent both sets of parents are identified. Birth parents(s) relinquish childrearing rights but may retain written contact or visitation rights.[14] Adoptive parents may even participate in the delivery of the infant they hope to adopt.

In certain programs a child may first be placed in a foster care family until legally free for adoption; the foster parents would be given first rights if and when the child were legally free. Placements of waiting children, often school-age or sibling groups, can occur rapidly, but court proceedings may take years, and this may not always meet the infertile couple's need for secure parenting.[15]

Specialized agencies may assist couples with strong international connections and language fluency to travel directly to the source and privately adopt overseas. This approach proceeds quite quickly, but may require 2 to 6 weeks' travel.

Single men and women, with or without a history of infertility, are increasingly interested in adoption. Accordingly, many more options and services address their needs, especially through foreign and special-needs adoptions. Long-standing opposition based on doubts that a single parent could manage the demands of career and adopted family have not proved valid on longitudinal study.[16]

Surrogate parent programs are an alternative offering the father a biologic child; his wife becomes the adoptive mother. The legalities of surrogacy vary widely across the country and have created a thicket of ethical dilemmas yet to be solved.[17,18]

Newer Policies and Procedures

The increased demands for adoption services have created new practices and procedures even in the most traditional agencies. Adoptive parents may find themselves writing appealing profile letters, assembling photographic albums, or producing videotapes of themselves to advertise their search for a child. Many agencies require applicants to write "Dear Birth Mother" letters to express their interests and gratitude to the biologic parent(s). Although such spontaneous exchange of correspondence can be both valuable and moving, the validity of mandated letters has been challenged.[19]

Nontraditional agencies have also begun to use aggressive advertising of their services to birth mothers through ads on billboards and in classified sections of newspapers. Even relatively traditional agencies that place special-needs children have successfully used the media and local celebrities to endorse programs and attract experienced parents. The high visibility of some adoption advertising strategies concerns infertile couples who are still cautious about adoption; many couples resent the increased costs these strategies incur, which are ultimately underwritten by the adoptive parents. Others express resistance to some procedures, such as housing a birth mother who plans to surrender a child to the chosen agency. To deal with these and other issues, some progressive agencies have offered group discussions and counseling services, but not all preadoptive couples find they can openly discuss issues with an agency that is also judging their readiness to adopt. Thus the need for collateral adoption support services has grown tremendously.

Cross-Cultural Adoptions

The decision to become a cross-cultural or cross-racial family presents the infertile couple with an additional set of issues. Adopting a young child in need has proved to be a most fulfilling and rewarding choice for many couples; but several issues must be considered in advance. Adopting through a licensed agency that obtains children through reputable sources overseas will minimize loss of an assigned child through faulty legal procedures. Even in the most stable international programs, however, there are risks that the placement may be delayed or denied by bureaucratic problems beyond agency control, such as loss of mailed records, social and political unrest, and internal policy changes in the source country. Most international adoptions proceed according to plan, but the couple may experience feelings of loss of control (again) when a country's politics interfere with the adoption of their child.

Couples often fear that a child will arrive with unusual medical conditions requiring extensive treatment. In a sampling of 128 foreign children, the following conditions were found: deficient immunizations, 37%; intestinal parasites, 29%; moderate to severe malnutrition, 20%; skin disease, 16%; questionable age estimates, 12%; and scabies and lice, 10%.[20] These conditions, including malnutrition, are treatable and reversible within reasonably short periods of treatment with the assistance of a knowledgeable pediatrician.[21]

All adoptees experience separation from their biologic heritage; a study of international adoptees with Colombian, Korean, and Afro-American heritage showed that a stable home over time can reverse the effects of previous deprivations.[22] Measurement of self-esteem and self-concept showed no significant differences between several subgroups of transracial adoptees and their nonadopted counterparts.[23]

Cross-racial adoption has been controversial in the United States, with many professionals opposing the placement of black children in white families. The issues extend beyond emotions to include ethics and economics; more longitudinal study is needed to identify the supposed ill effects, but cross-racial adoption remains an option for couples to consider. These families respond well and thrive when provided with supportive services and interaction with peer families (Fig. 40–1).[24]

Adoption Risks

Every approach to parenthood includes risks before the eventual benefits can be enjoyed. Pregnancy, labor, and delivery all pose formidable risk of loss; premature conception presents the unprepared mother with considerable risk of loss and disappointment. Adoptive parents face different risks depending on the type of adoption they choose.

In private or independent adoptions the couple identifies a birth mother they hope will surrender the child to them, but only from one third to one half of these birth mothers actually sign the surrender papers. The risk of financial loss should she not relinquish the child varies by state, but has been described as low in well-established programs with intensive supports.[25] In open adoption the extent of contact may eventually prove to be a great deal more or less intensive than anticipated. Contact with biologic parents may be easier for the child at certain stages than at others, necessitating renegotiation of visitation rights. Being foster parents incurs the legal and emotional risks that a court will order the child returned to its biologic family, perhaps several times, before final permission to adopt is granted. The risks of losing an assigned foreign-born child vary, but usually are modified by the knowledge that another child in need will be assigned.

The couple who pursues adoption without success suffers the same loss emotionally as the one who experiences a miscarriage. Family, friends, and medical practitioners may conclude that the adoption was "never meant to be" and try to reassure the couple that there will be another baby. At the time of the loss, however, the couple has suffered an adoptive miscarriage and they need none of the cliches indicating that the baby was never "really" theirs anyway. They grieve the loss of their potential child while trying to plan another approach to adopt.

THE ADOPTION PROCEDURE

Information Gathering

Couples often concentrate on finding a baby in the fastest or most economical way without first determining the characteristics of the child(ren) they can successfully parent over 20 or more years. Such shortsighted planning can place them at risk of many crises at later dates. When gathering information, a couple may apply to the only program known to them without fully exploring options available, or they may choose an agency more for its location than the quality of its service. Attending seminars and support group meetings, meeting with other adoptive families, and contacting numerous agencies can provide a wider range of possibilities from which to choose.

Application

Whether applying to a formal agency or establishing a contract with an intermediary, usually a physician

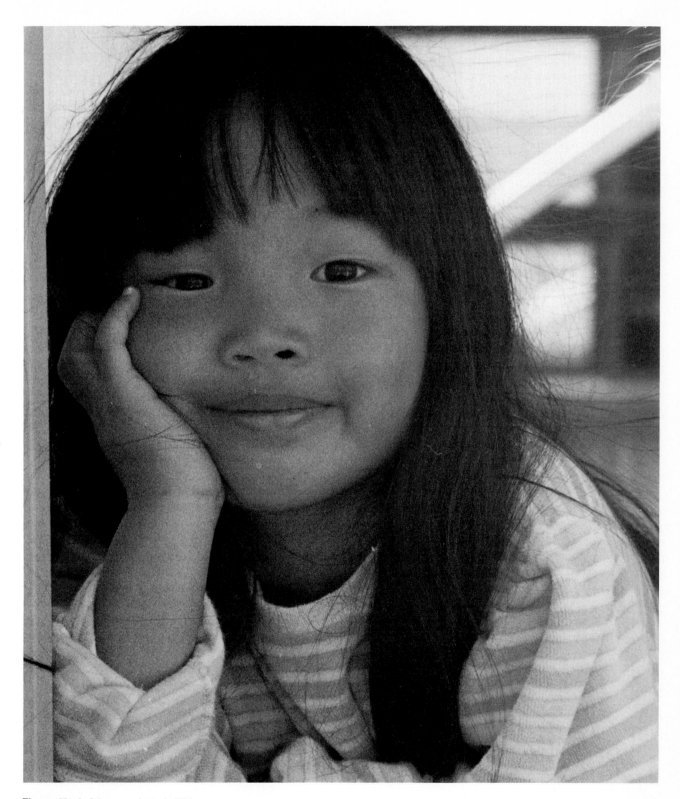

Figure 40–1. A happy adopted child.

or lawyer, the couple should first assume an attitude that they are entitled to first-quality professional services. The Adopting Parent's Bill of Rights outlines the entitlements of an educated consumer (Appendix 40–2).[26] When making any contact with adoption sources, the couple should project confidence and readiness in both verbal and written interactions; to do otherwise is to minimize their chance of success. Many couples find it helpful to gain assistance with applications and to rehearse for the interviews.

Preadoptive Counseling

The agency role during interviews is to determine whether the applicant couple is ready and able to provide a stable family life. The agency (or program director, in the case of a private adoption) conducts a series of interviews that attempts to establish the degree of the couple's readiness. Originally, the agency's investigation was called a home study because it did include a visit to check on the couple's residence; the focus has shifted to the prospective parents themselves, and away from their living arrangements. Preparation for the interviews can prevent unnecessary conflict with adoption workers and intermediaries. If couples recognize that agencies are, first and foremost, child welfare organizations designed to meet the needs of the child or birth parents before their own, much misunderstanding can be avoided.

Once accepted into a program, couples choosing a private or identified adoption may begin to advertise, trying to locate a birth mother by public announcement or private letters of inquiry. Couples report great satisfaction in this active inquiry process. In contrast, the more traditional approach presents the couple with an indefinite wait during which the agency may discourage further contact.

During the waiting period, the expectant adoptive parents may be hesitant to prepare for parenting lest the activity itself jinx the adoption. With more and more children being placed on short notice, however, it is advisable to begin some of the tasks in advance, namely, choosing health care providers; informing family, friends, other children, or employers as desired; attending classes on infant care, emergency procedures (first aid, CPR), or child development; learning cultural customs to incorporate; and acquiring safe, basic equipment.[27]

At the time of placement the ambivalences common to all new parents may surface and mix with euphoria. Before the adoption is final, agencies may require postplacement visits or reports. Adoptive parents consider this probation period to be an intrusion, but most realize that the agency must evaluate the family adjustment and the child's welfare during the initial custody period.

FAMILY BUILDING THROUGH ADOPTION

Adoptive family members typically have high expectations of themselves and of each other. The parents who have waited so long for a perfect child expect that the adoption will solve all accumulated problems. During the grief of infertility there is often a point of bargaining where they promise to be perfect parents if only they are granted a child.[28] The couple therefore must learn that adoption does not cure infertility or guarantee perfect parenthood.

Successful adjustment can be facilitated by several factors. The family's ability to develop attachment with a sense of identity and intimacy will support successful mutual adjustment.[29] Adoptive parents are encouraged to identify themselves as the real parents and to engage in honest dialogue with their children. Continued, open conversation can be the crucial factor in facilitating the adjustment.[30] Several specialists have described how best to explain adoption to children throughout their development.[11,31,32]

The Blended Family

A family with both biologic and adopted children is called a blended family. The blended family is increasingly more common as secondary infertility increases, as infertile couples in second marriages adopt, as couples fulfill their desire for large families by adopting after they have one or two biologic children, and as advanced reproductive technology gives adoptive parents the option of returning for infertility treatment.

Parents of blended families may be concerned that an adopted child and biologic sibling would perceive that they were treated differently. This variant of sibling rivalry closely follows the norm in all-biologic families and is not unique to adoption. The challenge is to relate to each child individually yet equitably despite the differences in their modes of arrival.

In the case of secondary infertility or infertility in a second marriage, the couple may consider adopting an older child or special-needs child. Also, age restrictions may limit the slightly older couple from adopting an infant. These adoptions were found to be more likely to succeed if parents could tolerate ambivalent or negative feelings during adjustment, refused to be rejected by the child, found satisfaction in small successes, and demonstrated flexible parenting.[33]

The Extended Family

Often couples raise the concern that the extended family will not accept the adopted child. The fear of bringing a child into the family only to face more rejection paralyzes many adoptive parents. Although families may hesitate to embrace the idea of adoption, few hold out when introduced to the child. Many relatives actually overindulge the adopted child, perhaps to compensate for guilt. Adoptive parents need eventually to heal wounds that infertility can create among family members; learning to forgive friends and families for their negative or insensitive comments is a crucial part of the process. Grandparents and other relatives will want to help when the newly adopted child arrives. Accepting help without holding grievance against them for past behavior will help the entire family adjust. Families also need support and educating in their new roles as adoptive relatives.[34]

REFERENCES

1. Bombardieri M: *The Twelve Stages of Adoption*. Belmont, MA, Fertility Counseling Associations, 1987.
2. Klerman LV: Adoption: A public health perspective. *Am J Public Health* 73(10):1158, 1983.
3. Jette SH: Adoption: Second choice or second best? *Resolve Newsletter*, April 1986.
4. Blum HP: Adoptive parents: Generative conflict and generational continuity. *Psychoanal Study Child* 38:141, 1983.
5. Kirk HD: *Shared Fate: A Theory and Method of Adoptive Relationships*. British Columbia, Canada, Ben-Simon, 1984.
6. Brodzinsky DM: Adjustment to adoption: A psychosocial perspective, *Clin Psychol Rev* 7(1):25, 1987.
7. Plomin R, DeFries JC: A parent–offspring adoption study of cognitive abilities in early childhood. *Intelligence* 9(4):341, 1985.
8. Thompson LA, Fulker DW, DeFries JC: Multivariate genetic analysis of environmental influences on infant cognitive development. *Br J Dev Psychol* 4(4):347, 1986.
9. Cadoret RJ: Adoptive studies: Historical and methodological critique. *Psychiatr Dev* 4(1):45, 1986.
10. Brodzinsky DM, Schechter DE, Braff AM, Singer LE: Psychological and academic adjustment in adopted children. *J Consul Clin Psychol* 52(4):582, 1984.
11. Melina LR: *Raising Adopted Children*. New York, Harper & Row, 1986.
12. Totty M: Balancing act: Private adoption agencies try a speedier and more open approach. *Wall Street Journal*, June 8, 1987.
13. Wells K, Reshotke P: Cooperative adoption: An alternative to independent adoption. *Child Welfare* 65(2):177, 1986.
14. Curtis PA: The dialectics of open vs closed adoption of infants. *Child Welfare* 65(5):437, 1986.
15. Lee RE, Hull RK: Legal, casework and ethical issues in risk adoption. *Child Welfare* 62(5):450, 1983.
16. Shireman J, Johnson PR: Single parent adoptions: A longitudinal study. *Child Youth Serv Rev* 7(4):321, 1985.
17. Andrews LB: *New Conceptions: A Consumer's Guide to the Newest Infertility Treatments*. New York, St Martin's, 1984.
18. Frankel MS: *Surrogate Motherhood: An Ethical Perspective*. Chicago, Illinois Institute of Technology, 1982.
19. Dukette R: Values issues in present-day adoptions. *Child Welfare* 63(3):233, 1984.
20. Jenista JA, Chapman D: Medical problems of foreign-born adopted children. *Am J Disabled Child* 141(3):298, 1987.
21. Cusminsky M, Azzarini LC, Dopchiz Z, et al: Malnutrition and adoption: Two variables in child development. *Early Child Dev Care* 15:45, 1984.
22. Feigelman W, Silverman AR: The long-term effects of transracial adoption. *Soc Serv Rev* 58:588, 1984.
23. McRoy RG, Zurcher LA: *Transracial and Inter-racial Adoptees: The Adolescent Years*. Springfield, IL, Charles C Thomas, 1983.
24. Feigelman W, Silverman A: *Chosen Children: New Patterns of Adoptive Relationships*. New York, Praeger, 1983.
25. Gradstein BD, Gradstein M, Glass RH: Private adoption. *Fertil Steril* 37(4):548, 1982.
26. Bombardieri M: *The Adopting Parents' Bill of Rights*. Belmont, MA, Fertility Counseling Associates, 1987.
27. Hallenbeck C: *Our Child: Preparation for Parenting in Adoption*. Wayne, PA, Our Child Press, 1983.
28. Jette SH: Adjusting to adoptive parenthood. *Resolve Newsletter*, Sept 1987.
29. Kraft AC: Some theoretical considerations on confidential adoptions. III. The adopted child. *Child Adolescent Social Work* 2(3):139, 1985.
30. Nickman SL: Losses in adoption: The need for dialogue. *Psychoanal Study Child* 40:365, 1985.
31. Jewett CL: *Helping Children Cope with Separation and Loss*. Harvard, MA, Harvard Common Press, 1982.
32. Brodzinsky DM, Singer LE, Braff AM: Children's understanding of adoption. *Child Devel* 55(3):869, 1984.
33. Katz L: Parental stress and factors for success in older child adoption. *Child Welfare* 65(6):555, 1986.
34. Holmes P: *Supporting and Adoption*. Gig Harbor, WA, Richlynn, 1982.

APPENDIX 40–1.

Major Organizations that Provide Information and Support for Adoption

Adopted Child Publications, LR Melina, editor, PO Box 9362, Moscow, ID 83843. Monthly newsletters publishing most current information.

Committee for Single Adoptive Parents, PO Box 15084, Chevy Chase, MD 20815. Information and referrals to local resources for single parents.

Families Adopting Children Everywhere (FACE), PO Box 28058, Baltimore, MD 21239. Support and programming for international families.

Latin American Parent's Association (LAPA), PO Box 72, Seaford, NY 11783. Information to guide successful adoptions from Latin America.

National Adoption Exchange, 1218 Chestnut Street, Philadelphia, PA 19107. Broad-based organization of adoption agencies with active legislative work.

National Committee for Adoption, 2025 M Street NW, Suite 512, Washington, DC 20036. Legislative group publishing current legal information.

Open Door Society, 867 Boylston Street, Boston, MA 02116. Largest of the parent support groups in the northeastern states.

OURS, Inc, 3307 Highway 100 North, Minneapolis, MN 55422. National organization of parent support groups with extensive publication.

RESOLVE, Inc, 5 Water Street, Arlington, MA 02174. National organization for education, advocacy, and support for infertile couples.

APPENDIX 40–2.
ADOPTING PARENTS'
BILL OF RIGHTS

1. The right to courteous, respectful treatment by all adoption, social service, medical, and legal personnel involved in adoption, including telephone receptionists.
2. The right to receive appropriate referrals for identified and international adoptions from all traditional agencies with long waiting lists. Rather than, "Sorry, we can't help you unless you're willing to wait 7 years," followed by a click: "I'm sorry we can't help you directly, but I *can* send you a list of agencies that can help you get a child in 2 years or less via international or identified adoption."

From Gradstein et al.[25] Reprinted with permission of the publisher, the American Fertility Society.

3. The right to become parents without being perfect. Most parents with biologic children are not perfect.
4. The right to adopt a healthy baby without being accused of selfishness that they do not adopt special needs children.
5. The right to become parents after age 40 if they are in good health.
6. The right to accurate, reasonable estimates of total expected costs for an identified adoption. Fees should be normal legal, medical, and counseling fees rather than clearly exploitive arrangements.
7. The right to adoption agency personnel and lawyers, and doctors who are knowledgeable enough about infertility to have compassion for them and not to inflict remarks such as, "What's the big rush?" "So what if the adoption takes another 6 months?" or, "Still trying for pregnancy? Why not just adopt? Why are you so hung up on pregnancy?"

PART XI

Statistics

CHAPTER 41

Statistical Analysis of Infertility Data

David S. Guzick

Statistical Analysis of Infertility	
Special Features of Infertility Data	**Statistical Techniques**
Measurements of Outcome	Analysis When Follow-Up Is Not
Dependent Versus Independent	Uniform
Variables	Analysis When Follow-Up Is
Dichotomous Versus Continuous	Uniform
Variables	Computer Software
Impact of Nonuniform Follow-Up	**Summary**
After Treatment	

For clinicians who do not have a background in statistics, it is a formidable task to acquire a general understanding of statistical theory and methods before applying them. By restricting the focus to a specific area of interest such as infertility, however, one can become familiar with a few key principles and procedures.

The word *statistics* originally meant the collection of population and economic information vital to the state. A statistic in this sense has come to mean an item of data. More generally, the subject area is now considered to encompass the entire science of decision making in the face of uncertainty. This covers enormous ground; uncertainties are present when we experiment with a new drug, determine life insurance premiums, inspect manufactured products, rate the abilities of human beings, make business decisions, and so forth.

The practice of clinical medicine almost continuously involves making decisions in the face of uncertainties. In the case of infertility, clinical decisions must often be made in the absence of definitive information: for example, how to treat mild or moderate endometriosis; whether to recommend *in-vitro* fertilization (IVF) or fimbrioplasty for women

with moderate to severe distal tubal disease; how many cycles of intrauterine insemination to perform when the husband has severe oligospermia before recommending IVF or therapeutic insemination by donor (TID); and how optimally to induce ovulation in a particular anovulatory patient.

Statistical methods can help with these decisions because they allow us to make inferences about an entire population based on information gathered from a sample. For example, before investing in equipment needed for laser tubal surgery, we may wish to know whether pregnancy rates after tuboplasties performed with the aid of a laser are higher than those performed using microcautery. What we really want to know is whether this is true in general, that is, for the entire population of women undergoing tuboplasty. Because there are only limited numbers of patients to study in a given geographic location, however, we collect information on a sample of patients undergoing one procedure or the other. The method of sampling is critical; ideally, patients sampled from two surgical treatment groups should differ in no important respect other than the type of procedure performed. Underlying the sampling method is the assumption that the pregnancy rate observed after a specified period of follow-up in the laser-treated sample approximates the pregnancy rate in the entire population of women treated with a laser. We make the same assumption about the pregnancy rate in the microcautery-treated group.

Reformulating these concepts in statistical language, we note that the population is fixed, so the pregnancy rate, although unknown, is a constant; it is called a *population parameter*. The pregnancy rate observed in our sample is a *random variable* because it varies from sample to sample. Such a random variable, calculated from observations in a sample is a *sample statistic*. The sample pregnancy rate observed in our particular group of patients is an estimate of the population pregnancy rate. As a random variable, it has a certain *probability distribution* associated with it. Given estimates of pregnancy rates in our two treated patient samples (laser and microcautery), and given estimates of the associated probability distributions, it is then possible to test the *null hypothesis* that there is no difference in pregnancy rates between the two groups. This statistical test, which is representative of virtually all statistical tests, is based on estimates of the probability that the difference observed between the two groups is reflective of a true difference in the population rather than the particular variability of the samples chosen.

Suppose that after a prolonged period of follow-up one treatment group has a higher pregnancy rate than another. Several explanations are possible. Perhaps the group that had the higher rate was composed of patients who would have conceived easily with either treatment. Perhaps one treatment is truly better. The concept of statistical significance simply means that the experimenter has made an *a priori* decision about his or her willingness to be wrong when stating that one treatment is "truly" better. A 5% level of significance (that is, a *p* value of 0.05) means that the researcher has decided that the likelihood of finding the observed difference when none exists in nature is 1 in 20, and that this is a comfortable margin of error.

As noted above, our ability to make statistical judgments about whether one treatment group has a better outcome than another hinges on the assumption that there are no differences between the two groups other than treatment. The best way to protect against a violation of this assumption is to assign individual subjects to treatments prospectively on a random basis. Randomization ensures that the distributions of age, severity of disease, parity, and other potentially confounding factors, are essentially the same for the two groups. Often in the infertility literature, treatments are compared by examining the outcome of patients who received one or another treatment in the course of clinical practice. The very process of clinical decision making that results in a

patient being treated one way or another may lead to selection of more favorable patients for a particular therapy. If this treatment is found to be associated with a higher pregnancy rate, it cannot be known whether this is due to a better treatment or a group of patients selected for a better prognosis. Thus good research design is an absolute prerequisite for sound hypothesis testing. Data obtained from a poor design cannot be used to make reliable inferences no matter how sophisticated the statistical method. Conversely, rigorous research design leads to definitive conclusions with the simplest of statistical tests.

SPECIAL FEATURES OF INFERTILITY DATA

Measurements of Outcome
The obvious measurement of outcome in an infertility investigation is pregnancy—yes or no. There are, however, variations on this theme. First, one must decide whether the outcome of interest is conception, clinical pregnancy, or term delivery. In the case of TID, for example, conception may be a useful end point, because it has been well documented that pregnancies resulting from donor insemination do not differ from normal pregnancies in the rates of spontaneous abortion, ectopic pregnancy, and prematurity. On the other hand, in studies of tubal surgery we must pay close attention to the distribution of outcomes among pregnancies that are achieved, especially the proportion that is ectopic.

Another important issue is the duration of follow-up against which the outcome measure is defined. Suppose the outcomes of infertile women undergoing tubal surgery over a number of years were reviewed as of September 1988. Should a patient operated on in June 1988 who is not pregnant at the time of review be classified as "not pregnant" just the same as a woman operated on 2 years earlier? Clearly, such a policy would introduce bias into the analysis, because the patient who is not pregnant after 3 months of follow-up may become pregnant after 6 or 12 months. This problem can be handled by performing a life-table analysis, as discussed later in the chapter, or by requiring that all patients have a specified duration of follow-up (such as years) to be included in the analysis.

Finally, some measurements of outcome other than pregnancy are pertinent to certain types of infertility investigations. The occurrence of ovulation is an obvious one in an investigation of the efficiency of an ovulation-induction protocol. The numbers of oocytes retrieved under different protocols of ovarian stimulation, and the proportion of oocytes fertilized under different protocols of sperm processing, are appropriate measurements of outcome for studies of

IVF. The average number of cycles required to achieve conception among patients having TID is another example.

Dependent Versus Independent Variables

In statistical terms, outcome is the *dependent* variable. It is variation in this dependent variable that one is trying to explain with one or more *independent* or *explanatory* variables. In a study of pregnancy success after tubal reanastomosis, for example, we might wish to explain the probability of pregnancy (dependent or outcome variable) on the basis of length of tube, type of tubal ligation, luminal discrepancy, and age (independent or explanatory variables). Although it may seem obvious, the distinction between dependent and independent variables is a critical one, and establishing explicit definitions in advance of the planned comparison provides a logical framework for the analysis.

Dichotomous Versus Continuous Variables

In general, the dependent variables in infertility investigations tend to be *dichotomous*, or *binary* (conception/no conception, fertilization/no fertilization, ovulation/no ovulation). Unfortunately, many of the statistical methods available were developed for continuous dependent variables. Blood pressure, serum cholesterol concentration, temperature, tensile strength of suture material, birth weight, and blood loss at surgery are all continuous variables that commonly serve as measurements of outcome in medical investigations. Standard statistical techniques, such as analysis of variance and multiple linear regression, can be used appropriately when the dependent variable is continuous. When the dependent variable is dichotomous, however, as in most infertility investigations, other techniques should be used.

Impact of Nonuniform Follow-Up After Treatment

A fundamental problem in evaluating the outcome of infertility therapy is incomplete or variable follow-up. It is often difficult, for reasons unrelated to the study, to maintain contact with patients over a prolonged period. Furthermore, because patients receive therapy at different times, the duration of follow-up varies even among those who are successfully followed until completion of the study.

For these reasons, the pregnancy rate commonly reported in infertility research—defined as the number of patients who conceive divided by the number of patients treated—is a poor measurement of treatment success. It may underestimate the true success of therapy, because an unknown fraction of nonpreg-

nant patients who are lost to follow-up early in the study, or who enter the study at a point close to its completion, become pregnant at a later date. Moreover, as some infertility centers have more successful patient follow-up than others, pregnancy rates after a particular treatment modality reported by different centers cannot be compared reliably. Similarly, if there is variability in the follow-up of patients who differ in severity of disease or other characteristics, a comparison of pregnancy rates according to these patient characteristics is also unreliable.

STATISTICAL TECHNIQUES

Analysis When Follow-Up Is Not Uniform

Over the years, many infertility researchers have recognized the importance of adjusting pregnancy rates for incomplete and variable follow-up. Consensus has grown for uniformity in reporting the results of infertility therapy using a life-table method to adjust for variability in follow-up.

Data appropriate for the life table method are presented graphically in Figure 41–1. Figure 41–1a shows that patients were treated at various times and that those who became pregnant (P) did so after varying periods of observation. Of the nonpregnant group, some patients were lost to follow-up (L). The remaining patients were followed nonpregnant to the time that the study was completed (O). Those who were either L or O are described as "censored." Figure 41–1b displays the same data after recording the time of entry into the study (that is, the time of treatment) as time zero. This is the starting point for the pregnancy life-table calculation.

The following life-table calculations are based on the original description by Berkson and Gage.[1] Table 41–1 is a life table constructed from 214 patients with endometriosis who were treated with conservative surgical management at the Johns Hopkins Hospital.[2] Each row represents data for a given interval of time after therapy. During the first 12 months after therapy, 68 patients conceived (column 2). None were censored (column 3), so all 214 patients who entered the study (column 4) were exposed to the possibility of pregnancy (column 5). The probability of pregnancy during this interval was equal to the number of pregnancies (68) divided by the number of women exposed (214), or 31.8% (column 6).

Because 68 patients became pregnant during the first 12 months, 146 (214 minus 68) entered the second interval (column 4). Of these, 21 conceived (column 2). During this period, however, 39 patients were censored (column 3). We assume uniform dropout of these patients over the 12-month interval; that is, half of them, or 19.5, were exposed. Thus, a

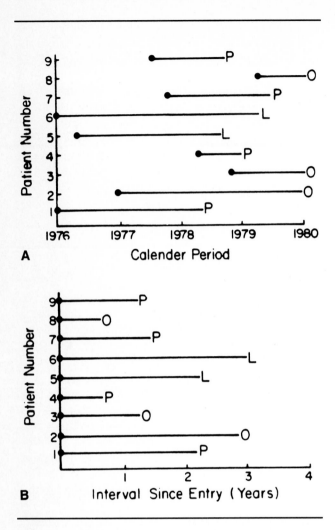

Figure 41-1. Graphic representation of data needed for life-table analysis of 9 hypothetical patients treated for infertility. Solid circles = time of treatment; P = pregnancy; L = loss to follow-up; 0 = nonpregnant at termination of study. **A.** Patients are treated at various times, and those who become pregnant do so after varying periods of observation. **B.** Patients are displayed after recording the time of entry into the study (i.e., the time of treatment) as time zero.

total of 146 − 19.5 = 126.5 patients were exposed (column 5), giving a probability of pregnancy for this interval of 21 ÷ 126.5 = 16.6% (column 6).

The cumulative probability of pregnancy was then obtained by successively applying the probabilities of pregnancy in each interval to a starting figure of 0% pregnant. Thus the probability of pregnancy during the first interval was 31.8%, and because none of the patients conceived prior to therapy, the cumulative pregnancy rate was also 31.8% (column 7). In the second interval we noted that 16.6% of the remaining 68.2% of nonpregnant patients conceived, adding an estimated 11.3% patients (0.166 × 0.682) to the pregnancy rate. Thus in the second interval the cumulative pregnancy rate was 31.8% +

11.3% = 43.1%. This process continued successively for the remaining intervals.

The cumulative pregnancy curve can be plotted graphically (closed circles in Fig. 41-2). Certain features of the curve can be inferred by examining the plot; that is, the curve seems to level off at a cumulative pregnancy rate of 60 to 65%, as compared with a crude pregnancy rate of 54% for these same data. To describe the curve more precisely, or to compare two or more such curves for different patient groups, however, a mathematical model is needed.

One model that has been advanced involves the assumption that the pregnancy rate per month (that is, the hazard rate) for all patients is constant over time.[3] Given a constant monthly pregnancy rate, the predicted cumulative pregnancy rate (CPR) can easily be calculated: assuming a 20% monthly pregnancy rate, CPR = 20% the first month. During the second month, 20% of the remaining 80% of patients conceive, or an additional 16%. Thus CPR = 36% after two months; similarly, it is 49% after 3 months, 59% after 4 months, and so on.

Applying such a model is straightforward. One simply calculates the average monthly pregnancy rate (or fecundability) by dividing the number of pregnancies by the total months of follow-up, and then predicts CPR as above. Indeed, estimates of fecundability after treatment are now commonly reported in the infertility literature. Interpretation of such estimates is difficult, however, because the underlying assumption of a constant hazard rate is often incorrect. From the endometriosis data in Table 41-1, for example, it can be seen that the hazard rate declines rather markedly over time, as shown in Figure 41-3. It is not surprising, therefore, that the predicted cumulative pregnancy curve based on this model fits the observed data poorly (Fig. 41-4). The CPR predicted by the model initially underestimates and then overestimates the observed CPR.

To develop a model of CPR that better approximates the observed data in a wide variety of infertility investigations, let us assume that the observed cumulative pregnancy curve is a weighted average of two curves, one for patients who will ultimately conceive (the "cured" group) and the other for those who will never conceive (the "uncured" group).[2] The curve for the uncured patients is a horizontal line at 0%. The proportion of patients in the uncured group increases as follow-up advances and pregnant patients in the cured group are progressively deleted from the sample, thus providing greater weight to the overall curve. This concept is shown graphically in Figure 41-5.

More formally, consider a group of women treated for a given, well-documented infertility problem at time zero. The proportion of patients who are

TABLE 41–1. CALCULATION OF CUMULATIVE PREGNANCY RATES BY THE LIFE TABLE METHOD

Interval After Treatment (mos)	Last Report		Number Not Pregnant at Beginning of Interval	Number Exposed to Pregnancy	Probability of Pregnancy in Interval	Cumulative Pregnancy Rate (%)
	Pregnant	Not Pregnant				
0–12	68	0	214	214.0	0.318	0.318
13–24	21	39	146	126.5	0.166	0.431
25–36	15	14	86	79.0	0.190	0.539
37–48	7	10	57	52.0	0.135	0.601
49–60	2	10	40	35.0	0.057	0.624
61–72	1	4	28	26.0	0.038	0.639

cured by treatment can be denoted by c. By "cure" we mean that a patient has the potential, after treatment, to conceive. Depending on the type of infertility problem, this potential may remain lower than that of a nontreated woman without a history of infertility, but the comparison is not relevant to this analysis. The cumulative probability of pregnancy to time t, denoted by $P(t)$, is equal to a weighted average of the cumulative probabilities of pregnancy in the cured $P_c(t)$ and uncured $P_\ell(t)$ groups:

$$P(t) = (1-c)P_\ell(t) + cP_c(t). \qquad (41-1)$$

It has been observed that couples with long-standing infertility problems occasionally become pregnant without treatment. In the context of our model, such couples would be included in the cured group, because they obviously had the potential, both before and after treatment, to conceive. The probability of pregnancy in the uncured group,

however, is 0, that is, $P_\ell(t) = 0$. This causes the term $(1-c)P_\ell(t)$ in equation 41–1 to drop out. We are now left with

$$P(t) = cP_c(t) \qquad (41-2)$$

If we make the assumption that the probability of pregnancy from month to month in the cured group is the same (that is, if a couple does not conceive 1 month after therapy, this does not change their probability of pregnancy the next month), the second term $P_c(t)$ can be expressed as[2]:

$$P_c(t) = 1 - exp(-\lambda t),^* \qquad (41-3)$$

where λ = the hazard rate or monthly probability of pregnancy.

Substituting equation 41–3 into equation 41–2,

---

*Notation: $exp(-\lambda t) = e^{-\lambda t}$.

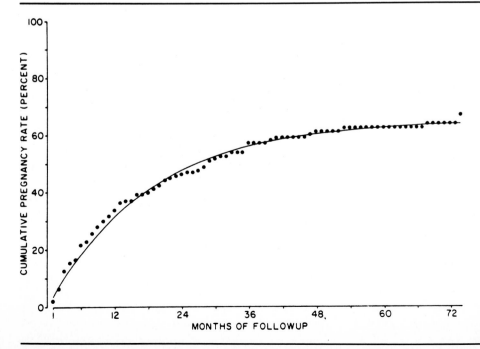

Figure 41–2. Comparison of the observed cumulative pregnancy curve (solid circles) after conservative surgery for endometriosis with that predicted by the model of Guzick and Rock[2] (solid line).

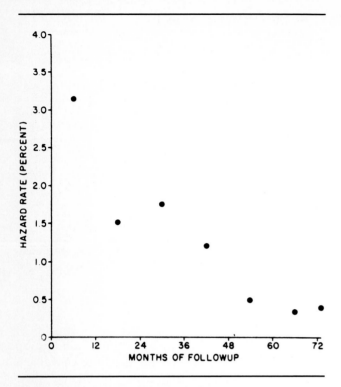

Figure 41–3. Hazard rate (i.e., probability of pregnancy) after conservative surgery for endometriosis as a function of months of follow-up.

we arrive at a simple expression for the cumulative pregnancy rate of the entire population:

$$P(t) = c[1 - exp(-\lambda t)]. \qquad (41-4)$$

Thus the cumulative pregnancy curve derived from life-table analysis for a cohort of treated infertil-

ity patients can be expressed in terms of two parameters: the cure rate (c) and the hazard rate (or monthly probability of pregnancy) among those cured (λ). This model can be estimated using nonlinear least squares,[2] or by a maximum-likelihood technique.[4]

We have estimated the model for data sets on endometriosis,[2] polycystic ovary syndrome,[5] artificial insemination by donor,[6,7] tubal reanastomosis,[8,9] and in-vitro fertilization.[10] In these studies and in other examples where the model has been used,[11,12] the fit has been uniformly excellent. For example, the results for the endometriosis data set are as follows:

$$P(t) = 0.645[1 - exp(0.056t).$$

Thus it is estimated that 64.5% of patients were "cured" of their infertility problem, and among those the monthly probability of pregnancy was 5.6%. The estimated model fits the observed data quite well (see Fig. 41–2). In Figure 41–5 it can be seen graphically that the predicted cumulative pregnancy curve for the sample is the weighted average of two curves, one for the patients who ultimately conceive and one for those who will never conceive. As follow-up advances and pregnant patients in the cured group are deleted from the sample, the relative proportion of patients in the uncured group increases, thus contributing more weight to the probability of pregnancy in the total group.

We have described the life-table method as a procedure to adjust for nonuniformity in the follow-up of patients, and have presented a method for estimating the cure rate and monthly probability of pregnancy represented by a given pregnancy curve.

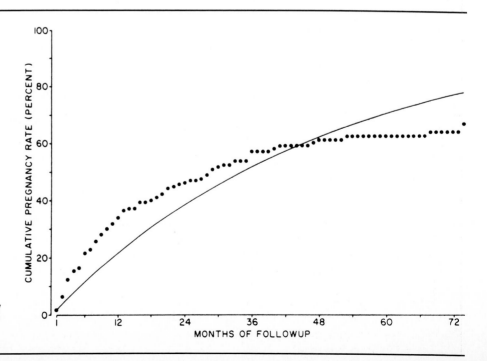

Figure 41–4. Comparison of the observed cumulative pregnancy curve (solid circles) after conservative surgery for endometriosis with that predicted by the model of Cramer et al[3] (solid line).

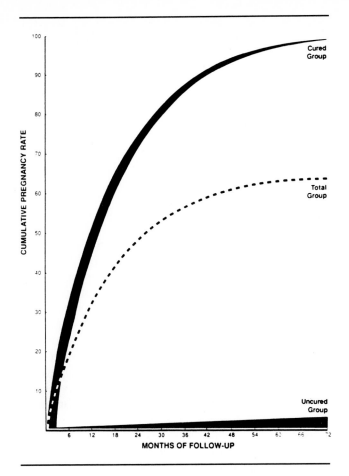

Figure 41–5. Schematic description of cumulative pregnancy model. Relative proportions of patients in the cured and uncured groups over time are represented by the caliber of the line.

It is often of interest to compare two or more groups of patients with respect to pregnancy after infertility therapy. Is there a difference between a newly proposed form of treatment and the conventionally accepted one? Is there a difference among women of different ages, or among women who differ in severity of disease?

Whenever follow-up is nonuniform, patient dropout or censoring may be different for the different groups. For this reason, the appropriate method of comparing pregnancy success between patient groups is to compare their entire cumulative pregnancy curves or the parameters that describe these curves, rather than their crude pregnancy rates. This can be accomplished by estimating the cumulative pregnancy curve for each patient group using the model described above, and then performing a statistical comparison of the estimated curves. We have developed a likelihood-ratio method for making such comparisons.[4] Unfortunately, the sample size required for this type of estimation (a minimum of 30 to 40 subjects in each group) is often not available. Nonparametric methods of comparing life tables[13,14] are available in such instances.

Analysis When Follow-Up Is Uniform

If follow-up of patients is uniform, complete, and of sufficiently long duration, the crude pregnancy rate closely approximates the asymptotic pregnancy rate of the life table or the cure rate of the model. Under this circumstance, some simple and powerful statistical methods can be applied.

Suppose, for example, that it was of interest to study factors associated with pregnancy success after tubal reanastomosis, and that 60 patients with at least 2 years of follow-up were available. Potential factors that may be associated with pregnancy can be identified on the basis of a theoretical model or previous research findings. From these considerations, suppose that the particular factors hypothesized to be associated with pregnancy success were tubal length at the completion of the operation, type of tubal ligation performed, type of anastomosis (such as isthmic–isthmic), and patient age.

How can we assess the association between pregnancy success and each of these potentially prognostic variables? There are two broad categories of such independent or explanatory variables: categorical (type of tubal ligation, type of anastomosis) and continuous (age, tubal length). In our example, the dependent or outcome variable (pregnancy/no pregnancy) is, of course, categorical.

In general, to determine whether a relationship exists between one categorical variable and another, it is appropriate to perform a chi-square test. To determine whether a relationship exists between a dichotomous and a continuous variable, the appropriate test is a *t* test. Each of these tests allows us to make a decision about whether the observed relationship is greater than would have been expected by some predetermined chance level. That is, we can infer a "statistically" significant association between the variables.

Chi-Square Test. The data for a chi-square test of the relation between pregnancy outcome (pregnant/nonpregnant) after 2 years of follow-up and type of tubal ligation procedure performed are shown in Table 41–2. Each cell represents a frequency count of the number of patients who fall into a particular category (for example, 5 patients who had a tubal cauterization conceived). Shown in parentheses below these observed frequencies are the expected frequencies that would occur if the null hypothesis (no difference in pregnancy rate among types of tubal ligation) were true. These expected frequencies can be calculated from the row and column totals. For example, 70% of the patients conceived (42 of 60). Thus if the null hypothesis were true and there were no differences in pregnancy rates among tubal ligation procedures, the proportion pregnant for each procedure type

TABLE 41–2. ILLUSTRATIVE CHI-SQUARE ANALYSIS FOR PREGNANCY VS. TUBAL LIGATION TYPE*

Clinical Pregnancy	Tubal Ligation Type			Totals
	Banding	Cautery	Pomeroy	
No	3 (6)	7 (3.6)	8 (8.4)	18
Yes	17 (14)	5 (8.4)	20 (19.6)	42
Totals	20	12	28	60

*Each cell contains the actual frequency observed and the expected frequency below it in parentheses.

would also be 70%. For example, since 20 patients had tubal banding, it would be expected that 14 of these patients would have conceived.

After the observed (o) and expected (e) frequency counts in each cell have been tabulated, the chi-square statistic can be calculated as follows:

$$\chi^2 = \sum_{i=1}^{6} \frac{(o_i - e_i)^2}{e_i} = 6.76. \qquad (41-6)$$

To determine whether this χ^2 value is statistically significant at the 5% level, we consult a χ^2 probability distribution and determine the value of χ^2 that represents a 5% probability of falsely rejecting the null hypothesis. Because our calculated χ^2 value of 6.76 exceeds this critical value of 4.6, we reject the null hypothesis of no association between tubal ligation and pregnancy success.

Student's *t* Test. One use for a *t* test is to examine the relation between a dichotomous and a continuous variable. Suppose we were interested in the relationship between tube length (continuous variable, in centimeters) and pregnancy success (dichotomous variable, yes/no). Student's *t* test can be used to compare the mean tube length of the pregnant group with that of the nonpregnant group.

The formula for the Student's *t* statistic is as follows:

$$t = \frac{\text{difference between means}}{\text{standard error of difference between means}}$$

Conceptually, the *t* statistic is the ratio of the difference between two samples and the variability between them. If the difference between the means of the two samples were high and variability low, the *t* statistic would be high, and it would be reasonable to conclude that the observed difference between the means reflects a true difference in tube length between the populations of women who do and do not conceive. If the difference between the observed sample means were small and the standard error of the difference large, the *t* statistic would be low, and we could not reject the null hypothesis that there was no difference between the means—that is, the differ-

ence observed would probably be due to sampling variation.

In our example, the observed sample mean of tube length in the pregnant group was 6.10, the sample mean of tube length in the nonpregnant group was 4.83, and the standard error of difference between the means was 0.44. The *t* statistic is thus (6.10 − 4.83)/0.44 = 2.88. This value exceeds the critical value of 2.0 for a 0.05 level of significance (as determined from a table of critical points for Student's *t*). Thus we conclude that tube length at completion of the operation was significantly higher in the pregnant group than in the nonpregnant group.

Multivariate Analysis—Logistic Regression. From the univariate analyses performed thus far, it appears that type of ligation and tube length are both directly associated with the likelihood of pregnancy after anastomosis. It is possible, however, that part of the reason higher pregnancy rates occur after anastomosis of a banded tube than a burned tube is that banding destroys less tissue, so that final tube length is longer. If this were true, can we tease out the true independent contributions to the probability of pregnancy of tube length and ligation type? The answer lies within the general framework of multivariate analysis.

The simplest type of multivariate analysis is cross-classification. Tube length could be rounded to whole numbers in centimeters and a separate chi-square table of tubal ligation type (cautery, resection, banding) with pregnancy (yes, no) could be analyzed for each tube length. If a statistically significant relationship were found between ligation type and pregnancy at each tube length, we could conclude that ligation type has an effect on the probability of pregnancy even after controlling for tube length.

The cross-classification approach is simple but cumbersome. As the number of variables included in the analysis grows, so does the number of subjects required to address the question with meaning. Even with only the two explanatory variables in our example, one with three levels (tubal ligation type), and the other with six levels (tube length 3 to 8 cm), there are 18 subgroups. Given a sample size of 60, there are only about three subjects, on average, with which to calculate a pregnancy rate for each subgroup. If we were then to add additional variables, such as type of anastomosis and age, the situation would be even more difficult.

The general purpose of multivariate analysis is to obtain estimates of the effect of a particular explanatory variable on outcome while statistically adjusting for other explanatory variables in an efficient way. Let Y represent the outcome or dependent variable, and let X_1, X_2, X_3, and X_4 represent four explanatory or independent variables. The most commonly used multivariate model in medical research is that of *multiple linear regression:*

$$Y = b_0 = b_1 X_1 + b_2 X_2 + b_3 X_3 + b_4 X_4. \quad (41-5)$$

where b_0 is the intercept that obtains when all Xs equal 0, and b_1, b_2, b_3, and b_4 are the regression coefficients of the independent variables. A particular regression coefficient (for example, b_2) represents an estimate of the slope of the relation between Y and X_2 when "all other things" (X_1, X_3, and X_4) are equal.

The difficulty with using this linear model in infertility research is that it is based on the assumption that the dependent variable is continuous and normally distributed rather than dichotomous. Use of dichotomous dependent variables such as pregnancy (yes/no) in this model has been shown to lead to inaccurate estimates of the b's when the probability of outcome deviates much from 50%.

Multiple logistic regression[15] is a technique that was developed in the early 1960s to handle multivariate analysis with a dichotomous dependent variable. As applied to our example where the dependent variable is pregnancy (yes = 1/no = 0), the logistic model specifies that the probability of pregnancy $P = Prob(Y=1)$ depends on the four explanatory variables X_1, X_2, X_3, and X_4 in the following way:

$$P = Prob(Y = 1) = 1/[1 + exp- (b_0 + b_1 X_1 + b_2 X_2 + b_3 X_3 + b_4 X_4)]. \quad (41-6)$$

Figure 41–6 shows the general shape of the logistic function, which may be viewed as a basic model for dose–response relationships. The higher the X (tube length, or dose) the greater the probability of Y (pregnancy, or response).

Two transformations of equation 41–6 are helpful. First, let Q represent the probability of no pregnancy. From equation 41–6 a little algebraic manipulation leads to:

$$\frac{P}{Q} = \frac{Prob\ (Y=1)}{Prob\ (Y=0)} =$$
$$exp\ (b_0 + b_1 X_1 + b_2 X_2 + b_3 X_3 + b_4 X_4).$$

The term P/Q represents the likelihood or odds of a pregnancy occurring with a particular combination of X's.

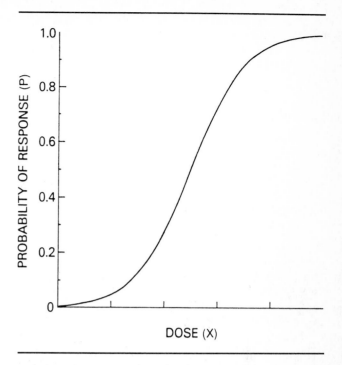

Figure 41–6. General shape of the logistic function.

Taking natural logarithms of both sides of equation 41–7 so as to linearize the right side of the expression, we have:

$$ln(P/Q) = b_0 + b_1 X_1 + b_2 X_2 + b_3 X_3 + b_4 X_4. \quad (41-8)$$

The term $ln(P/Q)$ is the log odds, or logit, of pregnancy. The parameters b_i (b_0, b_1, b_2, b_3, and b_4) are called *logistic regression coefficients.* It can be shown that for a dichotomous independent variable X_i, the antilog of b_i is equivalent to the *odds ratio* of pregnancy attributable to X_i, controlling for all other X's. The odds ratio for a given X_i is the odds of pregnancy if X_i were present ($X_i = 1$) divided by the odds of pregnancy if X_i were absent ($X_i = 0$).

The term *logistic model* is used to refer to either equation 41–6 or 41–8, which are algebraically equivalent. Equation 41–8 is also called a *logit model.* Expressed in terms of logit, a unit change in the variable X_i changes the logit of pregnancy ($1n\ P/Q$) by the amount of b_i.

The set of explanatory variables X_i can be dichotomous, continuous, or both. When a categorical variable contains more than two levels, such as anastomosis type, we can create dichotomous variables. Thus we might create the variable "isthmic–isthmic" or "ii" (yes = 1/no = 0). This variable would be entered into the logit model and its coefficients would be interpreted in relation to the other types of anastomoses (ampullary–ampullary and isthmic–ampullary) that were not entered. A coefficient of 1.01 for ii means that women who had an isthmic–isthmic anastomosis have a logit of pregnancy after

TABLE 41–3. LOGISTIC REGRESSION RESULTS FOR ILLUSTRATIVE DATA ON TUBAL REANASTAMOSIS (DEPENDENT VARIABLE IS CLINICAL PREGNANCY)

Independent Variables (X_i)	Estimated Logistic Coefficients*			
	Eq. 1	Eq. 2	Eq. 3	Eq. 4
Intercept	0.43	1.98	−0.29	−0.31
Cautery (y = 1/n = 0)	−0.77	−0.69	−0.67	−0.78
	(0.02)	(0.06)	(0.07)	(0.05)
ii (yes = 1/no = 0)		1.01	0.18	
		(0.02)	(0.53)	
Tube length (cm)			0.36	0.38
			(0.02)	(0.02)

*p values are in parentheses below the estimated coefficients.

surgery that is 1.01 units higher than that for women who had other types of anastomoses. Since the antilog of 1.01 is 2.75, we conclude that the odds of pregnancy in the ii group is 2.75 times higher than that in the non-ii groups.

Using our illustrative data set, estimation of the logistic model (using a method of estimation called maximum likelihood that is beyond our present scope) yields results that can be summarized as shown in Table 41–3. Age was not found to be related to pregnancy and thus was deleted from the logistic model. The p value shown below each coefficient estimate represents a test of whether the coefficient is significantly different from 0.

The first equation in Table 41–3 is analogous to the univariate analysis. When cautery (yes or no) is entered as the only variable to explain pregnancy success (equation 41–1, Table 41–3) it has a highly significant negative coefficient. This means that it is associated with a *lower* probability of pregnancy after reversal than either banding or Pomeroy tubal ligations. When type of anastomosis (ii) is added (equation 41–2, Table 41–3), it can be seen that the probability of pregnancy is significantly higher for ii anastomosis than for ia or aa, controlling for ligation type. But when tube length is added to the model (equation 41–3, Table 41–3), ii loses its significance, while tube length enters with a strongly positive coefficient. This implies that the apparent importance of ii was mainly due to its association with tube length; when tube length was controlled for, ii was no longer that important. Tube length appears to be highly important, however, even after controlling for type of ligation and type of anastomosis. Because ii was not found to be significant after tube length was controlled for, a final model was estimated (equation 41–4, Table 41–3) that excluded ii.

An additional benefit of logistic analysis is that it provides a method for estimating the probability of an outcome given particular combinations of prognostic factors.[15] Using our example as an illustration, we can calculate from equation 41–4 and Table 41–3 that an individual who was sterilized by tubal banding and who had 6 cm of tube after anastomosis would have a logit score (S) of $0.31 - 0.78(0) + 0.38(6) = 1.97$. The probability of pregnancy in this situation is estimated to be $exp(S)/[1+exp(S)] = exp(1.97)[1+exp(1.97)] = 7.17/8.17 = 0.878$. Similar calculations can be made for patients with other combinations of characteristics.

Computer Software

Fortunately, once the conceptual framework for the statistical techniques is understood, calculations by hand are unnecessary. All that one needs are the raw data organized in a format that is acceptable as input into preprogrammed computer software. Three major statistical packages for mainframe computers—SAS, SPSS, and BMDP—are widely available at most universities. These packages have been adapted for use with personal computers. Consultation with a statistician is advisable prior to implementing a research design so that suitable statistical methods can be chosen, and so that the data can be collected in a manner appropriate for the software available at a particular site.

SUMMARY

Certain features of infertility investigations lend themselves to particular statistical techniques. Life-table methods are useful because follow-up after treatment is often nonuniform, and logistic regression (or a similar technique) is useful because of dichotomous outcome measures such as pregnancy/nonpregnancy.

The importance of sound research design prior to data collection is worthy of reemphasis. Valid conclusions can not be drawn from statistical tests unless the data are based on research design that is without intrinsic bias. In this context, the importance of randomized clinical trials cannot be overstated.

REFERENCES

1. Berkson I, Gage RP: Calculation of survival rates for cancer. *Mayo Clin Proc* 25:270, 1950.
2. Guzick DS, Rock JA: Estimation of a model of cumulative pregnancy following infertility therapy. *Am J Obstet Gynecol* 140:573, 1981.
3. Cramer DW, Walker AM, Schiff I: Statistical methods in evaluating the outcome of infertility therapy. *Fertil Steril* 32:80, 1979.
4. Guzick DS, Bross DS, Rock JA: A parametric method for comparing cumulative pregnancy curves following infertility therapy. *Fertil Steril* 37:503, 1982.
5. Adashi EY, Rock JA, Guzick DS, et al: Fertility following bilateral ovarian wedge resection: A critical analysis of 90 consecutive cases of the polycystic ovary syndrome. *Fertil Steril* 35:320, 1981.
6. Bergquist CA, Rock JA, Miller J, et al: Artificial Insemination with fresh donor semen using the cervical cap technique: A review of 278 cases. *Obstet Gynecol* 60:195, 1982.
7. Bradshaw KD, Guzick DS, Gun B, Johnson N, Ackerman GA: Cumulative pregnancy rates for donor insemination according to ovulatory functions and tubal status. *Fertil Steril*, in press.
8. Rock JA, Chang YS, Limpaphayom K, et al: Microsurgical tubal reanastomosis: A controlled trial in four Asian centers. *Microsurgery* 5:95, 1984.
9. Rock JA, Guzick DS, Katz E, Zacur HA, King TM: Tubal anastomosis: Pregnancy success following reversal of Falope ring or monopolar cautery sterilization. *Fertil Steril* 48:13, 1987.
10. Guzick DS, Hinkle C, Jones HW: Cumulative clinical pregnancy rates for in vitro fertilization and embryo transfer. *Fertil Steril* 46:663, 1986.
11. Olive DL, Stohs GF, Metzger DA, Franklin RR: Expectant management and hydrotubations in the treatment of endometriosis-associated infertility. *Fertil Steril* 44:35, 1985.
12. Olive DL, Martin DC: Treatment of endometriosis-associated infertility with CO_2 laser laparoscopy: The use of one- and two-parameter exponential models. *Fertil Steril* 48:18, 1987.
13. Mantel N: Evaluation of survival data and two new rank order statistics arising in its consideration. *Cancer Chemother Rep* 50:163, 1966.
14. Breslow N: A generalized Kreuskil-Willis test for comparing K samples subject to unequal patterns of censorship. *Biometrika* 57:579, 1974.
15. Schiesselman JJ: *Case Control Studies*. Oxford: Oxford University Press, 1982.

Epilogue

Machelle M. Seibel, Claude Ranoux

Why write an epilogue? Surely 41 chapters ought to convey sufficient information. Nevertheless, while reading the galley proofs it occurred to me (MMS) that during the gestation of this book several changes from both a scientific and philosophical perspective had occurred. Therefore, rather than trying to weave these thoughts into existing text, it seemed preferable to comment briefly as a summary.

Infertility is more than a medical diagnosis; it has evolved into an industry. Delayed child bearing has condensed the fertile years into a shorter time interval. In addition, a scarcity of children available for adoption and aging of the baby-boom generation has resulted in infertility reaching crisis proportions.[1] Nearly 2 million office visits related to infertility occurred in 1984 and the annual cost for infertility services in 1987 was $1 billion.[2] All of this is occurring at a time when our national resources are unable to keep pace with society's demands. Furthermore, a lack of scientific integrity by a small percentage of medical providers has cast a shadow on medicine per se and led to an intensified effort by congress to control the practice of medicine. During a 12-month period in 1988–1989, verification of in vitro fertilization results through extensive audits have been requested by the American Fertility Society, the In Vitro Fertilization Registry, the Congress of the United States, the Federal Trade Commission, and the United States General Accounting Office. The raging war surrounding abortion has also been revived. In its wake, some of the reproductive technologies are placed at risk as segments of our society struggle to keep pace with the ethical and religious aspects of new advances.

Having said all this, what conclusions can be drawn? There is, at present, insurance coverage for infertility available in Arkansas, Hawaii, Maryland, Massachusetts, and Texas. Surely more states will follow. Along with this obvious benefit, restrictions on age, diagnosis, and length of treatment will no doubt fall under regulation because of cost. Because limited resources are available for research, it is likely that most of the monies provided for scientific advances will come from industry and not government. The goal will be to make medical technology "user friendly." Let us use the example of a new technique for in vitro fertilization, intravaginal culture (IVC).[3]

Despite the overwhelming acceptance of IVF as a procedure, personal and religious objections have been raised concerning fertilization in vitro per se. A new method of fertilization, intravaginal culture (IVC), allows fertilization to occur in vivo.

Following ovulation induction and oocyte retrieval, the oocytes are identified and consolidated into one petri dish. A 3 mL plastic IVC tube is filled completely with culture medium and all oocytes are placed within it. The oocytes sink to the bottom of the tube. Approximately 30,000 to 60,000 motile spermatozoa are added to the top of the 3 mL tube. The tube is then hermetically closed without air or CO_2 and wrapped tightly in a cryoflex envelope sealed at both ends to prevent vaginal contamination. The tube is then inserted into the vagina for 44 to 50 hours where it is kept in place by a diaphragm. Activities are not restricted. As a result of this process, fertilization occurs in vivo within the woman's body. Following the intravaginal culture, the tube is removed, wiped of vaginal secretions, and the contents poured into a petri dish. The embryos are then transferred into the uterus. Over 500 cases using IVC have now been performed. Results are comparable to IVF with a birth rate per retrieval of 13.5%.[3]

We believe the IVC technique is the type of infertility research that will be seen in the future. From a biologic perspective, IVC uses sperm concentrations for insemination that are much lower than those usually used for IVF which proves that a relatively low volume of motile sperm are capable of achieving fertilization. The current practice of IVF also requires that mature oocytes be preincubated 4 to 6 hours and immature oocytes be preincubated 24 to 26 hours prior to insemination in order that full maturity can be achieved. However, IVC clearly demonstrates that human fertilization can routinely occur without preincubation. In addition, the IVC technique requires neither CO_2 nor air whereas these gases are always used in the atmosphere of the incubator for IVF. These observations require biologists to rethink current dogma concerning the fertilization process.

From a psychologic perspective, the availability of the IVC technique resulted in patients discussing their anxiety about potential laboratory error or congenital anomalies which they feared might result from gamete manipulation. These types of concerns were rarely discussed prior to the introduction of IVC.

Perhaps the most potentially far reaching aspect of IVC concerns a religious and ethical perspective. Objections have been raised to IVF because conception excludes the conjugal act and because fertilization occurs outside of the body. IVC may obviate these objections. If a perforated sialastic sheath were used to collect the semen during intercourse, neither contraception nor masturbation would be involved. A portion of the semen could be placed into the vagina and the remainder used for IVC. It has been shown that no matter how mature the oocyte, fertilization of human oocytes following insemination requires at least 45 minutes to 3 hours to occur.[4] Because the IVC tube is placed within the patient's vagina in less than 15 minutes, fertilization definitely occurs within the woman and not external to the body. Therefore, the IVC technique would make it possible for all couples to benefit from advances in infertility treatment by taking in vitro out of fertilization.[5]

In addition to the perspectives listed above, "user friendly" advances in infertility such as IVC can also have a socioeconomic impact. The cost of the procedure is reduced making it more affordable and the simplified steps allow it to be performed outside of a hospital setting where overhead is lower. For all of these reasons, IVC typifies the scientific and philosophical changes which have occurred in reproductive medicine.

REFERENCES

1. Seibel MM, Taymor ML: The emotional aspects of infertility. *Fertil Steril* 37:127, 1982.
2. Congress of the United States, Office of Technology Assessment: Infertility: Medical and Social Choices. 1988.
3. Ranoux C, Aubriot FX, Dubuisson JB, Cardon V, Foulot H, Poirot C, Chevallier O. A new in vitro fertilization technique: intravaginal culture. *Fertil Steril* 49:654, 1988.
4. Plachot M, Junca AM, Mandelbaum J, Cohen J, Salat-Baroux J, DaLage C: Timing of in vitro fertilization of cumulus-free and cumulus-enclosed human oocytes. *Hum Reprod* 1:237, 1986.
5. Ranoux C, Seibel MM: Taking in vitro out of fertilization through intravaginal culture. The Hastings Center Report. In press.

Index

---

t indicates table; *f* indicates figure

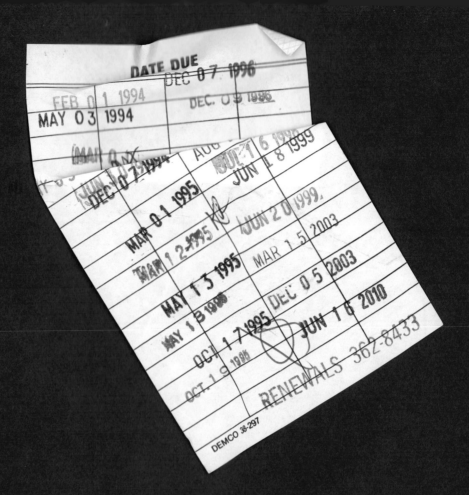